DETERMINATION	REFERENCE RANGE		NOTES
	Conventional	SI*	
HEMATOLOGY *(continued)*			
Leukocyte count	Newborn: 9000–30,000/μl 1 week: 5000–21,000/μl 1 month: 5000–19,500/μl 6–12 months: 6000–17,500/μl 2 years of age: 6200–17,000/μl Child/adult: 4800–10,800/μl		Hemacytometer
Erythrocyte count	Newborn: 4.4–5.8 million/μl Infant/child: 3.8–5.5 million/μl Adult male: 4.7–6.1 million/μl Adult female: 4.2–5.4 million/μl		Hemacytometer
Eosinophil count	50–400/μl		
Reticulocyte count	Newborn (0–2 weeks): 2.5–6.0% Adult: 0.5–2.0% red cells		New Methylene Blue
Absolute reticulocyte count	60,000 μl		
Erythrocyte sedimentation rate (ESR)	Male: 0–9 mm/hr Female: 0–15 mm/hr		Use EDTA as anticoagulant; Winthrobe and Landsberg Method
Osmotic fragility of erythrocytes	Initial hemolysis: 0.45% Complete hemolysis: 0.30–0.35%		Use heparin as anticoagulant
Acidified serum test (Ham test) for paroxysmal nocturnal hemoglobinuria (PNH)	No hemolysis		
Sugar water test for PNH	Lysis at 48 hrs: without added dextrose: 0.2%, with added dextrose: 0–0.9%, with added ATP: 0–0.8%		
Heinz body induction test	1 Heinz body per RBC		
Erythrocyte enzymes: Glucose–6–phosphate dehydrogenase	5–15 U/g Hb	5–15 U/g	Use special anticoagulant (ACD solution)
Pyruvate kinase	13–17 U/g Hb	13–17 U/g	Use special anticoagulant (ACD solution)
Ferritin (serum)			
Iron deficiency	0–12 ng/ml 13–20 borderline	0–4.8 nmol/liter 5.2–8 nmol/liter borderline	
Iron excess	>400 ng/liter	>160 nmol/liter	
Folic acid			
Normal	>3.3 ng/liter	>7.3 nmol/liter	
Borderline	2.5–3.2 ng/ml	5.75–7.39 nmol/liter	
Haptoglobin	40–336 mg/100 ml	0.4–3.6 g/liter	

*SI—System of International Units.

Clinical Hematology and Fundamentals of Hemostasis
Second Edition

Denise M. Harmening, Ph.D., M.T. (ASCP), C.L.S.(NCA)
Editor
Chairman and Professor
Department of Medical and Research Technology
School of Medicine
University of Maryland at Baltimore
Baltimore, Maryland

 F. A. DAVIS COMPANY • Philadelphia

F. A. Davis Company
1915 Arch Street
Philadelphia, PA 19103

Printed in the United States of America

Last digit indicates print number: 10 9 8 7 6 5 4

NOTE: As new scientific information becomes available through basic and clinical research, recommended treatments and drug therapies undergo changes. The author(s) and publisher have done everything possible to make this book accurate, up-to-date, and in accord with accepted standards at the time of publication. The authors, editors, and publisher are not responsible for errors or omissions or for consequences from application of the book, and make no warranty, expressed or implied, in regard to the contents of the book. Any practice described in this book should be applied by the reader in accordance with professional standards of care used in regard to the unique circumstances that may apply in each situation. The reader is advised always to check product information (package inserts) for changes and new information regarding dose and contraindications before administering any drug. Caution is especially urged when using new or infrequently ordered drugs.

Library of Congress Cataloging-in-Publication Data

Clinical hematology and fundamentals of hemostasis/edited by
  Denise M. Harmening—2nd edition

    Includes bibliographical references and index.
    ISBN 0-8036-4603-8 (hardbound : alk. paper)
    1. Hematology.   2. Blood—Diseases.   3. Hemostasis.
  I. Harmening, Denise.
    [DNLM: 1. Hematologic Diseases.   2. Hemostasis. WH 100 C6413]
  RB145.C536   1991
  616.1′5—dc20

                                                              91-20053

To all students, full-time, part-time, past, present, and future, who have touched and will continue to touch the lives of so many educators . . .

It is to you this book is dedicated in the hope of inspiring an unquenchable thirst for knowledge and love of mankind.

Preface

The second edition of this text has been designed to be a thorough and concise guide to clinical hematology and fundamentals of hemostasis. It is a practical and applied approach to the subject matter, and illustrative case histories have been incorporated to provide the reader with an up-to-date working knowledge of contemporary hematology and coagulation. Two hundred and sixty color plates demonstrating peripheral smears, bone marrow aspirates, gross morphology, and clinical manifestations enhance the text, as the foundation for the interpretation and practice of clinical medicine. This edition emphasizes the teaching of normal and abnormal morphology by presenting characteristic laboratory profiles for each major pathologic condition.

The first five chapters serve as an introduction to clinical hematology by focusing on red cell metabolism, hematopoiesis and bone marrow examination, evaluation of red cell morphology, and the pathogenesis of anemia. Ann Bell of the University of Tennessee has supplied a collection of striking illustrations depicting erythrocytic, myelocytic, lymphocytic, monocytic, plasmocytic, and megakaryocytic cell lines of maturation. The next ten chapters are devoted to the subject of anemias, presenting the disease processes leading to abnormal red cell morphology. The following section of nine chapters focuses on white blood cell disorders, including both benign and malignant states. An in-depth discussion of leukemias presents both the morphologic and immunologic classifications supported by the cytochemical profiles. A review of myelodysplastic syndromes, myeloproliferative disorders, plasma cell dyscrasias, lymphomas, and lipid storage disease completes this section.

The final section provides an overview of hemostasis, including platelet structure and function, vascular and platelet disorders, defects of plasma-clotting factors, von Willebrand's disease, and disseminated intravascular coagulation (DIC), followed by an introduction to thrombosis and anticoagulant therapy. Laboratory diagnosis and treatment of these hemorrhagic processes are presented and reinforced by illustrative case histories. The final chapter consists of four sections on laboratory methods and serves as a ready guide to procedures routinely performed in the clinical hematology and hemostasis laboratory.

Several features of this textbook have proved to have great appeal to both students and educators. Comprehensive outlines and educational objectives precede each chapter. The study-guide questions at the end of each chapter are accompanied by answers cross-referenced to the appropriate text page. An extensive glossary provides easy access to hematologic terms. Case histories throughout the text exemplify actual clinical situations, further illustrating key pathologic conditions. The tables of normal values on the inside covers of this book have proved to be an invaluable time-saver in the interpretation of patient laboratory data.

This new edition, like the first, is a culmination of dedicated efforts of a group of prominent professionals. They committed to this project by donating their time and expertise out of a concern for our common goal: improving patient care by providing a high-quality practical and usable textbook. In particular, I would like to express my thanks to Janice Hundley of the Medical University of South

Carolina and Carol LeCrone of the University of Washington for their editorial comments.

My sincere appreciation also goes to the following educators and clinicians for their thorough and thoughtful review of the manuscript: Cheryl Burns, M.S. M.T.(ASCP), Assistant Professor, Medical Technology Program, University of Texas at San Antonio; Kathleen A. Clark, M.S., M.T.(ASCP) S.H., Program Director, School of Medical Technology, Childrens Hospital Los Angeles; Nancy Geier, M. T.(ASCP) S.H., manager of the Hematology Laboratory of the University of Minnesota Hospital; Karen L. Hay, M.S., M.T.(ASCP), Clinical Instructor, School of Allied Health Professions, Loma Linda University; Karen Lofness, M.S., C.L.Sp.H.(NCA), Assistant Professor, Division of Medical Technology at the University of Minnesota; Betty Murphy, M.Ed., M.T.(ASCP), Emeritus Professor, Department of Medical Technology, State University of New York at Buffalo; Kathy V. Waller, Ph.D., Assistant Professor, Medical Technology Division, Ohio State University; and J. Lynne Williams, Ph.D., M.T.(ASCP), Associate Professor and Director, Medical Laboratory Sciences, Oakland University School of Health Sciences, Rochester, Michigan.

Finally, I would like to acknowledge the contribution of Sharon Kutt, M.H.E., M.T.(ASCP), Department of Medical Technology of the Medical College of Georgia, Augusta, Georgia, who functioned as reviewer and educational consultant throughout the book's preparation.

In summary, this book has been designed to inspire an unquenchable thirst for knowledge in every medical technologist, hematologist, and practitioner whose knowledge, skills, and ongoing education provide the public with excellence in health care.

D. M. Harmening, Ph.D., M.T.(ASCP), C.L.S.(NCA)

Contributors

Educational Consultant

Sharon Kutt, M.H.E , M.T.(ASCP)
Assistant Professor
Department of Medical
  Technology
Medical College of Georgia
Augusta, Georgia

Ann Bell, M.S., S.H.(ASCP),
C.L.SP.H.(NCA)
Professor of Clinical Laboratory
  Sciences
Assistant Professor
Department of Medicine
Division of Hematology/
  Oncology
The Health Science Center
University of Tennessee
Memphis, Tennessee

Michele L. Best, B.S.,
M.T.(ASCP)
Director, Laboratory Quality
  Assurance and Human
  Resources
Program Director, Medical
  Technology Program
Washington Hospital Center
Washington, D.C.

Barbara S. Caldwell,
M.T.(ASCP) S.H.
Instructor
Department of Medical and
  Research Technology
School of Medicine
University of Maryland at
  Baltimore
Baltimore, Maryland

Michel M. Canton, Pharm.D.
Director, Clinical and Business
  Development
American Bioproducts Company
Parsippany, New Jersey

Betty E. Ciesla, M.S.,
M.T.(ASCP) S.H.
Assistant Professor
Department of Medical and
  Research Technology
School of Medicine
University of Maryland at
  Baltimore
Baltimore, Maryland

Armand B. Glassman, M.D.
Vice President and Laboratory
  Director
National Reference Laboratory
Clinical Professor of Pathology
Vanderbilt University
Nashville, Tennessee

Clinical Professor of Pathology
  and Laboratory Medicine
Clinical Professor of Radiology
  (Nuclear Medicine)
Medical University of South
  Carolina
Charleston, South Carolina

Ralph Green, B.App.Sci.
(MLS), F.A.I.M.L.S.
Principal Lecturer in Medical
  Laboratory Science
Department of Applied Biology
Royal Melbourne Institute of
  Technology
Melbourne, Victoria, Australia

Kathryn Ann Grenier, M.T.(ASCP), C.L.S.(NCA)
Senior Clinical Research Associate
Becton Dickinson Immunocytometry Systems
San Jose, California

Sandra Gwaltney-Krause, M.A., M.T.(ASCP)
Former Instructor
Department of Medical Technology
University of South Alabama
Mobile, Alabama

Chantal Ricaud Harrison, M.D.
Associate Professor of Pathology
University of Texas Health Science Center at San Antonio
San Antonio, Texas

Laurel Krewson Holmer, M.Ed., M.T.(ASCP) S.H.
Educational Coordinator
Department of Clinical Laboratory Science
University of Nevada School of Medicine
Reno, Nevada

Ellen Hope, M.S., S.H.(ASCP) H.
Associate Professor of Clinical Sciences
Department of Clinical Sciences School of Health
California State University at Dominguez Hills
Carson, California

Dan M. Hyder, M.D.
Director, Department of Pathology and Laboratory Medicine
Medical Director, Eric and Ronna Hoffman Cancer Immunology Laboratory
Good Samaritan Hospital and Medical Center
Portland, Oregon

Joette Kizer, M.L.T.(ASCP)
Supervisor, Hematology Section
Department of Pathology and Laboratory Medicine
Medical University of South Carolina
Charleston, South Carolina

John Lazarchick, M.D.
Professor
Director of Hemostasis Laboratory
Medical University of South Carolina
Charleston, South Carolina

Susan J. Leclair, M.S., C.L.S.(NCA)
Associate Professor
Department of Medical Laboratory Science
University of Massachusetts/ Dartmouth
North Dartmouth, Massachusetts

James M. Long, M.D., Major, USAF, MC
Staff, Hematology and Medical Oncology
David Grant USAF Medical Center
Travis Air Force Base, California

Joe Marty, M.S., M.T.(ASCP)
Research Instructor of Pathology
Technical Director of Hematopathology Laboratory
Department of Pathology
University of Utah School of Medicine
Salt Lake City, Utah

David L. McGlasson, M. S., C.L.S.(NCA)
Clinical Investigation Directorate
Wilford Hall USAF Medical Center
Lackland Air Force Base, Texas

Jeannine R. Meloon, M.S., M.T.(ASCP)
Program Director, Assistant Professor, Chairperson
Department of Medical Technology
West Liberty State College
West Liberty, West Virginia

Milka Montiel, M.D.
Professor and Director of Clinical Laboratories
Department of Pathology
University of Texas Health Science Center at San Antonio;
San Antonio, Texas

Ellinor I.B. Peerschke, Ph.D.
Associate Professor of Pathology
Head, Clinical Hematology Laboratories
State University of New York at Stony Brook
Stony Brook, New York

Mary Loring Perkins, M.S., M.T.(ASCP) S.H.
Medical Technologist
Eric and Ronna Hoffman Cancer Immunology Laboratory
Good Samaritan Hospital and Medical Center
Portland, Oregon

Lloyd A. Simandl, A.R.T. (CSLT)
Subject Head, Hematology
Division of Diagnostic Services
British Columbia Institute of Technology
Burnaby, British Columbia, Canada

Catherine M. Spier, M.D.
Associate Professor of Pathology
Department of Pathology
University of Arizona College of Medicine
Tucson, Arizona

Ronald G. Strauss, M.D.
Medical Director, DeGowin Blood Center
Professor of Pathology and Pediatrics
University of Iowa Hospitals and Clinics
Iowa City, Iowa

Janis Wyrick-Glatzel, M.S., M.T.(ASCP)
Assistant Professor
Department of Clinical Laboratory Science
University of Nevada at Las Vegas
Las Vegas, Nevada

S. Zail, M.B., B.Ch., M.D., FRCPath(London)
Director, Hemolytic Anemia Research Unit
Department of Hematology School of Pathology
South African Institute for Medical Research and the University of the Witwatersrand
Johannesburg, South Africa

Hallye Zeringer, B.S., M.T.(ASCP) S.H.
Medical Technologist
Southern Baptist Hospital
New Orleans, Louisiana

Contents

Left column: Macrocytic erythrocytes (megalocytic, megaloblastic) of the type seen in pernicious anemia and related B$_{12}$-folic acid deficient states

Middle column: Normal erythrocytic sequence

Right column: Microcytic, hypochromic cells of type seen in iron deficient states

Rubriblasts

Prorubricytes

Rubricytes

Metarubricytes

Diffusely basophilic erythrocytes

Erythrocytes

Color Plate 1. Erythrocytic system. (From Diggs, LW, Sturm, D, and Bell, A: Morphology of Human Blood Cells. Abbott Laboratories, Abbott Park, IL, 1985, with permission.)

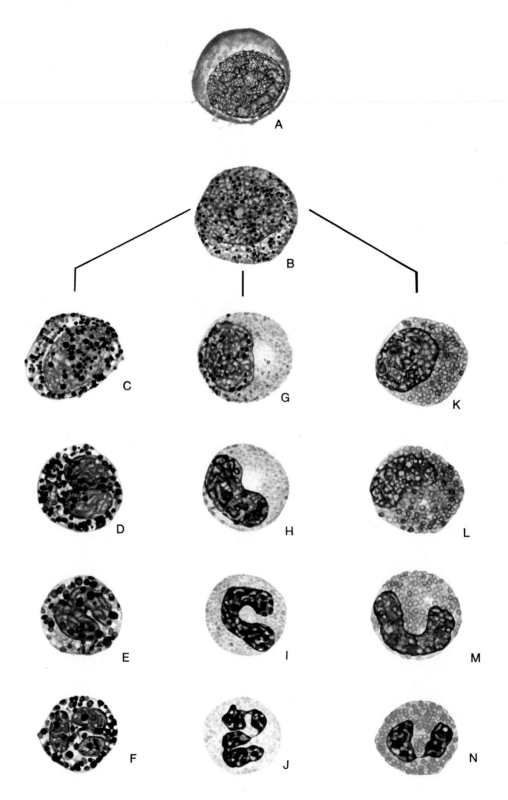

Color Plate 2. Granulocytopoiesis; Myelocytic (granulocytic) system. (*A*) Myeloblast; (*B*) promyelocyte (progranulocyte); (*C*) basophilic myelocyte; (*D*) basophilic metamyelocyte; (*E*) basophilic band; (*F*) basophilic segmented; (*G*) neutrophilic myelocyte; (*H*) neutrophilic metamyelocyte; (*I*) neutrophilic band; (*J*) neutrophilic segmented; (*K*) eosinophilic myelocyte; (*L*) eosinophilic metamyelocyte; (*M*) eosinophilic band; (*N*) eosinophilic segmented. (From Diggs, LW, Sturm, D, and Bell, A: Morphology of Human Blood Cells. Abbott Laboratories, Abbott Park, IL, 1985, with permission.)

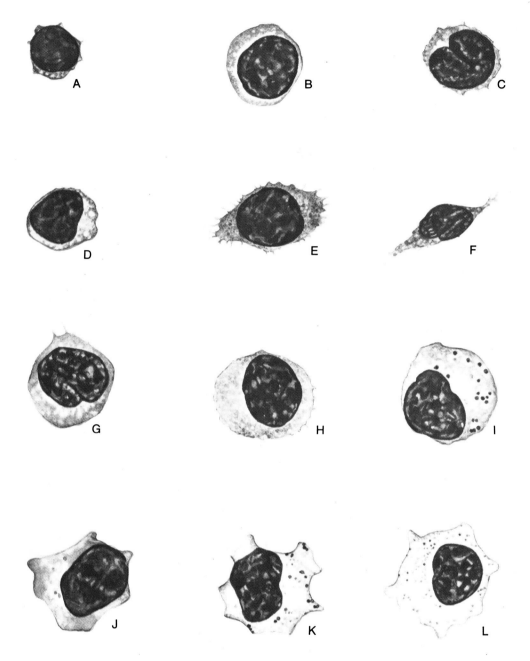

Color Plate 3. Lymphocytes. (*A*) Small mature lymphocyte; (*B*) lymphocyte of intermediate size; (*C*) lymphocyte with indented nucleus; (*D*) lymphocyte of intermediate size; (*E*) lymphocyte with pointed cytoplasmic projections (frayed cytoplasm); typical nucleus; (*F*) spindle-shaped and pointed cytoplasmic projections; (*G*) large lymphocyte with indented nucleus and pointed cytoplasmic projections; (*H*) large lymphocyte; (*I*) large lymphocyte with purplish-red (azurophilic) granules; (*J*) large lymphocyte with irregular cytoplasmic contours; (*K*) large lymphocyte with purplish-red (azurophilic) granules and with indentations caused by pressure of erythrocytes; (*L*) large lymphocyte with purplish-red (azurophilic) granules. (From Diggs, LW, Sturm, D, and Bell, A: Morphology of Human Blood Cells. Abbott Laboratories, Abbott Park, IL, 1985, with permission.)

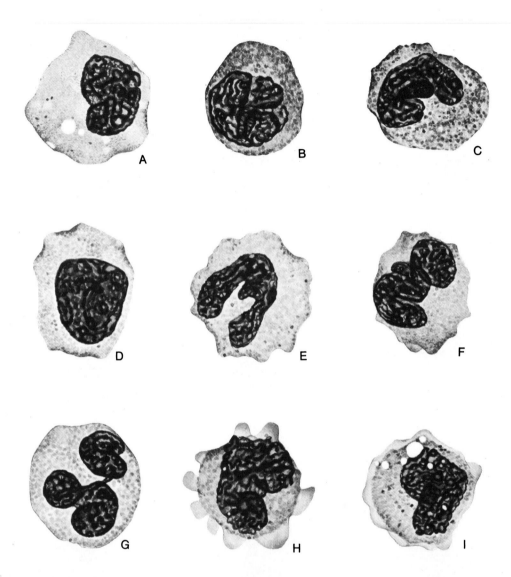

Color Plate 4. Monocytes. (*A*) Monocyte with "ground-glass" appearance, evenly distributed fine granules, occasional azurophilic granules, and vacuoles in cytoplasm; (*B*) monocyte with opaque cytoplasm and granules and with lobulation of nucleus and linear chromatin; (*C*) monocyte with prominent granules and deeply indented nucleus; (*D*) monocyte without nuclear indentations; (*E*) monocyte with gray-blue color, band type of nucleus, linear chromatin, blunt pseudopods, and granules; (*F*) monocyte with gray-blue color, irregular shape, and multilobulated nucleus; (*G*) monocyte with segmented nucleus; (*H*) monocyte with multiple blunt nongranular pseudopods, nuclear indentations, and folds; (*I*) monocyte with vacuoles and with nongranular ectoplasm and granular endoplasm. (From Diggs, LW, Sturm, D, and Bell, A: Morphology of Human Blood Cells. Abbott Laboratories, Abbott Park, IL, 1985, with permission.)

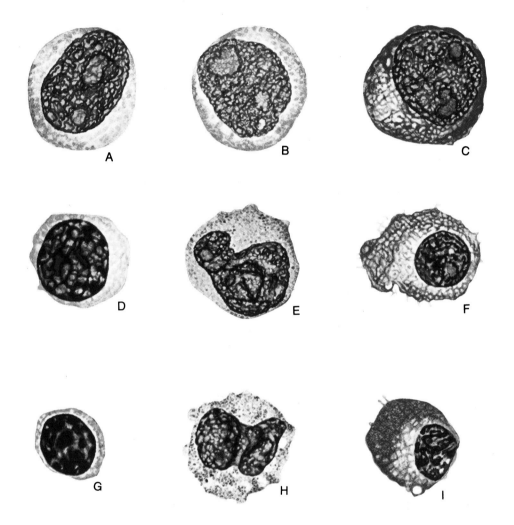

Color Plate 5. Lymphocytic, monocytic, and plasmocytic systems. (*A*) Lymphoblast; (*B*) monoblast; (*C*) plasmoblast; (*D*) prolymphocyte; (*E*) promonocyte; (*F*) proplasmocyte; (*G*) lymphocyte with clumped chromatin; (*H*) monocyte; (*I*) plasmocyte. (From Diggs, LW, Sturm, D, and Bell, A: Morphology of Human Blood Cells. Abbott Laboratories, Abbott Park, IL, 1985, with permission.)

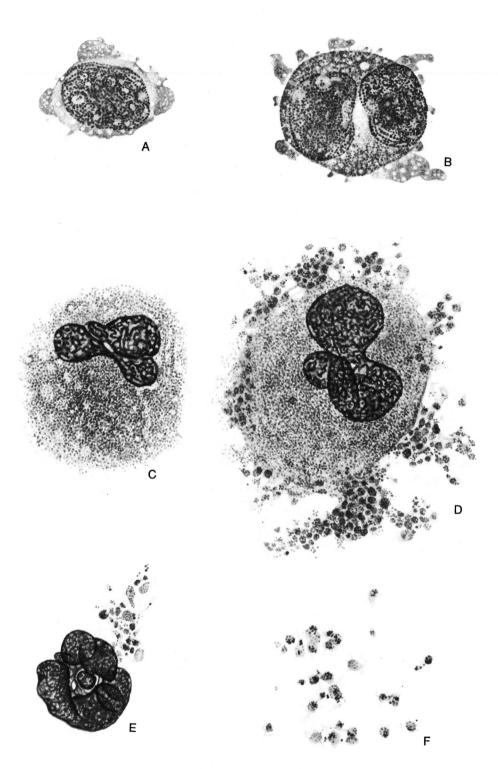

Color Plate 6. Megakaryocytic system. (*A*) Megakaryoblast with single oval nucleus, nucleoli, and bluish foamy marginal cytoplasmic structures; (*B*) promegakaryocyte with two nuclei, granular blue cytoplasm, and marginal bubbly cytoplasmic structures; (*C*) megakaryocyte with granular cytoplasm and without discrete thrombocytes (platelets); (*D*) metamegakaryocyte with multiple nuclei and with thrombocytes (platelets); (*E*) metamegakaryocyte nucleus with attached thrombocytes; (*F*) thrombocytes (platelets). (From Diggs, LW, Sturm, D, and Bell, A: Morphology of Human Blood Cells. Abbott Laboratories, Abbott Park, IL, 1985, with permission.)

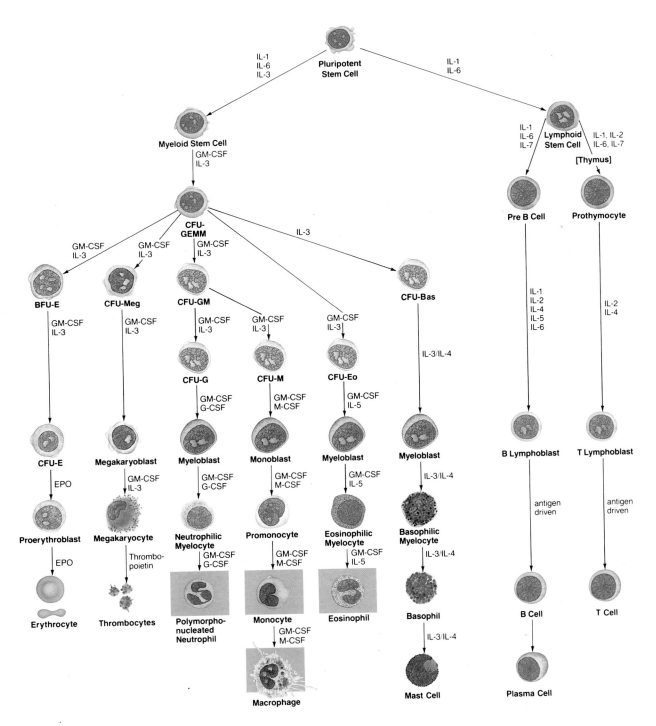

Color Plate 7. Regulation of hematopoiesis by colony stimulating factors (CSFs) and interleukins. (Reprinted from Sandoz Pharmaceuticals Corporation and Schering-Plough, with permission.)

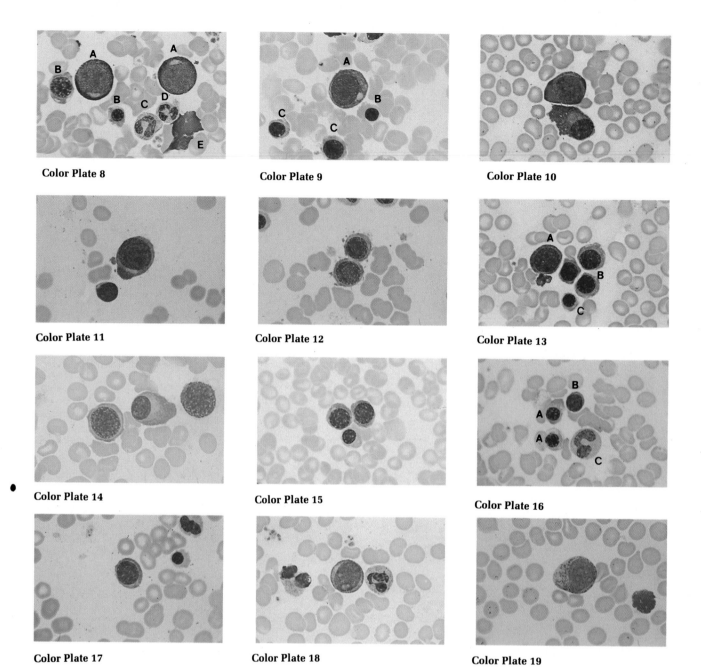

Color Plate 8

Color Plate 9

Color Plate 10

Color Plate 11

Color Plate 12

Color Plate 13

Color Plate 14

Color Plate 15

Color Plate 16

Color Plate 17

Color Plate 18

Color Plate 19

Color Plate 8. Two rubriblasts: (*A*) note the perinuclear halo, two rubricytes (*B*) N. band (*C*) N. segmented (*D*) and (*E*) smudge cell.

Color Plate 9. Rubriblast (*A*), metarubricyte (*B*), two rubricytes (*C*).

Color Plate 10. Rubriblast (*center*), plasmocyte (*lower center*).

Color Plate 11. Rubriblast (*center*), lymphocyte (*lower center*).

Color Plate 12. Prorubricytes.

Color Plate 13. Prorubricyte (*A*), three rubricytes (*B*), metarubricyte (*C*).

Color Plate 14. Prorubricyte (*left*), plasmocyte (*center*).

Color Plate 15. Rubricytes: early and late stages.

Color Plate 16. Rubricytes (*A*), lymphocyte (*B*), N. segmented (*C*).

Color Plate 17. Prorubricyte (*center*), metarubricyte (*right*).

Color Plate 18. Myeloblast (*center*), N. segmented (*right*), disintegrated neutrophil (*left*).

Color Plate 19. Progranulocyte.

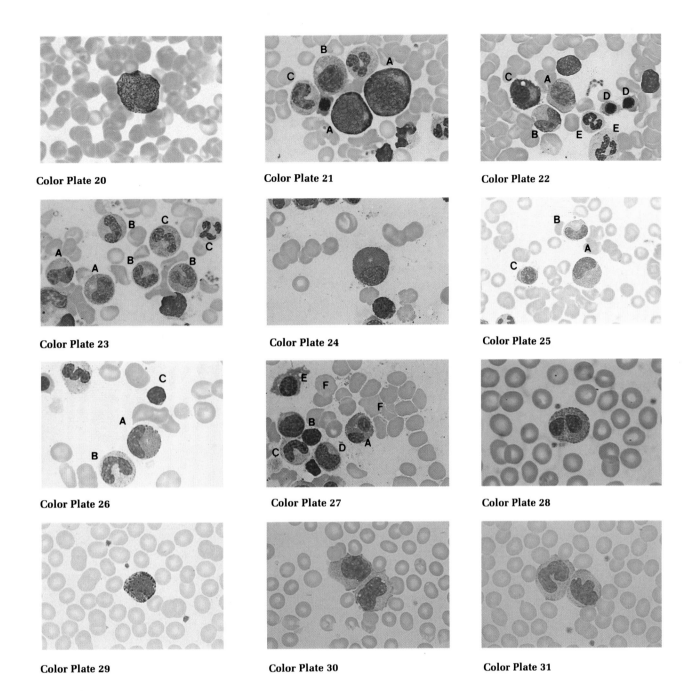

Color Plate 20

Color Plate 21

Color Plate 22

Color Plate 23

Color Plate 24

Color Plate 25

Color Plate 26

Color Plate 27

Color Plate 28

Color Plate 29

Color Plate 30

Color Plate 31

Color Plate 20. Progranulocyte.

Color Plate 21. Rubriblasts (*A*), N. myelocyte (*B*), N. metamyelocyte (*C*).

Color Plate 22. N. myelocyte (*A*), N. metamyelocyte (*B*), plasmocyte (*C*), metarubricytes (*D*), segmented neutrophils (*E*).

Color Plate 23. Two N. metamyelocytes (*A*), three N. bands (*B*), two N. segmented (*C*).

Color Plate 24. Eosinophilic myelocyte (*center*), basophil (*below*).

Color Plate 25. E. metamyelocyte (*A*), N. band (*B*), rubricyte (*C*).

Color Plate 26. E. band (*A*), N. band (*B*), lymphocyte (*C*).

Color Plate 27. E. segmented (*A*), lymphocyte (*B*), N. band (*C*), N. metamyelocyte (*D*), plasmocyte (*E*), two diffusely basophilic red cells (*F*).

Color Plate 28. Eosinophil (segmented).   **Color Plate 29.** Basophil (*center*).   **Color Plate 30.** Monocytes.

Color Plate 31. Monocytes.

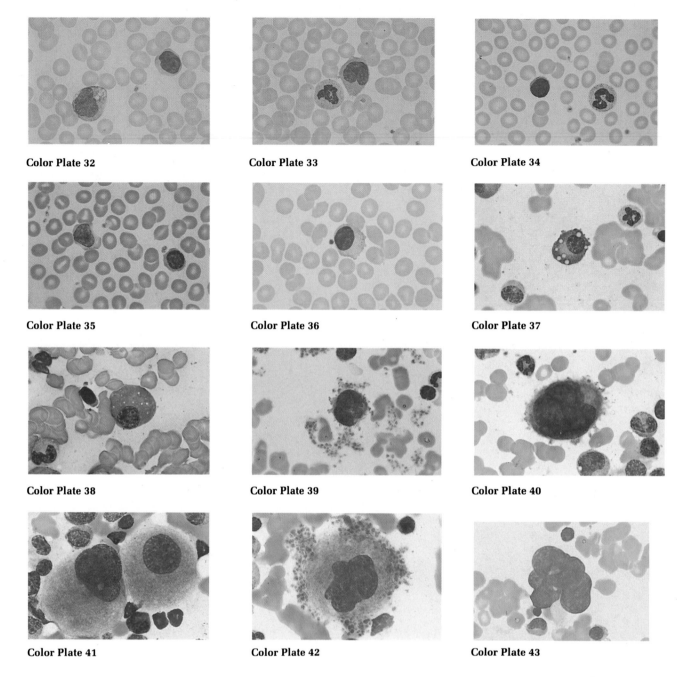

Color Plate 32. Monocyte (*left*), lymphocyte (*right*).

Color Plate 33. Monocyte (*right*), N. segmented (*left*).

Color Plate 34. Lymphocyte (*left*), N. segmented (*right*).

Color Plate 35. Lymphocytes: large, (*left*) and small, (*right*).

Color Plate 36. Lymphocyte, large.

Color Plate 37. Plasmocyte (*center*), N. segmented (*upper right*), resting monocyte (*lower left*).

Color Plate 38. Plasmocyte (*center*), small lymphocyte (*left center*).

Color Plate 39. Early megakaryocyte.

Color Plate 40. Early megakaryocyte (*center*), segmented neutrophil (*top left*), N. metamyelocyte (*bottom center*).

Color Plate 41. Megakaryocytes without platelets.   **Color Plate 42.** Megakaryocyte with platelets.

Color Plate 43. Naked nuclei, megakaryocyte.

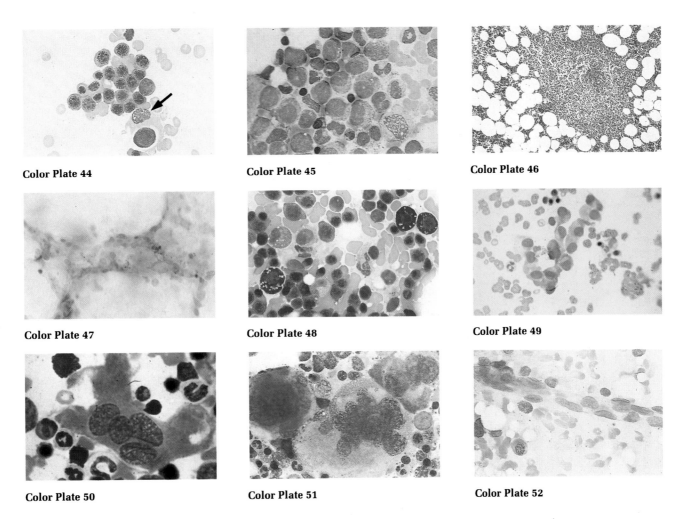

Color Plate 44

Color Plate 45

Color Plate 46

Color Plate 47

Color Plate 48

Color Plate 49

Color Plate 50

Color Plate 51

Color Plate 52

Color Plate 44. Erythropoietic island composed mainly of polychromatophilic normoblasts. The nutrient-histiocyte (*arrow*) is slightly displaced of its central position by smearing of the particle. Its cytoplasmic slender processes envelop a basophilic normoblast establishing intimate contact with the maturing red cell precursor. (magnification ×640)

Color Plate 45. Compartment of granulopoiesis. A reticular cell (*arrow*) with open reticulated chromatin and light blue cytoplasm containing dust-like fine granules is situated among numerous granulocytic precursors, especially myelocytes. (magnification ×640)

Color Plate 46. A lymphocytic nodule (follicle) in bone marrow as shown here may alter very significantly the marrow differential count when aspirated and give a false impression of lymphocytic malignancy. (magnification ×250)

Color Plate 47. Iron stain of bone marrow smear shows the processes of the nutrienthistiocytes surrounding the erythrocyte precursors (magnification ×640)

Color Plate 48. Three mast cells (*arrows*), known also as tissue basophils, are shown in this marrow aspirate on a background of erythroid hyperplasia. Numerous regular round granules fill their cytoplasm and obscure the nucleur details. (magnification ×640)

Color Plate 49. Group of osteoblasts (*center*) aspirated from the marrow of a child. (magnification ×400)

Color Plate 50. Osteoclast usually is seen as a single giant cell with multiple and separated nuclei and basophilic granular cytoplasm (*center*). (magnification ×640)

Color Plate 51. Megakaryocytes, compared with osteoclasts, tend to be in small groups with multilobated single nuclei. Mature megakaryocytes have numerous fine cytoplasmic granules and occasionally platelet units can be seen at their periphery. (magnification ×640)

Color Plate 52. A string of endothelial cells aspirated from hypocellular marrow. The nuclei are elongated and slightly tapered. The cytoplasm is transparent and barely visible. (magnification ×640)

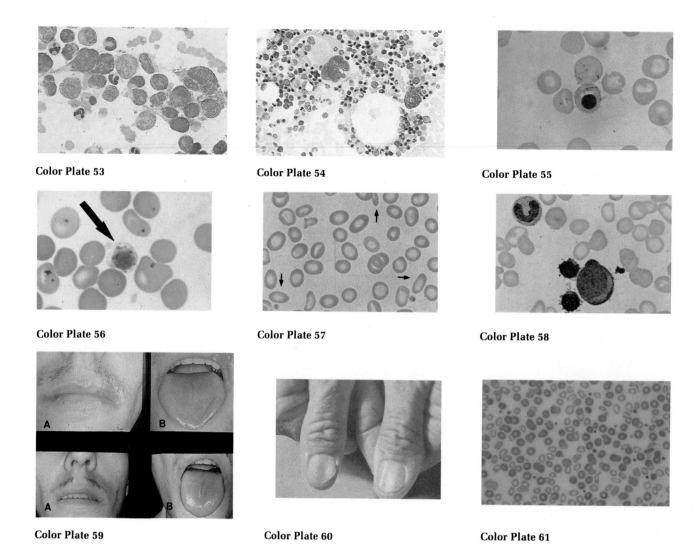

Color Plate 53

Color Plate 54

Color Plate 55

Color Plate 56

Color Plate 57

Color Plate 58

Color Plate 59

Color Plate 60

Color Plate 61

Color Plate 53. Metastatic tumor to the bone marrow. The tumor cells are usually pleomorphic and in groups with large nuclear:cytoplasmic ratios, irregular nuclear outline, and deep blue cytoplasm. (magnification ×640)

Color Plate 54. Smear of normal cellular marrow with normal maturation of erythropoietic, granulocytic, and megakaryocytic cells. (magnification ×250)

Color Plate 55. Erythropoietic porphyria. Note the precipitated porphyrins in the cytoplasm. (From Listen, Look, and Learn, vol 3: Coagulation, Hematology. The American Society of Clinical Pathologists Press, Chicago, 1973, with permission.)

Color Plate 56. Ringed sideroblast (*center*), siderocytes (*arrows*). (From Listen, Look, and Learn, vol 3: Coagulation, Hematology. The American Society of Clinical Pathologists Press, Chicago, 1973, with permission.)

Color Plate 57. Peripheral blood smear in iron-deficiency anemia showing microcytosis and hypochromia and poikilocytosis. Note the occasional thin ovalocyte or pencil cell. (From Listen, Look, and Learn, vol 3: Coagulation, Hematology. The American Society of Clinical Pathologists Press, Chicago, 1973, with permission.)

Color Plate 58. Bone marrow aspirate in iron-deficiency showing ineffective erythropoiesis, "ragged" erythroid precursors. (From Listen, Look, and Learn, vol 3: Coagulation, Hematology. The American Society of Clinical Pathologists Press, Chicago, 1973, with permission.)

Color Plate 59. Clinical manifestations of iron-deficiency anemia: cheilitis (*A*), and glossitis (*B*), before and after therapy.

Color Plate 60. Koilonychia, characteristic of iron deficiency: spooning of nails.

Color Plate 61. Peripheral blood of patient with iron-deficiency anemia following therapy. Note the two populations of red cells.

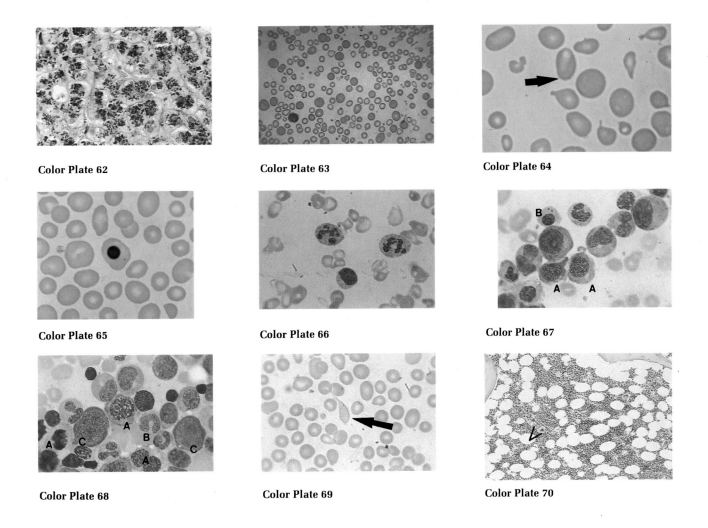

Color Plate 62

Color Plate 63

Color Plate 64

Color Plate 65

Color Plate 66

Color Plate 67

Color Plate 68

Color Plate 69

Color Plate 70

Color Plate 62. Liver biopsy of a patient with idiopathic hemochromatosis and cirrhosis. Note the excess deposits of iron (ferric ferricyanide stain).

Color Plate 63. Sideroblastic anemia (peripheral blood). Note the characteristic dimorphic blood picture. (magnification ×500)

Color Plate 64. Extreme degree of anisocytosis (+4) and poikilocytosis (+4) with oval macrocytosis (*arrow*) in a severe pernicious anemia case. (From Listen, Look, and Learn, vol. 3: Coagulation, Hematology. The American Society of Clinical Pathologists Press, Chicago, 1973, with permission.)

Color Plate 65. Howell-Jolly body in an orthochromic megaloblast in pernicious anemia (*center*). (From Listen, Look, and Learn, vol 3: Coagulation, Hematology. The American Society of Clinical Pathologists Press, Chicago, 1973, with permission.)

Color Plate 66. Neutrophil hypersegmentation in pernicious anemia.

Color Plate 67. Polychromatophilic megaloblasts (*A*); and orthochromic megaloblast with multiple Howell-Jolly bodies (*B*). Bone marrow.

Color Plate 68. Mitotic figures in megaloblastic marrow (*A*); large megaloblastic band neutrophil (*B*); and megaloblastic pronormoblast with open, sieve-like chromatin (*C*).

Color Plate 69. Cabot ring in pernicious anemia (*center*).

Color Plate 70. Normal bone marrow biopsy showing approximately 50 percent marrow cellularity. Note the megakaryocytes (low power).

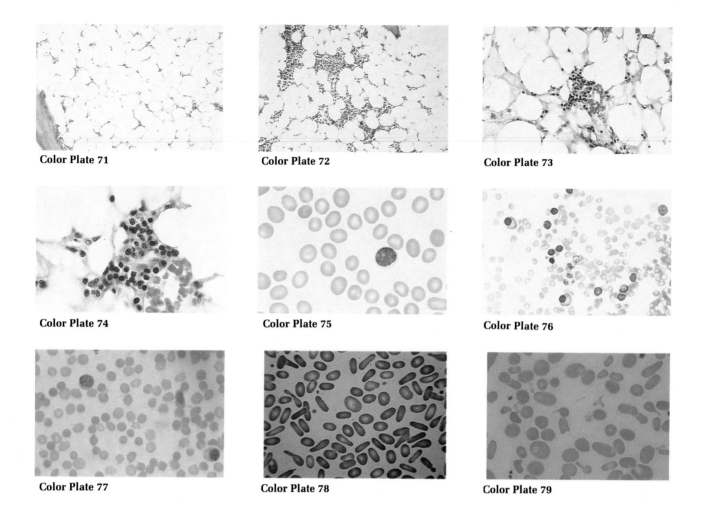

Color Plate 71. Markedly hypocellular bone marrow biopsy as commonly seen in severe aplastic anemia (low power).

Color Plate 72. Bone marrow biopsy showing variable cellularity (low power).

Color Plate 73. Bone marrow biopsy showing small lymphoid aggregate or nodule (low power).

Color Plate 74. Higher magnification of lymphoid aggregate depicted in Color Plate 73. (magnification ×400)

Color Plate 75. Wright-stained peripheral blood smear of a patient with aplastic anemia. Red cells are normochromic and slightly macrocytic, with slight anisocytosis. Note the absence of reticulocytes and platelets.

Color Plate 76. Wright-stained bone marrow touch preparation. Aspirate was a "dry tap." Present are a few scattered lymphocytes and plasma cells. (magnification ×400)

Color Plate 77. Hereditary spherocytosis (peripheral blood). Note the small condensed spherocytes with no central pallor.

Color Plate 78. Hereditary elliptocytosis (peripheral blood). Note the high percentage of elliptocytes or ovalocytes.

Color Plate 79. Hereditary pyropoikilocytosis (peripheral blood). Note the bizarre micropoikilocytosis, red cell budding, microspherocytes, and elliptocytes.

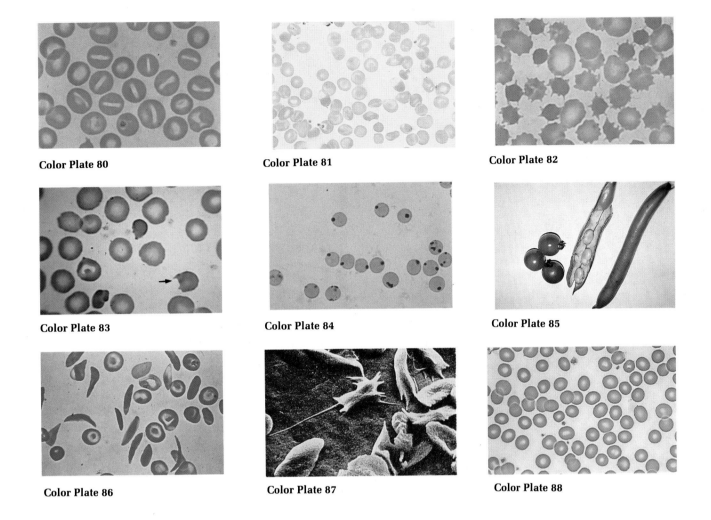

Color Plate 80

Color Plate 81

Color Plate 82

Color Plate 83

Color Plate 84

Color Plate 85

Color Plate 86

Color Plate 87

Color Plate 88

Color Plate 80. Hereditary stomatocytosis (peripheral blood). Note the high percentage of red cells with a central slit of pallor. (From Listen, Look, and Learn, vol 3: Coagulation, Hematology. The American Society of Clinical Pathologists Press, Chicago, 1973, with permission.)

Color Plate 81. Hereditary xerocytosis (peripheral blood).

Color Plate 82. Acanthocytosis from a patient with abetalipoproteinemia. (From Hyun, BH, Ashton, JK, and Dolan, K: Practical Hematology. A Laboratory Guide with Accompanying Filmstrip. WB Saunders, Philadelphia, 1975, with permission.)

Color Plate 83. Peripheral blood smear from a patient with a G6PD deficiency. Note the small condensed "bite" or "helmet" cells.

Color Plate 84. Heinz bodies. (From Listen, Look, and Learn, vol 3: Coagulation, Hematology. The American Society of Clinical Pathologists Press, Chicago, 1973, with permission.)

Color Plate 85. Fava beans (Note: the tomatoes were added for color and contrast.)

Color Plate 86. Sickle cell disease (peripheral blood). Note the sickle-shaped red cells and target cells. (From Listen, Look, and Learn, vol 3: Coagulation, Hematology. The American Society of Clinical Pathologists Press, Chicago, 1973, with permission.)

Color Plate 87. Scanning electron micrograph (SEM) of sickle cells. (From Listen, Look, and Learn, vol 3: Coagulation, Hematology. The American Society of Clinical Pathologists Press, Chicago, 1973, with permission.)

Color Plate 88. Sickle trait (peripheral blood). Note the normal-appearing smear.

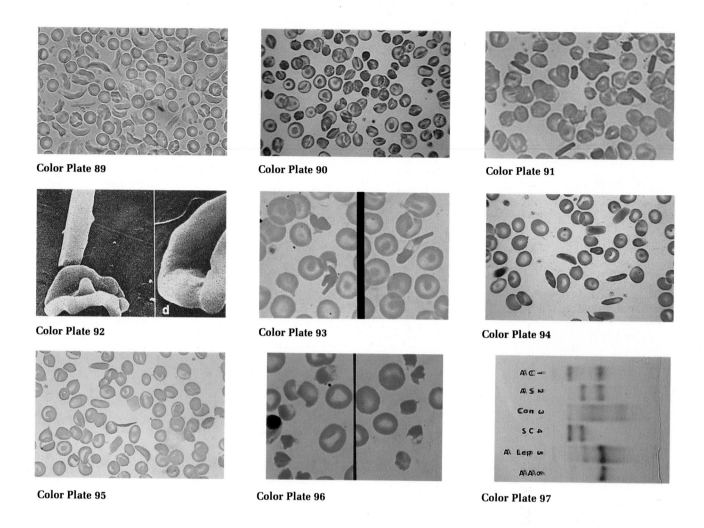

Color Plate 89

Color Plate 90

Color Plate 91

Color Plate 92

Color Plate 93

Color Plate 94

Color Plate 95

Color Plate 96

Color Plate 97

Color Plate 89. Sodium metabisulfite sickle preparation.

Color Plate 90. Hemoglobin C disease (pre-splenectomy). Note the numerous target and envelope forms.

Color Plate 91. Hemoglobin C disease (peripheral blood). Note the particular crystals: "bar of gold" and numerous target cells (post-splenectomy). (From Listen, Look, and Learn, vol 3: Coagulation, Hematology. The American Society of Clinical Pathologists Press, Chicago, 1973, with permission.)

Color Plate 92. SEM of hemoglobin C crystals. (From Listen, Look, and Learn, vol 3: Coagulation, Hematology. The American Society of Clinical Pathologists Press, Chicago, 1973, with permission.)

Color Plate 93. SC disease (peripheral blood). Note the type of "Washington monument" crystals and target cells. (From Listen, Look, and Learn, vol 3: Coagulation, Hematology. The American Society of Clinical Pathologists Press, Chicago, 1973, with permission.)

Color Plate 94. SC disease (peripheral blood). (From Listen, Look, and Learn, vol 3: Coagulation, Hematology. The American Society of Clinical Pathologists Press, Chicago, 1973, with permission.)

Color Plate 95. Sickle thalassemia syndrome (peripheral blood).

Color Plate 96. Unstable hemoglobin: hemoglobin Zurich (peripheral blood). (From Listen, Look, and Learn, vol 3: Coagulation, Hematology. The American Society of Clinical Pathologists Press, Chicago, 1973, with permission.)

Color Plate 97. Hemoglobin electrophoretic patterns (1) Hemoglobin (Hb) A/C, (2), Hb A/S, (3) commercial control; (4) Hb S/C, (5) HbA/Lepore, and (6) Hb A/A normal control.

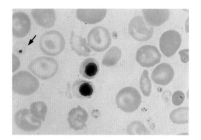

Color Plate 98

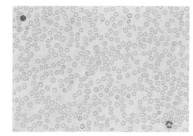

Color Plate 99

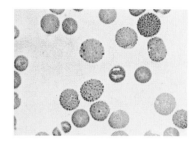

Color Plate 100

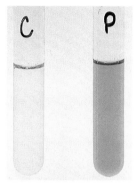

Color Plate 101

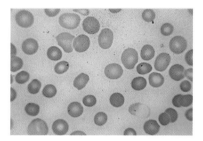

Color Plate 102

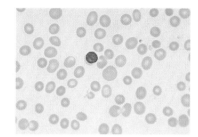

Color Plate 103

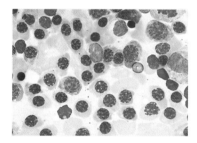

Color Plate 104

Color Plate 105

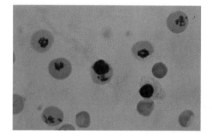

Color Plate 106

Color Plate 98. Peripheral smear in B-thalassemia major. Note the nucleated red cells, the Howell-Jolly body in the hypochromic microcyte (*arrow*), the numerous target cells and the moderate anisocytosis and poikilocytosis (Wright's stain). (From Listen, Look, and Learn, vol 3: Coagulation, Hematology. The American Society of Clinical Pathologists Press, Chicago, 1973, with permission.)

Color Plate 99. Peripheral smear in thalassemia minor. Note the microcytosis and the hypochromia with mild anisocytosis and poikilocytosis. A few target cells and basophilic stippling are present. (Wright's stain, magnification ×400)

Color Plate 100. Hemoglobin H inclusions (supravital stain). (From Listen, Look, and Learn, vol 3: Coagulation, Hematology. The American Society of Clinical Pathologists Press, Chicago, 1973, with permission.)

Color Plate 101. Sugar water test: the tube on the left represents the control (C), and the tube on the right represents the patient (P) with a positive sugar water test. Ten to 80 percent hemolysis will be seen in PNH.

Color Plate 102. Ham's test. Positive results will occur in patients with PNH. A positive test is reported when hemolysis occurs in tube number 1, containing fresh normal serum and patient cells; tube number 2, containing acidified normal serum and patient cells; and tube number 3, containing acidified patient serum and patient cells.

Color Plate 103. Peripheral blood smear from a patient with paroxysmal nocturnal hemoglobinuria. (magnification ×600)

Color Plate 104. Bone marrow aspirate smear from a patient with paroxysmal nocturnal hemoglobinuria demonstrating erythroid hyperplasia. (magnification ×500)

Color Plate 105. Autoimmune hemolytic anemia (peripheral blood). Note spherocytes and polychromasia.

Color Plate 106. Reticulocytes. New methylene blue stain of peripheral blood. Note *non-nucleated* reticulocytes with varying amounts of stained reticulum (RNA). Reticulocytosis is associated with increased erythropoietic activity reflected by polychromasia on the Wright's stain of the peripheral smear (see Color Plate 105). (From Listen, Look, and Learn, vol 3: Coagulation, Hematology. The American Society of Clinical Pathologists Press, Chicago, 1973, with permission.)

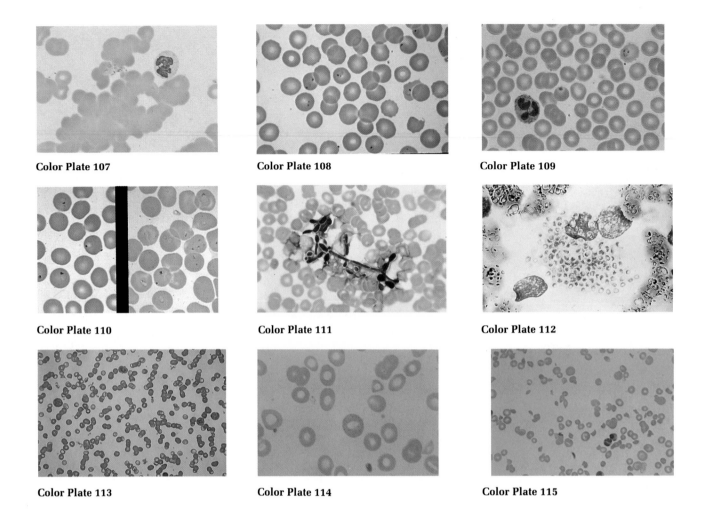

Color Plate 107

Color Plate 108

Color Plate 109

Color Plate 110

Color Plate 111

Color Plate 112

Color Plate 113

Color Plate 114

Color Plate 115

Color Plate 107. Cold agglutinin disease (peripheral blood). Note the autoagglutination of red cells, polychromasia, anisocytosis, and poikilocytosis.

Color Plate 108. Ringed forms of Plasmodium falciparum in red blood cells (RBCs). Note that the same RBCs may be infected with more than one ring.

Color Plate 109. Late stages of P. vivax malaria. Note and contrast the platelet on the RBC (*center*) and the ring form of malaria toward the periphery (*upper right*).

Color Plate 110. Comparison of parasitemia of malaria (*left*) and babesiosis (*right*).

Color Plate 111. Candidemia: peripheral blood. Candida albicans in the peripheral blood demonstrating both hyphae, psuedohyphae, and yeast forms. Note that some of the organism has broken out of the cytoplasm of disintegrating monocytes, of which nuclear remnants are still visible.

Color Plate 112. Histoplasma capsulatum (peripheral blood).

Color Plate 113. Hook worm information (*arrow*).

Color Plate 114. Basophilic stippling in lead poisoning (*left*) and coarse basophilic stippling (*arrows*).

Color Plate 115. Peripheral blood showing red cell fragmentation with thrombocytopenia and nucleated RBCs from a case of thrombotic thrombocytopenic purpura (TTP). (magnification ×500)

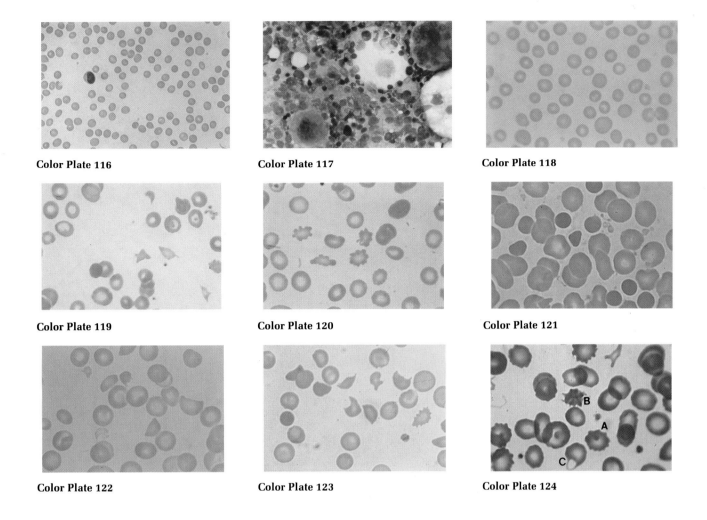

Color Plate 116   Color Plate 117   Color Plate 118

Color Plate 119   Color Plate 120   Color Plate 121

Color Plate 122   Color Plate 123   Color Plate 124

Color Plate 116. Idiopathic thrombocytopenic purpura (ITP), peripheral blood.

Color Plate 117. Idiopathic thrombocytopenic purpura (ITP), bone marrow.

Color Plate 118. Post-transfusion purpura, note the absence of platelets.

Color Plate 119. RBC fragmentation in microangiopathic hemolysis from a patient with prosthetic cardiac valve (mechanical hemolysis), note the presence of schistocytes.

Color Plate 120. Burr cells (peripheral blood).

Color Plate 121. Peripheral blood from a patient with extensive burns. Note typical microspherocytes and membranous fragments. (From Listen, Look, and Learn, vol 3: Coagulation, Hematology. The American Society of Clinical Pathologists Press, Chicago, 1973, with permission.)

Color Plate 122. Peripheral blood from a patient with disseminated carcinoma. Note presence of schistocytes and helmet cells. (From Listen, Look, and Learn, vol 3: Coagulation, Hematology. The American Society of Clinical Pathologists Press, Chicago, 1973, with permission.)

Color Plate 123. Peripheral blood from a patient with malignant hypertension. Note presence of schistocytes, helmet cells, and a burr cell. (From Listen, Look, and Learn, vol 3: Coagulation, Hematology. The American Society of Clinical Pathologists Press, Chicago, 1973, with permission.)

Color Plate 124. Renal disease (peripheral blood). Note presence of burr cells (A), thorn cell (B), and blister cell (C). (From Listen, Look, and Learn, vol 3: Coagulation, Hematology. The American Society of Clinical Pathologists Press, Chicago, 1973, with permission.)

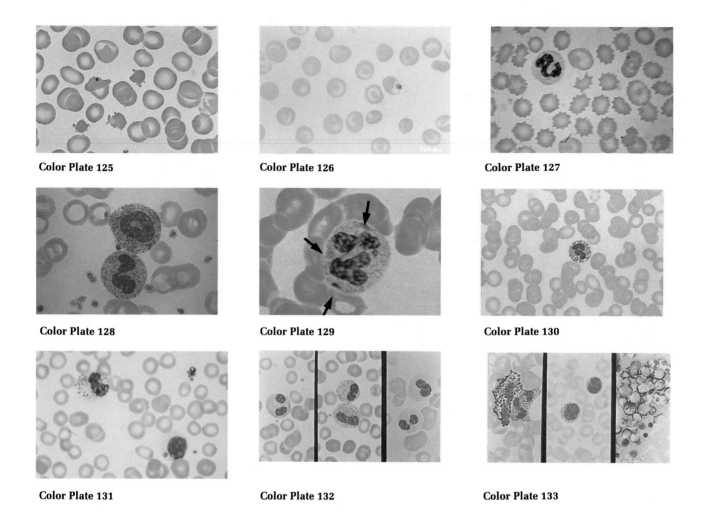

Color Plate 125

Color Plate 126

Color Plate 127

Color Plate 128

Color Plate 129

Color Plate 130

Color Plate 131

Color Plate 132

Color Plate 133

Color Plate 125. Peripheral blood of a patient after kidney transplant and splenectomy. Note small, condensed, irregularly shaped cells and presence of a Howell-Jolly body. (From Listen, Look, and Learn, vol 3: Coagulation, Hematology. The American Society of Clinical Pathologists Press, Chicago, 1973, with permission.)

Color Plate 126. Target cells seen on the peripheral blood smear of a patient with liver disease.

Color Plate 127. "Spur cell anemia" (acanthocytosis) associated with severe liver disease.

Color Plate 128. Toxic granulation (peripheral blood). Note the prominent dark-staining granules.

Color Plate 129. Dohle bodies (*arrows*). Note the large bluish bodies in the periphery of the cytoplasm.

Color Plate 130. Vacuolated neutrophils suggesting the presence of infection or a severe inflammation.

Color Plate 131. Chediak-Higashi. (*Right*) lymphocyte in peripheral blood; (*left*) neutrophil in peripheral blood. (From Listen, Look, and Learn, vol 3: Coagulation, Hematology. The American Society of Clinical Pathologists Press, Chicago, 1973, with permission.)

Color Plate 132. Pelger-Huet anomaly. Peripheral blood. (From Hyun, BH, Ashton, JK, and Dolan, K: Practical Hematology. A Laboratory Guide with Accompanying Filmstrip. WB Saunders, Philadelpha, 1975, with permission.)

Color Plate 133. Alder-Reilly anomaly, (*Left and middle*) note azurophilic granulation in cells from peripheral blood; (*right*), bone marrow. (From Hyun, BH, Ashton, JK, and Dolan, K: Practical Hematology. A Laboratory Guide with Accompanying Filmstrip. WB Saunders, Philadelphia, 1975, with permission.)

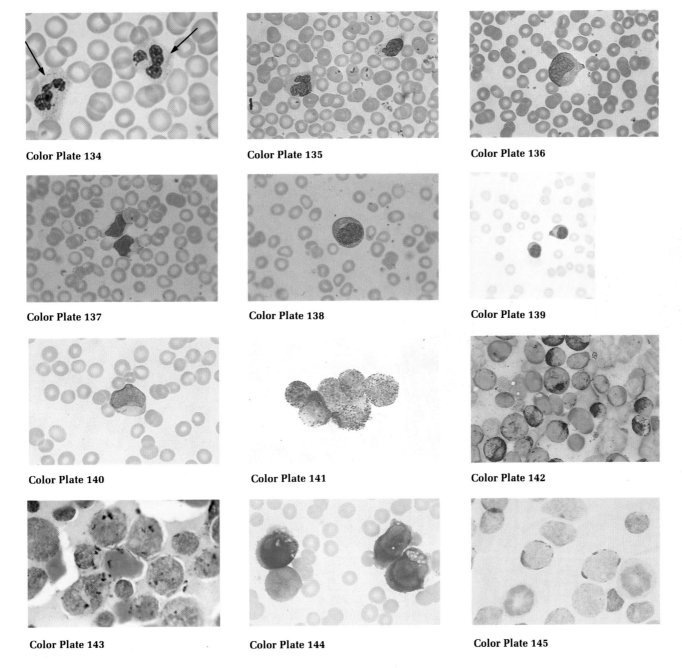

Color Plate 134

Color Plate 135

Color Plate 136

Color Plate 137

Color Plate 138

Color Plate 139

Color Plate 140

Color Plate 141

Color Plate 142

Color Plate 143

Color Plate 144

Color Plate 145

Color Plate 134. May-Hegglin anomaly. Note the Dohle body present in each neutrophil (*arrows*) not shown in the slide but associated with May-Hegglin anomaly is the presence of giant platelets. (From Listen, Look, and Learn, vol 3: Coagulation, Hematology. The American Society of Clinical Pathologists Press, Chicago, 1973, with permission.)

Color Plate 135. Normal monocyte (*left*) and medium-size lymphocyte (*right*).

Color Plate 136. Large reactive lymphocyte with prominent perinuclear halo in infectious mononucleosis.

Color Plate 137. Reactive lymphocytes in infectious mononucleosis.

Color Plate 138. Plasmacytoid reactive lymphocyte in a drug reaction.

Color Plate 139. Plasmacytoid lymphocytes, note the red staining accumulation of immunoglobulin in the cytoplasm.

Color Plate 140. Auer rod in myeloblast.

Color Plate 141. Myeloperoxidase positivity in acute promyelocytic leukemia.

Color Plate 142. Sudan black B positivity in AML (M2).

Color Plate 143. Specific esterase Naphtol AS-D Chloracetate positivity in AML (M2).

Color Plate 144. Nonspecific esterase (alpha-naphthyl butyrate) positively in acute monocytic leukemia (M5).

Color Plate 145. Periodic acid–Schiff positivity in ALL. Note the "block" staining pattern.

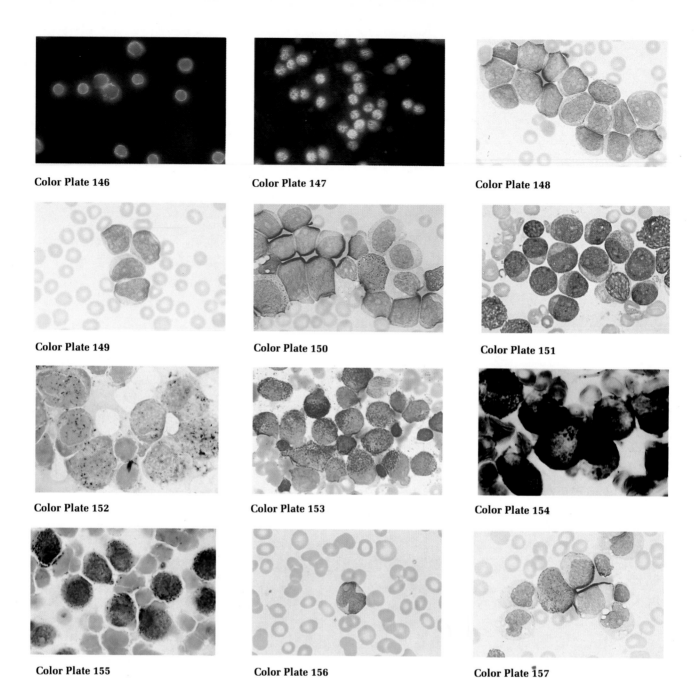

Color Plate 146. Surface immunoglobulin (SIg) positive cells in B-cell ALL (L3).

Color Plate 147. TdT positivity in ALL using immunofluorescence method.

Color Plate 148. Acute myeloblastic leukemia (AML) without maturation, MI, bone marrow.

Color Plate 149. AML, M1, peripheral blood.

Color Plate 150. Acute myeloblastic leukemia with maturation, M2, bone marrow.

Color Plate 151. AML (M2).

Color Plate 152. AML, M2 (myeloperoxidase stain)

Color Plate 153. Acute promyelocytic leukemia, (APL) M3, bone marrow.

Color Plate 154. APL, M3 (sudan black B stain).

Color Plate 155. APL, M3 (chloroacetate esterase).

Color Plate 156. Acute ''microgranular'' promyelocytic leukemia, M3m, peripheral blood.

Color Plate 157. Acute myelomonocytic leukemia, AMML M4, bone marrow.

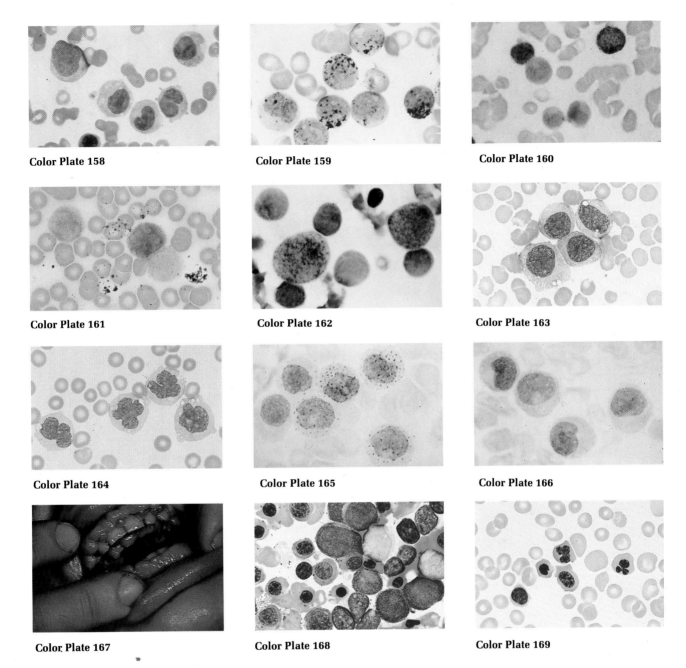

Color Plate 158

Color Plate 159

Color Plate 160

Color Plate 161

Color Plate 162

Color Plate 163

Color Plate 164

Color Plate 165

Color Plate 166

Color Plate 167

Color Plate 168

Color Plate 169

Color Plate 158. Acute myelomonocytic leukemia, M4, peripheral blood.

Color Plate 159. AMML, M4 (sudan black B stain).

Color Plate 160. AMML, M4 (chloroacetate esterase stain).

Color Plate 161. AMML, M4 (alpha naphthyl butyrate stain).

Color Plate 162. AMML, M4 (combined esterase stain). Note the red staining granules in the monocytes and blue staining granules in the granulocytes.

Color Plate 163. Acute monocytic leukemia (AMoL), poorly differentiated, M5a, peripheral blood.

Color Plate 164. Acute monocytic leukemia, well-differentiated, M5b, peripheral blood.

Color Plate 165. AMoL, M5b (naphthol AS-D chloracetate stain).

Color Plate 166. AmoL, M5b (NASDA stain with sodium fluoride inhibition).

Color Plate 167. Gum hypertrophy: a clinical manifestation of acute leukemia.

Color Plate 168. Erythroleukemia, M6, bone marrow.

Color Plate 169. Erythroleukemia, M6, peripheral blood.

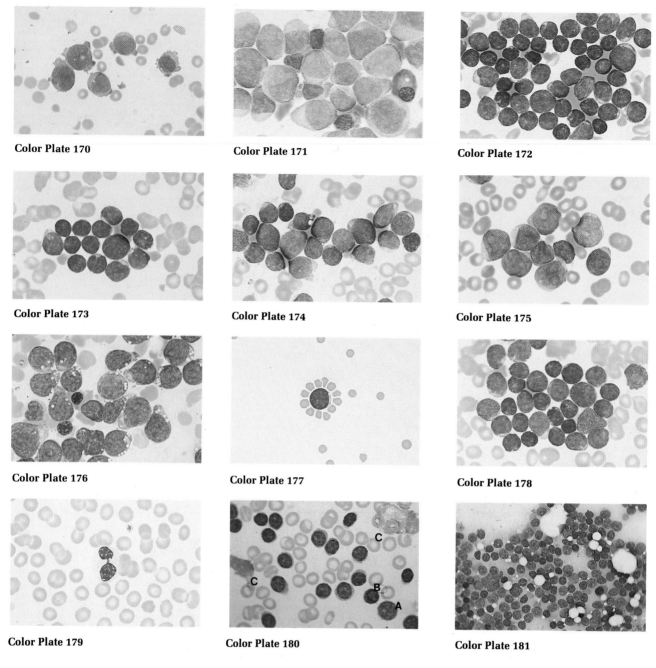

Color Plate 170. Acute megakaryoblastic leukemia, (AMegL) M7.

Color Plate 171. Case study bone marrow (AML).

Color Plate 172. Acute lymphoblastic leukemia (ALL), L1, bone marrow.

Color Plate 173. Acute lymphoblastic leukemia, L1, peripheral blood.

Color Plate 174. Acute lymphoblastic leukemia, L2, bone marrow.

Color Plate 175. Acute lymphoblastic leukemia, L2, peripheral blood.

Color Plate 176. Acute lymphoblastic leukemia, L3, bone marrow.

Color Plate 177. E-rosette formation in T-cell ALL.

Color Plate 178. Case study: bone marrow (ALL).

Color Plate 179. Pseudo–Pelger-Huët cell in peripheral blood of patient with myelodysplastic syndrome. Note that the cytoplasm is hypogranular.

Color Plate 180. Chronic lymphocytic leukemia (CLL). Note lymphoblasts (*A*), lymphocytes (*B*), and smudge cells (*C*).

Color Plate 181. CLL: bone marrow aspirate (magnification ×10). Note monotonous appearance of cell population and lack of megakaryocytes.

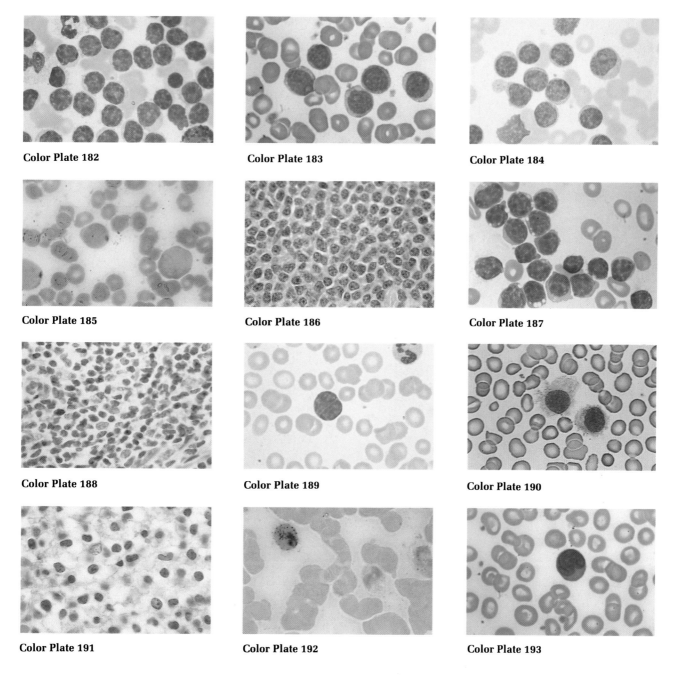

Color Plate 182

Color Plate 183

Color Plate 184

Color Plate 185

Color Plate 186

Color Plate 187

Color Plate 188

Color Plate 189

Color Plate 190

Color Plate 191

Color Plate 192

Color Plate 193

Color Plate 182. CLL: bone marrow aspirate (magnification ×100).

Color Plate 183. Prolymphocytic leukemia (PL), peripheral blood.

Color Plate 184. CLL with occasional prolymphocyte, peripheral blood.

Color Plate 185. Naphthol acetate esterase (ANAE) stain showing localized "dot-like" positivity in two T lymphocytes.

Color Plate 186. Well-differentiated lymphocytic lymphoma (WDLL), lymph node.

Color Plate 187. WDLL in leukemic phase, peripheral blood.

Color Plate 188. Poorly differentiated lymphocytic lymphoma (PDLL), lymph node.

Color Plate 189. PDLL, peripheral blood.

Color Plate 190. Hairy cell leukemia (HCL): peripheral blood. (From Hyun, BH: Morphology of Blood and Bone Marrow. American Society of Clinical Pathologists, Workshop 5121, Philadelphia, September 7, 1983, with permission.)

Color Plate 191. HCL: bone marrow aspirate

Color Plate 192. Tartrate-resistant acid phosphatase (TRAP) stain of peripheral blood showing positivity in hairy cell and no staining in neutrophils.

Color Plate 193. Sezary cell, peripheral blood.

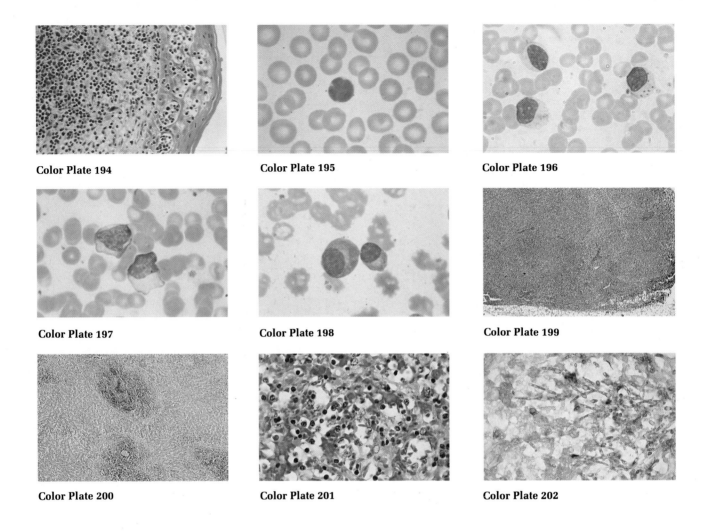

Color Plate 194   **Color Plate 195**   **Color Plate 196**

Color Plate 197   **Color Plate 198**   **Color Plate 199**

Color Plate 200   **Color Plate 201**   **Color Plate 202**

Color Plate 194. Infiltration of the epidermis and upper dermis by lymphocytes, many with convoluted (cerebriform) nuclei, histiocytes, and formation of Pautrier microabcesses, characteristic of the cutaneous T-cell lymphoma mycosis fungoides.

Color Plate 195. Abnormal lymphocyte with "cloverleaf" nucleus in a patient with adult T-cell leukemia/lymphoma (ATLL), peripheral blood.

Color Plate 196. Large granular lymphocytes (LGL) in a patient with chronic T-gamma lymphoproliferative disease, peripheral blood.

Color Plate 197. Atypical lymphocytes in patient with infectious mononucleosis, peripheral blood.

Color Plate 198. Plasma cells in patient with multiple myeloma, peripheral blood.

Color Plate 199. Hematoxylin and eosin (H&E) section of lymph node showing infiltration by well-differentiated lymphocytes in a patient with CLL. Normal nodal architecture is obliterated and no lymphoid nodules are seen.

Color Plate 200. H&E section of liver showing infarction of liver parenchyma, hemorrhagic congestion and a dense lymphocyte infiltrate consisting of well-differentiated lymphocytes from a patient with CLL.

Color Plate 201. H&E section of spleen showing hemorrhagic congestion, a monomorphic lymphocytic infiltrate consisting of well-differentiated lymphocytes and sickled red blood cells in a patient with CLL and sickle cell anemia (SS).

Color Plate 202. H&E section of pyloric region of the stomach showing necrotic tissue and colonization of an ulcerated area with fungus in a patient with adenocarcinoma, CLL and SS.

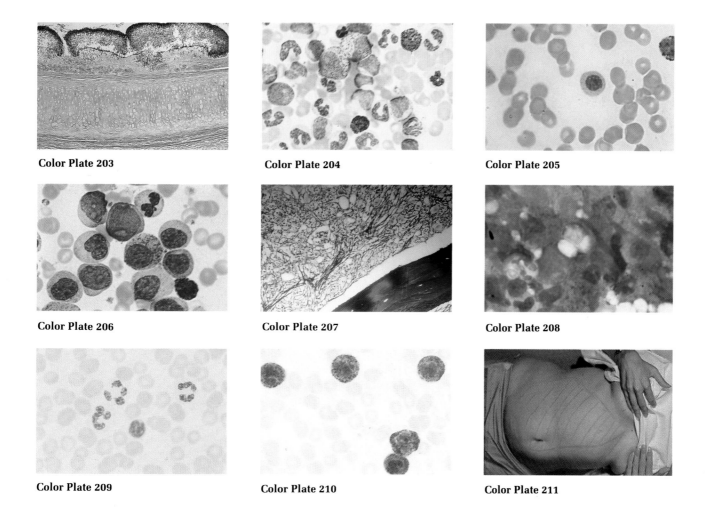

Color Plate 203. Gomori methenamine silver (GMS) stain of section of trachea showing multiple colonies of fungus with hyphae present along the tracheal epithelium and invading the tracheal mucosa in a patient with CLL.

Color Plate 204. Peripheral smear: chronic myelogenous leukemia (CML). (From Listen, Look, and Learn, vol 3: Coagulation, Hematology. The American Society of Clinical Pathologists Press, Chicago, 1973, with permission.)

Color Plate 205. Pelgeroid granulocyte (pseudo Pelger cell) in a patient with CML, peripheral blood. Note that the nucleus is round with condensed chromatin and should not be mistaken for a normal myelocyte or a nucleated red blood cell.

Color Plate 206. CML: bone marrow aspirate.

Color Plate 207. Silver stain for reticulin and collagen fibers on bone marrow biopsy in a patient with CML and secondary myelofibrosis.

Color Plate 208. Sea-blue histiocytes (pseudo Gaucher cells) in the bone marrow aspirate of a patient with CML.

Color Plate 209. LAP stain of peripheral blood showing little or no activity in CML.

Color Plate 210. Leukemoid reaction: increased LAP activity.

Color Plate 211. Hepatosplenomegaly: a characteristic finding in patients with idiopathic myelofibrosis with myeloid metaplasia (IMF-MM).

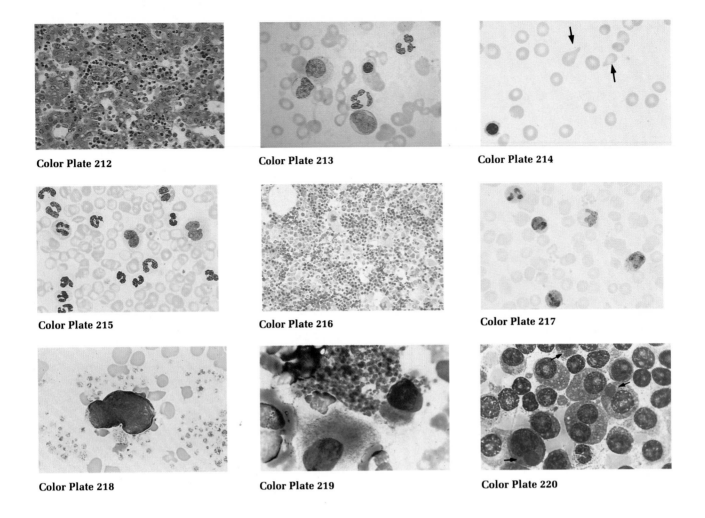

Color Plate 212

Color Plate 213

Color Plate 214

Color Plate 215

Color Plate 216

Color Plate 217

Color Plate 218

Color Plate 219

Color Plate 220

Color Plate 212. Extramedullary hematopoiesis in the liver of a patient with IMF.

Color Plate 213. "Leukoerythroblastosis," a peripheral blood picture that often accompanies marrow infiltration by tumors (myelophthisic anemia). Note the presence of immature red and white cells.

Color Plate 214. Tear drops (*arrows*): peripheral blood in a patient with myelofibrosis.

Color Plate 215. Polycythemia vera (PV) (peripheral blood). Note hypochromia and increased cellularity. (magnification ×400)

Color Plate 216. Bone marrow showing panhyperplasia in PV. Note increased number of megakaryocytes (*arrow*). Hematoxylin and eosin stain (low power).

Color Plate 217. LAP stain of peripheral blood showing increased activity in PV (red staining).

Color Plate 218. Essential thrombocythemia: peripheral blood megakaryocyte and numerous platelets. (From Hyun, BH: Morphology of Blood and Bone Marrow. American Society of Clinical Pathologists, Workshop 5121, Philadelphia, September 7, 1983, with permission.)

Color Plate 219. Essential thrombocythemia: bone marrow. Note increased megakaryocytes. (From Hyun, BH: Morphology of Blood and Bone Marrow. American Society of Clinical Pathologists, Workshop 5121, Philadelphia. September 7, 1983, with permission.)

Color Plate 220. Bone marrow aspirate showing atypical and binucleate plasma cells and Russell bodies (*arrow*).

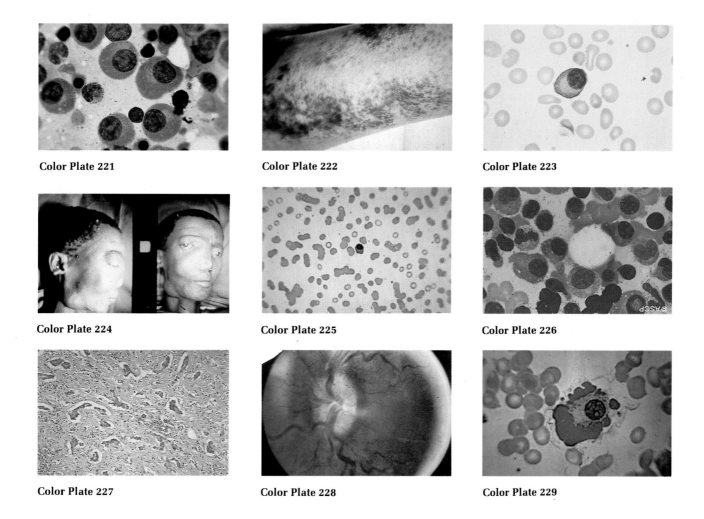

Color Plate 221. Bone marrow biopsy showing replacement of marrow by plasma cells.

Color Plate 222. Patient with cryoglobulinemic purpura. Note the skin manifestations.

Color Plate 223. Peripheral blood in plasma cell leukemia showing presence of circulating plasma cells. (From Listen, Look, and Learn, vol 3: Coagulation, Hematology. The American Society of Clinical Pathologists Press, Chicago, 1973, with permission.)

Color Plate 224. Plasmacytomas of the face and jaw in a patient with multiple myeloma.

Color Plate 225. Peripheral blood showing marked rouleaux formation. Note the "stacked-coin" appearance of the red cells.

Color Plate 226. Plasmacytoid lymphocytes in marrow aspirate from a patient with Waldenstrom's macroglobulinemia. (From Listen, Look, and Learn, vol 3: Coagulation, Hematology. The American Society of Clinical Pathologists Press, Chicago, 1973, with permission.)

Color Plate 227. Amorphous amyloid deposits replacing normal liver architecture.

Color Plate 228. Tortuous veins with sausage-linked appearance present in the fundus of the eye.

Color Plate 229. Flame cell: sometimes associated with IgA myeloma.

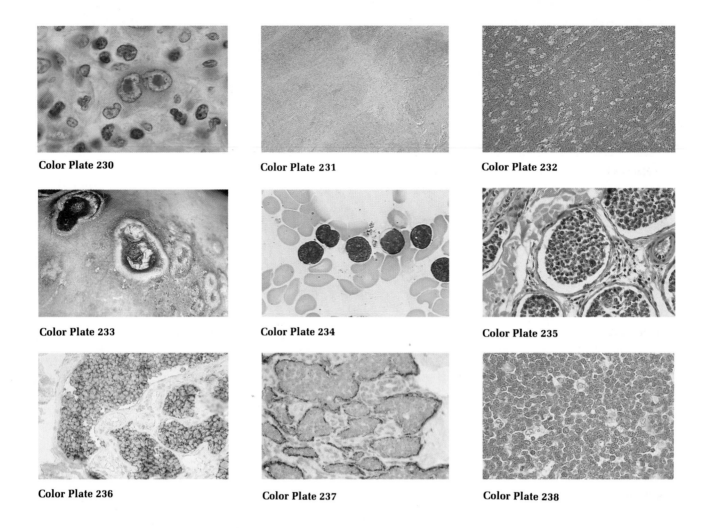

Color Plate 230. Classical Reed-Sternberg (RS) cell (*center*). Characterized by large size, multi-lobed nucleus, and inclusion-like nucleoli.

Color Plate 231. Nodular sclerosing Hodgkin's disease: orderly bands of collagen subdivide the tissue into cellular nodules containing a mixture of cell types including large numbers of lacunar cells.

Color Plate 232. Malignant lymphoma, small non-cleaved cell type. "Starry sky" pattern is produced by the clear cytoplasm of numerous tingible body macrophages which are admixed with the neoplastic small non-cleaved cells.

Color Plate 233. Mycosis fungoides, tumor stage. Tumor nodules are produced by massive local infiltrates of the skin by the characteristic cerebriform cells of mycosis fungoides.

Color Plate 234. Sezary cells in peripheral blood. Note large abnormal T lymphocytes with prominent nuclear folds and clefts giving the nucleus a cerebriform shape. (From Hyun, BH: Morphology of Blood and Bone Marrow. American Society of Clinical Pathologists, Workshop 5121. Philadelphia, September 7, 1983, with permission.)

Color Plate 235. Angiotropic large-cell lymphoma, malignant cells are confined to vascular spaces.

Color Plate 236. Angiotropic large cell lymphoma: immunoperoxidase stain demonstrates positive staining (*red*) of the malignant cells for leukocyte common antigen.

Color Plate 237. Angiotropic large cell lymphoma: staining for factor VIII antigen is confined to the endothelial cells lining the vascular spaces.

Color Plate 238. Undifferentiated lymphoma: Burkitt's type. Note the prominent histiocytes give a "starry sky" pattern. (Courtesy of Dr. John Sutherland.)

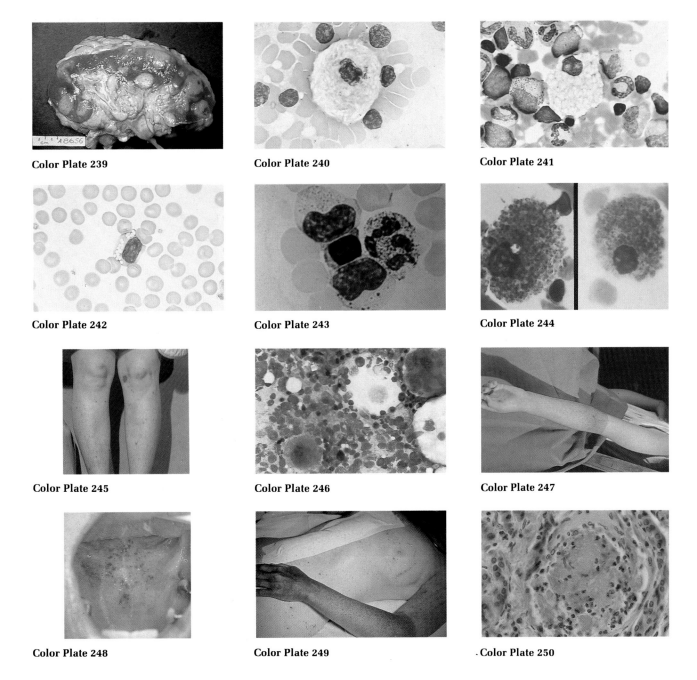

Color Plate 239

Color Plate 240

Color Plate 241

Color Plate 242

Color Plate 243

Color Plate 244

Color Plate 245

Color Plate 246

Color Plate 247

Color Plate 248

Color Plate 249

Color Plate 250

Color Plate 239. Gross anatomy of a kidney involved in metastatic lymphoma. Note the white nodular lymphocytic infiltration. (Courtesy of Dr. John Sutherland.)

Color Plate 240. Gaucher's cell: bone marrow aspirate.

Color Plate 241. Neimann-Pick cell: bone marrow aspirate.

Color Plate 242. Tay-Sachs disease: vacuolated lymphocytes.

Color Plate 243. Hurler's anomaly.

Color Plate 244. Sea-blue histiocytes. Note the abnormally coarse azurophilic granules present in neutrophils, lymphocytes, and monocytes. (From Listen, Look, and Learn, vol 3: Coagulation, Hematology. The American Society of Clinical Pathologists Press, Chicago, 1973, with permission.)

Color Plate 245. Petechial bleeding of the lower extremities in a patient with idiopathic thrombocytopenic purpura (ITP).

Color Plate 246. ITP: bone marrow aspirate. Note increased number of megakaryocytes with normal cellularity (M/E 3:1).

Color Plate 247. Positive tourniquet test in a patient with ITP.

Color Plate 248. Oral cavity, patient with ITP.

Color Plate 249. Post-transfusion purpura (PTP).

Color Plate 250. Renal biopsy from a case of thrombotic thrombocytopenic purpura (TTP) showing glomerular deposits of platelet-fibrin microvascular occlusion.

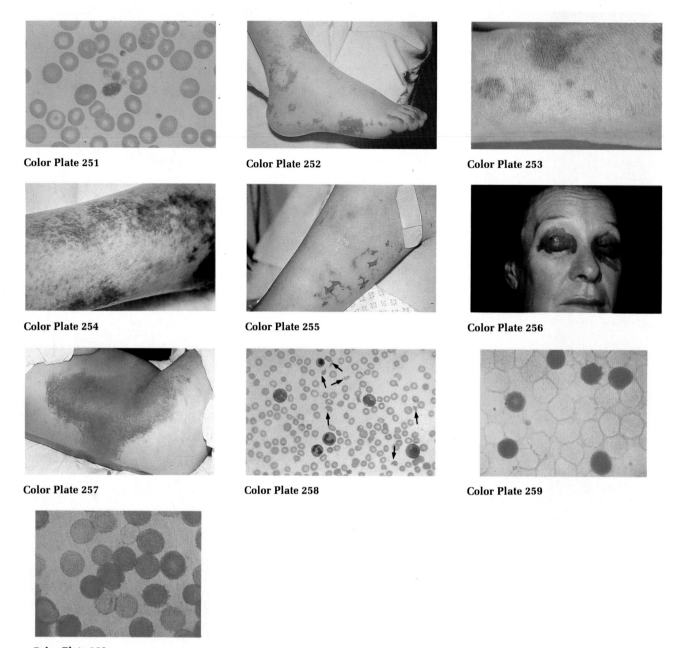

Color Plate 251

Color Plate 252

Color Plate 253

Color Plate 254

Color Plate 255

Color Plate 256

Color Plate 257

Color Plate 258

Color Plate 259

Color Plate 260

Color Plate 251. Giant platelet from a patient with myeloproliferative disease with thrombocytosis.

Color Plate 252. Anaphylatoid (Henock-Schonlein) purpura. Purpuric lesions of the foot.

Color Plate 253. Senile purpura (skin manifestations).

Color Plate 254. Steroid purpura (skin manifestations).

Color Plate 255. Cryoglobulinemic purpura (skin manifestations).

Color Plate 256. Amyloid purpura, note characteristic periorbital distribution.

Color Plate 257. Diffuse hemorrhage: a clinical manifestation of a patient with disseminated intravascular coagulation (DIC). Note the multiple cutaneous ecchymoses.

Color Plate 258. DIC (peripheral blood). Note presence of schistocytes (*arrows*) and nucleated red cell (*top border*).

Color Plate 259. Betke-Kleihauer stain of blood from a newborn. Red-staining cells contain hemoglobin F; clear staining cells contain hemoglobin A. (From Listen, Look, and Learn, vol 3: Coagulation, Hematology. The American Society of Clinical Pathologists Press, Chicago, 1973, with permission.)

Color Plate 260. Betke-Kleihauer stain of blood from a patient with hereditary persistence of fetal hemoglobin (HPFH). Note that all the red cells stain red, owing to the varying amounts of hemoglobin F. (From Listen, Look, and Learn, vol 3: Coagulation, Hematology. The American Society of Clinical Pathologists Press, Chicago, 1973, with permission.)

PART ONE

INTRODUCTION TO CLINICAL HEMATOLOGY

CHAPTER 1

DENISE M. HARMENING, Ph.D., M.T.(ASCP), C.L.S.(NCA)

The Red Blood Cell: Structure and Function

RED BLOOD CELL METABOLISM

RED BLOOD CELL MEMBRANE
RED BLOOD CELL MEMBRANE LIPIDS
Phospholipids
Glycolipids and Cholesterol
RED BLOOD CELL MEMBRANE PROTEINS
Integral Membrane Proteins
Peripheral Proteins
DEFORMABILITY
PERMEABILITY

HEMOGLOBIN STRUCTURE AND FUNCTION
HEMOGLOBIN SYNTHESIS
Iron Delivery and Supply
Synthesis of Protoporphyrins
Globin Synthesis
Hemoglobin Function
ABNORMAL HEMOGLOBINS OF CLINICAL IMPORTANCE

MAINTENANCE OF HEMOGLOBIN FUNCTION: ACTIVE RED BLOOD CELL METABOLIC PATHWAYS
ERYTHROCYTE SENESCENCE

CONCLUSION

OBJECTIVES

At the end of this chapter, the learner should be able to:
1. Identify three areas of red blood cell (RBC) metabolism crucial for normal erythrocyte survival and function.
2. State the function of biochemical substances that compose the outer, central, and inner portion of the RBC membrane.
3. Describe the consequences of structural membrane defects that lead to RBC deformity.
4. List the criteria for normal hemoglobulin synthesis.
5. Describe the assembly of the protoporphyrin ring.
6. Name the number and type of globin chains found in adults.
7. List the types of hemoglobin composing the normal adult hemoglobin.
8. Describe the cellular manifestations of iron accumulation.
9. Characterize the oxygen affinity of the tense (T) form and the related (R) form of the hemoglobin molecule.
10. Define "shift to the left" in relation to the hemoglobin-oxygen dissociation curve.
11. Define "shift to the right" in relation to the hemoglobin-oxygen dissociation curve.
12. Name the abnormal hemoglobins that are unable to transport oxygen.
13. Name the metabolic pathway that generates most of RBC ATP.
14. List the steps in the extravascular breakdown of senescent RBCs.
15. List the steps in the intravascular breakdown of senescent RBCs.

RED BLOOD CELL METABOLISM

Three areas of red blood cell (RBC) metabolism are crucial for normal erythrocyte survival and function: the RBC membrane, hemoglobin structure and function, and cellular energetics. Defects or problems associated with any of these areas will result in impaired RBC survival.[1] A thorough working knowledge of these areas of RBC physiology will ensure basic understanding of the various complex erythrocyte functions.

RED BLOOD CELL MEMBRANE

The actual biochemical structure and organization of the RBC membrane still remains to be elu-

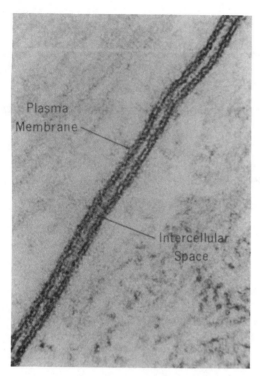

Figure 1–1. TEM plasma membrane.

cidated; however, our general knowledge of all plasma membranes has been expanded. The RBC membrane viewed by transmission electron microscopy (TEM) appears as a trilaminar structure consisting of a dark–light–dark band arrangement of layers (Fig. 1–1). These layers represent (1) an

outer hydrophilic portion chemically composed of glycolipid, glycoprotein, and protein; (2) a central hydrophobic layer containing protein, cholesterol, and phospholipid; and (3) an inner hydrophilic layer containing protein.

The RBC membrane represents a semipermeable lipid bilayer supported by a protein meshlike cytoskeleton structure (Fig. 1–2). This fluid lipid matrix contains equal amounts of cholesterol and phospholipids with a mosaic of proteins interspersed throughout at various intervals. Those proteins that extend from the outer surface and traverse the entire membrane to the inner cytoplasmic side of the RBC are termed *integral* membrane proteins. The other class of RBC membrane proteins, called *peripheral* proteins, is limited to the cytoplasmic surface of the membrane, which is beneath the lipid bilayer and forms the RBC cytoskeleton. Both the protein and the lipids are organized asymmetrically within the RBC membrane. The chemical composition of the membrane mass is approximately 42 percent lipids, 50 percent proteins, and 8 percent carbohydrates.[2]

Red Blood Cell Membrane Lipids

Phospholipids

The erythrocyte membrane lipid consists of a bilayer of phospholipids interspersed with molecules of unesterified cholesterol and glycolipids. Two groups of phospholipids are known to possess a distinct asymmetry within the bilayer matrix of the RBC: choline phospholipids and amino phospholipids.[3]

Choline phospholipids, consisting of phosphati-

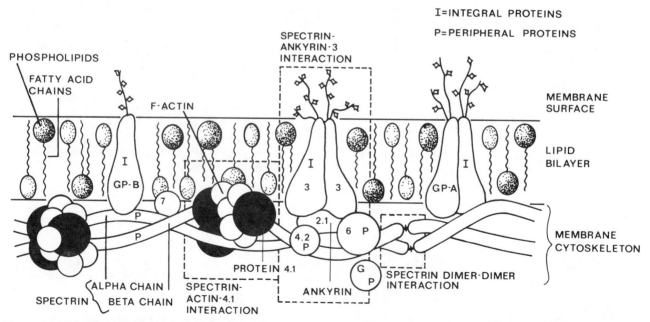

Figure 1–2. Schematic illustration of red blood cell membrane depicting the composition and arrangement of red cell membrane proteins. GP-A = glycophorin A; GP-B = glycophorin B; G = globin. Numbers refer to pattern of migration on SDS (sodium, dodecyl, sulfite) polyacrylamide gel pattern stained with Coomassie brilliant blue. Relations of protein to each other and to lipids are purely hypothetical; however, the positions of the proteins relative to the inside or outside of the lipid bilayer are accurate. (Note: proteins are not drawn to scale and many minor proteins are omitted.)

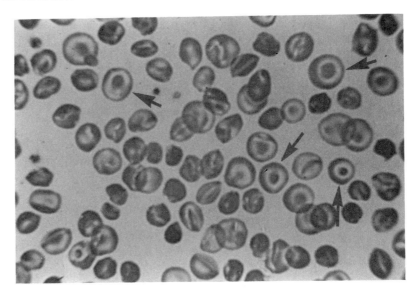

Figure 1–3. Target cells.

dyl choline and sphingomyelin, are primarily located on the outside half of the lipid bilayer readily accessible to the external environment.[3] Because of their outward orientation in the lipid bilayer, the choline phospholipids may represent controlling points in the major pathways of lipid renewal as there is an exchange between plasma fatty acids and the RBC membrane. Fatty acids are incorporated through an energy-dependent process into membrane phospholipids.[4] Therefore, changes in body lipid transport and metabolism may cause abnormalities in the plasma phospholipid concentration, which may alter the RBC membrane composition, resulting in a decreased RBC survival in circulation. In addition, it is suggested that the interaction of these phospholipids with cholesterol may play a role in cholesterol homeostasis in the RBC membrane.[4]

In contrast, amino phospholipids, consisting of phosphatidylethanolamine and phosphatidylserine, are located almost exclusively on the inside half or cytoplasmic side of the RBC membrane along with phosphatidylinositol.[5] This specific orientation of these phospholipids maintains a precise lipid pattern that is critical to normal RBC survival in circulation. Alteration of this arrangement leading to the abnormal appearance of these amino phospholipids on the outer surface of the lipid bilayer promotes activation of the clotting cascade and may result in extravascular hemolysis.[6] Stabilization of this phospholipid asymmetry in the erythrocyte membrane is maintained through the interaction with specific peripheral proteins (see section on RBC membrane proteins).[7]

Glycolipids and Cholesterol

The majority of the glycolipids are located in the outer half of the lipid bilayer and interact with glycoproteins to form many of the RBC antigens. Cholesterol is approximately equally distributed, being located on both sides of the lipid bilayer

inserted between the choline and amino phospholipids.[3] Cholesterol composes 25 percent of the RBC membrane lipid and is present in a 1:1 molar ratio with phospholipids. Red blood cell membrane cholesterol is in continual exchange with plasma cholesterol and is therefore affected by changes in body lipid transport.

Accumulation of cholesterol results in morphologic changes in the RBC, such as target cells, (Fig. 1–3) and may cause RBC membrane damage. Acanthocytes, RBCs with irregular, spiny projections called spicules (Fig. 1–4), have also been associated with an excess accumulation of membrane cholesterol in association with liver disease and particular lipid disorders such as abetalipoproteinemia.[8] All of these RBCs have a decreased survival rate because the excess lipid makes the cell membrane less deformable.

Another example, the congenital deficiency of the plasma enzyme LCAT (lecithin-to-cholesterol acyltransferase), leads to an excess of free cholesterol in both the plasma and the RBC membrane, resulting in, among other problems, a chronic hemolytic anemia.[8] In general, all of these lipids are mobile within the plane of the erythrocyte membrane, and, as a result of this phenomenon, the

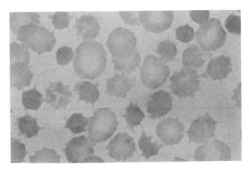

Figure 1–4. Acanthocytes.

RBC membrane is characteristically a viscous, two-dimensional fluid. This lipid bilayer also acts as an impenetrable barrier. Consequently, most transport across the RBC membrane is to occur through transport protein globules.

Red Blood Cell Membrane Proteins

It is estimated that 10 major and 200 minor proteins are asymmetrically organized within the RBC membrane. After solubilization of the RBC membrane with the detergent sodium dodecyl sulfite (SDS), membrane proteins can be separated by polyacrylamide gel electrophoresis and stained. The separated RBC membrane proteins are numbered 1 through 8 when stained with Coomassie blue and 1 through 4 when stained with periodic acid–Schiff (PAS) stain, which is the basis of their nomenclature (Fig. 1–5). The proteins range in molecular weight from 16,000 to 244,000 daltons.[9]

Two of the most important protein constituents include glycophorin, an integral membrane protein, and spectrin, a peripheral membrane protein.

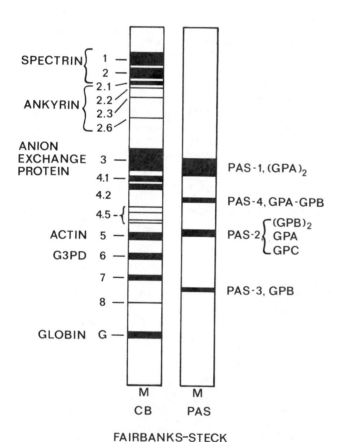

Figure 1–5. Schematic illustration of SDS (sodium, dodecyl, sulfite) polycrylamide gel electrophoresis patterns of red cell membrane proteins stained with Coomassie brilliant blue (CB) and sialoglycoproteins stained with periodic acid–Schiff (PAS) stain. GPA, GPB, and GPC refer to glycophorins A, B, and C, respectively. (GPA)₂ and (GPB)₂ are the dimers, and GPA-GPB is the heterodimer of GPA and GPB.

Integral Membrane Proteins

Glycophorin, the major integral membrane protein, is the principal RBC glycoprotein, representing approximately 10 percent of the total membrane protein.[10] The molecule contains approximately 60 percent carbohydrate and accounts for most of the membrane sialic acid, which gives the erythrocyte its negative charge. Glycophorin, similar to other integral membrane proteins, spans the entire thickness of the lipid bilayer and appears on the external surface of the RBC membrane, accounting for the location of many RBC antigens. Three types of glycophorins have been described—glycophorin A, B, and C (see PAS bands 1, 2, and 3).[10] In addition, all glycoproteins are exposed on the outer RBC membrane surface and migrate primarily in band 3 of the SDS gel electrophoretic pattern stained with Coomassie blue (Fig. 1–5).[11] The majority of these proteins, as mentioned previously, carry RBC antigens and are receptors (such as the glycophorins) or are transport proteins (such as band 3, the anion exchange channel glycoprotein). It is speculated that band 3 and the glycophorins play a major role in anchoring the RBC membrane cytoskeleton to the lipid bilayer.[12] As a result, lateral mobility of these integral proteins within the lipid bilayer is relatively restricted.

Peripheral Proteins

Spectrin, the principal peripheral protein, is a large molecule that represents approximately 75 percent of the peripheral protein and 25 percent of the total membrane protein.[13]

Spectrin is composed of a helix of two polypeptide chains, an alpha chain (band 1, molecular weight 240,000 daltons) and a beta chain (band 2, molecular weight 225,000 daltons).[11] These chains form dimers, which link together with other alpha-beta chains to form tetramers.[12] Spectrin is intimately related to RBC membrane integrity as it binds with other peripheral proteins such as actin (band 5), ankyrin (band 2.1), and band 4.1 to form a skeleton of microfilaments on the inner surface of the RBC membrane [13] (see Fig. 1–2). These microfilaments strengthen the membrane, protecting the cell from being broken by circulatory shear forces, and also control the biconcave shape and deformability of the cell.[14] Two sets of spectrin complexes tie the RBC cytoskeleton network together: a spectrin–actin–band 4.1 complex and a spectrin-ankyrin complex that binds to the integral protein, band 3, to anchor the skeleton to the overlaying lipid bilayer (see Fig. 1–2).[13,15] In addition, spectrin is also linked to the RBC lipid bilayer through the bonding between band 4.1 and the integral protein, glycophorin C.[16,17] The preservation of the spectrin–actin–band 4.1 and spectrin-ankyrin network, and thus the integrity of the RBC membrane, requires phosphorylation of spectrin by a protein kinase present in the membrane, which is energy dependent, being catalyzed by adenosine triphosphate (ATP).[17] Other peripheral membrane proteins that lack carbohydrates and are confined to the cytoplasmic membrane surface include certain enzymes such as glyceraldehyde-3-phosphate dehydrogenase (band 6) and structural proteins such as hemoglobin.[18]

As mentioned earlier, the normal chemical composition, structural arrangement, and molecular interactions of the erythrocyte membrane are crucial to the normal RBC survival in circulation of 120 days. In addition, they play a critical role in two important RBC characteristics: deformability and permeability.[19]

Deformability

It has already been mentioned that a loss of ATP (energy) levels leads to a decrease in the phosphorylation of spectrin and, in turn, a loss of membrane deformability. An accumulation or increase in deposition of membrane calcium also results, causing an increase in membrane rigidity and loss of pliability. These cells are at a marked disadvantage when they pass through the small (3 to 5 μm diameter) sinusoidal orifices of the spleen, one of whose functions is extravascular sequestration and removal of aged, damaged, or less deformable RBCs or fragments of their membrane (Fig. 1–6).[1] The loss of RBC membrane is exemplified by the formation of spherocytes (Fig. 1–7), cells with a reduced surface-to-volume ratio, and "bite cells" (Fig. 1–8), in which the removal of a portion of membrane has left a permanent indentation in the remaining cell membrane. The survival time of these forms is also shortened.

Permeability

The RBC membrane is freely permeable to water and anions; chloride (Cl^-) and bicarbonate (HCO_3^-) traverse the membrane in less than a second. It is speculated that this massive exchange of HCO_3^- and Cl^- ions occurs through a large number of

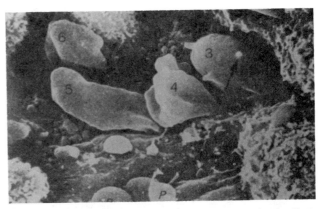

Figure 1–6. SEM (scanning electron micrograph) of red cells (3 to 6) squeezing through fenestrated wall in transit from splenic cords to sinus. Epithelial linings of sinus wall, to which platelets (P) adhere, along with "hairy" white cells, probably macrophages, are shown. (From Weiss, L: A scanning electron microscopic study of the spleen. Blood, 43:665, 1974, with permission.)

exchange channels formed by the integral membrane protein, band 3, a glycoprotein previously described (see section on RBC integral membrane proteins).[20] In contrast, the RBC membrane is relatively impermeable to cations, with a half-time exchange of sodium (Na^+) and potassium (K^+) of more than 30 hours. It is primarily through the control of the sodium and potassium intracellular concentrations that the RBC maintains its volume and water homeostasis. The erythrocyte intracellular-to-extracellular ratios for sodium and potassium are 1:12 and 25:1, respectively.[21] The passive influx of sodium and potassium is controlled by as many as 300 cationic pumps, which actively transport sodium out of the cell and potassium into the cell. Like other cationic pumps, these sodium-potassium pumps are energy-dependent, requiring ATP. The functional active transport of these particular cations by these cationic pumps also re-

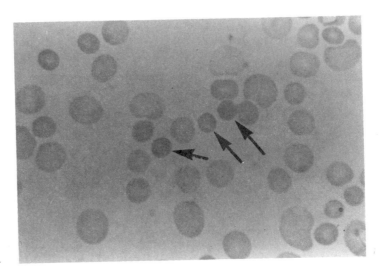

Figure 1–7. Spherocytes.

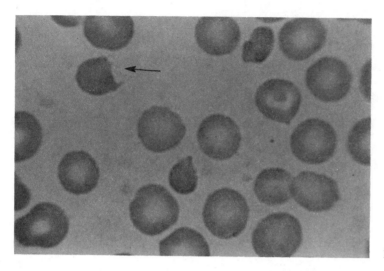

Figure 1-8. Bite cells.

quires the membrane enzyme sodium-potassium ATPase. It is interesting to note that full activation of the sodium-potassium ATPase pumps requires the presence of the RBC membrane amino phospholipid, phosphatidyl serine.[22] Similarly, calcium (Ca^{2+}) is also actively pumped from the interior of the RBC through the energy-dependent calcium-ATPase cationic pump.[23] Calmodulin, a cytoplasmic calcium-binding protein, is speculated to control these calcium-ATPase pumps, preventing excessive intracellular calcium buildup, which is deleterious to the RBC, resulting in shape changes and loss of deformability.[24] The permeability properties of the RBC membrane, as well as active cation transport, are crucial to the prevention of colloid osmotic hemolysis and controlling the volume of the red blood cell. In addition, ATP-depleted cells allow the accumulation of excess intracellular calcium and sodium, followed by potassium and water loss, resulting in a dehydrated, rigid cell subsequently sequestered by the spleen.[25] The energy required for active transport and maintenance of membrane electrochemical gradients is provided by ATP. Any abnormality that increases membrane permeability or alters cationic transport may lead to a decrease in RBC survival.

HEMOGLOBIN STRUCTURE AND FUNCTION

Hemoglobin, a conjugated protein with a molecular weight of approximately 68,000, constitutes 95 percent of the RBC's dry weight or 33 percent of the RBC's weight by volume.[26] Approximately 65 percent of the hemoglobin synthesis occurs during the nucleated stages of RBC maturation, and 35 percent occurs during the reticulocyte stage. Normal hemoglobin consists of globin (a tetramer of two pairs of polypeptide chains) and four heme groups, each of which contains a protoporphyrin ring plus iron (Fe^{2+}).

Hemoglobin Synthesis

Normal hemoglobin production is dependent on three processes (Fig. 1-9):
1. Adequate iron delivery and supply
2. Adequate synthesis of protoporphyrins (the precursor of heme)
3. Adequate globin synthesis

Iron Delivery and Supply

Iron is delivered to the membrane of the RBC precursor by the protein carrier transferrin. The majority of the iron that crosses the membrane and enters the cytoplasm of the cell is committed to hemoglobin synthesis and thereby proceeds to the mitochondria for insertion into the protoporphyrin ring to form heme. Excess iron in the cytoplasm aggregates as ferritin, the amount of which is dependent on the ratio between the level of plasma iron and the amount of iron required by the erythrocyte for hemoglobin synthesis. Two thirds of the total body iron supply is bound to heme in the hemoglobin molecule (see Chapter 6 for a discussion of iron kinetics).

Synthesis of Protoporphyrins

Protoporphyrin synthesis begins in the mitochondria with the formation of delta aminolevulinic acid (δALA) from glycine and succinyl CoA, which is the major rate-limiting step in heme biosynthesis. The mitochondrial enzyme δALA synthetase, which mediates this reaction, is influenced by erythropoietin and requires the presence of the cofactor pyridoxal phosphate (vitamin B_6).[27]

In the cytoplasm, condensation of two molecules of δALA, catalyzed by δALA dehydrase, produces the pyrrole porphobilinogen (PBG). Uroporphyrinogen (UPG) is formed by the condensation of four molecules of PBG. Because four molecules are involved in this reaction, the formation of four types of isomers is theoretically possible. However, only

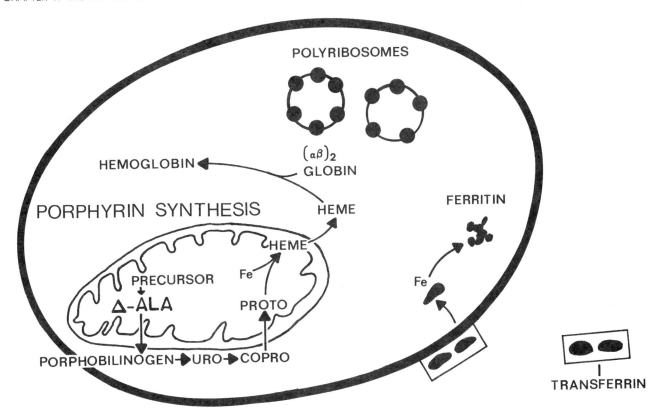

Figure 1–9. Hemoglobin synthesis in the reticulocyte.

two types of isomers have occurred physiologically—UPG I and III—and virtually all of the UPG is the Type III isomer. (The formation of UPG Type I isomer represents an enzymatic "dead-end" pathway; heme can only be derived from UPG III [Fig. 1–10]. This abnormal pathway is associated with a rare inherited disorder known as *congenital erythropoietic porphyria*, resulting from large amounts of UPG I accumulating in the RBCs, bone marrow, and urine [see **Color Plate 55**]).[27]

Coproporphyrinogen (CPG) is formed next through decarboxylation reactions from UPG III. The final steps of heme synthesis are carried out in the mitochondria and involve the formation of protoporphyrinogen (PP) from CPG III. Because PP chemically has three types of side chains, 15 possible isomers of PP can form, compared with four possible UPG and CPG isomers. However, normal mitochondrial physiology leads to the formation of only one of these isomers, PP-IX, from CPG III. After further conversion of protoporphyrin IX, the incorporation of iron results in heme (ferroprotoporphyrin IX) formation (Fig. 1–10).

Porphyrinogens, not porphyrins, are the intermediate of heme synthesis. Porphyrinogens are unstable tetrapyrroles that are readily and irreversibly oxidized to form porphyrins. In contrast, porphyrins are highly stable resonating molecules that are normally found in small quantities in the urine as the result of normal RBC catabolism.[21]

Excessive formation of porphyrins can occur if any one of the normal enzymatic steps in heme synthesis is blocked and can result in one of a number of metabolic disorders collectively called the porphyrias.

Globin Synthesis

Globin chain synthesis occurs on RBC-specific cytoplasmic ribosomes, which are initiated from the inheritance of various structural genes. Each gene results in the formation of a specific polypeptide chain. Each somatic diploid cell, including the RBC, contains four alpha (α), two zeta (ζ), two beta (β), two delta (δ), two epsilon (ϵ), and four gamma (γ) genes. The alpha and zeta genes are located on chromosome 16, and the beta, delta, epsilon, and gamma genes on chromosome 11 (Fig. 1–11). The resulting gene products formed have been called alpha, zeta, beta, delta, epsilon, and gamma globin chains. Throughout embryonic and fetal development, activation of the globin genes progresses from the zeta to the alpha gene and from the epsilon to the gamma, delta, and beta genes.

The epsilon and zeta chains normally appear only during embryonic development (Table 1–1). These two chains, plus the alpha and gamma chains, are constituents of embryonic hemoglobins: Hb Gower 1 ($\zeta_2 \epsilon_2$), Hb Gower 2 ($\alpha_2 \epsilon_2$), and Hb Portland ($\zeta_2 \gamma_2$). The epsilon and zeta chains are produced up to approximately 3 months following

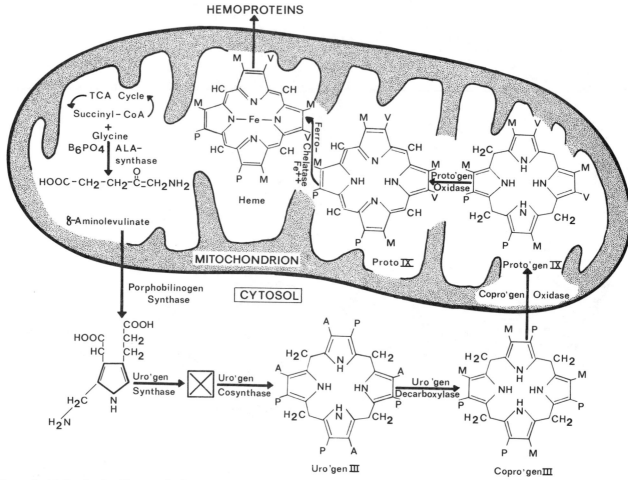

Figure 1–10. Synthesis of heme. The heme biosynthetic pathway showing the distribution of enzymes between the mitochondria and the cytoplasm. Intermediates between uroporphyrinogen and coproporphyrinogen, designated by X, remain unidentified. B_6PO_4 = pyridoxal phosphate. (From Tietz, MW: Textbook of Clinical Chemistry. WB Saunders, Philadelphia, 1986, with permission.)

conception. The alpha chain is always present. Gamma chain production is active from the third fetal month until 1 year postnatally. In the fetus, the major hemoglobin is $\alpha_2\gamma_2$ (hemoglobin F). The gamma chains occur as a mixture of two types of chains, differing only by one amino acid at position 136. G-gamma ($^G\gamma$) contains glycine, whereas A-gamma ($^A\gamma$) has alanine at that position. The ratio of G-gamma to A-gamma is approximately 3:1 at birth and 2:3 by 1 year of age. By the age of 2 years, hemoglobin F composes less than 2 percent of the total hemoglobin. Beta-chain production rises gradually prenatally and reaches adult percentages between 3 and 6 months postnatally.[2-5] Figure 1–12 depicts the time sequence of globin chain synthesis during fetal development, birth, and infancy.

All normal adult hemoglobins are formed as tetramers consisting of two alpha chains plus two (nonalpha) globin chains. Normal *adult* RBCs contain the following types of hemoglobin:

95 to 97% of the hemoglobin is HbA, which consists of $\alpha_2\beta_2$ chains

2 to 3% of the hemoglobin is HbA$_2$, which consists of $\alpha_2\delta_2$ chains

2% of the hemoglobin is HbF (fetal hemoglobin), which consists of $\alpha_2\gamma_2$ chains

Each synthesized globin chain links with heme (ferroprotoporphyrin 9) to form hemoglobin, which primarily consists of two alpha chains, two beta chains, and four heme groups. Normal alpha chains consist of 141 amino acid residues linked together in a linear fashion, whereas normal beta chains consist of 146 amino acid residues.[27] Table 1–1 shows the composition of hemoglobin found during normal human development. The precise order of amino acids is critical to the hemoglobin molecule's structure and function. The substitution of even one amino acid, such as valine for the normal glutamic acid at the sixth position on the beta chain, can result in such functional abnormalities as a hemoglobin that tends to polymerize when deoxygenated (sickle hemoglobin). An adequate amount of globin chain synthesis is also important because decreased production of one of the polypeptide chains leads to a group of disorders

GENE PRODUCTS (GLOBIN CHAINS)
HEMOGLOBINS (Hb)

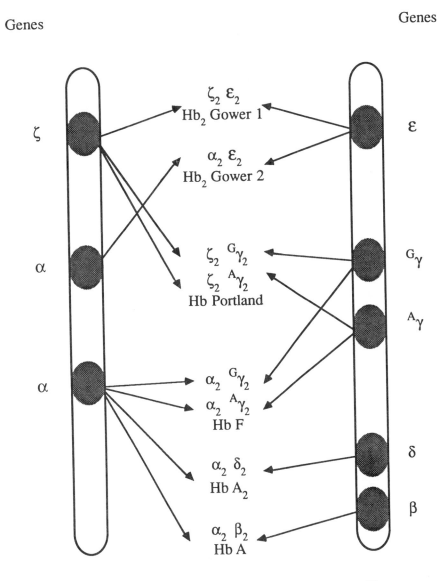

Figure 1–11. Genetic control and formation of human hemoglobins.

Chromosome 16

Chromosome 11

Table 1–1. **COMPOSITION OF HEMOGLOBIN FOUND IN NORMAL HUMAN DEVELOPMENT**

Globin Chains	Hemoglobin	Stage of Development
$\alpha_2\epsilon_2$	Gower 2	
$\zeta_2\epsilon_2$	Gower 1	Embryo
$\zeta_2\gamma_2$	Portland	
$\alpha_2{}^A\gamma_2$	F	
$\alpha_2{}^G\gamma_2$	F	Fetus
$\alpha_2\beta_2$	A	
$\alpha_2\delta_2$	A_2	Adult

known as thalassemia. Beta thalassemia, the more common form, refers to a decrease in beta chain production, and alpha thalassemia refers to a decrease in alpha chain production (see Chapter 12).

The rate of globin synthesis is directly related to the rate of porphyrin synthesis, and vice versa: protoporphyrin synthesis is reduced when globin synthesis is impaired. There is, however, no such relationship with iron uptake when either globin or protoporphyrin synthesis is impaired; iron accumulates in the RBC cytoplasm as ferritin aggregates. The iron-laden, nucleated RBC is termed a *sideroblast*, and the anucleated form a *siderocyte*, when stained with Prussian blue for visualization

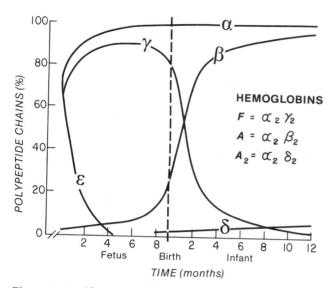

Figure 1–12. Changes in globin chain synthesis during fetal development, birth, and infancy. (From Hillman, RF and Finch, CA: Red Cell Manual, ed 5. FA Davis, Philadelphia, 1985, with permission.)

of iron (**see Color Plate 56**). When protoporphyrin synthesis is impaired, the mitochondria become encrusted with iron, which is visible around the nucleus of the RBC precursor when stained with Prussian blue. Such an RBC is termed a *ringed sideroblast* and is diagnostic for indicating a pathogenesis linked to deficient protoporphyrin synthesis (**see Color Plate 56**).[27]

Hemoglobin Function

Hemoglobin's primary function is gas transport (oxygen and carbon dioxide): delivery and release of oxygen to the tissues and facilitation of carbon dioxide excretion. Owing to hemoglobin's multichain structure, the molecule is capable of a considerable amount of allosteric movement as it loads and unloads oxygen. One of the most important controls of hemoglobin affinity for oxygen is the RBC organic phosphate 2,3-diphosphoglycerate (2,3-DPG). The unloading of oxygen by hemoglobin is accompanied by the widening of the space between beta chains and the binding of 2,3-DPG, on a mole-for-mole basis, with the formation of anionic salt bridges between the beta chains. The resulting conformation of the deoxyhemoglobin molecule is known as the tense (T) form, which has a lower affinity for oxygen. When hemoglobin loads oxygen and becomes oxyhemoglobin, the established salt bridges are broken and beta chains are pulled together, expelling 2,3-DPG. This relaxed (R) form of the hemoglobin molecule has a higher affinity for oxygen.

These allosteric changes that occur as the hemoglobin loads and unloads oxygen are referred to as the *respiratory movement*. The dissociation and binding of oxygen by hemoglobin are not directly proportional to the pO_2 of its environment but instead exhibit a sigmoid-curve relationship—the hemoglobin-oxygen dissociation curve depicted in Fig. 1–13. The shape of this curve is very important physiologically, as it permits a considerable

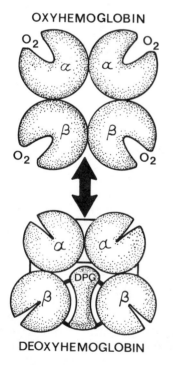

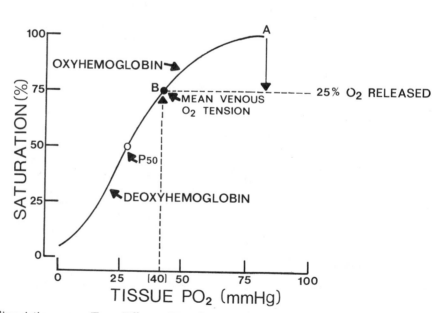

Figure 1–13. Normal hemoglobin-oxygen dissociation curve. (From Hillman, RF and Finch, CA: Red Cell Manual, ed 5. FA Davis, Philadelphia, 1985, with permission.)

amount of oxygen to be delivered to the tissues with a small drop in oxygen tension. For example, in the environment of the lungs, where the pO_2 (oxygen tension), measured in millimeters of mercury (mmHg), is nearly 100 mmHg, the hemoglobin molecule is almost 100 percent saturated with oxygen (Fig. 1–13, point A). As the RBCs travel to the tissues where the pO_2 drops to an average 40 mmHg (mean venous oxygen tension), the hemoglobin saturation drops to approximately 75 percent saturation, releasing approximately 25 percent of the oxygen to the tissues (point B).

This is the normal situation of oxygen delivery at basal metabolic rate. In conditions such as hypoxia, a compensatory "shift to the right" of the hemoglobin-oxygen dissociation curve (Fig. 1–14) occurs to alleviate a tissue oxygen deficit. This rightward shift of the curve, mediated by increased levels of 2,3-DPG, results in a decrease in hemoglobin's affinity for the oxygen molecule and an increase in oxygen delivery to the tissues. Note that the oxygen saturation of hemoglobin in the environment of the tissues (40 mmHg pO_2 [Fig. 1–13, point B]) is now only 50 percent; the other 50 percent of the oxygen is being released to the tissues. The RBCs thus have become more efficient in terms of oxygen delivery.

Therefore, a patient who is suffering from an anemia caused by a loss of RBCs may be able to compensate by shifting the oxygen dissociation curve to the right, making the RBCs, though fewer in number, more efficient. Some patients may be able to tolerate anemia better than others because of this compensatory mechanism. A shift to the right also may occur in response to acidosis or a rise in body temperature. The shift to the right of the hemoglobin-oxygen dissociation curve is only one way in which patients may compensate for various types of hypoxia; other ways include increases in total cardiac output and in erythropoiesis.

A "shift to the left" of the hemoglobin-oxygen

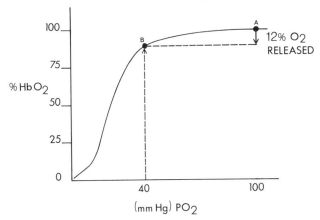

Figure 1–15. Left-shifted hemoglobin-oxygen dissociation curve.

dissociation curve results, conversely, in an increase in hemoglobin-oxygen affinity and a decrease in oxygen delivery to the tissues (Fig. 1–15). With such a dissociation curve, RBCs are much less efficient because only 12 percent of the oxygen can be released to the tissues (point B). Among the conditions that can shift the oxygen dissociation curve to the left are alkalosis; increased quantities of abnormal hemoglobins, such as methemoglobin and carboxyhemoglobin; increased quantities of hemoglobin F; or multiple transfusions of 2,3-DPG–depleted stored blood (attesting to the importance of 2,3-DPG in oxygen release).

Hemoglobin-oxygen affinity also can be expressed by P_{50} values, which designate the pO_2 at which hemoglobin is 50 percent saturated with oxygen under standard in vitro conditions of temperature and pH. The P_{50} of normal blood is 26 to 30 mmHg.[26] An increase in P_{50} represents a decrease in hemoglobin-oxygen affinity or a shift to the right of the oxygen dissociation curve. A decrease in P_{50} represents an increase in hemoglobin-oxygen affinity or a shift to the left of the oxygen dissociation curve. In addition to the reasons listed previously for shifts in the curve, inherited abnormalities of the hemoglobin molecule can result in either situation; these abnormalities are described by the P_{50} measurements. Abnormalities in hemoglobin structure or function can therefore have profound effects on the RBC's ability to provide oxygen to the tissues.

Abnormal Hemoglobins of Clinical Importance

The hemoglobins previously described—oxyhemoglobin and reduced hemoglobin—are physiologic hemoglobins because they function in the transport and delivery of oxygen within the circulation. Abnormal hemoglobins of clinical significance that are unable to transport or deliver oxygen include the following:

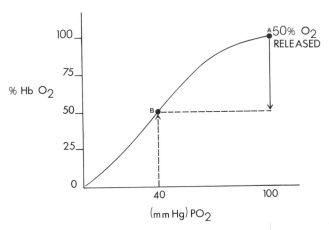

Figure 1–14. Right-shifted hemoglobin-oxygen dissociation curve.

1. Carboxyhemoglobin
2. Methemoglobin
3. Sulfhemoglobin

In carboxyhemoglobin, the oxygen molecules bound to heme have been replaced with carbon monoxide (CO). This replacement process is relatively slow and dependent upon the concentration of carbon monoxide in the blood. Once attached, however, the binding of carbon monoxide to the heme of the hemoglobin molecule is 200 times tighter than the binding of oxygen to heme.[22] The concentration of carbon monoxide can be increased in a number of conditions, including that of chronic heavy smokers.

Methemoglobin is formed when the iron of the hemoglobin molecule is oxidized to the ferric (Fe^{+++}) state. Normally, less than 1 percent of the total circulating hemoglobin is in the methemoglobin form.[27] Increased formation of methemoglobin can occur as a result of an overload of oxidant stress, owing to the ingestion of strong oxidant drugs or to an enzyme deficiency (see the following section on RBC metabolic pathways).

Sulfhemoglobin is formed when a certain situation or condition, such as ingestion of a sulfur-containing drug or chronic constipation, builds up the sulfur content of the blood. Sulfhemoglobin is incapable of carrying oxygen and represents an irreversible change of the hemoglobin molecule that persists until the RBCs are removed from the circulation. Both carboxyhemoglobin and methemoglobin, however, can be reverted back to oxyhemoglobin through the use of oxygen inhalation and the administration of strong reducing substances, respectively.

Table 1–2 lists the toxic levels for each abnormal hemoglobin at which cyanosis, anemia, and death may occur owing to a tissue oxygen deficit and increased concentration of circulating abnormal hemoglobin.

Table 1–2. **TOXIC LEVELS FOR ABNORMAL HEMOGLOBINS OF CLINICAL IMPORTANCE**

Abnormal Hemoglobin	Toxic Level (g%)
Carboxyhemoglobin	5.0
Methemoglobin	1.5
Sulfhemoglobin	0.5

MAINTENANCE OF HEMOGLOBIN FUNCTION: ACTIVE RED BLOOD CELL METABOLIC PATHWAYS

Active erythrocyte metabolic pathways are necessary for the production of adequate ATP levels. Such generated energy is crucial to RBC survival and function in that it is necessary for maintaining (1) hemoglobin function, (2) membrane integrity and deformability, (3) RBC volume, and (4) adequate amounts of reduced pyridine nucleotides.

Red blood cells generate energy almost exclusively through the anaerobic breakdown of glucose because the metabolism of the anucleated erythrocyte is more limited than that of other body cells. The adult RBC possesses little ability to metabolize fatty acids and amino acids. Additionally, mature RBCs contain no mitochondrial apparatus for oxidative metabolism (Table 1–3 compares RBC metabolism during various stages of maturation). The RBC's metabolic pathways are mainly anaerobic, fortunately, because the function of the RBC is to deliver oxygen and not to consume it. Four pathways of RBC metabolism will be considered: the anaerobic glycolytic pathway and three ancillary pathways that serve to maintain the function of hemoglobin (Fig. 1–16). All of these processes are essential if the RBC is to transport oxygen and

Table 1–3. **COMPARISON OF RED BLOOD CELL METABOLIC ACTIVITIES DURING VARIOUS STAGES OF MATURATION**

	Nucleated RBC	Reticulocyte	Adult RBC
Replication	+	0	0
DNA synthesis	+	0	0
RNA synthesis	+	0	0
Lipid synthesis	+	0	0
RNA present	+	+	0
Heme synthesis	+	+	0
Protein synthesis	+	+	0
Mitochondria	+	+	0
Krebs' tricarboxylic acid cycle	+	+	0
Embden-Meyerhof pathway	+	+	+
Pentose phosphate pathway	+	+	+
Maturation and/or senescence	+	+	+

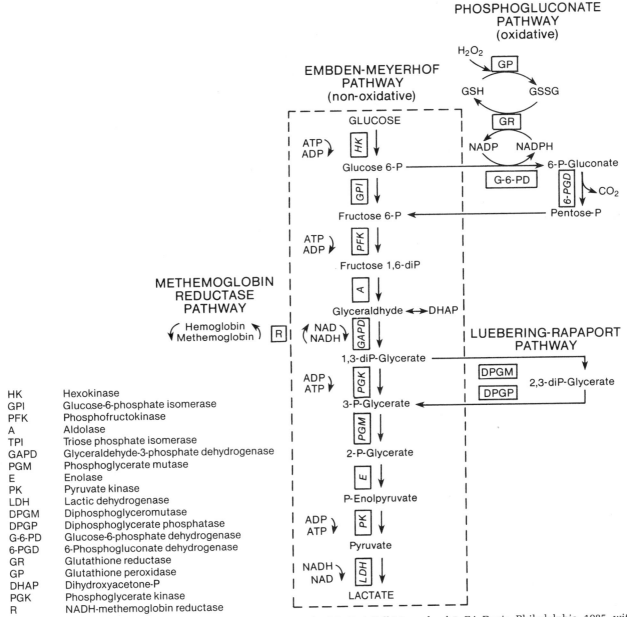

HK   Hexokinase
GPI   Glucose-6-phosphate isomerase
PFK   Phosphofructokinase
A   Aldolase
TPI   Triose phosphate isomerase
GAPD   Glyceraldehyde-3-phosphate dehydrogenase
PGM   Phosphoglycerate mutase
E   Enolase
PK   Pyruvate kinase
LDH   Lactic dehydrogenase
DPGM   Diphosphoglyceromutase
DPGP   Diphosphoglycerate phosphatase
G-6-PD   Glucose-6-phosphate dehydrogenase
6-PGD   6-Phosphogluconate dehydrogenase
GR   Glutathione reductase
GP   Glutathione peroxidase
DHAP   Dihydroxyacetone-P
PGK   Phosphoglycerate kinase
R   NADH-methemoglobin reductase

Figure 1–16. Red cell metabolism. (From Hillman, RF and Finch, CA: Red Cell Manual, ed 5. FA Davis, Philadelphia, 1985, with permission.)

maintain those physical characteristics required for its survival in circulation.

Ninety percent of the ATP needed by RBCs is generated by the Embden-Meyerhof glycolytic pathway, the RBC's main metabolic pathway. Here, the metabolism of glucose results in the net generation of two molecules of ATP. Although this ATP synthesis is inefficient when compared with cells that use the Krebs' cycle (aerobic metabolism), it provides sufficient ATP for the RBC's requirements. Glycolysis also generates NADH from NAD$^+$, important in some of the RBC's other metabolic pathways (see later discussion).

Another 5 to 10 percent of glucose is metabolized by the hexose monophosphate shunt (also called the *phosphogluconate pathway*). This pathway produces the pyridine nucleotide NADPH from NADP$^+$. NADPH, together with reduced glutathione, provides the main line of defense for the RBC against oxidative injury. Oxidant drugs, as well as infections, can cause the accumulation of hydrogen peroxide and other oxidants, which can be toxic to cell proteins. The sequence of biochemical reactions shown in Figure 1–17 occurs within the normal RBC with adequate levels of appropriate enzymes and substrate to prevent the accumulation of these agents.

When the hexose monophosphate pathway is

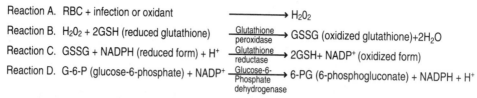

Reaction A. RBC + infection or oxidant $\longrightarrow$ H_2O_2

Reaction B. H_2O_2 + 2GSH (reduced glutathione) $\xrightarrow{\text{Glutathione peroxidase}}$ GSSG (oxidized glutathione)+$2H_2O$

Reaction C. GSSG + NADPH (reduced form) + H^+ $\xrightarrow{\text{Glutathione reductase}}$ 2GSH+ $NADP^+$ (oxidized form)

Reaction D. G-6-P (glucose-6-phosphate) + $NADP^+$ $\xrightarrow{\text{Glucose-6-Phosphate dehydrogenase}}$ 6-PG (6-phosphogluconate) + NADPH + H^+

Figure 1–17. Reactions within erythrocytes to prevent accumulation of oxidants.

functionally deficient, the amount of reduced glutathione becomes insufficient to neutralize intracellular oxidants.[28] This results in globin denaturation and precipitation as aggregates (Heinz bodies) within the cell. If this process sufficiently damages the membrane, cell destruction occurs.[29] Inherited defects in the pentose phosphate glutathione pathway, the most common of which is glucose-6-phosphate dehydrogenase (G6PD) deficiency, result in the formation of Heinz bodies with subsequent extravascular hemolysis. (Glutathione not only is crucial to keeping hemoglobin in a functional state but also is important in maintaining RBC integrity by reducing sulfhydryl groups of hemoglobin, membrane protein, and enzymes subsequent to oxidation.[28])

The methemoglobin reductase pathway is another important component of RBC metabolism. Two methemoglobin reductase systems are important in maintaining heme iron in the reduced (Fe^{2+}, ferrous) functional state.[28] Both pathways are dependent on the regeneration of reduced pyridine nucleotide and are referred to as the NADH and NADPH methemoglobin reductase pathways. In the absence of the enzyme methemoglobin reductase and the reducing action of the pyridine nucleotide NADH, there is an accumulation of methemoglobin, resulting from the conversion of the ferrous iron of heme to the ferric form (Fe^{+++}). Methemoglobin is a nonfunctional form of hemoglobin, having lost oxygen transport capabilities, as the metheme portion cannot combine with oxygen. Normal efficiency of the methemoglobin reductase pathway is exemplified by the fact that usually no more than 1 percent of RBC hemoglobin exists as methemoglobin in the RBCs of healthy individuals.

Another important pathway that is crucial to RBC function is the Leubering-Rapaport shunt. This pathway causes an extraordinary accumulation of the RBC organic phosphate 2,3-DPG, important because of its profound effect on hemoglobin's affinity for oxygen and also because its stores can serve as a reserve for additional ATP generation.

Erythrocyte Senescence

The RBC, a 6- to 8-μm biconcave disc, travels 200 to 300 miles during its 120-day lifespan. During this time, circulating RBCs undergo the process of senescence or aging. Various metabolic and physical changes associated with the aging of RBCs are listed in Table 1–4. Each day 1 percent of the old RBCs in circulation are taken out by a system

Table 1–4. CHANGES OCCURRING DURING AGING OF RBC

Increases	Decreases
Membrane-bound IgG	Several enzyme activities
Density	Sialic acid
Spheroidal shape	Deformability
MCHC	MCV
Internal viscosity	Phospholipid
Agglutinability	Cholesterol
Na^+	K^+
Methemoglobin	Protoporphyrin
Oxygen affinity	

MCHC = mean cell hemoglobin concentration.
MCV = mean cell volume.
Source: Garratty, G: Basic mechanisms of in vivo cell destruction. In Bell, C (ed): A Seminar in Immune-Mediated Cell Destruction. American Association of Blood Banks, 1981, with permission.

of fixed macrophages in the body known as the reticuloendothelial system (RES). These RBCs are replaced by the daily release of 1 percent of the younger RBCs reticulocytes, from the bone marrow storage pool.[7] As erythrocytes become old, certain glycolytic enzymes decrease in activity, resulting in a decrease in the production of energy and loss of deformability. At a certain critical point, the RBCs are no longer able to traverse the microvasculature and are phagocytized by the RES cells. Although RES cells are located in various organs and throughout the body, those of the spleen, called *littoral cells*, are the most sensitive detectors of RBC abnormalities. This is primarily due to the microanatomic arrangement of the spleen for a longer time. Ninety percent of the destruction of senescent RBCs occurs by the process of extravascular hemolysis (Fig. 1–18). During this process, old or damaged RBCs are phagocytized by the RES cells and digested by their lysosomes. The hemoglobin molecules are disassembled—broken down into their various components. The iron recovered is salvaged and returned by the plasma protein carrier, transferrin, to the erythroid precursors in the marrow for synthesis of the new hemoglobin. Globin is broken down into amino acids and redirected to the amino acid pool of the body. Finally, the protoporphyrin ring of heme is disassembled, its alpha carbon exhaled in the form of carbon monoxide. The opened tetrapyrrole, biliverdin, is converted to bilirubin and carried by the plasma protein albumin to the liver. In the liver, bilirubin is conjugated to bilirubin

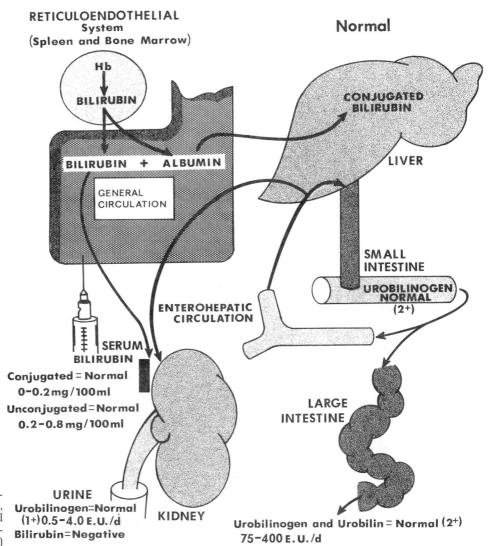

Figure 1–18. Normal extravascular hemolysis. (From Tietz, MW: Textbook of Clinical Chemistry. WB Saunders, Philadelphia, 1986, with permission.)

glucuronide and excreted along with bile into the intestines. Here it is further converted through bacterial action into urobilinogen (stercobilinogen) and excreted in the stool. A small amount of urobilinogen is reabsorbed through enterohepatic circulation, filtered by the kidneys, and excreted in small amounts in the urine. Both unconjugated, (prehepatic) and conjugated (posthepatic) bilirubin can be measured in the plasma as indirect and direct bilirubin, respectively, and used to monitor the amount of hemolysis.

Only 5 to 10 percent of normal RBC destruction occurs through the process of intravascular hemolysis (Fig. 1–19).[27] During this process, RBC breakdown occurs within the lumen of the blood vessels. The RBC ruptures, releasing hemoglobin directly into the bloodstream. The hemoglobin molecule dissociates into alpha-beta dimers and is picked up by the protein carrier, haptoglobin. The haptoglobin-hemoglobin complex prevents renal excretion of hemoglobin and carries the dimers to the liver cell for further catabolism. The hepato-

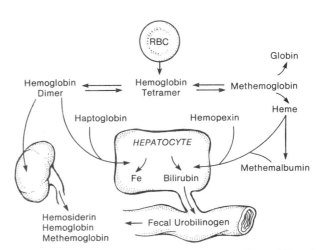

Figure 1–19. Intravascular hemolysis. (From Hillman, RF and Finch, CA: Red Cell Manual, ed 5. FA Davis, Philadelphia, 1985, with permission.)

cyte uptake and processing is identical at this point to the process previously described for extravascular hemolysis (see Fig. 1–18). Haptoglobin levels, therefore, fall in plasma as it is removed as the hemoglobin-haptoglobin complex. It is estimated that as little as 1 to 2 ml of RBC intravascular hemolysis can totally deplete the amount of plasma haptoglobin. Normally, 50 to 200 mg/dl of plasma haptoglobin is available and represents the hemoglobin-dimer binding capacity. As haptoglobin is depleted, unbound hemoglobin dimers appear in the plasma (hemoglobinemia) and are filtered through the kidneys and reabsorbed by the renal tubular cells. The renal tubular uptake capacity is approximately 5 g per day of filtered hemoglobin.[27] Beyond this level, free hemoglobin appears in the urine (hemoglobinuria).

Hemoglobinuria is always associated with hemoglobinemia. A normal plasma hemoglobin level is approximately 2 to 5 mg/dl, which is released as a result of excessive intravascular hemolysis.[27] Depending on the amount of hemolysis and type of hemoglobin, the plasma may be pink, red, or brown. Likewise, in hemoglobinuria the urine also may be pink, red, brown, or black. Two hemoglobin pigments, oxyhemoglobin and methemoglobin, are produced by auto-oxidation of the hemoglobin in the urinary tract when the urine is acidic. Oxyhemoglobin is bright red and methemoglobin dark brown. The color of the urine, therefore, depends on the amount of hemolysis and concentration and relative proportions of these two pigments. Oxyhemoglobin predominates in alkaline urine, and methemoglobin predominates in acidic urine.

Hemoglobin, that is neither processed by the kidneys nor bound to haptoglobin is oxidized to methemoglobin, which is further disassembled as metheme groups are released and globin degradated. Free metheme is quickly bound by another transport protein, hemopexin, and is carried to the liver cell to be catabolized, as previously described. The heme-binding capacity of hemopexin is approximately 50 to 100 mg/dl; when this is exceeded, the metheme groups combine with albumin to form methemalbumin. Albumin cannot transfer the metheme across the membrane of the hepatocyte for subsequent degradation. As a result, the methemalbumin circulates until additional hemopexin is produced by the liver to serve as the protein carrier. It is this circulating methemalbumin that imparts a brown tinge to the plasma or blood. (Table 1–5 provides a review of the various protein carriers discussed regarding hemolysis.) In-

travascular hemolysis, as a result of RBC senescence, is so minimal that it is limited to the involvement of only haptoglobin, which is rarely depleted. Hemoglobinemia and hemoglobinuria, as well as the other processes discussed, come into play only with excessive intravascular hemolysis, which can occur in patients having various hemolytic anemias (see Chapters 9 through 14).

CONCLUSION

This chapter has outlined and described three important areas of RBC structure and metabolism: the red cell membrane, hemoglobin structure and function, and red-cell metabolic pathways. An understanding of these aspects of the RBC is important to appreciating the development and pathogenesis of the many forms of inherited and acquired RBC defects that result in hemolytic anemias.

REFERENCES

1. Mohandas, N and Groner, W: Cell membrane and volume changes during red cell development and aging. Ann NY Acad Sci 554:217, 1989.
2. Chasis, JA, et al: Membrane assembly and remodeling during reticulocyte maturation. Blood 74(3):1112, 1989.
3. Butikofer, P, et al: Erythrocyte phospholipid organization and vesiculation in hereditary high red cell membrane phosphatidylcholine hemolytic anemia. J Lab Clin Med 113(3):278, 1989.
4. Rybczynska, M and Csordas, A: Chain length-dependent interaction of free fatty acids with the erythrocyte membrane. Life Sci 44(9):625, 1989.
5. Rybicki, AC, et al: Human erythrocyte protein 4.1 is a phosphatidylserine binding protein. J Clin Invest 81(1):255, 1988.
6. Butikofer, P, et al: Chlorpromazine inhibits vesiculation, alters phosphoinositide turnover and changes deformability of ATP-depleted RBCs. Blood 73(6):1699, 1989.
7. Butterfield, DA: ESR studies of transmembrane signaling processes: Modulation of skeletal protein-protein interactions and their influence on the physical state of cell-surface carbohydrates in human erythrocyte membranes. Progr Clin Biol Res 292:53, 1989.
8. Clark, MR, et al: Red cell deformability and lipid composition in two forms of acanthocytosis: Enrichment of acanthocytic populations by density gradient centrifugation. J Lab Clin Med 113(4):469, 1989.
9. Woods, CM and Lazarides, E: The erythroid membrane skeleton: Expression and assembly during erythropoiesis. Annu Rev Med 39:107, 1988.
10. Lisowska, E: Antigenic properties of human erythrocyte glycophorins. Adv Exp Med Biol 228:265, 1988.
11. Schubert, D: The relationships between oligomeric structure and function of band 3 protein from human erythrocyte membranes: Present knowledge and suggestions for further experiments. Mol Aspects Med 10(3):233, 1988.
12. Di Stasi, AM, et al: Interactions of skeletal proteins with red blood cell membrane. Ann Inst Super Sanita 24(4):591, 1988.
13. Bennett, V: The spectrin-actin junction of erythrocyte membrane skeletons. Biochem Biophys Acta 988(1):107, 1989.
14. Fortier, N, et al: The relationship between in vivo generated hemoglobin skeletal protein complex and increased red cell membrane rigidity. Blood 71(5):1427, 1988.
15. McGuire, M and Agre, P: Clinical disorders of the erythrocyte membrane skeleton. Hematologic Pathology 2(1):1, 1988.
16. Liu, ZY, Sanders, ME, and Hu, VW: Effect of complement on the lateral mobility of erythrocyte membrane proteins.

Table 1–5. **PROTEIN CARRIERS**

Protein	Substance Carried
Transferrin	Iron
Haptoglobin	Hemoglobin dimers
Hemopexin	Metheme
Albumin	Bilirubin

Evidence for terminal complex interaction with cytoskeletal components. J Immunol 142(7):2370, 1989.

17. Boivin, P: Role of the phosphorylation of red blood cell membrane proteins. Biochem J 256(3):689, 1988.
18. Chasis, JA, et al: Membrane assembly and remodeling during reticulocyte maturation. Blood 74(3):1112, 1989.
19. Chasis, JA, Agre, P, and Mohandas, N: Decreased membrane mechanical stability and in vivo loss of surface area reflect spectrin deficiencies in hereditary spherocytosis. J Clin Invest 82(2):617, 1988.
20. Krupka, RM: Role of substrate binding forces in exchange-only transport systems: II. Implications for the mechanism of the anion exchange of red cells. J Membr Biol 109(2):159, 1989.
21. Halperin, JA, Brugnara, C, and Nicholson-Weller, A: Ca^{2+}-activated K^+ efflux limits complement-mediated lysis of human erythrocytes. J Clin Invest 83(5):1466, 1989.
22. Donahue, HJ, Penniston, JT, and Heath, H, III: Kinetics of erythrocyte plasma membrane (Ca^{2+}, Mg^{2+}) ATPase in familial benign hypercalcemia. J Clin Endocrinol Metab 68(5):893, 1989.
23. James, PH, et al: Primary structure of the cAMP-dependent phosphorylation site of the plasma membrane calcium pump. Biochemistry 28(10):4253, 1989.
24. Takakuwa, Y and Mohandas, N: Modulation of erythrocyte membrane material properties by Ca^{2+} and calmodulin. Implications for their role in regulation of skeletal protein interactions. J Clin Invest 82(2):394, 1988.
25. Waugh, RE and Agre, P: Reductions of erythrocyte membrane viscoelastic coefficients reflect spectrin deficiencies in hereditary spherocytosis. J Clin Invest 81(1):133, 1988.
26. Krueger, S and Nossal, R: SANS studies of interacting hemoglobin in intact erythrocytes. Biophys J 53(1):97, 1988.
27. Kjeldsberg, C: Practical Diagnosis of Hematologic Disorders. American Society of Clinical Pathologists, Chicago, 1989.
28. Chiu, D and Lubin, B: Oxidative hemoglobin denaturation and RBC destruction: The effect of heme on red cell membranes. Semin Hematol 26(2):128, 1989.
29. Platt, OS and Falcone, JF: Membrane protein lesions in erythrocytes with Heinz bodies. J Clin Invest 82(3):1051, 1988.

QUESTIONS

1. *Which of the following is not a crucial area of RBC survival and function?*
   a. Integrity of RBC cellular membrane
   b. Cell metabolism
   c. Intravascular hemolysis
   d. Hemoglobin structure

2. *Which of the following is not a function of the RBC membrane?*
   a. Transport and exchange of metabolic substances
   b. Synthesis of hemoglobin molecule
   c. Maintenance of cellular integrity
   d. Cellular communication and interaction through antigens and receptors

3. *Which abnormal RBC is not caused by a structural membrane defect?*
   a. Spherocytes
   b. Target cells
   c. Siderocytes
   d. Acanthocytes

4. *Which list represents the complete set of processes necessary for normal hemoglobin production?*
   a. Iron delivery and supply, synthesis of protoporphyrins, globin synthesis
   b. Iron salvage, synthesis of conjugated bilirubin, haptoglobin synthesis
   c. Iron accumulation, synthesis of hemoplexin, globin catabolism
   d. Iron catabolism, synthesis of uroporphyrinogen, ferritin synthesis

5. *What is the proper order of assembly of the protoporphyrin ring?*
   a. ALA, porphobilinogen, uroporphyrinogen, coproporphyrinogen, protoporphyrinogen
   b. Protoporphyrinogen, coproporphyrinogen, uroporphyrinogen, ALA
   c. ALA, protoporphyrinogen, porphobilinogen, coproporphyrinogen, protoporphyrinogen
   d. Porphobilinogen, ALA, uroporphyrinogen, coproporphyrinogen, protoporphyrinogen

6. *What is the correct list for the number and type of globin chains in normal adult hemoglobin?*
   a. 4 alpha, 2 beta, 2 delta chains
   b. 2 alpha, 2 nonalpha chains
   c. 2 alpha, 4 beta, 1 delta, and 1 epsilon chain
   d. 4 alpha, 2 beta, 2 delta, and 1 epsilon chain

7. *What is the composition of normal adult hemoglobin?*
   a. 92–95% HbA; 5–8% HbA_2; 1–2% HbF
   b. 90–92% HbA; and HbA_2
   c. 80–85% HbA; 2–3% HbA_2
   d. 92–95% HbA; 2–3% HbA_2; 1–2% HbF

8. *Which of the following cells is caused by iron accumulation?*
   a. Acanthocyte
   b. Ringed sideroblast
   c. Burr cell
   d. Bite cell

9. *Which form of the hemoglobin molecule has the highest affinity for oxygen?*
   a. Tense (T) form
   b. Tissue form
   c. Relaxed (R) form
   d. Venous form

10. *What happens during a shift to the right of the hemoglobin-oxygen dissociation curve?*
    a. Increased 2,3-DPG results in decrease of hemoglobin oxygen affinity and increase in oxygen delivery to tissues.
    b. Decreased 2,3-DPG results in increase of hemoglobin oxygen affinity and decrease in oxygen delivery to tissues.
    c. Increased 2,3-DPG results in increase of hemoglobin oxygen affinity and increase in oxygen delivery to tissues.
    d. Decreased 2,3-DPG results in decrease of hemoglobin oxygen affinity and decrease in oxygen delivery to tissues.

11. *What happens during a shift to the left of the hemoglobin-oxygen dissociation curve? (Use answer choices for question 10.)*

12. *Which of the following is a complete list of*

abnormal hemoglobins that are unable to transport or deliver oxygen?
a. Carboxyhemoglobin and methemoglobin
b. Methemoglobin and fetal hemoglobin
c. Carboxyhemoglobin, sulfhemoglobin, and fetal hemoglobin
d. Carboxyhemoglobin, methemoglobin, and sulfhemoglobin

13. *Which metabolic pathway generates 90 percent of the ATP needed by RBCs?*
a. Methemoglobin reductase pathway
b. Hexose monophosphate shunt
c. Embden-Meyerhof pathway
d. Leubering-Rapaport shunt

14. *What steps occur in the extravascular breakdown of senescent RBCs?*
a. RES cells phagocytize red cells; iron is coupled to transferrin and returned to marrow; globin is returned to amino acid pool; biliverdin is converted to bilirubin; bilirubin is coupled to albumin and transported to liver; bilirubin glucuronide is converted to urobilinogen and excreted.
b. RBCs break down in lumen of vessel; haptoglobin picks up dissociated hemoglobin; haptoglobin-hemoglobin complex goes to liver; unbound hemoglobin dimers are excreted through kidney as hemosiderin, hemoglobin, or methemoglobin; haptoglobin is broken down to be excreted as urobilinogen.
c. RES cells phagocytize red cells; iron is coupled to transferrin and returned to marrow; globin is returned to amino acid pool; haptoglobin-hemoglobin complex goes to liver; unbound hemoglobin dimers are excreted through kidney as hemosiderin, hemoglobin, or methemoglobin; haptoglobin is broken down to be excreted as urobilinogen.
d. RBCs break down in lumen of vessel; haptoglobin picks up dissociated hemoglobin; haptoglobin-hemoglobin complex goes to liver; biliverdin is converted to bilirubin; bilirubin is coupled to albumin and transported to liver; bilirubin glucuronide is converted to urobilinogen and excreted.

15. *What steps occur in the intravascular breakdown of senescent RBCs? (Use answer choices for question 14.)*

ANSWERS

1. c (p. 3)
2. b (p. 4)
3. c (p. 5)
4. a (p. 8–9)
5. a (p. 8–9)
6. b (p. 10)
7. d (p. 10)
8. b (p. 11)
9. c (p. 12)
10. a (p. 13)
11. b (p. 13)
12. d (p. 14)
13. c (p. 15)
14. a (p. 16)
15. b (p. 17–18)

CHAPTER 2

ANN BELL, M.S., S.H.(ASCP), C.L.SP.H.(NCA)

Hematopoiesis: Morphology of Human Blood and Marrow Cells

OBJECTIVES

At the end of this chapter, the learner should be able to:
1. Name organs responsible for hematopoiesis in the fetus.
2. Describe the various phases of the cell cycle.
3. Trace cellular development from the multipotential stem cell to a single committed cell line.
4. Describe the functions of colony-stimulating factors.
5. Describe the functions of various interleukins.
6. List the proper cell maturation sequence of erythropoiesis.
7. Recognize each cell in the erythrocytic series.
8. List the maturation pool sequence for granulocyte production.
9. List the proper cell sequence for granulocytopoiesis.
10. Recognize each cell in the granulocytic series.
11. Distinguish between eosinophils and basophils.
12. List the proper cell sequence for the monocyte-macrophage phagocytic system.
13. List characteristics of lymphocytes.
14. Explain the process of platelet release.
15. Distinguish between osteoblasts and osteoclasts.

HEMATOPOIESIS

Hematopoiesis is the dynamic process of blood cell production and development. The hematopoietic system continuously maintains a cell population through a complex network of tissues, organs, stem cells, and controlling factors. This network is responsible for the maturation and division of undifferentiated cells into the operational cell lines that perform immune functions, transport oxygen and carbon dioxide, and maintain hemostasis.

All cells derive from a pool of multipotential hematopoietic stem cells found in the bone marrow. Under the influence of factors such as colony-stimulating factors and interleukins, stem cells divide and differentiate to form the mature cellular elements of the blood. The hematopoietic system consists of the bone marrow, liver, spleen, lymph nodes, and thymus. All these tissues and organs are involved in the production, maturation, and destruction of blood cells. The entire process of hematopoiesis involves an intricate structure of tissues, organs, cellular elements, and factors which result in the maintenance and function of blood cells.

Ontogeny of Hematopoiesis

During the first weeks of embryonic life, hematopoiesis begins in the mesoderm of the yolk sac (Fig. 2–1) with mesenchymal stem cells forming large primitive nucleated erythroid cells.[1] Yolk sac production of these nucleated erythroid cells begins to decline in about 6 weeks and ends in about 2 months.[1-5]

The fetal liver assumes responsibility for hematopoiesis about the second month, with the yolk sac nucleated red blood cells migrating to the liver and remaining in the liver until the seventh month.[1,2] From the third to the sixth month, splenic hematopoiesis also occurs. At around 7 months of fetal life, the responsibility for hematopoiesis shifts from the liver to the marrow, which then becomes the major site of blood cell development in the fetus.[1] Production of hematopoietic cells in the marrow is termed *medullary hematopoiesis*. Fetal marrow becomes filled with red blood cells during hematopoiesis. Bones of the toes, fingers, vertebrae, ribs, pelvis, long bones, and cranium are filled with erythroid cells. In addition to primitive erythroid cells, early lymphocytic cells also may be formed during fetal life. A few megakaryocytes first appear at approximately 3 months of fetal life, and granulocytes are observed at about 5 months.[4]

At birth, the liver and spleen have ceased hematopoietic cell development and the active sites of hematopoiesis are in bone cavities (red marrow). Bone seems to provide a microenvironment most appropriate for proliferation and maturation of cells.[1] Hematopoiesis occurs in the extravascular part of the red marrow with a single layer of epithelial cells separating the extravascular marrow compartment from the intravascular compartment (venous sinuses). When new blood cells produced in the marrow are almost mature and ready to circulate in the peripheral blood, the migrating cells leave the marrow parenchyma by squeezing through cytoplasmic fenestrations in sinus endothelial lining cells and emerging into venous sinuses.[1-5]

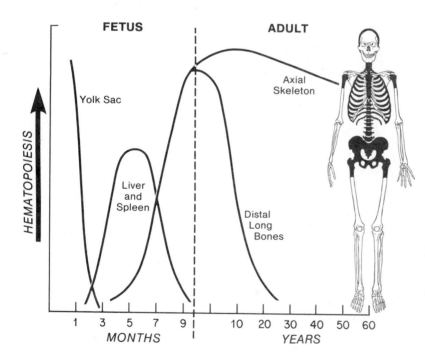

Figure 2–1. Location of active marrow growth in the fetus and adult. During fetal development, hematopoiesis is first established in the yolk sac mesenchyme, later moves to the liver and spleen, and finally is limited to the bony skeleton. From infancy to adulthood, there is a progressive restriction of productive marrow to the axial skeleton and proximal ends of the long bones, shown as the shaded areas on the drawing of the skeleton. (From Hillman, RF and Finch, CA: Red Cell Manual, ed 5. FA Davis, Philadelphia, 1985, with permission.)

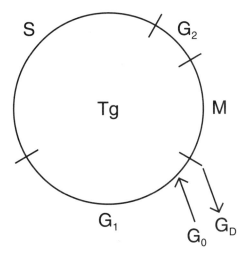

Figure 2-2. Cell cycle kinetics. Tg-one complete mitotic division cycle. G_0 = resting or dormant phase; G_1 = postmitotic rest period; S = active DNA synthesis phase; G_2 = premitotic rest period; M = mitotic period; G_d = nondividing cell.

During infancy and early childhood hematopoiesis takes place in the entire medullary space, with the volume of marrow in the newborn infant almost equaling the hematopoietic marrow space of adults. Hematopoiesis gradually decreases in the shaft of the long bones, and after age 4 fat cells begin to appear in the long bones.[1]

Around age 18 to 20, hematopoietic marrow is found in the sternum, ribs, pelvis, vertebrae, and skull. Other bones contain fat primarily (yellow marrow). Past the age of 40, marrow in the sternum, ribs, pelvis, and vertebrae is composed of equal amounts of hematopoietic tissue and fat.[1] Generally hematopoiesis is sustained in a steady state as production of mature cells equals blood cell removal. When there is increased demand for blood cells, active hematopoiesis may again be found in the spleen, liver, and other tissues as a compensatory mechanism known as *extramedullary hematopoiesis*.[1-5]

Cell Cycle Kinetics

When stimulated by hematopoietic growth factors (see section on colony-stimulating factors and interleukins), hematopoietic cells undergo a continuous cell cycle in which the cells divide, differentiate, or remain dormant (Fig. 2-2). The bone marrow contains cell populations in all phases of cell development. Cells have two mitotic divisions, and the cell cycle is generally described as the cell activity between the mitotic divisions. After the first mitotic division, the cell enters a resting or dormant phase (G_0). When the cell is suitably activated, it enters a postmitotic rest period (G_1), which is a phase directly preceding deoxyribonucleic acid (DNA) synthesis. The cell proceeds into the S (synthesis) phase of active DNA synthesis, where the DNA content is doubled. The next phase is the premitotic rest period (G_2) as the cell prepares to enter the mitotic period (M). T_g is the

HEMATOPOIESIS

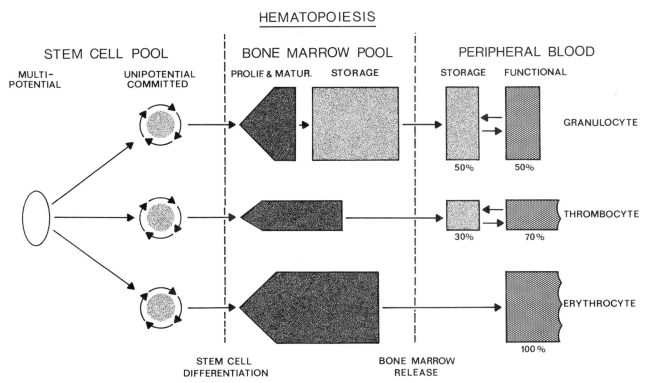

Figure 2-3. A dynamic model of hematopoietic activity. (From Erslev, AJ and Gabuzda, TG: Pathophysiology of Blood, ed 3. WB Saunders, Philadelphia, 1985, with permission.)

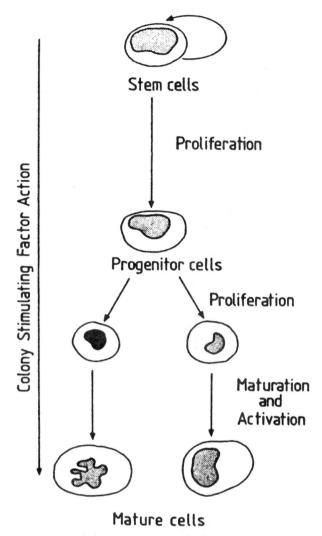

Figure 2–4. Scheme for the organization of the hematopoietic system. Colony-stimulating factors stimulate not only the proliferation and differentiation of cells in the myeloid lineages but also the activation of the mature cells. (From Morstyn, G and Burgess, AW: Hemopoietic growth factors: a review. Cancer Res 48:5624, 1988, with permission.)

cycle of one complete mitotic division. After final differentiation, the cell will leave the cycle as a nondividing cell (G_D) (Fig. 2–2).

Multipotential Stem Cell

Residing in the bone marrow is a pool of multipotential hematopoietic stem cells (Fig. 2–3) that, through cell kinetics, produce mature circulating blood cells that have the capacity not only for self-renewal but also the proliferation and differentiation (Fig. 2–4) into progenitor cells committed to one cell lineage.[7–10,32] The process of formation and development of mature blood cells from a marrow multipotential stem cell is not only under the con-

trol of a complex network of growth factors and inhibitors but is also influenced by the microenvironment.[11]

The multipotential stem cell was shown to exist in a classic experiment in 1961 by Till and McCullock[12] who irradiated mice to empty the hematopoietic organs and then injected a suspension of marrow cells intravenously. About a week later, nodules of injected marrow could be observed on the cut surface of the spleen and in splenic tissue. The nodules were named spleen colonies. All cell lines found in normal marrow were generated from the multipotential stem cells in the marrow suspension. The term colony-forming unit–spleen (CFU-S) was applied to the multipotential stem cell in these colonies.[2–4] The multipotential stem cell also has been referred to as the colony-forming unit–blast (CFU-blast).

Because the splenic colonies were noted to be mixtures of cell lines, the progenitor cell giving rise to these multiple lineages was called colony-forming unit–granulocyte, erythrocyte, macrophage/monocyte, and megakaryocyte (CFU-GEMM).[2–4] The multipotential stem cell provides a cellular reserve for the progenitor stem cells committed to the two major cell lines: myeloid and lymphoid.[1–4] These committed stem cells are genetically destined to make irreversibly differentiated cells and are recognized primarily by morphologically distinct progeny. Daughter cells formed in in vitro clonal assays serve to identify the committed cell.[6]

The CFU-GEMM in a colony assay forms a series of committed myeloid progenitor cells (CFU-GM, CFU-Eo, CFU-Bs, CFU-Meg, BFU-E) (Table 2–1), each of which in turn can produce a colony of one hematopoietic lineage under appropriate growth conditions (Fig. 2–5).[9,10] For example, the committed progenitor colony-forming unit–granulocyte macrophage/monocyte (CFU-GM) makes colonies of granulocytes and macrophages/monocytes. The CFU-Eo forms colonies of eosinophils, the CFU-Bs forms early basophils in colonies, and the committed progenitor cell CFU-Meg forms megakaryocyte colonies. Bursts of primitive erythroid cells are formed by the committed progenitor cell burst-forming unit–erythroid (BFU-E).

The lymphoid stem cell is also derived from the multipotential stem cell. The lymphoid progenitor cell has the potential to differentiate into a T or B cell. T cells participate in immune functions of a cellular nature, either directly cytotoxic or in helping or suppressing immune activities through interaction with other immunocompetent cells. B cells differentiate into plasmacytes, which secrete specific immunoglobulins important in the host's defense against infection. Another population of lymphocytes, called null cells, have neither the characteristics of the T nor the B cells. Killer (K) cells interact with antibody to cause destruction of antibody-coated targets, and natural killer (NK) cells can lyse target cells through direct cytotoxic activity. Their differentiation is uncertain.[1]

Table 2–1. **HEMATOPOIETIC PROGENITOR CELLS**

CFU-GEMM	Colony-forming unit – Granulocyte, erythrocyte, macrophage/monocyte, megakaryocyte
CFU-GM	Colony-forming unit – granulocyte, macrophage/monocyte
CFU-Eo	Colony-forming unit – eosinophil
CFU-Bs	Colony-forming unit – basophil
CFU-Meg	Colony-forming unit – megakaryocyte
CFU-E	Colony-forming unit – erythrocyte
BFU-E	Burst-forming unit – erythrocyte

Colony-Stimulating Factors and Interleukins

Human hematopoietic growth factors or col-ony-stimulating factors (CSFs) and interleukins regulate blood cell development by mediating proliferation, differentiation, and maturation of hematopoietic progenitor cells (**see Color Plate 7**). In addition, they regulate survival and function of mature blood cells (Table 2–2).[13,14]

Colony-stimulating factors initiating myeloid differentiation were first discovered in semisolid matrix cultures in which marrow, spleen, or blood cells formed colonies of myeloid progenitor cells.[13,15] Simultaneously, the growth factors, termed interleukins (ILs), also were discovered while using various liquid culture systems to study T- and B-cell proliferation and differentiation.[15]

One of the first hematopoietic growth factors dis-covered was found to stimulate the production of progenitor cells capable of differentiation into neutrophils, eosinophils, and macrophages/mono-cytes. This CSF was named granulocyte-macro-phage colony-stimulating factor (GM-CSF).[8–11,13–17] Granulocyte-macrophage CSF is produced by acti-vated vascular endothelial cells, fibroblasts, T lym-phocytes, and macrophages (Fig. 2–6). Granulo-cyte-macrophage CSF induces early myeloid progenitor cells to proliferate and differentiate.

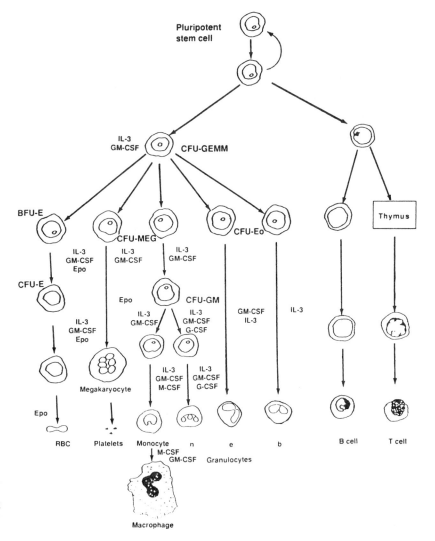

Figure 2–5. Interactions of the CSFs with he-matopoietic cells. The pathways of hemato-poiesis are as described by Metcalf and Ni-cola.[4] The different progenitor cells that are identified in the in vitro culture systems are CFU-GEMM (colony-forming unit, granulo-cyte-erythrocyte-monocyte-megakaryocyte), CFU-Meg (CFU-megakaryocyte), CFU-Eo (CFU-esosinophil), CFU-GM (CFU-granulo-cyte/monocyte), CFU-E (CFU-erythroid), and BFU-E (burst-forming unit-erythroid). The abbreviations for the hematopoietic lineages (as proposed at a UCLA symposium) are n, neutrophil; e, eosinophil; b, basophil; m, monocyte/macrophage; E, erythrocyte; and M, megakaryocyte. The interactions of the different CSFs with the various lineages are as indicated. These interactions are based on analysis of mature cells found in colonies grown in the presence of the CSFs as dis-cussed in the text. The sites of action are intended to indicate that at least some, but not necessarily all, of the progenitors of that lineage are responsive to the indicated CSF. Erythropoietin (EPO) is essential for develop-ment of erythroid cells[9] and can promote the differentiation of megakaryocyte progenitors in vitro. (From Clark, SC and Kamen, R: The human hematopoietic colony-stimulating factors. Science 236:1229, 1987, with permis-sion.)

Table 2–2. **HEMATOPOIETIC GROWTH FACTORS**

Name		Source	Target	Gene Location
Epo	Erythropoietin	Kidney, liver	Erythroid progenitors	7q
G-CSF	Granulocyte colony-stimulating factor	Macrophages, endothelial cells, fibroblasts	Stem cells, neutrophil precursors	17q
GM-CSF	Granulocyte-macrophage colony-stimulating factor	T lymphocytes, macrophages, endothelial cells, fibroblasts	Progenitors for neutrophils, eosinophils, monocytes	5q
M-CSF	CSF-1	Many cell types	Mononuclear phagocytes	5q
IL-1α	Endogenous pyrogen	Mononuclear phagocytes	Many	
IL-1β	Lymphocyte-activating factor	Endothelial cells	T cells and others	2q
IL-2	T-cell growth factor	T lymphocytes	T cells, B cells, macrophages	4q
IL-3	Multi-CSF	T lymphocytes	Precursors of neutrophils, platelets, monocytes, eosinophils, basophils, stem cells	5q
IL-4	B-cell stimulatory factor I	T lymphocytes	B cells, mast cells	5q
IL-5	B-cell growth factor II Eosinophil differentiation factor	T lymphocytes	B cells, eosinophils	5q
IL-6	Interferon β2 Hybridoma growth factor Hepatocytic growth factor	T lymphocytes, macrophages	Stem cells, B cells	7p
IL-7		Stromal cells	Pre-B cells, T cells	—

Source: From Golde, DW: Hematopoietic growth factors—an overview. Int J Cell Cloning 8 (Suppl) I: 4, 1990, with permission.

The effects of the CSFs are mediated by specific surface receptors present on precursor cells and mature cells.[17] Granulocytes and macrophages/monocytes retain GM-CSF receptors even when mature.

Granulocyte–colony-stimulating factor (G-CSF) is a growth and differentiation factor for marrow progenitor cells committed only to neutrophil lineage. It also primes neutrophils for enhanced function with regard to oxidative metabolism, phagocy-

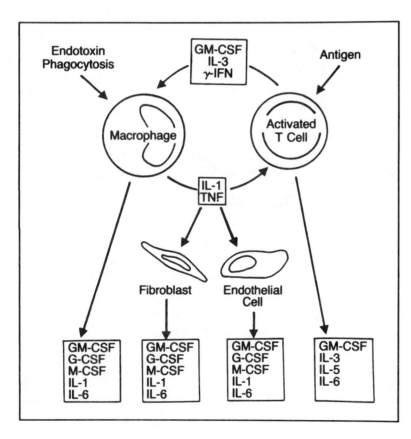

Figure 2–6. Regulation of production and cellular sources of colony-stimulating growth factors. Interleukin-3 (IL-3), gamma-interferon (γ-IFN), interleukin-1 (IL-1), tumor necrosis factor (TNF), GM-CSF, G-CSF, M-CSF, interleukin-5 (IL-5), and interleukin-6 (IL-6). (From Groopman, JE, Molina, JM, and Scaddon, DT: Hematopoietic growth factors. N Engl J Med 321(21):1449, 1989, with permission.)

tosis, and cytotoxicity.[8,9,18] Granulocyte-CSF acts by stimulating growth and proliferation of neutrophil precursors. It is released by macrophages after stimulation with endotoxin and endothelial cells. Bone marrow stromal cells, epithelial cells, and fibroblasts, which are major constituents of the bone marrow microenvironment, also produce G-CSF (Fig. 2–6).[18]

The production of macrophage/monocyte late progenitor cells is stimulated by macrophage/monocyte colony-stimulating factor (M-CSF).[8,10,15,16,19] Macrophage/monocyte CSF does not appear to affect the first divisions of the progenitor cells in other lineages. Endothelial cells, macrophages, fibroblasts, as well as placental tissue, are sources of human M-CSF (Fig. 2–6). Mature macrophages/monocytes have M-CSF receptors and respond to M-CSF. Macrophage/monocyte CSF regulates every aspect of the phagocytic cell function of monocytes and enhances the production of tumor necrosis factor (TNF) by monocytes (Fig. 2–6).[15]

Another growth factor, erythropoietin (EPO), regulates the growth of erythroid progenitor cells into mature erythrocytes and acts with other growth factors to stimulate burst-colony formation.[15,26] Erythropoietin, a hormonal glycoprotein, is produced primarily by the kidney. Recently, a peritubular interstitial cell was identified as the probable site of synthesis.[15] The principal stimulus for the production of erythropoietin is tissue hypoxia.

Thrombopoietin is comparable in action to erythropoietin. Thrombopoietin stimulates thrombopoiesis by stimulating megakaryocytic maturation and the subsequent release of platelets.

Protein molecules that work in conjunction with CSFs to stimulate particular cell lineages to proliferate and differentiate marrow progenitor cells are the interleukins (ILs); IL-1, IL-2, IL-3, IL-4, IL-5, IL-6, and IL-7.[11,12,15,21] Interleukins are cytokines that act separately or in combination to support hematopoietic growth. Interleukin-1 (IL-1) is called a response modulator molecule because it appears to influence hematopoiesis indirectly or in synergy with IL-3, M-CSF, G-CSF, and GM-CSF to stimulate different progenitor cells.[8,15] Interleukin-1 stimulates the lymphoid stem cell and enhances B-cell response and proliferation of T cells. Interleukin-1 is derived from macrophages and endothelial cells.[15]

Interleukin-2 (IL-2), a T-cell growth factor from activated mature helper T lymphocytes and NK cells, affects the proliferation and regulation of T cells, B cells, NK cells, and monocytes.[8,15] Interleukin-2 is secreted from stimulated T cells, which interact with IL-2 receptors to mediate cell growth. This interleukin acts upon activated B cells as an influential growth and differentiation factor. Interleukin-2 can also metabolically activate NK cells and monocytes.

Interleukin-3 (IL-3) is one of the primary colony-stimulating factors supporting the growth and development of normal hematopoietic cells in culture.[20,21] Interleukin-3 (or multi-CSF) preferentially supports proliferation of CFU-GEMM, CFU-M, CFU-Meg, CFU-Eo, and CFU-Bs colonies from bone marrow.[9,11,20] The developing cells eventually lose their response to IL-3, and the final developmental stages in most of the lineages are supported by lineage-specific factors such as G-CSF, GM-CSF, or other interleukins.[20] Interleukin-3 interacts with other growth factors to stimulate early progenitor cells of the myeloid lineages. For example, IL-3 is not as effective in supporting granulocytic colony formation as is G-CSF, but the combination of IL-3 and G-CSF provides a more potent stimulus for hematopoiesis than does either factor alone.[20] There are similar interactions of IL-3 with M-CSF to enhance macrophage/monocyte colonies IL-3 with GSF and MEG-CSF to augment megakaryocyte colonies,[23] and IL-3 with erythropoietin in stimulating BFU-E and CFU-E colonies.[19] Interleukin-3 has also been found to be a primary hormone supporting the CFU-blast in vitro, as long as this cell is in the G_0 phase of the cell cycle.[20] Interleukin-3 acts with M-CSF to stimulate proliferation of monocytes and macrophages. It also stimulates granulocytes, monocytes, eosinophils, and mast cell production in vivo and induces basophil histamine release. Lymphoid cells are not influenced by IL-3, but T lymphocytes are induced to produce IL-3 by activation of antigen, lectin, or IL-1.[15] Mature monocytes have IL-3 receptors and are responsive to IL-3, but mature neutrophils do not have these receptors and thus do not respond to IL-3.[8,10,20]

Interleukin-4 (IL-4) affects the T- and B-lymphocyte pathways and the mast cells. Interleukin-4 assists B-cell maturation, stimulates growth of T helper cells, enhances growth of mast cells in response to IL-3, and interacts with G-CSF to proliferate myeloid progenitor cells.[15]

Interleukin-5 (IL-5) promotes differentiation of B cells, and IgM secretion and proliferation by B cells. It also stimulates eosinophil colony and differentiation and interacts with GM-CSF and IL-3 in eosinophil induction.[8,15,24,25]

Interleukin-6 (IL-6) induces differentiation of B cells and enhances Ig secretion by B lymphocytes.[15,21] Interleukin-7 (IL-7) is active in the development of immature B cells and stimulates T lymphocytes.[15]

Combinations of two or more of the hematopoietic growth factors can support proliferation and differentiation more effectively than can the individual growth factors. Growth factors interact with one another to provide additive or synergistic effects.[15] Cross-lineage stimulation between CSFs and ILs affects multiple lineages.[15] The whole system of CSFs functions in a regulatory manner to producing enough cells to maintain a constant number of cells.

Each hematopoietic growth factor is encoded by a single gene. The genes for GM-CSF, IL-3, and M-CSF are on chromosome 5; G-CSF is on chromosome 17.[14] The gene for erythropoietin is located on chromosome 7.[14]

MORPHOLOGY OF HUMAN BLOOD AND MARROW CELLS

After stimulation by growth factors, stem cells differentiate and become committed to production of one cell line, and progenitor cells mature to develop into morphologically recognizable cell lines with distinctive features. The stages of maturation are classified according to cellular characteristics and staining properties such as size, nuclear chromatin pattern, presence of nucleoli, amount and color of cytoplasm, and ratio of nucleus to cytoplasm. Recognition and classification can be made between different cell lines, as well as between different maturational stages in the same cell line.

Erythropoiesis (Color Plate 1)

The Erythron

The erythron is the total population of mature erythrocytes and their precursors in blood and bone marrow and other sites. The use of this term indicates that the widely distributed red blood cells function as a unit.[1]

In response to erythropoietin, erythropoiesis occurs in the central sinus beds of medullary marrow over a period of about 5 days through at least three successive reductions-divisions from rubriblast to prorubricyte to rubricyte, and finally to metarubricyte (orthochromatic normoblast). With successive developmental stages, there is a reduction in cell volume, condensation of chromatin, loss of nucleoli, decrease in ribonucleic acid (RNA) in the cytoplasm, decrease in mitochondria, and gradual increase in synthesis of hemoglobin. The nucleus of the metarubricyte is extruded, leaving a non-nucleated polychromatophilic erythrocyte, which is released into the circulating blood to mature in 1 to 2 days. From 14 to 16 erythrocytes are produced from one rubriblast (Fig. 2–7).[1]

Rubriblast (Pronormoblast, Proerythroblast) (Color Plates 8 to 11 and 21)

The rubriblast, the earliest recognizable cell of the erythrocytic series, has a round primitive nucleus with visible nucleoli and chromatin strands that are indistinct and dispersed. There is no evidence of clumped chromatin. The nucleus stains

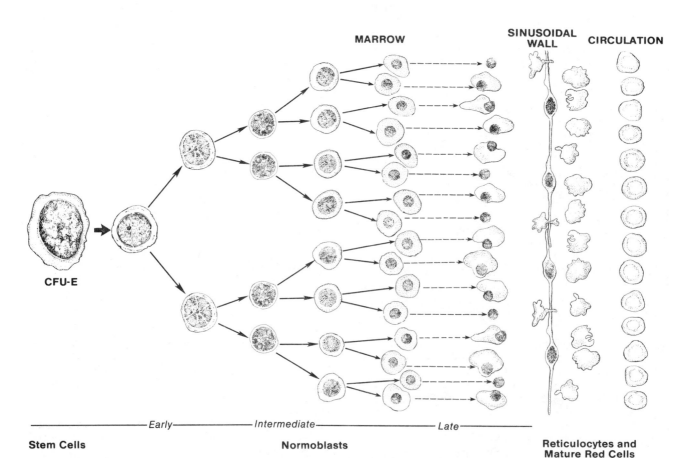

Figure 2–7. Proliferation and maturation of the CFU-E to form adult red cells. Each primitive erythroid cell undergoes four mitoses, during which time there is a progressive increase in hemoglobin content. These steps in proliferation and maturation are divided into early, intermediate, and late stages of normoblast development. From each red cell precursor are produced 14 to 16 progeny, which then lose their nuclei to become marrow reticulocytes, and, subsequently, circulating reticulocytes and adult red blood cells. Red cells normally enter circulation as reticulocytes, containing a small amount of residual RNA for approximately another 24 hours. (From Hillman, RF and Finch, CA: Red Cell Manual, ed 5. FA Davis, Philadelphia, 1985, with permission.)

Table 2-3. **BONE MARROW CELLS: NORMAL ADULT VALUES**

Stem cell	0–0.01%
Myeloblast	0–1
Promyelocyte	1–5
N. myelocyte	2–10
N. metamyelocyte	5–15
N. band	10–40
N. segmented	10–30
Eosinophil	0–3
Basophil	0–1
Lymphocyte	5–15
Plasmacyte	0–1
Monocyte	0–2
Other cells	0–1
Megakaryocyte	0.1–0.5
Rubriblast	0–1
Prorubricyte	1–4
Rubricyte	10–20
Metarubricyte	5–10
WBC:Nucleated RBC Ratio = 4:1	

Source: From Diggs,[31] with permission.

reddish-blue with Wright's stain. The cytoplasm stains royal or larkspur blue owing to the presence of RNA and to the superimposed slightly pinkish tinge of hemoglobin over the blue; this imparts to the cytoplasm a dark blue or royal blue similar to that seen in some plasmocytes.[1,31]

Rubriblasts range in size between 18 and 25 μm. Usually a rubriblast is slightly larger than a myeloblast and has more cytoplasm which stains a deeper blue. Rubriblasts constitute 1 percent or less of the cells observed in normal bone marrow (Table 2-3). Rubriblasts usually divide within 12 hours to make two daughter cells (prorubricytes).[1,31]

Prorubricyte (Basophilic Normoblast, Basophilic Erythroblast) (Color Plates 12 to 14 and 17)

Prorubricytes, the daughter cells of rubriblasts, require about 20 hours to develop. In normal bone marrow there are about four times as many prorubricytes as rubriblasts.[1,31] In the prorubricyte the nuclear chromatin pattern has begun to coarsen and the nucleoli are ill-defined or not visible. As the prorubricyte matures, it accumulates more RNA and hemoglobin. The predominant color of the cytoplasm is the blue, due to the staining of RNA, but there is a pinkish tinge reflecting the presence of varying amounts of hemoglobin.[31]

A prorubricyte is normally smaller than a rubriblast. Normal marrow contains from 1 to 4 percent prorubricytes (Table 2-3). The division of the prorubricyte forms cells (rubricytes) that are smaller than prorubricytes but that have twice the amount of hemoglobin.[31]

Rubricyte (Polychromatic Normoblast, Polychromatic Erythroblast (Color Plates 15 and 16)

Rubricytes are smaller than prorubricytes. Rubricytes have relatively more cytoplasm with a smaller nucleus than a prorubricyte. The cytoplasm contains varying mixtures of the pink of hemoglobin and the blue of RNA; in the late rubricytes, the pinkish stain is usually predominant.[1,31]

Nuclear chromatin is thickened and irregularly condensed in the rubricyte. Light-staining parachromatin areas are visible among the dark blue–staining, pyknotic areas. Nucleoli are no longer visible.[31]

The transit time for rubricytes is about 30 hours, and there are approximately three times as many rubricytes as prorubricytes in marrow. Marrow in a normal adult contains 10 to 20 percent rubricytes (Table 2-3). Rubricytes are not present in normal blood of adults but may appear in blood of newborn infants.[1,31]

Metarubricyte (Orthochromatic Normoblast, Orthochromatic Erythroblast) (Color Plates 13 and 17)

Metarubricytes are formed from rubricytes and are recognized by the solid blue-black degenerated nucleus with a nonlinear clumped chromatin pattern. The metarubricyte nucleus is incapable of further DNA synthesis. The nucleus of the metarubricyte is destined to be extruded and will be phagocytized.

The cytoplasm is predominantly pinkish (or reddish) because of increasing hemoglobin synthesis, but there remain minimal amounts of blue cytoplasm due to RNA. Mitochondria are no longer evident.[31]

The transit time for metarubricytes is 48 hours. The number of metarubricytes in normal marrow varies between 5 and 10 percent (Table 2-3). Metarubricytes are not observed in normal adult peripheral blood but can be found in the blood of normal newborn infants.[1,31]

Diffusely Basophilic Erythrocyte (Polychromatophilic Erythrocyte) (Color Plate 27)

The condensed pyknotic nucleus of a metarubricyte is extruded, leaving a diffusely basophilic or polychromatophilic cell. The membrane of the erythrocyte reseals itself. Some of the bluish staining color remains due to the presence of RNA. The erythrocyte contains approximately two thirds of its total hemoglobin content by the time the nucleus is lost. There are decreases in RNA content and mitochondria.[1,31]

A diffusely basophilic erythrocyte is larger than a mature red cell. It is released in 2 to 3 days from the marrow and circulates for 1 or 2 days before maturing into an erythrocyte. Only occasionally are diffusely basophilic erythrocytes found in the blood of normal adults; however, polychromatophilic cells are frequently seen in the blood of normal newborn infants.[1,31]

When stained with new methylene blue, diffusely basophilic cells reveal ribosomes in a granulofilamentous arrangement and are classified as reticulocytes (**see Color Plate 106**). As ribosomes disappear, the diffusely basophilic cell changes into a mature erythrocyte.[31]

With anemia or hypoxia, erythropoietin stimulates erythroid precursors to proliferate and increase the number of early erythroid cells. An increased number of polychromatophilic cells are delivered early from the marrow and, therefore, the reticulocyte count is increased.[1,31]

Erythrocyte (Discocyte, Mature Red Blood Cell)

A normal mature erythrocyte is a biconcave disc that is 7 to 8 μm in mean diameter and 1.5 to 2.5 μm thick; it has a volume of 90 fl. After Wright's staining an erythrocyte appears as a circular cell with distinct and smooth margins. In the central portion where the cell is thinnest, the intensity of the stain is less than at the marginal area, creating an area of central pallor. At the thin end of the smear, red blood cells are flattened out, lack central pallor, and do not reveal their biconcavity.[31]

A mature erythrocyte is not able to synthesize protein, as it is without a nucleus and mitochondria, but it has a unique yet limited metabolism to sustain itself while traversing the microvasculature. The erythrocyte carries oxygen from the lungs to the tissues where it is exchanged for carbon dioxide. Erythrocytes are pliable or flexible and deformable, making them capable of unusual changes in shape that are necessary for passage through the microcirculation to transport oxygen.[1,31]

Granulocytopoiesis (Color Plate 2)

Granulocytopoiesis or myelopoiesis refers to the production of neutrophils, eosinophils, basophils, and monocytes. Mature neutrophils, eosinophils, and basophils have similar patterns of proliferation, differentiation, and division. Maturation and division of the myeloid series in the marrow demonstrate a continuum of development from the blast to the most mature cells (neutrophil segmented) requiring from 7 to 11 days.[1,32,37]

Granulocyte production proceeds after cell line commitment has determined the identity of the maturing cell as a member of the granulocytic series. The system moves cells through passages and compartments where various cellular stages occur in response to various stimuli. The mitotic or proliferative pool contains the committed stem cells, myeloblasts, promyelocytes, and myelocytes. These cells actively divide and mature, taking 1 to 2 days for each cellular cycle (T_g). The maturation pool is composed of metamyelocytes and bands, and represents the end of DNA synthesis. The transformation of myelocyte to metamyelocyte to band takes about 8 to 9 hours after entry into the maturation pool. The storage pool retains mature cells for release into peripheral circulation. These mature cells leave the marrow by moving through transiently formed pores in endothelial cells which separate marrow parenchyma from venous sinuses; when leaving blood for tissue, cells migrate between endothelial cells (diapedesis). After release, cells become part of the functional pool and reside as circulating cells or as marginated cells, which line blood vessel walls. Cells are released to enter the peripheral blood or vessel walls for a few hours, and then leave the blood to enter tissues and body cavities. Under normal circumstances the rate at which these cells enter the blood and the rate at which they egress to tissue are in equilibrium.[1,3] As these cells exit the blood for the tissues, they are replaced by other cells from the marrow. Once in the blood, half of the released cells freely circulate while the other half are in a marginating pool on the walls of blood vessels—particularly those in lungs, liver, and spleen.[1,7,32,33] These latter cells leave the peripheral vessels to be directed by chemotactic factors to inflammatory or infectious tissue.[1,32,33,35-37] After cells enter tissues, they do not reenter circulation or the marrow.[3,7,32,33]

Morphologic Changes

During maturation there is a reduction in nuclear volume, condensation of chromatin, appearance and disappearance of primary granules, appearance of secondary granules, color changes in cytoplasm from blue to pinkish red, and change in size of cells.[1,3,32-34]

Maturation of the granulocytic series of cells is characterized by the development of primary blue-staining granules which are replaced by secondary granules that differ in their affinity for various dyes.[31,34,35] Cells with an affinity for basic dyes are basophils; those cells that stain reddish-orange with the acid dye eosin are eosinophils; the cells that do not stain intensely with either acid or basic dyes are called neutrophils. As these motile cells mature, the nucleus undergoes progressive changes from round to multilobular forms.[31,35,36]

Granulocytopoiesis: Stages of Differentiation and Maturation

Myeloblast (Color Plate 18). The earliest recognizable cell in the granulocytic series is a myeloblast. A myeloblast usually has a round nucleus that stains predominantly reddish blue and has a smooth nuclear membrane. The interlaced chromatin strands are delicate, finely dispersed or granular, and evenly stained, but are not clumped. One or more nucleoli of uniform size are usually demonstrable, but occasionally nucleoli may be barely visible.[31] A slight to moderate amount of bluish nongranular cytoplasm stains lighter next to the nucleus than at the periphery of the cell (**see Color Plates 2, 19, and 20**). A myeloblast is smaller and has less blue cytoplasm than a rubriblast.

After about three to five mitotic divisions, the myeloblast matures into a progranulocyte as primary granules become visible.[1,31] Ultrastructural studies of myeloblasts reveal numerous mitochondria, a Golgi area and free ribosomes.[1]

Myeloblasts vary in size but are about 17 μm.[1] They are not observed in normal peripheral blood. Normal marrow contains 1 percent or less myeloblasts (Table 2–3). With the appearance of primary granules the myeloblast has matured into a promyelocyte.[31]

Promyelocyte (Progranulocyte) (Color Plates 19 and 20). Granules that stain dark blue or reddish blue may be round or irregular in shape. They appear throughout the cytoplasm and may lie over the nucleus.[31,34] Primary granules are filled with lysosomal granules, which contain myeloperoxidase, acid phosphatase, hydrolytic enzymes, elastase, and β-glucuronidase but not alkaline phosphatase.[1,3,33,34]

The nucleus of a promyelocyte is usually round and is large in relation to the cytoplasm. In young promyelocytes the chromatin is almost as finely granular as it is in a myeloblast. In older cells the chromatin structure is slightly coarser than that in a myeloblast. Nucleoli may be faintly visible but are not often distinct[31] **(see Color Plates 2 and 21 to 23).**

The cytoplasm is blue with a relatively light zone adjacent to the nucleus. The periphery of the cytoplasm is smooth and is not indented by neighboring cells.[31]

The size of a promyelocyte may vary depending on the stage of a given cell in the mitotic cycle, but this cell may often be 20 μm and may be larger than a myeloblast. Progranulocytes do not appear in normal peripheral blood. From 1 to 5 percent progranulocytes are observed in normal bone marrow[31] (Table 2–3).

As the progranulocyte matures, nucleoli begin to fade, the chromatin becomes more condensed, and the granules are not as intensely stained. Specific secondary neutrophilic granules begin to appear, and the synthesis of primary granules ceases.[1,31,34] Some primary granules remain through division and maturation and may even appear in segmented neutrophils.[1,31,34]

Neutrophil Myelocyte (Color Plates 21 and 22). When primary granules are no longer synthesized and smaller, less dense secondary neutrophilic granules can be identified, the cell then has matured into a myelocyte.[31] The first sign of neutrophilic differentiation has been called the "dawn of neutrophilia" or "beginning neutrophilia," which refers to a relatively light island of illdefined or barely visible reddish (or pinkish) secondary lysosomal granules that develop adjacent to the nucleus and in proximity to the remaining primary granules.[31,34] As myelocytes divide and age, the primary granules become fewer and the secondary neutrophilic granules predominate. Secondary granules are considered to be specific granules for neutrophils and they contain collagenase, lysozyme, lactoferrin, plasminogen activators, aminopeptidase, and alkaline phosphatase.[1,35,38]

The nuclei of myelocytes may be round, oval, or flattened on one side and usually are not centrally located.[31] Chromatin strands become condensed, partly clumped, and thickened, and are unevenly stained. Nucleoli are absent or indistinct in myelocytes **(see Color Plates 2 and 21).** The neutrophil myelocyte is the last myeloid precursor capable of division.[31]

Neutrophil myelocytes are often smaller than progranulocytes and have relatively larger amounts of cytoplasm, which gradually becomes less basophilic and more pinkish. Normal peripheral blood does not contain neutrophilic myelocytes. There are 2 to 10 percent myelocytes in normal bone marrow[31] (Table 2–3).

Neutrophil Metamyelocyte (Color Plates 21 to 23). As maturation proceeds, the nucleus becomes slightly indented (bean- or kidney-shaped), which serves to identify the cell as a metamyelocyte.[31] The indentation is less than half the width of the arbitrary round nucleus. There is noticeable condensation with clumping of the chromatin but the chromatin structure is not as dense as that of the neutrophilic segmented cell. Metamyelocytes do not divide, nor do they have nucleoli.[31]

Many small, pinkish secondary granules fill the cytoplasm, and there may be a few primary darker granules remaining **(see Color Plates 2, 24, 26, and 28).** These maturing cells remain in marrow and form a granulocytic reserve.

Metamyelocytes are minimally smaller than myelocytes and are larger than the neutrophilic band or segmented cell. These cells are rare or absent in normal peripheral blood. There are approximately 5 to 15 percent metamyelocytes in normal bone marrow[31] (Table 2–3).

Neutrophil Band (N. Nonsegmented, N. Nonfilamented) (Color Plates 23, 25, 26, and 27). When the stage is reached in which the nuclear indentation is greater than half the width of the nucleus, the cell is identified as a neutrophilic band.[31] The opposite edges of the nucleus become almost parallel for an appreciable distance giving the appearance of a horseshoe or a curved link of sausage.[31] The nuclear chromatin is clumped and shows degenerative changes and there is usually a dark pyknotic mass at each pole where the lobe is destined to be.[31] The secondary neutrophilic granules are small and evenly distributed, stain various shades of pink, and contain alkaline phosphatase.[1,31] There may be an occasional dark primary granule[31] **(see Color Plates 2, 25, 26, and 27).**

Neutrophilic band cells are often slightly smaller than metamyelocytes. Band forms constitute from 2 to 6 percent of the leukocytes in the peripheral blood of healthy individuals and 10 to 40 percent of the nucleated cells in bone marrow[31] (Tables 2–3 and 2–4).

Neutrophil Segmented (N. Filamented, N. Polymorphonuclear Leukocyte PMN) (Color Plates 22 and 23). In a neutrophilic segmented cell the nu-

Table 2-4. **PERIPHERAL BLOOD CELLS: NORMAL ADULT VALUES**

	Percent	Per mm³
N. band	2-6	96-648
N. segmented	50-70	2400-7560
Eosinophil	0-4	0-432
Basophil	0-2	0-216
Lymphocyte	20-44	960-4752
Monocyte	2-9	96-972

cleus is normally separated into two to five (usually three) lobes with a narrow filament or strand connecting the lobes. Nuclear chromatin is heavily clumped or pyknotic and stains purplish red. The cytoplasm in an ideal stain is light pink and the small, numerous, and evenly distributed secondary granules either stain pink or take a neutral stain.[31] Neutrophil secondary granules are lysosomes that contain alkaline phosphatase.

Mature neutrophils are approximately twice the size of normal erythrocytes. There are 50 to 70 percent segmented neutrophils in the peripheral blood of older children and adults and 10 to 30 percent in normal marrow.[31] Approximately 5 percent of the neutrophils have one lobe (N. band), 35 percent have two lobes, 41 percent three lobes, 17 percent four lobes, and 2 percent five lobes. Segmentation of the nucleus enables these motile cells to pass through an opening in endothelial lining cells of capillaries and to "home in on selected prey."[31]

Because there is a gradual transition between the various stages of granulocytes, the division of neutrophils into developmental stages is somewhat arbitrary but is necessary for morphologic evaluation. Borderline cells that are difficult to distinguish from each other may be present. The major difficulty arises in differentiating between bands and segmented cells and in deciding whether the link connecting the lobes is narrow enough to be called a filament or wide enough to be identified as a band. A filamented or segmented cell has a threadlike connection between two lobes, and there is no visible chromatin between the two sides. In a band cell there are two distinct margins with nuclear chromatin material visible between the margins. Lobes of nuclei often touch each other or overlap, and it is impossible to see the connecting filaments. If the margin of a lobe can be traced as a definite and continuing line from one side of the nucleus across the isthmus to the other side, then it may be assumed that a filament is present even though it is not visible. In attempting to differentiate between a segmented cell and a band cell, identification should not be made on a single morphologic characteristic but rather on combined features. In case of doubt regarding identifying a borderline cell, the questionable cell should be placed in the mature category.[31]

Tissue Neutrophil (Fig. 2-8). Tissue neutrophils are large narrow cells with ample cytoplasm that is irregular with blunt pseudopods and often multipointed and that has nebulous cytoplasmic streamers. These cells are readily indented by adjacent marrow cells or are squeezed between them. Often there are long and tenuous cytoplasmic extensions that seem to wrap around other cells. These cells are not phagocytic and seldom have vacuoles in the cytoplasm.[31,39]

The cytoplasm stains light blue and has a fine

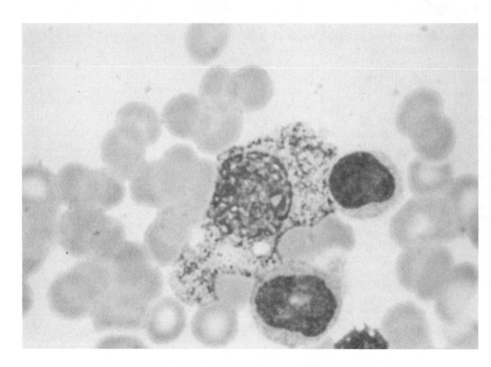

Figure 2-8. Tissue neutrophil, bone-marrow aspirate.

latticelike structure. Granules vary in number and stain varying shades of red to blue but the majority have a reddish purple stain. Many of the granules tend to be arranged in chains. The beadlike granular aggregates extend into the cytoplasmic projections.[39]

The large round or oval nucleus has a coarse chromatin structure with a distinct linear pattern. Nucleoli are usually conspicuous and stain light blue.[31,39]

Tissue neutrophils are fixed or semifixed tissue cells that have developed neutrophilic granules. They are immobile end-stage cells that are probably derived from the same progenitor cell as neutrophils (that is, CFU-GEMM).

Tissue neutrophils occur infrequently in normal bone marrow; however, they are found in increased numbers in bone marrow smears of patients having conditions in which there is a proliferation of neutrophilic cells such as myelocytic leukemia, myelocytic-monocytic leukemia, and myelofibrosis, as well as in neutropenic states in which there is an arrest in the maturation and delivery of cells into the circulating blood.[31,39]

Eosinophils (Color Plate 28)

Eosinophils are usually easily recognizable because of the large, round, secondary refractile granules that have an affinity for the acid eosin stain. With Wright's stain, normal eosinophil granules become orange to reddish orange. The granules are spherical, uniform in size, and evenly distributed. Because of the size and roundness of the granule, eosinophils may be recognized in unstained moist preparations of blood in light microscopy and in phase microscopy.[31] Eosinophil granules contain an electron-dense crystalloid core when observed in the electron microscope. This crystalloid core is composed mainly of major basic protein (MBP), which binds to acid aniline dyes and which may help to explain the staining qualities of the granule.[1,33,38,40] The granules of eosinophils contain various hydrolytic enzymes including peroxidase, acid phosphatase, aryl sulfatase, β-glucuronidase, phospholipase, cathepsin, and ribonuclease but lack lysozyme, cationic proteins, and alkaline phosphatase.[1,33,38,40,41]

Eosinophils pass through the same developmental stages as neutrophils: myelocyte, metamyelocyte, band, and segmented stages[1,40] (see Table 2–3; **see also Color Plates 2 and 24 to 28**). The earliest eosinophil has a few dark bluish primary granules intermingled with the few specific reddish orange granules. During development the bluish granules become less visible and disappear and the round specific secondary eosinophil granules fill the cytoplasm.[31]

Eosinophils spend 3 to 6 days in production in marrow before appearing in peripheral blood. Bone marrow provides a storage area for eosinophils so that they can be rapidly mobilized when needed.[1] The factors that regulate production and release eosinophils into blood are probably different from those of neutrophils. The mean transit time of these cells in the circulatory system of humans has been reported to be about 8 hours, but in some disease states with eosinophilia the time may be longer.[1] Much less is known about the stem cell kinetics of the eosinophils than of the neutrophil.[1] Eosinophils migrate from blood to tissue, with most eosinophils residing in tissue, such as bronchial mucosa, skin, gastrointestinal tract, and vagina for about 12 days. Eosinophils may migrate from tissue back into blood and marrow.[40]

Eosinophils which are motile, can migrate between endothelial cells into tissue or into an area of inflammation in the same manner as neutrophils.

Normal adult peripheral blood contains 0 to 4 percent eosinophils, with approximately the same number observed in normal bone marrow (Tables 2–3 and 2–4). In normal blood, eosinophils are about the size of or slightly larger than neutrophils and have a band or two-lobed nucleus with condensed chromatin; rarely does an eosinophil have three lobes.[31]

Tissue Eosinophil. In smears of bone marrow, occasionally there may be a large cell with elongate and tapering cytoplasmic extensions, containing typical reddish orange granules of the type seen in the eosinophils of the circulating blood.[31,39] The nucleus of such cells, instead of being indented or lobulated, is round or oval and has a well-defined reticular chromatin and often nucleoli. Such cells are identified as tissue eosinophils and are thought to be fixed tissue variants of the more motile eosinophils of the circulating blood.[31,39] Tissue eosinophils arise from the same progenitor cell as eosinophils in marrow and blood.

Basophils (Color Plate 29)

Although basophils constitute 0 to 2 percent of normal blood cells (Table 2–4), the large abundant violet-blue (or purple-black) granules aid in the immediate recognition of this cell. These granules are visible above the nucleus as well as lateral to the nucleus, and they obscure most of the nucleus. The granules vary in size from 0.2 to 1.0 μm. They are coarse, unevenly distributed; vary in number, shape, and color; and are less numerous than eosinophil granules. These granules have an affinity for blue or basic thiazine dyes. Basophil granules are also water soluble. In cells that are poorly fixed during staining, the center of the granules may disappear or the entire granule may be washed away, leaving a small colorless cytoplasmic area.[31]

Based on the shape of their nuclei, basophils may be identified as basophilic myelocytes, metamyelocytes, bands, and segmented cells. However, the shape of the nucleus is often masked by the granules[29] **(see Color Plates 2, 24, and 29).** The specific violet-blue granules of basophils are formed in the myelocyte stage and continue to be made during the later maturation stages. There are also some smaller granules that do not stain as darkly as the specific basophil granules but that tend to be more reddish blue.[31,42,43]

Maturation of basophils takes place over 7 days.[1]

Mature basophils rarely have more than two segments. Basophils circulate for a few hours in blood, then migrate into skin, mucosa, and other serosal areas.[1]

Basophils in all stages of maturation are smaller than promyelocytes and neutrophil myelocytes; their size approximates that of neutrophils. Basophils show diurnal variation similar to eosinophils, increasing at night and decreasing in the morning.[1]

Tissue Basophil (Mast Cell) (Fig. 2–9). Tissue basophils (mast cells) **(see Color Plate 48)** and blood basophils are closely related in their functions and biochemical characteristics, but the relationship between them is controversial.[1,31] Both cells participate in a similar manner in acute and delayed allergic reactions. The granules of both cells have similar morphologic characteristics and each contain histamine and heparin and are water soluble.[31]

Tissue basophils are derived from the multipotential undifferentiated stem cell and are fixed tissue cells. The cytoplasm of the tissue basophil is filled with large prominent intensely stained violet-blue granules. The granules are usually round and about the same size (0.1 to 0.3 μm). They may overlie the margins of the palely stained nucleus or obscure the nucleus completely. The nucleus is small and round or oval.[31]

Tissue basophils are widely scattered in connective tissue of various organs, bone marrow, and mucosal areas of serous membranes. In bone marrow tissue basophils are usually observed in the hypercellular area of a "squashed" smear made from a marrow particle. Some tissue basophils have spindle shapes and jagged margins due to trauma in the process of aspiration.[31]

Monoblasts and Promonocytes
(Color Plate 5)

Monoblasts have a large, eccentrically placed nucleus that may be slightly indented, one or two large prominent nucleoli, a fine lacy nuclear chromatin, and an agranular cytoplasm that stains a deep blue. Monoblasts are nonmotile and nonphagocytic cells. Monoblasts divide and give rise to promonocytes.[31]

Promonocytes also are large, have indented or folded nuclei and irregular margins, and sometimes contain a few peroxidase-positive granules. Promonocytes are slightly motile and may infrequently take part in phagocytosis.[31]

Promonocytes and monoblasts are not easily identifiable in bone marrow or peripheral blood smears except in disorders in which there is marked proliferation of monocytic cells. The identification of early monocytic cells is based on slightly indented or folded, large nuclei and on association with more mature cells that have pseudopods and brainlike convolutions in the nucleus.[31]

Monocytes and Macrophages
(Color Plate 4)

Monocytes and macrophages constitute the monocyte-macrophage phagocytic system. Monoblasts, found in the marrow, divide and develop into promonocytes, and then into monocytes. They enter the circulation for a short time, and migrate into tissue to transform into macrophages.[14,15,19,21,27]

In thin areas of the peripheral blood smear, the monocyte is about 15 to 18 μm and is larger than

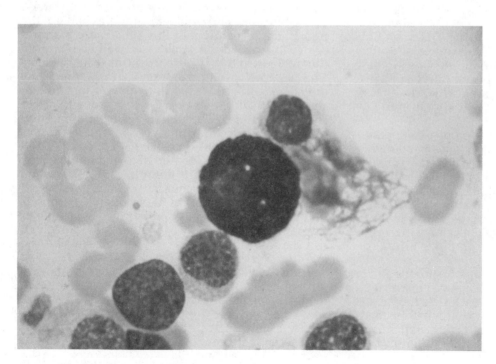

Figure 2–9. Tissue basophil, bone-marrow aspirate.

the neutrophil. Monocytes have abundant cytoplasm in relation to the nucleus. The scanning electron microscope shows the monocyte to have a ruffled plasma membrane with long, thin microvilli. With Wright's stain the cytoplasm turns a dull gray-blue, in contrast to the pink cytoplasm of neutrophils.[31] Numerous fine, small, reddish- or purplish-stained, evenly distributed granules in the cytoplasm give the cell a ground-glass appearance. There may be varying numbers of prominent granules in addition to the small granules. Some monocytes may appear nongranular, suggesting rapid turnover. Digestive vacuoles may be observed in the cytoplasm. In disease states phagocytized erythrocytes, nuclei, cell fragments, bacteria, fungi, and pigment may be present.

The nuclei of monocytes frequently may be kidney-shaped, deeply folded, or indented or occasionally lobular. One of the distinctive features of the monocyte is the appearance of brainlike convolutions in the nucleus. Another characteristic is the lacy chromatin network of fine strands intermingled with small chromatin clumps.[31]

The shape of the monocyte is variable. Many cells are round; other cells reveal blunt pseudopods which are manifestations of their slow mobility. These ameboid cells continue to move while the blood film is drying and become fixed before the cytoplasmic extensions are retracted. These pseudopods vary in size and number; the outer portion of the outstretched cytoplasm may have a hyaline appearance without granules in contrast to the inner granular cytoplasm.[31]

Three helpful characteristic features of the monocyte are brainlike nuclear convolutions, blunt pseudopods, and dull gray-blue cytoplasm[31] (see Color Plates 30 to 33).

Kinetic studies have revealed that the half-time clearance of monocytes in the circulation is an average of 8.4 hours.[1,33]

Monocytes account for 2 to 9 percent of normal blood leukocytes and for less than 2 percent of normal marrow cells (Tables 2–3 and 2–4). Monocytes are known to be in the marginating pool of cells. There is not a large reserve pool of monocytes in normal marrow. Monocytes leave the marrow when mature and enter the bloodstream, where they circulate for about 14 hours before entering tissue to transform into macrophages.[1] Macrophages are observed occasionally in normal marrow.

As monocytes grow they become too large to pass readily through capillaries, and so they move into tissue and convert into macrophages in many organs (for example, pulmonary alveolar macrophages, splenic macrophages, Kupffer's cells in the liver, and connective tissue macrophages).[1] This transformation involves rapid growth, enlargement, and intensified phagocytic activity. Macrophages do not normally reenter the bloodstream but may reenter the circulation during inflammation.[1]

Macrophages are large cells (25 to 50 μm) with a round or reniform nucleus and contain one or two nucleoli, clumped chromatin, abundant cytoplasm with vacuoles, and numerous azurophilic granules.[1]

Lymphopoiesis (Color Plate 5)

The common lymphoid progenitor cell can differentiate into either T or B cells, depending on the microenvironment. T cells differentiate in the thymus, the B cells in adult bone marrow. Null cells, or third-population cells, originate in the bone marrow, although the maturation sequence is unknown.

Interleukins and other cytokines stimulate proliferation of these cells in the cell cycle. In primary lymphoid organs such as the thymus and bone marrow, lymphocytes differentiate, proliferate, and mature into fully functional immune cells. In secondary lymphoid organs such as lymph nodes, spleen, and mucosal tissues (tonsils, Peyer's patches), lymphocytes communicate and interact with antigen-presenting cells (APCs), phagocytes, and macrophages in an active immune response.

Lymphoblasts and Prolymphocytes (Color Plate 5)

The earliest lymphocytes are identified as lymphoblasts and prolymphocytes. Lymphoblasts contain a large round nucleus with a small or moderate amount of basophilic cytoplasm. The nuclear chromatin strands in lymphoblasts are thin, evenly stained, and not clumped. One or several nucleoli are demonstrable usually.[27]

Prolymphocytes have an intermediate chromatin pattern that has clumps in some areas of the nucleus but does not appear as clumped as in mature lymphocytes. Nucleoli are less distinct than in lymphoblasts. Differences are subtle, and in case of doubt the cell should be called a lymphocyte.[31]

Lymphocytes (Color Plate 3)

Lymphocytes are the second most numerous cell in the blood; from 20 to 55 percent of blood cells are lymphocytes (Table 2–4). There are 5 to 15 lymphocytes in bone marrow smears (see Table 2–3). Most lymphocytes are small, varying from 7 to 10 μm compared with monocytes (15 to 18 μm). Large lymphocytes may be 12 to 15 μm or more. (see Color Plates 3, 5, 32, and 34 to 36). Between the small and large lymphocytes, there are many intermediate sizes. Size is not a reliable basis for determining the age or metabolic activity of lymphocytes because the size varies with the thickness of the smear. Lymphocytes tend to become spherical and small in thick areas of the smear; in the thinnest end of the smear, lymphocytes may be spread out and appear large.[31]

Small lymphocytes usually are round with smooth margins (see Color Plates 34 and 35). Rarely a lymphocyte may have a spindle form with an oval nucleus and cytoplasmic filaments extending outward at each end (see Color Plate 3F). The margin of large lymphocytes frequently is indented by neighboring erythrocytes causing them to have a serrated (holly-leaf) shape.[31]

With Wright's stain, the color of the cytoplasm is blue, with the intensity of the blue varying from light to dark in different cells. The color is evenly distributed in some cells and uneven in other cells. The intensity of the blue stain is greater at the periphery of the cell than near the Golgi area adjacent to the nucleus. The cytoplasm of some large lymphocytes that stain a pale sky blue has a structureless appearance; other large cells may reveal fine bluish interlacing fibrils with critical illumination.[31]

The majority of lymphocytes do not have granules. In some large cells there may be a variable number of a few well-defined granules that vary in size, are unevenly distributed, and may be easily counted. These granules are a purplish-red and have been called azurophilic; this term is misleading because these granules are predominantly red rather than blue.[31]

The diameter of the nucleus of the smallest lymphocyte in peripheral blood is slightly larger than or the same size as a normal erythrocyte in the same microscopic field. The lymphocyte's nucleus, in relation to its cytoplasm, is large, and the nuclei are round or slightly indented. Chromatin structure is lumpy or clumped and stains dark-purple with lighter bluish-purple areas between chromatin aggregates.[31]

Nucleoli are present in some lymphocytes but are not visible in light microscopy for they are obscured by the darkly stained chromatin masses. The fact that nucleoli may be present in small lymphocytes is evidence that these cells are capable of growth and replication.[31,32]

Null Cells. A third population of cells is that of the non-T, non-B cells, or null cells. T, B, and null cells cannot be separately identified morphologically but can be distinguished functionally and by immunologic marker studies.

Large Lymphocytes versus Monocytes. A monocyte is often mistaken for a large lymphocyte (**see Color Plate 32**) because the monocytic cytoplasm may be blue, granules may be indistinct, nucleus is round, and blunt pseudopods and digestive vacuoles are missing. To distinguish monocytes from large lymphocytes, nuclear chromatin structure, character of the cytoplasm, and shape of the cells are useful. The nucleus of a lymphocyte tends to be clumped rather than linear or lacy, as it is in a monocyte (**see Color Plates 34 to 36**). There is a greater tendency for the nuclear chromatin to be condensed at the periphery of the nucleus in the lymphocyte. Brainlike convolutions present in a monocyte are not observed in a lymphocyte.[31]

Large lymphocytes and monocytes may have distinct bluish red granules. In a monocyte the large bluish red granules are interspersed with numerous fine granules in the cytoplasm and cannot be enumerated (**see Color Plates 30 and 31**). In a lymphocyte these large granules are prominent

and can be counted easily because there are no other granules (**see Color Plate 36 and 135**). Because of the finely granular cytoplasm the monocyte has a ground-glass appearance, whereas the cytoplasm of the lymphocyte has a relatively clear nongranular background. Large lymphocytes are often deeply indented by neighboring red blood cells. Monocytes tend to project blunt pseudopods between cells or to compress cells, rather than being indented by them.[31]

Activated and Reactive Lymphocytes (Color Plates 136 to 138). In reaction to appropriate antigenic stimuli, lymphocytes have been shown to transform into cells that are immunologically competent. The size of activated lymphocytes varies, but usually these cells are large with abundant cytoplasm. The increase in size is due to an increase in DNA in the nucleus and of RNA in the cytoplasm. Nuclei may be oval and indented, with an intermediate chromatin pattern. Nuclei of some lymphocytes may have blastlike nuclei with nucleoli. Varying degrees of cytoplasmic basophilia may be present. There may be distinctive reddish granules. The cytoplasm may appear bubbly and vacuoles may be seen.[31]

Lymphocytes that respond to antigenic stimuli constitute a wide spectrum of morphologic variants. The most striking variants are observed in infectious mononucleosis (see Chapter 17), but reactive lymphocytes are also present, in lesser numbers, in other viral diseases, such as cytomegalo virus (CMV) and infectious hepatitis, and in conditions such as post-transfusion reactions, organ transplants, and serum sickness.

Plasmablasts and Proplasmacytes (Color Plate 5). Cells designated as plasmablasts are similar to blast cells of other series. The nuclei are large in relation to the cytoplasm, appear round with fine and linear chromatin strands, and have a clearly visible nucleolus. Plasmablasts are identified primarily in the presence of proplasmacytes and plasmacytes but cannot be differentiated easily from other blasts.[31]

Proplasmacytes and plasmacytes differ from plasmablasts in that the color of the cytoplasm is dark blue, the juxtanuclear light areas are prominent, and the nuclei are eccentric. The chromatin structure of the nuclei in proplasmacytes is intermediate between that of plasmablasts and plasmacytes. In proplasmacytes the nucleolus may be ill-defined or absent.[31]

Plasmablasts and proplasmacytes, although not observed in normal bone marrow, are seen in diseases associated with abnormal immunoglobulin production, especially multiple myeloma.[31]

Plasmacytes (Plasma Cells) (Color Plates 37 and 38). Plasmacytes represent the end stage of B-lymphocyte lineage. They are not observed in peripheral blood smears of normal individuals but constitute about 1 percent of the nucleated cells in normal marrow (see Table 2–3). Mature plasmacytes range in size from 15 to 25 μm.[1] They may be round or oval with slightly irregular margins. The cytoplasm is nongranular and usually stains a deep or vibrant blue that has been described as "cornflower" or "larkspur" blue. The cytoplasm adjacent to the nucleus is pale with a perinuclear clear zone containing the Golgi apparatus, and at the cell periphery there are secretory vesicles. Fibrillar structures which stain blue may be demonstrable in the cytoplasm. One or several small vacuoles may be observed. There is no evidence of phagocytosis of visible particles.

The nucleus of a plasmacyte is relatively small, round, or oval and eccentrically placed in the cell. The nuclear chromatin is clumped or coarse and lumpy, similar to that of a lymphocyte[31] (**see Color Plates 5, 10, 14, 27, 37, and 38**).

Plasmacytes in bone marrow are semifixed cells that are torn in the process of aspiration and appear in marrow smears with irregular spiculate margins. Plasmacytes may cluster around large nongranular or finely granular tissue cells. This contact of plasmacytes with tissue cells is probably a manifestation of the immune response in which antigenic material, processed by macrophages, is transferred to the plasmacytes, which in turn will manufacture immune globulins.[31]

Immune globulins manufactured by plasmacytes produce unusual morphologic variants. The proteinaceous material is in the form of round globules that may be red, pink, blue, or almost colorless and are called Russell bodies. The globules may fill the cytoplasm, giving the appearance of a bunch of grapes (berry, grape, or morula cells).[31]

In some cells, the globules are so numerous and so tightly packed that they assume a honeycomb configuration. In other cells, the redness has a diffuse distribution, producing cells called "flame cells,"[31] which are observed particularly in association with IgA (**see Color Plate 229**). The red-staining proteinaceous material may appear as granules or as pools at the margins; it also may crystallize and produce elongated crystalline structures that stain reddish.[31]

Megakaryocytopoiesis (Color Plate 6)

The megakaryocyte is the largest hematopoietic cell in the bone marrow and descends from the same multipotential stem cell as do the other blood cells. The mission of megakaryocytes is to proliferate and then fragment their cytoplasm into platelets when needed in order to maintain a normal number of platelets. Because of their size and volume, megakaryocyte precursors increase their amount of nuclear chromatin (or DNA doublings) without cytoplasmic division (process of endomitosis).[1,33] IL-3, G-CSF together with Meg-CSF, fosters megakaryocyte colonies in assay systems.[22,23]

Megakaryoblasts are moderately large cells in the range of 20 to 45 μm, with a single, round, primitive nucleus, one or two nucleoli, and basophilic protrusions that stain blue and contain chromophobic globules.[8,20]

Pathologic alterations in megakaryoblasts are observed in myeloproliferative diseases. The presence of micromegakaryoblasts is typical of acute megakaryocytic leukemia (classified as M7 in the French-American-British (FAB) classification of acute leukemia). They may also be found in the blast crisis of chronic granulocytic leukemia and other acute leukemias. Such cells are small and difficult to distinguish from myeloblasts, but cytoplasmic blebs or budding (suggesting early platelet formation) help identify micromegakaryoblasts.[31,33]

As the megakaryoblast matures into a promegakaryocyte, it increases both the amount of nuclear chromatin through division of the cytoplasm and the amount of cytoplasm itself (**see Color Plates 39 to 42**). A promegakaryocyte not only increases the size of the nucleus but also becomes lobed, with each lobe having a 2n complement of DNA. Reddish granules appear in the enlarging bluish cytoplasm. Electron micrographs reveal that demarcation membranes are beginning to develop as invaginations from the plasma membrane of the megakaryocyte. The demarcation membrane system establishes an outer limit of each platelet, which arises as a cytoplasmic fragment.[1,22,33]

As endomitosis and DNA synthesis cease and maximum ploidy is attained, the megakaryocyte has increased in volume with an abundant amount of cytoplasm and a polyploid nucleus (**see Color Plates 41 and 42**). The majority of the cells are of the 8n, 16n, and 32n ploidy classes (16n average represents eight lobes).[1,33] The chromatin is linear and coarse. Numerous small, uniformly distributed, dense granules that stain reddish blue are present. The demarcation membrane system is uniform and its lumen open; the cytoplasm is divided into partitions that define platelet limits.[1,33]

After maturation is completed, the megakaryocyte membrane ruptures, the entire megakaryocyte cytoplasm fragments, and thrombopoiesis occurs. The polyploid naked nucleus (**see Color Plate 43**) is soon to be engulfed by a macrophage.[1]

In addition, some mature megakaryocytes are located adjacent to marrow sinuses and extend portions of their cytoplasm through the basement membrane and between endothelial cells of the marrow sinusoids in order to put platelets into the sinus. Membrane-bound platelets are released and swept into the flowing blood stream from these cytoplasmic projections. Further fragmentation to form individual platelets occurs after release into the sinus. Some fragments swept into the circulation may become lodged in the capillary beds of the lung. One megakaryocyte can release several thousand platelets.[1,33]

In the past, megakaryocytes were believed to shed platelets from their outer surface. However, transmission electron micrographs demonstrate that mature megakaryocytes have a well-defined marginal zone and that there are only a few channels of the demarcation membrane system in which platelets could be shed from the surface.

Therefore, during thrombocytopoiesis, the entire megakaryocyte cytoplasm fragments to form platelets.[1,33]

Ultrastructural features and marker studies on megakaryocytes aid in their identification at all stages. Ultrastructural features are the demarcation membrane, alpha granules, and platelet peroxidase activity.[1] Monoclonal antibodies for platelet glycoproteins Ib, IIb, and IIIa, factor VIII antigen, beta thromboglobulin; and factor V are markers for all stages of megakaryocytes.[1]

Platelets (or thrombocytes) are cytoplasmic fragments and have no nucleus. In peripheral smears of normal adults, platelets vary in size from 1 to 4 μm. Platelets stain light blue and contain a variable number of small reddish blue granules.[31]

Platelets tend to adhere to each other and may form small aggregates in a well-made normal smear. In the thin area of the blood smear where erythrocytes are separated or gently touching each other but not overlapping, the number per oil immersion field varies from 7 to 25.[31]

In marrow smears of normal individuals, there are approximately one to four megakaryocytes per 1000 nucleated cells, and these cells are in the late stage of maturation.[31]

Osteoblasts (Color Plate 49)

An osteoblast is a large cell with ample cytoplasm and a small, round, eccentrically placed nucleus. These cells may be traumatized in the process of marrow aspiration and smearing and often have irregular shapes and cytoplasmic streamers. The cells may have comet or tadpole shapes. The nucleus may be partially extruded, similar to a small round head on a round body. The nuclear chromatin strands and nuclear margins are well defined and stain purple-red. Usually there is a distinct blue nucleolus.[31]

Throughout the blue cytoplasm, there are small spherical bodies that are colorless and give a bubbly appearance to the cytoplasm. Within the cytoplasm, there is a prominent round or oval chromophobic zone that stains lighter than the rest of the cytoplasm. This area is usually away from the nucleus but may be adjacent to the nucleus.[31]

Osteoblasts, most often seen in marrow from young children, are responsible for the formation, calcification, and maintenance of trabeculae and cancellous bone.[31] Osteoblasts morphologically resemble plasmacytes, both having irregular shapes, cytoplasmic protrusions, blue cytoplasm, eccentric nuclei, spherical bodies within the cytoplasm, chromophobic areas, cytoplasmic fibrils, and vacuoles. The relatively unstained zone of the plasmacytes is adjacent to the nucleus and partially surrounds the nucleus like a collar, whereas the chromophobic zone of the osteoblast is often distinctly separate from the nuclear margin and, when adjacent to the nucleus, does not surround or enclose the nucleus. The protein secretions of the plasmacytes impart a reddish background color to the cells which is not demonstrable in osteoblasts.[31]

Osteoblasts occurring in clusters or aggregates may be misinterpreted as malignant cells. Malignant cells in a cluster are crowded and distorted and their margins indistinct, rendering it impossible to identify individual cells. The size, shape, structure, and color of malignant cells are variable, whereas osteoblasts are more orderly and uniform. Chromophobic areas in the cytoplasm of osteoblasts are seldom demonstrable in malignant cells.[31]

Osteoclasts (Color Plate 50)

Osteoclasts are giant, multinucleated, irregularly shaped marrow phagocytes that are capable of absorption of bone. Osteoclasts have from 2 to 50 nuclei, which are separate, usually round or oval, all about the same size, and haphazardly distributed within the cytoplasm; they have visible nucleoli.[31] The lineage of osteoclasts has been established as fusion of precursor cells—CFU-M—derived from monocyte-macrophages.

The abundant cytoplasm with ragged margin is bluish with numerous reddish lysosomal granules containing acid phosphatase. In thin marrow smears it may be possible to demonstrate a ruffled cytoplasmic fringe consisting of diaphanous veils, fingerlike protrusions, and saccular invaginations.[31]

Osteoclasts and megakaryocytes are sometimes difficult to differentiate, for both cells are large with granular cytoplasm, irregular shapes, and multiple nuclei. The nuclei of megakaryocytes are connected by a nuclear strand, have irregularly nuclear shapes, and may be superimposed (**see Color Plate 51**), whereas the nuclei of osteoclasts are separated, uniform in size, and have no visible connections to each other. The number of nuclei in normal megakaryocytes is even, whereas in osteoclasts it may be uneven.[31]

Osteoclasts secrete enzymes that aid in dissolution of osteoid tissue and calcific bone. Osteoclastic activating factor (OAF), secreted by plasmacytes in myeloma, is a lymphokine that stimulates osteoclastic activity in the endosteum near groups of myeloma cells. The presence of OAF helps to explain the development of osteolytic bone lesions observed in myeloma.[1,31]

TRENDS IN THERAPEUTIC MANIPULATION OF HEMATOPOIESIS

Many growth factors have been isolated, biochemically characterized, purified, genetically cloned, and produced through recombinant DNA technology.[8–11,13–16] During the last 5 years, growth factors G-CSF, GM-CSF, EPO, and the interleukins have been used for preclinical study and for clinical application. Colony-stimulating factors have been employed to strengthen patients with cancer and acquired immunodeficiency syndrome (AIDS) and to guard against infection for bone marrow transplant patients. These factors have also been used to treat those with anemia due either to surgery or to kidney failure. The blood count of autologous donors can be raised for donation prior to surgical procedures. Interleukins are used clinically for wound healing, activating lymphocytes, and assisting in the growth of transplanted or damaged bone marrow.[9,26-30]

Recombinant Colony-Stimulating Factors (CSFs)

Granulocyte-macrophage CSF has been purified to homogeneity from a human cell line and also from murine lung conditioned medium.[9,27] These purified proteins have been amino acid sequenced and their mRNAs identified so that complementary sequences of DNA (cDNA) of both human and murine GM-CSFs, and the genes encoding these factors, have been cloned.[9,10,27] The recombinant human GM-CSF (rHuGM-CSF) has been produced in yeast, bacteria, and mammalian systems and is now available in large amounts, thus allowing the biologic specificity of GM-CSF to be studied in vitro and in vivo.[8,9,27] This recombinant growth factor has been shown not only to produce neutrophilic and monocytic lineages but also eosinophilic, megakaryocytic, and erythrocytic lineages.[8-10,27]

Human G-CSF has been purified to homogeneity from human cell lines and placenta, and the amino acid sequence has been determined. The gene for G-CSF has been expressed in bacterial and mammalian cells, and recombinant human granulocyte colony-stimulating factor (rHuG-CSF) has been produced.[11,14] There appears to be no difference in vivo between the natural G-CSF and the synthesized G-CSF with respect to stimulating production of neutrophils.

The gene for EPO has been cloned, and almost pure recombinant human EPO (rHuEpo) is available in large quantities. The amino acid sequence of EPO has been determined and the protein part of the hormone and the recombinant EPO are similar.[30]

Clinical Trials of Recombinant Human Colony-Stimulating Factors

Clinical trials of recombinant CSFs using biologic substances similar to those in the human body have provided new opportunities for evaluating their clinical usefulness in the treatment of hematologic and oncologic disorders.[12,13,28,29] Investigations have shown that rHuG-CSF accelerates recovery from neutropenia induced by myelotoxic chemotherapy for different types of carcinoma.[18] Recombinant human G-CSF has been given to patients receiving myelosuppressive chemotherapy and undergoing autologous bone marrow transplantation, to accelerate the rate of neutrophil recovery.[12,28] Clinical trials are being conducted to determine whether rHuG-CSF is effective in correcting severe neutropenia in hematopoietic malignancies, such as hairy-cell leukemia, and also in

non-neoplastic hematopoietic diseases, such as aplastic anemia and cyclic neutropenia.[18,28] Recombinant human GM-CSF appears to offer useful therapy with graft failure after bone marrow transplantation.[14,15,17,26] There is hope that hematopoietic growth factors can be combined with chemotherapy in treatment of patients with advanced malignancies and bone marrow transplant patients by increasing production of granulocytes and platelets.[14,15] There is also hope that CSFs can augment mechanisms of host defense in patients with AIDS.[14,15] Granulocyte-macrophage CSF has been evaluated in HIV-infected (AIDS) patients and has been shown to increase the leukocyte count and to be effective when combined with antiretrieval agents such as AZT (azydothymidine or zidovudine — also, Retrovir).[14,15] Interleukin-3 together with M-CSF stimulates myelocytes, erythrocytes, and platelet production in aplastic anemia, myelodysplastic syndrome, and prolonged chemotherapy for malignancy. Chronic anemia due to renal failure has shown that treatment with recombinant human erythropoietin (rHuEpo) has increased RBC production and alleviated the anemia in more than 97 percent of patients.[14,15,26,30] The rise in hematocrit is dose-dependent and is in proportion to the increase in RBC mass.[30]

Clinical trials using other synthesized CSFs are currently in progress to determine their activity in controlling hematopoiesis. Each factor needs to be purified and its function determined before the interactions between hematopoietic growth factors in the marrow microenvironment can be completely understood.

REFERENCES

1. Jandl, JH: Blood. Textbook of Hematology. Little, Brown, Boston, 1987.
2. Beck, WS: Hematology, ed 4. MIT Press, Cambridge, MA, 1985.
3. Spivak, JL: Fundamentals of Clinical Hematology, ed 2. Harper & Row, Philadelphia, 1984.
4. Hillman, RF and Finch, CA: Red Cell Manual, ed 5. FA Davis, Philadelphia, 1985.
5. Nathan, DG: The benificence of neonatal hematopoiesis. N Engl J Med 321(17):1190, 1989.
6. Ogawa, M: Effects of hemopoietic growth factors on stem cells in vitro. Hematol Oncol Clin North Am 3(3):453, 1989.
7. Erslev, AJ and Gabuzda, TG: Pathophysiology of Blood, ed 3. WB Saunders, Philadelphia, 1985.
8. Morstyn, G and Burgess, AW: Hemopoietic growth factors: A review. Cancer Res 48:5624, 1988.
9. Clark, SC and Kamen, R: The human hematopoietic colony-stimulating factors. Science 236:1229, 1987.
10. Griffin, JD: Clinical applications of colony-stimulating factors. Oncology 2(1):15, 1988.
11. Platzer, E: Human hemopoietic growth factors. Eur J Haematol 42:1, 1989.
12. Till, TE and McCulloch, EA: A direct measurement of the radiation sensitivity of normal mouse bone marrow cells. Radiat Res 14:213, 1961.
13. Gabrilove, JL: Introduction and overview of hematopoietic growth factors. Sem Hematol 26(2):1, 1989.
14. Groopman, JE, Molina, JM, and Scaddon, DT: Hematopoietic growth factors. N Engl J Med 321(21):1449, 1989.
15. Quesenberry, P, Souza, L, and Krantz, S: Growth Factors.

American Society of Hematology, Education Program, Atlanta, 1989, pp 98–113.

16. Weisbart, RH, Gasson, JC, and Golde, DW: Colony-stimulating factors and host defense. Ann Intern Med 110(4):297, 1989.

17. Weisbart, RH and Golde, DW: Physiology of granulocyte and macrophage colony-stimulating factors in host defense. Hematol Oncol Clin North Am (3):401, 1989.

18. Gabrilove, JL and Jakubowski, A: Granulocyte colony-stimulating factor: Preclinical and clinical studies. Hematol Oncol Clin North Am 3(3):427, 1989.

19. Rettenmier, CW and Sherr, CJ: The mononuclear phagocyte colony-stimulating factor (CSF-1, M-CSF). Hematol Oncol Clin North Am 3(3):479, 1989.

20. Yang, YC and Clark, SC: Interleukin-3: Molecular biology and biologic activities. Hematol Oncol Clin North Am 3(3):441, 1989.

21. Garnick, MB and O'Reilly, RJ: Clinical promise of new hematopoietic growth factors: M-CSF, Il-3, Il-6. Hematol Oncol Clin North Am 3(3);495, 1989.

22. Murphy, MJ: Megakaryocyte colony-stimulating factor and thrombopoiesis. Hematol Oncol Clin North Am 3(3):465, 1989.

23. McNiece, IK, McGrath, E, and Quesenberry, PJ: Granulocyte colony-stimulating factor augments in vitro megakaryocyte colony formation by interleukin-3. Exp Hematol 16:807, 1988.

24. Sonoda, V, Arai, N, and Ogawa, M: Humoral regulation of eosinophilopoiesis in vitro: Analysis of the targets of interleukin-3, granulocyte-macrophage colony-stimulating factor (GM-CSF) and interleukin-5. Leukemia 3(1):14, 1989.

25. Siberstein, DS, Austin, KF, and Owen, WF: Hemopoietins for eosinophils: Glycoprotein hormones that regulate the development of inflammation in eosinophilia-associated disease. Hematol Oncol Clin North Am 3(3):511, 1989.

26. Grabor, SE and Krantz, SB: Erythropoietin: Biology and clinical use. Hematol Oncol Clin North Am 3(3):369, 1989.

27. Mitsuyasu, RT and Golde, RW: Clinical role of granulocyte-macrophage colony-stimulating factor. Hematol Oncol Clin North Am 3(3):411, 1989.

28. Applebaum, FR: The clinical use of hematopoietic growth factors. Semin Hematol 26(3):7, 1989.

29. Groopman, JE: New directions in hematologic biotherapy. Semin Hematol 26(3) (Suppl):1, 1989.

30. Adamson, JW: The promise of recombinant human erythropoietin. Semin Hematol 26(2) (Suppl):5, 1989.

31. Diggs, LW, Sturm, D, and Bell, A: The Morphology of Human Blood Cells, ed 5. Abbott Laboratories, Abbott Park, IL, 1985.

32. Boggs, DR and Winkelstein, A: White Cell Manual, ed 4, FA Davis, Philadelphia, 1983.

33. Williams, WW, et al: Hematology, ed 3. McGraw-Hill, New York, 1989.

34. Bainton, DF and Farquher, MG: Origin of granules in polymorphonuclear leucocytes; two types derived from opposite faces of the Golgi complex of developing granulocytes. J Cell Biol 28:277, 1966.

35. Boggs, DR: Physiology of neutrophil proliferation, maturation and circulation. Clin Haematol 4:535, 1975.

36. Murphy, P: The Neutrophil. Plenum Press, New York, 1976.

37. Stossel, TP and Cohen, HJ: Neutrophil function normal and abnormal. In Gordon, AS, et al (eds): The Year in Hematology. Plenum Press, New York, 1977.

38. Zucker-Franklin, D, et al: Atlas of Blood, Function and Pathology. Vol 1. Lea & Fibiger, Philadelphia, 1988.

39. Diggs, LW and Shibata, S: Ferrata cells—Tissue neutrophils, not artifacts. Laboratory Medicine 14:50, 1970.

40. Beeson, PB and Bass, DA: The eosinophil. In Smith, LH (ed): Major Problems in Internal Medicine. Vol 14. WB Saunders, Philadelphia, 1977.

41. Zucker-Franklin, D: Eosinophil function and disorders. Adv Intern Med 19:1, 1974.

42. Parwaresch, MR: The Human Blood Basophil. Springer-Verlag, Berlin, 1976.

43. Dvorak, JF and Dvorak, AM: Basophilic leukocytes: Structure, function, and role in disease. Clin Haematol 4:651, 1975.

QUESTIONS

1. *Which organ(s) is (are) the primary site(s) for hematopoiesis in the fetus?*
   a. Liver
   b. Spleen
   c. Bone marrow
   d. All of the above

2. *In which phase of the cell cycle does the cell emerge as a nondividing cell after final differentiation?*
   a. G_0
   b. G_1
   c. S
   d. G_D

3. *At what stage of differentiation will cells become committed to one cell line?*
   a. Stem cell
   b. Colony-forming unit (CFU)
   c. Blast
   d. Mature cell

4. *What growth factors are lineage-specific?*
   a. Colony-stimulating factors
   b. Interleukins
   c. Interferons
   d. Cytokines

5. *Which interleukin primarily supports proliferation of CFUs?*
   a. IL-1
   b. IL-4
   c. IL-3
   d. IL-5

6. *Which listing represents the proper cell sequence of erythropoiesis?*
   a. Rubriblast, prorubricyte, rubricyte, metarubricyte, reticulocyte, erythrocyte
   b. Rubriblast, rubricyte, prorubricyte, metarubricyte, reticulocyte, erythrocyte
   c. Rubriblast, prorubricyte, metarubricyte, rubricyte, reticulocyte, erythrocyte
   d. Rubriblast, reticulocyte, prorubricyte, rubricyte, metarubricyte, erythrocyte

7. *What is the best description of a metarubricyte?*
   a. Solid, blue-black degenerated nucleus with nonlinear clumped chromatin pattern; no nucleoli; pink cytoplasm
   b. Round nucleus with visible nucleoli; indistinct and dispersed chromatin; blue cytoplasm
   c. Coarse chromatin; ill-defined or absent nucleoli; predominately blue cytoplasm with pink tinge
   d. Small nucleus; thick and condensed nuclear chromatin; no nucleoli; mixture of pink and blue cytoplasm

8. *What is the sequence for the maturation pools of granulocyte production?*
   a. Maturation, proliferation, storage, functional (or marginated) pool
   b. Proliferation, maturation, storage, function (or marginated) pool
   c. Storage, maturation, proliferation, functional (or marginated) pool
   d. Functional (or marginated) pool, storage, proliferation, maturation

9. *Which listing represents the proper cell sequence of granulocytopoiesis?*
   a. Myeloblast, myelocyte, promyelocyte, metamyelocyte, band, segmented cell
   b. Myeloblast, metamyelocyte, myelocyte, promyelocyte, segmented cell, band
   c. Myeloblast, promyelocyte, myelocyte, metamyelocyte, band, segmented cell
   d. Myeloblast, band, promyelocyte, myelocyte, metamyelocyte, segmented cell

10. *Which granulocytic cell has a kidney-shaped nucleus with clumped chromatin and small, pink secondary granules with a few primary dark granules?*
    a. Band
    b. Myelocyte
    c. Promyelocyte
    d. Metamyelocyte

11. *Which granulocytic cell has large, abundant violet-blue or purple-black granules?*
    a. Eosinophil
    b. Basophil
    c. Neutrophil

12. *What is the proper cell sequence for the monocyte-macrophage phagocytic system?*
    a. Monoblast, macrophage, promonocyte, monocyte
    b. Monoblast, monocyte, promonocyte, macrophage
    c. Monoblast, promonocyte, monocyte, macrophage
    d. Monoblast, promonocyte, macrophage, monocyte

13. *Which cell classification is described by the following: Second most numerous cell in the blood; usually small and round; intensely blue cytoplasm; and nucleus with clumped dark purple chromatin?*
    a. Monocyte
    b. Lymphocyte
    c. Null cell
    d. Plasmacyte

14. *How are platelets released?*
    a. Megakaryoblast proceeds through various maturation changes and eventually mature platelets are released
    b. Megakaryoblast releases mature platelets from cytoplasm by a budding process
    c. Megakaryocyte matures to individual platelets, which are then released from bone marrow
    d. Megakaryocyte membrane ruptures and releases platelets

15. *Which bone marrow cell is a giant, multinucleated, phagocytic cell with visible nucleoli?*
    a. Osteoblast
    b. Osteoclast

ANSWERS

1. d (p. 22)
2. d (p. 23)
3. b (p. 24)
4. a (p. 27)
5. c (p. 27)
6. a (p. 28)
7. a (p. 29)
8. b (p. 30)
9. c (p. 30–31)
10. d (p. 31)
11. b (p. 33)
12. c (p. 34–35)
13. b (p. 35–36)
14. d (p. 37)
15. b (p. 38)

CHAPTER 3

MILKA MONTIEL, M.D.

Bone Marrow

OBJECTIVES

At the end of this chapter, the learner should be able to:
1. Name the bones that participate in active hemopoiesis in adults.
2. List conditions that indicate bone marrow studies.
3. Name the most common skeletal sites for hematologic studies.
4. Explain the role of the technologist during a bone marrow aspiration.
5. Describe the preparation of marrow aspirate for laboratory examination.
6. List stains used for dried bone marrow smears.
7. Name some advantages and disadvantages of a bone marrow biopsy.
8. Explain how to calculate the myeloid-to-erythroid (M:E) cell ratio.
9. List conditions for which a bone marrow differential count has diagnostic value.
10. List conditions for which the evaluation of marrow iron stores is essential for diagnosis.

BONE MARROW STRUCTURE

The bone marrow is one of the body's largest organs, representing 3.4 to 4.6 percent of total body weight and averaging about 1500 g in adults. The hematopoietic marrow is organized around the bone vasculature.[1,2] An artery entering the bone branches out toward the periphery to specialized vascular spaces called sinuses (Fig. 3–1). Several sinuses combine in a collecting sinus, forming a central vein that enters the systemic circulation. Hematopoietic cords, in which the development of the hematopoietic cells takes place, lie just outside of the sinuses. Following maturation in the cords, the hematopoietic cells cross the walls of the sinuses and enter the blood.[3–5]

Hematopoietic processes are compartmentalized in the cords. Erythropoiesis takes place in distinct anatomic units called erythropoietic islands[6] (**see Color Plate 44**). Each "island" consists of a macrophage surrounded by a cluster of maturing erythroblasts. Granulopoiesis is less conspicuously oriented toward a distinct reticular cell, yet still is recognizable as a unit[7] (**see Color Plate 45**). Early granulocytic precursors are located about the bone trabeculae. Megakaryopoiesis occurs adjacent to the sinus endothelium. The megakaryocytes protrude small cytoplasmic processes through the vascular wall, delivering platelets directly to the sinusoidal blood.[8] Marrow immunocytes consist of lymphocytes and plasma cells. Lymphocyte production is compartmentalized in lymphocytic nod-

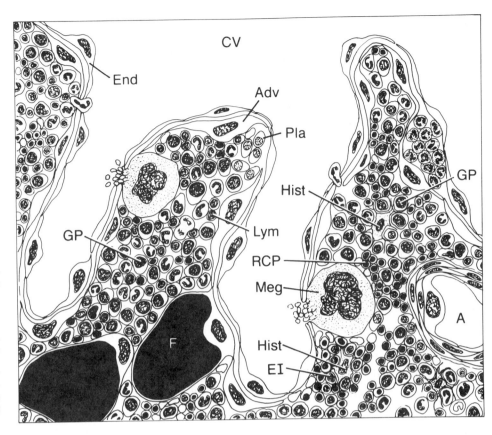

Figure 3-1. Graphic presentation of hemopoietic tissue. The vascular compartment consists of arteriole (*A*) and central sinus (*CV*). The venous sinusoids are lined by endothelial cells (*End*), and their wall outside is supported by adventitial-reticulum cells (*Adv*). Fat tissue (*F*) is part of the marrow. The compartmentalization of the hematopoiesis is represented by areas of granulopoiesis (*GP*), areas of erythropoiesis (*RCP*), and erythropoietic islands (*EI*) with its nutrient histiocyte (*Hist*). The megakaryocytes protrude with small cytoplasmic projections through the vascular wall (*Meg*). Lymphocytes (*Lym*) are randomly scattered among the hemopoietic cells while plasma cells are usually situated along the vascular wall (*Pla*).

ules and lymphocytes are randomly dispersed throughout the cords. The lymphocytic nodules are unevenly distributed and tend to influence the lymphocyte count in bone marrow samples (**see Color Plate 46**). Plasma cells are situated along the outside of vascular walls.

The bone marrow is also the source of immune stem cells, which on Wright's stain smears are indistinguishable from small lymphocytes. These stem cells, when mature, perform humoral immune functions, respectively. Some cellular and immune progenitor cells produced in the marrow mature in the thymus as T lymphocytes[9]; others are produced and continue their maturation and differentiation in bone marrow as B lymphocytes from the 12th gestational week throughout life.[10] Therefore, the bone marrow and thymus are primary lymphoid organs of *antigen-independent* progenitor immune cell division and differentiation, which give rise to new lymphocytes. These new lymphocytes may then populate the secondary lymphoid organs, lymph nodes, spleen, and lymphoid apparatus of the gastrointestinal tract, where *antigen-dependent* effector cells proliferate and antibody production takes place.

The meshwork of stromal cells in which the hematopoietic cells are suspended is in a delicate semifluid state and is composed of reticulum cells, histiocytes, fat cells, and endothelial cells. The reticulum cells are associated with fibers that can be visualized after silver staining. They are adjacent to the sinus endothelial cells forming the outer part of the walls as an adventitial reticular cell. Their fine cytoplasmic projections are extended deep into the cords, making contact with similar projections of other cells. Occasionally, the nuclear region of these cells can be seen deep in the cords surrounded by granulopoiesis. Cytochemically, these cells test alkaline-phosphatase positive. The histiocyte macrophage is seen as a perisinusoidal cell related to the bone marrow–blood barrier and as a central storage macrophage part of the erythropoietic islands. In the role of storage nutrient cell delivering iron to the growing immature erythroblasts, the storage macrophage sends out long, slender cytoplasmic processes that envelope the erythroid precursors (**see Color Plate 47**). This extensive and intimate contact with the maturing erythropoietic cells is necessary in transferring iron from the macrophage to the red cell precursors. Histochemically, the macrophages test acid-phosphatase positive.

Tissue mast cells (**see Color Plate 48**), 6 to 12 μm in diameter, are connective tissue cells of mesenchymal origin, normally present in the bone marrow in varying numbers. They have a round or oval reticular nucleus and abundant blue-purple granules that obscure the nucleus. Their granules contain serotonin and proteolytic enzymes in addition to all other substances that are present in the granules of basophils. Mast cells increase in number in chronic infections, autoimmune diseases, and especially systemic mastocytosis.

The stromal cells produce an extracellular matrix[11] composed of collagens, glycoproteins, proteoglycans, and other proteins. This extracellular matrix is essential in sustaining normal renewal and differentiation of marrow cells. The fat cells vary in amount according to the age of the individual and the location from which the marrow is obtained. Only a few fat cells are seen in children. Their numbers gradually increase after 4 years of age; in adults fat cells average about 50 percent of the total marrow volume. The marrow fat and the extracellular matrix are dynamic tissues similar to the hematopoietic tissue, and these are altered rapidly in disease.

In marrow aspirates, cells are occasionally seen originating from bone tissue. Osteoblasts are bone matrix synthesizing cells usually found in groups. They may be as large as 30 μm in diameter, and they resemble plasma cells. The osteoblast nucleus has a fine chromatin pattern with a prominent nucleolus. A perinuclear halo, detached from the nuclear membrane with a cytoplasmic bridge, represents the Golgi apparatus area (**see Color Plate 49**). Osteoblasts, which stain alkaline-phosphatase positive, are characteristically seen in children and patients with metabolic bone diseases.

Osteoclasts, bone remodeling cells, are multinucleated giant cells larger than 100 μm in diameter that resemble megakaryocytes. The nuclei of the osteoclasts are separated from each other and may have nucleoli (compared with the megakaryocyte nucleus which is lobated). The acidophilic or basophilic cytoplasm is granular and well delineated (**see Color Plates 50 and 51**).

The bone marrow is a highly vascularized tissue from which endothelial cells can occasionally be aspirated. Endothelial cells are more visible in hypoplastic marrows and should not be mistaken for metastatic tumors (**see Color Plate 52**).

The main function of the marrow is to supply mature hemopoietic cells for the circulating blood in a steady-state condition as well as to respond to increased demands. Self-renewal is maintained by a semidormant pool of pluripotential stem cells. Still, little is known of the mechanisms governing the physiology of stem cells commitment to progenitor cells. However, a progenitor is a cell committed to a single line of proliferation and differentiation. Granulocytic, monocytic, eosinophilic, erythroid, and megakaryocyte committed cells are governed by colony-stimulating factors (CSFs).[12–14] Colony-stimulating factors are produced by T lymphocytes as well as stromal cells, fibroblasts, endothelial cells, and macrophages when stimulated by monocyte interleukin-1 (IL-1) and tumor necrosis factor (TNF). Some CSFs, such as interleukin-3 (IL-3) and granulocyte-monocyte, have broad influence and are required throughout proliferation and differentiation of progenitor cells. Others, which include granulocyte, monocyte, and eosinophil CSFs, are lineage specific and regulate division and differentiation only of corresponding committed progenitor cells. The erythropoiesis is influenced in addition by erythropoietin[15,16] pro-

duced in the kidney (for more information, see Chapter 1). It is apparent that the bone marrow is subjected to a complex regulation by many cellular systems of the body and any disease affecting these systems is likely to affect hematopoiesis.

INDICATIONS FOR BONE MARROW STUDIES

Bone marrow study in the diagnosis of hematopoietic disorders was introduced by Arinkin.[17] Although once a formidable task, with current improved techniques obtaining bone marrow tissue has now become a standard procedure. Several techniques have been devised, each having its own merits and limitations. Bone marrow aspiration and bone marrow biopsy are usually performed concurrently.

Although obtaining bone marrow for examination carries little procedural risk for the patient, the procedure is costly and can be quite painful. For this reason, bone marrow studies should be done only when clearly indicated or whenever the physician expects a beneficial diagnostic result for his or her patient.

Hematologic diseases, which primarily affect the bone marrow, causing a decrease or increase of any cellular blood element, are among the most common indications. These conditions typically include the following:

1. Anemias, erythrocytosis, polycythemia
2. Leukopenia and unexplained leukocytosis
3. Appearance of immature or abnormal cells in the circulation
4. Thrombocytopenia and thrombocytosis

It is not rare for more than one blood element to be increased or decreased, as occurs in leukemias and some refractory anemias. In these situations, bone marrow study affords specific information and usually precedes any other diagnostic procedure.

Systemic diseases may affect the bone marrow secondarily and require bone marrow studies for diagnosis or for monitoring the patient's condition. These diseases include the following:

1. Solid malignant tumors arising somewhere else in the body, such as lymphomas, carcinomas, and sarcomas, may metastasize to the bone marrow. Patients having any of these solid malignant tumors may undergo bone marrow studies when the initial diagnosis is established for evaluation of the degree of tumor spread and clinical staging of disease. On occasion the bone marrow study may be the site of first diagnosis of unsuspected disseminated solid tumor. During the course of malignant disease, additional studies are performed periodically for monitoring the status of tumor spread and its therapeutic response.
2. Infections manifested clinically as "fever of unknown origin" may exhibit granulomas, focal necrosis, or histiocytic proliferation

with intracytoplasmic organisms within the marrow. Material for morphologic studies and bacterial cultures may be obtained simultaneously during a single procedure. The suspected diagnoses of disseminated tuberculosis, fungal infections (particularly histoplasmosis, cryptococcosis), and some protozoan infections are frequently confirmed through such studies.

3. Hereditary and acquired histiocytoses occasionally involve the bone marrow histiocyte (for example, Gaucher's disease, sea blue histiocytosis, and others). A simple procedure such as bone marrow aspiration or biopsy may establish diagnosis.

OBTAINING AND PREPARING BONE MARROW FOR HEMATOLOGIC STUDIES

The most common sites for bone marrow studies in adults are the posterior superior iliac crest, sternum, anterior superior iliac crest, and (very rarely) spinal processes or vertebral bodies (Fig. 3–2). Occasionally, when a localized bone lesion is visualized on roentgenogram or computed tomographic (CT) scan, a directed or "open" bone marrow biopsy of the lesion may be done by a surgeon in an operating room with the patient anesthetized. In newborns and infants, marrow for studies can be obtained from the upper end of the tibial bone.

Before performing the procedure, the physician should inform the adult patient or the parent or guardian of a child about the procedure, its risks, and its benefits for the diagnostic process. An authorized permission form, the so-called informed consent form, is then signed, allowing the physician to perform the procedure. Signature of the permission form is witnessed by a second person, in many instances the patient's nurse. The actual procedure is often performed with the assistance of a medical technologist. While the physician performs the procedure and the nurse attends to the patient, the medical technologist gives full attention to processing the specimens. It is the medical technologist's responsibility to see that the samples are adequate. If they are not, the physician is informed immediately so that the procedure can be repeated before the patient is released. Samples are preserved appropriately for histologic, electron microscopic, cytogenetic, immunologic, microbiologic, and other studies as they are indicated in each particular case.

Equipment

The instrument tray used to perform a bone marrow procedure should contain enough equipment to complete the procedure and to prepare the tissues obtained (Table 3–1). A hematology laboratory that routinely assists in performing bone marrow procedures should always have at least two

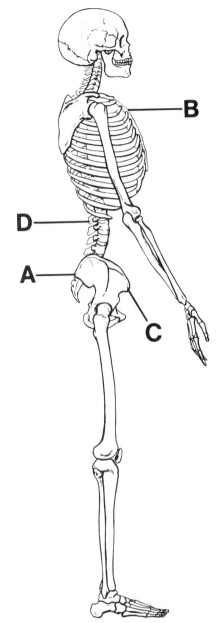

Figure 3–2. Common sites for bone marrow studies. Posterior superior iliac crest (A), sternum (B), anterior superior iliac crest (C), and spinal processes (D) indicate the site of the skeleton in descending order of frequency from which bone marrow tissue is obtained for studies.

sterile bone marrow trays ready, as well as a basic inventory of equipment and reagents to handle samples. Complete bone marrow trays are sold as disposable equipment, which may be convenient for some laboratories performing few bone marrow procedures. The disposable tray's convenience is offset by its higher cost and lack of versatility.

Several different styles of aspiration and trephine bone biopsy needles are commonly used (Fig. 3–3). Examples include the University of Illinois sternal needle, with its adjustable guard for

Table 3–1. **EXAMPLE OF AN INVENTORY OF A TRAY FOR BONE MARROW ASPIRATION AND BIOPSY**

Required Materials

1. 30-ml syringes
2. 20-ml syringes
3. 10-ml syringes
4. 5-ml syringes
5. 2% lidocaine
6. Prepodyne prep
7. Alcohol (70%) or prep
8. 23-gauge needles
9. 21-gauge needles
10. Filter papers
11. Buffered formalin 10% or other fixative for histologic processing of bone biopsy and marrow particles
12. Tube containing liquid EDTA anticoagulant
13. One box of slides
14. One slide folder
15. One rubber bulb
16. Pasteur pipette
17. Petri dish
18. Sterile blades
19. Gloves (several pairs of different sizes)
20. Sterile gauze and cotton balls
21. Sterile bone marrow aspiration and trephine biopsy needles
22. Applicator sticks
23. Bandage
24. One culture bottle (*not* biphasic) for bacterial culture
    (Note: Save some bone marrow specimen in syringe for tuberculosis and fungal cultures, when indicated.)
25. Pencil to label slides
26. Bard Parker blades No. 11

aspiration, and various modifications of the Vim-Silverman trephine needle for bone biopsy. Examples of such modified trephine needles are the Westerman-Jensen, Jamshidi, and others. There are also smaller needles designed for use with infants and children. Modifications of these original aspiration and trephine needles have been adapted by different companies and are manufactured as disposable equipment.

Aspiration

Bone marrow aspiration may be performed as an independent procedure or in conjunction with bone biopsy. It is favored by hematologists in ambulatory and office practice. As a rule, very apprehensive patients and children receive a mild sedative prior to the procedure. The site selected is shaved, if hairy, and washed with soap. Then an antiseptic is applied, and the area is draped with sterile towels. A local anesthetic such as 1 to 2 percent lidocaine (Xylocaine) is infiltrated in the skin, in the intervening tissues between the skin

and bone, and in the periosteum of the bone from which the marrow is to be obtained. A cut of about 3 mm is made through the skin with a Bard-Parker blade to facilitate piercing skin and subcutaneous tissue.

The physician penetrates the bone cavity with an aspiration needle, assembled with guard and stylet locked in place. When the marrow cavity is penetrated, the stylet is removed, a syringe is attached to the free end of the needle, and the plunger is quickly pulled, drawing 1.0 to 1.5 ml of marrow particles and sinusoidal blood in the syringe. Because the vacuum created in the syringe is important for rapid and efficient suctioning of cells and particles, the syringe should be 10-ml or larger with a well-fitting plunger. Despite the use of local anesthesia, the patient normally experiences discomfort during the aspiration process (aspiration pain). Accomplishing the aspiration with a quick and continuous pull on the plunger diminishes the patient's discomfort and decreases the chance of clotting the specimen. A clotted specimen is useless for smear preparation because the fibrin threads strip the cytoplasm from the cells and hamper their spreading.

Keeping the volume of the initial aspirate small also prevents dilution of the sample with large amounts of sinusoidal blood, which diminishes the quality of the aspirate. This first-aspirated material is used immediately for preparing smears. More aspirate may be obtained in additional syringes if needed for chromosome studies, bacterial cultures, and other tests. Once an adequate aspirate is obtained, the quality of the smear depends entirely on the technologist's skill and speed in preparing the smears and preserving the morphology of the marrow cells. Part of the first aspirate is used for the preparation of direct and marrow particle smears. The other part is placed in an ethylene diamine tetraacetic acid (EDTA) anticoagulant-containing tube for use later in the laboratory. If some aspirate still remains, it can be left to clot. The clot may be fixed in 5 percent buffered formalin or other chosen fixative and processed for histologic sections.

Preparation of Bone Marrow Aspirate

All necessary materials, preservatives, and slides should be meticulously clean and in readiness, to avoid any delay. The aspirate in the first syringe contains mostly blood admixed with fat, marrow cells, and particles of marrow tissue, which should be used for smears. Several direct smears can be prepared immediately, using the technique for blood film preparation. A small drop is placed on a glass slide, and the blood and particles are dragged behind a spreading slide with a technique similar to that for preparing blood film. Although this method of preparation preserves the cell morphology well, it is inadequate for the evaluation of the

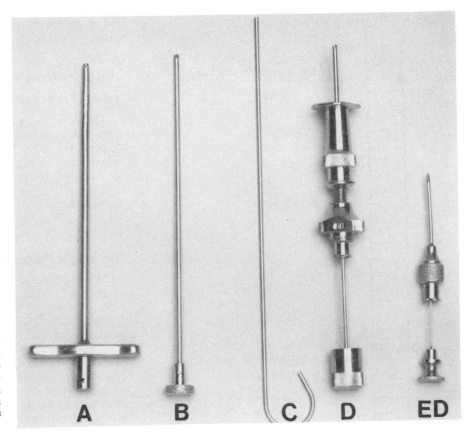

Figure 3–3. Trephine biopsy and aspiration needles. Jamshidi trephine needle biopsy (A) includes a stylet (B) and probe (C). University of Illinois sternal aspiration needle with an adjustable guard and stylet (D). A smaller-sized pediatric aspiration needle and trephine biopsy (ED) is also shown.

cells in relationship to each other and for the estimation of marrow cellularity.

Smears of marrow particles are prepared by pouring a small amount of the aspirate on a glass slide. The marrow tissue is seen as gray particles floating in blood and fat droplets. The particles are aspirated selectively with a plastic dropper or Oxford pipette and are transferred to a clean glass slide, which is then covered gently with another slide. The two slides are pulled in opposite and parallel directions, to smear the particles without crushing the cells. Some techniques recommend using two cover glasses instead.[18] In this process, the marrow particles are squashed between two coverslips, which are then gently pulled apart.

Techniques for preparing particle smears vary from person to person and from laboratory to laboratory. The aspirate may be transferred into a watch glass and the particles collected with a capillary pipette or with the broken end of a wooden stick applicator. With experience, technologists usually adapt a technique that best suits them to produce high-quality slides.

Marrow particle smears are used in the evaluation of cellularity and the relationship of the cells to each other. In well-prepared smears there is the added advantage of excellent cell morphology so that subtle changes in cell maturation and cytoplasmic inclusions can be easily recognized.

All direct and particle smears should be labeled with the patient's name, identification number, and date at the bedside, and then quickly air dried.

Measurement of Bone Marrow Aspirate

The EDTA-anticoagulated aspirate can be used for quantitative studies.[19] About 1 ml of this aspirate is transferred to a Wintrobe tube and is centrifuged at 2800 rpm (at 850 g) for 8 minutes. The fluid is separated into four layers representing fat and perivascular cells, plasma, buffy coat of myeloid-erythroid cells, and erythrocytes (Fig. 3–4). Each layer is measured and read as a percentage directly from the Wintrobe tube, its volume correlating with a given basic element of the marrow. Smears can be prepared from fat-perivascular and buffy coat layers and used accordingly to study iron and hematopoietic cell and myeloid-to-erythroid (M:E) cell ratio. Such quantitative studies may be useful in estimating cellularity (fat versus buffy coat) when no histologic sections of bone biopsy and marrow particles are available.

Bone Biopsy

A bone biopsy is especially indicated when bone marrow cannot be aspirated (known as "dry tap"), owing to pathologic alterations encountered in acute leukemias, myelofibrosis, hairy-cell leuke-

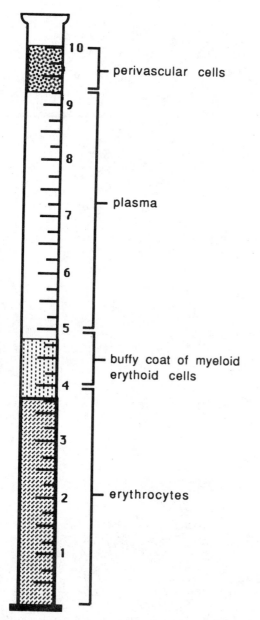

Figure 3-4. Quantitative measurement of bone marrow aspirate. A schematic presentation of the four marrow layers formed by centrifugation of aspirate in a Wintrobe tube.

through a new puncture site in the anesthetized area.

Preparation of Trephine Biopsy

Touch Preparation

The bone core is supported lightly without pressure between the blades of a forceps and touched several times on two or three clean slide surfaces. The biopsy core should not be rubbed on the slide, as rubbing destroys the cells. The slides are air dried rapidly. The touch preparations may be fixed in absolute methanol and stained with Wright-Giemsa stain or other histochemical stains as needed.

Histologic Preparation

The biopsy specimen is immersed without delay in B-5 or 5 percent buffered formalin fixative. Histology laboratories may have a choice of other preferred fixatives such as Zenker's solution, Carnoy's solution, and others.[21] After fixation the biopsy undergoes standard histologic processing of decalcification, dehydration, embedding in paraffin blocks, and section of 2- to 3-μm thick sections for staining. The advantage of bone marrow biopsy is that it represents marrow structures in their natural relationships. A variety of different stains can be used to demonstrate marrow iron, reticulum, and collagen. Acid-fast organisms and fungi in granulomatous diseases may be detected quickly with specific stains, offering great advantages in diagnosing these infections. For instance, mycobacterial cultures may require weeks of incubation to show growth of organisms, whereas on tissue sections the histologic and etiologic diagnosis may be made within 10 to 12 hours. At present, when metastatic tumors and lymphomas are found in the bone marrow, monoclonal hybridoma antibodies can be used on histologic material to demonstrate specific tumor markers. Thus, a very precise diagnosis of the origin of a tumor can be made.

A disadvantage of the bone biopsy is that fine cellular details are lost in the processing; therefore, it is of little value in the diagnosis of leukemias and of some refractory anemias. In these situations, the touch preparation from the biopsy may supply the missing morphologic details. Multiple touch preparations also offer an opportunity for histochemical stains (Sudan Black B, naphthol AS-D chloracetate esterase, alpha-naphthyl butyrate esterase, and so on) which are essential in diagnosis and classification of leukemias.

Trephine bone marrow biopsy may be embedded in methyl methacrylate, synthetic plastic media, and sectioned into 1- to 2-μm thin sections without decalcification. The morphologic quality of the cells is extremely well preserved and a differential count can be done on hematoxylin-eosin– or Giemsa-stained slides.[22] However, this technique requires specially trained personnel, equipment, and separate handling in the histology

mia, and other conditions. Trephine bone biopsy is also performed for the diagnosis of neoplastic and granulomatous diseases. For clinical staging of lymphomas and carcinomas, bilateral posterior superior iliac crest biopsies are recommended, which increase the chance to diagnose a focal process. In adults, an 11-gauge Jamshidi biopsy needle is used, whereas in children a 13-gauge needle is preferred. An adequate biopsy is at least 15 mm long.[18-20] When bone biopsy is performed in conjunction with marrow aspirate, it customarily follows the aspirate. This is performed by changing the direction of the needle to avoid the aspiration site. It is better yet for the marrow biopsy to be done laboratory, which increases expenses. The processing time of the tissue also increases, which may not be acceptable for rapid diagnosis. In addition, tissue embedded in plastic media, instead of paraffin, may not be suitable for immunologic studies of bone marrow.

BONE MARROW EXAMINATION

The examination of the bone marrow aspirate smears should start at low magnification with a dry objective of ×10. A scan over the slide permits selection of a suitable area for examination and differential count. "Bare nuclei" due to destruction of the marrow cells by squashing them or stripping their cytoplasm by fibrin thread should be avoided. An area is selected in which the cells are well spread, intact, and not diluted by sinusoidal blood. When marrow particles are examined, such areas are found at the periphery of the particles. On this low magnification, marrow cellularity is also evaluated. The number and the distribution of the megakaryocytes is usually noted adjacent to a spicule, about five per low magnification field. Nonhematopoietic tumor cells infiltrating the bone marrow could also be seen at this magnification. These are usually larger than the granulocytic or erythropoietic precursors, and are scattered in small groups and clusters (see Color Plate 53).

After the initial scan, immersion oil is applied on the slide and the examination continues on high magnification (oil immersion objective ×50 or ×100). The high magnification provides details of the nuclear and cytoplasmic maturation process. The iron in histiocytes is visualized as brown-blue granules. Cytoplasmic inclusions of a diagnostic nature can be seen in histiocytes, erythroblasts, and granulocytes. Differential counts of bone marrow are also done with the oil immersion objective.

ESTIMATION OF BONE MARROW CELLULARITY

The cellularity is reflected in the ratio of nucleated hematopoietic cells to fat cells. Overall marrow cellularity in adults is about 50 percent (±10 percent). The bone biopsy is the most reliable for assessment of cellularity, because it offers a large amount of tissue for evaluation. However, the evaluation of the cellularity can also be done on good aspirate smears. The best areas for examination of cellularity in smears is the areas between two uncrushed particles. The ratio of cells to fat is evaluated on low magnification (objective ×10), so that larger areas are included in the field of observation. The empty spaces that result from the spreading of the cells but are not occupied by fat cells are disregarded and treated as artifacts (see Color Plate 54). "Decreased" or "increased" cellularity is implied when less or more than the expected normal number of cells is seen. Precise evaluation can be achieved with experience, and

good reproducibility can be attained among several observers. The marrow cellularity can be expressed in percentages, but this is best done on histologic sections of biopsy specimens. Marrow cellularity has diagnostic value when it is related to the M:E ratio, which is calculated after a differential count is performed.

BONE MARROW DIFFERENTIAL COUNT

A bone marrow differential count is an excellent tool for training a novice in bone marrow morphology and is widely used in diagnosing and following patients with leukemias, refractory anemias, and myelodysplastic syndromes. Because of the compartmentalization of the hematopoietic cells and high cellularity of marrow, at least 500 to 1000 nucleated cells need to be classified for a representative differential count.[23]

In infants during the first month after birth, dramatic alterations occur in the distribution of the different marrow compartments.[24] At birth there is a predominance of granulocyte precursors, which switches within a month to a predominance of lymphoid elements. In early infancy many lymphocytes have fine chromatin, high nucleus-to-cytoplasm ratio, and distinct nucleoli. They can be misinterpreted as blasts if the observer is unfamiliar with these characteristics. These lymphoid cells may represent stem cells in the infant marrow.[25] In children up to 3 years old, one third or more of the marrow cellularity is made up of lymphocytes. The lymphocyte number gradually declines to the normal adult level thereafter.

In adult marrow the lymphocytes are distributed both at random among the hematopoietic cells and in lymphocytic follicles. This can introduce significant variation in the differential count from sample to sample in the same patient. The great mass of the adult marrow is composed of granulopoietic and erythropoietic precursors. For the purpose of the differential count, these are enumerated into different categories according to their stage of maturation (see Chapter 2). When adequate numbers of cells are tabulated, the percentage of each category is calculated. The ratio between all granulocytes and their precursors and all nucleated red cell precursors represents the M:E ratio.

Some hematologists prefer to exclude the segmented neutrophils from the differential count as being part of the neutrophil storage pool of the marrow. The normal M:E ratio in this case is between 1.5:1 and 3:1. However, pathologists and hematologists who interpret the bone marrow histologic sections of particle clot and biopsies in conjunction with marrow smears include the segmented neutrophils in the differential counts, because these cannot be excluded in the evaluation of histologic specimens and are part of the marrow cellularity. The normal M:E ratio then is slightly higher, and ranges between 3:1 and 4:1. The granulopoietic tissue occupies two to four times greater marrow space than the erythropoie-

Table 3–2. **DIFFERENTIAL CELL COUNT OF BONE MARROW IN PERCENT OF TOTAL NUCLEATED CELLS***

	AT BIRTH	UP TO 1 MO	CHILDREN	ADULTS
Undifferentiated cells	0–2	0–2	0–1	0–1
Myeloblast	0–2	0–2	0–2	0–2
Promyelocyte	0–4	0–4	0–4	0–4
Myelocytes				
Neutrophilic	2–8	2–4	5–15	5–20
Eosinophilic	0–5	0–3	0–6	0–3
Basophilic	0–1	0–1	0–1	0–1
Metamyelocytes and bands				
Neutrophilic	15–25	5–10	5–15	5–35
Eosinophilic	0–5	1–5	1–8	0–5
Basophilic	0–1	0–1	0–1	0–1
Segmented neutrophils	5–15	3–10	5–15	5–15
Pronormoblast	0–3	0–1	0–2	0–1.5
Basophilic normoblast	0–5	0–3	0–5	0–5
Polychromatophilic normoblast	6–20	5–20	5–11	5–30
Orthochromatic normoblast	0–5	0–2	0–8	5–10
Lymphocytes	5–15	5–50	5–35	10–20
Plasma cells	0–2	0–2	0–2	0–2
Monocytes	0–5	0–2	0–4	0–5
M:E ratio based on 500-cell count	3–4.5	3–4.5	1.5–4	2–4

* Normal reference range from the laboratory computing resources of the University of Texas Health Science Center and the Medical Center Hospital, San Antonio, Texas.

tic precursors, owing to the shorter survival of the granulocytes in the circulation (neutrophils' survival of 5 to 10 hours versus erythrocytes' survival of 120 days). Changes in the survival of granulocytes and erythrocytes is reflected in changes of the M:E ratio.

Megakaryocytes are unevenly distributed, and a differential count is a poor means for their evaluation. Usually 5 to 10 megakaryocytes are seen per microscopic field on low magnification (objective ×10). When clusters of megakaryocytes and promegakaryocytes are seen in every field, it is an indication of megakaryocytic hyperplasia. In a normal cellular marrow, finding less than two megakaryocytes per field on screening may indicate megakaryocytic hypoplasia. Marked increases or decreases in the number of megakaryocytes are easy to evaluate, whereas slight to moderate changes are difficult to judge and are better estimated on histologic sections of biopsy and particle specimens.

Table 3–2 represents the data of normal marrow reference ranges used by the computer resources of the University of Texas Health Science Center and the Medical Center Hospital at San Antonio.

BONE MARROW AND BLOOD INTERPRETATION BASED ON CELLULARITY AND M:E RATIO CHANGES

A bone marrow aspirate or biopsy sample represents a minute part of a very large and dynamic organ, whose activity and responses are reflected in blood changes; therefore, evaluation of the bone marrow should always be done in conjunction with evaluation of the peripheral blood. In adult humans with 50 percent marrow cellularity, about 30 to 40 percent represents granulopoiesis and 10 to 15 percent erythropoiesis, with an average M:E ratio of 4:1. When marrow cellularity increases or decreases preserving the normal M:E ratio, it is indicative of a balanced granulocytic and erythrocytic hyperplasia or hypoplasia, correspondingly. However, if cellularity change occurs simultaneously with M:E ratio change, the interpretation requires a broader understanding of hematopoietic tissue physiology and its reactions during disease.

Cell morphology and the M:E ratio are well represented in random bone marrow specimens. The variations are not significant even when samples are compared with sternal and iliac crest aspirates.[26] But marrow cellularity is poorly represented in random smears; thus, this interpretation should be considered with some degree of reservation. Even large biopsy specimens may have a great degree of variation in cellularity.[27] For this reason, in diseases in which marrow cellularity is crucial for the diagnosis (aplastic anemia, marrow hypoplasia), more than one bone biopsy sample may be needed.

Table 3–3 is to be used only as a simple guide to provide the reader with some basic information; it is not intended to be a diagnostic tool without the patient's clinical history and clinical evaluation of the disease. Also, the variety of problems frequently presented by different patients with the same disease may not fit in such a schematic concept.

Table 3-3. **MARROW AND BLOOD INTERPRETATION BASED ON CELLULARITY AND M:E RATIO**

COMPLETE BLOOD COUNT	BONE MARROW CELLULARITY	M:E RATIO	BONE MARROW INTERPRETATION
Normal	Increased or decreased*	Normal range	Normal
Neutropenia	Decreased	Decreased	Granulocytic hypoplasia
Neutropenia	Normal or increased	Increased	Decreased neutrophilic survival or ineffective granulopoiesis
Neutrophilia	Normal or increased	Increased	Granulocytic hyperplasia
Anemia	Normal or decreased	Increased	Red cell hypoplasia
Anemia	Normal or increased	Decreased	Erythrocytic hyperplasia or ineffective erythropoiesis†
Erythrocytosis (polycythemia)	Normal or increased	Decreased	Erythrocytic hyperplasia
Pancytopenia	Decreased	Normal range	Marrow hypoplasia
Pancytopenia	Increased	Normal, increased, or decreased	Ineffective myelopoiesis or hypersplenism

* Because of poor presentation of cellularity in random specimen.
† Reticulocyte count is necessary to differentiate between erythrocytic hyperplasia and ineffective erythropoiesis.

BONE MARROW IRON STORES

The storage iron of the bone marrow is in the form of hemosiderin. The iron content of hemosiderin is higher than that of ferritin. Other components of hemosiderin are protein, ferritin aggregates, some lipids, and membranes of cellular organelles. Hemosiderin can be seen on unstained smears as golden-yellow granules. On Wright-Giemsa–stained smears, it appears as brownish-blue granules. However, for more precise evaluation Prussian blue reaction is used to demonstrate the intracytoplasmic iron of histiocytes and red cell precursors. The evaluation of marrow iron stores is essential in the diagnosis of anemias and especially in refractory and dyserythropoietic anemias. When the morphologic characteristic of the iron particles in the storage nutrient histiocyte and erythroblastic precursors is an important diagnostic consideration (such as sideroblastic anemias), an iron stain is done on a particle smear. If the overall distribution of the amount of iron is of clinical importance (iron deficiency anemia, anemia of chronic diseases, hemochromatosis and others), then histologic sections of bone marrow biopsy and marrow clotted particles are stained for iron. The biopsy and the particles are a more reliable source of information, because they represent a large sample of hematopoietic tissue. Bone biopsy for iron studies should be decalcified by the EDTA chelating method, which does not affect the storage iron. Rapid acid decalcifying solutions extract iron and must not be used in these cases.

Hemosiderin and some ferritin aggregates are seen after staining, as bright-blue specks and granules **(see Color Plate 47).** Hemoglobin iron and dispersed ferritin do not stain. Normal marrow iron is seen as fine cytoplasmic granules in histiocytes. Thirty to 50 percent of marrow erythroblasts contain iron specks and are called sideroblasts. Clumps of iron easily seen on scanning magnification (×10) indicate increased storage. If specks of iron are not found after searching several microscopic fields (×50 or ×100 magnification), this indicates decreased iron storage. The storage iron may be reported as "absent," "decreased," "adequate," "moderately increased," or "markedly increased," or it can be given corresponding numeric values from 0 to 4, with 2 representing the normal or adequate iron stored in an adult.

BONE MARROW REPORT

The bone marrow report usually encompasses the following:
1. The laboratory or physician's office from which the report originates
2. Patient's addressograph data, including age and relevant clinical summary
3. Description of material received for studies, such as smears of aspirate, marrow particles, and/or bone biopsy(ies)
4. Data of the complete blood count (CBC) and white blood cell (WBC) differential count, as well as a description of the blood smear preferably from the day on which the bone marrow specimen is obtained; platelet count and reticulocyte count
5. Bone marrow differential count
6. Description of cellularity, M:E ratio, granulopoiesis, erythropoiesis, and megakaryopoiesis, including any change of the nonhematopoietic elements of marrow, such as histiocytic hyperplasia, erythrophagocytosis, or metastatic tumor cells; the status of iron stores
7. Description of histologic sections of bone marrow biopsy, if done
8. Diagnostic conclusion, which may encompass separate diagnoses of blood and bone marrow if necessary or a single diagnosis when applicable to both (for example, blood: pancytopenia; bone marrow left posterior iliac spine aspirate: aplasia, or blood and bone marrow

left posterior iliac spine [LPIS], aspirate: acute myelogeneous leukemia, FAB-M1).

The medical technologist's contribution in this phase is to perform the blood and bone marrow differential counts. The examination of the blood and bone marrow, the correlation with clinical presentation, and the diagnostic conclusions on each specimen is the responsibility of a physician who has adequate training and experience to integrate all available clinical and laboratory information for the purpose of reaching the correct diagnosis.

REFERENCES

1. Tavassoli, M and Jossey, JM: Bone Marrow, Structure and Function. Alan R Liss, New York, 1978, p 43.
2. Lichtman, MA: The ultrastructure of the hematopoietic environment of the marrow: A review. Exp Hematol 9:391, 1981.
3. Tavassoli, M and Shaklai, M: Absence of tight junctions in endothelium of marrow sinuses: Possible significance for marrow cell egress. Erythropoiesis in BM. Br J Haematol 41:303, 1979.
4. Aoki, M and Tavassoli, M: Dynamics of red cell egress from bone marrow after blood letting. Br J Haematol 49:337, 1981.
5. Aoki, M and Tavassoli, M: Red cell egress from bone marrow in state of transfusion plethora. Exp Hematol 9:231, 1981.
6. Bessis, M: L'ilot erythroblastique, unite fonctionelle de la moelle osseuse. Rev Hematol 13:8, 1958.
7. Western, H and Bainton, DF: Association of alkaline-phosphatase-positive reticulum cells in bone marrow with granulocytic precursors. J Exp Med 150:919, 1979.
8. Lichtman, MA, et al: Parasinusoidal location of megakaryocytes in marrow. A determinant of platelet release. Am J Hematol 4:303, 1978.
9. Claman, HN, Chaperon, EA, and Triplett, RF: Immunocompetence of transferred thymus—marrow cell combinations. J Immunol 97:828, 1966.
10. Hassett, JM: Humoral immunodeficiency: A review. Pediatr Ann 16:404, 1987.
11. Gordon, MY: Annotation. Extracellular matrix of the marrow microenvironment. Br J Haematol 70:1, 1988.
12. Clark, SC and Kamen, R: The human hematopoietic colony-stimulating factors. Science 236:1229, 1987.
13. Neinhuis, AW: Hematopoietic growth factors. Biologic complexity and clinical practice. N Engl J Med 318:916, 1988.
14. Iscove, NN: Erythropoietin-independent stimulation of early erythropoiesis in adult marrow cultures by conditioned media from lactin-stimulated mouse spleen cells. In Golde, DW, et al (eds): Hematopoietic Cell Differentiation. Academia, New York, 1978, p 25.
15. Erslev, AJ: Humoral regulation of red cell production. Blood 8:349, 1953.
16. Erslev, AJ: Erythropoietin coming of age. N Engl J Med 316:101, 1987.
17. Arinkin, MJ: Intravitale Untersuchungsmethodik der Knochenmarks. Folia Haematol (Leipz) 38:233, 1929.
18. Wintrobe, MM: Clinical Hematology. Lea & Febiger, Philadelphia, 1981, p 58.
19. Nelson, DA: Hematopoiesis. In Henry, JB (ed): Clinical Diagnosis and Management by Laboratory Methods. WB Saunders, Philadelphia, 1979, p 956.
20. Brynes, RK, McKenna, RW, and Sundberg, RD: Bone marrow aspiration and trephine biopsy, an approach to a thorough study. Am J Clin Pathol 70:753, 1978.
21. Sheeham, DC and Hrapchak, BB: Theory and Practice of Histotechnology. CV Mosby, St Louis, 1980, pp 46, 94.
22. Wilkins, BS and O'Brien, CJ: Techniques for obtaining differential cell counts from bone marrow trephine biopsy specimens. J Clin Pathol 41:558, 1988.
23. Williams, WJ and Douglas, AN: Examination of the marrow. In Williams, WJ, et al (eds): Hematology, ed 4. McGraw-Hill, Health Professions Div, New York, 1990, p 28.
24. Rosse, C, et al: Bone marrow cell population of normal infants: The predominance of lymphocytes. J Lab Clin Med 89:1225, 1977.
25. Oski, FA and Naiman, LJ: Hematologic Problems of the Newborn. WB Saunders, Philadelphia, 1982, p 21.
26. Rubinstein, MA: Aspiration of bone marrow from iliac crest comparison of iliac crest and sternal bone marrow studies. JAMA 137:1821, 1948.
27. Hartsock, RJ, Smith, EB, and Petty, SC: Normal variations with aging of the amount of hematopoietic tissue in bone marrow from anterior iliac crest. Am J Clin Pathol 43:326, 1965.

QUESTIONS

1. *Which bone(s) does not participate in active hematopoiesis in adults?*
   a. Ribs
   b. Pelvic bones
   c. Skull
   d. Sternum

2. *Which condition would not be an indication for bone marrow examination?*
   a. Thrombocytopenia
   b. Aplastic anemia
   c. Acute lymphocytic leukemia
   d. Histoplasmosis
   e. Bone marrow examination useful for all above conditions

3. *What skeletal site is not used for hematologic studies in adults?*
   a. Tibial bone
   b. Posterior superior iliac crest
   c. Sternum
   d. Anterior superior iliac crest

4. *Which of the following is not a responsibility of the medical technologist during a bone marrow aspiration?*
   a. Obtaining an adequate sterile bone marrow tray
   b. Acquiring patient consent for procedure
   c. Checking quantity and quality of aspirate
   d. Making proper smears

5. *How is the bone marrow aspirate prepared for laboratory studies?*
   a. First aspirated material is used for preparation of smears; other part is placed in EDTA tube for further studies.
   b. All aspirated material is allowed to clot and processed later for histologic sections.
   c. First aspirated material is placed in EDTA tube; other part is used for preparation of smears.
   d. Aspirated material is placed in EDTA tube; smears and other studies are performed later in laboratory.

6. Which of the following stains is not routinely used for dried bone marrow smears?
   a. Wright's
   b. Wright-Giemsa
   c. Sudan Black B
   d. May-Grunwald-Giemsa

7. What is not an advantage of a bone marrow biopsy?
   a. Represents marrow structures in their natural relationships
   b. Useful for detection of fine cellular details for diagnosis of leukemias and refractory anemias
   c. Useful for detection of bacterial and fungal infections
   d. Useful in evaluation of metastatic tumors and lymphomas

8. What is the formula for calculation of M:E ratio?
   a. Divide the number of nucleated red cells by the number of granulocytes and precursor cells.
   b. Multiply the number of granulocytes and precursor cells by the number of nucleated red cells.
   c. Divide the number of granulocytes and precursor cells by the number of nucleated red cells.
   d. Multiply the number of nucleated red cells by the total number of cells, then divide the result by the number of granulocytes and precursor cells.

9. In which condition is performing a bone marrow differential not essential?
   a. Chronic lymphocytic leukemia
   b. Dysmyelopoiesis
   c. Metastatic carcinoma
   d. Chronic erythemic myelosis

10. In which anemia is bone marrow iron store evaluation not essential for diagnosis?
    a. Sideroblastic anemia
    b. Iron-deficiency anemia
    c. Dyserythropoietic anemia
    d. Aplastic anemia

ANSWERS

1. c (p. 43)
2. e (p. 44)
3. a (p. 45)
4. b (p. 46)
5. a (p. 46–47)
6. c (p. 48)
7. b (p. 47–48)
8. c (p. 49)
9. c (p. 49)
10. d (p. 51)

CHAPTER **4**

ARMAND B. GLASSMAN, M.D.

Anemia: Diagnosis and Clinical Considerations

OBJECTIVES

At the end of this chapter, the learner should be able to:
1. Name laboratory diagnostic criteria for anemia.
2. List causes of anemia.
3. Describe clinical signs of anemia.
4. Explain the most common method for the measurement of hemoglobulin.
5. Explain how hematocrit is calculated on automated hematology instruments.
6. Calculate and state the significance of red blood cell indices as related to the diagnosis of anemia.
7. Describe appearance of the peripheral blood smear in anemia.
8. Explain the diagnostic value of the reticulocyte count.
9. List factors to be evaluated in interpretation of a bone marrow aspirate smear.
10. Explain the diagnostic value of hemoglobulin electrophoresis.
11. Explain why antiglobulin testing would be important in the diagnosis of hemolytic anemia.
12. List two laboratory tests useful to determine the sensitivity of red blood cell lysis.
13. Name the two most commonly measured red blood cell enzymes.
14. Explain the use of measuring erythropoietin levels in the evaluation of anemias.
15. Discuss the value of performing a bone marrow culture.
16. Explain why the measurement of haptoglobin binding is of limited use in the evaluation of hemolytic anemia.
17. List tests useful in evaluation of iron-deficient states.

DEFINITION OF ANEMIA

Anemia in its broadest sense is a functional inability of the blood to supply the tissue with adequate oxygen for proper metabolic function.[1] Clinically, the diagnosis of anemia is made by patient history, physical examination, signs and symptoms, and hematologic laboratory findings. Determining the specific etiology of an anemia is important to the physician so that the appropriate therapy and prognosis related to the natural history of the disease can be applied for the patient. Anemia is usually associated with decreased levels of hemoglobin or a decreased packed red blood cell (RBC) volume, also known as the hematocrit. Under rare circumstances, abnormal hemoglobins have very strong oxygen-binding capacities or oxygen is not released normally to tissue, resulting in all the clinical signs and symptoms of anemia and yet a normal or even raised hemoglobin or hematocrit value. From a practical laboratory standpoint, however, the usual diagnostic criterion for a patient with anemia is a decreased hemoglobin (Hgb), hematocrit (Hct), or RBC count.

Because most patients with anemia have lowered hemoglobin levels, the anemia may be classified arbitrarily as either moderate (7 to 10 g of hemoglobin/dl) or severe (less than 7 g of hemoglobin/dl).[2] Moderate anemias are not usually accompanied by clinically evident signs or symptoms, especially if the onset is slow. However, depending on the patient's age or cardiovascular condition, even moderate amounts of anemia may be associated with exertional dyspnea (difficulty breathing), light-headedness, vertigo, muscle weakness, headache, or general lethargy. Anemia of rapid onset, such as that resulting from gastrointestinal hemorrhage, may be associated with significant clinical symptoms such as hypotension, tachycardia, and dyspnea. These symptoms are associated with the precipitous loss of intravascular volume as well as the oxygen-carrying capacity of the RBCs.

CONSIDERATIONS BY AGE, GENDER, AND OTHER FACTORS

Newborn infants (less than 1 week old) have a hemoglobin of 18 ± 4 g/dl as a reference range. At approximately 6 months of age the reference range is 12.5 ± 1.5 g/dl. Childhood levels from the ages of 1 to 15 years have a reference range of approximately 13.0 ± 2 g/dl. Adult hemoglobin reference ranges are approximately 15.0 ± 2 g/dl for men and 14.0 ± 2 g/dl for women (Table 4–1). Individual laboratories' reference ranges should be obtained reflecting the patient population served. In the geriatric age group, the difference between hemoglobin levels of men and women narrows. Hemoglobin levels of geriatric men usually decrease slightly and begin to approach those of the postmenopausal woman. Many other factors influence individual "normal" hemoglobin levels, including

Table 4–1. REFERENCE RANGE VALUES FOR HEMOGLOBIN

Age Group	Hemoglobin g/dl
Infants	
Newborns (<1 wk old)	14.0–22.0 g/dl
6 mo old	11.0–14.0 g/dl
Children (1–15 yr old)	11.0–15.0 g/dl
Adults	
Men	13.0–17.0 g/dl
Women	12.0–16.0 g/dl

one's residential geographic elevation. Persons living at elevations above 8000 feet may have persistently increased hemoglobin values secondary to decreased oxygen saturation in the ambient atmosphere.[3] Lung diseases may alter oxygen diffusion at the lung alveolar membranes, resulting in increased hemoglobin levels (secondary polycythemia) as an attempt to compensate for this.[4] Various other diseases and disorders are associated with lower than usual hemoglobin levels; these conditions include nutritional deficiencies, external or internal blood loss, accelerated destruction of RBCs, ineffective or decreased production of RBCs, abnormal hemoglobin synthesis, bone marrow replacement by infection or tumor, and bone marrow suppression by toxins, chemicals, or radiation.[5]

CAUSES OF ANEMIA

There are many causes of anemia. Usually these are classified as nutritional deficiency, blood loss, accelerated destruction, bone marrow replacement, infection or toxicity, hematopoietic stem cell arrest or damage, and hereditary or acquired. Categories may be simplified to embrace conditions of decreased production, increased destruction, or some combination thereof.

SIGNIFICANCE OF ANEMIA AND COMPENSATORY MECHANISMS

RBC and Hemoglobin Production

In a healthy ambulatory individual, approximately 1 percent of the senescent circulating RBCs are lost daily. The bone marrow of such an individual continues to produce replacement red blood cells. A laboratory measure of this replacement is the reticulocyte count. Reticulocytes, early circulating RBCs containing residual ribonucleic acid (RNA), account for 0.5 to 1.5 percent of the circulating RBCs.[6] In order to produce this number of RBCs with normal RBC maturation processes, one needs a bone marrow with adequate functioning stem cells and the ability to release mature RBCs from the bone marrow. Proper hemoglobin and RBC production require a variety of nutritional factors including iron, vitamin B_{12}, folic acid, and normal hemoglobin synthesis pathways. The role of hemoglobin synthesis in anemias is covered in greater detail in the chapter on hemoglobinopathies (see Chapter 11).

In severe anemias (less than 7 g hemoglobin/dl) symptoms of functional impairment of a number of organ systems may be evident. With minimal exercise, the patient's cardiac and respiratory rates may increase dramatically. If the anemia is secondary to blood loss and decreased intravascular volume, the patient's blood pressure may drop significantly when he or she is raised from the reclining to a sitting or standing position. The heart rate will be increased in order to elevate the cardiac output to keep pace with peripheral tissue oxygen demands in the face of a decreased oxygen-carrying capacity of the lowered hemoglobin level. Respiratory symptoms, including dyspnea on exertion, also may occur with anemia. An interesting compensatory mechanism that occurs is an increase in the 2,3-diphosphoglycerate (2,3-DPG) levels. This compound is a remarkable physiologic regulator of normal hemoglobin as it relates to its oxygen-carrying capacity and tissue oxygen delivery.[7] In the presence of 2,3-DPG, hemoglobin can more readily release the oxygen it is carrying to peripheral tissues. This enhanced release of oxygen occurs regardless of pH or blood arterial oxygen level.

Rapid blood loss of large volumes (greater than 10 percent of the total blood volume) may cause the aforementioned symptoms as well as hypotension and syncope. When the hemoglobin level is decreased without external blood loss, there is a compensatory increase in plasma in order to maintain the intravascular volume. A person can have a moderately low hemoglobin level and yet have few of the effects of the depleted intravascular volume because of these fluid shift mechanisms.

A normal individual responds to anemia with elevated levels of erythropoietin (see Chapter 1). Erythropoietin levels are sometimes used as ancillary diagnostic aids in the differential diagnosis of anemia. Responses of the bone marrow to produce new RBCs when given proper nutrients, vitamins, and other factors may be evaluated by the reticulocyte count.

CLINICAL DIAGNOSIS OF ANEMIA

The clinical diagnosis of anemia is made by a combination of factors including patient history, physical signs, and changes in the hematologic profile. The signs and symptoms of anemia are generally nonspecific, such as fatigue and weakness, and may include gastrointestinal symptoms such as nausea, constipation, diarrhea, or increased gas. The patient may complain of dypsnea after a level of exertion that previously had not caused any problems. For example, a man who had been able to climb two flights of stairs with neither difficulty nor significant shortness of breath might report that now he must stop after climbing one

flight of stairs and is then very short of breath. Subsequent information indicates that the patient has passed very dark stools (melena), and measurement of his hemoglobin reveals a level of 8 g/dl. The diagnostic impression from the clinical information is that the patient's anemia is being caused by gastrointestinal bleeding.

Physical signs of anemia are usually not specific for the underlying disease. Occasionally, in patients who have certain physical findings, the underlying diagnosis may be suspected. One example would be signs of malnutrition and neurologic changes with loss of proprioception and vibration sense in a patient with vitamin B_{12} deficiency.[8] Another example would be severe pallor, smooth tongue, and an esophageal web seen in a patient with severe iron-deficiency anemia.[9] Patients who are anemic may appear to have pale coloration of mucosal membranes, nailbeds, and skin in light-skinned individuals. Occasionally, a mild temperature elevation may be present, particularly in patients having certain types of hemolytic anemia. In the presence of anemia, heart murmurs may be heard, sometimes secondary to the cause of the anemia and sometimes related to the increased cardiac workload required to bring oxygen to the tissues. Patients with bacterial endocarditis have fever, heart murmurs, and anemia.[10] Bacterial endocarditis is a clinical example in which the damaged myocardial valve and heart murmur are related etiologically to the anemia.

CLASSIFICATION OF ANEMIA

The individual types of anemias can be classified according to several different criteria. A functional classification would be hypoproliferative, accelerated destruction (hemolytic), or a combination thereof (sometimes called ineffective hematopoiesis). Anemias are often classified clinically according to their associated causes such as blood loss, iron deficiency, hemolysis, infection, metastatic bone marrow replacement, or nutritional deficiency. Anemias can also be categorized quantitatively by assessing hematocrit, hemoglobin, blood cell indices, and/or the reticulocyte count.[11] The laboratory technologist most frequently is involved in these quantitative measurements and in subsequent evaluations.

Hemoglobin and Hematocrit

Measurement of the hemoglobin or hematocrit level is the usual method of determining anemia. As discussed earlier, reference ranges may vary by age, gender, state of hydration, patient positioning and local laboratory patient population determinations (Table 4–1). Hemoglobin methods are based on the spectrophotometric absorbance readings of cyanmethemoglobin compared with known amounts. Several companies manufacture automated instruments that include these determinations as part of a hematologic profile. The hematocrit, or packed red blood cell volume (PCV), is determined by centrifugation of blood from either capillary or venous origin. The reference PCV for adult men varies by institution (ours is 45 ± 5 percent). For adult women during the reproductive years, the PCV reference range is 42 ± 4 percent. On the basis of hemoglobin or PCV values and the duration of onset, anemias may be classified as mild, moderate, or severe and as either acute or chronic. The approximate relationship of the hemoglobin to hematocrit is 1:3, a ratio that may vary with the cause of the anemia and the effect of that cause on the RBC indices.

RBC Indices

The RBC indices are the mean corpuscular volume (MCV), mean cell hemoglobin (MCH), and mean cell hemoglobin concentration (MCHC). The MCV is used as an estimation of the average size of the RBC, and may be calculated by dividing the hematocrit by the number of RBCs or measured directly using automated cell counters. If the MCV is within the reference range, then the RBCs are referred to as being normocytic. When the MCV is less than normal, the RBCs are referred to as microcytic; when greater than normal, macrocytic. Both MCH and MCHC values are used to determine the content of hemoglobin in RBCs.[12] Some automated hematology instruments also provide a RBC distribution width (RDW) value. The reference range for RDW is 11.5 to 14.5 percent for both men and women. The RDW is an index of size variation used to quantitate the amount of anisocytosis seen on a peripheral blood smear. The MCH is not dependable when RBCs vary markedly in size. If there is a normal MCHC, then the RBCs are referred to as normochromic. Hypochromic RBCs have a less than normal MCHC; there are no truly hyperchromic RBCs.

RBC Indices and Other Tests

The RBC indices are accurately calculated by the automated blood profiling machines. These instruments provide precise numeric values of the Hgb, the numbers of RBCs, and the MCV. Although less precise, careful microscopic examination of a peripheral blood smear can tell the examiner whether the RBCs are normocytic, microcytic, macrocytic, normochromic, or hypochromic. Red blood cell index calculations and reference ranges are:

MCV equals Hct (%) × 10, divided by RBC count (millions/μl); reference range: 90 ± 10 fl.

$$MCV = \frac{Hct \times 10}{RBC\ count\ (in\ millions/\mu l)}$$

MCH equals Hgb (g/dl) × 10, divided by RBC count (millions/μl); reference range: 29 ± 2 pg

$$MCH = \frac{Hgb\ (in\ grams\ per\ liter)}{RBC\ count\ (in\ millions\ per\ \mu l)}$$

MCHC equals Hgb (g/dl) × 100, divided by Hct (%); reference range: 34 ± 2%

$$MCHC = \frac{Hgb\ (g/dl) \times 100}{Hct\ (as\ a\ percentage)}$$

Use of the RBC indices in the differential diagnosis of anemia can provide a general idea as to what is occurring clinically (Table 4–2). A normocytic normochromic anemia may be the result of bone marrow failure, hemolytic anemia, or some subset of either of these conditions. The differential diagnosis of bone marrow failure includes the concern for whether there was normal or decreased RBC production. A reticulocyte count indicates whether there is bone marrow capacity for increased RBC production. RBC destruction may exceed the amount of production. The reticulocyte count measures effective RBC production. Hemolytic anemia occurs when there is decreased RBC survival and may be the result of extravascular elimination, intravascular elimination, or a combination of the two.

Macrocytic normochromic anemias usually occur in association with folate or vitamin B_{12} deficiency. The most commonly encountered anemias are the microcytic hypochromic anemias usually

Table 4–2. **CLASSIFICATION OF ANEMIA BY RBC INDICES**

Size (MCV) (μ^3 or fl)	Hgb Content (MCHC) (g/dl)	May Be Associated with
Normocytic (80–100)	Normochromic (32–36)	Bone marrow failure, hemolytic anemia, chronic renal disease, leukemia, metastatic malignancy
Macrocytic (>100)	Normochromic (32–36)	Megaloblastic, nonmegaloblastic macrocytic anemias (e.g., liver disease, myelodysplasias)
Microcytic (<80)	Hypochromic (<32)	Iron deficiency, sideroblastic anemia, thalassemia, lead poisoning, chronic diseases, chronic infection or inflammation, unstable hemoglobins

related to iron-deficiency anemia. Beta-thalasse-mia, an inherited defect of hemoglobin synthesis, is another cause of microcytosis. Less frequently seen are the sideroblastic anemias, which are associated also with decreased mean corpuscular volume. Microscopic examination of a properly prepared peripheral blood smear is a requirement for the clinical and laboratory evaluation of anemia. This technique is discussed later under the tests in the diagnosis of anemia. Histologic examinations of the bone marrow smear and aspirate are adjuncts to fully elucidate the etiology of anemia.

DIFFERENTIAL DIAGNOSIS OF ANEMIA

The differential diagnosis of anemia is based on a combination of the clinical and laboratory findings (Table 4–2, Fig. 4–1). An abbreviated flow chart for the diagnosis of anemia using the RBC indices is provided (Fig. 4–1).

GENERAL COMMENTS ON TREATMENT OF ANEMIAS

Anemia is treated according to its etiology. Anemias must be evaluated as to their cause before beginning either supportive therapy (such as a transfusion) or replacement therapy (such as iron for iron-deficiency anemia). Table 4–2 and Figure 4–1 represent only some of the possible causes for anemia. More than one cause of anemia can exist in a patient. Obtaining the proper diagnostic studies in the shortest and most cost-effective manner is the responsibility of the attending physician and the laboratory professionals. More details concerning the appropriate treatment of anemias are provided in Chapters 6 to 15.

The natural history of anemia depends on its etiology. For example, an iron-deficiency anemia associated with carcinoma of the colon may present first as simply an iron-deficiency anemia associated with blood loss from the tumor. Later, with more extensive tumor involvement and possible replacement of the bone marrow, there may be a bone marrow failure component to the anemia because of bone marrow replacement (a myelophthisic anemia). Patients with pernicious anemia will require a lifetime of parenteral vitamin B_{12} supplementation. Patients with other forms of megaloblastic anemia may need only a balanced diet and replacement of folic acid.

Transfusions can obscure and confuse the findings of diagnostic tests in patients with anemia. Transfusions can suppress erythropoiesis; alter vitamin B_{12}, folate, and iron levels; and thwart the interpretation of diagnostic tests seeking the specific cause of the anemia.

TESTS IN THE DIAGNOSIS OF ANEMIA
Hemoglobin

Hemoglobin is the main component of the RBC. It is the physiologic carrier of oxygen to tissues and acts as a buffer to handle carbon dioxide formed in metabolic activities. There are three methods for measuring hemoglobin: the cyanmethemoglobin method, the oxyhemoglobin method, and the

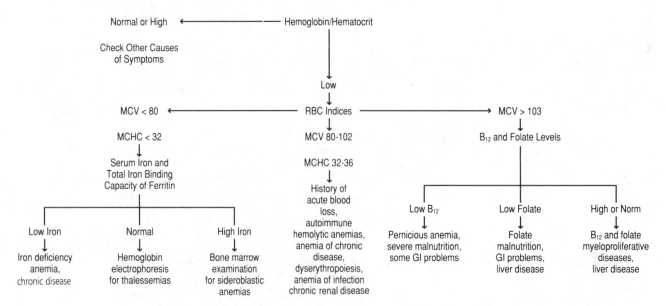

Figure 4–1. Anemia: abbreviated diagnostic tests and clinical possibilities.

method in which iron content is measured. The cyanmethemoglobin method is the one recommended by the International Committee for Standardization in Hematology as modified in 1978, and will be the only one discussed. In this technique, blood is diluted in a solution of potassium ferricyanide and potassium cyanide. The hemoglobin is oxidized to methemoglobin and subsequently, in the presence of the potassium cyanide, forms hemoglobincyanide. The absorption maximum is at wavelength 540 nm. The absorbance of the solution is read in a spectrophotometer at 540 nm and compared with a standard cyanmethemoglobin solution. The advantages of this method are that most forms of hemoglobin are measured, the sample can be directly compared with a standard, the solutions are stable, and the coefficient of variation for the method is less than 2 percent at physiologic ranges.

Errors that can occur in the measurement of hemoglobin include improperly obtaining a specimen, improper handling of the specimen, and difficulties with the reagents, equipment, or operator.

Hematocrit

The hematocrit, or packed RBC volume, is the ratio of the volume of RBCs to the volume of whole blood. Hematocrit is usually expressed as a percentage (for example, 42 percent) but is expressed in Système International d'Unités as a decimal fraction (for example, 0.42). The venous hematocrit agrees closely with the central blood hematocrit but is greater than the total body hematocrit. Anticoagulants—usually ethylenediaminetetraacetic acid (EDTA), oxalate, or heparin—are used to prevent the blood from clotting.

Measurement of the hematocrit may be done by centrifugation or through calculations, as done on many automated hematology instruments. The calculated hematocrit is the result of the mean corpuscular volume (MCV) times the RBC count.

The adult reference range for hematocrit is 40 to 50 percent in men and 38 to 46 percent in women. Different reference ranges are required, particularly for neonatal and early pediatric age groups, and may vary among institutions.

Problems in the measurement of hematocrit include incorrect centrifugation calibration, poor sample site, alteration of proper anticoagulant to blood ratio owing to amount of blood drawn, and reading error—particularly for centrifuged hematocrits. In our laboratory the coefficient of variation for hematocrit, within the reference range, is approximately 2 percent. With centrifuge hematocrit techniques, the lower hematocrit values are associated with the higher coefficients of variation.

RBC Indices

Red blood cell indices have been introduced earlier. The mean cell volume (MCV) is the average volume of RBCs and is measured directly or calcu-

lated from the hematocrit and RBC count expressed in femtoliters. The MCH is the content of hemoglobin in the average RBC. Mean cell hemoglobin is calculated from the hemoglobin concentration and the RBC count. Mean cell hemoglobin concentration, the average concentration of hemoglobin in a volume of packed RBCs, is calculated from the hemoglobin concentration and the hematocrit.

Red blood cell indices are readily available from the newer automated hematology counting devices. In those devices where the MCV is derived from the voltage changes formed during the RBC count and the hemoglobin is measured by spectrophotometric determination of the cyanmethemoglobin, the values are calculated as follows: The hematocrit equals the MCV times the RBC count, the MCH is measured by the hemoglobin divided by the RBC count, and the MCHC is measured by the hemoglobin divided by the hematocrit. The reference range for MCV in our institution is 80 to 100 fl; for the MCH 27 to 31 pg; and for the MCHC 32 to 36 percent.

In various anemic states, the indices may be altered as follows: Microcytic anemia: from an MCV of less than 80 fl down to a low of approximately 50 fl; from MCH less than 25 pg to approximately 15 pg; and from MCHC less than 30 percent to 22 percent. In the macrocytic anemias, MCV values are usually greater than 100 fl and may be as high as, or higher than, 120 fl; the MCHC may be normal or decreased. The MCHC may increase only in spherocytosis, if at all.

Peripheral Blood Smear

Much information concerning the etiology of an anemia can be determined from a peripheral blood smear. The size and shape of the RBCs can be noted. Alteration in size of the RBCs results in anisocytosis; alterations in their shape results in poikilocytosis. The hemoglobin (chromatic) content of the RBCs can be inspected visually on the peripheral smear. In addition, the peripheral smear may provide a clue to the etiology of the anemia or the bone marrow response, or both. The white cells may be evaluated. For example, excess lobulations of the polymorphonuclear leukocytes are seen in the hypersegmented granulocytes of macrocytic anemias (**see Color Plate 66**). Coexistent neutropenia, thrombocytopenia, and anemia may indicate that there is bone marrow failure or a lack of a nutritional substance to provide adequate bone marrow production.

The presence of basophilic stippling in the RBCs may suggest the presence of increased bone marrow production and reticulocytosis (**see Color Plates 106 and 114**). Basophilic stippling of RBCs indicates remnants of ribonucleic acid (RNA) and may be associated with lead poisoning and some malignancies. Howell-Jolly bodies (**see Color Plates 65 and 67**), small, round, blue inclusions seen in RBCs, are the result of leftover fragments of deoxyribonucleic acid (DNA). Howell-Jolly bodies are often seen in hyposplenism or asplenism, pernicious anemia, and some hemoglobinopathies — particularly thalassemia.[13] The Pappenheimer body appears as a purplish-blue granule with Wright's stain and as a coarse blue granule with Prussian blue iron stain. Pappenheimer bodies are iron-containing or siderotic granules. The clinical disorders associated with Pappenheimer bodies include sideroblastic anemia, alcoholism, thalassemia, and some preleukemic states.[14] Nucleated RBCs with iron granules are known as sideroblasts. Red blood cells containing iron granules without a nucleus are referred to as siderocytes. Ringed sideroblasts occur where there are more than five granules in a ring around the nucleus of an orthochromatic normoblast (**see Color Plate 56**). Ringed sideroblasts are indicative of ineffective erythropoiesis.

A threadlike blue ring entirely contained within an abnormal RBC, which may or may not have a "figure-8" and a round or oval configuration, is known as a Cabot's ring[15] (**see Color Plate 69**). This is a remnant of the nuclear membrane. This infrequent finding may be seen in several clinical disorders including severe anemia. Heinz bodies (**see Color Plate 84**) are small, rounded, angular inclusions about 1 μm in diameter that are aggregates of denatured hemoglobin and are negative when stained with Prussian blue or other iron stains. Heinz bodies can be demonstrated only by using supravital stains (for example, methylene blue) and are not visible with the usual Wright's stain. The clinical disorders that have been associated with the Heinz bodies include postsplenectomy, glucose-6-phosphate dehydrogenase (G6PD) deficiency after exposure to oxidizing drugs, a variety of unstable hemoglobinopathies, and α-thalassemia.

Reticulocyte Count

The reticulocyte count is of great use in determining the response and potential of the bone marrow. Reticulocytes are non-nucleated RBCs that still contain RNA.[16] Reticulocytes may be visualized after incubation with a variety of so-called supravital dyes, including new methylene blue or brilliant cresyl blue (**see Color Plate 106**). Ribonucleic acid is recipitated as a dye protein complex. Reticulocytes under normal circumstances lose their RNA a day or so after reaching the bloodstream from the marrow. Reticulocyte activity can be expressed as an absolute count, a production index, or a percentage.

Interpretation of the reticulocyte count must take into account the age and nutritional status of the patient. Normal adults have a reticulocyte count of between 0.5 and 1.5 percent, or from 24 to 84×10^9 reticulocytes per liter. The newborn infant has a higher reticulocyte count, which falls to the adult range usually by the second or third week of life. Sources of error in the reticulocyte count are associated with the sampling error of counting relatively few reticulocytes in a large number of erythrocytes. The 95 percent confidence level when counting 100 RBCs, where the true reticulocyte count is 1 percent, ranges from 0.4 to 1.6 percent; obviously, there is a very high coefficient of variation.

Bone Marrow Smear and Biopsy

Bone marrow aspiration and biopsy are important diagnostic tools in the determination of anemia. Bone marrow interpretation and evaluation is covered earlier in this book. Factors to be evaluated in interpretation of a bone marrow aspirate smear and biopsy include maturation of the red and white cell series, presence of megakaryocytes, ratio of myeloid to erythroid series, abundance of iron stores, presence or absence of granulomas, tumor cells, and overall estimate of bone marrow activity.

Interpretation requires a differential count of the myeloid and erythroid series, an iron stain, and other appropriate stains if a differential diagnosis of lymphoproliferative or myeloproliferative disorders is entertained. Other appropriate specific stains may be indicated if metastatic tumor or infection is suspected or being evaluated.

Hemoglobin Electrophoresis

Hemoglobin electrophoresis is used to identify hemoglobinopathies and thalassemia syndromes. There are a variety of techniques in hemoglobin electrophoresis, including standard cellulose acetate and barbital buffer methods and specific isoelectric focusing techniques. Cellulose acetate and starch agar gel techniques using both barbital and citrate buffers should be available, as some hemoglobinopathies are not determined by one method and will be picked up by the other. Isoelectric focusing of hemoglobins is becoming a more widely accepted analytical technique. Additional identification such as column separation of fetal and hemoglobin A_2 can be extremely useful. Interpretation of hemoglobin electrophoresis will be discussed further in Chapter 11.

Antiglobulin Testing

The presence or absence of immune globulin, immune globulin fragments, and complement and complement products on the RBC may be useful in the differential evaluation of hemolytic anemias. These techniques and reagents are often available in immunohematology (blood banking) laboratories. The presence of immune globulin or complement, or both, on the RBC surface in the proper clinical context can support a diagnosis of autoimmune hemolytic anemia.

Osmotic Fragility

The osmotic fragility test is used to determine whether RBCs are more sensitive to lysis when they are introduced to solutions of hypotonic saline. A series of tubes containing the patient's blood and solutions of saline from 0.0 to 0.9 percent are incubated at room temperature. Percent hemolysis is measured and plotted for each concentration. Spherical cells have a limited capacity to expand in these hypotonic solutions and lyse at a lower concentration of sodium chloride than do either normal RBCs or cells from patients with a hemoglobinopathy or iron-deficiency anemia. In hereditary spherocytosis, RBCs have an increased osmotic fragility. This also may be seen in acquired spherocytic anemias. Patients with hereditary spherocytosis have increased autohemolysis as well. Red blood cells from patients with severe iron deficiency, sickle-cell disease, or β-thalassemia have great resistance to osmotic lysis or marked reduction in their osmotic fragility.

The test for RBC hemolysis in sucrose solutions (so-called sucrose hemolysis test) assesses membrane fragility in the presence of complement (**see Color Plate 101**). It is used to aid in the differential diagnosis of paroxysmal nocturnal hemoglobinuria (PNH) (see Chapter 13). Sucrose provides a low ionic strength solution that promotes the binding of complement to the RBCs. In PNH and some hypoplastic anemias, as well as in some preleukemic states, the RBCs are abnormally sensitive to this kind of complement-mediated hemolysis. Some overlap in positive results is occasionally seen in megaloblastic anemias and some autoimmune hemolytic anemias. If a serum lacks complement activity, a false-negative test result can occur.

The acidified serum test (Ham's test) is the definitive test in the diagnosis of PNH (**see Color Plate 102**). In acidified serum, the complement is activated by the alternate pathway, binds to the RBCs, and lyses the abnormal cells of PNH. In PNH 10 to 50 percent of the cells may be lysed in acidified serum. A positive test result also occurs in congenital dyserythropoietic anemia type II (CDA-II) (see Chapter 8). Lysis occurs in CDA-II not with the patient's own serum but with the addition of most other normal sera (with some, but not all, normal sera), and the sucrose hemolysis test result is negative in CDA-II.

RBC Enzymes and Metabolic Activities

Evaluation of a variety of enzymes in the carbohydrate aerobic and anaerobic metabolic pathways is possible. These enzyme deficiencies are associated with hemolytic anemias. The mature RBC lacks a nucleus and a mitochondria. Ninety percent of the energy production occurs through the Embden-Meyerhof pathway.[17] Abnormalities in this pathway result in impaired high-energy phosphate generation and a chronic hemolytic anemia.

Heinz bodies are usually not seen. The most common RBC enzyme deficiency is G6PD deficiency, which is present in about 10 percent of black American men and which is also found in much smaller percentages of whites and Asians. The deficiency exists in X-linked and non–X-linked varieties. Other enzyme deficiencies occur. Pyruvate kinase (PK) deficiency is an RBC enzyme deficiency involving the Embden-Meyerhof glycolytic pathway.[18] It can result in a mild to moderately severe hemolytic anemia and splenomegaly. Inheritance is autosomal recessive, but PK mutants are thought to occur relatively frequently. A fluorescent spot test, in which the blood is mixed with the proper substrate plus coenzyme and buffer, can be used for qualitative identification of enzyme cellular deficiencies. Quantitative assays can be performed on a variety of spectrophotometric instruments. Other enzyme and metabolic abnormalities of RBCs do occur but tend to be much rarer. (For a more detailed discussion of enzyme deficiencies, see Chapter 10).

RBC Protein and Membrane Studies

Various emerging techniques can evaluate the lipid and protein makeup of the RBC membrane; at present, however, these techniques are not readily available as routine clinical laboratory tests. They may be of great value in the differential diagnosis of some of the dyserythropoietic anemias. Assays of RBC membranes and proteins such as spectrin may aid in the understanding of spherocytic anemias and other related hemolytic anemias. Chapter 9 discusses the hemolytic anemias caused by membrane defects.

Other Tests

Erythropoietin (EPO) levels may be useful in determining a proper response of the bone marrow in disorders in which a high reticulocyte count is expected. A high EPO level in the presence of a high hemoglobin level may indicate that there is an abnormal hemoglobin level that is binding oxygen and is not releasing it at the level of the tissues, or that some other oxygen transfer abnormality exists. Deficient levels of erythropoietin may indicate a congenital absence of EPO, changes that cause decreased production of EPO, or both. The kidney is the site of EPO production. Erythropoietin deficiencies and anemia may be seen in patients with severe renal disease. A clinically available injectable form of EPO is now being produced by recombinant molecular biology techniques that can be used for treatment of appropriate anemias. Erythropoietin can be measured by an immunologic or a biologic method. The most frequently used technique for measuring EPO is radioimmunoassay (RIA).

Bone Marrow Culture

This is an expanding technology in which bone marrow precursor cells are grown in culture to determine the viability of stem cells.[19]

There is increasing interest in the effect of growth factors on pluripotential stem cells of the bone marrow. Various growth factors, including erythropoietin and platelet growth factor, are known to have an impact on RBC production. Sophisticated techniques of tissue culture are available to evaluate colony-forming units of erythrocytes (CFU-E), burst-forming units of erythrocytes (BFU-E), and colony-forming units of granulocytes and monocytes (GFU-GM).

The use of this technique for differential diagnosis of aplastic anemias and anemias of bone marrow failure is yet to be fully exploited. It is apparent that some of the aplastic anemias may be associated with bone marrow stem cell failure, suppression of bone marrow stem cells by cells of the lymphocyte series or humoral antibody, or alterations in the bone marrow milieu that prevent maturation of the precursor cells.[20]

Haptoglobin

Rapid hemolysis leads to free hemoglobin in the plasma. There are tests to measure circulating haptoglobin, a protein that binds to free hemoglobin and permits removal via the reticuloendothelial system. Clinical measurements of haptoglobin binding are of limited use in the evaluation of hemolytic anemias. Massive rapid intravascular hemolysis of greater than 15 ml of RBCs will overwhelm the capacity of haptoglobin and its backup systems, resulting in free plasma hemoglobin which can be measured directly.[21]

Serum Iron and Iron-Binding Capacity and Other Tests

Iron and iron-binding capacity tests are extremely important for differential diagnosis and definitive evaluation of iron in patients who have iron-deficiency anemia. The usual ratio of serum iron to iron-binding capacity is roughly 30 percent. Levels below 20 percent for serum iron in relation to serum iron-binding capacity are indicative of iron-deficiency anemia. Reference ranges for serum iron are approximately 50 to 150 μg/dl with an iron-binding capacity of 200 to 300 μg/dl. Transferrin and ferritin levels, which can be measured by enzyme-linked immunoassays, nephelometry, or RIAs, can be useful in evaluation of iron-deficiency states. Ferritin level measurement is recommended for following bone marrow iron stores and can be a helpful test, particularly when there is severe iron deficiency or iron overload. Ferritin is the major protein associated with body stores of iron. Circulating ferritin is in equilibrium with tissue levels. Although ferritin is replacing serum iron measurements in some laboratories, it

should be noted that serum ferritin may be falsely elevated in some patients with acute infections or liver disease. Transferrin level measurement is not usually as useful.

The direct measurement of folate and vitamin B_{12} levels by either RIAs or bioassays is useful for providing a definitive diagnosis in assessing the differential diagnosis of megaloblastic anemias. Controversy continues as to whether folate and vitamin B_{12} levels should be measured in the serum alone or whether sensitivity would be enhanced by measuring intraerythrocytic levels.

SUMMARY

Anemia has physiologic, functional, and quantitative parameters that may be related to hemoglobin or hematocrit levels. The differential diagnosis of anemia requires careful consideration of a wide variety of marrow, extramedullary, and interrelating disease states. A large armamentarium of tests is available to aid in the differential diagnosis of the spectrum of anemias. To study anemia requires broad knowledge of clinical laboratory techniques and the practice of medicine.

PATIENT STUDIES IN ANEMIA

Individual patient studies of anemia are addressed in Chapters 6 to 15, respectively.

REFERENCES

1. Beck, WS: Hematology, ed 3. MIT Press, Cambridge, MA, 1981, p 16.
2. Wintrobe, M, et al: Clinical Hematology, ed 8. Lea & Febiger, Philadelphia, 1981, pp 529–558.
3. Isselbacher, KJ, et al: Harrison's Principles of Internal Medicine. McGraw-Hill, New York, 1980, pp 262–263.
4. Erslev, AJ: Polycythemia. In Wyngaarden, JB and Smith, LH (eds): Cecil's Textbook of Medicine. WB Saunders, Philadelphia, 1982, pp 937–943.
5. Rifkind, RA, et al: Fundamentals of Hematology, ed 2. Year Book Medical Publishers, Chicago, 1980, pp 19–22.
6. Woodson, RD, et al: Introduction to hemopoiesis. In MacKinney, AA, Jr (ed): Pathophysiology of Blood. John Wiley & Sons, New York, 1984, pp 12–15.
7. Wintrobe, MM, et al: Clinical Hematology, ed 8. Lea & Febiger, Philadelphia, 1981, pp 94–95.
8. Kupp, MA and Chatton, MJ: Current Medical Diagnosis and Treatment. Lange Medical Publications, CA, 1980, p 293.
9. Nelson, DA and Davey, FR: Erythrocytic disorders. In Henry, JB (ed): Todd, Sanford, and Davidson: Clinical Diagnosis and Management by Laboratory Methods, ed 17. WB Saunders, Philadelphia, 1984, p 665.
10. Kaye, D: Infective endocarditis. In Kay, D and Rose, LF (eds): Fundamentals of Internal Medicine. CV Mosby, St Louis, 1983, pp 168–172.
11. Ravel, R: Clinical Laboratory Medicine: Clinical Application of Laboratory Data, ed 3. Year Book Medical Publishers, Chicago, 1978, pp 1–8.
12. Maile, JB: Laboratory Medicine Hematology, ed 6. CV Mosby, St Louis, 1982, pp 379–380.
13. Williams, WJ, et al: Hematology, ed 3. McGraw-Hill, New York, 1983, pp 270–271.

14. Miale, JB: Laboratory Medicine Hematology, ed 6. CV Mosby, St Louis, 1982, pp 488–489, 582.
15. Henry, JB (ed): Todd, Sanford, and Davidsohn: Clinical Diagnosis and Management by Laboratory Methods, ed 17. WB Saunders, Philadelphia, 1984, pp 609–610.
16. Wintrobe, MM, et al: Clinical Hematology, ed 8. Lea & Febiger, Philadelphia, 1981, p 112.
17. Nelson, DA and Davey, FR: Erythrocytic disorders. In Henry, JB (ed): Todd, Sanford, and Davidsohn: Clinical Diagnosis and Management by Laboratory Methods, ed 17. WB Saunders, Philadelphia, 1984, p 87.
18. Wintrobe, MM, et al: Clinical Hematology, ed 8. Lea & Febiger, Philadelphia, 1981, p 773.
19. Nelson, DA and Davey, FR: Erythrocytic disorders. In Henry, JB (ed): Todd, Sanford, and Davidsohn: Clinical Diagnosis and Management by Laboratory Methods, ed 17. WB Saunders, Philadelphia, 1984, pp 626–629.
20. Erslev, AJ and Weiss, L: Structure and function of hemopoietic organs. In Williams, WJ, et al: (eds): Hematology, ed 3. McGraw-Hill, New York, 1983, pp 78–81.
21. Hillman, RF and Finch, CA: General characteristics of the erythron. In Hillman, RS and Finch, CA (eds): Red Cell Manual, ed 5. FA Davis, Philadelphia, 1985, pp 19–21.

QUESTIONS

1. Which of the following laboratory results would not be part of the usual diagnostic criterion for a patient with anemia?
   a. Decreased hemoglobin
   b. Decreased hematocrit
   c. Decreased platelet count
   d. Decreased RBC count

2. What condition is not a cause for anemia?
   a. Dietary deficiency
   b. Moderate exercise
   c. Decreased RBC production
   d. Increased RBC destruction or loss

3. Which response represents the most complete and correct listing of the most common clinical signs of anemia?
   a. Fatigue, weakness, gastrointestinal symptoms, dypsnea, pallor
   b. Urticaria, hypertension, inflammation, nausea
   c. Nausea, hypertension, temperature elevation, melena
   d. Rapid pulse, inflammation, temperature elevation, dehydration

4. What is the most commonly accepted method for measuring hemoglobulin?
   a. Conversion of hemoglobulin to oxyhemoglobin, followed by spectrophotometric measurement
   b. Iron content measured by RIA technique
   c. Copper sulfate by specific gravity
   d. Conversion of hemoglobulin to cyanmethemoglobin followed by spectrophotometric measurement

5. How is hemocrit measured on automated hematology instruments?
   a. Centrifugation
   b. Photometrically
   c. Calculation (MCV × RBC count)
   d. Calculation (MCH × Hgb)

6. A patient had the following results: Hct 26%; Hgb 8 g/dl; and RBC count 3.5×10^6 mm³. Calculate the RBC indices—MCV, MCH, and MCHC—and determine the classification of the anemia.
   a. MCV 88 M³; MCH 30 pg; MCHC 33 g/dl; normocytic, normochromic
   b. MCV 101 M³; MCH 33 pg; MCHC 35 g/dl; macrocytic, normochromic
   c. MCV 74 M³; MCH 22 pg; MCHC 31 g/dl; microcytic, hypochromic

7. Which of the following would not be characteristically found on a peripheral blood smear in a case of anemia?
   a. Anisocytosis and/or poikilocytosis
   b. Basophilic stippling, Howell-Jolly bodies, and Pappenheimer bodies
   c. Cabot's rings and Heinz bodies
   d. Rouleaux and Döhle bodies

8. What is the diagnostic value of the reticulocyte count in the evaluation of anemia?
   a. Determines response and potential of the bone marrow
   b. Determines compensation mechanisms for anemia
   c. Determines the corrected RBC count after calculation
   d. Determines the potential sampling error for RBC count

9. Which of the following is not a factor to be evaluated in the interpretation of a bone marrow aspirate smear?
   a. Maturation of red and white blood cell series
   b. M:E ratio
   c. Type and amount of hemoglobin
   d. Estimate of bone marrow activity

10. When does hemoglobin electrophoresis have greatest diagnostic value?
    a. In cases of G6PD and PK deficiency
    b. In cases of hemoglobinopathies and thalassemia syndromes
    c. In cases of hemolytic anemias
    d. In cases of hereditary spherocytosis and iron-deficient anemia

11. When is antiglobulin testing important in the diagnosis of anemias? (Use answer choices for question 10.)

12. What laboratory tests are useful to determine RBC sensitivity to lysis?
    a. Antiglobulin tests for anti-IgG and anti-C3b
    b. Tests for RBC enzymes
    c. EPO levels and RBC membrane studies
    d. Osmotic fragility and sucrose hemolysis

13. What are the two most commonly measured RBC enzymes?
    a. G6PD and PK
    b. EPO and LDH
    c. Methemoglobin reductase and enolase
    d. NADH and GSH

14. *What is the value of measuring EPO?*
    a. May indicate congenital absence or decreased production of EPO
    b. May indicate RBC enzyme deficiency
    c. May indicate severe liver disease
    d. May indicate the presence of an abnormal hemoglobin as the result of deficient EPO

15. *What test allows the determination of stem cell viability?*
    a. Haptoglobin binding
    b. Iron-binding capacity
    c. EPO levels
    d. Bone marrow culture

16. *Why is haptoglobin measurement of limited value in the evaluation of anemias?*
    a. It is usually found in very small quantities in anemias.
    b. It is difficult to detect when not bound to free hemoglobin.
    c. Free hemoglobin may be found in larger quantities than haptoglobin.
    d. Haptoglobin levels do not change as a result of anemias.

17. *Which test(s) would not be useful in cases of iron-deficiency anemia?*
    a. Iron and iron-binding capacity
    b. Folate and vitamin B_{12} levels
    c. Transferrin levels
    d. Ferritin levels

ANSWERS

1. c (p. 55)
2. b (p. 55)
3. a (p. 56)
4. d (p. 56)
5. c (p. 57)
6. c (p. 57)
7. d (p. 59–60)
8. a (p. 60)
9. c (p. 60)
10. b (p. 60)
11. c (p. 60)
12. d (p. 61)
13. a (p. 61)
14. a (p. 61)
15. d (p. 62)
16. c (p. 62)
17. b (p. 62)

CHAPTER 5

BETTY E. CIESLA, M.S., M.T.(ASCP)S.H.

Evaluation of Red Cell Morphology and Summary of Platelet and White Cell Morphology

OBJECTIVES

At the end of this chapter, the learner should be able to:
1. Define anisocytosis and poikilocytosis.
2. List cell parameters for classification of macrocytes and microcytes.
3. Identify clinical conditions that show oval macrocytes.
4. Name disease states that produce a microcytic blood picture.
5. List cell parameters for classification of cell hypochromia.
6. Specify conditions showing hypochromia.
7. List diseases that may produce polychromatophilic cells.
8. Indicate which clinical conditions may show target cells, spherocytes, ovalocytes, elliptocytes, and stomatocytes.

9. Describe the physiologic mechanism for formation of sickle cells.
10. List diseases that may show acanthocytes, fragmented RBCs (schistocytes, burr cells, and helmet cells), and teardrop cells.
11. Identify the composition of RBC inclusions such as Howell-Jolly bodies, basophilic stippling, Pappenheimer bodies, Heinz bodies, and Cabot's rings.
12. Specify conditions showing leukocyte cytoplasmic changes such as toxic granulation, toxic vacuolization, or Döhle bodies.

It is the purpose of hematology atlases to guide the student through red cell morphology in a step-by-step fashion, but that is not the intent of this chapter. Although some basic mechanics in estimating morphology are discussed, the emphasis is on interpretative morphology and its relevance to clinical conditions. By explaining physiologic mechanisms, an attempt is made to demonstrate the cause of a particular morphologic picture. In this way the student can more readily associate the underlying disease with the peripheral smear observation. This approach to blood cell morphology should facilitate the overall assessment of the patient's condition.

ANISOCYTOSIS AND POIKILOCYTOSIS

By definition, anisocytosis implies a variation in size of erythrocytes seen in a well-stained, well-dispersed smear. Poikilocytosis implies a variation in shape seen in a well-stained, well-dispersed smear. The majority of institutions use either qualitative remarks or a numeric grading (1 to 4+) to describe anisocytosis and poikilocytosis; they proceed to quantitate the red cell changes observed. It is recommended that a simple statement ("aniso and poik observed") be adopted when applicable and that the quantitation or use of qualitative adjectives be reserved only for the more important assessment of the actual numbers and types of morphologic abnormal cells. What is paramount in the examination of the peripheral smear is the *type of cells* seen, as they provide the morphologic clues to the hematology diagnostics.

Why is a new approach to red cell morphology necessary? It is difficult to explain to the new student what a 1+ variation in size of red blood cells is as opposed to a 2+ variation in size. Proponents of the quantitative methods instruct students to use an analysis of size and shape changes in 10 oil immersion fields, by tallying up these changes, dividing by 10, and then assessing anisocytosis. Likewise, the qualitative genre applies the adjective "slight," "moderate," or "marked" to the words "aniso" and "poik." Either one of these procedures invites subjectivity and is confusing for new learners and clinical practitioners. It becomes apparent that time spent in either of these endeavors in a differential (for the purpose of recording the presence of anisocytosis or poikilocytosis) might be better spent in assessing the numbers and types of cells that make these variations obvious.

THE NORMAL RED BLOOD CELL

The mature red blood cell (RBC, erythrocyte, normocyte) is a remarkable structure, and its simple appearance is deceiving. It is a cell that passes from a nucleated to a non-nucleated state upon maturity, with decreasing size and a dramatic change in cytoplasmic color. On a Wright-stained blood smear, this mature RBC has a reddish orange appearance. The red cell has an average range of 6.0 to 8.0 μm and an average volume of 90 μm^3. The area of central pallor is approximately 2 to 3 μm in diameter, and the size variation of RBCs from a healthy person is approximately 5 percent.

Fundamental to the RBC is the formation of hemoglobin, which functions primarily as the oxygen-carrying element of the cell. Additionally, human qualitative hemoglobin is required for maintenance of structural integrity. The red cell membrane is a lipid bilayer whose skeleton is composed of actin and spectrin. Spectrin, the dominant membrane protein, consists of two high molecular weight polypeptides and functions prominently in the maintenance of cell shape and deformability. (See Chapter 1 for more detailed information on the normal red cell.)

SIZE VARIATIONS
Macrocytes (Color Plates 64 and 65)

Physiologic Mechanism

Macrocytes are cells with a diameter of approximately 9 μm or larger, having a mean cell volume (MCV) of greater than 100 μm^3. Additionally, the red cell distribution width (RDW) is high in the heterogenous macrocytic population (see inside cover for Système International d'Unités (SI). Macrocytes may arrive in the peripheral circulation by several mechanisms. Three of the most distinct are (1) impaired deoxyribonucleic acid (DNA) synthesis leading to a decreased number of cellular divisions consequently a larger cell (megaloblastic erythropoiesis), (2) accelerated erythropoiesis yielding a reticulocytosis which in the Wright-stained smear is manifested as polychromatophilic macrocytes; and (3) increased membrane cholesterol and lecithin, although this mechanism may not be reflective of a true macrocytosis (obstructive liver disease).

Peripheral Blood Findings

A careful examination of the type of macrocyte seen in the peripheral blood smear can give many clues to the underlying mechanism. Macrocytes should be evaluated for shape (oval versus round), color (red versus blue), presence or absence of pallor, and the presence or absence of inclusions.

Common clinical conditions in which macrocytes, particularly oval macrocytes, can be found include the megaloblastic anemias (those due to vitamin B_{12} or folate deficiency) and myelodysplasia. Thin macrocytes with some targeting may be seen in liver disease, postsplenectomy, or hyposplenic conditions. In patients undergoing chemotherapy a macrocytosis invariably develops, as these drugs interfere with folate metabolism or DNA synthesis. Additionally, macrocytes may be seen in scurvy, metastatic marrow infiltration in neonatal blood, and hypothyroidism.

Microcytes (Color Plate 57)

Physiologic Mechanism

A microcyte is a small cell having a diameter of less than 7 μm and an MCV of less than 80 μm³. The RDW is high in the heterogenous microcytic population. Any defect that results in impaired hemoglobin synthesis causes a microcytic hypochromic blood picture. When developing erythroid cells are deprived of any of the essentials in hemoglobin synthesis, the result is increased cellular divisions and, consequently, a smaller cell in the peripheral blood. Hemoglobin synthesis involves multiple steps, and microcytosis develops from (1) ineffective iron utilization, absorption, or release; and (2) decreased or defective globin synthesis. Effective porphyrin synthesis is, of course, vital for hemoglobination; however, the porphyrias usually do not cause a microcytic erythrocyte.

Peripheral Blood Findings

Only three clinical conditions produce a microcytosis: iron-deficiency anemia, thalassemia syndromes, and anemia of chronic disease. A significant number of microcytes may be seen in patients with lead poisoning and iron-loading anemias. However, the number of microcytes in these conditions is not in large enough numbers to cause microcytic blood indices.

COLOR VARIATIONS
Hypochromia (Color Plate 57)

Physiologic Mechanism

Any RBC having a central area of pallor of greater than 3 μm is said to be hypochromic. There is a direct relationship between the amount of hemoglobin produced in the RBC and the appearance of the RBC when properly stained. For this reason an aberration of hemoglobin synthesis will lead to some degree of hypochromia. Most clinicians choose to assess hypochromia based on the mean cell hemoglobin concentration (MCHC), which measures hemoglobin content in a given volume of cells (100 ml). This value is derived from a calculated hematocrit, which is not as sensitive as a manual hematocrit. Although this calculation is usually reliable, it does not account for situations in which a true hypochromia is observed in the presence of a normal MCHC. Not all hypochromic cells are microcytic. Target cells possess some degree of hypochromia, and some macrocytes and normocytes can be distinctly hypochromic.

Peripheral Blood Findings

The most common and severe hypochromia is found in patients with iron deficiency anemia. In severe cases of iron deficiency, red cells exhibit an inordinately thin band of hemoglobin. Patients with iron deficiency have many hypochromic cells, depending on the magnitude of the deficiency. Hypochromia in thalassemia syndromes is much less pronounced. In α-thalassemia and β-thalassemia, the MCHC is normal. The sideroblastic anemias show a dimorphic blood picture: macrocytic, normocytic, and microcytic cells together, only some of which show true hypochromia. Some hypochromic cells may be seen in lead poisoning; however, the association of microcytosis with lead poisoning irrespective of other underlying processes is being questioned.

The morphologist should not be unduly influenced by the RBC indices in the evaluation of hypochromia. In some cases the MCHC will be concordant with what is observed on the peripheral blood smear. True hypochromia will appear as a delicately shaded area of pallor, whereas in pseudohypochromia (the water artifact) the area of pallor is distinctly outlined.

Polychromasia

Physiologic Mechanism

When RBCs are delivered to the peripheral circulation prematurely, their appearance on the Wright-stained smear is distinctive. Red cells showing polychromatophilia are gray-blue and are usually larger than normal red cells. The basophilia of the RBC is the result of the residual ribonucleic acid (RNA) involved in hemoglobin synthesis. Polychromatophilic macrocytes are actually reticulocytes; however, the reticulum cannot be visualized without supravital staining.

Peripheral Blood Findings

It is not uncommon to find a few polychromatophilic (diffusely basophilic) cells in a normal peripheral blood smear because RBC regeneration is a dynamic process. In the blood smear, polychromatophilic red cells come in varying shades of blue (see Color Plate 27). Any clinical condition in which the marrow is stimulated—particularly RBC regeneration—produces a polychromatophilic blood picture. This represents effective erythropoiesis. The degree of polychromasia in a peripheral blood smear can serve as a quality control to the reticulocyte count, and most laboratories look for agreement between these values. Examples of several conditions in which polychromasia is observed include acute and chronic hemorrhage, hemolysis, and any regenerative RBC process. The degree of polychromasia is an excellent indicator of therapeutic effectiveness when a patient is given iron or vitamin therapy as a treatment for the anemia.

SHAPE VARIATIONS

Target Cells (Codocytes) (Color Plates 90 and 126)

Physiologic Mechanism

Target cells appear in the peripheral blood as a result of increase in RBC surface membrane. Their true circulating form is a bell-shaped cell. In air-dried smears, however, they appear as "targets," with a large portion of hemoglobin displayed at the rim of the cell and another portion of hemoglobin shown as central, eccentric, or banded. Target cells are always hypochromic.

The mechanisms of targeting are related to excess membrane cholesterol and phospholipid and decreased cellular hemoglobin. This is well documented in patients with liver disease, whose cholesterol-to-phospholipid ratio is altered. Mature red cells are unable to synthesize cholesterol and phospholipid independently. As cholesterol accumulates in the plasma, as is the case with liver dysfunction, the RBC membrane is expanded by increased lipid, resulting in increased surface area. Consequently, the osmotic fragility is also decreased.

Peripheral Blood Findings

The presence of target cells is a common clinical finding in any of the conditions in which hemoglobin synthesis is abnormal: thalassemia major and minor, sickle-cell anemia, and homozygous and heterozygous hemoglobin C disease. Target cells may also be observed in patients with iron deficiency or liver disease, and following splenectomy.

Spherocytes (Color Plate 77)

Physiologic Mechanism

Spherocytes have several distinctive properties and, in contrast to the target cell, they have the lowest surface area–to–volume ratio. They are smaller in diameter than normal red cells, and their hemoglobin content is relatively concentrated. Because these cells have no visible central pallor, they are easily distinguished in a peripheral blood smear. Their shape change is irreversible.

There are several mechanisms for the production of spherocytes, each sharing the mutual defect of loss of membrane. In the normal aging process of

RBCs, spherocytes are produced as a final stage before senescent RBCs are detained in the spleen and trapped by the reticuloendothelial system (RES). Coating of the red cells with antibodies and the detrimental effect of complement activation will produce spherocytes as the RBC membrane loses cholesterol and, consequently, surface area owing to splenic sequestration.

Perhaps the most complex mechanism for sphering is seen in the congenital condition known as hereditary spherocytosis (HS). An autosomal dominant, inherited condition, this intrinsic defect in the RBC membrane causes the spheroid RBC to be prematurely trapped and destroyed in the spleen. Erythrocytes from patients with HS have a mean influx of sodium twice that of normal cells. It is thought that this increased permeability to sodium results from some sort of membrane lesion. Because spherocytes have 35 times the ability of normal cells to metabolize glucose, these cells can handle their increased sodium content as they travel through plasma, by producing enough energy to pump sodium from the cell. However, once these cells reach the microenvironment of the spleen where glucose is deficient, the active-passive transport system is invariably injured, causing the cells to swell and hemolyze (see Chapter 9).

Peripheral Blood Findings

Spherocytes may be seen in immune hemolytic anemias, in the hemoglobinopathies, in hereditary spherocytosis, and in severe burns. They may also be observed in any of the splenic states— hypersplenism or postsplenectomy.

Ovalocytes/Elliptocytes (Color Plate 78)

Physiologic Mechanism

The ovalocyte is a cell of many capabilities. It can appear normochromic or hypochromic; normocytic or macrocytic. Its exact physiologic mechanism is not well defined. When ovalocytes are incubated in vitro, they reduce adenosine triphosphate (ATP) and 2,3-diphosphoglycerate (2,3-DPG) more rapidly than do normal cells. Hemoglobin seems to have a bipolar arrangement in these cells, and they seem to have a reduction in membrane cholesterol.

Although many investigators consider "ovalocyte" and "elliptocyte" as interchangeable terms, these two items will be dealt with distinctly and separately. Ovalocytes are egg-shaped and have a greater tendency to vary in their hemoglobin content. Elliptocytes, on the other hand, are pencil-shaped and invariably not hypochromic.

Peripheral Blood Findings

Ovalocytes may be found in patients with megaloblastic anemias, and in this condition they appear as oval macrocytes. They may be seen in patients with sickle-cell anemia, myelodysplasia, and thalassemia major, as well as following postsplenectomy. Elliptocytes are seen in those patients with hereditary elliptocytosis, iron-deficiency anemia, and myelofibrosis.

Stomatocytes (Color Plate 80)

Physiologic Mechanism

The stomatocyte is a normal-sized red cell that, in wet preparation, appears bowl-shaped. This peculiar shape is manifested in air-dried smears as a slitlike area of central pallor. The exact physiologic mechanism of stomatocytosis in vivo has yet to be clarified. Many chemical agents may induce stomatocytosis in vitro (phenothiazine and chlorpromazine), but these changes are reversible. Stomatocytes are known to have an increased permeability to sodium; consequently, their osmotic fragility is increased.

Peripheral Blood Findings

Stomatocytes are more often artifactual than a true manifestation of a particular pathophysiologic process. The artifactual stomatocyte will have a distinct slitlike area of central pallor, whereas the area of pallor in the genuine stomatocyte will appear shaded. Stomatocytes may be found in patients with hereditary spherocytosis (the stomatospherocyte, viewed best in wet preparations), which is usually a benign condition but occasionally is hemolytic; in those with acute alcoholism; and in individuals with the Rh$_{null}$ phenotype.

Sickle Cells (Drepanocytes) (Color Plate 86)

Physiologic Mechanism

Sickle cells, or drepanocytes, are red cells that have been transformed by hemoglobin polymerization into rigid, inflexible cells with at least one pointed projection. These patients may be homozygous or heterozygous for the presence of the abnormal hemoglobin known as hemoglobin S. Conditions of low oxygen tension (in vivo or in vitro) cause the abnormal hemoglobin to polymerize, forming tubules that line up in bundles to deform the cell. The surface area of the transformed cell is much greater, and the normal elasticity of the cell is severely restricted. Most sickle cells possess the ability to revert to the discocyte shape when oxygenated, but approximately 10 percent of these cells are incapable of reverting to their normal shape. These irreversibly sickled cells (ISC) are the result of repeated sickling episodes. In the peripheral blood smear, they appear as crescent-shaped cells with long projections. When reoxygenated, ISCs may undergo fragmentation.

Classically sickle cells are best seen in wet preparations. Many of the cells observed in the Wright-Geimsa stain are oat cells, or the boat-shaped form of the sickle cell. In this form, the projections are much less pronounced, and the central area of the cell is fairly broad. This shape is reversible. During a symptomatic period the percentage of ISCs varies tremendously and consequently does not correlate with symptomatology.

Peripheral Blood Findings

Sickle cells are naturally seen in patients homozygous for hemoglobin S and are rarely seen in the heterozygous states. Several other hemoglobinopathies may exhibit sickling (for example, hemoglobin C Harlem and hemoglobin I). Hemoglobin O Arab does not sickle, but it facilitates the sickling process and therefore increases the severity of the S heterozygous state. Varying numbers of sickle cells may be seen in combination with other hemoglobinopathies and with the thalassemias.

Acanthocytes (Color Plate 82)

Physiologic Mechanism

An acanthocyte is a cell of normal or slightly reduced size, possessing 3 to 12 blunt-ended spicules of uneven lengths, distributed along the periphery of the cell membrane. The acanthocyte can easily be distinguished from the peripheral blood smear background because it appears to be saturated with hemoglobin.

The specific mechanism related to the formation of acanthocytes is unknown. Some details concerning these peculiar cells are of interest, however. Acanthocytes contain an excess of cholesterol and have an increased cholesterol-to-phospholipid ratio. Their surface area is increased. The lecithin content of acanthocytes is decreased. The only inherited condition in which numerous acanthocytes are seen is congenital abetalipoproteinemia. Most conditions in which acanthocytes are present are acquired, such as the deficiency of lecithin-cholesterol acyltransferase (L-CAT), which has been well documented in patients with severe hepatic disease. This enzyme, which is synthesized by the liver, is directly responsible for esterifying free cholesterol; consequently, a deficiency of this enzyme causes cholesterol to build up in the plasma.

The RBC responds to this excess cholesterol in one of two ways, depending on the balance of other lipids in the membrane: it will become either a target cell or an acanthocyte. The fluidity of the membrane is directly affected once an acanthocyte is formed; the membrane then is very liable to splenic sequestration and fragmentation.

Peripheral Blood Findings

As previously mentioned, acanthocytes are seen in high percentages in congenital abetalipoproteinemia. Variable numbers of acanthocytes may be observed in severe liver disease, hypothyroidism, and vitamin E deficiency, and in splenectomized patients. In patients in whom acanthocytes are acquired, some type of plasma factor may be operative. Evidence for this is suggested by the fact that blood cells transfused to these patients showed some acanthocyte formation within 5 days.

The Fragmented Cells (Burr Cells, Helmet Cells, Schistocytes) (Color Plates 119 to 124)

Physiologic Mechanism

Although it may seem unusual to group these three RBC forms under the same heading, the reason becomes clear with an expanded definition of fragmentation. As Cooper stated in 1980, fragmentation may be defined as "loss from the cell of a piece of membrane which may or may not contain hemoglobin." These events may occur repeatedly without the loss of hemoglobin; however, each successive loss of membrane (each fragmentation that occurs) leaves the red cell more rigid and more likely to become entrapped in the splenic sinuses. It is recognized that not all membrane alterations occur pathologically. Indeed, the echinocytic transformation of normal RBC in stored plasma is known to be reversible. Likewise, discocyte to echinocyte transformation is part of normal RBC senescence. However, certain triggering events in disease invariably lead to fragmentation.

Two mechanisms for fragmentation are recognized. First, alteration of normal fluid circulation occurs, which may predispose to fragmentation. Examples of this include vasculitis, malignant hypertension, thrombotic thrombocytopenic purpura, and heart valve replacement.

Second, intrinsic defects of the RBC make it less deformable and therefore more likely to be fragmented as it traverses the microvasculature of the spleen. Spherocytes, antibody-altered red cells, and red cells containing inclusions have significant alterations that decrease their RBC survival; these serve as examples of the second mechanism.

Peripheral Blood Findings

Burr cells (echinocytes) are red cells with approximately 10 to 30 spicules evenly placed over the cell surface. Burr cells are normochromic and mostly normocytic. They may be observed as an artifact, but can also occur in small numbers in uremia, heart disease, stomach cancer, bleeding peptic ulcer, immediately following an injection of heparin, and in a number of patients with untreated hypothyroidism. In general, burr cells may occur in situations that cause a change in tonicity of the intravascular fluid (for example, dehydration and azotemia).

Helmet cells are recognized by their distinctive projections—usually two—surrounding an empty area of the RBC membrane that looks as if it has been bitten off. In hematologic conditions in which large inclusion bodies (Heinz bodies) are formed, helmet cells are visible in the peripheral blood smear. Fragmentation occurs by the pitting mecha-

nism of the spleen. Helmet cells may also be seen in pulmonary emboli, myeloid metaplasia, and disseminating intravascular coagulation (DIC).

Schistocytes represent the extreme form of RBC fragmentation. Whole pieces of RBC membrane seem to be missing, and very bizarre RBCs are apparent. Schistocytes may be seen in patients with microangiopathic hemolytic anemia, DIC, heart valve surgery, hemolytic uremic syndrome, thrombotic thrombocytopenic purpura, and severe burns.

Teardrop Cells (Color Plate 214)

Physiologic Mechanism

Teardrop cells appear in the peripheral circulation as pear-shaped red cells. The extent to which a portion of the red cells forms a tail is variable, and these cells may be normal, reduced, or increased in size. The exact physiologic mechanism is unknown, yet teardrop formation from inclusion-containing red cells is well documented. As cells containing large inclusions attempt to pass through the microcirculation, the portion of the cells containing the inclusion gets pinched, leaving a tailed end, as it continues its journey. For some reason, the red cell is unable to maintain the discoid shape once this has occurred. The teardrop shape may also result from pulling the RBC membrane beyond its limit of deformability. In any of the pathologic conditions showing a congested spleen there may be the association of teardrop cells.

Peripheral Blood Findings

Teardrop cells are seen especially in myelofibrosis with myeloid metaplasia. This type of morphologic finding can also be seen in the thalassemia syndrome, in iron deficiency, and in conditions in which inclusion bodies are formed.

VARIATIONS IN RED CELL DISTRIBUTION

Agglutination (Color Plate 107)

If an erythrocyte antibody is present in a patient's plasma and if a corresponding erythrocyte antigen is represented, agglutination will take place. Such is the case with cold antibody syndromes such as cold hemagglutination disease and paroxysmal cold hemoglobinuria. The agglutination occurs at room temperature and will appear as interspersed areas of clumping throughout the peripheral blood smear. The use of saline will not disperse these agglutinated areas; however, warming the sample helps to break up the agglutination.

Rouleaux (Color Plate 225)

Rouleau formation is the result of elevated globulins or fibrinogen in the plasma. Red cells that are constantly bathed in this abnormal plasma have the appearance of a stack of coins, when observed in the peripheral blood smear. These stacks are rather evenly dispersed throughout the smear. The use of a saline dilution of the plasma will disperse rouleaux. Rouleau formation correlates well with a high erythrocyte sedimentation rate and occurs as a direct result of protein disposition or adsorption to the erythrocyte membrane. This lowers the zeta potential, thereby facilitating the stacking effect. Patients with multiple myeloma, Waldenström's macroglobulinemia, chronic inflammatory disorders, and some lymphomas will show rouleaux.

RED CELL INCLUSIONS
Howell-Jolly Bodies (Color Plate 65)

Howell-Jolly bodies are nuclear remnants containing DNA. They are 1 to 2 μm in size and may appear singly or doubly in an eccentric position on the periphery of the cell membrane. They are thought to develop in periods of accelerated or abnormal erythropoiesis. A fragment of chromosome becomes detached and is left floating in the cytoplasm after the nucleus has been extruded. Under ordinary circumstances the spleen effectively pits these nondeformable bodies from the cell. However, during periods of erythroid stress the pitting mechanism cannot keep pace with inclusion formation. Howell-Jolly bodies may be seen following splenectomy and in thalassemic syndromes, hemolytic anemias, megaloblastic anemias, and functional hyposplenia.

Basophilic Stippling (Color Plate 114)

Red cells that contain ribosomes can potentially form stippled cells; however, it is believed that the actual stippling is the result of the drying of cells in preparation for microscope examination. Coarse, diffuse, or punctate basophilic stippling may occur and consist of ribonucleoprotein and mitochondrial remnants. Diffuse basophilic stippling appears as a fine blue dusting, whereas coarse stippling is much more outlined and easily distinguished. Punctate basophilic stippling is a coalescing of smaller forms and is very prominent and easily identifiable. Stippling may be found in any condition showing defective or accelerated heme synthesis, in lead intoxication, and in thalassemia syndrome.

Sideroblastic Granules/ Pappenheimer Bodies (Color Plate 56)

Sideroblastic granules are small, irregular magenta inclusions seen along the periphery of RBCs. They usually appear in clusters, as if they have been gently placed upon the red cell membrane. Their presence is presumptive evidence for the presence of iron. However, the Prussian blue stain is the confirmatory test for determining the presence of these inclusions. These granules in red blood cells consist of nonheme iron caused by an excess of available iron throughout the body. They are designated "Pappenheimer bodies" when seen in a Wright-stained smear and "siderotic granules" when seen in Prussian blue stain.

Siderotic granules are found in sideroblastic anemias and in any condition leading to hemochromatosis or hemosiderosis. They may also be seen in the hemoglobinopathies, such as sickle-cell anemia and thalassemia, as well as following splenectomy.

Heinz Bodies (Color Plate 84)

Heinz bodies are formed as a result of denatured or precipitated hemoglobin. They can be formed experimentally by incubation with phenylhydrazine. They are large (0.2 to 2 μm) inclusions that are rigid and severely distort the cell membrane. Upon initial exposure to phenylhydrazine, small crystalline bodies appear, coalesce, and migrate to an area beneath the cell membrane. They may not be visualized in Wright's stain but may be seen with crystal violet and brilliant cresyl blue.

Heinz bodies may be seen in the thalassemia syndrome, in glucose-6-phosphate dehydrogenase (G6PD) deficiency under oxidant stress, and in any of the unstable hemoglobin syndromes. They may also be seen in RBC injury resulting from chemical insult.

Cabot's Rings (Color Plate 69)

The exact physiologic mechanism in Cabot's ring formation has yet to be elucidated. It is known that they appear in a "figure-eight" conformation like the beads of a necklace. They are not composed of DNA but do contain arginine-rich histone and nonhemoglobin iron.

Cabot's rings are rare morphologically but may be found in megaloblastic anemias, in homozygous thalassemia syndromes, and following splenectomy. Figure 5–1 pictorially summarizes the normal and abnormal RBC morphology previously discussed in this chapter.

PLATELET MORPHOLOGY
General Comments

The normal platelet has several morphologic characteristics. It is approximately 2 to 4 μm, with a discoid shape and evenly spaced blue granules dispersed throughout a light blue cytoplasm. In pathologic states platelets may appear as blue granular blobs; they may be extremely large; and they may show tailing or streaming of the cytoplasm. In rare instances, one may see megakaryocytic fragments in the peripheral circulation.

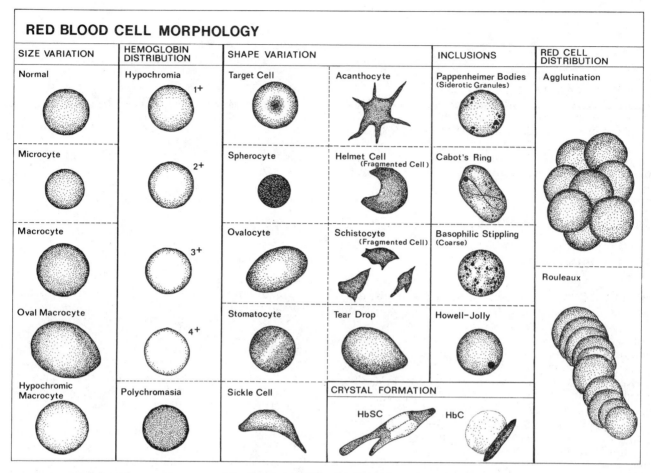

Figure 5–1.   Red blood cell morphology.

A thorough examination of platelet morphology will provide important information regarding the patient's hemostatic capability. Gross variation in platelet morphology may be seen in infiltrative disease of the bone marrow, such as myelofibrosis or metastatic infiltrates. Large platelets may occur in any disorder associated with increased platelet turnover as may occur with idiopathic thrombocytopenic purpura (ITP) or bleeding disorders. In addition to the elevated platelet count, morphologic changes also may occur after splenectomy.

WHITE BLOOD CELL MORPHOLOGY

White blood cells (WBCs, leukocytes) may exhibit several morphologic changes, with neutrophils as the cell type primarily affected. Most of these neutrophilic changes originate in the cytoplasm in response to various pathologic processes. Severe infections, inflammatory conditions, or other leukemoid reactions may be accompanied by toxic granulation, toxic vacuolization, or the presence of Döhle bodies (see Chapter 16). Toxic granulation and Döhle bodies are generally considered nonspecific reactive changes, whereas vacuolization strongly indicates a serious bacterial infection **(see Color Plates 128 to 130).**

Toxic granulation describes medium to large granules that are evenly scattered throughout the cytoplasm of segmented polymorphonuclear neutrophil leukocytes (PMNs). These granules are seen in metabolically active neutrophilia and are composed of peroxidases and acid hydrolases. Although nonspecific, they may occur in patients with severe bacterial infections, toxemia of pregnancy, or vasculitis, or in patients receiving chemotherapy. Toxic vacuolization refers to the round, clear unstained areas that are dispersed randomly throughout the cytoplasm of neutrophils in patients with overwhelming infections. Additional cytoplasmic inclusions—Döhle bodies—are oval, blue, single or multiple inclusions originating in RNA, and are 1 to 3 μm in diameter. Döhle bodies may be seen in peripheral blood smears of patients with severe infections, in patients with severe burns, in pregnant women, and in patients receiving chemotoxic drugs. In these conditions, they represent toxic changes; however Döhle bodies are also characteristically observed in certain congenital qualitative WBC disorders such as the May-Hegglin anomaly and the Chédiak-Higashi disorder (see Chapter 16) **(see Color Plates 131 and 134).**

In addition to these morphologic changes, severe

bacterial infections are also commonly associated with a moderate leukocytosis and a shift to the left in granulocytes. Mild infections are characterized by a slight leukocytosis, with or without the shift to the left. "Shift to the left" implies a release of younger granulocytes—specifically bands and metamyelocytes—from the bone marrow storage pool. These particular cell populations may often be observed during an infection or inflammatory process. The presence of more immature forms such as promyelocytes or myeloblasts, in the absence of severe infection, strongly suggests direct marrow architectural involvement. This may indicate an infiltrative, neoplastic, or myeloproliferative process.

The degree of leukocytosis or neutrophilia is useful in discriminating among bacterial, viral, or fungal conditions. Leukocytosis commonly refers to an increase in peripheral blood leukocyte (WBC) concentration of greater than 10,000 cells/mm. Because acute infection can rapidly mobilize the neutrophilic nondividing marrow storage pool, the patient usually has a WBC count below 50,000 cells/mm (average 25,000 cells/mm). A shift to the left is seen in the peripheral blood smear; however, it is unusual to see cells as immature as myelocytes in the peripheral blood. Fungal infections may also be associated with neutrophilia and an increased WBC count, but a monocytosis is more commonly observed. Viral infections usually are not associated with neutrophilia but rather with lymphocytosis (see Chapter 17).

Leukemoid reactions are characterized by a peripheral neutrophilia that may resemble an emerging leukemia. The WBC count is between 50,000 and 100,000 cells/mm, with immaturity observed in one or more cell types. However, a high blast count is not part of the WBC differential picture, which can be helpful in eliminating leukemia as part of the differential diagnosis. Acute infections, chronic infections such as tuberculosis (TB) and chronic osteomyelitis, as well as severe metabolic inflammatory and neoplastic processes have all been associated with leukemoid reactions. Extremely elevated WBC counts (greater than 100,000 cells/mm) are more suggestive of a myeloproliferative process (see Chapter 21), although exceptions have been reported.

Physiologic leukocytosis is defined as an increased WBC count without a shift to the left or any associated morphologic changes previously described for granulocytes. This transient condition may be associated with such stimuli as exercise, intense emotional stress, or the administration of epinephrine or glucocorticoids.

BIBLIOGRAPHY

Aarts, PA, et al: Red blood cell size is important for adherence of blood platelets to artery subendothelium. Blood 62(1):214, 1983.

Backman, L: Shape control in the human red cell. J Cell Sci (80):281, 1986.

Bacus, JW: Quantitative red cell morphology. Monogr Clin Cytol (9):1, 1984.

Bartels, PC and Roijers, AF: Effects of aging on preserved red blood cell populations as measured by light scattering. J Clin Chem Clin Biochem 26(1):29, 1988.

Bator, JM, et al: Erythrocyte deformability and size measured in a multiparameter system that includes impedance sizing. Cytometry 5(1):34, 1984.

Bauer, JD: Clinical Laboratory Methods. CV Mosby, St Louis, 1982.

Beck, WS: Hematology. MIT Press, Cambridge, MA, 1981.

Bessis, M, Weed, RI, and Leblond, PF: Red Cell Shape Physiology, Pathology, Ultrastructure. Springer-Verlag, New York, 1973.

Beutler, E, et al: The Woronets trait: a new familial erythrocyte anomaly. Blood Cells 6(2):281, 1980.

Buchanan, GR, Holtkamp, CA, and Horton, JA: Formation and disappearance of pocked erythrocytes: Studies in human subjects and laboratory animals. Am J Hematol 25(3):243, 1987.

Boggs, DR and Winkelstein, A: White Cell Manual, ed 4. FA Davis, Philadelphia, 1983.

Bolton, FG, Street, MS, and Pace, AJ: Changes in erythrocyte volume and shape in pregnancy. Br J Obstet Gynecol 89(12):1018, 1982.

Branton, D: Erythrocyte membrane protein associations and erythrocyte shape. Harvey Lect 77:23, 1981–1982.

Chasis, JA and Schrier, SL: Membrane deformability and the capacity for shape change in the erythrocyte. Blood 74(7):2562, 1989.

Christensen, RL and Triplett, DA: Neutrophil dysfunction: Quantitative and qualitative disorder. Lab Med 13(11):666, 1982.

Cohen, AR, Trotzky, MS, and Pincus, D: Reassessment of the microcytic anemia of lead poisoning. Pediatrics 67(6):904, 1981.

Cooper, RA: Hemolytic syndromes and red cell membrane abnormalities in liver disease. Semin Hematol 17:103, 1980.

Crouch, JY and Kaplow, LS: Relationship of reticulocyte age to polychromasia, shift cells, and shift reticulocytes. Arch Pathol Lab Med 109(4):325, 1985.

DeHaan, LD, et al: Alteration in size, shape and osmotic behavior of red cells after splenectomy: a study of their age dependence. Br J Hematol 69(1):71, 1988.

Florance, RK: Hemolytic manifestations of an RBC defect. Diagn Med 6(3):99, 1983.

Giraud, J, et al: Changes in morphology and in poly phosphoinositide turnover of human erythrocytes after cholesterol depletion. Biochem Biophys Res Commun 125(1):90, 1984.

Groner, W, et al: Variability of erythrocyte size and hemoglobin content observed in man and four selected mammals. Blood Cells 12(1):65, 1986.

Howard, J: Myeloid series abnormalities: Neutrophilia. Lab Med 14(3):147, 1983.

Inauen, W, et al: Erythrocyte deformity in dialysed and nondialysed uraemic patients. Eur J Clin Invest 12(2):173, 1982.

Johnson, CS, Tegos, C, and Beutler, E: Thalassemia minor: Routine erythrocyte measurements and differentiation from iron deficiency. Am J Clin Pathol 80:31, 1983.

Kapff, CT: Blood Atlas and Sourcebook of Hematology. Little, Brown, Boston, 1981.

Koeffler, HP and Golde, DW: Human preleukemia. Ann Intern Med 93:347, 1980.

Lange, Y and Stech, TL: Mechanism of red blood cell acanthocytosis and echinocytosis in vivo. J Membr Biol 77(2):153, 1984.

Leiter, SS: The human blood platelet: Its derivation from the red cell. Folia Haematol 111(6):60, 1984.

Lloyd, EM: How flowcharts improve RBC morphology reporting. Medical Laboratory Observer 49, 1982.

O'Conner, BH: A Color Atlas and Instruction Manual of Peripheral Blood Cell Morphology. Williams & Wilkins, Baltimore, 1984.

Pearson, HA: Red cell "rubbish" as a key to splenic function. Lab Man 25, 1982.

Rao, KR and Patel, AR: Erythrocytic ecdysis in shears of EDTA venous blood in eight patients with sickle cell anemia. Blood Cells 12(3):543, 1987.

Reich, PR: Hematology: Physiopathologic Basis for Clinical Practice. Little, Brown, Boston, 1984.

Reinhart, WH, and B'artsch, P: Red cell morphology at high altitude. Br Med J (Clin Res) 293(6542):309, 1986.

Reinhart, WH and Chien, S: Red cell vacuoles: Their size and distribution under normal conditions and after splenectomy. Am J Hematol 27(4):265, 1988.

Salt, HB and Wolf, OH: On having no beta lipoprotein: A syndrome comprising a beta-lipoproteinemia acanthocytosis and steatorrhea. Lancet 2:323, 1968.

Silinsky, JJ: Understanding red cell morphology. RN 47(11):99, 1984.

Smith, CM II, et al: Variable deformability of irreversibly sickled erythrocytes. Blood 58(1):71, 1981.

Spivak, JL: Fundamentals of Clinical Hematology. Harper & Row, Philadelphia, 1984.

Stewart, GW, et al: Stomatocytosis, abnormal platelets and pseudohomozygous hypercholesterolemia. Eur J Hematol 38 (4):376, 1987.

Takashima, S, Chang, S, and Asakura, T: Shape change of sickled erythrocytes induced by pulsed rf electrical fields. Proc Natl Acad Sci USA 82(20):6860, 1985.

Westerman, MP and Bacus, JW: Red blood cell morphology in sickle cell anemia as determined by image processing analysis: The relationship to painful crisis. Am J Clin Pathol 79:667, 1983.

Williams, WJ, et al: Hematology. McGraw-Hill, New York, 1990.

QUESTIONS

1. A peripheral blood smear showed some very small and some very large red cells. How would this finding be reported?
   a. Poikilocytosis
   b. Anisocytosis
   c. Both poikilocytosis and anisocytosis
   d. Marked poikilocytosis

2. How would a red cell be classified that has a diameter of 9 μm and an MCV of 104?
   a. Macrocyte
   b. Microcyte
   c. Normal
   d. Either normal or slightly microcytic

3. Which of the following conditions would show oval macrocytes?
   a. Iron-deficiency anemia
   b. Lead poisoning
   c. Megaloblastic anemia
   d. Hereditary spherocytosis

4. Which condition would not produce a microcytic blood picture?
   a. Thalassemia syndrome
   b. Iron-deficiency anemia
   c. Anemia of chronic disorders
   d. Myelodysplasia

5. How is a cell classified when the area of central pallor is increased beyond 3 μ?
   a. Microcytic
   b. Spherocytic
   c. Polychromatophilic
   d. Hypochromic

6. Which condition is most commonly associated with hypochromia? (Use answer choices for question 4.)

7. What type of disease may produce polychromatophilic cells?
   a. Condition that stimulates regenerative RBC processes
   b. Condition that produces abnormal hemoglobin
   c. Condition that produces a deficiency in RBC maturation process
   d. Condition that shows abnormal concentrations of cholesterol

8. Which of the following statements is true?
   a. Target cells are commonly found in myelofibrosis.
   b. Spherocytes are normally produced as a final stage of senescent RBCs.
   c. Ovalocytes are seen in thalassemia major.
   d. Stomatocytes may be found in patients with the Rh$_{null}$ phenotype.
   e. b and d are true statements.

9. What causes transformation of normal RBCs into sickle cells?
   a. Increased oxygen tension
   b. Exposure to certain antibiotics
   c. Low oxygen tension
   d. Enzyme deficiency

10. What type of cell is seen in myelofibrosis with myeloid metaplasia?
    a. Acanthocytes
    b. Burr cells
    c. Schistocytes
    d. Teardrop cells

11. Which type of red cell inclusion is a DNA remnant?
    a. Heinz bodies
    b. Howell-Jolly bodies
    c. Pappenheimer bodies
    d. Cabot's rings

12. What leukocyte cytoplasmic changes may be seen in severe infections or inflammatory conditions?
    a. Toxic granulation
    b. Toxic vacuolization
    c. Döhle bodies
    d. All of the above

ANSWERS

1. b (p. 66)
2. a (p. 66)
3. c (p. 67)
4. d (p. 67)
5. d (p. 67)
6. b (p. 67)
7. a (p. 68)
8. b (p. 68–69)
9. c (p. 69)
10. d (p. 70)
11. b (p. 71)
12. d (p. 72)

PART **TWO**

ANEMIAS

CHAPTER **6**

SUSAN J. LECLAIR, M.S., C.L.S.(NCA)

Iron Metabolism and Hypochromic Anemias

OBJECTIVES

At the end of this chapter, the learner should be able to:
1. State the primary function of iron in the body.
2. List factors that influence iron absorption.
3. Trace iron transport from ingestion to tissue and hemoglobin incorporation.
4. Name three stages of iron deficiency and describe findings associated with each stage.
5. List two major categories of iron deficiency.
6. Name the most diagnostic laboratory finding for iron-deficiency anemia.
7. List laboratory test results that help to distinguish iron-deficiency anemia from anemia of chronic disease.
8. Define hemosiderosis.
9. Describe typical laboratory findings for patients with sideroblastic conditions.
10. List three major classifications for porphyrias.
11. Specify characteristic findings in lead poisoning.

Because of its importance, there are many ways to evaluate hemoglobin. One method is to look at the molecule as a set of three independent, yet interdependent, components: iron, protoporphyrin IX, and globin chains. Disorders involving any of these three components will result in the development of a hemoglobin-deficient state and microcytic erythrocytes demonstrating hypochromia. In this chapter, the roles of iron and protoporphyrin are discussed. The first part of the chapter is a consideration of normal iron metabolism. In the second part, iron-deficiency anemia and iron utilization dysfunction are covered. The third part of the chapter presents a discussion of the hereditary porphyrias and the most common acquired heme disorder, lead poisoning (or intoxication). The chapter ends with case histories that illustrate some of these conditions. Globin chain abnormalities are presented in Chapter 12.

NORMAL IRON METABOLISM

The primary function of iron in the body is oxygen transport. A lesser function is participation in catalytic energy transfer and reactions. The average adult has a total body iron content between 3500 and 4000 mg. Found in a variety of sites in the human body, approximately two thirds (2500 mg) of this iron is bound to heme in hemoglobin. The remainder is found in storage pools of the marrow, spleen, and liver and in such compounds as myoglobin, myeloperoxidase, and some electron transfer proteins. Figure 6–1 illustrates the continuous process of daily iron turnover. Iron's importance in humans cannot be overstated, for studies have indi-

cated that damage caused during gestation by iron deficiency may be lifelong and that iron deficiency in adults is a major cause of morbidity and mortality—a statement of significance because 10 to 30 percent of the world's population is believed to be iron deficient.[1]

Biochemistry Review

The biochemical role of iron within human metabolism is to serve as a complex builder.[2] In most of

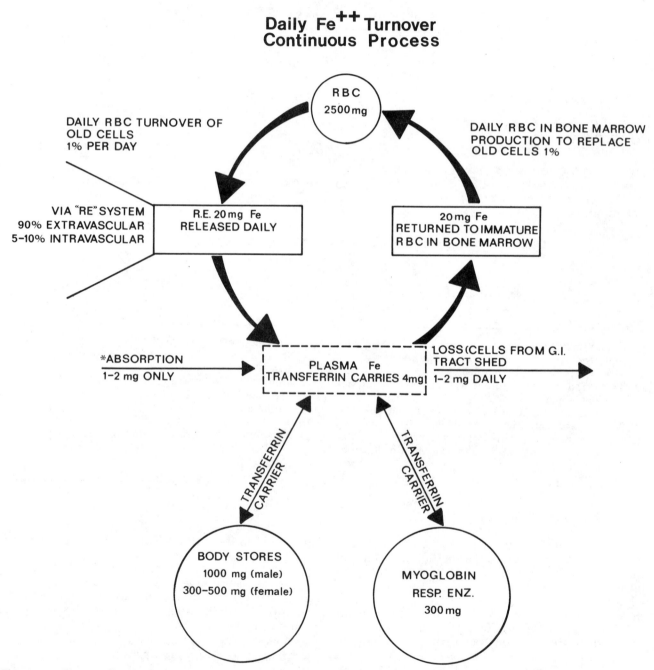

Figure 6–1. Diagram illustrating daily iron turnover and pathways of internal iron exchanges. (From Pittiglio, DH and Sacher, RA: Clinical Hematology and Fundamentals of Hemostasis, ed. 1. FA Davis, Philadelphia, 1987, p 42.)

these reactions, iron serves as a Lewis acid (electron pair acceptor). Transitional elements such as iron always try to attain electron stability by accepting electrons from ligands or electron pair donors. In hemoglobin, iron tries to become more stable by binding three molecules of oxygen. The relationship between iron as a Lewis acid and any available Lewis bases is dynamic and beyond the scope of this chapter. Simply put, increasing the strength of an available Lewis base will result in a more stable iron-containing complex. This is why carbon monoxide has a higher affinity for hemoglobin than oxygen and why oxygen is more acceptable to hemoglobin than water.[3]

Iron is more stable in the ferric (Fe^{3+}) state than in the ferrous (Fe^{2+}) state. Most of the iron in organic compounds, such as protein, is in the ferric state. Reduction of iron from the ferric to the ferrous state and its subsequent maintenance in human hemoglobin requires energy derived from the reduced form of nicotinamide adenine dinucleotide phosphate (NADPH) and a number of enzymatic reactions. The mechanisms involved in this are discussed more fully in Chapter 3.

Iron-Containing Compounds

Iron is found in a wide variety of animal and plant tissues. A significant iron concentration exists in both vegetables and meats. Plant tissue is a less accessible source of iron because vegetables contain less iron on a weight basis. In addition, many food items such as spinach and other green leafy vegetables contain substances such as phytates and phosphates that greatly interfere with iron absorption. Iron is in a more accessible form in meats because this source contains few insoluble complexes. Foods considered high in available iron include organ meats, wheat germ, brewer's yeast, and certain legumes. Foods with a moderate amount of iron include most muscle meats, fish, fowl, prunes, some green vegetables, and most cereals. Milk and non-green vegetables contain little available iron. Preparation of foods may also affect iron content. For example, pasta cooked in an iron container will contain more iron than pasta cooked in glass. Low molecular weight compounds such as fructose, amino acids, and other organic acids such as ascorbic acid (vitamin C) facilitate iron absorption.[4] However, despite the abundance of dietary iron, iron deficiency is the world's most common cause of anemia.

Iron-containing compounds are typically divided into two categories: heme and nonheme. The term "heme compound" refers to those proteins in which iron is complexed to a porphyrin. The most important of these are the oxygen carriers, hemoglobin and myoglobin. Figure 6-2 illustrates the iron-porphyrin bond (A) and compares it to a compound in which iron is not bound to a porphyrin (B). Nonheme iron-containing compounds include a large number of transfer and storage compounds such as transferrin, lactoferrin, and ferritin. Nonheme iron

M = methyl
V = vinyl

(A)

(B)

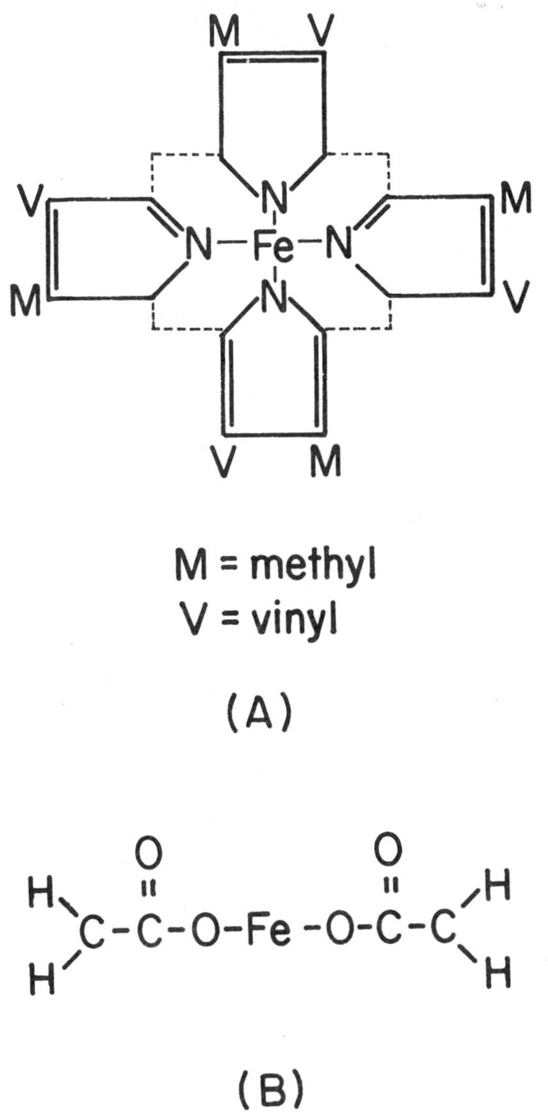

Figure 6–2. *A* is a representation of a *heme* iron compound; *B* is a representation of a *nonheme* iron compound.

is sometimes visible in developing erythroid cells. Inclusions that morphologically appear to correspond to nonheme iron are sometimes called Pappenheimer bodies. Only when these inclusions have been stained positively with an iron-specific stain, such as Perl's Prussian blue, are they called siderotic granules. Nucleated red cells containing stainable nonheme iron are called sideroblasts; non-nucleated red cells containing stainable iron are called siderocytes (**see Color Plate 56**).

Iron Requirements

A minor though sometimes confusing point is that of nomenclature. Iron is expressed in milligrams when the element is being described, whereas erythroid cells (that contain iron) are usually quantified in milliliters. Because 1 mg of iron is needed to produce 1 ml of erythrocytes, it is easy to become

Table 6–1. **MINIMUM DAILY REQUIREMENTS (MDR) FOR IRON***

	MDR (mg)	Iron Content of Food Required (mg)
Infants	1.0	10
Children	0.5	5
Women	2.0	20
Pregnant women	3.0	30
Men	1.0	10

confused about whether one is speaking of iron or hemoglobin. The average 1 percent (approximately 20 to 25 ml) red cell loss each day translates into 20 to 25 mg of iron needed to maintain homeostasis. However, humans typically absorb only 1 mg of dietary iron, or 5 percent of the required amount each day. Therefore, homeostasis requires that 95 percent of the total iron used for new red cell development each day must be recycled from normal RBC senescence. Iron recycling in the normal individual is extraordinarily efficient and recovers all iron except that lost through sweating, desquamated skin or fecal/urinary excretion, and, in women, menstruation.

Iron requirements vary with age and sex. Assuming adequate prenatal care and maternal stores, the typical neonate has approximately 300 mg in total body iron, all of which was transferred to the developing fetus from maternal stores during pregnancy. There is an increased need for iron during the growth spurt of the first 2 years of life and, particularly in males, during peak adolescent growth years. In males, this need for daily replacement levels off after adolescence and remains a constant requirement of 1 mg/day. The total body iron content for a man remains at approximately 2.5 to 4.0 g throughout adult life. The need for iron in premenopausal adult women is more variable because it is affected by both menstrual blood loss and pregnancy. In menstruating women, approximately 60 to 80 ml of blood is lost per month; therefore, an additional 1 to 1.5 mg of iron is needed daily to maintain iron balance. Approximately 2 mg of iron is lost daily during an uncomplicated pregnancy.[5] Compared with adult men and postmenopausal women, premenopausal women typically have both decreased iron ingestion and increased loss and, as a result, have lower storage iron concentrations ranging from 100 to 400 mg (Table 6–1). Because postmenopausal women do not have these increased losses, they have the same iron requirements as adult men, although they often have lower iron stores than men of the same age.

Iron Absorption and Storage

Iron absorption responds to daily need and is influenced by (1) the amount and type of iron accessible from food, (2) the functional state of the gastrointestinal mucosa and pancreas, (3) current iron stores, and (4) erythropoietic needs. As mentioned previously, iron exists in a wide variety of foods, although it may be more or less accessible for human absorption. Absorption is increased by ingestion of acidic foods such as citrus fruit juices along with the iron-containing foods.[6] Conversely, absorption is decreased by eating foods containing phosphates, phytates, or other compounds that form insoluble iron complexes.[7] Large amounts of dairy products also interfere with the conversion of ferric iron to ferrous iron. Although both the ferric (Fe^{+++}) and ferrous (Fe^{++}) states of iron are biologically active, the small intestine preferentially absorbs ferrous iron. The entire gastrointestinal (GI) tract has the capacity to absorb iron, but optimal absorption occurs in the duodenum and jejunum. The strongly acidic pH of the stomach in conjunction with pancreatic enzymes contribute to a favorable microenvironment for increased iron absorption in the duodenum and jejunum. Thus, iron absorption can be increased by maintaining a healthy gastric pH or decreased by an injudicious use of antacids.

In most developed countries, a typical diet contains less than 20 mg of elemental iron. Because only 10 percent of ingested iron is actually absorbed, the average daily absorption does not reach more than 2 mg of iron. Most well-nourished adult men absorb at least 1 mg of iron per day. Premenopausal women absorb approximately the same amount of iron but do so as a result of different conditions. They tend to eat less than men, but because the typical premenopausal woman's iron stores are lower than normal, the GI tract increases iron absorption. Circumstances such as pregnancy or recovery from anemia can cause the GI tract to absorb as much as 20 percent of ingested elemental iron. Supplementing foods with iron helps to prevent dietary iron deficiency. However, the tendency toward heavy supplementation of basic foodstuffs, such as wheat, must be balanced against the possibility of iron overload in susceptible people.

Though the dietary form of iron is usually in the ferric state, it is converted to the ferrous state when the gastric acid pH is less than 4.0 and in the presence of reducing substances such as ascorbic acid or glutathione. This ferrous form is absorbed through the mucosal cells of the duodenum and jejunum. Once in the bloodstream, ferrous iron is reconverted to the ferric state by serum ferroxidases. This reconversion allows iron to be carried by transferrin, a β-globulin with a molecular weight of 80,000 daltons that is synthesized in the liver and is a transport protein specific for iron. Two atoms of ferric iron can bind to each transferrin molecule, giving the protein a total iron binding capacity of 240 to 280 mg/dl. Because transferrin has a short half-life (8 to 10 days), any hepatic dysfunction that interferes with the liver's synthetic pathways will result in a relatively quick decrease in serum transferrin. Usually saturation of transferrin is approximately 30 percent; saturation of both of the two available binding sites, however, occurs in only 10 percent of transferrin. Figure 6–3 illustrates the relationship

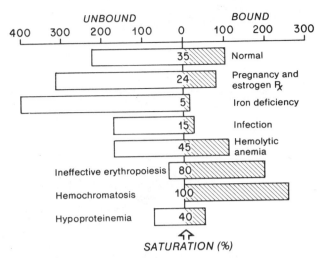

Figure 6-3. Transferrin and its iron. The reference range for serum iron ranges from 50 to 150 $\mu g/dl$ of plasma, with 10 $\mu g/dl$ being an average normal value. This represents only about one third of the binding capacity of transferrin so that the saturation (%) is about 30 percent. Both the serum iron and the total iron binding capacity are altered by disease states. Pregnancy is associated with a modest reduction in the serum iron and an increase in the total iron binding capacity. Iron deficiency shows an even more striking change with a major reduction in the serum iron and a dramatic increase in the total iron binding capacity, giving a percent saturation below 10 percent. In contrast, infection reduces both the serum iron and the total iron binding capacity. The pattern observed with most hemolytic anemias is quite different from that observed with marked ineffective erythropoiesis. In the hemolytic anemias, the plasma iron is relatively normal, while with ineffective erythropoiesis there may be an increase in the serum iron with near total saturation of the iron binding capacity. A similar pattern is seen with hemochromatosis. Severe starvation, nephrotic syndrome, and chronic inflammatory disease can result in marked hypoproteinemia with pronounced reductions in transferrin. (From Hillman, RS and Finch, CA: Red Cell Manual, ed. 5. FA Davis, Philadelphia, 1985, p 53, with permission.)

of iron and transferrin in a variety of conditions. Following absorption and transferrin binding, iron is delivered to body tissues because transferrin is freely distributed in extravascular fluids.[8] Transferrin can also directly release its iron content to developing red cells.

Once all immediate iron needs are satisfied, transferrin releases iron in the liver, where it is bound to ferritin, the major storage compound. An equilibrium between intracellular ferritin and serum ferritin exists. Thus, serum ferritin reflects the dynamic equilibrium of total iron stores and cellular requirements.[9] Quantitative serum ferritin assays were once thought to be a sensitive measure of iron metabolism. However, experience suggests that this test is an unreliable indicator if the patient is experiencing an acute inflammatory condition or hepatic injury.[10] In either situation, ferritin levels are unusually elevated and values may be misleading.

Another compound involved in iron storage is hemosiderin. Hemosiderin is a water-insoluble ferric hydroxide and partial apoferritin complex in a

pseudocrystalline form. It can be found in lysosomal membranes of macrophages. Temporary hemosiderin storage occurs commonly during hemoglobin degradation after senescent red cells have been phagocytized by macrophages. Less commonly, a more prolonged storage occurs after ferritin capacity has been reached. Hemosiderin can be visualized in bone marrow aspirates by staining with Prussian blue (**see Color Plate 47**).

Since only 1 mg of elemental iron is absorbed from dietary sources each day and approximately 20 mg of iron is needed to synthesize hemoglobin in replacement red cells, it is clear that the major source of the daily iron requirement is recycled iron liberated from senescent red cells. Dying red cells are phagocytized by cells of the mononuclear phagocytic system (MPS) and hemoglobin's degradation into bilirubin is begun. Microsomal enzymes within the macrophage allow the now nonheme iron to bind to transferrin, which in turn transfers it back to developing erythroid cells. This efficient system allows for the recycling of approximately 80 percent of iron released from hemoglobin. Ferric iron released from hemoglobin through hemolysis rather than phagocytosis is converted to ferrous iron by serum ferroxidases. This ferrous iron is then bound to transferrin, and the cycle continues. Figure 6-4 illustrates some normal sites and concentrations of iron utilization and storage over a 24-hour period.

CLINICAL SYNDROMES OF IRON METABOLISM

Iron Deficiency and Iron-Deficiency Anemia (IDA) (Color Plates 57 to 61)

Iron deficiency is a state in which iron stores in the body are inadequate to preserve homeostasis. Because this condition is acquired and progressive, the signs and symptoms range from asymptomatic to severe. As a result, three stages can be defined in the development of IDA (Table 6-2).

At the mildest extreme (stage I), in the face of a negative iron balance, iron stores are mobilized first and then body iron is depleted. In stage I, iron depletion, the hemosiderin content of the cells of the MPS in the marrow aspirate is decreased or absent. Serum ferritin levels (the storage form of iron) are decreased during this stage. An individual may not have any iron reserves yet be able to maintain a minimum equilibrium by increasing mucosal absorption of iron. This person is capable of maintaining homeostasis by mobilizing all available iron but is incapable of responding to any alteration in demand. As soon as this person fails to respond adequately to a challenge that increases iron utilization, a series of physiologic corrections is initiated.

Stage II is known as iron-deficient erythropoiesis. During this stage, transferrin levels, reflected in total serum iron binding capacities (TIBC), are increased in order to increase the absorption of di-

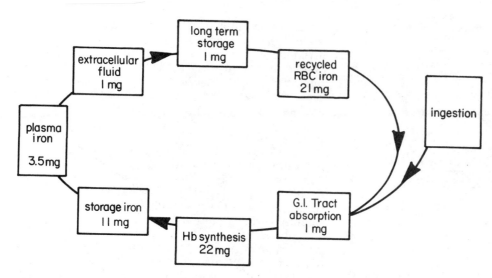

Figure 6-4. Brief overview of iron storage showing sites and concentrations of iron over a 24-hour period. Iron is absorbed by the intestinal mucosa, added to iron reclaimed from senescent red cells, and distributed to the developing normoblasts, plasma, intracellular fluids, and both long- and short-storage compounds, such as hemosiderin.

etary iron. In addition there is a fall in plasma iron, and transferrin saturation drops to less than 15 percent with an accompanying increase in red cell protoporphyrin levels. Free RBC protoporphyrin concentration increases because there is insufficient iron to convert protoporphyrin to heme. The decreased available iron limits hemoglobin synthesis even though there is no recognizable anemia

present on the peripheral blood smear; the red cells still appear normocytic and normochromic.

Stage III, iron-deficiency anemia, represents the very last stage and is characterized by a decrease in hemoglobin, hematocrit, and mean corpuscular volume (MCV). As a result, the process of red cell development becomes less efficient and is termed "ineffective erythropoiesis." Hemoglobin forma-

Table 6-2. **THREE STAGES IN THE DEVELOPMENT OF IRON-DEFICIENCY ANEMIA**

Tests	Normal	Stage I: Iron Depletion	Stage II: Iron-Deficient Erythropoiesis	Stage III: Iron-Deficiency Anemia
Peripheral Blood				
Hgb	N	N	>10 g/dl	<10 g/dl
Hct	N	N	N	DEC
RBC count	N	N	N	DEC
RBC morphology	N/N	N/N	M/N	M/N to M/H
Reticulocyte count (%)	N	N	SLT↑	INC 2-5%
Bone Marrow				
Stainable iron stores	N	N to DEC	0	0
Erythrocyte cellularity	N	N	HYPER	HYPER/INEFF
Sideroblasts (%)	40-60	N	DEC	DEC
Fe Studies				
Serum iron	N	N	DEC	DEC
TIBC	N	N	N/INC	N/INC
% Saturation	N	N	DEC	DEC
Ferritin	N	DEC	DEC	DEC
Hemosiderin	N	DEC	DEC	DEC
FEP	N	N	INC	INC
Iron absorption (%)	5-10	INC	INC	INC
Ferrokinetics*	N	N	Shortened	Shortened

*Half-life plus clearance from plasma.
N = within expected limits; DEC = decreased; SLT = slight; INC = increased; M = microcytic; HYPER = hyperplastic; H = hypochromic; INEFF = ineffective.

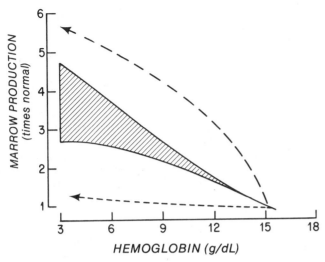

Figure 6-5. The role of iron supply and the degree of anemia in determining the erythroid marrow response. Moderate reductions in the hemoglobin level are largely compensated for by a shift in hemoglobin-oxygen affinity and do not elicit a maximal marrow response. With more severe anemia, the most important factor in determining the marrow production is the level of iron supply. When iron stores are exhausted (*lower dashed curve*), the erythroid marrow will not proliferate despite increased erythropoietin stimulation. In the presence of moderate to abundant iron stores, marrow production can increase from as little as two to as much as four times basal (*shaded area*). In contrast, patients with acute hemolytic anemia who have an ample iron supply from catabolized red cells will show production levels in excess of five times basal. With chronic hemolysis, sustained higher production levels with only moderate anemia are seen (*upper curve*). (From Hillman, RS and Finch, CA: Red Cell Manual, ed. 5. FA Davis, Philadelphia, 1985, p 31, with permission.)

tion is delayed, additional red cell division occurs during development, and microcytes result (**see Color Plates 57 and 58**). The anemia of iron deficiency is morphologically classified as microcytic hypochromic anemia with a decrease in red cell indices. Iron-deficiency anemia is also characterized by an increased red cell distribution width (RDW) and eventually a microcytic MCV calculation.[11] Eventually the diminished number of RBC will stimulate an increase in erythropoietin activity and a slight to moderate reticulocytosis will occur. Figure 6-5 illustrates the relationship of iron, anemia, and bone marrow response capability. If the primary cause of the condition is bleeding, leukocytosis and thrombocytosis are possible. If the anemia continues to progress beyond this point, abnormal shapes of RBC (poikilocytosis) will appear in the circulation. In the bone marrow, normoblasts will show decreased hemoglobinization and ragged cytoplasm (**see Color Plate 58**).

Clinical Signs and Symptoms

At some point in the progression of this condition, the clinical disease state begins. Patients begin to experience the classic signs and symptoms of anemia. Clinical symptoms of fatigue, lethargy, and dizziness are common. Elderly patients complain of palpitations, shortness of breath, and possibly chest pain. Clinical signs might include pallor of mucous membranes, cheilitis, koilonychia (spooning of the nails), and/or an apical systolic, or "hemic," heart murmur (**see Color Plates 59 and 60**). Occasionally, neurologic signs and symptoms are seen. Peculiar craving for unusual "foods" such as ice (pagophagia), clay (pica), dirt (glophagia), starch, or pickles is common in patients with iron-deficiency anemia. This manifestation is also seen in certain cultural subpopulations, however, and therefore cannot be used as evidence of an iron-deficient state.

Although the initial red cell values are within normal limits, they eventually become the classic hematologic values of moderate to severe anemia (Hgb less than 10 g/dl) and microcytic (MCV less than 80 fl), hypochromic (MCHC less than 30 percent) red cell morphology.

As one of the most common deficiency states seen, iron deficiency may have many different causes. However, all causes can be grouped into one of two major categories: low availability of iron and increased loss of iron-containing compounds or cells (Table 6-3). Low iron availability in children would include dietary inadequacy during times of growth and/or stress occurs in premature births, immediately postpartum, and during growth spurts in infancy.[12] Low availability also includes those conditions that interfere with the absorption of iron from the GI tract, such as celiac disease, defective gastric function, or achlorhydria, or following gastrectomy. Less common causes include copper deficiency, inherited or acquired inadequate production of transferrin, and steatorrhea.

Both children and adults commonly fail to achieve adequate dietary iron intake during weight reduction diets, particularly fad-type diets. Pregnant women are especially vulnerable to iron deficiency because they lose some maternal iron stores to the developing fetus. Finally, many older people,

Table 6-3. **COMMON CAUSES OF IRON DEFICIENCY**

Neonates	*Premenopausal Women*
Maternal iron deficiency	Menstrual blood loss
Fetomaternal hemorrhage	Inadequate diet and malabsorption
Multiple birth (e.g., twins)	Pregnancy
Adult Males and Post-Menopausal Women	*Not Specifically Age- or Sex-Related Causes*
Blood loss—typically chronic	Celiac disease
Inadequate diet	Inherited or acquired bleeding disorders
GI tract disease	Atransferrinemia
	Repeated blood donations and phlebotomies
Infants and Children	
Growth spurts	
Inadequate diet and malabsorption	

especially those living alone, find it difficult to cook an adequate diet and fall into the habit of a diet of tea and toast or milk and crackers.

The two most common conditions that result in iron deficiency due to increased loss are menstrual bleeding and chronic bleeding, most often in, but not limited to, the GI tract. Menstrual bleeding is the most common cause of iron deficiency in American premenopausal women. One common problem in confirming the etiology of iron-deficiency anemia due to menstrual blood loss is the inability of women to estimate normality of menstrual flow. Although the "normal" menstrual flow range is as large as 35 to 80 ml of blood per day, approximately 60 to 80 ml is considered average. In adult men and postmenopausal women the most common cause of increased iron loss is GI bleeding.[13] Indeed, a commonly held rule of thumb is to assume GI bleeding in any male with hematologic values suggesting an iron-deficient state. Gastrointestinal bleeding occurs commonly in all of the following intestinal diseases and disorders: malignancy, ulceration, inflammation, diverticulosis, infestation of certain parasites, and hemorrhoids. Causes of blood loss unrelated to the GI tract include parasite infestation or infection due to *Plasmodium* sp., *Babesia* sp., or *Bartonella bacilliformis* (these organisms produce chronic hemolysis). Other conditions that lead to increased blood loss include all of the bleeding disorders (inherited or acquired), hemoptysis (expectoration of blood), nosebleeds, and hematuria. Other, normal activities that can result in increased loss include repeated pregnancies, lactation, hemodialysis, and repeated blood donations.

Laboratory Values

Clinically iron deficiency can be characterized by two levels of severity. In the first, iron stores may be unacceptably low or even absent, while no clinical state of anemia exists. Unless the patient is investigated for some other complaint, the condition is typically not recognized by the physician or identified by the laboratory. There is adequate iron to maintain almost-normal red cell production. This subtle condition often goes undetected, for it would be difficult to know a priori that a person's hemoglobin value of 13.5 g/dl really should be 15.0 g/dl. The traditional laboratory-based definition of iron deficiency includes the absence of stainable iron in the bone marrow as the sine qua non of the condition. This is an important point because many premenopausal women have no stainable iron, yet do not have iron-deficiency anemia. Physicians treating patients who are at risk for iron deficiency without anemia are left with two unacceptable alternatives: prophylactic intervention with supplemental iron on the assumption of iron deficiency or no intervention until the condition becomes severe enough to demonstrate RBC numeric abnormalities.

Unless there is some intervention, the patient will eventually proceed from iron deficiency without anemia to the more serious state of IDA. Though anemia is a major consequence of the iron-deficient state, there are many other deficits that occur as a result of iron lack. Patients with IDA may show decreased or inefficient activity of other compounds that require iron for biologic activity. For example, decreased myeloperoxidase activity or a diminished T-cell function may be seen in conjunction with IDA. These deficits are usually not seen as critical in making the diagnosis or determining treatment. Moreover, many of the nonerythroid iron compounds are difficult to sample or measure. From the laboratory's standpoint, it becomes useful then to evaluate a patient's overall condition by the use of a few narrowly defined aspects (such as hemoglobin value, erythrocyte morphology, iron stores in the marrow) of iron deficiency.

Using these quantitative aspects as a guide, parameters available in modern hematology instruments can identify iron-deficient states at a much earlier stage of progression. An elevated red cell distribution width (RDW) in the absence of any other RBC numerical abnormalities is seen as a major diagnostic tool in the evaluation of iron-lack states. Classic laboratory values for iron deficiency anemia include a hemoglobin value of less than 10 g/dl and an RBC morphology consistent with an elevated RDW and low MCV, MCH, and MCHC values. Peripheral blood morphology should demonstrate microcytic hypochromic cells and a mild to moderate poikilocytosis (ovalocytes, elliptocytes, folded forms, and so on). The reticulocyte count will be within normal range to slightly elevated providing the end test result of the ineffective erythropoiesis of the bone marrow. Serum iron concentration is usually below 50 mg/dl. Total iron binding capacity may be normal to elevated with the percent saturation usually decreased below 15 percent (Table 6–4).

Evaluation of the bone marrow is not necessary for the diagnosis of iron deficiency. When performed, however, the bone marrow aspirate illustrates morphologic changes associated with faulty hemoglobin synthesis and increased cell death resulting in ineffective erythropoiesis. The aspirate shows a moderate increase in cellularity with erythroid hyperplasia that decreases the myeloid-to-erythroid (M:E) ratio in favor of the erythroid component. Normoblasts are smaller than normal. The cytoplasm is typically described as scanty. The usual comparison of hemoglobin content to nuclear maturity reveals an increase in the number and variety of cellular abnormalities as well, including karyorrhexis and nuclear fragmentation. As stated before, in iron deficiency sideroblasts are reduced or absent and the corresponding special stain for iron (Prussian blue) will be negative.

Treatment

Therapy of IDA demands the correction of the underlying cause. Dietary deficiencies can be corrected through nutrition counseling or oral medication. Malabsorption syndromes may or may not be corrected by diet alone. Correction of the primary disease state is the first choice, but if uncorrectable

Table 6–4. **DIFFERENTIAL DIAGNOSIS OF MICROCYTIC HYPOCHROMIC ANEMIAS**

	Iron Deficiency	Chronic Disease of Infection	Sideroblastic Anemia
Marrow iron	Decreased	Normal to increased	Increased
Sideroblasts	Decreased	Decreased	Increased (ringed sideroblasts)
Serum ferritin	Decreased	Normal or increased	Increased
Serum iron	Decreased	Decreased/increased	Normal or increased
TIBC	Increased	Normal or decreased	Normal or increased
% Iron saturation of transferrin	Decreased	Decreased	Normal or increased
FEP	Increased	Increased	Increased
Anisopoikilocytosis	Variable	Usually absent	Variable
Target cells	Few	Absent	Absent
Basophilic stippling	Absent	Usually absent	Mild to moderate

(for example, because of surgical loss of duodenal or jejunal tissue from some other disease), then supplementary iron in oral or intramuscular form is required. Recovery from anemia is first seen on the peripheral blood smear by the presence of a dual population of red cells: older cells that are microcytic and hypochromic as a result of iron deficiency and a younger, normochromic normocytic cell group able to make use of supplemental iron (**see Color Plate 61**). The second stage of recovery is equated with the reestablishment of normal hemoglobin concentration and marrow iron stores.

Whenever iron supplements are given, they should be considered as part of the therapeutic regimen. Any underlying disorders must be corrected if iron supplementation is to be effective. Typically, appropriate therapy consists of ferrous sulfate tablets or elixir. Parenteral therapy is available but not frequently used. Because iron absorption in the iron-deficiency patient is increased, as much as 20 percent absorption should occur, provided absorption is not impaired. Iron supplements can cause side effects (for example, nausea, diarrhea, constipation) and many patients prefer to take the medication with meals rather than before eating. Assuming the absorption is adequate, quantifiable changes will be seen quickly, regardless of the route of administration.[14]

Dysfunction of Iron Utilization

Usually secondary to another disease, iron deficiency may be caused by an inability of erythroid cells to access iron stored within macrophages. One common cause involves a blockage within mitochondria that prevents nonheme iron from being used by the developing red cell. Known as the anemia of chronic disease, this condition is thought to be influenced by the strong inflammatory component and suppressive effect found in diseases such as rheumatoid arthritis or increased immune hemolysis through cold agglutinins such as those found in infectious mononucleosis (anti-i) and infections by *Mycoplasma pneumoniae* (anti-I). Much

less frequently, ironlike deficiency can be caused by direct infection of red cell precursors by hepatitis B virus or parovirus. A primary chronic inflammatory disease with secondary microcytic hypochromic anemia is important to distinguish from a microcytic hypochromic anemia caused by iron deficiency due to nutritional deficit or blood loss. A more thorough discussion of anemia of chronic disease is found in Chapter 15.

Laboratory values for an ironlike anemia are less dramatic than those of iron deficiency. Typically, the whole blood hemoglobin is between 9 and 12 g/dl. The red cells are normocytic, normochromic, with some anisocytosis. The RDW is usually within reference limits. Important biochemistry test results include a decreased serum iron and a decreased TIBC. The decreased TIBC is important inasmuch as it helps distinguish this condition from iron-deficiency anemia, which typically has a high-normal to elevated TIBC.

Iron Excess/Sideroblastic States

Although the absorption of iron is carefully regulated to prevent overload, the sideroblastic state still occurs. Increased iron absorption and storage are seen in patients with inherited disorders and malignancies, and in those following food fad diets. Regardless of cause, similarities in morphology and hemogram values exist.

Hemosiderosis

Hemosiderosis is the accumulation of excess iron in macrophages in varying tissues. Most often, hemosiderosis has no significant signs or symptoms of its own but can occur secondary to bleeding into an organ such as the lungs or kidneys. For example, pulmonary hemosiderosis results from an accumulation of iron in the pulmonary macrophages after episodes of bleeding into the lungs and is found as a complication of the primary condition. This iron is bound to hemosiderin but is unavailable to the recycling process. The hemosiderin found in patients with primary or secondary hemochromatosis has an altered molecular structure compared with the hemosiderin found in healthy persons.[15]

Hemochromatosis

Hereditary hemochromatosis, on the other hand, is a significant and common disease in its own right.[16] This autosomal recessive disease is characterized by an iron absorption rate of up to 4 g daily.[17] Though this disease may actually begin early in childhood, the accumulation of iron occurs slowly and the complications of that accumulation often take time to become apparent. As a consequence, most patients with hemochromatosis are adults in their 50s or 60s. Men are more often afflicted than women. It is unknown whether this is due to some genetic predisposition or to the fact that women typically ingest less iron and eliminate more iron through menstrual bleeding or pregnancy or both. The major concern is the location of the iron deposits. Hemosiderosis occurs in the reticuloendothelial system (RES); hemochromatosis occurs in the parenchymal tissues of organs such as the pancreas, liver, and spleen, where it initiates a fibrotic process. This disease is often referred to as "bronze diabetes" because a major presenting syndrome consists of a type of adult-onset diabetes caused by fibrosis in the pancreas and a peculiar skin discoloration. The signs of "bronze diabetes" include weakness and weight loss (probably due to the diabetes) and excessive melanin deposits in the skin most frequently exposed to sun light. These patients can also develop cirrhosis of liver and heart failure (**see Color Plate 62**). Therapeutic removal of iron, either by phlebotomy or chelating agents, may lessen the degree of diabetes or heart failure. Repeated phlebotomies are the treatment of choice in patients with a hemoglobin value greater than 10 g/dl. Fewer donations are needed once an acceptable serum iron level is reached. The frequency is regulated by the need to keep the serum iron within acceptable limits. For patients who have a hemoglobin level of less than 10 g/dl or who show a decreased marrow response, the chelating agent deferoxamine is the treatment of choice.[18]

Sideroblastic States (Color Plate 63)

Primary sideroblastic anemia may be either inherited or acquired (Table 6-5). Hereditary sideroblastic anemia is a sex-linked disorder usually affecting men, though women also may develop some abnormalities. Some patients demonstrate hepatosplenomegaly. Approximately 50 percent of these patients respond to vitamin B_6 (pyridoxine) therapy. Idiopathic or acquired sideroblastic anemia, a type of myelodysplastic disorder, is discussed in Chapter 19.

Secondary sideroblastic anemia actually comprises a group of diseases with several different acquired mechanisms of iron overload. Some are acute, others chronic. Acute iron intoxication may be found in suicide attempts or accidental poisoning in children and will not be discussed here.

Table 6-5. CATEGORIES OF SIDEROBLASTIC ANEMIAS

Primary
Sideroblastic anemia—autosomal recessive
Congenital sideroblastic anemia—sex linked
Idiopathic sideroblastic anemia (RARS)

Secondary
Secondary to Other Disease States
  Infections
  Neoplasms
  Acute or chronic inflammation
Secondary to Toxic Exposure
  Chronic alcohol abuse
  Unusual dietary habits or culture
  Lead poisoning
Iatrogenic
  Chronic transfusion support
  Antitubercular medications (e.g., isoniazid)
  Antiparkinsonian medications
  Antibiotics (e.g., choramphenicol)

Clinical Signs and Symptoms

An iatrogenic secondary sideroblastic state is seen in patients taking antitubercular antimicrobial or antiparkinsonian drugs (inhibitors of pyridoxine metabolism). Chloramphenicol treatment also causes iron overload due to the combined aplasia and cytosol abnormalities found in the p10 region of the 50s subunit of ribosomes. Iatrogenic sideroblastosis occurs also in patients who need chronic transfusions such as those with aplastic anemia, thalassemia, and leukemia. Because these patients usually have a normal dietary intake of iron, the combination of normal intake and increased iron from transfusions results in increased absorption and storage.

Chronic iron overload is achieved by an increased iron uptake accompanied by increased iron absorption. Although seen among such cultural groups as the Bantu tribe of South Africa (due to use of iron utensils) and certain tribes of Mancurian hunters (due to Kashin-Beck disease, iron utensils, and heavy concentration of iron in well water), this condition is much more commonly seen in the developed countries in persons who are food faddists and take megavitamins or mineral supplements. Alcoholics too may have an increased iron absorption (alcoholic beverages have an iron content that ranges from 5 to 20 mg/liter), although their condition may be complicated by folate deficiency, cirrhosis, or lead poisoning.

Laboratory Values

A patient with any of these sideroblastic conditions typically presents with mild to moderate anemia, variable red cell indices, and an elevated RDW with a significant widening of the RBC histogram. This suggestion of a dual population is borne out in the evaluation of the peripheral blood smear, in which anisopoikilocytosis and Pappenheimer bodies are seen (**see Color Plate 56**). Care must be used to differentiate Pappenheimer bodies from basophilic stippling, which also occurs in these patients. Reticulocyte counts are decreased. Microscopic examination of the bone marrow aspiration shows erythroid hyperplasia resulting from ineffective erythropoiesis. Since mitochondria are usually located around the nucleus of developing normoblasts and the iron is entrapped within them, Prussian blue staining will sometimes create the halolike effect around the negatively stained nucleus. Ringed sideroblasts are found in normal bone marrow aspirates, but patients with any of the sideroblastic anemias will commonly have a significant increase in the number of ringed sideroblasts. Furthermore, these patients will have a significant number of siderotic granules in peripheral blood erythrocytes. Greater than 10 percent positive-staining cells is common. In addition to the increased iron absorption seen in many of these patients, there is also an ineffective erythropoiesis due to the failure to utilize nonheme iron trapped in the mitochondria. As a consequence of the engorgement of the normal iron deposits, the serum iron and marrow iron stores are elevated and additional deposit sites in the liver and spleen occur. Table 6–4 compares these microcytic hypochromic states.

Treatment

Treatment of these secondary disease states must be directed at the primary disturbance. Simple steps include diet modification or changes in therapeutic regimens requiring antimicrobial agents or transfusions. More difficult to implement are regimens involving cultural mores or addictive behaviors. Aggressive therapies include repeat phlebotomies or chelation agents, or both.

Lead Poisoning (Acquired Sideroblastic Anemia or Acquired Porphyria) (Color Plate 114)

Similar to both porphyria and sideroblastic anemia, lead intoxication produces a microcytic hypochromic anemia, skin lesions, and neurologic dysfunctions.[19] Lead consumption produces two coincidental and synergistic effects: first, it interferes with iron storage in the mitochondria, thus producing a classic sideroblastic anemia. When severe enough, the mitochondrial buildup of iron can be shown by Prussian blue staining.[20] Second, lead has a damaging effect on the activity of at least six of the enzymes used in heme synthesis: δ-aminolevulinic acid (ALA) dehydrogenase synthetase, ALA dehydrase, porphyrinogen oxidase, uroporphyrinogen decarboxylase, coproporphyrinogen oxidase, and heme synthetase. Delta-aminolevulinic dehydrase is most sensitive to the presence of lead, and the resultant elevations in ALA is an early sign of

lead intoxication.[21] Although other precursors may also be elevated, measurement of increased quantities of zinc-bound protoporphyrin (also known as free erythrocyte protoporphyrin, or FEP) caused by dysfunctional heme synthetase within the red cell is widely used as a diagnostic tool.

It was hoped that lead poisoning as a major disease could be diminished through the enactment of laws regulating the manufacture of lead-based paint and other lead-based substances. Unfortunately this has not been the case, and the incidence of lead intoxication is still a concern, especially in large urban settings. Lead intoxication occurs in both children and adults, although the mechanism of exposure and clinical sequelae of that exposure are quite different. Children may be exposed to lead by eating sweet-tasting lead-based paint that is flaking or by inhaling the powdery residue from lead-based paint. This paint, sometimes hidden under several layers of newer paints, can often be found in older homes. Infants and toddlers are particularly sensitive to the effects of lead exposure, and moderate to severe mental retardation can result. There may also be abdominal pains and cramping (abdominal colic) following lead exposure of this type. Adults may be exposed to lead in the workplace (for example, in the manufacture of batteries or decoration of pottery in which lead is used in the underglazing processes. Adults tend to complain of peripheral neuropathy and skin lesions as well as abdominal pains, but mental retardation is not an issue in adult-onset lead poisoning. Another difference between adult and pediatric patients with lead intoxication is the complicating state of iron deficiency. Many infants and toddlers will also have iron deficiency due to poor nutrition during gestation and during the formative growth spurt of the first 2 years.[22]

The interference of lead with heme synthesis results in an ineffective erythropoietic state in which shortened red cell survival and difficulty in heme synthesis produce a mild hypochromic microcytic anemia. Basophilic stippling is found in many circulating RBCs and may occur due to other lead-induced enzyme dysfunctions. As a result of RBC inclusions, damaged enzymes, and inadequate hemoglobinization, erythrocyte osmotic fragility may be decreased. Reticulocytosis may or may not be present. Hemoglobin A_2 or F may be elevated and ineffective erythroid hyperplasia is seen in the marrow.

Both children and adult victims of lead poisoning are usually treated with chelation therapy. Ethylenediaminetetracetic acid (EDTA) binds irreversibly to lead to produce a lead chelate that is neurologically toxic but rapidly excreted in the urine. Therapy will eliminate the lead; however, those cells that have been damaged will remain in that state until senescence. Newest studies indicate that damage sustained during the acute phase of lead intoxication is never completely repaired, regardless of therapy.[23]

HEME SYNTHESIS AND RELATED DISORDERS

Normal Heme Synthesis

The term "heme synthesis" is reserved for those steps involving the synthesis of protoporphyrin IX (heme without the iron). Heme synthesis is a series of eight enzymatic reactions that involve time- and concentration-dependent equilibria among substrates, enzymes, and cofactors, with each product acting as the substrate for the next step. A defect causing a slower reaction rate or a lessened amount of product results in the accumulation of substrate. Some accumulated substrates are inherently unstable and metabolize into porphyrins, a class of stable but highly resonating compounds. Defects occurring in either of the first two steps result in the formation of compounds loosely called porphyrin precursors.

The intermediate substrates occurring after the second step in the pathway are forms of porphyrinogen,[24] which, if unused in normal heme synthesis, degrade into small amounts of porphyrins easily excreted in the urine. Excessive formation of porphyrins occurs if any one of the normal enzymatic steps in heme synthesis is blocked and results in one of a number of metabolic disorders collectively called the porphyrias. (For a more detailed explanation of heme synthesis, see Chapter 3.)

Abnormal Heme Synthesis

Disorders of heme synthesis (porphyrias) can be either inherited or acquired. In either case, abnormal accumulation of porphyrin precursors or porphyrins occurs in the two major sites of heme synthesis—the bone marrow and the liver, respectively. The inherited porphyrias are uncommon and are classically categorized by the mode of transmission, the defective enzyme, and the porphyrin allowed to accumulate. Clinically, these disorders are categorized by site of accumulation and major signs and symptoms.[25] Using this method, porphyrias are divided into three major classes: (1) erythropoietic porphyrias—accumulation of porphyrins in the bone marrow associated with high incidence of photosensitivity and dermatitis; (2) hepatic porphyrias—accumulation of porphyrin precursors in the liver associated with neurologic deficit; and (3) mixed porphyrias—accumulation in both bone marrow and liver resulting in both neurologic and dermatologic involvement (Table 6–6).

Inherited Porphyrias

These disorders are listed in chronologic sequence. There have been no reported instances of defective generation of ALA synthetase. Cases of defective ALA dehydrase have been reported, but the process has not been completely characterized. Defects in uroporphyrinogen I synthetase result in the buildup of porphobilinogen and ALA. Occur-

Table 6–6. **INHERITED HEME SYNTHESIS DISORDERS**

Erythropoietic porphyrias (hematology and/or skin manifestations)
  Congenital erythropoietic porphyria (congenital photosensitive porphyria)
  Porphyria cutanea tarda
Hepatic porphyrias (neurologic and/or hepatic manifestations)
  Acute intermittent hepatic porphyria (acute or Swedish-type porphyria)
  Hereditary coproporphyria (benign coproporphyria)
  Erythropoietic protoporphyria (congenital erythropoietic protoporphyria)
Mixed porphyrias (variable manifestations)
  Variegate porphyria (mixed hepatic porphyria)

ring after adolescence, this disease is characterized by attacks of abdominal colic of varying frequency and by chronic hypertension. Colic attacks can be initiated by the use of various medications such as aspirin. This disease with its acute exacerbations, hepatic accumulation of substrate, and neurologic problems is called acute intermittent hepatic porphyria.

Congenital erythropoietic porphyria (**see Color Plate 55**) is the least common of these rare disorders[26] and occurs when the defective enzyme is uroporphyrinogen III cosynthetase, with a resultant buildup of uroporphyrin II and III and coproporphyrin in the bone marrow, with onset in early childhood or infancy. Because this disease involves an accumulation of porphyrins in developing red blood cells, RBC survival time is shortened. The hemolytic process develops into a hemolytic anemia with splenomegaly and ineffective erythropoiesis. Dermal photosensitivity occurs as a result of the accumulation of fluorescing compounds such as coproporphyrin.

Porphyria cutanea tarda has the greatest variety of causes. Biochemically it results from functional loss of uroporphyrinogen decarboxylase, with an increase in urinary uroporphyrin and coproporphyrin. It can be inherited or acquired. Severe liver disease, usually related to exposure to toxic chemicals such as benzene or alcohol, is a common cause. There is no neurologic dysfunction because porphyrin precursors do not accumulate in the central nervous system (CNS), although there is sufficient accumulation of porphyrin precursors in the skin to cause lesions. These lesions include ulceration on exposed areas or in response to trauma, erythema, vesicles or bullae (sometimes hemorrhagic), scabs, and scarring. In addition, there may be areas of pigmentation or depigmentation, hirsutism, and sclerodermalike changes. Occasionally these patients have coexisting liver disease.

Hereditary coproporphyria is characterized by acute attacks of abdominal pain and neurologic involvement. This disease is caused by a loss of coproporphyrinogen oxidase, with a subsequent buildup of coproporphyrin. Remissions may be prolonged so that biochemical testing for porphobilinogen and ALA may be within expected ranges.

Variegate porphyria is inherited as an autosomal dominant disorder. One interesting aspect of this disease is its incidence in South Africa, where sufferers are all descendants of a single Dutch settler family. The clinical manifestations are remarkably like those of porphyria cutanea tarda, and many people refer to this disease as "porphyria cutanea tarda hereditaria." Biochemical testing of the urine is required for a differential diagnosis. Signs and symptoms include dermal photosensitivity and mechanical fragility of skin, along with possible attacks of abdominal colic and neurologic involvement. This disorder may be responsible for the mental instability of Mary, Queen of Scots, and of her indirect descendant, King George III. Onset of attacks is usually precipitated by drugs. It is caused by a loss of protoporphyrinogen oxidase and a buildup of coproporphyrin and protoporphyrin. Incidence of this disease is difficult to confirm because (1) there are geographic, familial, and drug considerations; and (2) the disease may be easily misdiagnosed.[27]

Finally, there is erythropoietic protoporphyria. Dermal photosensitivity and solar erythema, urticaria, and eczema with onset in childhood characterize the loss of heme synthetase and the buildup of protoporphyrin. Inherited as a possible autosomal dominant, it is seen throughout the world. Protoporphyria is usually considered a relatively benign disorder, concentrated in skin lesions, although many patients also have liver and biliary tract dysfunctions.

CASE STUDY 1

An 18-year-old woman came to her physician for a routine physical examination before entering college. Family history was unremarkable. Her personal history revealed that she had begun menstruation at the age of 13 and had experienced no complaints other than cramping. Other than an occasional cold, she stated that she was perfectly healthy.

On physical examination, she appeared to be well nourished and looked her stated age. Mucous membranes were pale. Her overall muscle tone was poor but she explained that "she just wasn't very athletic." Her pulse was 80 beats per minute, and her blood pressure within normal limits. A grade I apical murmur was noted.

Results of laboratory tests included WBC 11.4 × 10^9/liter, Hgb 10.0 g/dl, MCV 79 fl, RDW 14.8, PLT 400 × 10^9/liter. Microcytes, some hypochromic cells, and polychromatophilic RBCs were seen on the peripheral blood smear. The reticulocyte count was 2.5%.

Questions: Case Study 1

1. *What is the most likely explanation of this presentation?*
   a. Iron-deficiency anemia
   b. Lead poisoning
   c. Hemochromatosis
   d. Acute intermittent porphyria

2. *What are the next laboratory tests that need to be performed? (see p. 84)*
   a. Bone marrow aspiration
   b. Hemoglobin electrophoresis
   c. Serum iron and TIBC
   d. Serum lead and FEP

3. *If the serum iron was abnormally low and the TIBC slightly elevated, what would you conclude about the state of iron storage in the bone marrow?*
   a. Iron stores are adequate.
   b. Iron stores are absent.
   c. Bone marrow hemosiderin is adequate.
   d. Insufficient information is given to answer the question.

4. *What questions need to be asked before initiation of any therapy?*
   a. Questions concerning her dietary habits
   b. Questions concerning exposure to any chemicals, lead, and so forth
   c. Questions that would elicit more detailed information concerning the frequency, duration, and severity of menstrual blood loss
   d. Questions regarding possible allergy or extreme sensitivity to ferrous sulfate medication

5. *Assuming that the correct medications have been given and it is 1 month later, what statement could be made about this young woman's condition?*
   a. Her hemoglobin concentration is now above 12.0 g/dl.
   b. Iron stores have been replenished in the bone marrow.
   c. Serum ferritin is increased but plasma iron is not.
   d. The TIBC is completely saturated.

CASE STUDY 2

A 36-month-old male of Sicilian ancestry was seen by his pediatrician to investigate a complaint of irritability and "coliclike pain." The child's birth weight was 7 pounds, 9 ounces. The mother's pregnancy and delivery had been without complication. Early developmental milestones were achieved without incident. Approximately 1 month earlier, the child had become unusually irritable in response to otherwise normal activity. This had been accompanied by signs of abdominal discomfort and diarrhea.

Physical findings included pale mucous membranes and a thin dark line around the gums. Neurologic examination showed increased irritability and decreased ability to maintain normal concentration. The rest of the examination was unremarkable.

Hematologic test results included WBC 14.5 × 10^9/liter, Hgb 9.7 g/dl, MCV 77 fl, and RDW of 15.5. Peripheral blood morphology demonstrated the presence of microcytic hypochromic cells, normocytic normochromic cells, basophilic stippling, and nonspecific poikilocytosis. Rare nucleated RBCs were seen on microscopic scan of Wright-stained peripheral blood smear.

Questions: Case Study 2

1. *What is the best explanation of this child's condition?*
   a. Iron-deficiency anemia
   b. Lead poisoning
   c. Hemochromatosis
   d. Acute intermittent porphyria

2. *What are the next laboratory tests that need to be performed?* (see p. 87)
   a. Bone marrow aspiration
   b. Hemoglobin electrophoresis
   c. Serum iron and TIBC
   d. Serum lead and FEP

3. *If the serum lead and FEP were elevated, what would you conclude about the state of iron storage in the bone marrow?*
   a. Iron stores are adequate.
   b. Iron stores are absent.
   c. Bone marrow hemosiderin is adequate.
   d. Insufficient information is given to answer the question.

4. *Which of the following enzymes needed for heme synthesis is altered in lead poisoning?*
   a. δ-Aminolevulinic acid synthetase
   b. Uroporphyrinogen decarboxylase
   c. Coproporphyrinogen oxidase
   d. Heme synthetase
   e. All of the above

5. *Why does treatment of lead poisoning involve chelation therapy and iron supplements?*
   a. Chelation drugs always interfere with iron metabolism.
   b. Many children who have lead poisoning also have a dietary iron deficiency.
   c. Iron supplements help to reestablish the normal iron concentrations.
   d. Iron supplements bind to excess chelation agents.

Answer Key: Case Studies

Case Study 1
1. a (see p. 82–83)
2. c (see p. 84)
3. b (see p. 82)
4. c (see p. 84)
5. b (see p. 85)

Case Study 2
1. b (see p. 87)
2. d (see p. 87)
3. d (see p. 87)
4. e (see p. 87)
5. b (see p. 87)

REFERENCES

1. Dallman, PR: Iron deficiency: Does it matter. J Intern Med 226(5):367, 1989.
2. Weinberg, ED: Cellular regulation of iron assimilation. Q Rev Biol 64(3):261, 1989.
3. Bhagavan, NV: Biochemistry, ed 2. JB Lippincott, Philadelphia, 1978, 676.
4. Bothwell, TH, et al: Nutritional iron requirements and food iron absorption. J Int Med Res (England) 226(5):357, 1989.
5. Beck, WS (ed): Hematology. MIT Press, Cambridge, MA, 1985.
6. Hallberg, L, Brune, M, and Rossander, L: The role of vitamin C in iron absorption. Int J Vitam Nutr Res (Suppl)30:103, 1989.
7. Conrad, ME and Barton, JC: Factors affecting iron balance. Am J Hematol 10:199, 1981.
8. Nimeh, N and Bishop, RC: Disorders of iron metabolism. Med Clin North Am 64:631, 1980.
9. Finch, CA and Huebers, H: Perspectives in iron metabolism. N Engl J Med 306:1520, 1981.
10. Ahmadzadeh, N, Shingu, M, and Nobunaga, M: Iron-binding proteins and free iron in synovial fluids of rheumatoid arthritis patients. Clin Rheumatol (Belgium) 8(3):345, 1989.
11. Qurtom, HA, et al: The value of red cell distribution width in the diagnosis of anaemia in children. Eur J Pediatr 148(8):745, 1989.
12. Dallman, PR, Siimes, MA, and Stekel, A: Iron deficiency in infancy and childhood. Am J Clin Nutr 33:86, 1980.
13. Fairbanks, VF and Beutler, E: Iron deficiency. In Williams, WWJ, et al (eds): Hematology, ed 3. McGraw-Hill, New York, 1983, p 300.
14. McCurdy, PR: Oral and parenteral iron therapy: A comparison. JAMA 191:859, 1965.
15. Ward, RJ, et al: Biochemical studies of the iron cores and polypeptide shells of haemosiderin isolated from patients with primary or secondary haemochromatosis. Biochem Biophys Acta 993(1):131, 1989.
16. Haddy, TB, Castro, OL, and Rana, SR: Hereditary hemochromatosis in children, adolescents, and young adults. Am J Pediatr Hematol Oncol 10(1): 23, 1988.
17. Lynch, SR, Skikne, BS, and Cook, JD: Food iron absorption in idiopathic hemochromatosis. Blood 74(6):2187, 1989.
18. Pippard, MJ: Desferrioxamine-induced iron excretion in humans. Baillieres Clinica Haematology 2(2):232, 1989.
19. Dagg, JG, et al: The relationship of lead poisoning to acute intermittent porphyria. Q J Med 34:163, 1965.
20. Albahary, C: Lead and hemopoiesis. Am J Med 52:369, 1972.
21. Lichtman, HC and Feldman, F: In vitro pyrrole and porphyrin synthesis in lead poisoning. Pediatrics 31:996, 1963.
22. Wintrobe, MM, et al (eds): Clinical Hematology, ed 8. Lea & Febiger, Philadelphia, 1981, pp 662–664.
23. Needleman, HL, et al: The long term effects of exposure to low doses of lead in childhood. N Engl J Med 322(2):83. 1990.
24. Robinson, SH and Glass, J: Disorders of heme metabolism: Sideroblastic anemia and the porphyrias. In Nathan, DG and Oski, FA (eds): Hematology of Infancy and Childhood, ed 2. WB Saunders, Philadelphia, 1981, pp 336–391.
25. Thompson, RB and Procter, SJ: A Concise Textbook of Hematology, ed 6. Urban & Schwarzenberg, Baltimore, 1984, p 48.
26. Meyers, US and Schmid, R: The porphyrias. In Stanbury, JB, Wyngaarden, JB, and Frederickson, DS (eds): The Metabolic Basis of Inherited Disease, ed 4. McGraw-Hill, New York, 1978, p 1166.
27. Dean, G and Barnes, HB: The Porphyrias: A Story of Inheritance and Environment. Pitman, London, 1963.

QUESTIONS

1. *What is the primary function of iron?*
   a. Molecular stability
   b. Oxygen transport
   c. Cellular metabolism
   d. Cofactor

2. *Which of the following influence(s) iron absorption?*
   a. Amount and type of iron in food
   b. Function of GI mucosa and pancreas
   c. Erythropoietic needs and iron stores
   d. All of the above

3. *What is the correct sequence for iron transport?*
   a. Ingestion, conversion to ferrous state in stomach, reconversion to ferric state in bloodstream, transport by transferrin, incorporation into cells and tissues
   b. Ingestion, transport by transferrin to liver, conversion in liver to ferric state, transport in ferrous state to cells and tissues for incorporation
   c. Ingestion, conversion to ferrous state in stomach, transport in bloodstream to cells and tissues, conversion to ferric state prior to incorporation into cells and tissues
   d. Ingestion, transport by transferrin to cells and tissues, conversion to ferrous state prior to incorporation into cells and tissues

4. *Which of the following is not consistent with the finding for a stage of iron deficiency?*
   a. Stage I: iron depletion; decreased serum ferritin levels; depletion of stored iron; equilibrium maintained through compensation mechanisms
   b. Stage II: iron-deficient erythropoiesis; increased TIBC; decreased plasma iron and transferrin saturation; normocytic, normochromic RBCs
   c. Stage III: iron-deficiency anemia; decreased hemoglobin, hemocrit, and MCV; microcytic, hypochromic anemia; increased RDW
   d. Stage IV: chronic iron-deficiency anemia; decreased hemoglobin, hemocrit; increased MCV; macrocytic, hypochromic anemia; decreased RDW

5. *What are the two major categories of iron deficiency?*
   a. Defects in globin synthesis and iron incorporation
   b. Low availability and increased loss of iron
   c. Defective RBC catabolism and recovery of iron
   d. Problems with transport and storage of iron

6. *What is (are) the most diagnostic laboratory finding(s) for IDA?*
   a. Increased RDW
   b. Decreased MCV, MCH, MCHC
   c. Ovalocytes, elliptocytes, microcytes
   d. Increased TIBC

7. *Which laboratory test results would be most helpful in distinguishing IDA from anemia of chronic disease?*
   a. Decreased MCV, MCH; marked poikilocytosis
   b. Increased MCV, MCH, MCHC; decreased RDW
   c. Increased RDW and TIBC
   d. Decreased RDW and TIBC

8. *What term refers to the accumulation of excess iron in macrophages?*
   a. Sideroblastic anemia
   b. Hemosiderosis
   c. Porphyria
   d. Thalassemia

9. *Which of the following findings would not be seen in sideroblastic conditions?*
   a. Increased RDW
   b. Pappenheimer bodies
   c. Ringed sideroblasts
   d. Decreased serum iron

10. *Which of the following is not a classification of porphyrias?*
    a. Erythropoietic porphyria
    b. Hepatic porphyria
    c. Dysfunctional porphyria
    d. Mixed porphyria

11. *What is a chracteristic finding in lead poisoning?*
    a. Basophilic stippling
    b. Target cells
    c. Sideroblasts
    d. Spherocytes

ANSWERS

1. b (p. 77)
2. d (p. 80)
3. a (p. 80–81)
4. d (p. 81–83)
5. b (p. 83)
6. a (p. 84)
7. c (p. 84–85)
8. b (p. 85)
9. d (p. 86–87)
10. c (p. 88)
11. a (p. 87)

CHAPTER 7

MICHELE L. BEST, B.S., M.T.(ASCP)

Megaloblastic Anemias

HISTORY AND DEFINITIONS

BIOCHEMICAL BASIS OF MEGALOBLASTIC DYSPOIESIS
ABSORPTION AND METABOLISM OF VITAMIN B$_{12}$ AND FOLIC ACID

CAUSES OF MEGALOBLASTIC ANEMIA
FOLIC ACID DEFICIENCY
VITAMIN B$_{12}$ DEFICIENCY
Pernicious Anemia

CLINICAL MANIFESTATIONS

MORPHOLOGY OF PERIPHERAL BLOOD AND BONE MARROW

MEGALOBLASTIC CHANGES IN NONDEFICIENT PATIENTS

NONMEGALOBLASTIC CAUSES OF MACROCYTOSIS

LABORATORY TESTS IN DIFFERENTIAL DIAGNOSIS OF MACROCYTOSIS

TREATMENT
VITAMIN B$_{12}$ DEFICIENCY
FOLIC ACID DEFICIENCY

CASE STUDY

OBJECTIVES

At the end of this chapter, the learner should be able to:
1. Define megaloblastic anemia.
2. List causes for megaloblastic dyspoiesis.
3. Describe clinical manifestations for vitamin B$_{12}$ and folate deficiencies.
4. Identify morphologic abnormalities seen on peripheral blood smears in cases of megaloblastic anemias.

5. Describe the appearance of the bone marrow in megaloblastic anemia.
6. Evaluate laboratory test results in the differential diagnosis of macrocytosis.
7. Compare the treatment of vitamin B$_{12}$ and folic acid deficiencies.

HISTORY AND DEFINITIONS

Megaloblastic anemia is anemia associated with defective deoxyribonucleic acid (DNA) synthesis and abnormal red cell maturation in the bone marrow. This abnormal maturation pattern is sometimes referred to as megaloblastic change, in contrast to normal, or normoblastic, maturation. Megaloblastic change also describes the characteristic maturation abnormality in the absence of anemia. Furthermore, megaloblastic maturation also affects granulocytic and megakaryocytic maturation. Megaloblastic dyspoiesis and megaloblastosis are other terms describing the same maturation defect. A similar term, megaloblastoid, has been used to describe malignant or premalignant changes in the bone marrow that are morphologically similar yet etiologically different from megaloblastic change.

Megaloblast was first used by Ehrlich[1] in 1880 to describe a distinctly abnormal cell seen in the bone marrow of a patient with pernicious anemia. This extremely large, deeply basophilic, immature erythroid cell was thought by Ehrlich and others to represent a cell type unique to the disease process rather than a morphologically and functionally abnormal counterpart of the normal erythroid precursor cell that it is known to represent today. For years, megaloblast and normoblast have been used to describe these abnormal and normal counterparts. Specific members of the normoblastic series are called pronormoblast, deeply basophilic normoblast, polychromatophilic normoblast, and orthochromic normoblast. The counterparts in megaloblastic maturation are described similarly by substituting "megaloblast" for "normoblast" (as in polychromatophilic megaloblast) (**see Color Plate 67**).

Pernicious anemia, the prototype of megaloblastic anemia, was initially described in 1855 by Addison,[2] who reported on a patient with an idiopathic persistent anemia that progressed to death. Addisonian anemia was used for many years to describe this disorder. The name pernicious anemia was first used by Biermer[3] in 1872.

Macrocytic anemia describes any anemia associated with an elevated mean corpuscular red cell volume (MCV). This is a morphologic category of anemia that includes but is not restricted to megaloblastic anemia. Unfortunately macrocytic anemia is sometimes used as a synonym for megaloblastic anemia. One term denotes a morphologic category of anemia (macrocytic) with several different causes, whereas the other denotes an etiologic category (megaloblastic).

BIOCHEMICAL BASIS OF MEGALOBLASTIC DYSPOIESIS

Megaloblastic dyspoiesis is the result of a slowdown in DNA synthesis in the developing cells of the bone marrow and other rapidly proliferative cells in the body. The primary defect is in DNA replication owing to a depletion of thymidine triphosphate, an immediate DNA precursor.[4] This deficiency causes retarded nuclear maturation and mitosis, which is responsible for both the enlargement of cells and the morphologic abnormalities

observed. The ratio of ribonucleic acid (RNA) to DNA in megaloblastic cells is higher than normal because RNA synthesis and therefore cytoplasmic maturation are not affected.

Impaired DNA synthesis can be caused by a variety of conditions, among them vitamin B_{12} deficiency, folic acid deficiency, and administration of drugs that interfere with DNA metabolism. The most common categories of drugs involved are chemotherapeutic agents and anticonvulsants. The exact role that vitamin B_{12} and folic acid play in DNA synthesis will be examined in the next section.

Absorption and Metabolism of Vitamin B_{12} and Folic Acid

Vitamin B_{12} and folic acid must be present in adequate dietary amounts and effectively absorbed to be available for DNA synthesis in the bone marrow.

Vitamin B_{12}, also called cyanocobalamin, has a chemical structure similar to that shown in Figure 7–1. There are also a number of other cobalamin compounds in which the -CN molecule is replaced with other types of side chains. The term "vitamin B_{12}" is often used collectively to describe cyanocobalamin and its analogues.

The richest dietary sources of vitamin B_{12} are meats, eggs, dairy products, and liver. The mini-

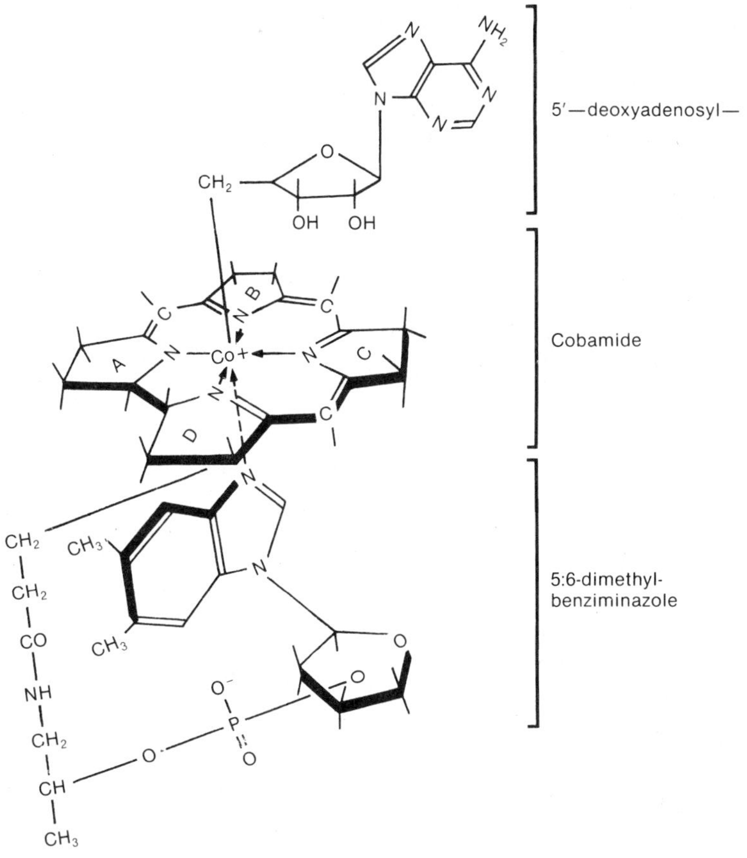

Figure 7–1. Structure of deoxyadenosyl cobalamin, a physiologically active form of vitamin B_{12}. (From Chanarin, I: The Megaloblastic Anemias. Blackwell Scientific Publications, Boston, 1969, with permission.)

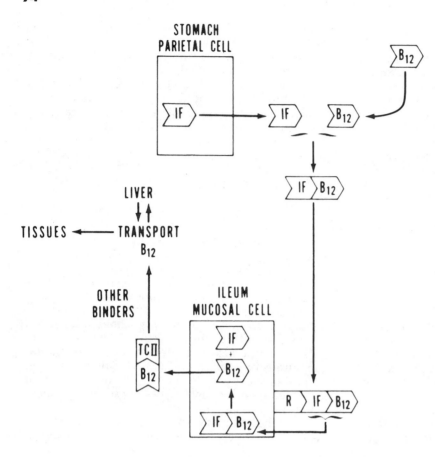

Figure 7–2. Absorption, transport, and storage of vitamin B_{12}. IF = intrinsic factor, R = tissue binders, TC II = transcobalamin II. (From Miale, JB: Laboratory Medicine: Hematology, CV Mosby, St. Louis, 1982, p 425, with permission.)

mum daily requirement is thought to be approximately 1 to 3 μg. Vitamin B_{12} is absorbed via a binding protein called intrinsic factor (IF), a glycoprotein produced by the gastric parietal cells. This IF binds vitamin B_{12}, producing an IF-B_{12} complex that attaches to receptors on the ileal mucosal cells allowing for its absorption (Fig. 7–2). Vitamin B_{12} is then released from the ileal cell and bound to a transport protein in the bloodstream, transcobalamin II. Transcobalamin II, like IF, is a fairly selective binder of cyanocobalamin and does not bind the other vitamin B_{12} analogues.[5]

Two other vitamin B_{12}–binding proteins, transcobalamin I and III, appear to play a minor role in transporting true vitamin B_{12} (cyanocobalamin) but a major role in transporting the other vitamin B_{12} analogues.[6]

As Figure 7–2 illustrates, transcobalamin II and other binders transport vitamin B_{12} to the bone marrow and other tissues to be used or to the liver to be stored. The quantity of vitamin B_{12} stored in the liver of the average person is large enough to last for approximately 3 years.

Folic acid, folate, and pteroylglutamic acid are synonyms for the compound shown in Figure 7–3. Pteroylglutamic acid is the parent compound of a large number of closely related compounds often referred to as folates.

Folic acid is present as folate polyglutamate in high concentration in leafy green vegetables, liver, meats, and certain fruits. The minimum daily adult requirement for folate is approximately 50 μg.[7]

Folate is absorbed in the mucosal cells of the duodenum and jejunum, where three biochemical reactions (hydrolysis, reduction, and methylation) convert the ingested polyglutamates into 5-methyl-tetrahydrofolate (5-methyl THF) (Fig. 7–4). This monoglutamate form is readily and completely absorbed into portal circulation where it is transported by α_2-macroglobulin, albumin, and transferrin[5] to the tissues and the liver. Folate stores in the liver are minimal. This explains why it takes only a few months of inadequate dietary intake to become folate deficient.

Once effectively absorbed and transported, vitamin B_{12} and folic acid become available to the actively dividing cells of the body to perform their key roles in DNA synthesis.

Vitamin B_{12} and a group of folic acid derivatives are required as cofactors in several key reactions leading to the synthesis of thymidine triphosphate and subsequently to DNA. A simplified diagram of these reactions is presented in Figure 7–5. Vitamin B_{12} is required for the conversion of homocysteine to methionine, during which a methyl group is transferred from 5-methyl THF to yield tetrahydrofolate (THF).[8] Folic acid and related folate compounds including THF participate in the conversion of deoxyuridine monophosphate to thymidine monophosphate, which eventually converts to thymidine triphosphate — one of the pyrimidine building blocks of DNA. It is evident from this diagram that a deficiency of vitamin B_{12} or folate has a serious impact on DNA synthesis.

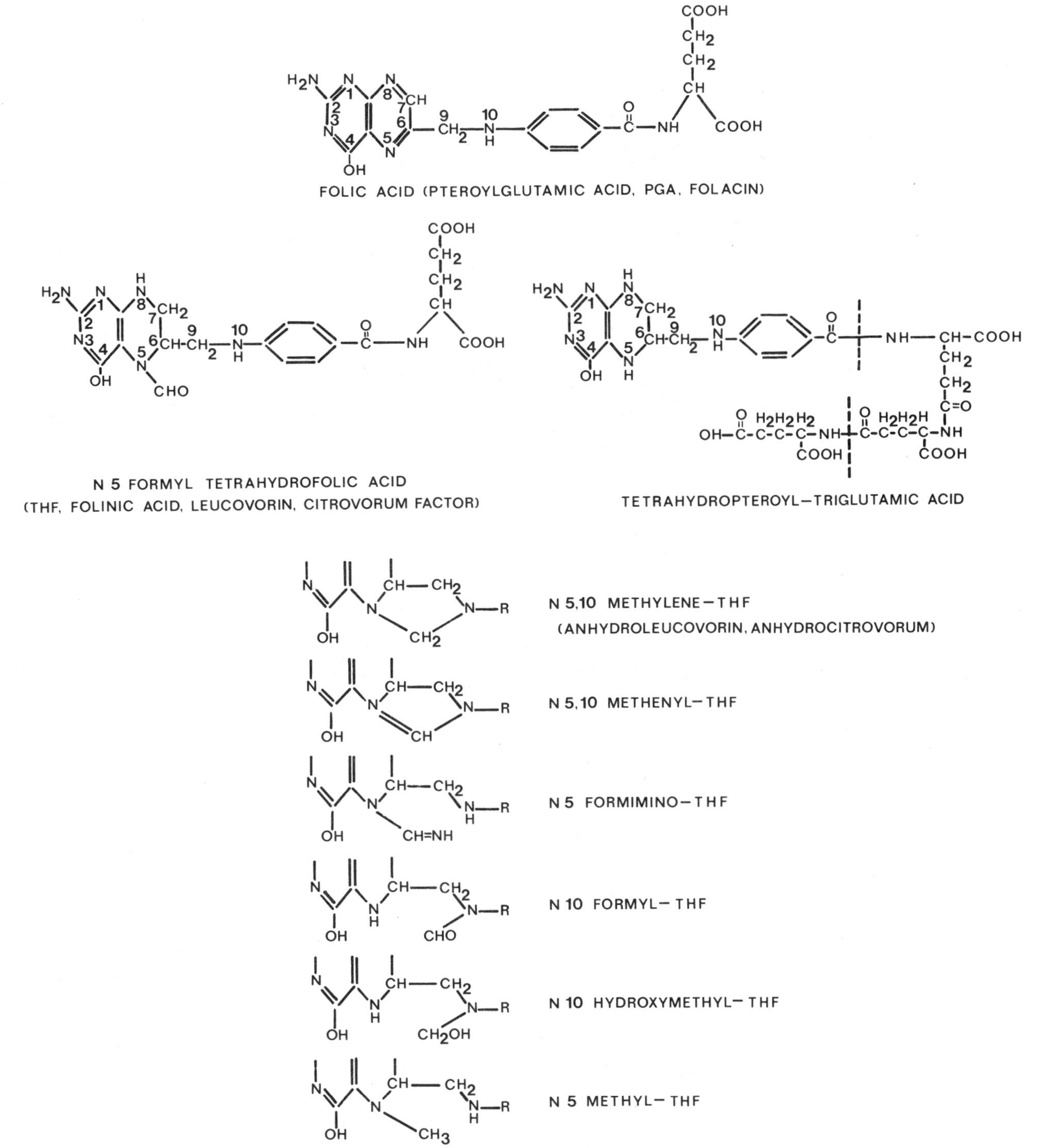

Figure 7–3. Structure of folic acid and its derivatives. THF = tetrahydrofolate. (From Harris, JW and Kellerman, RW: The Red Cell. Harvard University Press, Cambridge, MA, 1970, p 395, with permission.)

CAUSES OF MEGALOBLASTIC ANEMIA

When the normal cycle of adequate diet, absorption, transport, and cellular utilization of these vitamins is broken, a cellular deficiency and megaloblastic dyspoiesis result. Despite the fact that both deficiencies have very similar cellular consequences, the conditions that lead to these deficiencies are quite different. Folic acid deficiency is discussed first because it is the more common deficiency.

Folic Acid Deficiency

By far, the leading cause of folic acid deficiency is dietary. The major etiologic categories of folic acid

ERYTHROCYTES

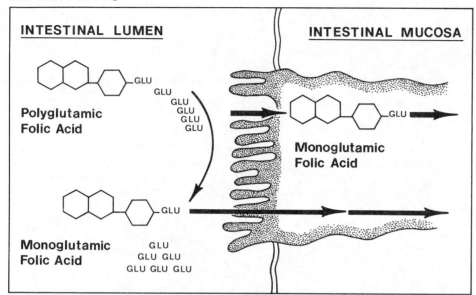

Figure 7–4. Intestinal absorption of the folate derivatives of food. (From Streiff, RR: Intestinal absorption of the folate derivatives of food. JAMA 214:105, 1970, fig. 48, with permission.)

deficiency are outlined in Table 7–1. Dietary deficiency results from a poor diet, usually owing to alcoholism, poverty, old age, or consistent overcooking of vegetables. In the alcoholic, folate deficiency is the leading cause of anemia.[9] Inadequate dietary intake has usually been regarded as the primary cause; however, a study by Sullivan and Herbert[10] suggests that alcohol ingestion has a direct antagonistic effect on folic acid metabolism. In this study, patients with untreated megaloblastic anemia were given folic acid together with alcohol. The alcohol prevented a hematologic response to folate in these patients.

Inadequate dietary intake in the face of increased physiologic need occurs in young infants and pregnant women. Good vitamin supplementation in infancy and pregnancy can eliminate this cause of folate deficiency.

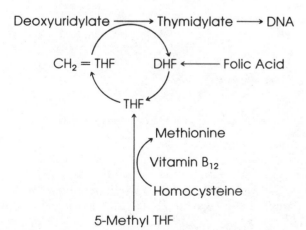

Figure 7–5. The roles of vitamin B_{12} and folic acid in DNA synthesis. THF = tetrahydrofolate, DHF = dihydrofolate, CH_2 = THF = methylene tetrahydrofolate. (Adapted from Waxman, Metz, and Herbert.[24])

Table 7–1. **CAUSES OF FOLIC ACID DEFICIENCY**

Inadequate intake
  Alcoholism
  Poor diet
  Overcooking vegetables
Increased utilization
  Pregnancy
  Infancy
  Hemolytic anemia
  Acute leukemia
  Metastatic cancer
  Multiple myeloma
  Hyperthyroidism
  Exfoliative dermatitis
Impaired absorption
  Tropical and nontropical sprue
  Drug-related
  ? Alcohol
  Anatomic and functional intestinal abnormalities
Increased loss
  Hemodialysis
Drug-related
  Folate antagonists (e.g., methotrexate)
  Isoniazid
  Cycloserine
  Phenytoin
  Oral contraceptives

Increased utilization and consumption of folate occurs in the bone marrow itself if a chronic proliferation of cells such as hemolytic anemia, leukemia, or multiple myeloma is present. Although rarely the cause of the anemia in these patients, folate deficiency can cause a megaloblastic change in the cellular morphology of the bone marrow and peripheral blood.

The third major reason for folic acid deficiency is malabsorption. The most notable malabsorption syndromes are tropical and nontropical sprue.

Sprue has traditionally referred to a chronic wasting disorder common in the tropics and associated with diarrhea, idiopathic steatorrhea (fatty stools), and glossitis.[9] The cause of sprue in the tropics remains a mystery, as it may respond simply to antibiotic treatment. Nontropical sprue is a similar clinical syndrome associated with a sensitivity of the intestinal tract to gluten, a wheat protein. It is sometimes called gluten-induced enteropathy and adult celiac disease. Childhood celiac disease is a related malabsorption syndrome seen in children. Malabsorption syndromes can result in a combined deficiency of folate plus vitamin B_{12} or iron deficiency.

Certain drugs such as methotrexate are used in cancer chemotherapy because they act as folate antagonists and inhibit pyrimidine synthesis. Other drugs associated with depressed serum folate levels for unclear reasons include certain anticonvulsants[11] and antituberculosis agents.[12]

Vitamin B_{12} Deficiency

In contrast to folate deficiency, vitamin B_{12} deficiency is almost always due to some type of malabsorption.[13] Table 7–2 summarizes the causes of vitamin B_{12} deficiency. Pernicious anemia represents one cause of malabsorption of vitamin B_{12}. Unfortunately pernicious anemia has often been used as a synonym for vitamin B_{12} deficiency and even for megaloblastic anemia, which is clearly incorrect. A resection of the stomach will result in a situation similar to that seen in pernicious anemia — that is, a lack of IF production. A variety of other intestinal disorders may also lead to malabsorption of vitamin B_{12}. Less common causes of vitamin B_{12} deficiency include fish tapeworm infection and abnormalities in the major vitamin B_{12} transport protein in the blood, transcobalamin II. Dietary deficiency of vitamin B_{12} is extremely rare and occurs only in very strict vegetarians who eat no meat, eggs, or dairy products.

There are progressive stages of vitamin B_{12} deficiency, beginning with a negative vitamin B_{12} balance and progressing to vitamin B_{12} depletion, then to vitamin B_{12}–deficient erythropoiesis, and finally to vitamin B_{12}–deficient macrocytic anemia. Vitamin B_{12}, as measured by the serum cobalamin level, is decreased as an early sign of vitamin B_{12} depletion before clinical symptoms and anemia develop. Therefore, a low serum vitamin B_{12} (cobalamin) level should be clinically regarded as the earliest sign of a vitamin B_{12}–deficiency state.

Pernicious Anemia

Pernicious anemia was named by Biermer[3] because of its persistent, inevitably fatal nature. It was originally believed to be a dietary deficiency of vitamin B_{12}, which might be corrected by feeding liver to patients. Castle[14] in 1929 described the presence of an intrinsic factor in gastric contents, which was required for the absorption of vitamin B_{12}. It is now known that deficient production of this intrinsic factor by the parietal cells of the stomach is the

Table 7–2. **CAUSES OF VITAMIN B_{12} DEFICIENCY**

Impaired absorption
  Lack of intrinsic factor (pernicious anemia)
  Gastrectomy
  Chronic gastritis
  Tropical and nontropical sprue
  Inflammatory bowel disease (e.g., regional ileitis)
  Ileal resection
Microorganism competition
  Diphyllobothrium latum (fish tapeworm)
  Bacteria in blind loop syndrome
Transport protein defects
  Hereditary lack of transcobalamin II
  Abnormal transcobalamin II
  Abnormal vitamin B_{12}–binding protein
Dietary deficiency
  Strict veganism

cause of pernicious anemia. Without this important substance, vitamin B_{12} cannot be absorbed into the body. The exact cause of the IF deficiency in pernicious anemia is still unknown, but a combination of genetic predilection and autoimmune factors is probably involved. The evidence for an autoimmune etiology centers on the fact that these patients produce autoantibodies to parietal cells and, to a lesser extent, to IF. It is believed that the antibody to parietal cells causes an atrophy of these cells, resulting in deficient production of both hydrochloric acid and IF. The discovery of these autoantibodies has led to the advent of new tests for pernicious anemia based on the detection of anti-IF and antiparietal cell antibodies.

Pernicious anemia is most common in persons of Scandinavian and northern European ancestry but is also seen in a variety of other races and nationalities. The peak age at diagnosis is 60 years.[5] The clinical manifestations of pernicious anemia are the same as those present in other types of vitamin B_{12} deficiency and will be discussed subsequently. Fortunately, pernicious anemia is no longer pernicious, and can be treated with lifelong injections of vitamin B_{12}. Pernicious anemia is also associated with autoimmune syndromes involving other tissues and organs (for example, hypothyroidism, Hashimoto's disease, and diabetes).

CLINICAL MANIFESTATIONS

The clinical manifestations of megaloblastic anemia are grouped into two categories: (1) those present in both vitamin B_{12} and folate deficiencies, and (2) those present only in vitamin B_{12} deficiency.

Clinical manifestations common to both vitamin B_{12} and folate deficiencies include pallor, weakness, light-headedness, and shortness of breath due to anemia; a lemon-yellow pallor (slight jaundice) due to increased bilirubin; and epithelial abnormalities such as a smooth, sore tongue. The anemia in both cases is usually insidious in onset and well compensated for by the patient.

Table 7 – 3. **THE P's OF NEUROLOGIC MANIFESTATIONS IN PERNICIOUS ANEMIA**

Peripheral neuropathy
Pyramidal tract signs
Posterior spinal column degeneration
Psychosis ("megaloblastic madness")

The neurologic manifestations (Table 7 – 3) found in pernicious anemia are unique to vitamin B_{12} deficiency and distinguish it from folate deficiency. These manifestations result in the numbness and tingling of extremities, gait abnormality, and difficulty with fine motor coordination that these patients experience. If left untreated, these abnormalities can progress to permanent neurologic damage. It is important to note that neurologic abnormalities may be present prior to macrocytosis and anemia in numerous patients with pernicious anemia.

Clinical signs and symptoms, although helpful in distinguishing vitamin B_{12} from folic acid deficiency, cannot differentiate with certainty the exact etiology without the aid of the laboratory.

MORPHOLOGY OF PERIPHERAL BLOOD AND BONE MARROW

Megaloblastic anemia is a classic example of how the deficiency of a single vitamin or cofactor (B_{12} or folic acid) can cause a cascade of destructive events affecting different cell types and tissues throughout the body. Although thought of as affecting mainly hematopoietic cells, these events affect all rapidly dividing cells in the body. The bone marrow in a megaloblastic anemia reveals the actual abnormality in maturation, whereas the peripheral blood reflects the effects of that abnormal maturation on the differentiated cells.

This section focuses on the morphologic effects on hematopoiesis observed in these two deficiencies. It is important to remember that the exact same morphologic abnormalities are present in both vitamin B_{12} and folic acid deficiencies and that the etiology of a megaloblastic anemia cannot be distinguished morphologically. Morphologic examination only determines that the anemia is megaloblastic in type; further laboratory tests are required to determine the specific etiology.

The peripheral blood finding most commonly associated with megaloblastic anemia is macrocytosis. In the years before the advent of the electronic particle counters, macrocytosis was visually detected by the enlargement of red cells on a peripheral blood smear. Red cell indices (MCV, MCH, MCHC) based on manual blood cell counts and calculations were also available but were somewhat inaccurate. Both mechanisms were very insensitive means of detecting slight increases in red cell size. The multiparameter electronic cell counters provided the hematology laboratory with the first accurate and precise measurement of red cell size — the electronically measured MCV. Mean corpuscular red cell volume is a very sensitive means of detecting macrocytosis. Macrocytosis is important to detect as it is often one of the earliest peripheral blood abnormalities in megaloblastic anemias. Most patients with a megaloblastic anemia will have an MCV greater than 100 fl but rarely greater than 150 fl; however, it must be remembered that the MCV is not always elevated in megaloblastic anemia. An MCV of less than 100 fl is reported in about one third of patients with documented vitamin B_{12} deficiency (low vitamin B_{12} level). There are various reasons for this lack of macrocytosis, including cases with striking anisocytosis or red cell dimorphism and cases of megaloblastic anemia coexistent with iron deficiency. The MCV is also not elevated in megaloblastic anemia patients who have a coexisting α- or β-thalassemia. This is particularly true of black patients, who may have a form of α-thalassemia trait about 30 percent of the time.

Examination of the peripheral smear is valuable in evaluating the etiology of an elevated MCV. Several types of macrocytes occur: (1) oval macrocytes, resulting from a megaloblastic (most commonly associated with vitamin B_{12} and folate deficiencies) or megaloblastoid dyspoiesis; (2) round, blue-gray macrocytes — polychromatophilic red cells due to reticulocytosis; and (3) round, pink macrocytes, most commonly associated with liver disease, alcoholism, and hypothyroidism.

The oval macrocyte is the most important red cell abnormality present in megaloblastic anemia (**see Color Plate 64**). Oval macrocytes are dyspoietic red cells formed in the bone marrow as a result of megaloblastic or megaloblastoid dyserythropoiesis. The peripheral blood morphology in a severe case of megaloblastic anemia is depicted in **Color Plates 64 to 66**. The severity of the red cell abnormalities in megaloblastic anemia correlates directly with the severity of anemia. In a severely anemic patient, striking anisocytosis and poikilocytosis are seen, with an interesting mix of different types of poikilocytes including oval macrocytes, target cells, schistocytes, spherocytes, and tailed red cells (teardrops). If the oval macrocytes are not recognized for their diagnostic importance, this mix of poikilocytes can be quite confusing. In a milder case with slight anemia, the oval macrocytosis may be minimal and difficult to detect, with slight degrees of anisocytosis and poikilocytosis.

When any degree of anisocytosis is present in megaloblastic anemia, it will result in an increased red cell distribution width (RDW) on the S Plus series of Coulter instruments. The red cell histogram in a severe case will reflect the wide disparity in red cell size in these cases, which at times generate a perfectly normal MCV because the extremes in size average out. The histogram will also reveal red cell dimorphism, which may be seen occasionally in megaloblastic anemia when iron deficiency coexists with a vitamin B_{12} or folate deficiency. Red cell trimorphism may even be seen when these dimorphic patients get transfused with a third, normal, red cell population. These different-sized populations of red cells create very interesting red cell histograms in some cases of megaloblastic anemia.

Red cell inclusions are regularly present in megaloblastic anemia. The most common is the Howell-Jolly body (**see Color Plate 65**). The two major clinical situations in which Howell-Jolly bodies are present on peripheral blood smears are megaloblastic anemia and asplenia (often due to splenectomy or sickle-cell disease). The Howell-Jolly bodies present in megaloblastic anemia are not numerous on the smear but are significant. There may occasionally be several Howell-Jolly bodies in a single red cell (**see Color Plate 67**). These multiple Howell-Jolly bodies strongly suggest a megaloblastic etiology, because they are formed as a result of nuclear fragmentation of karyorrhexis in the bone marrow nucleated red cells. This fragmentation occurs readily in megaloblastic nucleated red cells because their nuclei are defective. Other inclusions present less regularly in megaloblastic anemia are basophilic stippling and Cabot's rings. Cabot's rings (**Color Plate 69**) are an extremely rare occurrence in the hematology laboratory; however, when present, severe megaloblastic anemia is a definite possibility.

Occasionally polychromatophilic red cells and nucleated red cells are seen in an untreated patient. The relative percentage of reticulocytes may be slightly increased owing to the severe decrease in the total red cells, but the absolute reticulocyte count is decreased (less than 50 to 100 $\times 10^9$/liter), because erythropoiesis in these cases is ineffective in generating needed red cells. The absolute reticulocyte count is always a more accurate measure of red cell production by the bone marrow than is the reticulocyte percentage. The nucleated red cells noted in the peripheral blood may exhibit the same abnormal nuclear features as the cells in the bone marrow and should be identified as megaloblastic nucleated red cells. With treatment, polychromatophilia and nucleated red cells become more numerous, and polychromatophilic oval macrocytes may be seen.

The triad of an elevated MCV, oval macrocytes, and hypersegmented neutrophils constitutes strong evidence of megaloblastic dyspoiesis. Hypersegmentation of the neutrophil may sometimes be the only clue to a megaloblastic process. Hypersegmentation of polymorphonuclear neutrophils is defined as an increase in the average lobe number of the circulating neutrophils (**see Color Plate 66**). It should be reported as present when 5 percent of the neutrophils have five or more lobes. Rare numbers of neutrophils with six or more lobes and eosinophils with four or more lobes should also be reported as hypersegmented. Miale[15] has reported neutrophil lobe counts as high as 13 in megaloblastic anemia. Hypersegmented neutrophils are often larger than normal (macropolycytes) and their lobes tend to appear very detached with a longer, stringy-looking filamentation. This peculiar-looking lobulation and the size often alert the morphologist to the presence of hypersegmentation. Hypersegmentation is usually the first sign of megaloblastic dyspoiesis to appear in the peripheral blood smear and is present in 98 percent of the patients with megaloblastic anemia.[16] It is also the last smear abnormality to disappear in treated patients. Hypersegmented neutrophils may persist in the peripheral blood for about 10 days to 2 weeks after specific therapy has been initiated.[17]

The final key element of the peripheral blood in many cases is pancytopenia. Pancytopenia is defined as the combination of a decreased white cell count, a decreased red cell count, and a decreased platelet count. The diagnostic importance of pancytopenia in hematology cannot be overemphasized. Megaloblastic anemia is just one of a variety of hematologic disorders that present with pancytopenia. Pancytopenia in megaloblastic anemia is the direct result of the megaloblastic dyspoiesis and its resultant ineffective cell production that involves all three cell lines produced in the bone marrow. The precursors of these cell lines are numerous in the marrow, yet their mature products—red cells, white cells (granulocytes), and platelets—are decreased in number in the peripheral blood. This is known as ineffective hematopoiesis and, specifically for red cells, ineffective erythropoiesis. Megaloblastic hematopoiesis is ineffective, because, despite the fact that bone marrow is actively producing nucleated precursors, mature cells are not effectively manufactured and released. This is thought to occur because the defective nucleated precursors die prematurely in the bone marrow.

The degree of total cytopenia (cell reduction) is variable, but the white cell counts are usually between 2.0 and 4.0 $\times 10^9$/liter, with a relative lymphocytosis due to granulocytopenia. There may be a mild shift to the left, with myelocytes noted on the smear in some cases. The platelet count is usually between 50 and 150 $\times 10^9$/liter, but platelet counts as low as 15 $\times 10^9$/liter have been recorded. The red cell count, hemoglobin, and hematocrit are reduced to varying levels, dependent on the severity of the deficiency. As already noted, the MCV is increased, as is the MCH; however, the MCHC is normal in most cases.

The bone marrow morphology in a megaloblastic anemia (**see Color Plates 67 and 68**) reveals the actual abnormality in maturation that results from vitamin B_{12} or folic acid deficiency. Although the morphology is very interesting and valuable from an educational standpoint, the examination of the bone marrow is not required in order to diagnose the typical case of megaloblastic anemia. If the peripheral smear reveals the characteristic abnormalities described, testing the level of serum vitamin B_{12} (cobalamin), folic acid, and red cell folate will establish the diagnosis in most cases. However, since megaloblastic peripheral blood features can occur in myelodysplastic syndromes and in other disease states, a bone marrow aspirate is usually performed prior to the institution of therapy.

Megaloblastic change describes a morphologic abnormality in the bone marrow called asynchrony, the lack of normal coordinated nuclear and cytoplasm development of hematopoietic cells in the bone marrow. This is also called nuclear-cytoplasmic dissociation. In normoblastic red cell development, the hemoglobinization and pinking of the cytoplasm occur "in time" with nuclear maturation and changes in the nuclear chromatin clumping pattern. In megaloblastic red cell precursors, the nuclear maturation is lagging well behind the hemoglobinization in the cytoplasm because of the impaired DNA synthesis. The cells are also visibly larger than normal, owing to the lag in DNA replication and cell division. Megaloblastic change is most noticeable in the later stages of red cell development—the polychromatophilic (rubricyte) and orthochromic (metarubricyte) stages. The metarubricyte stage of normoblastic maturation normally shows a dense pyknotic nuclear chromatin with a very hemoglobinized pink-to-gray cytoplasm. The metarubricyte stage, if megaloblastic, shows the nuclear clumping pattern of a younger cell like a rubricyte with the cytoplasmic pinking expected of the metarubricyte stage. A corresponding abnormality in maturation is seen at every stage of the red cell series. The megaloblast initially described by Ehrlich[1] was a pronormoblast with a much more open, sievelike chromatin pattern than is normally seen. These very immature megaloblastic pronormoblasts are abundant in the more severe cases but not in mild cases of magaloblastic anemia. In milder cases, megaloblastic change in the metarubricyte stage is much easier to identify. Other abnormalities present in the later nucleated stages include multiple Howell-Jolly bodies and nuclear karyorrhexis.

Megaloblastic change is not restricted to the erythroid precursors. It is also present in the other rapidly dividing cell lines of the bone marrow, especially the granulocytic precursors. The most typical granulocytic abnormalities are the giant band and giant metamyelocyte (**see Color Plate 68**). These cells, as in the case of the erythroid precursors, exhibit giantism and nuclear maturation lagging behind cytoplasmic maturation; in other words, the nuclear chromatin is not clumping as much as a band or metamyelocyte should. In some cases, megaloblastic change in the granulocytes is more evident than in the erythroid cells. The megakaryocytes, when abnormal, are hyperlobulated and the lobes may appear somewhat detached and peculiar. This hypersegmentation of megakaryocytes may be the earliest detectable abnormality in the bone marrow.

The bone marrow is very hypercellular, with erythroid hyperplasia and a reversed myeloid-to-erythroid (M:E) ratio. The normal M:E ratio is 3:1 or 4:1, whereas in megaloblastic anemia it is often 1:1 or 1:3. The increased cellularity reflects the futile and ineffective attempt of the bone marrow to respond to the anemia by regenerating red cells. Increased numbers of mitoses and atypical-appearing mitoses are common in megaloblastic bone marrows and may be confused with malignant disorders. The bone marrow iron is normal to increased, and if increased, numerous macrophages laden with iron will be seen. Excess iron is present owing to the accelerated death of erythroid precursors in the marrow, a process that releases large amounts of heme iron.

MEGALOBLASTIC CHANGES IN NONDEFICIENT PATIENTS

Megaloblastic dyspoiesis is not limited to situations in which vitamin B_{12} or folic acid deficiency exist. It can sometimes be an indicator that the bone marrow is developing a clone of neoplastic cells. This is the case in myelodysplastic syndromes (preleukemia), in which a megaloblastic dyserythropoiesis is the most common finding in the bone marrow.[18] This dyserythropoiesis (abnormal erythropoiesis) will result in the exact same red cell abnormality present in megaloblastic anemia: the oval macrocyte. Oval macrocytosis is present in the peripheral blood in 74 percent of patients with myelodysplastic syndrome.[18] Myelodysplastic syndromes frequently exhibit cytopenias that are more severe than that present in megaloblastic anemia—that is, the white cell counts are lower (1.0 to 2.5×10^9/liter range) and the platelet counts are lower (less than 50×10^9/liter).

Another disease that shows marked megaloblastic dyserythropoiesis and that morphologically can resemble megaloblastic anemia is erythroleukemia (FAB class M_6). In the peripheral blood smear, erythroleukemia may appear similar to myelodysplastic syndrome or may show a flagrant erythroblastosis with bizarre megaloblastic nucleated red cells and accompanying myeloblasts.

Myelodysplasia and erythroleukemia show a megaloblastic-like change in the erythroid precursors of the bone marrow that is often referred to as "megaloblastoid" to distinguish the very different malignant or premalignant etiology. Many hematologists dislike "megaloblastoid," because of the difficulty in morphologically distinguishing megaloblastic from megaloblastoid. Megaloblastoid nuclear chromatin patterns tend to be more erratically clumped than do those in megaloblastic anemia due to vitamin B_{12} or folic acid deficiency.

A more detailed discussion of myelodysplastic syndromes and erythroleukemia may be found in Chapter 19.

NONMEGALOBLASTIC CAUSES OF MACROCYTOSIS

Macrocytosis is a hematologic abnormality that is common in large hospital centers. One study of Breedveld, Bieger, and van Wermeskerken[19] noted that an MCV greater than 100 fl was present in 2.3 percent of 10,000 blood counts performed at Bronova Hospital in the Netherlands. This percentage is

Table 7-4. **CAUSES OF MACROCYTOSIS**

Cause	Percentage of Patients
Vitamin B_{12} or folic acid deficiency	38.500
Alcoholism	27.000
Chronic hepatitis	0.030
Hematologic disease	18.600
Hematologic malignancy	12.900
Hemolytic anemia	5.700
Hypothyroidism	0.030
Unknown	0.085

Source: Adapted from Breedveld et al.[19]

probably somewhat higher (3 to 4 percent) in a large urban medical center in the United States owing to the frequency of alcohol-related macrocytosis. Table 7-4 summarizes the causes of macrocytosis in 70 of the patients studied by Breedveld. This table illustrates that the causes of macrocytosis are quite variable, and very important diagnostically. Megaloblastic anemia is the most common cause of an elevated MCV, but the nonmegaloblastic causes such as alcoholism account for many of the increased MCVs encountered in the laboratory. Patients receiving certain immunosuppressive agents consistently show elevated MCVs; these cases were excluded from the Breedveld study.

The two major causes of nonmegaloblastic macrocytosis are alcoholism and hematologic disease. Macrocytosis is such a common finding in alcoholics that the MCV has been recommended as a sensitive screening test for this condition. This form of macrocytosis in alcoholism appears to be related to a direct effect of alcohol on the red cell, rather than to folic acid deficiency. A patient history and liver function tests can be used to substantiate alcoholism as the cause of the elevated MCV.

Hematologic diseases associated with macrocytosis come under two major categories: (1) hematologic malignancy and (2) hemolysis. The most common hematologic malignancies involved are chronic myeloproliferative disorders, myelodysplastic syndromes, acute nonlymphocytic leukemias, and multiple myeloma. Hemolysis can be associated with macrocytosis if the reticulocyte count is greater than 5 percent because for each 1 percent increase in the reticulocyte count, the MCV increases by 1 fl.[20] This is explained by the fact that the mean cell volume (size) of a reticulocyte is greater than that of a mature red cell. This cause of red cell enlargement can be detected on the peripheral blood smear as polychromatophilia.

Sideroblastic (refractory, idiopathic, or hereditary) and aplastic anemia can also result in macrocytosis. Sideroblastic anemia frequently shows a dimorphic red cell population, one portion of the population being macrocytic and the other portion microcytic, hypochromic. This may result in a normal or slightly elevated MCV, depending on the size of the cells in the particular case. Both sideroblastic and aplastic anemias require a bone marrow examination for diagnosis.

Occasionally an elevated MCV occurs as a laboratory artifact — that is, the elevation is not truly due to increased red cell size. Two such situations are the presence of cold autoagglutinins and a very elevated white cell count. These two situations can easily be detected by looking carefully at the results of other instrument parameters and the peripheral blood smear.

LABORATORY TESTS IN DIFFERENTIAL DIAGNOSIS OF MACROCYTOSIS

The presence of abnormal hematologic findings, usually an elevated MCV, necessitates a logical and cost-effective scheme of laboratory evaluation and testing. As mentioned before, peripheral blood morphology, especially the type of macrocyte present on the smear and the presence or absence of hypersegmented neutrophils, only helps to determine whether the anemia is megaloblastic or nonmegaloblastic in nature. The exact cause of the anemia must be determined by further laboratory testing owing to the many different causes of vitamin B_{12} and folic acid deficiencies. Figure 7-6 illustrates a logical scheme of laboratory testing in cases of macrocytosis.

The first determination to be made is whether the macrocytosis is strictly due to an increased reticulocyte count. If the reticulocyte count is sufficiently increased to cause the degree of MCV elevation seen, no other laboratory tests are required to evaluate the macrocytosis. Checking for a possible hemolytic state or blood loss is more appropriate in this case. If the macrocytes are not reticulocytes, the serum vitamin B_{12} (cobalamin) and folate level, as well as the red cell folate level, should be measured. These three tests must be performed simultaneously for correct interpretation of the results. Measurement of the serum vitamin B_{12} level and the red cell folate level are the two best tests to identify accurately any deficiencies in the tissues. The serum vitamin B_{12} level in particular is the most sensitive and reliable means of detecting vitamin B_{12} deficiency at a very early stage. The serum folate level is less reliable than the red cell folate level in assessing tissue folate levels because of its tendency to be falsely normal if the patient has had a recent intake of folate-rich foods. Nevertheless, the serum folate level is important in the correct interpretation of serum vitamin B_{12} results.

Prior to the 1970s, serum vitamin B_{12} and folate levels were performed by microbiologic assay. The principle of either procedure was that if a microorganism requires either vitamin B_{12} or folic acid for growth and if this organism is incubated with patient's serum as the sole source of the vitamin, the amount of bacterial growth will directly correlate with the concentration of the vitamin in the serum.

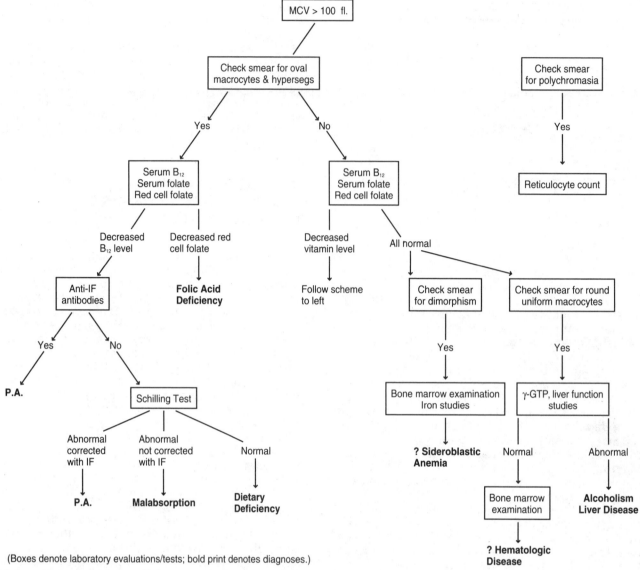

(Boxes denote laboratory evaluations/tests; bold print denotes diagnoses.)

Figure 7–6. Logical scheme of laboratory testing in cases of macrocytosis. Boxes denote laboratory evaluations and/or tests; boldface type denotes diagnoses.

Bacterial growth was measured spectrophotometrically by the turbidity produced and compared with serum standards with known amounts of vitamin B_{12} or folic acid to determine the serum concentration. These methods were accurate but time-consuming, cumbersome, and impossible to use if the patient was taking antibiotics.

The radioisotope dilution methods for vitamin B_{12} and folate became the methods of choice in the 1970s because they were quick, precise, and presumably accurate procedures for determining serum levels as well as the red cell folate level. In retrospect, it is now believed that these new methods were introduced into routine clinical use too early, with insufficient validation of their accuracy.[21] It was noted by various centers around the country that vitamin B_{12} levels by isotopic methods were inappropriately high; that is, patients had normal vitamin B_{12} levels with clinical signs of megaloblastic anemia due to vitamin B_{12} deficiency. Radioisotope dilution methods are based on the principle of competitive binding; that is, the isotope-labeled vitamin competes with the unlabeled vitamin present in the patient's serum for a limited number of binding sites on a specific binding protein. The vitamin level in the patient's serum can be calculated based on the radiometrically measured amount of labeled vitamin bound to the binder or alternatively on the amount left unbound in the supernatant. The more labeled vitamin bound, the lower the patient's serum vitamin level, as less unlabeled vitamin was present in the patient's serum to compete for the sites.

The binding protein currently used in the vitamin B_{12} assay is IF. For accuracy, the binder used must specifically bind vitamin B_{12} and no other substance. The binders initially used in many vitamin B_{12} kits were neither purified nor specific enough and bound cobalamin analogues as well as vitamin B_{12} itself. A 1978 study by Kolhouse and coworkers[22] demonstrated that 10 to 20 percent of patients with pernicious anemia showed false-normal vitamin B_{12} levels by radioisotope methods. In recent years, these binders have been modified to correct this problem; however, kits being considered for use should be evaluated carefully regarding their ability to differentiate normal from abnormal patients.

A variety of kits for measuring serum and red cell folate levels by radioisotope methods have been introduced recently. These methods seem to be reliable in detecting folic acid deficiency. It is uncertain whether any of these folate radioisotope dilution methods is superior or inferior to the microbiologic methods.[21] There is no question, though, that measuring the red cell folate level is a better test for tissue folate levels than the serum folate level. Determining the serum folate level is useful in interpreting the results of the serum vitamin B_{12} level. It is well known that the serum vitamin B_{12} level will decrease in folic acid deficiency and that if both serum levels are decreased, the deficiency is either a folic acid deficiency or a rare combined vitamin B_{12}–folate deficiency. It is also true that patients with low serum vitamin B_{12} levels tend to show increased levels of serum folic acid. These corresponding fluctuations are a result of the interrelationship of these two cofactors in normal metabolism.

Once vitamin B_{12} deficiency has been established (serum cobalamin level less than 250 pg/ml), the specific cause of the deficiency must be determined by further laboratory testing. Because pernicious anemia and other types of malabsorption are the leading causes of vitamin B_{12} deficiency, laboratory testing has centered on the diagnosis of these states.

A new highly specific but somewhat insensitive test for pernicious anemia is the test for the "blocking" type of antibodies to IF. Such antibodies are present in 50 to 60 percent of patients with pernicious anemia.[21] This test, if its result is positive, is diagnostic for pernicious anemia and probably eliminates the need for the much more cumbersome Schilling test. However, if these antibodies are not present, a Schilling test must be performed. The other antibody detectable in the serum of patients with pernicious anemia is parietal cell antibody. Tests for parietal cell antibodies are rarely useful in pernicious anemia because of low specificity. These antibodies can be found in the sera of normal healthy individuals and in the sera of patients with a variety of disorders other than pernicious anemia (particularly other autoimmune syndromes).

The Schilling test is a procedure to evaluate the ability of the patient's intestinal tract to absorb vitamin B_{12}. It involves the oral administration of a standardized dose of B_{12} labeled with ^{57}Co or ^{58}Co. Simultaneously, an intramuscular flushing dose of unlabeled vitamin B_{12} is given to the patient to bind all available storage sites for vitamin B_{12}. In this way, if IF is present and normal absorption occurs, greater than 7 to 10 percent of the oral, labeled 1-μg dose will be excreted in the patient's urine, collected over a 24-hour period. The excreted urine can then be assayed for radioactivity (part 1). If malabsorption of vitamin B_{12} occurs, a decreased amount of labeled vitamin B_{12} will be excreted. In the two-stage Schilling test, IF may then be given with the oral dose of vitamin B_{12} and the Schilling test repeated to see if the Schilling test is corrected to normal with addition of IF (part 2). If so corrected, the patient has pernicious anemia. If the Schilling test does not correct with the addition of IF, other causes for the vitamin B_{12} malabsorption must be investigated. New techniques use simultaneous administration of vitamin B_{12} and the B_{12}-IF complex (each labeled with a different isotope) to shorten the time required for the two-stage Schilling test. It is important to remember that the accuracy of the Schilling test is dependent on (1) a complete urine collection and (2) normal renal function.

Another new test, the deoxyuridine (DU) suppression test, can be used to measure the degree of functional metabolism of vitamin B_{12} or folic acid or both. This sophisticated radioisotope technique measures the ability of cells to convert deoxyuridine monophosphate to thymidylate, a step that requires adequate levels of vitamin B_{12} and folic acid. This test, unlike the Schilling test, is not routinely available in most hospital laboratories.

In the patient with a decreased red cell folate and documented folic acid deficiency, a careful evaluation of diet and drug history and alcohol intake, as well as tests for malabsorption, will usually identify the cause.

Cases of macrocytosis in patients having normal vitamin B_{12} and folate levels require careful investigation. The major causes of nonmegaloblastic macrocytosis have been previously discussed. If the macrocytic red cells are round, pink, uniform, and possibly targeting, then liver function tests should be performed. These tests will confirm whether alcoholism or liver disease is the cause. If no evidence of alcoholism or liver disease is present, a bone marrow examination is required, which will pinpoint the presence of various hematologic malignancies, myelodysplastic syndromes, and disease states such as sideroblastic anemia that can cause macrocytosis. It may also detect the presence of a mild megaloblastic anemia that exhibited falsely normal vitamin B_{12} and folate levels. If red cell dimorphism is noted on the peripheral blood smear, serum iron studies will complement the bone marrow iron stain in identifying the presence of sideroblastic anemia.

Two routine chemistry tests of special interest in the diagnosis of megaloblastic anemia are the serum lactic dehydrogenase (LD) level and the bilirubin level. The serum LD is often strikingly elevated in patients with megaloblastic anemia, regardless of its cause. The fractions responsible for the elevation are LD_1 and LD_2, with LD_1 greater than LD_2 (flipped pattern).[23] The serum bilirubin is usually only slightly elevated, owing to an increase in the indirect fraction. The results described for these two tests are usually associated with a hemolytic process. Megaloblastic anemia is in reality a hemolytic process because of the massive intramedullary destruction of red cell precursors in the bone marrow. This destruction has the exact same chemical results as the destruction of red blood cells peripherally (that is, hemolytic anemia).

TREATMENT

Vitamin B$_{12}$ Deficiency

The majority of patients who develop vitamin B$_{12}$ deficiency are maintained on lifelong vitamin B$_{12}$ therapy. During treatment, all patients require initial saturation of the body stores with vitamin B$_{12}$. In the United States, usually a minimum of six intramuscular injections of 1000 μg of cyanocobalamin given at 2- or 3-day intervals is required for initial saturation. In situations when the underlying disease process is irreversible, as in pernicious anemia, lifelong maintenance therapy is administered following the replenishment of the body stores of vitamin B$_{12}$.

Maintenance therapy varies in concentration given and intervals administered from one institution to another, depending on the severity of the deficiency and preference of the clinician. A dosage of 100 μg per month is usually considered adequate maintenance therapy. It should be noted that hydroxocobalamin may be preferred over cyanocobalamin for treatment of vitamin B$_{12}$ deficiencies because the former derivative is retained in the body three times as well as cyanocobalamin and binds more tightly to body proteins. Hydroxocobalamin, however, is a more expensive product and its extra cost may not be justifiable inasmuch as both products correct the anemia.

A rise in the reticulocyte count should be seen 3 to 4 days following treatment. This is followed by a reversal of the clinical abnormalities to normal in most patients. The complete blood count (CBC) and peripheral blood smear will completely normalize in about 4 to 6 weeks. It should be noted that treatment with folic acid will also partially correct the anemia of a patient with vitamin B$_{12}$ deficiency if given in very large doses (5 mg/day). However, neurologic deterioration will still progress in vitamin B$_{12}$ deficiency, if folate alone is given. As a result, simultaneous treatment of megaloblastic anemia with vitamin B$_{12}$ and folate is usually administered as a therapeutic trial if the exact pathogenesis has not been definitively established.

Folic Acid Deficiency

Physiologic daily doses for the treatment of folic acid deficiency range from 100 to 400 μg of folate, which is most commonly administered orally for a given period of time, usually several months. Larger doses of folate (1 to 5 mg daily) are also used to treat this deficiency; however, it is necessary to confirm that vitamin B$_{12}$ deficiency is not present before these large doses are prescribed. Lifelong therapy is usually unnecessary because it is often possible to correct the cause of the folate deficiency, thus preventing its recurrence. Table 7-5 compares the treatment of vitamin B$_{12}$ and folic acid deficiencies.

CASE STUDY

A 50-year-old white woman was referred to the hospital from an outpatient clinic because her hematocrit was 13 percent. Although she had recently lost 40 pounds (18 kg), she felt fairly well at the time. She had noted a lack of appetite (anorexia) and shortness of breath on exertion (dyspnea) in the past few weeks. She had had a previous history of iron-deficiency anemia 10 years earlier.

Physical examination revealed a thin, pale woman with a slightly yellow tinge to her skin color and icteric sclerae. Her tongue was very smooth and slightly reddened.

Laboratory data were as follows:
CBC:
WBC	= 7 $\times$ 10^9/liter
RBC	= 1.26 $\times$ 10^{12}/liter
Hemoglobin	= 3.7 g/dl
Hematocrit	= 11.2%

Table 7-5. **TREATMENT OF MEGALOBLASTIC ANEMIA**

	Vitamin B$_{12}$ Deficiency	Folic Acid Deficiency
Initial	1000 μg cyanocobalamin IM 6 times over 2-3 wk	1 mg folic acid daily for 3-4 mo
Maintenance	100 μg cyanocobalamin IM once/mo	Correct underlying cause; then 1 mg folic acid daily or weekly
Indications for prophylactic treatment	Total gastrectomy, ileal resection	Pregnancy, chronic hemolytic anemia, autoimmune hemolytic anemia, myelodysplastic syndromes, dialysis, parenteral feeding

IM = intramuscular.
*Other therapy that may be needed initially in severe megaloblastic anemia includes administration of diuretics, potassium supplements, and platelet concentrates. Blood transfusion is best avoided.

MCV	=	87 fl
MCH	=	29.8 pg
MCHC	=	32.9%
Platelet count	=	37×10^9/liter
Differential	=	60% segmented neutrophils
	=	37% lymphocytes
	=	1% monocytes
	=	2% eosinophils
Reticulocyte %	=	2.6% (0.5–1.5)
Serum LD	=	8700 U/liter (60–250)
Total bilirubin	=	3.2 mg/dl (0.2–1.0)
Indirect fraction	=	2.6 mg/dl (0.2–0.8)
Serum iron	=	204 μg/dl (42–166)
TIBC	=	204 μg/dl (239–380)
% Saturation	=	100% (20–50)
Serum ferritin	=	400 ng/ml (10–100)
Serum vitamin B_{12}	=	<50 pg/ml (200–900)
Red cell folate	=	375 ng/ml (160–640)

The peripheral blood and bone marrow morphology pertaining to this case may be seen in **Color Plates 64 to 69.**

Questions: Case Study

1. What is the probable etiology of the anemia?
2. What are the morphologic abnormalities in the blood and bone marrow?
3. What is the correct interpretation of the reticulocyte count?
4. What further test(s) should be performed?
5. What is unusual about this case's clinical presentation or laboratory findings?
6. Are all chemistry test results compatible with the diagnosis?

This case represents a classic example of a severe degree of anemia, well compensated for by the patient because of its insidious onset. This patient had relatively few complaints despite having a 3.7 g/dl hemoglobin level. Her physical signs pointed to the possibility of a hemolytic anemia or liver disease. In this particular case, the answer was indeed in the red cell. The red cell morphology was very striking, with a 4+ degree of anisocytosis and poikilocytosis. The types of poikilocytes were quite diverse and confusing, varying from spherocytes and schistocytes to tailed cells (teardrops) and ovalocytes. The diagnostically significant poikilocyte in this case was the oval macrocyte, which indicated a probable megaloblastic etiology. This was an important finding because, since the MCV was normal, a macrocytic anemia was not at all suggested by the CBC. Hypersegmented neutrophils were present on the smear, as were multiple Howell-Jolly bodies and rare Cabot rings **(see Color Plates 65, 66, and 69).** The classic signs of megaloblastic anemia were all present on the smear, even though the MCV was not elevated. The absence of an elevated MCV is not rare in megaloblastic anemia and can be seen in severely anemic patients, such as this woman, in whom the anisocytosis is very striking. The reticulocyte percentage in this case appears slightly elevated, but this is due to the very decreased red cell count. The absolute reticulocyte count is severely decreased at 32.8×10^9/liter.

Pancytopenia was not present in this case, because the white blood cell (WBC) count was normal, but the degree of thrombocytopenia was more severe than is usually seen. The patient had no hemorrhagic problems despite the thrombocytopenia.

The bone marrow aspiration was performed and predictably showed a flagrant megaloblastic dyspoiesis.

The chemistry results were entirely compatible with megaloblastic anemia. The LD level of 8700, although striking, is not at all unexpected. The iron studies and serum bilirubin level revealed results typical of chronic hemolysis (that is, elevated serum iron, percent saturation, serum ferritin, and indirect bilirubin fraction). As explained in the text, megaloblastic anemia shows chemical findings identical to those seen in hemolytic anemia.

Based on the peripheral blood and bone marrow morphology, serum vitamin B_{12} and red cell folate tests were performed. These results clearly pointed to a vitamin B_{12} deficiency. One of two tests had to be performed at this point—either the Schilling test or the anti-IF antibody test. In this case, the two-part Schilling was performed. The patient excreted a decreased amount of labeled dose (2.66 percent) in 24 hours. The vitamin B_{12} excretion increased to normal (12 percent) with the addition of IF. These results were diagnostic of pernicious anemia.

This case is somewhat unusual in that (1) the patient had not reported neurologic abnormalities and (2) the MCV was perfectly normal.

REFERENCES

1. Ehrlich, P: Farbenanalytische Untersuchungen zur Histologie und Klinik des Blutes. Hirschwald, Berlin, 1891.
2. Addison, T: On the constitutional and local effects of diseases of the suprarenal capsules. S Highly, London, 1855.
3. Biermer, A: Uker eine Form vow progressiver pernicioser anamie. Correspondenzbl Schweix Anzte 2:15, 1872.
4. Hoffbrand, AV, et al: Megaloblastic anemia: Initiation of DNA synthesis in excess of DNA chain elongation as the underlying mechanism. Clin Haematol 5(3):727, 1976.
5. Hardisty, RM and Weatherall, DJ: Blood and Its Disorders, Blackwell Scientific, 1982, pp 206, 225.
6. Kolhouse, JT and Allen, RH: Absorption, plasma transport and cellular retention of cobalamin analogues in the rabbit. J Clin Invest 60:1381, 1977.
7. Hillman, RS and Finch CA: Red Cell Manual. FA Davis, Philadelphia, 1985, p 80.
8. Chanarin, I, et al: How vitamin B_{12} acts. Br J Haematol 47(4):487, 1981.
9. Williams, W, et al: Hematology. McGraw-Hill, New York, 1983, p 448.
10. Sullivan, IW and Herbert, V: Suppression of hematopoiesis by alcohol. J Clin Invest 43:2048, 1964.
11. Dahlke, MD and Mertens-Roesler, E: Malabsorption of folic acid due to diphenylhydantoin. Blood 30:341, 1967.
12. Klipstein, FA, Berlinger, FG, and Reed, LJ: Folate deficiency associated with drug therapy for tuberculosis. Blood 29:697, 1967.
13. Castle, WB: Megaloblastic anemia. Postgrad Med 64:117, 1978.

14. Castle, WB: Observations on the etiologic relationship of achylia gastrica to pernicious anemia. The effect of administration to patients with pernicious anemia of the contents of the normal human stomach recovered after the ingestion of beef muscle. Am J Med Sci 178:784, 1929.

15. Miale, JB: Laboratory Medicine Hematology. CV Mosby, St Louis, 1982, pp 425, 432.

16. Lindenbaum, J: Folate and B_{12} deficiencies in alcoholism. Semin Hematol 17:119, 1980.

17. Nath, BJ and Lindenbaum, J: Persistence of neutrophil hypersegmentation during recovery from megaloblastic granulopoiesis. Ann Intern Med 90:757, 1979.

18. Pierre, RV and Hoagland, HC: Preleukemic States: Differential Diagnosis of Refractory Anemia, Dysmyelopoietic States and Early Leukemias. ASCP Workshop Publication, 1980.

19. Breedveld, FC, Bieger, R, and van Wermeskerken, RKA: The clinical significance of macrocytosis. Acta Med Scand 209:319, 1981.

20. Friedman, EW: Reticulocyte counts: How to use them, what they mean. Diagnostic Medicine 7:29, 1984.

21. Lindenbaum, J: Status of laboratory testing in the diagnosis of megaloblastic anemia. Blood 61(4):624, 1984.

22. Kolhouse, JF, et al: Cobalamin analogues are present in human plasma and can mask cobalamin deficiency because current radioisotope dilution assays are not specific for true cobalamin. N Engl J Med 299:785, 1978.

23. Winston, RM, Warburton, FG, and Stott, A: Enzymatic diagnosis of megaloblastic anemia. Br J Haematol 19:587, 1970.

24. Waxman, S, Metz, J, and Herbert, V: Defective DNA synthesis in human megaloblastic bone marrow: Effects of homocysteine and methionine. J Clin Invest 48:284, 1969.

QUESTIONS

1. *What is megaloblastic anemia?*
   a. Anemia associated with defective RNA synthesis and abnormal red cell maturation
   b. Anemia associated with defective DNA synthesis and abnormal red cell maturation
   c. Anemia associated with intracellular red cell hemolysis
   d. Anemia associated with a decrease in erythropoietin production

2. *Which of the following is not a cause of megaloblastic anemia?*
   a. Folic acid deficiency due primarily to low dietary intake
   b. Vitamin B_{12} deficiency due primarily to malabsorption
   c. Deficient production of IF
   d. Production of cold agglutinins

3. *Which clinical symptom is unique to vitamin B_{12} deficiency found in pernicious anemia and is often used to distinguish it from folate deficiency?*
   a. Neurologic manifestations
   b. Epithelial abnormalities
   c. Pallor, weakness, light-headedness, and shortness of breath
   d. Slight jaundice

4. *Which morphologic finding on the peripheral blood smear is not characteristic for megaloblastic anemia?*
   a. Oval macrocytes
   b. Howell-Jolly bodies
   c. Rubriblasts
   d. Hypersegmented neutrophils

5. *What is the appearance of the bone marrow in megaloblastic anemia?*
   a. Hypocellular with normal M:E ratio
   b. Hypercellular with erythroid hyperplasia and reversed M:E ratio
   c. Normocellular with myeloid hyperplasia and reversed M:E ratio
   d. Hypercellular with both erythroid and myeloid hyperplasia and normal M:E ratio

6. *What condition is indicated by the following test results: low serum folate level, low vitamin B_{12} level, negative for antibodies to IF, and normal Schilling test?*
   a. Folic acid deficiency
   b. Vitamin B_{12} deficiency other than pernicious anemia
   c. Pernicious anemia
   d. Nonmegaloblastic macrocytic anemia

7. *What are the most common treatments for vitamin B_{12} and folic acid deficiencies?*
   a. Administration of IF
   b. Administration of steroids and immunosuppressive drugs
   c. Administration of cyanocobalamin and folic acid
   d. Modification of dietary intake

ANSWERS

1. b (p. 92)
2. d (p. 93)
3. a (p. 98)
4. c (p. 99)
5. b (p. 100)
6. a (p. 103)
7. c (p. 104)

CHAPTER **8**

JOE MARTY, M.S., M.T.(ASCP)

Aplastic Anemia (Including Pure Red Cell Aplasia and Congenital Dyserythropoietic Anemia)

DEFINITION

HISTORY

PATHOPHYSIOLOGY

ETIOLOGY
ACQUIRED
Ionizing Irradiation
Chemical Agents
Idiosyncratic Reaction to Drugs
Infections
IDIOPATHIC

CONGENITAL DISORDERS
Fanconi's Anemia

CLINICAL MANIFESTATIONS

LABORATORY EXAMINATION

TREATMENT, CLINICAL COURSE, AND PROGNOSIS

RELATED DISORDERS
PURE RED CELL APLASIA
CONGENITAL DYSERYTHROPOIETIC ANEMIA

CASE STUDY

OBJECTIVES

At the end of this chapter, the learner should be able to:
1. Define aplastic anemia.
2. List three classifications of causes for aplastic anemia.
3. List four causes for acquired aplastic anemia.
4. Name and describe the most common congenital disorder of aplastic anemia.
5. List laboratory results that are used as transplantation guidelines in cases of aplastic anemia.
6. Describe the typical appearance of the bone marrow in aplastic anemia.
7. List clinical treatments for aplastic anemia.
8. Define pure red cell aplasia and list characteristics associated with this condition.
9. Describe common characteristics that define all types of congenital dyserythropoietic anemia (CDA).

DEFINITION

Aplastic anemia is a severe, life-threatening syndrome in which production of erythrocytes, platelets, and leukocytes has failed. Both genders and all age groups are affected. This disorder may result from a varied pathogenesis and etiology. Radiation, chemicals, drugs, infections, and autoimmune mechanisms are known to be associated with aplastic anemia. The incidence varies considerably but is approximately 1 per 500,000.[1]

HISTORY

The first reported case of aplastic anemia was described in 1888 by Ehrlich.[2] He described a young woman with a fatal case of severe anemia and leukopenia with hemorrhage. The autopsy findings showed little evidence of marrow development and led Ehrlich to conclude that the anemia was due to a depression of marrow function. A descriptive name was first applied in 1904 when Chauffard introduced the term "aplastic anemia."[3]

Reports and reviews increased in number, and in 1934, after a report by Thompson and colleagues,[4] aplastic anemia was first considered a distinct clinical entity. However, conceptual difficulties persisted, and criteria for diagnosis are becoming more clearly defined and accepted only now.

PATHOPHYSIOLOGY

The primary defect in aplastic anemia is a reduction or depletion of hematopoietic precursor cells. This decreased production of erythrocytes, leukocytes, and platelets results in peripheral pancytopenia **(see Color Plates 70 to 76)**. Most data suggest quantitative damage to pluripotential stem cells as the primary event in bone marrow failure.[5] Information on these stem cells, called spleen colony-forming cells (CFU-S), has been obtained from murine studies.[6] If bone marrow is infused into a lethally irradiated mouse, hematopoietic colonies will form in the spleen. These colonies are formed from single progenitor cells capable of self-renewal and production of granulocytes, erythrocytes, and megakaryocytes. Evidence suggests the existence of a similar stem cell in humans. Successful bone marrow transplantation in identical twins also implicates a stem cell aberration in aplastic anemia. Stem cell numbers or their ability to replicate, or both, are decreased in aplastic anemia. It is uncertain how stem cells are damaged. Direct damage by radiation, chemicals, drugs, and infections is suspected, particularly when previous exposure has occurred. Marrow hypoplasia and aplasia may possibly have an immunologic basis.[7]

Cellular and humoral abnormalities in hematopoietic regulation and an altered marrow microenvironment[8] have also been implicated as possible factors in aplastic anemia. Studies have suggested that in some cases T lymphocytes may suppress hematopoiesis.[9] Thomas and Storb[10] suggested an autoimmune mechanism in which a foreign agent attaches to a stem cell. The foreign substance acts as a hapten, and the stem cell becomes an innocent bystander in an autoimmune reaction.

The influence of genetic factors in the pathogenesis of aplastic anemia is supported by the association with Fanconi's anemia, which has a familial basis.

ETIOLOGY

Aplastic anemia may be (1) acquired as a result of exposure to ionizing radiation, chemical agents, drugs, and infections; (2) idiopathic; or (3) congenital due to a disorder such as Fanconi's anemia (Table 8–1).

Evidence for determining the causative agents in aplastic anemia is often circumstantial. Even regarding agents that are known to cause aplastic anemia, the number of individuals affected is small in relation to the number of individuals exposed. This makes epidemiologic studies difficult and results in ambiguity and inconclusiveness in determining the

Table 8–1. **CAUSES OF APLASTIC ANEMIA**

Acquired, from exposure to:	Chemical agents
	Drugs
	Infections
	Ionizing irradiation
Idiopathic	
Congenital:	Fanconi's anemia

true cause of the illness. Why certain individuals are abnormally susceptible to causative agents and develop aplastic anemia is not known. No method for predicting individual sensitivity to drug or chemical exposure has been discovered. Metabolic defects, such as primaquine-induced hemolysis in glucose-6-phosphate dehydrogenase (G6PD)-deficient individuals, have not been identified as causes of aplastic anemia. It is important to establish whether a causative agent may exist, so that continued exposure can be eliminated.

Acquired

Ionizing Irradiation

The acute results of radiation injury on cells have been well studied and documented. Radiation effects are consistent and predictable, depending on the dose of radiation received and the tissue involved. Hematopoietic cells are particularly sensitive to these effects. If the dosage is high, the marrow may become completely acellular. Whole-body irradiation with 300 to 500 rads can result in complete loss of hematopoietic activity. Sublethal exposure results in severe leukopenia, thrombocytopenia, and anemia. Aplasia from sublethal exposure lasts approximately 4 to 6 weeks, after which time the bone marrow recovers and cell counts return to normal. Only very penetrating forms of external radiation, such as those caused by x-rays and gamma rays, are likely to damage hematopoietic cells. Low-energy radiation—that from alpha and beta particles—may damage cells if ingested. The effects of continuous low-energy radiation became apparent in radium dial painters, who ingested radium when they wetted their brushes by mouth.[11] When exposure to radiation has been minimal or low, the immediate toxic effects on hematopoiesis are usually reversible. However, with both acute and chronic radiation exposure, the delayed or long-term effects are less predictable. Aplastic anemia can occur many years after initial exposure. The incidence of leukemia and carcinoma is increased in exposed individuals. Cancer patients may also be affected as a result of radiation therapy.

Chemical Agents

Various chemical agents have been associated with development of aplastic anemia, including benzene, trinitrotoluene, insecticides and weed killers, and arsenic. Chemical agents containing a benzene ring with a nitro or nitroso group are particularly implicated. Benzene, an organic solvent obtained from coal and petroleum, was the first recognized and is the most common cause of aplastic anemia. It has been widely used as a solvent in many different industries. Exposure is primarily from inhalation of vapor, although absorption through the skin can occur.

Aplastic anemia may develop shortly after exposure or as long as 10 years afterward. Most cases of benzene toxicity are reversible after exposure has been eliminated. The reversible anemia may have a hemolytic component resulting in reticulocytosis. Benzene has also been implicated as a cause of leukemia. Animal studies suggest that benzene may inhibit RNA and DNA synthesis and interfere with cell division and maturation.[12]

Idiosyncratic Reaction to Drugs

Idiosyncratic reactions to drugs that produce aplastic anemia are uncommon.[13] Often the etiology is assumed on the basis of epidemiologic data and temporal relationship to exposure. In the literature there are many long lists of drugs that may be implicated in aplastic anemia. However, a true relationship has been established in only a small number of cases, and unfortunately no definitive tests are available to predict or document the drug association. Drugs that have been implicated in idiosyncratic aplastic anemia are chloramphenicol, phenylbutazone, oxyphenbutazone, among others (Table 8–2). This individual sensitivity to a particular drug is poorly understood. A possible explanation for these idiosyncratic reactions is that the individual may have a genetic defect. This defect could affect the processing of the drug or increase the vulnerability of the stem cells, or both.

Chloramphenicol and phenylbutazone are drugs that most frequently cause aplastic anemia. The effects of chloramphenicol have been well studied and documented.[1] Approximately 1 in 40,000 individuals exposed to chloramphenicol will develop aplastic anemia. This is about 10 times more frequent than the incidence of aplastic anemia in the general population. The effects of chloramphenicol are either reversible, dose-dependent, and predictable or irreversible, dose-independent, and unpredictable. Reversible bone marrow suppression most commonly affects erythropoiesis and is due to decreased heme and hemoglobin formation. The morphologic finding of prominent cytoplasmic vacuolization in erythroblasts is common. In contrast, the irreversible effects of chloramphenicol are less predictable. The age of the individual and the dosage of the drug have no apparent relationship to the incidence or occurrence.

Table 8–2. **AGENTS ASSOCIATED WITH APLASTIC ANEMIA**

Those Regularly Producing Marrow Hypoplasia if Dose Sufficient
Ionizing irradiation
Benzene and derivatives (e.g., toluene)
Cytostatic agents (e.g., 6-mercaptopurine, busulfan, melphalan, vincristine)
Other poisons (inorganic arsenic)

Those Occasionally Associated with Marrow Hypoplasia

Class	Relatively Frequent	Infrequent
Antimicrobial	Chloramphenicol Organic arsenicals Penicillin, tetracyclines	Streptomycin Amphotericin B Sulfonamides Sulfisoxazole (Gantrisin)
Anticonvulsant	Methylphenylethylhydantoin (Mesantoin) Trimethadione (Tridione)	Methylphenylhydantoin Diphenylhydantoin (Dilantin) Primidone
Analgesic	Phenylbutazone	Aspirin
Antithyroid		Carbimazole Tapazole KClO$_4$
Hypoglycemic		Tolbutamide (Orinase) Chlorpropamide (Diabinese)
Antianxiety		Chlorpromazine (Thorazine) Chlordiazepoxide (Librium)
Insecticide		Chlorophenothane (DDT) Parathion
Miscellaneous		Colchicine Acetazolamide (Diamox) Hair dyes CCl$_4$, Bi, SCN

Source: Beck, WS: Hematology, ed. 3. MIT Press, Cambridge, MA, 1982, p 39, with permission.

Another well-studied marrow depressant is quinacrine. During World War II, quinacrine was given routinely to soldiers in the South Pacific for malaria prophylaxis. Custer analyzed the cases of aplastic anemia occurring there during the years 1943 and 1944 and found the incidence of aplastic anemia to be 3 per 100,000.[14]

Table 8-2 lists other drug categories that are associated with aplastic anemia. Clearly, as new drugs are developed, the associations and incidences will change. Indiscriminate use of drugs should be avoided. In particular, potentially toxic drugs should be used only when alternative therapy is unavailable. Drugs implicated in hematopoietic suppression are listed in Table 8-3.

Infections

Not infrequently, aplastic anemia is associated with hepatitis—particularly with types B and non-A, non-B. Reports of aplastic anemia following viral hepatitis have been increasing.[15] Possible mechanisms in viral hepatitis–associated aplastic anemia include (1) prolonged serum levels of drugs or their metabolites because of liver damage, (2) direct damage to stem cells by the virus, (3) depressed hematopoiesis by the viral genome, and (4) virus-induced haptogenic autoimmune damage. The possibility exists that subclinical viral infections may contribute to the incidence of aplastic anemia. Another possibility is that viral infections are secondary to marrow aplasia or dysfunction. Other infections such as Epstein-Barr virus, cytomegalovirus, miliary tuberculosis, and dengue fever also have been associated with aplastic anemia.

Idiopathic

Most patients have no history of exposure to any known or suspected causative agents. Detailed clinical histories have probably implicated many agents that have little to do with aplastic anemia. It is often difficult to determine the cause of aplastic anemia, because, by the time the damage is apparent, the causative agent may be absent or present in too small an amount to be detectable. It is hoped that in the future more specific environmental factors will be identified.

Congenital Disorders

Fanconi's Anemia

Assessment of family history and physical and hematologic abnormalities, as well as chromosome analysis, is helpful in making a diagnosis of congenital marrow aplasia. Fanconi's anemia is the most common and best described congenital disorder.[16,17] The inheritance pattern is autosomal recessive. Disorders that may be confused with Fanconi's anemia include dyskeratosis congenita, pure red cell aplasia, Shwachman's syndrome, and thrombocytopenia–absent radius (TAR) syndrome. Patients

Table 8-3. DRUGS IMPLICATED IN HEMOPOIETIC SUPPRESSION*

Acetophenetidin (1,3)	Iproniazid (1)
Acetyl sulfisoxazole (3)	Isoniazid (1,3,4)
Acetylsalicylic acid (aspirin) (1,2,3)	Lead (1)
Aminosalicylic acid (3,4)	Lithium carbonate (1)
Ammonium thioglycolate (3)	Meprobamate (1,2,3)
Amodiaquin HCl (3)	Methaminodiazepoxide (Librium) (3)
Arsenicals (1,2,3,4)	Methapyrilene HCl (4)
Arsphenamine (1,2)	Methylpromazine (3)
Atabrine (1,2)	Mezapine (2)
Benzene (1,2,3,4)	Nitrofurantoin (4)
Betanaphthoxyacetic acid (2)	Novobiocin (4)
Bishydroxycoumarin (3,4)	Nystatin (2)
Carbamide (2)	Oxyphenbutazone (2)
Carbon tetrachloride (1)	Para-aminosalicylic acid (3,4)
Carbutamide (Orabetic) (2)	Penicillin (1,2,3,4)
Chloramphenicol (1,2,3,4)	Phenobarbital (1,2,3,4)
Chlordane (1)	Phenylbutazone (Butazolidin) (1,2,3)
Chlorophenothane (DDT) (1,2)	Pipamazine (1)
Chlorothiazide (3)	Primidone (1)
Chlorpheniramine maleate (3)	Prochlorperazine (Compazine) (2,3)
Chlorpromazine (Thorazine) (3)	Pyrimethamine (Daraprim) (1,2,3)
Chlorpropamide (2)	Quinidine (2)
Chlortetracyline (1,3)	Quinine (2,3)
Cinophen (3)	Reserpine (2)
Coldricine (2,3)	Stibophen (2)
Cycloheximide (3)	Streptomycin (1,2,3)
Dextromethorphan HBr (2)	Sulfamethoxypyridazine (Kynex) (2,3,4)
Diethylstilbestrol (2)	Tetracycline (3)
Diphenylhydantoin (Dilantin) (4)	Thenalidine tartrate (3)
Dipyrone (3)	Thioridazine HCl (3)
Ethinamate (2)	Tolazoline HCl (1,2)
Fumagillin (3)	Tolbutamide (1,2,3)
Gamma benzene hexachloride (1,3)	Tolbutamide (Orinase) (2)
Hair lacquer (3)	Trifluoperazine (1,3)
Imipramine HCl (3)	Trifluoperazine (Stelazine) (3)
	Trimethadione (Tridione) (1,2)

Source: Miale, J: Laboratory Medicine: Hematology, ed. 6. CV Mosby, St Louis, 1982, with permission.

*More than 500 are listed in the latest report of the American Medical Association Subcommittee on Blood Dyscrasias. The drugs listed in this table are those that have produced dyscrasias when given alone. 1 = pancytopenia; 2 = thrombocytopenia; 3 = leukopenia; 4 = anemia.

with Fanconi's anemia have physical abnormalities including cutaneous hyperpigmentation, skeletal disorders (most common of which is aplasia or hypoplasia of the thumb), poor growth, renal anomalies, microcephaly, mental retardation, and strabismus. Not all of these abnormalities are always present. The most common findings are skin hyperpigmentation and short stature. Chromosome analysis usually reveals frequent chromatid breaks and exchanges. The extent of initial pancytopenia is variable but progressive and becomes symptomatic at about 5 years of age. Initially the bone marrow may show normal cellularity or hypercellularity, but eventually hypocellularity develops. These patients also have an increased incidence of acute myelogenous leukemia. In the past, treatment consisted of chronic androgen therapy. Because of anabolic steroid use, the incidence of hepatocellular carcinoma has increased. The majority of patients die in the second decade of life, owing to hemorrhage or infection. More recently, some patients have been treated somewhat successfully with bone marrow transplantation.

CLINICAL MANIFESTATIONS

The onset of aplastic anemia is often insidious. Symptoms include fatigue, dyspnea, palpitation, and, to a lesser extent, infection. Physical examination may reveal pallor, purpura, ecchymoses, petechiae, and mucosal bleeding. These symptoms are due to anemia, thrombocytopenia, and granulocytopenia. Splenomegaly is unusual. Mild lymphadenopathy may be present.

LABORATORY EXAMINATION

Characteristically, the hemoglobin, white blood cell count, and platelet count are decreased to a varying extent in aplastic anemia. Criteria for severe aplastic anemia vary among institutions, but the following guidelines have been used for choosing patients for transplantation:[18]

1. No significant improvement in blood values during 3 weeks following diagnosis
2. At least two of the following blood values (presence of which defines severe aplastic anemia):
   a. Platelet concentration of less than 20×10^9/liter
   b. Neutrophil concentration of less than 0.5×10^9/liter
   c. Reticulocyte counts of less than 1 percent in the presence of anemia

An examination of the peripheral blood will reveal normochromic, normocytic red cells and decreased numbers of platelets and granulocytes **(see Color Plate 75)**. Some patients will have slightly macrocytic red cells. Occasionally normoblasts, small numbers of myelocytes and metamyelocytes, and a few reticulocytes may be seen. Prominent reticulocytosis, blasts, and abnormal platelets should not be seen. Relative lymphocytosis may be present. There is no peripheral morphologic abnormality that is diagnostic of aplastic anemia. Diseases likely to be mistaken for aplastic anemia are listed in Table 8–4.

Bone marrow aspiration often results in a dry tap **(see Color Plate 76)**. Bone marrow biopsy examination most commonly reveals a marked hypocellular marrow with a reduction in all myeloid, eryth-

Table 8–4. **DIFFERENTIAL DIAGNOSIS OF PANCYTOPENIA**

Anemia of pregnancy	Myelofibrosis
Chronic renal disease	Myelophthisic anemia
Overwhelming infection	Paroxysmal nocturnal hemoglobinuria (PNH)
Megaloblastic anemia	
Leukemia	Hypersplenism
Lymphoma	Autoimmune disease
Myelodysplastic syndrome	

roid, and megakaryocytic elements **(see Color Plate 71)**. Small numbers of scattered lymphocytes are usually present, and an occasional aggregate or nodule of lymphocytes may be seen **(see Color Plates 73 and 74)**. Other patients may have focal normocellular marrow or even hypercellular marrow.[19] In the presence of a hypercellular marrow, leukemia and myelodysplasia must be excluded. It is crucial to remember that there may be variations in cellularity within the same section and from one site to another **(see Color Plate 72)**. It is, therefore, important to make an overall assessment and perhaps obtain multiple biopsies when the diagnosis is uncertain. Ideally, the length of core biopsy should be 1 to 2 cm. It may be necessary to follow the patient's course of illness carefully to establish the diagnosis.

TREATMENT, CLINICAL COURSE, AND PROGNOSIS

The prognosis of untreated aplastic anemia is poor.[20] Most patients will die if untreated. However, some patients may recover spontaneously, and this unpredictability complicates treatment decisions. Patients with low counts who fall into the severe aplastic anemia category have the poorest prognosis. In general, simple supportive transfusion therapy in these cases produces only a 20 percent survival at 2 years.

Treatment for aplastic anemia in the past was mainly supportive, with administration of steroids and androgens. These drugs have been shown to have limited value and undesirable toxic side effects. Today, the treatment of choice for severe aplastic anemia in patients under 40 years of age is bone marrow transplantation,[21] if an HLA-identical sibling is available. For other patients, immunosuppressive therapy is recommended. An increasing amount of evidence has implicated immunologic mechanisms as being responsible for some cases of acquired aplastic anemia. Treatment with cyclophosphamide and antilymphocyte or antithymocyte globulin may work by inhibiting the immune suppression of stem cells.

Reports from bone marrow transplant centers have indicated survival rates of from 60 to 80 percent, with complete hematopoietic recovery. These encouraging results have occurred in selected patients. Important factors for survival are early transplantation and avoidance of blood products, especially products from potential marrow donors. There is a higher mortality in multiply transfused patients because of graft rejection, which reportedly is 25 to 60 percent in these patients.[22] If transfusions are necessary, leukocyte-depleted red blood cells (RBCs) and platelets are recommended to decrease the incidence of graft rejection. The main complications of bone marrow transplantation are graft rejection and acute or chronic graft-versus-host disease (GVHD). Early transplantation, avoidance of transfusions, and immunosuppressive therapy have greatly decreased the occurrence of these complications.

The prognosis in aplastic anemia is variable and primarily depends on the severity of the anemia, supportive care, and method of treatment. Patients who do poorly often die from progressive deterioration due to repeated bleeding and infection. Intracranial hemorrhage is common. Patients treated successfully with transplants may develop acute or chronic GVHD and interstitial pneumonitis. However, today the prospects for cure are good — a significant improvement over the last decade.

RELATED DISORDERS

Pure Red Cell Aplasia

Pure red cell aplasia is a disorder predominantly involving erythropoiesis. Leukocytes and platelets do not appear to be affected. Bone marrow examination usually reveals normal cellularity with absence of erythroid precursors. Reticulocytes and nucleated RBCs are not seen in the peripheral blood smear. RBCs are normocytic or slightly macrocytic. Evidence of hemolysis or hemorrhage is not present. Serum erythropoietin is usually increased.

This disorder can be acquired or constitutional. In some patients with hemolytic anemia and concomitant infection, erythropoiesis may suddenly halt. This has been termed an aplastic crisis. An example is a patient with hereditary spherocytosis who has asymptomatic disease and develops a crisis with sudden reticulocytopenia. If the patient does not recover, severe anemia will develop.

Anemia may also be seen after administration of certain drugs. This anemia usually disappears after withdrawal of the drug. Other causes of acquired pure red cell aplasia include malnutrition and neoplasia. In about half of the adults with pure red cell aplasia, a thymoma (tumor of the thymus gland) has been found. Removal of this tumor has benefited some patients. Immune suppression of erythropoiesis is believed to have played a role in this form of red cell aplasia. The immune etiology is supported by the fact that some patients respond to steroid treatment and that infants born to mothers with the condition may be anemic at birth.

A congenital form of red cell aplasia was defined in 1938 by Diamond and Blackfan.[23] The syndrome is characterized by a slowly progressive and refractory anemia detected early in infancy. Leukocytes and platelets are normal. Other minor congenital abnormalities may be present, but renal abnormalities are not observed, in contrast to Fanconi's anemia. About 25 percent of these patients will show a spontaneous remission. This disorder is believed to be a result of a defective stem cell.

In this group of disorders limited success has been observed by giving the patient steroids, androgens, or immunosuppressive therapy.

Another condition, transient erythroblastopenia of childhood (TEC), occurs in early infancy and is usually self-limited. It is believed to be a result of inhibitors — either humoral antibody or viral — to late erythroid precursors in the marrow. Bone marrows in these patients show absence of late erythroblasts.

Congenital dyserythropoietic anemia

Congenital dyserythropoietic anemia (CDA) was classified into three categories by Heimpel and Wendt.[24] A potential fourth type was described by Benjamin and associates.[25] All types of CDA are characterized by indirect hyperbilirubinemia, ineffective erythropoiesis, and bizarre multinuclear erythroblasts. Multinuclear erythroblasts are not unique to CDA and can occur in other situations in which ineffective erythropoiesis is a prominent feature, such as hemoglobinopathies, megaloblastic anemias, and leukemia.

Congenital dyserythropoietic anemia (CDA) type 1 is characterized by a mildly macrocytic anemia with prominent anisocytosis and poikilocytosis. Bone marrow smears show erythroblasts with multilobated nuclei, megaloblastic changes, and thin internuclear chromatin bridges between two erythroblasts. The disease is apparent at birth but does not seem to affect longevity. The inheritance is autosomal recessive.

Type 2 CDA is known as hereditary erythroblast multinuclearity with positive acidified serum test (HEMPAS). Erythrocytes are similar to those in paroxysmal nocturnal hemoglobinuria (PNH) in that they are susceptible to hemolysis in acidified normal serum. They differ from PNH erythrocytes by their failure to hemolyze in the "sugar water" test. Type 2 CDA cells carry increased amounts of blood group antigen i and are susceptible to hemolysis by anti-i alloantibodies. (For a review of PNH, see Chapter 13.) Erythroblasts show bizarre changes but differ from type 1 CDA cells in that megaloblastic features are not present. Most patients have a normocytic anemia with a relatively benign course. Physical findings may reveal jaundice and hepatosplenomegaly. The inheritance is autosomal recessive.

CDA type 3 is similar to type 1 and frequently has giant multinucleated erythroblasts. Megaloblastic changes are not prominent, and the nuclear chromatin does not have a spongy appearance, as may be seen in CDA type 1. Type 3 CDA cells are not susceptible to lysis by acidified normal serum. The anemia is normocytic or slightly macrocytic. Inheritance is autosomal dominant.

Cells in the proposed type 4 CDA are similar in appearance to cells in type 2 CDA but differ ultrastructurally and lack serologic abnormalities.

CASE STUDY

A 3-year-old white boy was taken to the physician because of easy bruising, persistent black eyes, nosebleeds, and pallor. Physical examination revealed oral ulcers, widespread petechiae, and a few slightly enlarged lymph nodes, but no hepatosplenomegaly. The past history was noncontributory.

The laboratory data revealed a WBC of 2.2×10^9/liter, hematocrit 18 percent, platelets 5×10^9/liter, reticulocytes 1.8 percent, and absolute neutrophil count of 286 per μl. A differential of the peripheral blood showed 13 percent granulocytes, 85 percent lymphocytes, and 2 percent monocytes. Bone marrow biopsy examination revealed a hypocellular marrow with increased numbers of lymphocytes and some myeloid cells, but no megakaryocytes or blasts.

The search for a human leukocyte antigen (HLA)–compatible marrow donor was unsuccessful. The patient was initially treated with platelets, RBCs, steroids, and androgens. The symptoms did not improve, and the patient developed resistance to platelet donors and needed HLA-matched platelets. Treatment with antithymocyte globulin was tried with no immediate success. The patient was maintained with blood products and antibiotics. He had had recurrent problems due to the pancytopenia, including cellulitis and an episode of major intracranial bleeding. After 14 months of careful supportive therapy, a gradual improvement was noted. This continued for several months, and his counts stabilized with a WBC of 5.7×10^9/liter, hematocrit 38.5 percent, platelets 99×10^9/liter, and absolute neutrophil count of 1596 per μl. The differential showed 28 percent granulocytes, 66 percent lymphocytes, 5 percent monocytes, reticulocytes 1.4 percent, and 1 percent eosinophils.

This is an unusual but not rare example of a spontaneous remission in an individual with severe idiopathic aplastic anemia. Typically, in those individuals who do improve, the counts never return completely to normal. It is believed that more individuals would experience remission if they could be maintained through their course of severe pancytopenia as this child was. Unfortunately hemorrhage and infection are still major problems, and not all individuals will show improvement in their counts. Therefore, the treatment of choice is bone marrow transplantation when an HLA-compatible bone marrow donor is available.

REFERENCES

1. Wallerstein, RO, et al: Statewide study of chloramphenicol therapy and fatal aplastic anemia. JAMA 208:2045, 1969.
2. Ehrlich, P: Ueber einen fall von anamic mit bemerkungen uber regenerative veranderungen des khochenmarks. Charite-Annalen 13:300, 1888.
3. Chauffard, M: Un cas d'anemie pernicieuse aplastique. Bull Soc Med Hop 21:313, 1904.
4. Thompson, WP, Richter, MN, and Edsall, KS: An analysis of so-called aplastic anemia. Am J Med Sci 187:77, 1934.
5. Boggs, DR and Boggs, SS: The pathogenesis of aplastic anemia: A defective pluripotent hematopoietic stem cell with inappropriate balance of differentiation and self-replication. Blood 48:71, 1976.
6. Worton, RG, McCulloch, EA, and Till, JE: Physical separation of hemopoietic stem cells from cells forming colonies in culture. J Cell Physiol 74:171, 1969.
7. Parkinson, R: The immunopathology of marrow failure. Clin Haematol 7:475, 1978.
8. Keating, A, et al: Donor origin of the in vitro haematopoietic microenvironment after marrow transplantation in man. Nature 298:280, 1982.
9. Good, RA: Aplastic anemia—suppressor lymphocytes and hematopoiesis. N Engl J Med 296:41, 1977.
10. Thomas, DE and Storb, R: Acquired severe aplastic anemia: Progress and perplexity. Blood 64:325, 1984.
11. Martland, HS: Occupational poisoning in manufacture of luminous watch dials. JAMA 92:466, 1929.
12. Moeschlin, S and Speck, B: Experimental studies on the mechanism of action of benzene on the bone marrow (radioautographic studies using ³H-thymidine). Acta Haematol 38:104, 1967.
13. Williams, DM, Lynch, RE, and Cartwright, GE: Drug-induced aplastic anemia. Semin Hematol 10:195, 1973.
14. Custer, RP: Aplastic anemia in soldiers treated with atabrine. Am J Med Sci 212:211, 1946.
15. Hagler, L, et al: Aplastic anemia following viral hepatitis: Report of two fatal cases and literature review. Medicine 54:139, 1975.
16. Fanconi, G: Die familiare panmyelopathie. Schweiz Med Wochenschr 94:1309, 1964.
17. Barosi, G, et al: Iron kinetics and erythropoiesis in Fanconi's anemia. Scand J Haematol 21:29, 1978.
18. Thomas, DE, et al: Current status of bone marrow transplantation for aplastic anemia and acute leukemia. Blood 49:671, 1977.
19. Frisch, B and Lewis, SM: The bone marrow in aplastic anaemia: Diagnostic and prognostic features. J Clin Pathol 27:231, 1974.
20. Lynch, RE, et al: The prognosis in aplastic anemia. Blood 45:517, 1975.
21. Storb, R, et al: Marrow transplantation for aplastic anemia. Semin Hematol 21:27, 1984.
22. Storb, R, et al: Marrow transplantation for treatment of aplastic anemia: An analysis of factors associated with graft rejection. N Engl J Med 296:61, 1977.
23. Diamond, LK, Allen, DM, and Magill, FB: Congenital (erythroid) hypoplastic anemia. Am J Dis Child 102:403, 1961.
24. Heimpel, H and Wendt, F: Congenital dyserythropoietic anemia with karyorrhexis and multinuclearity or erythroblasts. Helv Med Acta 34:103, 1968.
25. Benjamin, JT, et al: Congenital dyserythropoietic anemia—type IV. J Pediatr 87:210, 1975.

BIBLIOGRAPHY

Camitta, BM, Storb, R, and Thomas, ED: Aplastic anemia. Pathogenesis, diagnosis, treatment, and prognosis. N Engl J Med 306:645, 1982.
Geary, CG (ed): Aplastic anemia. Ballière Tindall, London, 1979.

Scott, JL, Cartwright, GE, and Wintrobe, MM: Acquired aplastic anemia: An analysis of thirty-nine cases and review of the pertinent literature. Medicine 38:119, 1959.

Wintrobe, MM: Clinical Hematology, ed 8. Lea & Febiger, Philadelphia, 1981.

QUESTIONS

1. *What is aplastic anemia?*
   a. Condition in which production of erythrocytes, platelets, and leukocytes has failed
   b. Condition in which production of erythrocytes has failed
   c. Condition in which production of leukocytes has failed
   d. Condition in which there is a failure of production of different cellular elements

2. *Which of the following represents a complete listing of the classifications of causes for aplastic anemia?*
   a. Acquired and congenital
   b. Idiopathic and acquired
   c. Acquired, congenital, and idiopathic
   d. Idiopathic, acquired, and ecologic

3. *Which of the following is not a cause for acquired aplastic anemia?*
   a. Chemical agents
   b. Abnormal chromatids
   c. Drugs
   d. Infections
   e. Ionizing irradiation

4. *What is the most common congenital disorder of aplastic anemia?*
   a. Shwachman's syndrome
   b. Thrombocytopenia–absent radius (TAR) syndrome
   c. Chédiak-Higashi syndrome
   d. Fanconi's anemia

5. *Which of the following blood values is not a guideline for choosing patients for transplantation is cases of severe aplastic anemia?*
   a. Platelet concentration of less than $20 \times 10^9/$liter (20,000 per μl)
   b. Leukocyte count of less than $4 \times 10^9/$liter (4000 per μl)
   c. Neutrophil concentration of less than $0.5 \times 10^9/$liter (500 per μl)
   d. Reticulocyte counts of less than 1 percent

6. *What is the typical appearance of the bone marrow in aplastic anemia?*
   a. Hypercellular
   b. Normocellular
   c. Hypocellular
   d. No cellular elements present

7. *What is the treatment of choice for severe aplastic anemia in patients under age 40?*
   a. Red blood cell transfusion
   b. Leukocyte-poor red blood cell transfusion
   c. Bone marrow transplantation
   d. Erythropoietin therapy

8. *What is pure red cell aplasia and the characteristics associated with this condition?*
   a. Absence of red cell precursors with leukocytes and platelets unaffected
   b. Absence of red cell and leukocyte precursors and platelets unaffected
   c. Absence of red cell and platelet precursors and leukocytes unaffected
   d. Absence of all cellular precursors

9. *What characteristics are common to all types of congenital dyserythropoietic anemia (CDA)?*
   a. Direct hyperbilirubinemia, effective erythropoiesis, and large erythroblasts
   b. Indirect hyperbilirubinemia, ineffective production of all cellular elements, and microcytes
   c. Hyperbilirubinemia, ineffective erythropoiesis, and macrocytes
   d. Indirect hyperbilirubinemia, ineffective erythropoiesis, and bizarre multinuclear erythroblasts

ANSWERS

1. a (p. 107)
2. c (p. 108)
3. b (p. 108)
4. d (p. 110)
5. b (p. 111)
6. c (p. 111)
7. c (p. 111)
8. a (p. 112)
9. d (p. 112)

CHAPTER 9

S. ZAIL, M.B., B.Ch., M.D., FRCPath(London)

Introduction to Hemolytic Anemias: Intracorpuscular Defects

I. Hereditary Defects of the Red Cell Membrane

OBJECTIVES

At the end of this chapter, the learner should be able to:
1. Define intracorpuscular and extracorpuscular red cell defects as related to hemolytic processes.
2. List laboratory tests that reflect increased red cell destruction.
3. Calculate a reticulocyte production index.
4. Name laboratory tests that help to classify the cause of red cell hemolysis.
5. Identify the red cell membrane abnormality associated with hereditary spherocytosis.
6. Recognize abnormal laboratory results associated with hereditary spherocytosis.
7. Name the functional abnormality affecting membrane skeleton proteins in hereditary elliptocytosis.
8. Recall laboratory findings associated with hereditary elliptocytosis.
9. Identify the abnormality that causes the severe fragmentation and microspherocytosis characteristic of hereditary pyropoikilocytosis.
10. List rare disorders of membrane cation permeability.

CLASSIFICATION OF HEMOLYTIC ANEMIAS

A hemolytic state exists when the in vivo survival of the red cell is shortened. The presence of anemia in an individual patient is, however, dependent on the degree of hemolysis and the compensatory response of the erythroid elements of the bone marrow. Normal bone marrow is able to increase its output about sixfold to eightfold, so that anemia is not manifest until this capacity is exceeded, corresponding to a red cell lifespan of about 15 to 20 days or less. Anemia may, however, occur with more moderate shortening of the red cell lifespan if there is an associated depression of bone marrow function, which may occur in certain systemic diseases or exposure to chemicals or drugs.

A useful classification of the hemolytic anemias entails their subdivision into those disorders associated with an intrinsic (intracorpuscular) defect of the red cell and those associated with an extrinsic (extracorpuscular) abnormality. Red cells from a patient with an intracorpuscular defect have a shortened survival in both the patient and in a healthy recipient, whereas normal donor red cells survive normally in the patient. In contrast, normal red cells, when transfused into a patient with an extracorpuscular abnormality, are destroyed more rapidly. The patient's red cells, when transfused into a healthy recipient, have normal survival, provided they have not been irreversibly damaged. Hemolytic states have also traditionally been regarded as being intravascular or extravascular—that is, sequestration occurs in reticuloendothelial tissue. However, vigorous extravascular hemolysis may often be associated with signs of hemoglobin release into the plasma such as hemoglobinemia and decreased haptoglobin levels. The distinction is still useful from a clinical standpoint as certain hemolytic states are associated with predominantly intravascular hemolysis (for example, paroxysmal nocturnal hemoglobinuria, infections due to *Clostridia* or *Plasmodium falciparum*).

Hemolytic anemias may be classified as follows:

1. Intracorpuscular defects
   a. Hereditary defects
      (1) Defects in the red cell membrane
      (2) Enzyme defects
      (3) Hemoglobinopathies
      (4) Thalassemia syndromes
   b. Acquired defects
      (1) Paroxysmal nocturnal hemoglobinuria
2. Extracorpuscular defects
   a. Immune hemolytic anemias
   b. Infections
   c. Chemicals and toxins
   d. Physical agents
   e. Microangiopathic and macroangiopathic hemolytic anemias
   f. Splenic sequestration (hypersplenism)
   g. General systemic disorders (in which hemolysis is not the dominant feature of the anemia)

APPROACH TO DIAGNOSIS OF A HEMOLYTIC STATE

The approach to diagnosis of a hemolytic state initially involves establishing that the rate of red cell destruction is increased and then determining the cause of hemolysis.

Establishing the Presence of Hemolysis

Diagnostic tests used to establish the presence of hemolysis rely on the fact that hemolysis is characterized by both increased cell destruction and increased production.

Tests Reflecting Increased Red Cell Destruction

The most frequently used tests in this category are the serum unconjugated (indirect) bilirubin and serum haptoglobin determinations. The serum unconjugated bilirubin level seldom exceeds 3 to 4 mg/dl in complicated hemolytic states and reflects the catabolism of heme derived from red cells phagocytosed by the reticuloendothelial system (Fig. 9–1. The test is, however, relatively insensitive, as is the measurement of fecal stercobilinogen and urine urobilinogen that represents further stages in the disposition of unconjugated bilirubin by the liver (Fig. 9–1). As the unconjugated bilirubin is bound to albumin it cannot pass the glomerular filter, and the jaundice is said to be acholuric. On the other hand, a decreased serum haptoglobin level is a very sensitive test of both intravascular and extravascular hemolysis, and reflects the rapid clearance by the reticuloendothelial system of a complex formed between liberated hemoglobin and circulatory haptoglobin. Drawbacks to the use of serum haptoglobin levels are that low levels may occur in hepatocellular disease, reflecting decreased synthesis by the liver, while some individuals, particularly in black populations, may have a genetically determined deficiency of haptoglobin. Increased synthesis of haptoglobin in acute inflammatory states or malignancy may also mask depletion of serum haptoglobin owing to hemolysis.

Other tests that reflect increased red cell destruction, particularly if it is primarily intravascular, are the presence of hemoglobinemia, hemoglobinuria, and hemosiderinuria. The assessment of hemoglobinemia requires stringent precautions in the prevention of hemolysis during blood collection. Once the hemoglobin-binding capacity of serum haptoglobin is exceeded, hemoglobin passes through the glomerulus as alpha-beta chain dimers, reassociate to α_2-β_2 tetramers in the tubule where the hemoglobin is reabsorbed and degraded. The liberated iron is conserved as ferritin and hemosiderin. When the tubular reabsorptive capacity for hemoglobin is exceeded, hemoglobinuria ensues and is detectable either by spectroscopic examination or by commercially available dipsticks that detect heme. Staining of the urine sediment for iron (for example, with

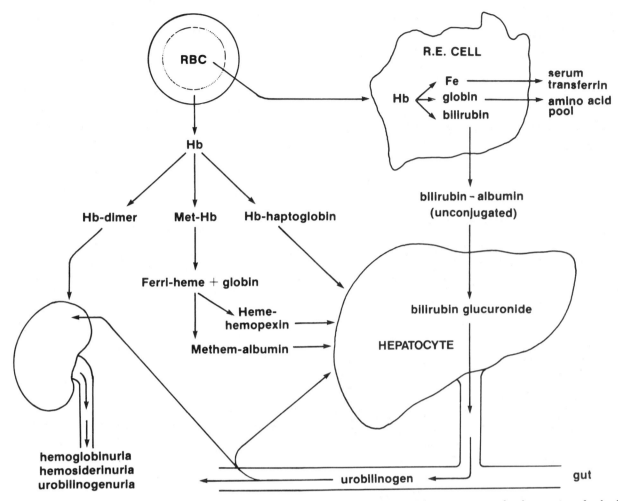

Figure 9-1. Diagrammatic representation of the disposition of hemoglobin after intravascular or extravascular destruction of red cells.

Prussian blue) will detect the hemosiderin- and ferritin-containing renal tubular cells that are sloughed several days after a hemolytic episode. Some of the free plasma hemoglobin may be oxidized to methemoglobin with subsequent dissociation of ferri-heme, which combines with albumin to form methemalbumin. Methemalbumin can be detected spectroscopically by the Schumm's test. This test is relatively insensitive and is seldom positive in mild hemolytic states. In routine practice, determination of red cell survival using ^{51}Cr-labeled red cells is seldom required to document an increased rate of red cell destruction. The fate of hemoglobin when processed intravascularly or extravascularly is shown diagrammatically in Figure 9-1.

Tests Reflecting Increased Red Cell Production

The compensatory bone marrow response to hemolysis results in the delivery of young red cells in the form of reticulocytes into the circulation. These young cells contain ribonucleic acid (RNA), which stains supravitally with dyes such as new methylene blue or brilliant cresyl blue. The normal reticu-locyte count ranges from 0.2 to 2.0 percent. This reflects the fact that each day approximately 1 percent of the red cell mass is destroyed and replaced by young red cells from the bone marrow, since red cell survival is approximately 120 days. The reticulocyte count is always elevated in a hemolytic state in which there is a normal compensatory bone marrow response. However, a more accurate assessment of red cell production is required because the percentage of reticulocytes may be "spuriously" elevated as the reticulocytes may be diluted into a lesser number of total circulating red cells. In addition, in response to the anemia, reticulocytes may leave the bone marrow prematurely and mature in the circulation for longer than the normal maturation time of one day, again leading to a falsely elevated reticulocyte count. These cells (so-called shift reticulocytes) are recognizable as large bluish-gray erythrocytes on Romanowsky stains.

The reticulocyte production index (RPI) corrects the hematocrit to a normal value of 45 percent and takes into account the maturation time of the reticulocyte at a particular hematocrit (approximately 1.0 day at a hematocrit of 45 percent, 1.5

days at 35 percent, 2.0 days at 25 percent, and 2.5 days at 15 percent).[1]

$$RPI = \frac{\% \text{ Reticulocytes}}{\text{Reticulocyte maturation time}} \times \frac{\text{Hematocrit}}{45}$$

For example, an RPI of 5.3 is calculated for a patient suspected of having a hemolytic state with the following indices: Hgb 12.0 g/dl, hematocrit 36 percent, reticulocyte count 10 percent, shift cells

$$\text{present} \left(\frac{10}{1.5} \times \frac{36}{45} \right)$$

An RPI of greater than 2.5 to 3.0 is generally regarded as indicative of a hemolytic state, but it is very important to exclude the presence of hemorrhage in a particular patient, as this too may lead to an elevated RPI. Although the RPI is probably the single most useful test to detect a hemolytic state, a cautionary note is in order, as the test may not be sensitive enough to detect mild hemolytic states (see Chapter 30).

Establishing Cause of Hemolysis

Once having documented the presence of hemolysis, it is our experience that the approach followed by Lux and Glader,[2] in establishing the cause of hemolysis, is pragmatic and logical and will be the technique followed in this chapter. The initial step consists of separating patients into Coombs' test–positive (that is, immunohemolytic anemias) and Coombs' test–negative groups. The latter group is then further divided into smear-positive and smear-negative subgroups (Table 9–1). It is fundamentally important to assess morphology in peripheral blood smears that are free of artifact. On the basis of the classification according to the predominant morphologic criteria associated with a particular disease state (Table 9–1), it is possible to narrow considerably the differential diagnosis and then institute further appropriate tests to make a definitive diagnosis.

It is also worth emphasizing that many hemolytic states are associated with an underlying disease, as will become apparent in the ensuing chapters, and this should not be lost sight of in the assessment of the individual patient.

HEREDITARY DEFECTS OF RED CELL MEMBRANE

Biochemistry and Structure of Red Cell Membrane

An understanding of the etiology and pathophysiology of hemolytic states due to defects of the red cell membrane requires some knowledge of the structure and biochemistry of the red cell membrane. In particular, the properties of the membrane

Table 9–1. **PREDOMINANT RED CELL MORPHOLOGY COMMONLY ASSOCIATED WITH NONIMMUNE HEMOLYTIC DISORDERS**

Spherocytes
Hereditary spherocytosis
Acute oxidant injury (HMP shunt defects during hemolytic crisis, oxidant drugs, and chemicals)
Clostridium welchii septicemia
Severe burns, other red cell thermal injuries
Spider, bee, and snake venoms
Severe hypophosphatemia

Bizarre Poikilocytes
Red cell fragmentation syndrome (microangiopathic and macroangiopathic hemolytic anemias)
Hereditary elliptocytosis in neonates
Hereditary pyropoikilocytosis

Elliptocytes
Hereditary elliptocytosis
Thalassemias

Stomatocytes
Hereditary stomatocytosis and related disorders
Stomatocytic elliptocytosis

Irreversibly Sickled Cells
Sickle-cell anemia
Symptomatic sickle syndromes

Intraerythrocytic Parasites
Malaria
Babesiosis
Bartonellosis
Unstable hemoglobins
Paroxysmal nocturnal hemoglobinuria
Dyserythropoietic anemias
Copper toxicity (Wilson's disease)
Cation permeability defects
Erythropoietic porphyria
Vitamin E deficiency
Hypersplenism

Prominent Basophilic Stippling
Thalassemias
Unstable hemoglobins
Lead poisoning
Pyrimidine-5-nucleotidase deficiency

Spiculated or Crenated Red Cells
Acute hepatic necrosis (spur cell anemia)
Uremia
Infantile pyknocytosis
Abetalipoproteinemia
McLeod blood group

Target Cells
Hemoglobins S, C, D, and E
Thalassemias
Hereditary xerocytosis

Nonspecific or Normal Morphology
Embden-Meyerhof pathway defects
HMP shunt defects
Adenosine deaminase hyperactivity with low red cell ATP

Source: Adapted from Lux and Glader.[2]

skeleton, which consists of a protein network connected to and lying just beneath the cell membrane, deserve special consideration, as several of the hemolytic states we shall discuss are associated with defective or absent membrane skeleton proteins. In its passage through the microcirculation and its ability to withstand the strong shear forces in the circulation, the structural integrity of the red cell is to a large extent dependent on its ability to deform during flow. This important property of the red cell depends on three main factors: (1) membrane deformability, which in turn depends heavily on the structural and functional integrity of the membrane skeleton; (2) cell surface area-to-volume ratio; and (3) cytoplasmic viscosity. Alterations in these properties occur to various degrees in several of the hereditary defects of the red cell membrane and contribute to the ultimate destruction of the red cell.

The structural organization of the red cell membrane and its underlying network of proteins has been reviewed in Chapter 2, and only some aspects of membrane skeleton structure will be emphasized here. The major components of the skeleton are spectrin, actin, and protein 4.1. Recent electron microscopic studies[3] using high-resolution negative staining reveal a hexagonal lattice in which junctional complexes of short F-actin filaments (approximately 15 monomers) are cross-linked to spectrin tetramers or three-armed hexamers at their tail ends (Fig. 9–2). The junctional complexes are thought to contain protein 4.1, which enhances the interaction of spectrin and actin, as well as the actin-binding proteins adducin, tropomyosin, and protein 4.9. The network is linked to the lipid bilayer by a high-affinity interaction between spectrin and ankyrin, which in turn binds to protein 3, a major integral protein in the lipid bilayer. Further linkage is provided by protein 4.1, which binds to glycophorins in the membrane (see Chapter 2).[4,5]

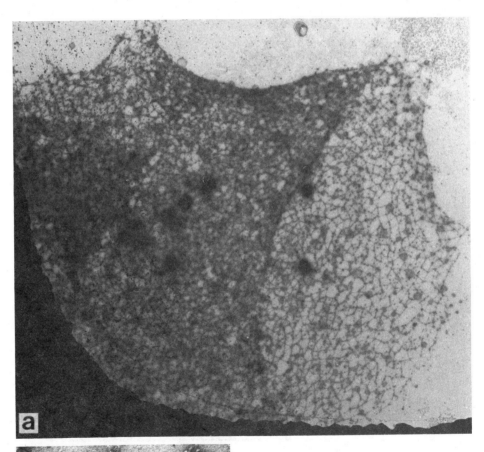

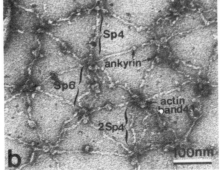

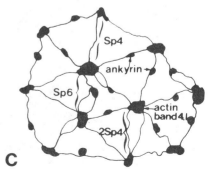

Figure 9–2. Transmission electron micrographs of negatively stained membrane skeletons. An area of spread skeleton network (a), the hexagonal lattice made up by spectrin tetramers (Sp 4), hexamers (Sp 6) or double tetramers (2 Sp4) (b) and (c), crosslinking junctional complexes thought to contain short F-actin filaments and protein 4.1. Globular ankyrin structures are bound to spectrin filaments about 80 nm from their distal ends. (From Liu et al,[3] with permission.)

Spectrin, a dimer of two highly flexible chains of 240,000 daltons (α chain) and 220,000 daltons (β chain), forms tetramers or higher oligomers by head-to-head associations between an N-terminal domain of the α chain and the phosphorylated C-terminal domain of the β chain (Fig. 9–3A). Nine trypsin-resistant domains, five on the α chain (αI–αV) and four on the β chain (βI–βIV), have been delineated[6] (Fig. 9–3A), and these currently form the basis for nomenclature of defects of the spectrin molecule (see farther on). Each chain is thought to consist of a number of homologous, triple-helical segments of about 12,000 daltons each (106 amino acids), linked together by nonhelical regions[7] (Fig. 9–3B, C). An important point relating to the biogenesis of the membrane skeleton is that during erythroid development α chains of spectrin are synthesized in threefold to fourfold excess over β spectrin chains, yet are assembled in stoichiometric amounts on the membrane, the excess of unassembled α chains being rapidly degraded.[8,9] These concepts are useful in understanding the expression of

the molecular defects in some forms of hereditary spherocytosis and elliptocytosis (see farther on).

Classification

Ideally, the classification of hereditary defects of the red cell membrane should be based on the delineation of specific defects of the membrane. The last few years have witnessed an explosive increase in knowledge in achieving this goal, particularly in the characterization of specific defects of the membrane skeleton. At present, however, all patients with clinical and morphologic evidence of a membrane defect cannot yet be categorized in this way, so that the classification used is still based on the prime morphologic features of the disorder (Table 9–2). Palek and Lux[10] have proposed the following nomenclature of known membrane skeleton defects (Table 9–2). Skeletal protein deficiencies or defective protein associations are shown in brackets following the disease state. Superscripts [+] and [0] indicate a partial or complete protein deficiency, re-

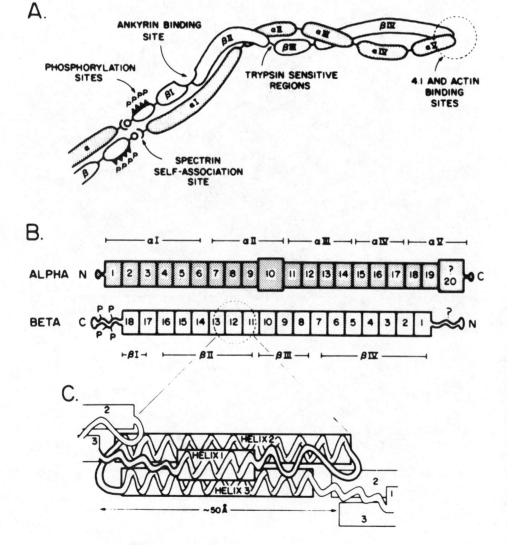

Figure 9–3. (A) The nine tryptic domains of α and β spectrin and the sites of self-association and also binding to ankyrin, 4.1, and actin. (B) The subunit structure of spectrin showing the homologous repeating units (106 amino acids, 12,000 daltons) of the α and β chains and their relationship to the tryptic domains. (C) The repeating subunit is thought to consist of three helical sequences (helix 1, 2, and 3) linked by short nonhelical sequences. The region between helix 3 and helix 1 is called the connecting region. (From Lux.[14])

Table 9–2. **HEREDITARY DEFECTS OF THE RED CELL MEMBRANE SKELETON***

	Known Defects	Prevalence	Usual Clinical Presentation
1. Hereditary Spherocytosis (HS)			
A. Autosomal recessive	HS (SP⁺)	±25% of HS patients	Moderate–severe HS
B. Autosomal dominant	HS (SP⁺)	Commonest variant	Mild–moderate HS
	HS (Sp-4.1)	±10% of HS patients	Mild–moderate HS
	HS (Ank⁺)	Rare	Moderate–severe HS
2. Hereditary Elliptocytosis (HE)			
A. Common HE			
(a) Heterozygous states			
α Chain mutants	$Sp\alpha^{I/74}$	Commonest variants in blacks	Mild HE
	$Sp\alpha^{I/65}$		Mild HE
	$Sp\alpha^{I/46}$	About 20% of assembly defects	Mild HE
β Chain mutants	Shortened β chain	Rare	Moderately severe HE
Protein 4.1 mutants	HE (4.1⁺)	Relatively common in whites in North and South Africa (20–30% of HE patients)	Mild HE
Glycophorin mutants	Glycophorin C deficiency	Rare	Mild HE
(b) Double heterozygous states			
Chain mutants	$Sp^{I/74}/?†$	Relatively rare	HPP
	$Sp^{I/46}/?†$	Relatively rare	HPP
	$Sp^{I/74}/Sp^{I/46}$	Rare	HPP
(c) Homozygous states			
Chain mutants	$Sp^{I/65}/Sp^{I/65}$	Rare	HE with mild–moderate hemolysis
Protein 4.1 mutants	HE (4.1⁰)	Rare	HE with severe hemolysis
B. Spherocytic HE			
Heterozygous states	Unknown	About 10% of HE in European and Japanese populations	Mild–moderate hemolysis with rounded elliptocytes and spherocytes
Homozygous states	Deficient Protein 4.2	Rare, recessively inherited	Mild–moderate hemolysis
C. Melanesian HE	Abnormal Protein 3	5–25% in Melanesian populations	Usually no hemolysis Elliptical stomatocytes Red cells resistant to malaria
3. Hereditary Stomatocytosis	Unknown	Rare	Mild–moderate hemolysis Stomatocytes due to influx of sodium and water
4. Hereditary Xerocytosis	Unknown	Rare	Mild–moderate hemolysis Xerocytes due to efflux of sodium and water

*Abetalipoproteinemia is a hereditary disorder (autosomal recessive) associated with abnormal red cell membrane lipid composition. However, the primary defect involves the plasma lipoproteins with secondary effects on the red cell membrane and will not be considered here (**see Color Plate 82**).

†Double heterozygotes for a spectrin mutant and a second presumed defect of spectrin synthesis.

spectively. For example, "HE (4.1⁰)" denotes homozygous hereditary elliptocytosis associated with absence of protein 4.1. In the case of defective skeletal protein interactions, the defective protein (or its subunit if relevant) is underlined. For example, HS (Sp-4.1) represents hereditary spherocytosis with a defective spectrin 4.1 interaction due to a spectrin defect; HE (SpDα-SpD) represents hereditary elliptocytosis due to defective spectrin dimer-dimer in-

teraction related to an abnormal α chain of spectrin. In some of the latter patients the defect has been ascribed to the 80,000-dalton αI domain of spectrin at the tetramer assembly site. Palek[11] has proposed that these spectrins should be designated by indicating in a superscript the largest tryptic peptide generated instead of the normal 80,000-dalton αI domain (SpD$\alpha^{I/74}$-SpD), which can be further abbreviated to $Sp\alpha^{I/74}$).

Hereditary Spherocytosis

Mode of Inheritance

Hereditary spherocytosis (HS) is the most common hereditary hemolytic anemia in white people **(see Color Plate 77)**. In the majority of cases (±75) percent) it follows a classic autosomal dominant pattern of inheritance, but in about a quarter of families there is no abnormality detectable in either parent, suggesting autosomal recessive inheritance or decreased penetrance of a dominant gene. Possible explanations for these two modes of inheritance, based on differing pathogenesis of spectrin deficiency, are discussed later.

Etiology and Pathophysiology of Membrane Disorder

The fundamental expression of the membrane defect in HS is a loss of surface area of the red cell, resulting in a decreased surface-to-volume ratio. This is manifested morphologically as spherocytosis and stomatocytosis (note that the majority of cells in HS are stomatocytic or spherostomatocytic rather than truly spherocytic). Such cells tolerate less swelling than normal red cells and are osmotically fragile. The decrease in surface-to-volume ratio also makes these cells less deformable than normal. This has a particularly deleterious effect on their survival in the spleen, and explains one of the hallmarks of HS, which is the excellent clinical response to splenectomy in most, but not all cases (see farther on). The exact pathogenesis of the loss of surface area of the HS cell is still an enigma. Most authorities favor actual physical fragmentation of the membrane, but contraction of the membrane surface by other mechanisms is a possibility. One finding that seems certain, however, is that almost all cases have a defective membrane skeleton.

An important advance in understanding the nature of the skeletal defect has recently come from the laboratory of Agre and co-workers.[12,13] Almost all patients with HS—whether autosomal dominant or recessive—have spectrin-deficient red cells. Moreover, the degree of spherocytosis, the severity of the disease, and the response to splenectomy correlate closely with the degree of spectrin deficiency. Autosomal recessive HS is associated usually with more severe spectrin deficiency and a poor response to splenectomy. The decrease in surface density of spectrin directly affects the elastic properties of the membrane. It has also been postulated that areas of the plasma membrane that are in excess of the contracted supporting spectrin network may be lost as microvesicles and lead to the observed decreased surface-to-volume ratio.

The excess synthesis of the α over the β chains of spectrin in erythroid development may afford an explanation for the finding of spectrin deficiency, which is common to both autosomal recessive and autosomal dominant HS. Asymptomatic carriers of recessively inherited HS (such as clinically unaffected patients) may be heterozygous for a defect of α chain synthesis but have normal amounts of membrane spectrin since there are still sufficient α chains to stoichiometrically bind to β spectrin.[13,14] Only in the homozygous state would the postulated defect of α chain synthesis be sufficient to lead to spectrin deficiency. Because β spectrin is rate limiting for tetramer assembly during erythroid development, a partial deficiency of β spectrin or ankyrin (which binds β spectrin) would be expected to manifest as a dominant trait with decreased membrane-bound spectrin. The recent demonstration of a linkage between an ankyrin gene polymorphism and the dominant transmission of HS in a large kindred suggests that ankyrin dysfunctions (as yet undefined) may turn out to be a common cause underlying spectrin deficiency in dominant HS.

In a minority of patients with HS, a specific defect affecting the tail end of the β chain of spectrin has been delineated.[15] This affects its interaction with protein 4.1 and is associated with mild spectrin deficiency. At present only a few patients with partial deficiency of ankyrin have been reported in one of whom the primary defect was due to a defect in synthesis of ankyrin.[9,16]

Hereditary spherocytosis cells with a decreased surface-to-volume ratio are selectively trapped and "conditioned" in the spleen, where the cells progressively lose more membrane surface and are ultimately destroyed. The exact mechanism of splenic conditioning and destruction of cells is again unclear. Previously held concepts that the HS cells undergo metabolic depletion with passive swelling and autohemolysis while they stagnate in the splenic cords are probably not correct, as it has been calculated that the average time HS cells spend in the spleen is too short for metabolic depletion to occur.[2] However, repeated metabolic stress in the "bywaters" of the spleen may contribute to the conditioning process. There is also indirect evidence that macrophage conditioning of HS cells may be of importance. In HS, peripheral red cells and particularly cells recovered from the splenic pulp are relatively dehydrated and have low concentrations of potassium and cell water, resulting in an elevated mean corpuscular hemoglobin concentration (MCHC) and increased cytoplasmic viscosity. Some of the possible mechanisms of splenic conditioning and destruction of HS cells are summarized in Figure 9–4.

Clinical Manifestations

The classic presenting features of patients with HS are the triad of jaundice, anemia, and an enlarged spleen, but many patients do not show all these signs. The age of presentation can vary from within a day or two after birth to old age and sometimes may only be diagnosed during family studies or investigation for other reasons. About two thirds of HS patients present with a mild uncompensated hemolytic state manifesting with the aforementioned classic signs. Characteristically the jaundice is acholuric, as unconjugated bilirubin cannot pass the glomerular filter. Many of these patients have pigment gallstones, presumably due to increased

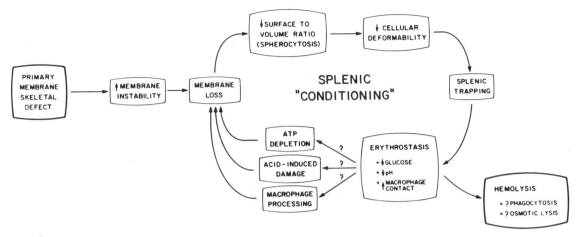

Figure 9-4. Postulated mechanisms of "conditioning" and destruction of HS red cells in the spleen. (From Lux and Glader,[2] with permission.)

concentrations of bilirubin in the bile. About a quarter of HS patients have a mild hemolytic state that is compensated for, and such patients are not anemic and are usually asymptomatic. A minority of patients (about 10 percent) have a severe hemolytic anemia that may require blood transfusion. Aplastic crises, in which erythropoiesis is suppressed leading to more pronounced anemia, occurs particularly in this group but may supervene in patients with milder forms of the disease. An uncommon complication of prolonged hemolysis, which is not limited to HS, is chronic leg ulceration.

Clinical Laboratory Findings

Evidence of Hemolytic Process. The laboratory features of extravascular hemolysis outlined earlier are usually apparent. Hyperbilirubinemia is found in about half the patients, and haptoglobins are variably reduced. Classic features of intravascular hemolysis such as hemoglobinemia, hemoglobinuria, or hemosiderinuria do not occur. The RPI is elevated above 2.5 in most cases (presplenectomy).

Red Cell Indices. Anemia is usually mild. The mean level of hemoglobin in several series is about 12 to 13 g/dl, but individual cases may vary widely depending on the severity of hemolysis and the degree of compensation. The mean corpuscular volume (MCV) is usually normal both before and after splenectomy but can be low, normal, or high. The mean corpuscular hemoglobin (MCH) tends to parallel the MCV. Although the MCV is usually normal, because of the red cell's spheroidal shape, the diameter of some cells is substantially decreased and these appear as dark, rounded microspherocytes on the peripheral smear (see later). In about 50 percent of cases the MCHC is elevated (higher than 36 percent), which probably reflects mild cellular dehydration, particularly of cells that have undergone splenic conditioning and that have low levels of cell water and potassium (see earlier section on etiology and pathophysiology).

Morphology of Peripheral Blood Smear. The morphologic hallmark of HS is the spherocyte **(see Color Plate 77)**. Although in many instances the detection of these cells may present no difficulty, in some patients their detection may provoke argument even among experienced hematologists. It is particularly important to examine well-prepared smears free of any artifact. In typical cases prior to splenectomy there may be varying degrees of polychromasia, poikilocytosis, and anisocytosis with many normal discoid cells, but the overriding impression is one of increased numbers of uniformly round cells (Fig. 9-5). Some of the cells appear as microspherocytes and are dark and round and lack a pale center.

Special Laboratory Tests

Osmotic Fragility Test. This test is essentially a measure of the surface-to-volume ratio of the red cell. If the test is performed on fresh red cells, it is then also a measure of the proportion of cells that have undergone splenic conditioning. When red cells are placed in a series of graded hypotonic salt solutions, water rapidly enters the cells and osmotic equilibrium is achieved. The cells swell and become spherical, and eventually a critical volume is reached, at which point the cellular contents (hemoglobin) leak out and ultimately the cell may burst. Red cells of patients with HS, because of their decreased surface-to-volume ratio, can tolerate less swelling than normal cells and lyse at higher concentrations of salt than do normal cells. It is important to note that about 25 percent of HS patients have normal osmotic fragility of fresh red cells, particularly in the group that is mildly affected and is difficult to diagnose on morphologic grounds. Patients in the latter group as well as patients with more typical cases, with very rare exception, have abnormal osmotic fragility of red cells that have been stressed by prior sterile incubation for 24 hours. During the 24-hour incubation, because of relative membrane instability, HS cells have greater loss of membrane surface. A corollary of the use of

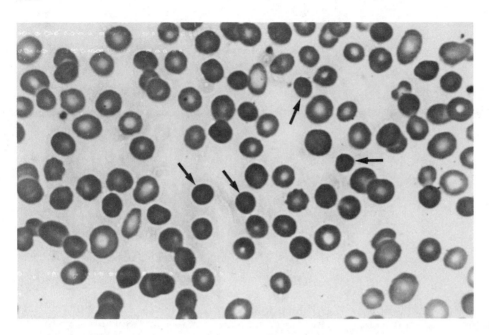

Figure 9-5. Photomicrograph of peripheral blood smear of patient with HS. Note the microsphero-cytes (*arrows*).

the incubated osmotic fragility test is that if the test result is normal, it is highly unlikely that one is dealing with a patient with HS. Representative osmotic fragility curves for fresh and incubated normal and HS red cells are shown in Figure 9–6. It is important to note that increased osmotic fragility is independent of the cause of spheroidal cells (for instance, it may be found in autoimmune hemolytic anemia, burns, and so on) (see Chapter 30).

Autohemolysis Test. This relatively sensitive test in the diagnosis of HS measures the structural and metabolic integrity of the HS red cell membrane under conditions of erythrostasis and relative glucose lack; that is, sterile incubation of red cells in their own plasma for 48 hours at 37°C. The HS red cell is leaky to sodium. To "keep its head above water," the cell utilizes adenosine triphosphate (ATP) and glucose to drive the cation pump to a greater extent than normal. Associated with the increased activity of the pump, there is a greater turnover of membrane phospholipids and associated membrane fragmentation with a decrease in surface-to-volume ratio until the critical hemolytic volume is reached and autohemolysis occurs. The usual range of autohemolysis in HS cells is variable and is about 10 to 50 percent, compared with control values of 0.2 to 2.0 percent. However, some patients show only minimally elevated autohemolysis or may even be within the normal range. In most HS patients, addition of glucose markedly diminishes autohemolysis but not usually to within the normal range of samples incubated with glucose (0 to 1.0 percent). A minority of patients show no correction of autohemolysis with glucose, a finding also obtained with many patients with spherocytosis associated with autoimmune hemolytic anemia. It should be noted that many laboratories do not use

this test routinely (see Chapter 30 for the procedure).

Spectrin Assay. Radioimmunoassay of spectrin is currently available in only a few specialized centers but is useful in predicting response to splenectomy. It may also help to distinguish HS from other acquired conditions associated with spherocytosis.

Treatment

From the foregoing discussion of the pathophysiology of the HS red cell and the central role of the spleen in conditioning such cells and ultimately leading to their destruction, it should not be surprising that splenectomy is functionally curative in most patients with this disease. In the relatively rare patient with severe spectrin deficiency (below 40 percent spectrin), clinical improvement occurs after splenectomy but ongoing hemolysis and anemia may continue. In the usual case, although spherocytosis persists, conditioned microspherocytes are no longer seen and red cell lifespan is normal or very near normal. At one time, many authorities recommended splenectomy uniformly in all patients with HS because of the risks of biliary tract disease and the development of aplastic crises, but this view has been considerably tempered in recent years. Patients with mild, compensated cases of HS are usually not offered splenectomy unless the previously mentioned complications intervene. An important consideration in infants and young children is the risk of postsplenectomy sepsis, particularly with *Streptococcus pneumoniae*, so that most authorities recommend deferment of splenectomy until about 6 years of age. In severe cases, however, splenectomy may have to be performed earlier; but in either event, treatment with pneumococcal vaccine is recommended, preferably starting before

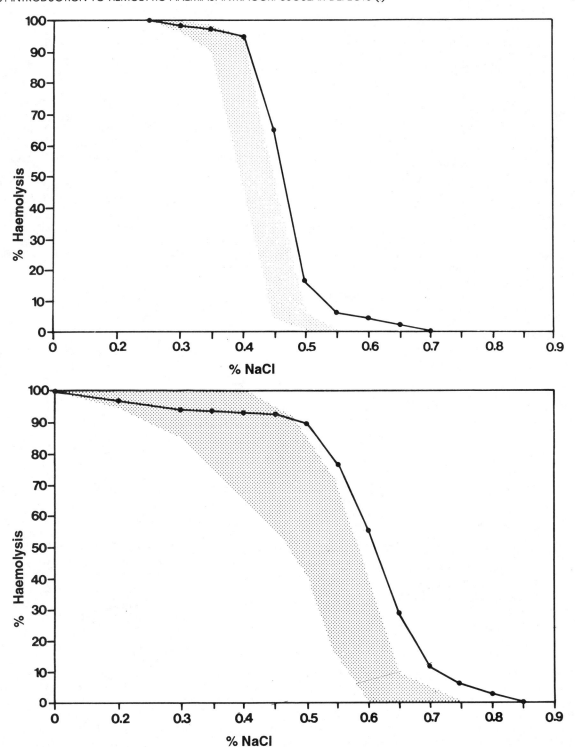

Figure 9-6. Osmotic fragility curves of fresh blood (*top*) and incubated blood (*bottom*) obtained from a HS subject. The normal range is shown by dotted areas. Note the increased fragility of the HS red cells to osmotic lysis.

splenectomy. Younger children may also require prophylactic penicillin or other antibiotics postsplenectomy, but the latter course is controversial. Failure of splenectomy is almost always associated with an accessory spleen not removed at surgery.

CASE STUDY

Mrs. T.P., aged 40 years, presented to her physician with an attack of acute cholecystitis. Physical examination revealed a palpable spleen in addition to the signs of acute cholecystitis. On investigation she was found to have numerous gallstones, and a routine blood count showed a mild, compensated hemolytic state: Hgb 13.8 g/dl, Hct 38 percent, MCV 80 fl, MCHC 36 percent, reticulocyte count 7 percent, shift cells present, RPI 3.9. The peripheral blood smear showed moderate numbers of spherocytes and a few microspherocytes. The Coombs' test result was negative. Unconjugated bilirubin was 2.5 mg/dl, and the conjugated bilirubin was 0.5 mg/dl. Haptoglobin concentration was less than 10 mg/dl (normal range: 25 to 180 mg/dl). Further investigation revealed that osmotic fragility of both fresh and incubated venous blood was increased. Autohemolysis was 25 percent after 48 hours' incubation, corrected to 3 percent in the presence of glucose. After the acute episode had settled, an elective cholecystectomy was performed. A diagnosis of hereditary spherocytosis was made and confirmed in a subsequent study of her family when two of her three children were found to have mild, compensated hemolytic states associated with spherocytosis. In view of the risk of recurrence of common bile duct calculi, an elective splenectomy was performed 6 months later, curing the hemolytic state.

Hereditary Elliptocytosis

Mode of Inheritance

Hereditary elliptocytosis is a disorder characterized by the presence of large numbers of elliptical red cells in the peripheral blood (see Color Plate 78). It has become clear over the past few years that this relatively common disorder (incidence about 1 in 4000, which shows variable linkage to the Rh gene, is genetically, biochemically, and clinically heterogeneous. Most of the variants are inherited in autosomal dominant fashion, including a morphologically and clinically distinct syndrome found almost exclusively in Melanesian populations. In addition, there is a close biochemical and genetic relationship to hereditary pyropoikilocytosis (HPP) (see farther on).

Clinical Phenotypes

Three major clinical and morphologic syndromes have been delineated by Palek and Lux[10,14] (Table 9–2). The most frequently occurring group is designated common HE, in which at least six subgroups have been categorized. The most common subgroup is mild HE, in which there is minimal or no hemolysis and in which one parent has mild HE. Some of these kindreds have members who exhibit mild to moderate hemolysis (HE with sporadic hemolysis). Rarely, both parents have mild HE and, depending on the nature of the molecular defect, the homozygous or double heterozygous offspring may present with a moderately severe hemolytic state (hemolytic HE) or with more severe hemolysis with gross fragmentation and poikilocytosis (HPP). Hereditary pyropoikilocytosis is considered in a separate section because historically it has been regarded as a distinct clinical entity, but it should be emphasized that it is a subgroup of common HE. Another subgroup is HE with poikilocytosis in infancy in which there is a transient neonatal state resembling HPP with gradual development of mild HE during the first 2 years of life. A rare variety of HE linked to families of Italian origin has associated ineffective erythropoiesis and erythroblast dysplasia.

The second major clinical category of HE is spherocytic HE, a phenotypic hybrid of mild HE and HS, in which the clinical course resembles HS and responds well to splenectomy. Most of these patients are of Northern European or Japanese origin.

Stomatocytic HE constitutes the last major category. It is common only in Melanesian populations in whom it may have a selective protective effect against malaria and is probably inherited in autosomal dominant fashion.

Etiology and Pathogenesis of Membrane Disorder

It is now well established that a defect in the red cell membrane skeleton exists in HE. A fundamental observation is that both red cell "ghosts" and membrane skeletons of HE subjects retain their elliptical shape and also show marked instability when subjected to mechanical stress. Several molecular lesions have been detected among the various phenotypic expressions of HE. (An abridged classification is shown in Table 9–2.) Of the known mutations the most common involve the 80,000-dalton αI domain at the N-terminus of α spectrin, resulting in a functional defect of tetramer assembly of varying degrees. These mutations are detected by tryptic peptide maps of isolated spectrin in which there is partial or complete replacement of the 80,000-dalton αI domain by peptides of lower molecular weight. At present, seven variants affecting this domain have been delineated, the most common being $Sp\alpha^{I/74}$, $Sp\alpha^{I/65}$, and $Sp\alpha^{I/46}$. In several of these variants the mutations seem to cluster around the connecting regions between different repeat units of spectrin[17-19] (Fig. 9–3C). These substitutions presumably exert their effect by critically altering the conformation of the head region of the α spectrin molecule, affecting its capacity to form tetramers; they also expose previously cryptic sites which become susceptible to trypsin cleavage.

In HE patients studied outside North America, a relatively common defect (± 20 percent of cases) is partial deficiency of protein 4.1 (HE 4.1$^+$). In two families, gene rearrangements (one upstream from the translation initiation codon, the other affecting the coding region) of the 4.1 gene have been described.[20,21]

In heterozygous states αI domain defects usually present with a mild functional defect of tetramer assembly and mild hemolysis, while in homozygous or double heterozygous forms a more pronounced functional defect and more severe hemolytic state with poikilocytosis ensues. The mutant gene dose thus affects the severity of the functional defect.

The intrinsic nature of the structural change also appears to affect the degree of functional impairment. For example, $Sp\alpha^{I/74}$ manifests with a more pronounced tetramer assembly defect than does $Sp\alpha^{I/65}$ or $Sp\alpha^{I/46}$. It is important to note that in patients with hemolytic HE there is no deficiency of membrane spectrin, in contrast to patients with HPP in whom there is a 30 to 40 percent deficiency of spectrin and in whom microspherocytosis is a hallmark of the condition (see farther on). These findings have led Palek and Lux[10] to propose a unifying hypothesis of the mechanism of red cell shape alterations in these conditions (Fig. 9–7). Mild defects lead to a weakened skeleton and to an alteration in the material properties of the HE membrane. This results in a greater tendency for the membrane to develop permanent plastic deformation (that is, to remain in an elongated elliptical form) when subjected to the repeated shear stresses in the microcirculation. This is in contrast to normal cells, which develop only transient elliptical deformation in traversing the microcirculation. More severe defects, such as may occur in homozygous HE states (or in double heterozygous states as in HPP), lead to greater membrane instability and actual fragmentation and poikilocytosis. In the presence of partial deficiency of spectrin, the contracted surface area of the skeleton leads to overlying lipid bilayer destabilization and the micropoikilocytosis and microspherocytosis characteristic of HPP. The altered characteristics of the red cells in hemolytic HE and HPP predispose them to destruction in the spleen, but the exact pathophysiologic mechanisms whereby the poikilocytes are destroyed are not yet understood.

With regard to spherocytic HE an almost complete absence of protein 4.2 has been found in some Japanese individuals with the recessively inherited variant of this disorder. These patients respond to splenectomy. The absence of protein 4.2 appears to

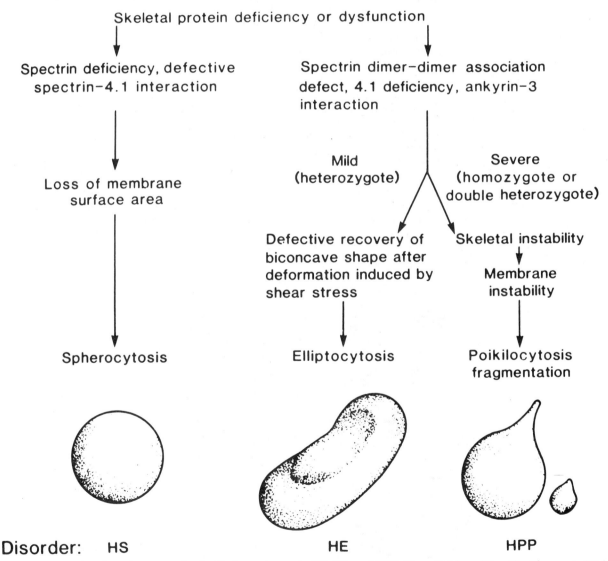

Figure 9–7. Postulated mechanisms of red cell shape change in HS, HE, and HPP. (From Palek and Lux,[10] with permission.)

destabilize ankyrin in the membrane,[22] but how this relates to splenic sequestration of these cells is at present unclear. The stomatocytic variant of elliptocytosis prevalent in Southeast Asian populations is of interest in that the membranes of these red cells are *more* rigid than normal and are resistant to malarial infection. Recently Palek and coworkers[23] have demonstrated a structural abnormality of protein 3 (the anion transporter) in tryptic digests of this protein which is associated with increased binding of ankyrin to the plasma membrane. This may lead to increased sites for, and increased density of, spectrin on the membrane and may account for the increased rigidity of these membranes.

Clinical Laboratory Findings

Evidence of Hemolytic Process. The usual picture in the most common variant (mild HE) is that of a very mild, compensated hemolytic anemia in which the only features may be a slight reticulocytosis and decreased haptoglobin levels. Many patients show no biochemical evidence of a hemolytic process. In the more severe cases, such as in spherocytic HE or in HE with infantile poikilocytosis, the usual features of extravascular hemolysis outlined earlier are found.

Morphology of Peripheral Blood Smear. The morphology of the peripheral blood smear obviously varies with the clinical phenotypes of HE. In the usual variant of mild HE with no hemolysis or a compensated hemolytic state, the red cells show prominent uniform elliptocytosis, the cells being elliptic rather than oval or egg-shaped (Fig. 9–8). Usually greater than 30 percent of the red cells are elliptocytic, but many patients have a higher proportion of elliptocytes (greater than 75 percent). Very elongated or rod-shaped cells are characteristic and often constitute more than 10 percent of the red cells. In patients with uncompensated hemolysis (mild HE with sporadic hemolysis) the red cells show more prominent poikilocytosis and a small proportion of elliptocytes may have budlike projections. The rare patient with homozygous HE presents with an even greater degree of poikilocytosis, as does the infant with mild HE and poikilocytosis of infancy. In such infants there is prominent poikilocytosis, microspherocytosis, fragmentation, budding of red cells, and a variable degree of elliptocytosis (Fig. 9–9). By the time the child reaches the age of 1 to 2 years, the morphology has changed to that characteristic of mild HE. In the neonatal period, the red cells show increased thermal sensitivity (which is also a characteristic of HPP), but the diagnosis is suggested by finding evidence of mild HE in one parent.

Red cell morphology in spherocytic HE is very variable, but the hallmarks are less prominent elliptocytosis with spherocytes and microspherocytes. The proportion of spherocytes and elliptocytes varies in different kindreds and even within the same kindred. Patients with stomatocytic or Melanesian HE have a characteristic red cell morphology. The elliptocytes are more rounded and have one or two transverse bars, giving them the appearance of double stomatocytes.

Red Cell Indices. In the common variants of mild HE with compensated and uncompensated hemolysis, the MCV is usually normal or slightly elevated, the latter finding probably reflecting an associated reticulocytosis. Usually the MCH and MCHC are also within the normal range. In infants with HE and poikilocytosis who have morphology representing that seen in HPP, the MCV may be decreased and the MCHC is either normal or slightly elevated.

Special Laboratory Tests. The osmotic fragility and autohemolysis tests are useful additional tests in delineating some of the HE phenotypes. In patients with mild HE (compensated and uncompensated) both the preincubation and the postincuba-

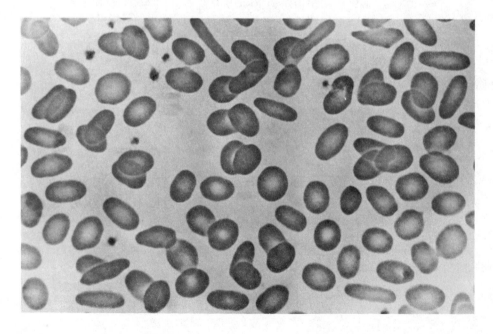

Figure 9–8. Photomicrograph of peripheral blood smear of a patient with mild HE (compensated hemolysis).

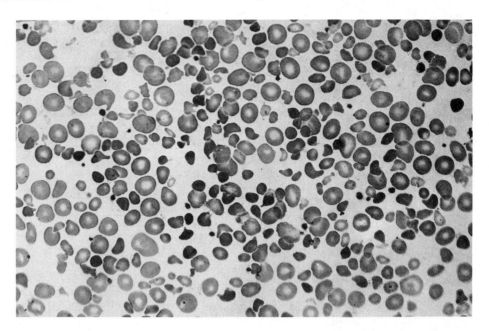

Figure 9-9. Photomicrograph of peripheral blood smear of a patient with mild HE and poikilocytosis of infancy. Note the bizarre poikilocytosis and fragmentation.

tion osmotic fragility and autohemolysis results are normal. Rarely patients with mild HE and uncompensated hemolysis may have increased autohemolysis corrected by glucose. Preincubation and postincubation osmotic fragility is uniformly increased in spherocytic HE, and autohemolysis is characteristically increased but corrected by glucose. Children with HE and infantile poikilocytosis have increased osmotic fragility and autohemolysis in the early neonatal period that reverts to normal with the development of more prominent elliptocytosis.

In laboratories with a specialized interest in HS and HE, further studies can be undertaken to define some of the structural and functional abnormalities of the membrane skeleton proteins, particularly of spectrin, outlined earlier. In brief, these involve one- and two-dimensional SDS-PAGE of membrane proteins as a screen for quantitating putative deficiencies of the skeletal proteins. Studies of the functional interactions of spectrin, actin, protein 4.1 ankyrin, and band 3 can be determined either in solution or, in some cases, with appropriately treated membrane vesicles. Structural studies of isolated skeletal proteins using techniques such as limited tryptic proteolysis and separation of tryptic peptides by one- and two-dimensional SDS-PAGE are powerful tools in delineating such defects (Fig. 9-10).

← Isoelectric Focusing

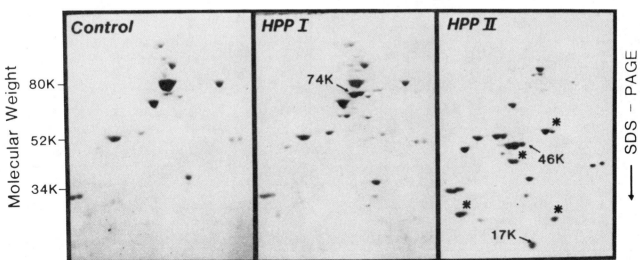

Figure 9-10. Two-dimensional SDS-PAGE of tryptic peptides of spectrin from patients with HPP. HPP I shows the defect seen in HPP (Spα$^{I/74}$), and HPP II represents the defect in HPP (Spα$^{I/46}$). The positions of the 74K peptide characteristic of HPP I and the 46K and 17K peptides characteristic of HPP II are arrowed. Peptides that are variable both in patients and controls are denoted by asterisks. (From Palek and Lux,[10] with permission.)

Treatment

Patients with mild HE (compensated) have a benign disorder with no splenomegaly and require no therapeutic intervention. Those with HE and uncompensated hemolysis usually benefit from splenectomy, which is also uniformly beneficial to patients with spherocytic HE. Patients with HE and infantile poikilocytosis should be recognized and treated symptomatically, as they will improve spontaneously with the development of a picture indistinguishable from mild HE.

CASE STUDY

Mrs. R.L., age 45, presented to her physician complaining of malaise and tiredness on mild exertion. On physical examination, she was found to have slight scleral icterus and a two-finger splenomegaly. A blood count revealed the following: Hgb 11.0 g/dl, Hct 32 percent, MCHC 34.3 percent, MCV 100 fl, reticulocyte count 12.0 percent, shift cells in peripheral blood smear, and RPI 5.7. The peripheral smear showed about 80 percent elliptocytes with some poikilocytosis consisting of a few fragmented cells and budding elliptocytes. Unconjugated bilirubin was 3.5 mg/dl, conjugated bilirubin 0.6 mg/dl, and haptoglobin 15 mg/dl (normal range 25 to 180 mg/dl). Preincubation and postincubation osmotic fragility and autohemolysis were within the normal range. Examination of her family showed striking elliptocytes with normal hemoglobin and reticulocyte count in her father and in one of her three children. A diagnosis of mild HE with sporadic hemolysis was made, and a good response to splenectomy was obtained.

Hereditary Pyropoikilocytosis

Hereditary pyropoikilocytosis, a relatively rare severe hemolytic state first recognized in 1975 as a distinct clinical entity, has subsequently been found to have a close genetic and biochemical relationship to mild HE. The hallmarks of the condition are (1) striking bizarre micropoikilocytosis in which red cell budding, fragments, microspherocytes, and elliptocytes are prominent (Fig. 9–11) **(see Color Plate 79)**; (2) thermal instability of red cells in which heparinized venous blood heated to 45°C in vitro for 15 minutes leads to striking fragmentation of the red cells in contrast to normal red cells which fragment only at 49°C; and (3) autosomal recessive inheritance.

The MCV is characteristically very low (55 to 70 fl), preincubation and postincubation osmotic fragility is markedly increased, and autohemolysis is increased and unaffected by glucose. The thermal instability of the red cells in HPP reflects thermal instability of the spectrin of the membrane skeleton and accounts for the in vitro fragmentation on heating to 45°C. However, as outlined earlier, the bizarre red cell picture found in vivo is thought to be a manifestation of spectrin deficiency and a functional defect in spectrin dimer-dimer association more severe than that found in HE. This leads to an unstable membrane skeleton that undergoes fragmentation on exposure to shear stresses in the circulation, with attendant decrease in surface-to-volume ratio and decreased cellular deformability (see Fig. 9–7). At present, three types of structural abnormalities have been described in different kindreds with HPP, affecting the 80,000-dalton αI domain of spectrin: $Sp\alpha^{I/74}$, $Sp\alpha^{I/46}$, and $Sp\alpha^{I/61}$. Figure 9–10 shows the tryptic peptides of spectrin obtained in two representative HPP kindreds.

Some HPP probands are doubly heterozygous for two of these structural mutants, one of the mutants, such as $Sp\alpha^{I/46}$, being unstable and resulting in a partial deficiency of spectrin. Others may have only one structural mutant of spectrin detectable (as in Fig. 9–10) but are thought to be doubly heterozygous for this mutant and a defect of spectrin synthesis.

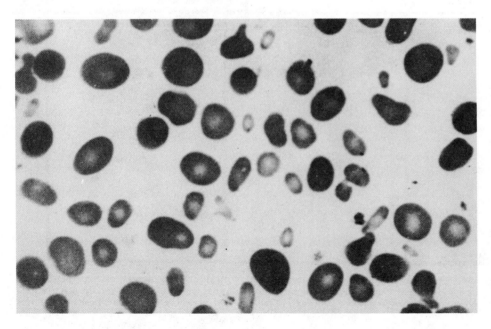

Figure 9–11. Photomicrograph of peripheral blood smear of a patient with HPP. Note the bizarre poikilocytosis and fragmentation similar to that seen in Figure 9–9. (From Palek and Lux,[10] with permission.)

Disorders of Membrane Cation Permeability: Hereditary Hydrocytosis (Stomatocytosis) and Hereditary Xerocytosis

This is a heterogeneous group of rare disorders characterized by alterations in the permeability of the red cell membrane to cations. Two main clinical and morphologic syndromes have been described and consist on the one hand of hereditary stomatocytosis (hydrocytosis) in which the red cells are swollen **(see Color Plate 80)** and on the other hand of hereditary xerocytosis in which the red cells are markedly dehydrated **(see Color Plate 81)**. A number of intermediate syndromes have been described, but these are not considered here.

Modes of Inheritance

Most reported cases of hereditary hydrocytosis are inherited in autosomal dominant fashion, but some patients who have a more severe degree of hemolysis show autosomal recessive inheritance. Hereditary xerocytosis is inherited by autosomal dominant transmission.

Etiology and Pathophysiology

An important determinant of the water content of red cells is their total content of sodium and potassium. To maintain osmotic equilibrium water enters cells in which the total cation content is increased, leading to swelling and hydrocyte formation. In contrast, a net loss of cations results in a movement of water out of the cell with formation of dehydrated cells or xerocytes.

The basic abnormality of hydrocytic red cells is a marked increase in the passive permeability of sodium into the cell and of potassium out of the cell. The defect in sodium permeability is greater than that for potassium. Although the sodium-potassium pump is stimulated by the influx of sodium, it cannot cope with the influx, and the total cation content of the cell increases with resultant water influx and formation of hydrocytes. There is some evidence of functional defects in the membrane skeleton of red cells with hydrocytosis (such as diminished phosphorylation of spectrin), but how these relate to the permeability defect is unknown. Recently a deficiency of one component of band 7 has been reported in red cell membranes of such patients, which may be important in determining the permeability lesion. Because of the influx of water, hydrocytes have an increased volume with a decreased surface-to-volume ratio and its attendant consequences of decreased red cell deformability and susceptibility to splenic sequestration. Although splenectomy is predictably of benefit in the majority of patients with hereditary hydrocytosis, paradoxically some patients with severe permeability defects do not have significant hemolysis, suggesting that other, as yet unknown factors may be important in the destruction of these cells.

Red cells from patients with hereditary xerocytosis have an increased efflux of potassium that is greater than the sodium influx. Although the influx of sodium leads to stimulation of the sodium-potassium pump, it is insufficient to correct the loss of potassium. Irreversible potassium and total cation loss occurs with resultant dehydration and formation of xerocytes that have an increased surface-to-volume ratio. These dehydrated cells, however, have an increased MCHC and presumably increased cell viscosity, which makes them less deformable and liable to sequestration in the reticuloendothelial system. The red cells are not specifically sequestrated in the spleen, so that splenectomy does not have a beneficial effect.

Clinical Laboratory Findings

Morphology of Peripheral Blood Smear. The characteristic morphologic features of hereditary hydrocytosis are a tendency to macrocytosis and the presence of increased numbers of stomatocytes on the peripheral blood smear. These are red cells with a central slit or stoma **(see Color Plate 80)**. On phase contrast or scanning electron microscopy the cells have a bowllike appearance. In hereditary xerocytosis there is an increase in the number of target cells (reflecting the greater surface-to-volume ratio of these cells). Small spiculated red cells and cells with hemoglobin concentrated in one part of the cell are also features of hereditary xerocytosis (Fig. 9–12).

Red Cell Indices. The MCV in both hereditary hydrocytosis and hereditary xerocytosis is elevated, notwithstanding the cellular dehydration in the latter condition. The MCHC is decreased in hereditary hydrocytosis and increased in hereditary xerocytosis.

Special Laboratory Tests. Osmotic fragility is increased in hereditary hydrocytosis and reflects the decreased surface-to-volume ratio. Red cell sodium concentration is elevated and potassium concentration is decreased. Total monovalent cation content is increased. In contrast, red cells in hereditary xerocytosis have strikingly decreased osmotic fragility, reflecting the increased surface-to-volume ratio. Red cell potassium concentration is markedly decreased, sodium concentration may be normal or slightly increased, and total cation concentration is decreased.

Treatment

Most patients with hemolysis due to hereditary stomatocytosis show a good response to a splenectomy. However, patients with hereditary xerocytosis, as stated earlier, do not benefit from splenectomy, presumably because of more generalized sequestration of these cells.

CASE STUDY

T.R., a 6-year-old boy, was noted to have slight scleral icterus by his mother and was referred for further investigation. He complained of some tiredness on exertion but was otherwise symptom-free. Physical examination showed only a one-finger splenomegaly. A blood count showed the following:

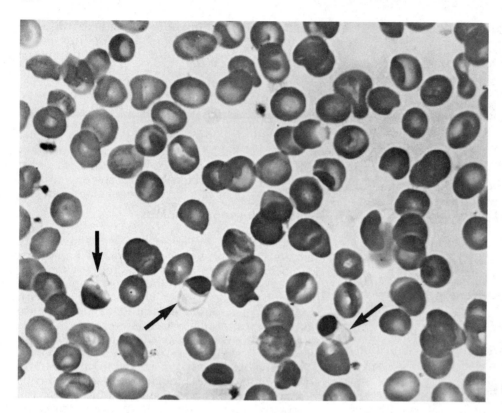

Figure 9–12. Photomicrograph of peripheral blood smear of a patient with hereditary xerocytosis. Note the characteristic target cells and cells with "puddle" hemoglobin (*arrows*).

Hgb 10.8 g/dl, Hct 29 percent, MCHC 37 percent, MCV 100 fl, and reticulocyte count 10 percent. Numerous target cells, some spiculated cells, and a few cells showing eccentric concentration of hemoglobin at one pole of the red cell were seen on the peripheral blood smear. The unconjugated bilirubin level was mildly elevated, and serum haptoglobins were decreased. There was no hemoglobinemia or hemosiderinuria. The osmotic fragility curve was strikingly decreased. Determination of red cell cation concentrations revealed a markedly decreased red cell potassium level of 65 mEq/LRBC (normal 90 to 104 mEq/LRBC) and a slightly elevated red cell sodium level of 15 mEq/LRBC (normal 5 to 12 mEq/LRBC). Similar findings were obtained in the child's father, who had previously been diagnosed at another center as having an "unusual" form of anemia. A diagnosis of hereditary xerocytosis was made. Splenectomy was not advised and the child has remained with a hemoglobin level varying between 9.5 and 11.0 g/dl over the past 2 years.

REFERENCES

1. Hillman, RS and Finch, CA: Red Cell Manual, ed 4. FA Davis, Philadelphia, 1974, p 60.
2. Lux, SE and Glader, BE: Disorders of the Red Cell Membrane. In Nathan, DG and Oski, FA (eds): Hematology of Infancy and Childhood, ed 2. WB Saunders, Philadelphia, 1981, p 456.
3. Liu, SC, Derick, LH, and Palek, J: Visualization of the hexagonal lattice in the erythrocyte membrane skeleton. J Cell Biol 104:527, 1987.
4. Marchesi, VT: Stabilizing infrastructure of cell membranes. Annu Rev Cell Biol 1:531, 1985.
5. Bennett, V: The membrane skeleton of human erythrocytes and its implications for more complex cells. Annu Rev Biochem 54:273,1985.
6. Speicher, DW, et al: A structural model of human spectrin: Alignment of chemical and functional domains. J Biol Chem 257:9093, 1982.
7. Speicher, DW and Marchesi, VT: Erythrocyte spectrin is comprised of many homologous triple helical segments. Nature (Lond)311:177, 1984.
8. Moon, RT and Lazarides, E: Beta-spectrin limits alpha-spectrin assembly on membranes following synthesis in a chicken. Nature 305:62, 1983.
9. Hanspal, M, et al: Synthesis and assembly of spectrin and ankyrin in atypical hereditary spherocytosis (HS) associated with spectrin and ankyrin deficiency. Blood (Suppl)70:53a, 1987.
10. Palek, J and Lux, SE: Red cell membrane skeleton defects in hereditary and acquired hemolytic anemias. Semin Hematol 10:184, 1983.
11. Palek, J: Hereditary elliptocytosis, spherocytosis and related disorders: consequences of a deficiency or a mutation of membrane skeletal proteins. Blood Reviews 1:147, 1987.
12. Agre, P, Orringer, EP, and Bennett, V: Deficient red cell spectrin in severe recessively inherited spherocytosis. N Engl J Med 306:1155, 1982.
13. Agre, P, et al: Inheritance pattern and clinical response to splenectomy as a reflection of erythrocyte spectrin deficiency in hereditary spherocytosis. N Engl J Med 315:1579, 1986.
14. Lux, SE and Becker, PS: Disorders of the red cell membrane skeleton: Hereditary spherocytosis and hereditary elliptocytosis. In Scriver, CR, et al (eds): The Metabolic Basis of Inherited Disease, ed 6. McGraw-Hill, New York, 1989, p 2367.
15. Becker, PS, Morrow, JS, and Lux, SE: Abnormal oxidant sensitivity and beta-chain structure of spectrin in hereditary spherocytosis associated with defective spectrin-protein 4.1 binding. J Clin Invest 80:557, 1987.
16. Coetzer, TL, et al: Partial ankyrin and spectrin deficiency in

severe atypical hereditary spherocytosis. N Engl J Med 318:230, 1988.

17. Roux, AF, et al: Molecular basis of Spα¹/⁶⁵ hereditary elliptocytosis in North Africa. Insertion of a TTG Triplet between codons 147 and 149 in the α-spectrin gene from five unrelated families. Blood 73:2196, 1989.

18. Lecomte, MC, et al: Spectrin Tunis (Spα¹/⁷⁸), an elliptocytogenic variant due to the CGG-TGG codon change (Arg-Trp) at position 35 of the αI domain. Blood 74:828, 1989.

19. Sahr, EK, et al: Sequence and exon-intron organization of the DNA encoding the αI domain of human spectrin. Application to the study of mutations causing hereditary elliptocytosis. J Clin Invest 84:1243, 1989.

20. Conboy, J, et al: Molecular basis of hereditary elliptocytosis due to protein 4.1 deficiency. N Engl J Med 315:680, 1986.

21. Lambert, S, Conboy, J, and Zail, S: A molecular study of heterozygous protein 4.1 deficiency in hereditary elliptocytosis. Blood 72:1926, 1988.

22. Rybicki, AC, et al: Deficiency of protein 4.2 in erythrocytes from a patient with a Coombs negative hemolytic anemia. Evidence for a role of protein 4.2 in stabilizing ankyrin on the membrane. J Clin Invest 81:893, 1988.

23. Zhai, S, et al: Molecular defect of the anion transporter in Southeast Asian ovalocytosis: Alterations of the cytoplasmic domain involved in ankyrin binding. Blood (Suppl)72:220a, 1989.

QUESTIONS

1. *What happens when normal donor red cells are transfused into a patient with an intracorpuscular red cell defect?*
   a. Donor cells are destroyed
   b. Donor cells have normal survival
   c. Depends on the severity of the defect
   d. Depends on the severity of the anemia

2. *Which of the following tests is not used to determine increased red cell destruction?*
   a. Unconjugated (indirect) bilirubin
   b. Serum haptoglobin
   c. Shumm's test
   d. Reticulocyte count

3. *An anemic patient investigated for a hemolytic state has the following laboratory findings: hemoglobin 8 g/dl, hematocrit 23%, reticulocyte count 8%, shift cells on peripheral smear. What is the RPI?*
   a. 8
   b. 4
   c. 2
   d. 1

4. *What tests are useful in the classification of the cause of red cell hemolysis?*
   a. Direct Coombs' test and peripheral smear examination
   b. Indirect Coombs' test and hemoglobin level
   c. Reticulocyte count and hemoglobin electrophoresis
   d. Red cell enzyme studies and iron-binding capacity

5. *Which of the following abnormalities of red cell membrane skeleton proteins is common to all cases of hereditary spherocytosis?*
   a. Deficiency of ankyrin
   b. Deficiency of protein 4.1
   c. Deficiency of spectrin
   d. Defective binding of spectrin to protein 4.1

6. *Which of the following laboratory test results would not be typical of hereditary spherocytosis?*
   a. Increased osmotic fragility
   b. Spherocytes on peripheral smear
   c. Decreased MCHC
   d. Increased RPI

7. *What is the functional abnormality affecting membrane skeleton proteins in common hereditary elliptocytosis?*
   a. Defective binding of spectrin to ankyrin
   b. Defective spectrin tetramer assembly
   c. Defective binding of ankyrin to protein 3
   d. Deficiency of protein 4.1

8. *What are the typical laboratory findings in hereditary elliptocytosis?*
   a. Elliptocytes on peripheral smear; normal red cell indices; osmotic fragility and autohemolysis may be increased
   b. Equal proportions of spherocytes and elliptocytes; decreased MCV, normal MCH and MCHC; decreased osmotic fragility
   c. Elliptocytes and microspherocytes on peripheral smear; decreased red cell indices; normal osmotic fragility and autohemolysis
   d. Greater than 90% elliptocytes; increased red cell indices; increased osmotic fragility; normal autohemolysis

9. *Which of the following abnormalities is thought to be a primary cause of the severe fragmentation and microspherocytosis characteristic of hereditary pyropoikilocytosis?*
   a. Susceptibility of spectrin to thermal denaturation
   b. Defective membrane spectrin tetramer assembly
   c. Unstable membrane lipids
   d. Membrane spectrin deficiency

10. *Which disorders are classified as disorders of membrane cation permeability?*
   a. Hereditary stomatocytosis and hereditary xerocytosis
   b. Sideroblastic anemia and myelofibrosis
   c. Autoimmune hemolytic anemia and microangiopathic hemolytic anemia
   d. Ehlers-Danlos syndrome and Bernard-Soulier syndrome

ANSWERS

1. b (p. 116)
2. d (p. 116–117)
3. c (p. 118)
4. a (p. 118)
5. c (p. 122)
6. c (p. 123–124)
7. b (p. 126)
8. a (p. 128–129)
9. d (p. 130)
10. a (p. 131)

CHAPTER 10

JEANNINE R. MELOON, M.S., M.T.(ASCP)

Introduction to Hemolytic Anemias: Intracorpuscular Defects

II. Hereditary Enzyme Deficiencies

GLUCOSE-6-PHOSPHATE DEHYDROGENASE DEFICIENCY
HISTORIC ASPECTS
MODE OF INHERITANCE
PATHOGENESIS
CLINICAL MANIFESTATIONS
LABORATORY TESTS

PYRUVATE KINASE DEFICIENCY
HISTORIC ASPECTS

MODE OF INHERITANCE
PATHOGENESIS
CLINICAL MANIFESTATIONS
LABORATORY TESTS

METHEMOGLOBIN REDUCTASE DEFICIENCY

OTHER ENZYME DEFICIENCIES

CASE STUDY

OBJECTIVES

At the end of this chapter, the learner should be able to:
1. Name the most common glycolytic enzyme deficiency associated with the pentose phosphate pathway.
2. Name the most common glycolytic enzyme deficiency associated with the Embden-Meyerhof pathway.
3. Identify the particles associated with oxidative denaturation of hemoglobulin.

4. List laboratory test results that would indicate a deficiency of G6PD.
5. Identify a laboratory test result that would indicate a PK deficiency.
6. Name the deficiency that causes hemoglobin to be oxidized from the ferrous to the ferric state.

Because anemia is not in itself a disease but rather the result of a disease process, treatment of an anemic condition depends on the accurate assessment of the underlying cause. In 1953 Dacie and his associates[1] reported on an apparently heterogeneous group of congenital hemolytic anemias that had several common characteristics. There was no detectable abnormal hemoglobin, the antiglobulin test result was negative, and the osmotic fragility was normal. The term "nonspherocytic" was used to describe this group of anemias. Investigators have since then been able to pinpoint specific

chemical explanations for many of these anemias.

The most commonly encountered anemia in this group is caused by deficiency of glucose-6-phosphate dehydrogenase (G6PD), an enzyme in the pentose phosphate pathway. The second most frequently encountered enzyme deficiency is that of pyruvate kinase (PK), an essential enzyme in the Embden-Meyerhof pathway. Many other enzyme deficiencies have also been identified, and laboratory testing is directed toward identification of the specific enzyme deficiency.

GLUCOSE-6-PHOSPHATE DEHYDROGENASE DEFICIENCY

Historic Aspects

In his review of some of the investigations that led to the discovery of G6PD deficiency, Beutler[2] cited a 1926 report of an individual who developed hemolytic anemia following the administration of the antimalarial drug primaquine. A few days after the drug was administered, the patient developed a dark urine and became jaundiced, as the red blood cell count and hemoglobin fell. Another report in 1928 noted the presence of Heinz bodies in the red blood cells of another patient with pamaquine-induced hemolysis. Although investigators had noted the connection between the drug administration and the hemolytic episodes, the reason for this apparently familial drug sensitivity remained unknown until after the introduction of the antimalarial drug primaquine.

The use of primaquine as an antimalarial treatment for soldiers in the Korean War enabled investigators to study the effects of the drug in controlled situations. In 1954, through the use of a new technique of radiolabeling erythrocytes, it was discovered that the susceptibility to hemolysis induced by primaquine was due to an intrinsic abnormality of the erythrocyte.[3] The intrinsic defect was shown to be an inborn error in erythrocyte glucose metabolism and was specifically identified as a deficiency of the enzyme G6PD.[4] The enzyme deficiency was first identified in American blacks, and a short time later a more severe form of the enzyme deficiency was found in Mediterranean populations.[5]

Mode of Inheritance

Glucose-6-phosphate dehydrogenase deficiency is transmitted by a mutant gene located on the X chromosome.[6] The disorder is fully expressed in men (hemizygote) who inherit the mutant gene. In women, full expression of the disorder occurs only when two mutant genes (homozygous) are inherited. The heterozygous woman has two populations of red blood cells — one population with normal enzyme activity and the other with deficient enzyme activity.

Distribution of the mutant gene for G6PD deficiency is worldwide; however, the highest incidence occurs in the darkly pigmented racial and ethnic groups. Normally active G6PD has been designated type Gd B. It is the most common form of the enzyme in all populations and exists in 99 percent of whites in the United States. Another variety of the G6PD enzyme that is commonly found in Africans also has normal activity but differs from Gd B by a single amino acid substitution that alters its electrophoretic mobility. This variant is designated as Gd A. The Gd A variant is found in about 20 percent of American black men. Among the American

Table 10–1. **DISTRIBUTION OF SOME COMMON G6PD VARIANTS**

Enzyme Type	Population Affected
Gd B (normal)	All
Gd A	Blacks
Gd A–	Blacks
Gd Med	Whites (Mediterranean area)
Gd Canton	Asians

blacks who possess the mutant gene, the type designated A– ([–] because of reduced activity) is the most common, occurring in approximately 10 to 15 percent of the men. Approximately 20 percent of the women are heterozygous for the Gd A– gene. Among whites, G6PD Mediterranean is the most common variant, although the overall prevalence is low. Among Kurdish Jews, however, the incidence of this enzyme may be as high as 50 to 60 percent. The variant Gd Canton is commonly found in the Chinese and in people of Southeast Asia. Table 10–1 lists the type of G6PD variant found in certain populations.

More than 300 variants of G6PD have been reported over the past 25 years.[7] These variants are generally designated by geographic names. The variants A and A– remain the exceptions, as these names are well-ingrained in the literature.

As G6PD amino acid sequence data become available, our perceptions concerning similarities and differences among the variants are changing. Beutler[8] suggests that this information be used in the nomenclature. Variants would be identified using superscripts to the geographic name to designate the substitution. For example, Gd A would be designated as G6PD A^{376G} to indicate the guanine substitution at nucleotide 376.

Pathogenesis

Glucose-6-phosphate dehydrogenase catalyzes the first step in the pentose phosphate pathway (aerobic glycolytic pathway). Oxidative catabolism of glucose is accompanied by reduction of NADP to NADPH (Fig. 10–1), which is subsequently required to reduce glutathione. Reduced glutathione (GSH) is an important source of reducing potential that protects hemoglobin from oxidative denaturation.

Activity of G6PD is highest in young erythrocytes and decreases with cell aging. Under normal conditions, the individual with G6PD deficiency compensates for the shortened lifespan of the erythrocytes. Oxidative stress, however, can lead to a mild to severe hemolytic episode. A deficiency of GSH results in oxidative destruction of certain erythrocyte components, including sulfhydryl groups of globin chains and the cell membrane.[9] More than 50 chemical agents may induce hemolysis in G6PD deficient erythrocytes. Table 10–2 lists the

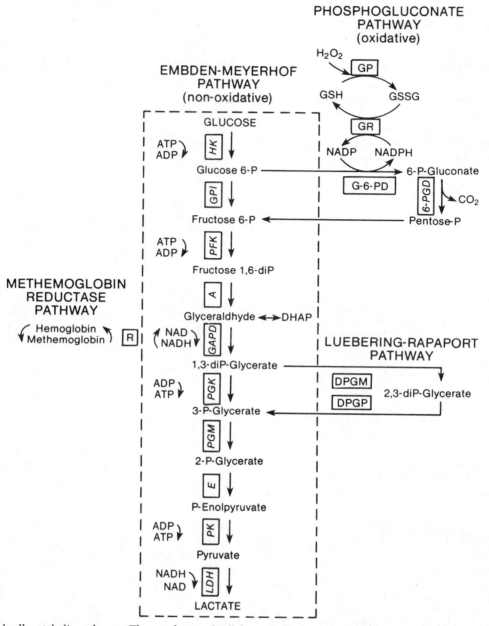

Figure 10–1. Red cell metabolic pathways. The anucleate red cell depends almost exclusively on the breakdown of glucose for energy requirements. The Embden-Meyerhof (nonoxidative or anaerobic) pathway is responsible for most of the glucose utilization and generation of ATP. In addition, this pathway plays an essential role in maintaining pyridine nucleotides in a reduced state to support methemoglobin reduction (the methemoglobin reductase pathway) and 2.3-diphosphoglycerate synthesis (the Leubering-Rapaport pathway). The phosphogluconate pathway couples oxidative metabolism with pyridine nucleotide and glutathione reduction. It serves to protect red cells from environmental oxidants. (From Hillman, RS and Finch, CA: Red Cell Manual, ed. 5, FA Davis, Philadelphia, 1985, with permission).

drugs commonly leading to hemolysis in individuals with G6PD deficiency. The drug-induced hemolytic episode results when G6PD-deficient erythrocytes fail to produce sufficient NADPH and subsequently fail to maintain adequate levels of GSH.[10] The resulting oxidation of hemoglobin leads to progressive precipitation of irreversibly denatured hemoglobin (Heinz bodies) **(see Color Plate 84).** The cells lack normal deformability when sulfhydryl groups are oxidized and consequently encounter difficulties navigating in the microcirculation. Premature destruction of the cells results when they undergo intravascular lysis or are sequestered and destroyed in the liver or spleen. This early destruction may sometimes be detected in the peripheral blood smear with the formation of small condensed bite- or helmet-shaped red cells **(see Color Plate 83).**

Certain G6PD-deficient individuals also exhibit a sensitivity to the fava bean (favism) **(see Color**

Table 10-2. **DRUGS AND CHEMICALS THAT HAVE CLEARLY BEEN SHOWN TO CAUSE CLINICALLY SIGNIFICANT HEMOLYTIC ANEMIA IN G6PD DEFICIENCY**

Acentanilid	Primaquine
Methylene blue	Sulfacetamide
Nalidixic acid (NegGram)	Sulfamethoxazole (Gantanol)
Naphthalene	Sulfanilamide
Niridazole (Ambilhar)	Sulfapyridine
Nitrofurantoin (Furadantoin)	Thiazolesulfone
Pamaquine	Toluidine blue
Pentaquine	Trintrotoluene (TNT)
Phenylhydrazine	

SOURCE: Beutler,[2] p 1631, with permission.

Plate 85). These individuals develop severe hemolysis after ingesting the fava bean or even after inhaling the plant's pollen. Favism is found in some individuals with G6PD deficiency of the Mediterranean and Canton types.

Clinical Manifestations

Stress, resulting from taking certain drugs or from infections, or occurring during the newborn period, challenges the G6PD-deficient erythrocytes, causing various degrees of hemolysis. Consequently, symptoms of the disorder are related to the severity of the hemolytic episode. Two to three days following the administration of the offending drug, the erythrocyte count decreases, along with the hemoglobin content. The anemia will appear normochromic and normocytic with an increase in reticulocytes. The patient may or may not experience back pain. Hemoglobinuria and jaundice may also be evidence of the hemolytic process. Table 10-3 compares the clinical features of the two most common variants.

The hemolytic episode is usually self-limiting. Young cells that are produced in response to the

Table 10-3. **COMPARISON OF CLINICAL FEATURES OF Gd A− AND Gd MED**

Clinical Feature	Gd A−	Gd Med
Cells affected by defect	Aging erythrocytes	All erythrocytes
Hemolysis with drugs	Unusual	Common
Hemolysis with infection	Common	Common
Favism	No	Occasionally
Degree of hemolysis	Moderate	Severe
Transfusions required	No	Occasionally
Chronic hemolysis	No	No
Hemolytic disease of newborn	Rare	Occasionally

anemia have levels of G6PD that are nearly normal.[11]

Laboratory Tests

Laboratory investigation of a hemolytic anemia when there is evidence (family history or drug sensitivity, or both) of G6PD deficiency may include several screening procedures. It has already been noted that oxidative denaturation of hemoglobin results in formation of Heinz bodies. These small particles of precipitated hemoglobin can be visualized by supravital staining using certain basic dyes such as crystal violet **(see Color Plate 84)**. Heinz bodies will appear as small (1 to 4 μm), purple inclusions, usually seen on the cell periphery. Heinz bodies will not be seen with Romanowsky stains such as Wright's stain. Although Heinz bodies may be seen in other enzyme deficiencies, they are not seen in pyruvate kinase deficiency. Some of the unstable hemoglobins will also form Heinz bodies when the erythrocytes have been incubated at 37°C for 48 hours.

Other test procedures that may be used to screen for G6PD deficiency include the methemoglobin reduction test[12] and the ascorbate-cyanide test.[13] The methemoglobin reduction test is a simple and sensitive screening procedure in which G6PD-deficient erythrocytes fail to reduce methemoglobin in the presence of methylene blue. The ascorbate-cyanide test measures perioxidative denaturation of hemoglobin. This test is not specific for G6PD deficiency, as it will yield moderately positive results in the presence of PK deficiency and of certain unstable hemoglobins.

The fluorescent spot test and the G6PD assay results will be positive only with G6PD deficiency. When a mixture of glucose-6-phosphate, NADP, saponin, and buffer is mixed with blood and placed on filter paper, G6PD acts to convert the NADP to NADPH. The filter paper is observed under fluorescent light. Erythrocytes deficient in G6PD fail to convert NADP to NADPH and will lack fluorescence. The quantitative assay of G6PD[14] is based on the measurement of the rate of reduction of NADP to NADPH measured at 340 nm.

It should be noted that diagnosis of G6PD deficiency during an acute hemolytic episode may be difficult. The deficiency may be obscured by a younger erythrocyte population as the older G6PD-deficient erythrocytes are destroyed.

PYRUVATE KINASE DEFICIENCY

Historic Aspects

Investigations of the nonspherocytic anemias pointed to a possible defect in erythrocyte glucose utilization. In 1961 Valentine, Tanaka, and Miwa[15] reported that three patients with congenital nonspherocytic anemia had a severe deficiency of PK. This enzyme catalyzes one of the steps in the Embden-Meyerhof pathway of glycolysis.

Mode of Inheritance

The deficiency of erythrocyte PK is inherited as an autosomal recessive trait[16] affecting both sexes equally. Individuals who are homozygous for the trait develop a hemolytic anemia, while those who are heterozygous remain clinically normal. One investigator has reported an apparently autosomal dominant inheritance of PK deficiency in one family.[17] The affected family members had PK activities of 20 percent of normal and exhibited nonspherocytic hemolytic anemia. Although studies have shown that the defect is distributed worldwide, there appears to be a predominance of the trait in individuals whose ancestors originated from Northern Europe.

Pathogenesis

Pyruvate kinase catalyzes the formation of pyruvate from phosphoenolpyruvate (PEP) with the generation of adenosine triphosphate (ATP) from adenosine diphosphate (ADP) (Fig. 10–1). Erythrocytes generate about 90 percent of their energy requirements through the anaerobic Embden-Meyerhof pathway of glycolysis. The PK-deficient erythrocyte fails to generate sufficient quantities of ATP to maintain normal erythrocyte membrane function. The cell membrane abnormalities result in a rigid, poorly deformable cell that is prematurely destroyed in the spleen and liver.

Clinical Manifestations

The severity of the hemolytic disease associated with PK deficiency varies widely. Because clinical features are related to the effects of the hemolysis and the severity of the anemia, clinical manifestations also vary. Onset may be during infancy or early childhood; however, some mild cases may not be detected until adulthood.

The peripheral blood smear will reveal varying degrees of polychromasia and poikilocytosis. Nucleated red blood cells may be seen. No significant leukocyte or platelet abnormalities are seen. Physical findings commonly include splenomegaly, and radiologic evaluation may demonstrate cholelithiasis.

Laboratory Tests

Several screening tests may be used to distinguish the nonspherocytic anemia of PK deficiency from the anemias of hereditary spherocytosis and the unstable hemoglobinopathies. These tests are nonspecific and serve only as a mechanism for classifying the type of anemia. Diagnosis is made on the basis of specific testing for the PK enzyme.

Screening tests may include the osmotic fragility test and the autohemolysis test (see Chapter 30), as well as the antiglobulin test and red blood cell survival tests. Erythrocytes that are PK deficient will show osmotic fragility that is near normal when the test is performed on freshly drawn blood. If the blood is incubated, some patients with nonspherocytic anemia exhibit an increase in osmotic fragility.[9] Sterile defibrinated blood is used to perform the test for autohemolysis. When normal erythrocytes are incubated in their own serum at 37°C they will gradually lyse, showing up to 3.5 percent lysis after 48 hours.[18] Erythrocytes from patients with nonspherocytic anemias, as well as those with hereditary spherocytosis, demonstrate an increased amount of autohemolysis. When glucose is added prior to incubation, erythrocytes from the patient with hereditary spherocytosis will show a normal amount of hemolysis. The addition of glucose does not correct the increased autohemolysis of PK-deficient erythrocytes (Fig. 10–2). The antiglobulin test in PK deficiency is negative and the red blood cell survival is decreased.

Differential diagnosis of PK deficiency is dependent on qualitative and quantitative assays for the specific enzyme. The fluorescent spot test[14] detects the decrease in fluorescence when PK catalyzes the reaction of PEP to pyruvate, and NADH is subsequently reduced to NAD by the pyruvate, with the formation of lactate. Erythrocytes that are PK deficient fail to produce this reaction, and the fluorescence of NADH persists even after 60 minutes. It should be noted that leukocytes contain a PK isoenzyme that will also catalyze the same reaction. Therefore, blood must be centrifuged and plasma

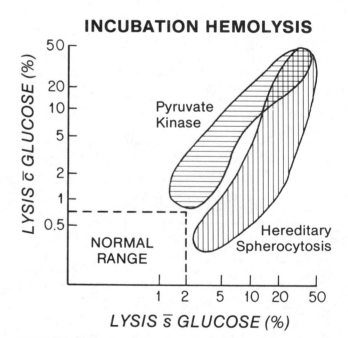

INCUBATION HEMOLYSIS

Figure 10–2. The incubation hemolysis test provides a further measure of cell resistance to hemolysis. Pyruvate kinase-deficient blood demonstrates an abnormal rate of hemolysis that is independent of the presence or absence of glucose in the incubation media. In contrast, the blood from a patient with hereditary spherocytosis shows more marked hemolysis when glucose is absent. (From Hillman, RS and Finch, CE: Red Cell Manual, ed. 5, FA Davis, Philadelphia, 1985, with permission.)

and buffy coat removed prior to testing the erythrocytes. In addition, patients who have recently been transfused may have enough donor cells remaining in circulation to give erroneous test results. A quantitative assay for PK is also available. The principle is the same as the fluorescent spot test, and the change in absorbance at 340 nm is measured to quantify PK activity.

In the orthocresol red test, the formation of lactic acid in the normal Embden-Meyerhof pathway is detected by the change of the indicator from red to yellow at an acid pH. Although the test has been proposed as a specific test for PK deficiency, it is probable that any enzyme deficiency in the Embden-Meyerhof pathway will result in decreased production of lactic acid. Therefore, the test may be useful as a nonspecific screening test for enzyme deficiencies.[19]

METHEMOGLOBIN REDUCTASE DEFICIENCY

Hemoglobin that is oxidized from the ferrous to the ferric state is called methemoglobin. Normally, about 1 percent of the circulating hemoglobin is in the form of methemoglobin. A balance is maintained between methemoglobin formation and reduction by the NADH-methemoglobin reductase (also called diaphorase) pathway. Methemoglobinemia may occur either when there is decreased enzyme activity or when production of methemoglobin exceeds the reducing capacity of the enzyme system. Hereditary deficiency of NADH-methemoglobin reductase results in increased levels of methemoglobin. This congenital deficiency is inherited as an autosomal recessive trait.[20] The heterozygote does not usually show signs of methemoglobinemia unless challenged with certain drugs.

The major clinical feature of methemoglobinemia is cyanosis. Because methemoglobin cannot carry oxygen, some patients exhibit symptoms similar to those of anemia. Some patients develop a compensatory mild polycythemia (see Chapter 21). The course of this disorder is generally benign, and patients are treated only for cosmetic reasons. In cases of severe cyanosis, methylene blue is administered intravenously to activate the NADH-methemoglobin reductase system.

In addition to the hereditary deficiency of NADH-methemoglobin reductase, methemoglobinemia may be due to the hemoglobin M diseases or to acute reaction to various drugs or toxic substances. The abnormality in the globin structure of hemoglobin that results in the hemoglobin M diseases is discussed further in Chapter 11. Hemoglobin may be oxidized by various substances such as nitrites, sulfonamides, and aniline derivatives. Toxic methemoglobinemia results when the methemoglobin-reducing system is unable to reduce the excess being formed.

The laboratory differentiation of the types of methemoglobinemia is shown in Table 10-4. Methemoglobin has a maximum absorbance band at 630 nm. The addition of cyanide causes the band to disappear, and the change in absorbance is directly proportional to the concentration of methemoglobin.[21] Although the concentration of methemoglobin is increased to varying degrees in all three disorders, enzyme activity is decreased only in hereditary NADH-methemoglobin reductase deficiency. Hemoglobin electrophoresis is normal except in the hemoglobin M diseases.

OTHER ENZYME DEFICIENCIES

Except for the deficiencies of G6PD and PK, reports of hereditary enzyme deficiencies have been limited to a few rare cases. In a study of 350 cases of suspected enzyme-deficient hemolytic anemia, Beutler[22] reported 13.9 percent G6PD deficiencies and 9.9 percent PK deficiencies. Glucose phosphate isomerase was the third most commonly identified enzyme deficiency (1.7 percent). Although there have been reports of other enzyme deficiencies (glycolytic and nonglycolytic), not all such deficiencies have been associated with hemolytic anemia. There is considerable controversy in the literature regarding the role of certain enzyme deficiencies in hemolytic anemia.

Laboratory tests are available to assay many of the specific enzymes. Some of these tests may be available only through reference laboratories. Most laboratories, however, will be able to screen patients with a suspected hemolytic anemia due to enzyme deficiency. The antiglobulin, erythrocyte survival, autohemolysis, osmotic fragility, and Heinz body tests can all be effectively used to distinguish the enzyme deficiencies from hereditary spherocytosis and the unstable hemoglobinopathies.

Table 10-4. **LABORATORY DIFFERENTIATION OF METHEMOGLOBINEMIA**

Methemoglobinemia Resulting From	Methemoglobin Level	Enzyme Activity	Hemoglobin Electrophoresis
Hereditary enzyme deficiency	Increased	Decreased	Normal
Toxic substance exposure	Increased	Normal	Normal
Hemoglobin M disease	Increased	Normal	Abnormal

CASE STUDY

A 26-year-old black man was referred to the clinical laboratory for investigation of reported hemoglobinuria. The patient had recently been diagnosed as having infectious mononucleosis. The following laboratory data were obtained:

RBC	3.7×10^{12}/liter
Hg	11.0 g/dl
Hct	0.32
MCV	86.0 fl
MCHC	34.0 g/dl
WBC	9.5×10^9/liter

Differential

Segs	40%
Bands	3%
Lymphs	48% (many atypical)
Monos	7%
Eos	2%
Platelets	Adequate
Reticulocytes	14.5% (uncorrected)

The RBC morphology was normochromic and normocytic. Polychromasia was noted. A slight poikilocytosis was also noted, with some red cells showing irregular protrusions. Upon further investigation, the anti–human globulin test result was found to be negative. The hemolytic process was not due to an immune reaction. A previously negative history would tend to rule out any of the hemoglobinopathies; this was confirmed by a normal hemoglobin electrophoresis.

The hematologist suggested that the patient return in 30 days for testing for erythrocyte enzyme deficiency. At that time, the patient was found to have an erythrocyte G6PD activity of 15 percent of normal.

Hemolysis can be induced in G6PD deficient individuals by infection with certain viral agents. Testing to confirm erythrocyte G6PD activity should be done after the patient has had sufficient time to recover from the hemolytic episode.

REFERENCES

1. Dacie, JR, et al: Atypical congenital haemolytic anemia. QJ Med 22:79, 1953.
2. Beutler, E: Glucose-6-phosphate dehydrogenase deficiency. In Stanbury, JB, et al (eds): The Metabolic Basis of Inherited Disease, ed 5. McGraw-Hill, New York, 1983, p 1630.
3. Dern, RJ, et al: The hemolytic effect of primaquine. I. The localization of the drug-induced hemolytic defect in primaquine-sensitive individuals. J Lab Clin Med 43:303, 1954.
4. Carson, PE, et al: Enzymatic deficiency in primaquine-sensitive erythrocytes. Science 124:484, 1956.
5. Beutler, E: The hemolytic effect of primaquine and related compounds. A review. Blood 14:103, 1959.
6. Desforges, JF: Genetic implications of G-6-PD deficiency. N Engl J Med 294:1438, 1976.
7. Beutler, E and Yoshida, A: Genetic variation of glucose-6-phosphate dehydrogenase: A catalog and future prospects. Medicine 67:311, 1988.
8. Beutler, E: Glucose-t-phosphate dehydrogenase: New perspectives. Blood 73:1397, 1989.
9. Beutler, E: Glucose-6-phosphate dehydrogenase deficiency. In Williams, WJ, et al (eds): Hematology, ed 2, McGraw-Hill, New York, 1977, p. 466.
10. Beutler, E: Glucose-6-phosphate dehydrogenase deficiency. In Stanbury, JB, et al (eds): The Metabolic Basis of Inherited Disease. McGraw-Hill, New York, 1978, p 1430.
11. Beutler, E, Dern, RJ, and Alving, AS: The hemolytic effect of primaquine. IV. The relationship of cell age to hemolysis. J Lab Clin Med 44:439, 1954.
12. Brewer, GJ, et al: The methemoglobin reduction test for primaquine-type sensitivity of erythrocytes: A simplified procedure for detecting a specific hypersusceptibility to drug hemolysis. JAMA 180:386, 1962.
13. Jacob, HS and Jandl, JH: A simple visual screening test for glucose-6-phosphate dehydrogenase deficiency employing ascorbate and cyanide. N Engl J Med 274:1162, 1966.
14. Beutler, E: Red Cell Metabolism. A Manual of Biochemical Methods, ed 2. Grune & Stratton, New York, 1975.
15. Valentine, WN, Tanaka, KR, and Miwa, S: A specific glycolytic enzyme defect (pyruvate kinase) in three subjects with congenital non-spherocytic hemolytic anemia. Trans Assoc Am Physicians 74:100, 1961.
16. Valentine, WN and Tanaka, KR: Pyruvate kinase deficiency hemolytic anemia. In Stanbury, JB, Wyngaarden, JR, and Frederickson, DS (eds): The Metabolic Basis of Inherited Disease, ed 2. McGraw-Hill, New York, 1966, p 1051.
17. Etiemble, J, et al: Erythrocytic pyruvate kinase deficiency and hemolytic anemia inherited as a dominant trait. Am J Hematol 17:251, 1984.
18. Beutler, E: Autohemolysis. In Williams, WJ, et al (eds): Hematology, ed 2. McGraw-Hill, New York, 1977, p 1610.
19. Miale, JB: Laboratory Medicine Hematology, ed 6, CV Mosby, St Louis, 1982, p 588.
20. Jaffe, ER: Hereditary methemoglobinemias associated with abnormalities in the metabolism of erythrocytes. Am J Med 41:786, 1966.
21. Evelyn, KA and Malloy, HT: Micro determination of oxyhemoglobin, methemoglobin and sulfhemoglobin in a single sample of blood. J Biol Chem 126:655, 1938.
22. Beutler, E: Red cell enzyme defects as nondiseases and as diseases. Blood 54:1, 1979.

QUESTIONS

1. *What is the most common glycolytic enzyme deficiency associated with the pentose phosphate pathway (aerobic pathway)?*
   a. Pyruvate kinase deficiency
   b. Glucose-6-phosphate dehydrogenase deficiency
   c. Hexokinase deficiency
   d. Glutathione reductase deficiency

2. *What is the most common glycolytic enzyme deficiency associated with the Embden-Meyerhof pathway (anaerobic pathway)? (Use answer choices for question 1.)*

3. *Oxidative denaturation of hemoglobin results in formation of small particles which are visualized with supravital staining. What is the term for these particles?*
   a. Basophilic stippling
   b. Howell-Jolly bodies
   c. Pappenheimer bodies
   d. Heinz bodies

4. *In the evaluation of a patient for G6PD deficiency, which of the following test results would indicate a deficiency of the enzyme?*
   a. Increased formation of Heinz bodies

b. Lack of fluorescence in the fluorescent spot test
c. Failure to reduce methemoglobin in the presence of methylene blue
d. All of the above

5. *Which laboratory test result would indicate a patient with PK deficiency?*
a. Abnormal rate of hemolysis that is independent of the presence or absence of glucose in the incubation media
b. Lack of flurorescence in the fluorescent spot test
c. A change in the indicator from red to yellow in the orthocresol red test
d. Increase in osmotic fragility

6. *What deficiency causes hemoglobin to be oxidized from the ferrous to the ferric state?*
a. G6PD deficiency
b. Pyruvate kinase deficiency
c. NADH-methemoglobin reductase deficiency
d. Lactate dehydrogenase deficiency

ANSWERS

1. b (p. 134)
2. a (p. 134)
3. d (p. 136)
4. d (p. 137)
5. a (p. 138)
6. c (p. 139)

CHAPTER 11

HALLYE ZERINGER, M.T.(ASCP), S.H.
DENISE M. HARMENING, Ph.D., M.T.(ASCP), C.L.S.(NCA)

Hemolytic Anemias: Intracorpuscular Defects

III. The Hemoglobinopathies

CLASSIFICATION

REVIEW OF NORMAL HEMOGLOBIN STRUCTURE

HEMOGLOBINOPATHIES
NOMENCLATURE
SICKLE-CELL ANEMIA
Historic Overview
Definition
Pathophysiology
Clinical Features
    Infarction
    Infections
Sickle-Cell Trait
Laboratory Diagnosis
Treatment
HEMOGLOBIN C DISEASE AND TRAIT

HEMOGLOBIN SC DISEASE
HEMOGLOBIN D DISEASE AND TRAIT
HEMOGLOBIN E DISEASE AND TRAIT
HEMOGLOBIN O ARAB AND HBS/HBO ARAB
    COMBINATION
HEMOGLOBIIN SD DISEASE
HEMOGLOBIN S/β-THALASSEMIA COMBINATION

METHEMOGLOBINEMIA

HEMOGLOBIN VARIANTS WITH ALTERED OXYGEN AFFINITY

UNSTABLE HEMOGLOBINS

SUMMARY OF LABORATORY DIAGNOSIS

CASE STUDY

OBJECTIVES

At the end of this chapter, the learner should be able to:
1. Characterize hemoglobinopathies.
2. Define qualitative and quantitative hemoglobin defects.
3. Explain the nomenclature for abnormal hemoglobins.
4. Name the amino acid substitution found in sickle-cell anemia.
5. List factors contributing to the sickling process.
6. Name and describe the three types of sickle-cell crises.
7. List tests useful in the laboratory diagnosis of sickle-cell disease.
8. Describe the effects on hemoglobin S cells when parasitized by *P. falciparum*.
9. List characteristics for sickle-cell trait.
10. Describe the goals of treatment for sickle-cell anemia.
11. Name the amino acid substitution found in hemoglobin C disease.
12. List findings for hemoglobin C disease.
13. Identify the laboratory finding that helps provide a diagnosis of hemoglobin SC disease.
14. List characteristics for hemoglobin D, hemoglobin E, and other variants and combinations such as hemoglobin O Arab and hemoglobin SD.
15. Identify causes of methemoglobinemia.
16. Recognize useful techniques for studying hemoglobin variants with altered oxygen affinity.

Hemoglobinopathies are defined in the broadest sense as conditions in which abnormal hemoglobins are synthesized. More than 700 known hemoglobin variants have been reported. The majority of these hemoglobin variants were discovered coincidentally and are of no clinical significance. However, there exist hemoglobinopathies that represent clinically significant hemolytic anemias in which the pathophysiologic basis of the red cell destruction is determined by the type of abnormal hemoglobin molecule present. The hemoglobinopathies are either inherited abnormalities or genetic mutations, resulting in a defect in the structural integrity or function of the hemoglobin molecule.

Greater than 90 percent of the hemoglobin variants are single amino acid substitutions in the alpha (α), beta (β), delta (δ), or gamma (γ) globin chain. Hemoglobin variants are inherited as codominant traits according to classic mendelian genetics (Fig. 11–1). Figure 11–2 depicts the eight genes on each one of two homologous chromosomes that code for polypeptide chains. The α and zeta (ζ) genes are located on chromosome 16, with two α and one ζ gene per chromosome. The β, δ, γ, and epsilon (ϵ) genes are located on chromosome 11, with one β, δ, and ϵ and two γ genes per chromosome.

CLASSIFICATION

Classification of hemoglobinopathies is somewhat arbitrary. Hemoglobin defects may be divided into two very broad categories: qualitative and

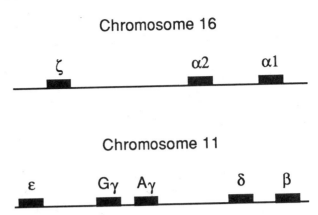

Figure 11–2. Location of the globin genes on chromosomes 16 and 11.

quantitative hemoglobinopathies. In the qualitative category are hemoglobins that are formed normally in structure ($\alpha_2\beta_2$) but differ in the *sequence* of the amino acids composing the globin chain. This category is the one usually referred to in the general discussion of hemoglobinopathies. Quantitative defects are those characterized by decreased production of hemoglobin with a decreased synthesis of one particular globin chain, which is commonly known as thalassemia (see Chapter 12).

A more inclusive method of classification allows division of the hemoglobinopathies into five major categories:
1. Abnormal hemoglobins without clinical significance
2. Aggregating hemoglobins
3. Unbalanced synthesis of hemoglobin
4. Unstable hemoglobins
5. Hemoglobins with abnormal heme function

Table 11–1 summarizes this classification of hemoglobinopathies.

REVIEW OF NORMAL HEMOGLOBIN STRUCTURE

A brief review of normal hemoglobin structure is provided here to aid in understanding the hemoglobinopathies; however, the reader is referred to Chapter 1 for a more detailed discussion.

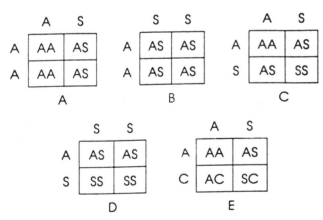

Figure 11–1. Inheritance of abnormal hemoglobins. (A) With one parent heterozygous for an abnormal hemoglobin, the offspring have a one in two chance of carrying the trait. (B) With one parent homozygous for an abnormal hemoglobin, all offspring will carry the trait, as that parent can contribute only an abnormal gene. (C) With both parents heterozygous for the abnormality, the chances are one in four normal, two in four heterozygous, and one in four homozygous. (D) With both parents carrying the same abnormal hemoglobin—one homozygous and one heterozygous—the offspring have a fifty-fifty chance of being either homozygous or heterozygous. (E) With parents carrying two different abnormal hemoglobins, offspring have a one in four chance of not inheriting an abnormality, a one in two chance of carrying the trait for one or the other abnormality, and a one in four chance of carrying both abnormalities in codominance.

Table 11–1. **CLASSIFICATION OF HEMOGLOBINOPATHIES**

Abnormal hemoglobins without clinical significance
Aggregating hemoglobins (structural abnormalities with amino acid substitution *away* from the crevice of the heme)
Unbalanced synthesis of hemoglobin (thalassemia)
Unstable hemoglobins
Hemoglobins with abnormal heme function (structural abnormalities with amino acid substitutions *near* the crevice of the heme)

Hemoglobin is a conjugated protein composed of iron, protoporphyrin IX type III, and globin. The combination of iron and porphyrin is referred to as the heme moiety. The globin portion of the molecule consists of four polypeptide chains, each with an attached heme group.[1] These heme moieties are positioned so that they are suspended in the center of the polypeptide chains. This provides an environment where iron can exist in the reduced (ferrous) state, a feature that is critical for oxygen transport.

There are six known polypeptide chains that make up the different globin portions of the hemoglobin molecule. These chains are alpha (α), beta (β), gamma (γ), delta (δ), epsilon (ϵ), and zeta (ζ). The latter two represent embryonic globin chains. The structure of the chains and the resulting hemoglobin molecule is described in the following four steps:

1. The primary structure relates to the number and sequence of amino acids constituting each chain. Alpha chains have 141 amino acids; the nonalpha chains have 146 amino acids. The sequence of amino acids is different in each chain.
2. The secondary structure occurs with the twisting of the amino acid chain around an axis in a helical conformation.
3. The tertiary structure consists of bending the twisted amino acid chain into a three-dimensional shape resembling an "irregular pretzel."[2] The polar groups are oriented outward, and the nonpolar groups are interior. The heme molecule is nestled in a nonpolar pocket and attached to a proximal histidine residue.
4. The quarternary structure is the assembling of the four three-dimensional chains with their respected heme groups. The result is a completed, functional hemoglobin molecule.[2,3,4]

Table 11–2 reviews the composition of normal physiologic hemoglobins.

HEMOGLOBINOPATHIES

The majority of hemoglobinopathies (hemoglobin variants) result from beta chain abnormalities. Many of these variants have no associated physiologic consequences. There also can be alpha, gamma, and delta chain abnormalities, but these conditions are usually clinically benign. Some individuals with beta chain abnormalities present with abnormal physical properties resulting in clinical disease. From the first description of a sickle cell by Herrick in 1910,[15] the work continues today to find, define, understand, and treat these abnormalities.

Most hemoglobin variants arise from a single amino acid substitution. For example, when valine substitutes for glutamic acid in the sixth position of the beta chain, HbS is produced rather than HbA. When lysine replaces glutamic acid at position six of the beta chain, HbC is produced. These changes truly represent a molecular alteration—a feature that was initially appreciated by Pauling in the late 1940s when he won the Nobel prize for defining sickle-cell anemia as a molecular disease.[6] The abnormality was demonstrated by electrophoresis to be located in the protein portion of the hemoglobin molecule. Other substitutions can cause instability of hemoglobin such as deformation of the three-dimensional structure, oxidation of the ferrous iron, or alteration in residues that interact with heme, with 2,3-diphosphoglycerate (2,3-DPG), or at subunit contact points.[3]

At the molecular level, a single-base DNA substitution in the corresponding triplet codon produces one amino acid change, which is the most common cause of a hemoglobinopathy. Other, rarer molecular changes include (1) multiple-base substitutions, (2) the production of long or short subunits, and (3) the occurrence of fusion subunits.[4]

Nomenclature

Investigators began naming the abnormal hemoglobins with capital letters, but with the end of the alphabet rapidly approaching, they changed to the use of names of places. A letter plus a place name indicates identical mobility on electrophoresis, but there are different substitutions. The description of the variant can also involve identifying the chains and the substitution. For example, homozygous HbS is $\alpha_2\beta_2^S$ or $\alpha_2\beta_2^{6val}$ or $\alpha_2\beta_2^{6glu\text{-}val}$. Hemoglobin G Philadelphia, the most common alpha chain variant in the black population, is written $\alpha_2^{G\ Phil}\beta_2^A$ or

Table 11–2. **COMPOSITION OF NORMAL PHYSIOLOGIC HEMOGLOBINS**

Globin Chains	Hemoglobin	Normal %	Stage of Development
$\alpha_2\epsilon_2$	Gower 2		
$\zeta_2\epsilon_2$	Gower 1		Embryo
$\zeta_2\gamma_2$	Portland		
$\alpha_2^A\gamma_2$	F	50–85	
$\alpha_2^G\gamma_2$	F		Fetus
$\alpha_2\beta_2$	A	95–97	
$\alpha_2\delta_2$	A_2	2	Adult

$\alpha_2^{68Lys}\beta_2$ or $\alpha_2^{68\,asn-Lys}\beta_2$. Additionally, the exact helix of the secondary structure and the position in that helix can be indicated. For example, the designations would be $\alpha_2\beta_2^{6(A3)}$ for HbS and $\alpha_2^{68(E17)}\beta_2$ for HbG Philadelphia. A limited list of hemoglobin variants can be found in Table 11–11.

Sickle-Cell Anemia (Color Plate 86)

Historic Overview

In 1910, a 20-year-old black student from the West Indies was described by Herrick[5] to be suffering from a severe hemolytic anemia in which peculiarly elongated, "sickled" red cells were found on his peripheral blood smear. The classic hematologic features included not only the presence of sickle cells on the peripheral blood smear but also nucleated red cells indicative of a severe anemia, cardiac enlargement, icterus, and leukocytosis. The presence of target cells as well as a normocytic, normochromic anemia is also generally associated with hemoglobinopathies. Sickle-cell anemia represents the most common type of severe hemoglobinopathy.

Definition

Sickle-cell anemia (SCA) is the homozygous form of the disease, in which the individual inherits a double dose of the abnormal gene that codes for hemoglobin S. This type of hemoglobin differs from normal hemoglobin by the single amino acid substitution of valine for glutamic acid in the sixth position from the NH$_2$ terminal end of the beta chain (Fig. 11–3). The structural formula for sickle-cell anemia (HbSS) is $\alpha_2\beta_2^{6Glu-Val}$. The formula alternatively may be written as $\alpha_2\beta_2^{S}$ or $\alpha_2\beta_2^{6Val}$. The gene for hemoglobin S occurs with greatest frequency in tropical Africa, particularly Central Africa. Many social and historic factors, such as slavery and conquest, are responsible for the appearance of this hemoglobin in the North American and Middle Eastern populations.[5] In the United States, the birth incidence of the homozygous state (HbSS), is approximately 0.16 percent.[3] It is estimated that 8 to 10 percent of American blacks carry the trait (one gene) for hemoglobin S.

Pathophysiology

Hemoglobin S is soluble and usually causes no problem when properly oxygenated. However, when the oxygen tension decreases, HbS polymerizes, forming tactoids or fluid polymers (Fig. 11–4).[7] As these polymers realign, they cause the red cell to deform into the characteristic sickle shape (Fig. 11–5 and **Color Plate 87**). The sickling process is dependent on the degree of oxygenation, pH, and dehydration of the patient. A decrease in oxygenation and pH as well as dehydration *promotes* sickling. Sickle cells in circulation increase the viscosity of the blood, which slows circulation, thereby increasing the time of exposure to a hypoxic environment, particularly in the small vasculature of the spleen. This then promotes further sickling. There are two types of sickle cells: reversible and irreversible. The sickling of the cell is reversible up to a point. However, repeated sickling eventually damages the RBC membrane permanently. The forma-

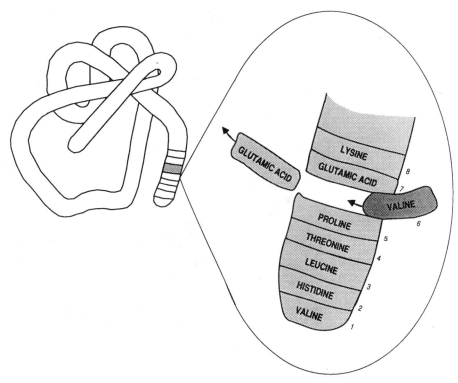

Figure 11–3. Amino acid substitution in hemoglobin S.

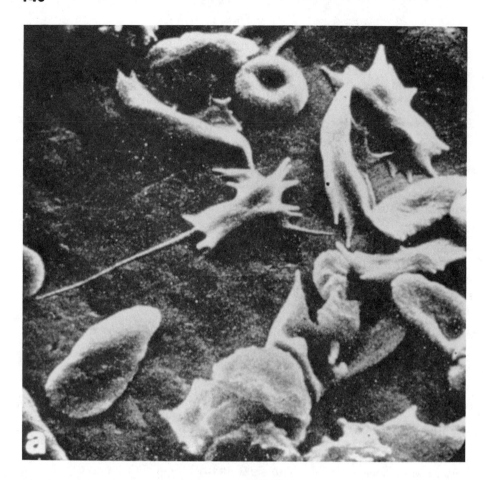

Figure 11–4. Scanning electron micrograph of hemoglobin S.

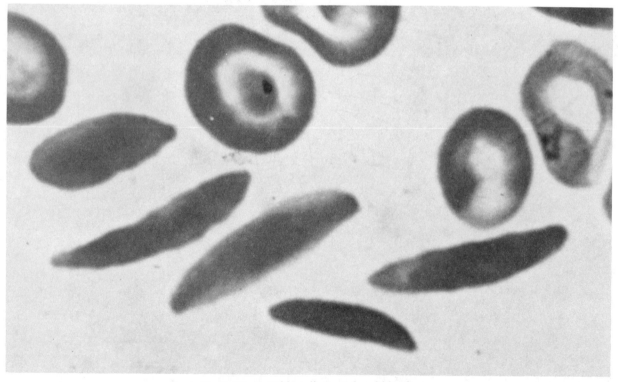

Figure 11–5. Sickle cells (peripheral blood).

Table 11–3. **FACTORS AFFECTING THE SEVERITY OF HbS**

Amount of HbS	Vascular stasis
Other hemoglobins	Temperature
Thalassemia	pH
G6PD deficiency	Viscosity
Deoxygenation	MCHC
Amount of HbF	Dehydration

G6PD = glucose-6-phosphate dehydrogenase

tion of rigid sickle cells is likely to plug small blood vessels, further lowering the pH and oxygen tension and increasing the number of sickled cells. All of this leads to hypoxia, painful crises, and infarction of organs.[8–11] It should be noted that the presence of HbA and HbF in RBCs with HbS modifies the degree or severity of the sickling.[12] Table 11–3 lists other factors affecting the severity of HbS.

Clinical Features

Sickle-cell anemia is usually diagnosed early in life, when the level of HbF declines. Hemoglobin SS typically presents as a severe chronic hemolytic anemia, with hemoglobin levels in the range of 6 to 8 percent. Characteristically the patient demonstrates an asthenic physique and is mildly jaundiced. Many complications are associated with the disease, with the major manifestations being "sickle crises." There are three types of crises: aplastic, hemolytic, and painful (vaso-occlusive).[13]

An aplastic crisis is usually associated with infections, particularly to parvovirus, which cause a temporary marrow aplasia reflected in a low reticulocyte count. The marrow is simply overworked as a result of the stress related to the continuous stimulus for production of new red cells. With an already shortened red cell lifespan, even a temporary decrease or arrest in red cell production causes a drastic anemia.

A hemolytic crisis reflects an acute exacerbation of the anemia with a resulting fall in hemoglobin and hematocrit, an increased reticulocyte count, and jaundice. Acute splenic sequestration causing a decrease in hemoglobin and hematocrit usually occurs in infants and young children between 5 months and 2 years of age. Intrasplenic pooling of vast amounts of blood results in enlarged spleens of some children with SCA. In contrast to this process, multiple infarctions and subsequent fibrosis leads to a process termed autosplenectomy in adult patients with SCA.

Vaso-occlusive or painful crisis is the hallmark of sickle-cell anemia. The crisis is usually associated with severe pain, caused by rigid sickle cells in the small blood vessels, resulting in tissue damage and necrosis. The decreased blood flow causes regional hypoxia and acidosis, further exacerbating the ischemic injury. A painful crisis usually lasts 4 to 6 days but sometimes persists for weeks. Painful crisis can be precipitated by infection, fever, acidosis, de-

hydration, and exposure to extreme cold. Some patients have reported that even emotional states such as anxiety, stress, and depression may cause their painful crises.

Generally, three principles of therapy are applied in the management of painful crisis: adequate rehydration, pain relief using sufficient analgesics, and antibiotic therapy to treat any precipitating or underlying illness such as infection. In severe cases, exchange transfusion may be necessary to reduce the hemoglobin S content in the blood of the patients with SCA. However, the mainstay of therapy for painful crisis is hydration (administration of fluid volumes) to correct fluid and electrolyte deficits in an attempt to maintain normal serum electrolyte concentrations.

Symptoms and clinical manifestations of SCA are many and varied. Table 11–4 lists the most prominent types of clinical manifestations associated with sickle-cell anemia. As mentioned previously, these clinical presentations represent the sequelae of repeated infarction. Table 11–5 provides a more comprehensive list, dividing the clinical features of SCA into hematologic and nonhematologic categories.

Infarction. Infarcts can occur virtually anywhere in the body: in bones, joints, lungs, liver, kidneys, eye, central nervous system, and spleen. Repeated splenic infarcts result in autosplenectomy by the adult years. These patients then become more prone to serious infections with encapsulated organisms such as pneumococcus and *Haemophilus influenzae*.[13] The most common cutaneous manifestation is the development of ulcers or sores on the lower leg (Fig. 11–6). Approximately 8 to 10 percent of patients develop leg ulcers, which are usually manifested between 10 and 50 years of age and are very difficult to resolve.

Bones and joints in sickle-cell disease are frequent sites of pathology, with musculoskeletal pain being the most common symptom. There can be bone marrow hyperplasia, infection, or infarction. Infarction is also commonly responsible for the symptoms of the hand-foot syndrome observed in sickle-cell anemia. Dactylitis (the painful swelling of the hands and feet) occurs commonly in infants

Table 11–4. **CLINICAL MANIFESTATIONS OF SICKLE-CELL ANEMIA**

Cutaneous manifestations (leg ulcers)
Cardiac enlargement
Joint and skeletal problems
Arthritis
Renal complications (renal papillary necrosis)
Bone marrow infarctions
Conjunctival vascular abnormalities
Gastrointestinal symptoms
Hepatomegaly
Autosplenectomy
Cholelithiasis
Priapism

Table 11–5. **CLINICAL FEATURES OF SICKLE-CELL ANEMIA BY CATEGORY**

I. Hematologic
  1. Aplastic crisis
  2. Hemolytic crisis
  3. Vaso-occlusive crisis
II. Nonhematologic
  1. Abnormal growth
  2. Bone and joint abnormalities
    a. Pain
    b. Salmonella infection
    c. Hand-foot dactylitis
  3. Genitourinary
    a. Renal papillary necrosis
    b. Priapism
  4. Spleen and liver
    a. Autosplenectomy
    b. Hepatomegaly
    c. Jaundice
  5. Cardiopulmonary
    a. Enlarged heart
    b. Heart murmurs
    c. Pulmonary infarction
  6. Eye
    a. Retinal hemorrhage
  7. Central nervous system
  8. Leg ulcers
  9. Risky pregnancy

and young children with SCA and is observed exclusively in patients in that age group. In many infants it is the first manifestation of the disease. The characteristic "hand-foot" syndrome develops later in life as a result of microinfarction of small bones of the hands and feet, which leads to unequal growth and bone deformities of the fingers and toes (Fig. 11–7).

In addition, episodes of painful swollen joints and aseptic necrosis of the femoral head and other articulating bones are caused by the process of infarction.

Patients with SCA have shortened life spans, usually dying by middle age.

Infections. Serious bacterial infections remain a major cause of morbidity and mortality in patients with SCA. Table 11–6 lists the organisms implicated in causing infections in these patients.

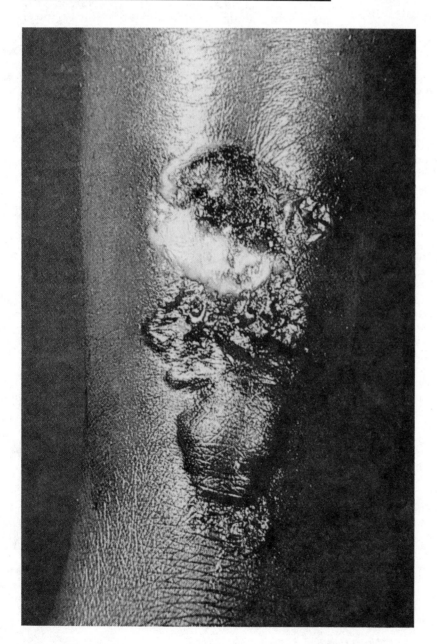

Figure 11–6. Leg ulcers in a patient with sickle-cell anemia. (Reproduced with permission from Sandoz Pharmaceuticals Corporation.)

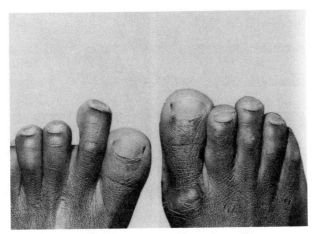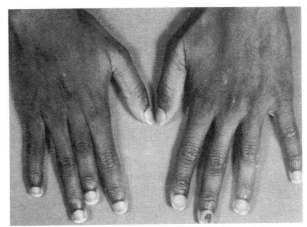

Figure 11–7. Hand-foot syndrome in a patient with sickle-cell anemia. (Reproduced with permission from Sandoz Pharmaceuticals Corporation.)

The most significant cause of death during early childhood is the severe overwhelming septicemia and meningitis due to *Streptococcus pneumoniae*. After the first decade of life, anaerobic and enteric organisms become important pathogens, causing infections in adult patients with SCA.

In comparison to healthy individuals, infections in patients with SCA cause greater morbidity, disseminate more rapidly, and are more difficult to resolve. In particular, pyelonephritis recurs regularly in these patients, is difficult to treat, and is often associated with septicemia. This infection results in a predisposition to sickling in the renal papilla, ultimately causing renal papillary necrosis, which frequently develops along with the pyelonephritis.

Table 11–7 outlines the multiple factors responsible for the increased susceptibility to infection in patients with SCA.

The relationship between the incidence of the malarial parasite and the frequency of the abnormal hemoglobin S gene requires further explanation. Malaria, caused by a parasite of the *Plasmodium* species, is still a serious disease in tropical areas, with *Plasmodium falciparum* being responsible for the most life-threatening situations. Cells carrying HbS, when parasitized by *P. falciparum*, will sickle more quickly than will nonparasitized cells. The

Table 11–6. **ORGANISMS IMPLICATED IN CAUSING INFECTIONS IN PATIENTS WITH SCA**

Bacterial	Viral
Streptococcus pneumoniae	Rubeola
Haemophilus influenzae	Cytomegalovirus
Neisseria meningitidis	Fungal
Mycoplasma pneumoniae	*Coccidioides immitis*
Staphylococcus aureus	*Histoplasma capsulatum*
Streptococcus pyogenes	Parasitic
Mycobacterium tuberculosis	*Plasmodium* species

Table 11–7. **FACTORS RESPONSIBLE FOR THE INCREASED SUSCEPTIBILITY OF SCA PATIENTS TO INFECTIONS**

Reticuloendothelial blockage due to increased hemolysis
Stasis of sickled RBCs in the sinusoids of the liver and spleen
Secondary splenic dysfunction
Deficiency of nonantibody serum opsonic activity

sickling affects the cycle of the parasite in one of two ways: directly, by killing the parasite; or indirectly, by causing the parasitized sickle cells to be sequestered in the spleen.[14] The fact that persons homozygous for the HbS gene often lack spleens by the time they reach adulthood (autosplenectomy or functional asplenia) may be one reason why malaria is exceptionally severe, and often fatal, in these cases.

Sickle-Cell Trait (Color Plate 88)

Sickle-cell trait, the heterozygous form of the disease, represents a combination of HbA and HbS. The structural formula is $\alpha_2\beta_1, \beta_1^{6glu-val}$. The frequency of this heterozygous condition in American blacks is approximately 8 percent.[3] Individuals with HbS trait are usually asymptomatic, but occasionally episodes of hematuria occur as a complication of the disorder. The potential for sickling exists, however, and the drastic lowering of pH or reduction in oxygen tension can precipitate a crisis. Causes for this include severe respiratory infections, air travel in unpressurized aircraft, anesthesia, and congestive heart failure. Even excessive exercise can lead to a significant buildup of lactic acid, resulting in sickling and subsequent infarction. Several deaths of American black soldiers with sickle-cell trait have been reported as a result of rigorous basic training at altitudes greater than 4000 feet, which led to a buildup of lactic acid, followed by acidosis and subsequent organic infarction.

Laboratory Diagnosis

The anemia of HbSS typically is quite severe, with hemoglobins ranging between 6 and 8 g/dl. The RBC indices are normochromic and normocytic. The peripheral red blood picture can be striking with numerous target cells, fragmented red cells, polychromasia, nucleated red cells, and usually sickle cells (Fig. 11–8). Siderotic granules and Howell-Jolly bodies may be seen in the red cells as a result of rapid RBC turnover and "stressed" erythropoiesis. An average reticulocyte count will be between 5 and 20 percent.[8] The reticulocyte count, however, will decrease during an aplastic crisis; indeed, a falling reticulocyte count may herald the onset of such a crisis. There may be a neutrophilic leukocytosis with a shift to the left and thrombocytosis. The bone marrow reflects a marked erythroid hyperplasia, except during an aplastic crisis.

There are screening procedures, referred to as solubility tests, that detect the presence of HbS. These tube tests either isolate HbS at an interface or cause the abnormal hemoglobin to precipitate (Fig. 11–9). An older screening test uses sodium metabisulfite to induce sickling (see **Color Plate 89**). It is important to remember that some rare hemoglobins also sickle, including HbC Georgetown (Harlem), HbC Ziguinchor, HbS Memphis, HbS Travis, Hb Alexandra, and Hb Porto-Alegre.[2]

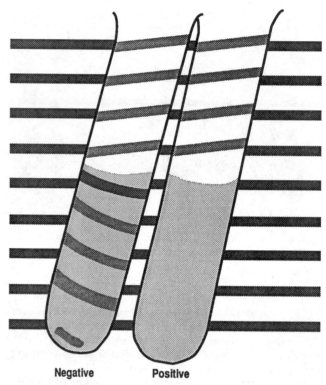

Negative   **Positive**

Figure 11–9. Tube solubility screening test for sickle-cell anemia.

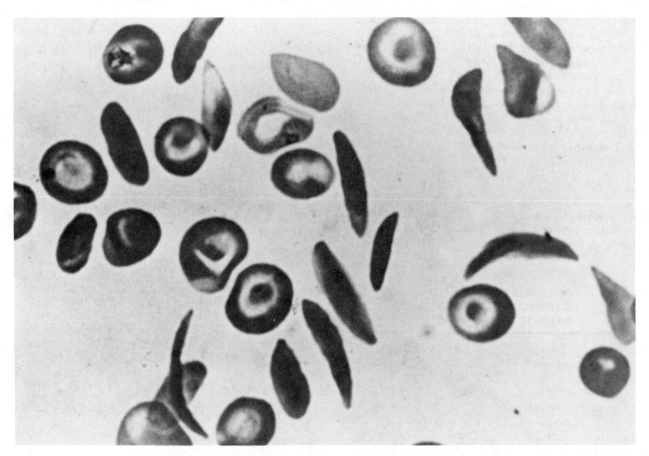

Figure 11–8. Peripheral smear of a patient with sickle-cell anemia.

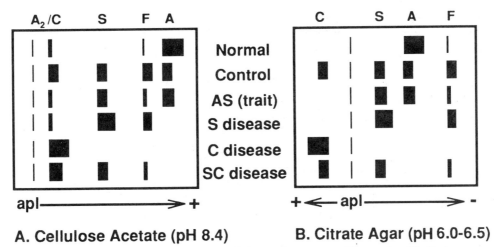

Figure 11–10. Electrophoretic patterns of hemoglobin on (*A*) cellulose acetate, run at pH 8.4 and on (*B*) citrate agar, run at pH 6.0 to 6.5 (apl = point of application.)

The definitive test for HbS is a hemoglobin electrophoresis at alkaline pH (see **Color Plate 97**), followed if necessary by electrophoresis at acid pH (Fig. 11–10). The patient with sickle-cell anemia produces no normal beta chains; therefore, there will be no HbA on electrophoresis (unless the patient has been recently transfused). Hemoglobin S constitutes 80 percent or more of hemoglobin, with HbF ranging from 1 to 20 percent. When HbF levels are higher than 20 percent, there is a mediating effect in the severity of the disease. This is seen in newborns and in a combination of HbS with hereditary persistence of fetal hemoglobin (HPFH).[12] In sickle-cell anemia, the HbA_2 level may be slightly increased with a mean of 3.4 percent.[15] Hemoglobins D and G both migrate to the same position as HbS at alkaline pH. Hemoglobin S will differentially separate from these two hemoglobins at acid pH. Additionally, HbS is the only hemoglobin of these three (S, D, G) that will have a positive solubility test.

The peripheral blood smear in sickle-cell trait is usually normal, with the exception of target cells. Solubility screening tests are positive. Hemoglobin electrophoresis at alkaline pH shows 60 percent HbA, 40 percent HbS, and usually elevated HbA_2 (mean 3.6 percent).[15] At acid pH one band is present in the A position ($HbA + HbA_2$), while the other band migrates to the S position.

It should be noted that most hemoglobin variant traits, without coexistent conditions such as iron deficiency, or thalassemia, have alkaline electrophoretic patterns with an approximate 60:40 ratio of normal to abnormal hemoglobin.

In individuals with the trait, sickle cells are *not* present in the peripheral blood smear. On *rare* occasions, however, sickle cells may be observed in the peripheral blood smear during a crisis episode.[16]

Treatment

A variety of drugs are being tested for their potential in ameliorating the effects of sickle-cell anemia.

At present, no single drug is completely effective, and there is controversy about most. Ideally the best drug or drug combination would inhibit polymerization of the abnormal hemoglobin while having little effect on the oxygen affinity of the hemoglobin molecule. Many drugs seem to increase the oxygen affinity, which increases the hemoglobin and hematocrit and thus the viscosity of the blood. Because increased viscosity would have a detrimental effect on the sickling process, such drugs should be avoided.

Because there is still no cure for HbSS, efforts must be made to try and keep the patients in as controlled a state as possible. Exchange transfusions are beneficial in certain situations. A good diet, early treatment of infection, and avoidance of situations that could precipitate a crisis still represent the mainstay of traditional treatment.

New therapeutic strategies are currently being tested on a multicenter scale. Table 11–8 lists the goals of these newer therapeutic approaches to the treatment of sickle-cell anemia.

One approach, using various pharmacologic agents to induce the production of hemoglobin F, is particularly interesting when combined with the use of erythropoietin. The combination of hydroxyurea and erythropoietin induces the production of F reticulocytes synergistically in adult patients with SCA. In addition, combination treat-

Table 11–8. **TREATMENT OF SCA: GOALS OF NEW THERAPEUTIC APPROACHES**

Decrease microvascular entrapment of sickle cells
Modify the oxygen affinity or solubility of sickle hemoglobin
Change the volume of the sickle erythrocyte
Alter expression of the abnormal sickle gene
Increase the production of fetal hemoglobin in the adult

Table 11–9. **EFFECTS OF APPROACHES TO SPECIFIC THERAPY**

Therapeutic Approach	Drugs	Effect
Inhibition of hemoglobin S polymerization	Urea / Ethanol / Peptides	Noncovalent hemoglobin modification
	Cyanate / Pyridoxal / Glyceraldehyde	Covalent hemoglobin modification
	DDAVP / Cetiedil / Hyponatremia	Erythrocyte modification (increase in red cell volume, decrease in 2,3-DPG)
	Hydroxyurea / 5-Azacytidine	Genetic modification (increase in gamma gene globin expression, bone marrow transplantation)
Decreased erythrocyte microvascular entrapment	Nifedipine	Vasodilator

ment (such as butyrate and 5-azacytidine) using doses that are less toxic to the patient also results in achieving therapeutic levels of HbF.

Table 11–9 lists various approaches to specific therapy with a specific drug.

Hemoglobin C Disease and Trait (Color Plates 90 to 92)

Hemoglobin C disease is found almost exclusively in the black population. Hemoglobin C differs from normal HbA by the single amino acid substitution of lysine for glutamic acid in the sixth position from the NH$_2$ terminal end of the beta chain (Fig. 11–11). This represents the exact same substitution point as HbS but with a different amino acid. The structural formula for HbC, the presence of which is often referred to as HbC disease, is $\alpha_2\beta_2^{6glu-lys}$. Hemoglobin C is seen with great frequency in West Africa, particularly Northern Ghana, where the incidence is 17 to 28 percent.[13] In the United States, only 0.02 percent of blacks have HbC disease. The clinical manifestations are mild chronic hemolytic anemia with associated splenomegaly and abdominal discomfort. The red cell morphology is typically normocytic, normochromic, with numerous target cells (50 to 90 percent) and occasionally microspherocytes, fragmented cells, and folded cells (Fig. 11–12). Hemoglobin C crystals (**see Color Plate 91**) or "bar of gold" crystals occur more often in the red cells of individuals who have been splenectomized than in those whose spleen is intact (Figs. 11–13 and 11–14).

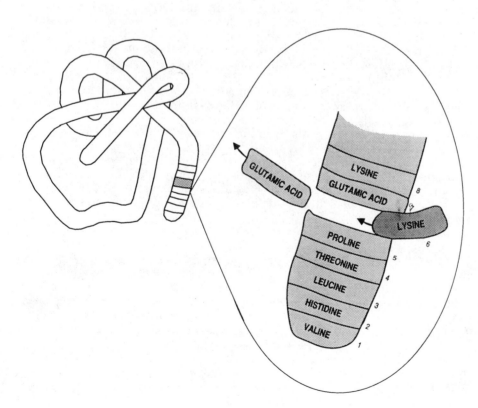

Figure 11–11. Amino acid substitution in hemoglobin C.

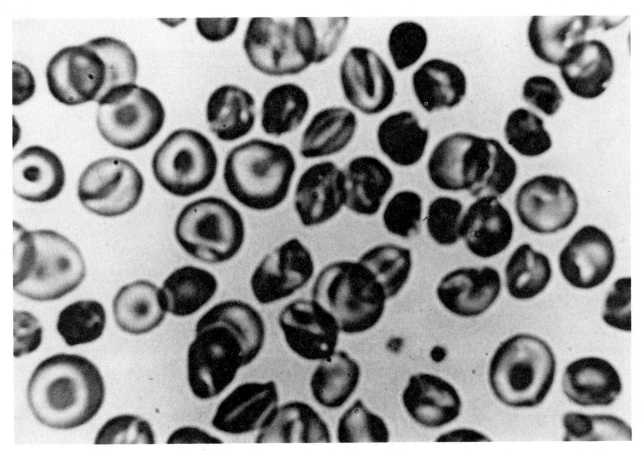

Figure 11–12. Peripheral smear of a patient with hemoglobin C disease.

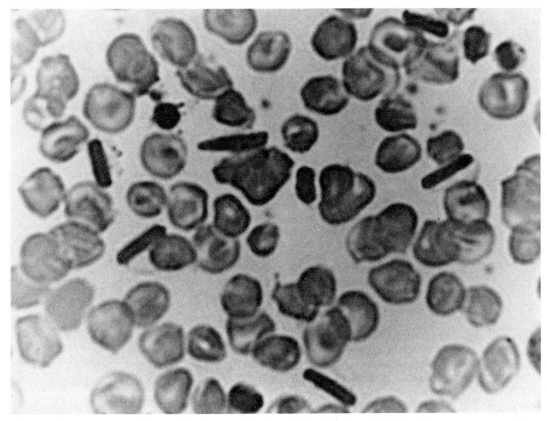

Figure 11–13. Hemoglobin C crystals in a splenectomized patient.

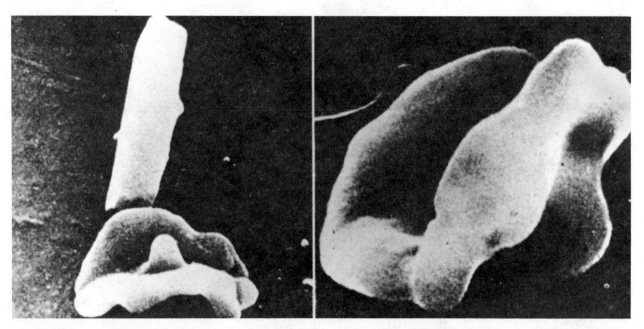

Figure 11–14. Scanning electron micrograph of hemoglobin C.

These crystals can be demonstrated in wet preparations by washing the red cells and then suspending them in a sodium citrate solution.[17] The reticulocyte count is slightly increased. Hemoglobin bands, at alkaline pH, are approximately 95 percent HbC plus A_2, less than 7 percent HbF, and no HbA. Hemoglobins E, O Arab, C, and A_2 all migrate to the same position at alkaline pH. Hemoglobin C can be separated from these other hemoglobins at acid pH (see Fig. 11–10).

Hemoglobin C trait, $\alpha_2\beta_1\beta^{6Glu\text{-}Lys}$, is present in 2 to 3 percent of American blacks, and these individuals are clinically asymptomatic.[7] The only significant finding on the peripheral blood smear is targeting. At alkaline pH, there is approximately 60 percent HbA and 40 percent HbC plus A_2.

Hemoglobin SC Disease (Color Plates 93 and 94)

Hemoglobin SC disease $(\alpha_2\beta_1^{6Val}\beta_1^{6Glu\text{-}Lys})$ occurs when the gene for HbS is inherited from one parent and that for HbC from the other. About 0.08 percent of black Americans have SC disease. Patients with HbSC disease are generally less anemic and experience a milder course than those with SCA. However, because of increased blood viscosity, this condition has a greater incidence of retinal hemorrhage, renal papillary necrosis, and necrosis of the femoral head.[18] Peripheral blood smear findings include target cells, folded red cells, and occasionally glove-shaped intracellular crystals (Fig. 11–15 and **Color Plate 93**). The solubility test results are positive owing to the presence of HbS. Hemoglobin electrophoresis at alkaline pH separates HbS and HbC in approximately equal amounts. Hemoglobin F is usually less than 2 percent compared with average HbF levels of about 6 percent in sickle-cell anemia.

Electrophoresis at acid pH will confirm the S and C hemoglobins (see Fig. 11–10). Table 11–10 compares the incidence of the most common hemoglobinopathies found in American blacks.

Hemoglobin D Disease and Trait

Hemoglobin D has several variants. The most common variant in American blacks is HbD Punjab, which is synonymous with HbD Los Angeles. Its frequency is less than 0.02 percent.[19] Both the homozygous $(\alpha_2\beta_2^{121Glu\text{-}Gln})$ and the heterozygous $(\alpha_2\beta_1\beta_1^{121Glu\text{-}Gln})$ states are asymptomatic. The peripheral blood smear is unremarkable, except for a few target cells. Hemoglobin D migrates electrophoretically to the same position as HbS and HbG at alkaline pH but migrates with HbA at acid pH. Hemoglobin D is a nonsickling soluble hemoglobin.

Hemoglobin E Disease and Trait

Hemoglobin E occurs with greatest frequency in Burma, Thailand, Cambodia, Laos, Malaysia, and Indonesia. This variant is now prevalent in the United States because of the influx of refugees from Southeast Asia. The homozygous state $(\alpha_2\beta_2^{26Glu\text{-}Lys})$ presents with little or no anemia, target cells, and microcytic, hypochromic red cell indices. On alkaline electrophoresis, there is approximately 95 to 97 percent HbE + A_2 and the remainder is HbF. Hemoglobin E migrates with HbC and HbO Arab at alkaline pH, and comigrates with HbA at acid pH. Hemoglobin E trait $(\alpha_2\beta_1\beta_1^{26Glu\text{-}Lys})$ is asymptomatic clinically. There is microcytosis, target cells, and approximately 70 percent HbA and 30 percent HbE + A_2 on routine electrophoresis. Hemoglobin E is slightly unstable and there is an associated thalas-

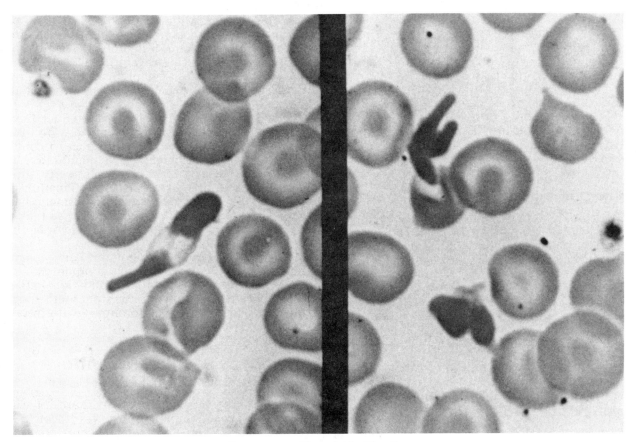

Figure 11-15. Hemoglobin SC cells.

semic component with this hemoglobin variant. This is responsible for the microcytosis, and the lower than expected quantified value of HbE in HbAE.[13,20]

It has been postulated that HbE may protect against malaria, because areas such as Thailand that are highly endemic for malaria also have a high incidence of the HbE gene.[21] Some authors attribute this effect to the fact that the parasite *P. falciparum* multiplies more slowly in HbE red cells than in the HbAE or HbAA red cells.[22]

Hemoglobin O Arab and HbS/HbO Arab Combination

Hemoglobin O Arab is a rare hemoglobin variant that occurs infrequently in black, Arab, and Sudanese populations.[23] Homozygous O Arab ($\alpha_2\beta_2^{121\text{Glu-Lys}}$) exhibits a mild hemolytic anemia with slight splenomegaly and target cells on the peripheral blood smear. This hemoglobin migrates electrophoretically with HbC, HbE, and HbA$_2$ at alkaline pH but separates at acid pH, migrating in the

Table 11-10. **INCIDENCE OF COMMON HEMOGLOBINOPATHIES IN AMERICAN BLACKS**

Condition	Genotype	Incidence (All Ages)	
Hemoglobin C disease	$\alpha_2\beta^C\beta^C$	0.02%	(1 in 4500)
Hemoglobin C trait	$\alpha_2\beta^A\beta^C$	3.0%	(1 in 33)
Sickle-cell disease	$\alpha_2\beta^S\beta^S$	0.16%	(1 in 1875)
Sickle-cell trait	$\alpha_2\beta^A\beta^S$	8.0%	(1 in 13)
Sickle C disease	$\alpha_2\beta^S\beta^C$	0.08%	(1 in 1250)

HbA position (see Chapter 30, Fig. 30–I–5). In the heterozygous state of HbO Arab $(\alpha_2\beta_1\beta_1{}^{121\text{Glu-Lys}})$ the patient is asymptomatic.

The combination of HbS and HbO Arab can have a clinical presentation that is similar in severity to that of SCA. The anemia is severe, with typical sickle cells seen on the peripheral blood smear.[4] This condition might initially be confused with HbSC on routine electrophoresis; however, differentiation can be made with acid electrophoresis (see Fig. 11–10).

Hemoglobin SD Disease

The combination of HbS and HbD, although rare, presents an interesting diagnostic problem. Because these hemoglobins migrate together at alkaline pH, the electrophoretic pattern is similar to that of SCA. Solubility tests are positive. The clinical severity of HbSD disease, however, falls between that of sickle-cell anemia and that of sickle-cell trait. Acid electrophoresis separates these two hemoglobins. Hemoglobin S has its own migration point, whereas HbD will comigrate with HbA (see Fig. 30–I–5 in Chapter 30).

Hemoglobin S/β-Thalassemia Combination (Color Plate 95)

The severity of HbS combined with β-thalassemia depends on the degree of suppression of β-globin chain synthesis. Hemoglobin S/β⁰ thalassemia is a severe condition that clinically resembles sickle-cell anemia; on the other hand, HbS/β⁺ thalassemia generally has a milder clinical presentation. The reader is referred to Chapter 12 for a detailed discussion of HbS/β-thalassemia and other hemoglobin variants that occur in combination with thalassemia.

METHEMOGLOBINEMIA

Methemoglobinemia is a clinical condition associated with methemoglobin levels greater than 1 percent of the total hemoglobin.[2,3,13,24] Methemoglobin contains the oxidized ferric form of iron (Fe^{3+}) rather than ferrous form (Fe^{2+}). In this state, the molecule is unable to bind oxygen and results in cyanosis. The blood is chocolate-brown. Generally there are three causes of methemoglobinemia:

1. Hemoglobin M variants (dominant inheritance)
2. NADH-diaphorase deficiency (recessive inheritance)
3. Toxic substance (acquired)

There are five variants of hemoglobin M (Table 11–11), which result from a single amino acid substitution in the globin chain that stabilizes iron in the ferric form. If the substitution occurs in the alpha chain, cyanosis is present at birth. Cyanosis does not occur with a beta chain substitution until approximately 6 months of age. This correlates with the switch from gamma to beta chains. The presumptive diagnosis of hemoglobin M is made from the absorption spectra of hemolysates, and hemoglobin electrophoresis on agar gel at pH 7.1. Patients have obvious cyanosis but otherwise are generally asymptomatic. No specific treatment is indicated or possible.[4]

The enzyme NADH-diaphorase reduces cytochrome b5 which converts the naturally occurring ferric iron back to the ferrous state. To confirm NADH-diaphorase deficiency, a quantitative enzyme assay is necessary. Although nearly all enzyme-deficient individuals are asymptomatic, some find their lifelong cyanosis to be a cosmetic hardship. The level of methemoglobin can be reduced with the administration of ascorbic acid or methylene blue.[4,13,24]

Acquired methemoglobinemia can occur in healthy individuals when drugs or other toxic substances oxidize hemoglobin in circulation. Patients who appear to be symptomatic from methemoglobinemia should be treated promptly with intravenous methylene blue.[4,24]

HEMOGLOBIN VARIANTS WITH ALTERED OXYGEN AFFINITY

High-affinity hemoglobins, which are inherited as an autosomal dominant disorder, are seen in the heterozygous state. These hemoglobins bind oxygen more readily and release it less easily to the tissues. The result is tissue hypoxia, which stimulates increased erythropoietin production. This, in turn, causes a compensatory increase in red cell mass, with increases in red count, hemoglobin and hematocrit, producing erythrocytosis and congenital polycythemia. Other hematologic parameters are normal. There is a shift to the left in the oxygen dissociation curve, and a diagnosis is established by measuring P_{50} levels (Fig. 11–16). Individuals with these hemoglobin variants are asymptomatic.[3,13,24]

Hemoglobins with decreased oxygen affinity release oxygen quite readily to the tissues. There is a shift to the right in the oxygen-dissociation curve (Fig. 11–16). As more oxygen is released per gram of hemoglobin, erythropoietin concentrations fall. This can result in decreased hemoglobin concentration with the development of a mild anemia. There may also be mild cyanosis associated with a decreased oxygen saturation level.[3,13,24]

Hemoglobins with increased or decreased oxygen affinities are listed in Table 11–12.

UNSTABLE HEMOGLOBINS (Color Plate 96)

Unstable hemoglobins are hemoglobin variants in which amino acid substitutions or deletions have weakened the binding forces that maintain the structure of the molecule. The instability may cause hemoglobin to denature and precipitate in the red cells as Heinz bodies.[25] Most unstable hemoglobin

Table 11–11. **FUNCTIONAL CLASSIFICATION OF HEMOGLOBIN VARIANTS**

I. Homozygous: Hemoglobin polymorphisms; the variants that are most common

HbS	$\alpha_2\beta_2^{6Val}$	Severe hemolytic anemia; sickling
HbC	$\alpha_2\beta_2^{6Lys}$	Mild hemolytic anemia
HbD Punjab	$\alpha_2\beta_2^{121Gln}$	No anemia
HbE	$\alpha_2\beta_2^{26Lys}$	Mild microcytic anemia

II. Heterozygous: Hemoglobin variants causing functional aberrations or hemolytic anemia in the heterozygous state

  A. Hemoglobins associated with methemoglobinemia and cyanosis
  1. HbM Boston $\alpha_2^{58Tyr}\beta_2$ 4. HbM Milwaukee $\alpha_2\beta_2^{67Glu}$
  2. HbM Iwate $\alpha_2^{87Tyr}\beta_2$ 5. HbM Hyde Park $\alpha_2\beta_2^{92Tyr}$
  3. HbM Saskatoon $\alpha_2\beta_2^{63Tyr}$

  B. Hemoglobins associated with altered oxygen affinity
  1. Increased affinity and polycythemia
    a. Hb Chesapeake $\alpha_2^{92Leu}\beta_2$
    b. HbJ Cape Town $\alpha_2^{92Gln}\beta_2$
    c. Hb Malmo $\alpha_2\beta_2^{97Gln}$
    d. Hb Yakima $\alpha_2\beta_2^{99His}$
    e. Hb Kemp $\alpha_2\beta_2^{99Asn}$
    f. Hb Ypsi (Ypsilanti) $\alpha_2\beta_2^{99Tyr}$
    g. Hb Hiroshima $\alpha_2\beta_2^{146Asp}$
    h. Hb Rainier $\alpha_2\beta_2^{145Cys}$
    i. Hb Bethesda $\alpha_2\beta_2^{145His}$
  2. Decreased affinity — may have mild anemia or cyanosis
    a. Hb Kansas $\alpha_2^{102Thr}\beta_2$
    b. Hb Titusville $\alpha_2^{94Asn}\beta_2$
    c. Hb Providence $\alpha_2\beta_2^{82Asn,Asp}$
    d. Hb Agenogi $\alpha_2\beta_2^{90Lys}$
    e. Hb Beth Israel $\alpha_2\beta_2^{102Ser}$
    f. Hb Yoshizuka $\alpha_2\beta_2^{108Asp}$

  C. Unstable hemoglobins
  1. Hemoglobins that may precipitate as Heinz bodies after splenectomy: congenital Heinz body hemolytic anemia

  a. α-chain abnormalities

Hb Torino	$\alpha_2^{42Val}\beta_2$
Hb L-Ferrara	$\alpha_2^{47His}\beta_2$
Hb Hasharon	$\alpha_2^{47His}\beta_2$
Hb Ann Arbor	$\alpha_2^{80Arg}\beta_2$
Hb Etobicoke	$\alpha_2^{84Arg}\beta_2$
Hb Dakar	$\alpha_2^{112Glu}\beta_2$
Hb Bibba	$\alpha_2^{136Pro}\beta_2$

  b. β-chain abnormalities

Hb Leiden	$\alpha_2\beta_2^{6or7}$	(Glu deleted)
Hb Sogn	$\alpha_2\beta_2^{14Arg}$	
Hb Freiburg	$\alpha_2\beta_2^{23}$	(Val deleted)
Hb Riverdale Bronx	$\alpha_2\beta_2^{24Arg}$	
Hb Genova	$\alpha_2\beta_2^{28Pro}$	
Hb Tacoma	$\alpha_2\beta_2^{30Ser}$	
Hb Philly	$\alpha_2\beta_2^{35Phe}$	
Hb Louisville	$\alpha_2\beta_2^{42Leu}$	
Hb Hammersmith	$\alpha_2\beta_2^{42Ser}$	
Hb Zurich	$\alpha_2\beta_2^{63Arg}$	
Hb Toulouse	$\alpha_2\beta_2^{66Glu}$	
Hb Bristol	$\alpha_2\beta_2^{67Asp}$	
Hb Sydney	$\alpha_2\beta_2^{67Ala}$	
Hb Shepherd's Bush	$\alpha_2\beta_2^{74Asp}$	
Hb Seattle	$\alpha_2\beta_2^{76Glu}$	
Hb Boras	$\alpha_2\beta_2^{88Arg}$	
Hb Santa Ana	$\alpha_2\beta_2^{88Pro}$	
Hb Gun Hill	$\alpha_2\beta_2^{91-97}$	(5 a.a. deleted)
Hb Sabine	$\alpha_2\beta_2^{91Pro}$	
Hb Köln	$\alpha_2\beta_2^{98Met}$	
Hb Kansas	$\alpha_2\beta_2^{102Thr}$	
Hb Wein	$\alpha_2\beta_2^{130Asp}$	
Hb Olmsted	$\alpha_2\beta_2^{141Arg}$	

  2. Tetramers of normal chains; appear in thalassemias

Hb Bart's	γ_4
HbH	β_4
Hbα_4^A	α_4

Source: From Henry,[7] with permission.

variants are inherited as autosomal dominant disorders. However, absence of a positive family history is not always helpful, as new mutations are common. Many of the unstable hemoglobins have high oxygen affinity and therefore may not cause anemia, making diagnosis in this group of patients particularly difficult. When anemia is present, the degree of hemolysis associated with an unstable hemoglobin varies considerably. Some patients experience severe chronic hemolysis with jaundice and splenomegaly. However, most patients have a mild compensated condition and seek medical attention only after exacerbation of the hemolysis caused by infection or exposure to oxidative drugs. Reticulocytosis is variable. Hypochromia may be apparent on the peripheral blood smear, and the mean red cell hemoglobin concentration (MCHC) can be low in some cases because the unstable hemoglobin

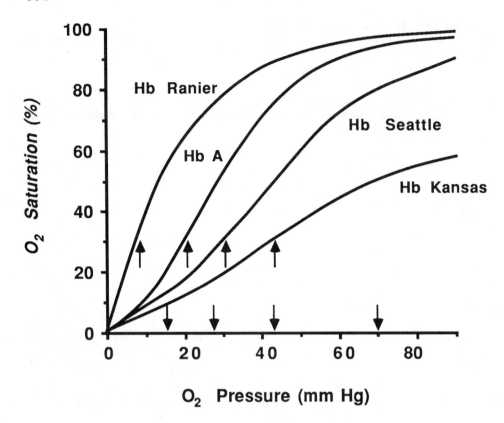

Figure 11–16. Oxygen equilibrium curve of whole blood from subjects with hemoglobin Ranier, Seattle, Kansas, and from normal controls.

may be denatured and "pitted" out of the cell by the mononuclear phagocytic cells of the spleen.

Hemoglobin electrophoresis is usually not a very helpful laboratory method to detect unstable hemoglobins. The isopropanol precipitation or heat denaturation test is the procedure of choice in this instance.

SUMMARY OF LABORATORY DIAGNOSIS

Hemoglobinopathies usually cannot be correctly diagnosed with a single laboratory procedure. It is usually necessary to correlate the results of a complete blood count and indices with additional laboratory tests. Selected patient information such as age, gender, ethnic background, family history, and physical symptoms is helpful.

Most abnormal hemoglobins are associated with RBC indices that are normocytic and normochromic. Microcytosis and hypochromia are seen in some variants (for example, HbE). Abnormal red cell morphology may or may not be noted on the peripheral blood smear, and reticulocyte counts are often elevated.

Solubility and sodium metabisulfite tests are quick screening procedures that can detect the presence of sickle hemoglobin. Confirmation of an abnormal variant must be made by hemoglobin electrophoresis.

One of the most informative tests is cellulose acetate electrophoresis at alkaline pH (Fig. 11–17 and

Table 11–12. **VARIOUS HEMOGLOBINS WITH ALTERED OXYGEN FACILITY**

Hemoglobins with Increased O$_2$ Affinity		Hemoglobins with Decreased O$_2$ Affinity
Chesapeake	Kohn	Torino
Rainer	Yakima	Seattle
Hiroshima	Bethesda	Kansas
Tacoma	Ypsi	Hammersmith
Zurich	Kempsey	Beth Israel
Gun Hill	J Capetown	Bristol
Freiberg		

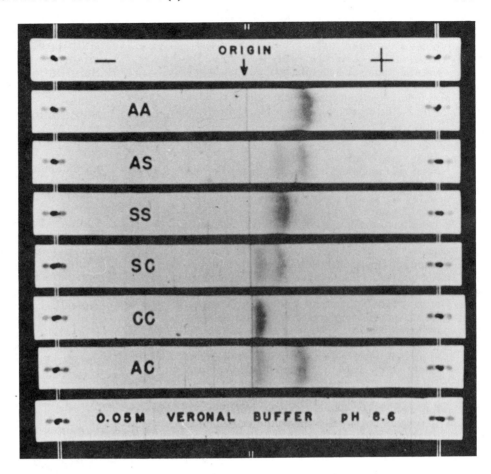

Figure 11–17. Hemoglobin electrophoresis on cellulose acetate at alkaline pH.

Color Plate 97). Electrophoresis on citrate agar at acid pH can further differentiate abnormal hemoglobins. Hemoglobin F quantitation should be done, following the newborn period, when this hemoglobin is seen on cellulose acetate.

A presumptive diagnosis of hemoglobin M can be made from absorption spectra and hemoglobin electrophoresis on agar gel at pH 7.1. In cases of unexplained erythrocytosis or cyanosis, oxygen affinity studies may be helpful. The isopropanol precipitation or heat denaturation test can be performed, if an unstable hemoglobin is suspected.

Another method worthy of mention is isoelectric focusing (IEF), a type of sensitive electrophoresis that separates hemoglobins according to their isoelectric points.[26] Though beyond the scope of this chapter, improved technology is providing systems that are applicable for routine laboratory usage. Superior IEF resolution differentiates some hemoglobins that migrate to the same electrophoretic point at alkaline and acid pH.

CASE STUDY

H.M., a 13-year-old black girl, was admitted to the hospital appearing acutely ill with fever and abdominal pain. On physical examination, an enlarged spleen was evident. Laboratory test results were as follows:

Hgb	5.0 g/dl
Hct	15%
RBC	1.4×10^{12}/liter
WBC	2.2×10^{9}/liter
Reticulocyte count	1%
Differential	
Segmented neutrophils	62%
Bands	12%
Lymphocytes	19%
Monocytes	4%
Eosinophils	2%
Basophils	1%
RBC indices	Normal
Platelet count	400×10^{9}/liter

Peripheral blood smear (see Color Plate 94)

Hemoglobin electrophoresis, alkaline pH, showed one band in the HbS position, and one band in the HbC position. The hemoglobins were quantified as 55 percent HbS and 45 percent HbC + A_2. Hemoglobins S and C were confirmed by electrophoresis at acid pH.

Questions: Case Study
1. Describe the morphologic features of this peripheral blood smear.
2. In reviewing the electrophoretic data, what diagnosis is suggested?
3. Comment on crystal formation in this condition.
4. Discuss the clinical presentation of the patient. Is it consistent with HbSC disease?

5. This young girl's parents have no hematologic problems; therefore, for her to have HbSC disease, what would be their most likely genotypes?
6. The inheritance of structurally abnormal hemoglobins follows simple mendelian laws. With parents having the trait form of HbS and HbC, what would be the expected genotypes in each of four children?

Answers: Case Study

1. Numerous target cells are present on the peripheral blood smear along with some cells that appear to have shadows of precipitating intraerythrocytic crystals.
2. The data suggest a diagnosis of HbSC disease.
3. The crystals in HbSC disease appear to be only partially formed, or there may be more than one formation. The crystals in the red cells often are described as having a glove-shaped appearance with several "fingers" protruding.
4. Generally HbSC disease has a milder presentation than SCA; however, this patient appears to be experiencing a severe episode of SC crisis. This is indicated by her acute illness, abdominal pain, and decrease in hemoglobin and hematocrit without an increase in the reticulocyte count.
5. With no hematologic problems, one parent would be expected to have HbS trait (HbAS), while the other would most likely have HbC trait (HbAC).
6. The probability for offspring would be one child with HbAA, one with HbAS, one with HbAC, and one with HbSC.

QUESTIONS

1. *Which of the following is not a characteristic of hemoglobinopathies?*
   a. Conditions in which abnormal hemoglobins are synthesized
   b. Result from inherited abnormalities or genetic mutations
   c. All are manifested in clinically significant conditions
   d. Result in a defect in structural integrity of function of the hemoglobin molecule

2. *What type(s) of hemoglobin defects is (are) normal in structure but differ(s) in the sequence of amino acids composing the globin chain?*
   a. Qualitative
   b. Quantitative
   c. Both qualitative and quantitative

3. *Which of the following are used in the nomenclature system for abnormal hemoglobins?*
   a. Capital letters
   b. Names of places
   c. Names of chains and substitutions
   d. All of the above

4. *What is the amino acid substitution found in sickle-cell anemia?*
   a. Substitution of valine for glutamic acid in the sixth position from the NH_2 terminal beta chain

   b. Substitution of lysine for glutamic acid in the sixth position from the NH_2 terminal beta chain
   c. Substitution of lysine for glutamic acid in the 26th position from the NH_2 terminal beta chain
   d. Substitution of valine for glutamic acid in the 121st position from the NH_2 terminal beta chain

5. *What factors contribute to the sickling of RBCs?*
   a. Increase in pH and oxygenation
   b. Decrease in pH and oxygenation and dehydration
   c. Increase in pH and decrease in oxygenation
   d. Decrease in dehydration and increase in pH and oxygenation

6. *Which of the following are crises associated with sickle-cell anemia?*
   a. Aplastic crisis with low reticulocyte count and infections
   b. Hemolytic crisis with splenic sequestration; decreased hemoglobin and hematocrit, increased reticulocyte count, and jaundice
   c. Vaso-occlusive/painful crisis with severe pain, tissue damage, and necrosis
   d. All of the above

7. *Which laboratory finding would be most useful in establishing a diagnosis of sickle-cell anemia?*
   a. Normocytic, normochromic anemia
   b. Increased reticulocyte count
   c. Finding of HbS on hemoglobin electrophoresis
   d. Target cells, Howell-Jolly bodies, siderocytes on peripheral blood smear

8. *What happens to hemoglobin S red cells when invaded by P. falciparum?*
   a. Resist invasion by the parasite
   b. Sickle quickly and kill the parasite
   c. Lose membrane integrity and fragment
   d. No response

9. *Which of the following are not true for sickle-cell trait?*
   a. Heterozygous form of sickle-cell disease
   b. Individuals may be asymptomatic
   c. Lower pH or reduction in oxygen tension may precipitate a crisis
   d. Sickle cells found routinely on peripheral blood smear

10. *What are therapeutic goals in the treatment of sickle-cell anemia?*
    a. To decrease microvascular entrapment of sickle cells or change the volume of RBCs
    b. Modify oxygen affinity or solubility of sickle hemoglobin
    c. Increase production of fetal hemoglobin
    d. All of the above

11. *What is the amino acid substitution found in hemoglobin C disease?*
    a. Substitution of valine for glutamic acid in the sixth position from the NH_2 terminal beta chain
    b. Substitution of lysine for glutamic acid in the sixth position from the NH_2 terminal beta chain
    c. Substitution of lysine for glutamic acid in the 26th position from the NH_2 terminal beta chain
    d. Substitution of valine for glutamic acid in the 121st position from the NH_2 terminal beta chain

12. *Which of the following is not true for hemoglobin C disease?*
    a. Mild anemia
    b. Numerous target cells
    c. Crystals in red cells
    d. Hemoglobin C can be separated from other hemoglobins at an alkaline pH

13. *Which finding would be most useful in establishing a diagnosis of hemoglobin SC disease?*
    a. Target cells and sickle cells on peripheral blood smear
    b. Severe anemia; increased reticulocyte count
    c. Hemoglobin electrophoresis at alkaline pH
    d. RBC indices

14. *Which hemoglobin disease occurs most frequently in Southeast Asians; is a mild anemia with target cells; and may confer some protection against P. falciparum?*
    a. Hemoglobin D
    b. Hemoglobin E
    c. Hemoglobin SD
    d. Hemoglobin OArab

15. *Which of the following is a cause for methemoglobinemia?*
    a. Hemoglobin M variants
    b. NADH-diaphorase deficiency
    c. Toxic substances
    d. None of the above

16. *What type of study is useful for cases of unexplained erythrocytosis or cyanosis?*
    a. Oxygen affinity; isopropanol or heat denaturation
    b. Examination of peripheral blood smear
    c. Hemoglobin electrophoresis
    d. RBC indices

ANSWERS

1. c (p. 143)
2. a (p. 143)
3. d (p. 144)
4. a (p. 145)
5. b (p. 145)
6. d (p. 147)
7. c (p. 150–151)
8. b (p. 149)
9. d (p. 149–151)
10. d (p. 151)
11. b (p. 152)
12. d (p. 152)
13. c (p. 154)
14. b (p. 154–155)
15. d (p. 156)
16. a (p. 159)

REFERENCES

1. Tietz, NW: Textbook of Clinical Chemistry. WB Saunders, Philadelphia, 1986.
2. Miale, JB: Laboratory Medicine Hematology, ed 6. CV Mosby, St Louis, 1982.
3. Spivak, JL: Fundamentals of Clinical Hematology, ed 2. Harper & Row, Philadelphia, 1984.
4. Bunn, HF and Forget, EG: Hemoglobin Molecular, Genetic and Clinical Aspects. WB Saunders, Philadelphia, 1986.
5. Herrick, JB: Peculiar elongated and sickle-shaped red corpuscles in a case of severe anemia. Arch Intern Med 6:517, 1910.
6. Pauling, L, et al: Sickle cell anemia, a molecular disease. Science 110:543, 1949.
7. Henry, JB: Clinical Diagnosis and Management by Laboratory Methods, ed 16. WB Saunders, Philadelphia, 1984.
8. May, A and Huehns, ER: The mechanism and prevention of sickling. Br Med Bull 32(3):223, 1976.
9. Noguchi, CT and Schechter, AN: The intracellular polymerization of sickle hemoglobin and its relevance to sickle cell disease. Blood 58(6):1057, 1981.
10. Nagel, RL, Fabry, ME, and Paul, DK: New insights on sickle cell anemia. Diagn Med 7:26, 1984.
11. Fabry, ME and Nagel, RL: The effect of deoxygenation on red cell density: Significance for the pathophysiology of sickle cell anemia. Blood 60(6):1370, 1980.
12. Powars, DR, et al: Is there a threshold level of fetal hemoglobin that ameliorates morbidity in sickle cell anemia? Blood 63(4):921, 1984.
13. Williams, WJ, et al: Hematology, ed 4. McGraw-Hill, New York, 1990.
14. Luzzatto, L: Genetics of red cells and susceptibility to malaria. Blood 54(5):961, 1979.
15. Wrightstone, RN and Huisman, T.H.J.: On the levels of hemoglobins F and A in sickle-cell anemia and some related disorders. Am J Clin Pathol 61:375, 1974.
16. Chang, H, et al: Comparative evaluation of fifteen antisickling agents. Blood 61(4):693, 1983.
17. Hyun, BH, Ashton, JK, and Dolan, K: Practical Hematology. WB Saunders, Philadelphia, 1975.
18. Ballas, SK, et al: Clinical, hematological, and biochemical features of hg SC disease. Am J Hematol 13(1):37, 1982.
19. McKenzie, SB: Textbook of Hematology. Lea & Febiger, Philadelphia, 1988.
20. Fairbanks, VF, et al: Hemoglobin E trait reexamined: a cause of microcytosis and erythrocytosis. Blood 53(1):109, 1979.
21. Cunningham, TM: Hemoglobin E in Indochinese refugees. West J Med 137:186, 1982.
22. Nagel, RL, et al: Impairment of the growth of P. falciparum in hgb EE erythrocytes. J Clin Invest 68(1):303, 1981.
23. Ramot, B: Haemoglobin O in an Arab family. Sickle cell Haemoglobin O trait. Br Med J 2:1262, 1960.
24. Liebhaber, SA and Mano, CS: Update on hemoglobinopathies. Disease-a-Month 29(10):1, 1983.
25. Vichinsky, EP and Lubin, BH: Unstable hemoglobins, hemoglobins with altered oxygen affinity, and M hemoglobin. Pediatr Clin North Am 27(2):421, 1980.
26. Basset, P, et al: Isoelectric focusing of human hemoglobins: Its application to screening, to the characterization of 70 variants, and to the study of modified fractions of normal hemoglobins. Blood 51(5):971, 1978.

BIBLIOGRAPHY

Benjamin, LJ, Kokkini, G, and Peterson, CM: Cetiedil: Its potential usefulness in sickle cell disease. Blood 55(2):265, 1980.

Carache, S, Lubin, B, and Reid, CD: Management and Therapy of Sickle Cell Disease. US Dept of Health and Human Services, Sept 1985.

Eaton, JW, Jacob, HS, and White, JG: Membrane abnormalities of irreversibly sickled cells. Semin Hematol 16(1):52, 1979.

Fairbanks, VF and Pierre, RV: Hemoglobin E/Alpha Thalassemia. ASCP Check Sample. (H-122) 1982 (H 82-3).

Hoffman, GC: Thalassemia Minor—Hg Lepore Trait. ASCP Check Sample, (H-75) 1975.

Inchausti, BC, Levin, B, and DiBolla, J: Hemoglobin C Disease (Hgb CC). ASCP Check Sample. (H-139) 1983 (H 83-8).

International Committee for Standardization in Hematology: Recommendations of a system for identifying abnormal hemoglobins. Blood 52(5):1065, 1978.

International Committee for Standardization in Hematology: Simple electrophoretic system for presumptive identification of abnormal hemoglobins. Blood 52(5):1058, 1978.

Mears, JG, et al: Alpha thalassemia is related to prolonged survival in sickle cell anemia. Blood 62(2):286, 1983.

Richardson, MA: Hemoglobin SC Disease. ASCP Check Sample. (H-134), 1983 (H 83-3).

Schechter, AN, et al: New approaches to the treatment of the hemoglobinopathies. Hematology 1989: The Education Program of the American Society of Hematology, Atlanta, Dec 2, 1989.

Simmons, A: Technical Hematology, ed 2. JB Lippincott, Philadelphia, 1976.

Steinberg, MH and Hibbel, RP: Clinical diversity of sickle cell anemia: Genetic and cellular modulation of disease severity. Am J Hematol 14(4):405, 1983.

Sunshine, HR: Effects of other hemoglobins on gelation of sickle cell hemoglobin. Tex Rep Biol Med 40:233, 1981.

Ward, PCJ, et al: Hgb Lepore: Diagnosis by Differential Electrophoresis and Isoelectric Focusing. ASCP Check Sample, (H-93) 1978.

White, JM: The unstable hemoglobins. Br Med Bull 32(3):219, 1976.

CHAPTER 12

CHANTAL RICAUD HARRISON, M.D.

Hemolytic Anemias: Intracorpuscular Defects

IV. Thalassemia

GENETICS OF HEMOGLOBIN SYNTHESIS

PATHOPHYSIOLOGY OF THALASSEMIA
BETA-THALASSEMIA
β^0-Thalassemia
β^+-Thalassemia
Clinical Expression of the Different Gene Combinations
ALPHA-THALASSEMIA
(Alpha-Thalassemia 1)
α^0-Thalassemia
(Alpha-Thalassemia 2)
α^+-Thalassemia
Clinical Expression of the Different Gene Combinations
DELTA-BETA THALASSEMIAS AND HEMOGLOBIN LEPORE SYNDROME
HEREDITARY PERSISTENCE OF FETAL HEMOGLOBIN
THALASSEMIA ASSOCIATED WITH HEMOGLOBIN VARIANTS
Beta-Thalassemia/Hemoglobin S
Beta-Thalassemia/Hemoglobin C
Beta-Thalassemia/Hemoglobin E
Alpha-Thalassemia with Sickle Cell Anemia

CLINICAL COURSE AND THERAPY

BLOOD TRANSFUSION IN THALASSEMIA

LABORATORY DIAGNOSIS OF THALASSEMIA
ROUTINE HEMATOLOGY PROCEDURES
Automated Blood Cell Analyzer
Peripheral Blood Smear Examination
    Wright's Stain
    Supravital Stains
    Acid Elution Stain
Osmotic Fragility
HEMOGLOBIN ELECTROPHORESIS
Cellulose Acetate
Starch Gel
Citrate Agar Gel
HEMOGLOBIN QUANTITATION
Hemoglobin A_2 Quantitation
Hemoglobin F Quantitation
ROUTINE CHEMISTRY
MISCELLANEOUS
Alpha/Beta Globin Chain Synthesis
Gene Analysis

DIFFERENTIAL DIAGNOSIS OF MICROCYTIC HYPOCHROMIC ANEMIA

CASE STUDY

OBJECTIVES

At the end of this chapter, the learner should be able to:
1. Name the hemoglobin defect of thalassemia.
2. List the type of globin chains and hemoglobin found in alpha- and beta-thalassemia.
3. Describe the clinical expression of different gene combinations of alpha- and beta-thalassemia.
4. Describe delta-beta thalassemia and hemoglobin Lepore syndrome.
5. Describe the condition known as hereditary persistence of fetal hemoglobin (HPFH).
6. Describe thalassemia associated with hemoglobin variants.
7. Describe alpha-thalassemia associated with sickle-cell anemia.
8. List risks for patients with thalassemia major who are on a regular blood transfusion program.
9. Name the most characteristic laboratory finding for the diagnosis of thalassemia.
10. List red cell indices that help to distinguish thalassemia from iron deficiency.
11. Describe the appearance of the peripheral smear in thalassemia.
12. Explain the use of the Betke-Kleihauer acid elution test in the diagnosis of thalassemia.

13. Name the test used as a population screening test for thalassemia carriers.
14. Explain the primary usage of different types of hemoglobin electrophoresis.
15. Explain how hemoglobin electrophoresis can detect abnormal hemoglobins.
16. Explain why hemoglobin quantitation is important in defining the diagnosis of thalassemia.
17. List conditions in which quantitation of hemoglobin F is important.
18. Describe the use of routine chemistries for differentiation of thalassemia from iron deficiency anemia.

The thalassemia syndromes consist of a diverse group of inherited disorders, which clinically manifest themselves as anemia of varying degrees. These disorders are the result of a defective production of the globin portion of the hemoglobin.

In 1925 Thomas B. Cooley and Pearl Lee described the first case of severe thalassemia in several North American children of Mediterranean origin. *Cooley's anemia* is still a commonly used term for this form of severe thalassemia, which is also known as thalassemia major. The name *thalassemia* was actually applied to these clinical syndromes a few years later. The term is derived from the Greek word *thalassa*, which means "sea," because at that time all of the cases described were from the Mediterranean coastal region. It is now well known that the distribution of thalassemia is worldwide and not restricted to the Mediterranean Sea area. It was later realized that the original severe clinical disease described by Cooley was the result of a homozygous defect in hemoglobin production, whereas many milder cases described as "thalassemia minima" or "thalassemia minor" were manifestations of a heterozygous defect.

The thalassemia syndromes are often considered part of a larger category of hematologic disorders called hemoglobinopathies (disorders in hemoglobin synthesis or production). Hemoglobinopathies are further divided into two main categories. One group is the result of an inherited structural defect in one of the globin chains resulting in an abnormal hemoglobin (true hemoglobinopathies), which may have abnormal physical or physiologic properties. Examples of these structural abnormalities are hemoglobin S, hemoglobin C, hemoglobin E, and so on. The second group consists of the thalassemia syndromes, which are caused by an abnormality in the rate of synthesis of the globin chains. With a few minor exceptions, the globin chains produced are structurally normal, but there is an imbalance in production of the two different types of chain resulting in an absolute decrease in the amount of normal hemoglobin formed, as well as an excess production of one type of chain that may precipitate and induce hemolysis.

The globin portion of hemoglobin is formed by four polypeptide chains consisting of two identical dimers. Ninety-five to ninety-seven percent of adult hemoglobin consists of hemoglobin A, which contains two alpha (α) chains and two beta (β) chains (see Chapter 1). There are two major types of thalassemia: α-thalassemia, which is caused by a defect in the rate of synthesis of alpha chains; and β-thalassemia, caused by a defect in the rate of synthesis of beta chains. The original cases described by Cooley were cases of homozygous β-thalassemia. In the Old World thalassemia was present in a wide tropical geographic band originating in Portugal, Spain, and North Africa, surrounding the Mediterranean Sea, including southern Italy, Greece, Bulgaria, Turkey, and the Middle East, continuing through Afghanistan, Pakistan, India, Southeast Asia, China, Malaysia, and the Philippines, and extending as far as New Guinea. Another pocket of β-thalassemia is found in West Africa. Whereas β-thalassemia appears to have its highest frequency in the Mediterranean area, α-thalassemia has its highest frequency in Southeast Asia, particularly in Thailand. Alpha-thalassemia is also common throughout Africa. In the New World thalassemia has been imported and is present in immigrant populations, mostly those originating in Italy, Greece, West Africa, and Southeast Asia. For all practical purposes thalassemia is absent from native American (Indian) populations. The world distribution of thalassemia is summarized in Figure 12–1. The marked similarity in worldwide distribution of thalassemia to that of malignant malaria caused by *Plasmodium falciparum* has given rise to the hypothesis that persons who are heterozygous for the thalassemia gene are resistant to *Plasmodium falciparum* infections and that the high frequencies of thalassemia can be explained by the process of gene selection by malaria.

Because the hemoglobin structural variants (such as hemoglobin S and hemoglobin C in West African and North American blacks or hemoglobin E in Southeast Asians) occur in the same population where α- or β-thalassemia is frequent, the two types of genetic defects may be found in the same person, resulting in variability of clinical expression of the two defects.

GENETICS OF HEMOGLOBIN SYNTHESIS

All normal human hemoglobins have a general tetrametric structure consisting of two alphalike (α or zeta [ζ]) and two betalike (β, delta [δ], A-gamma [$^A\gamma$], G-gamma [$^G\gamma$], or epsilon [ϵ] chains. During embryonic and fetal development there is a progression in activation of the globin genes from the zeta to the alpha gene and from the epsilon to G-gamma to

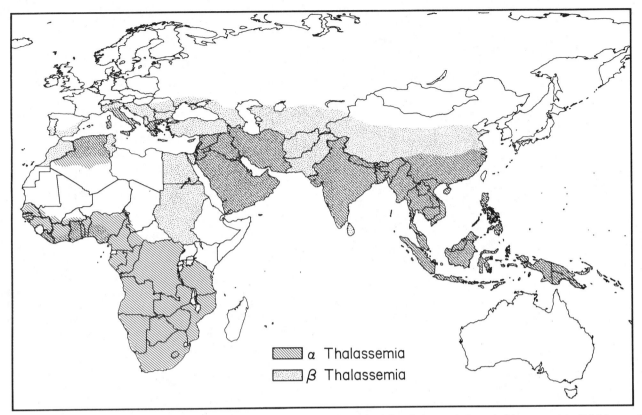

Figure 12–1. World distribution of alpha- and beta-thalassemia. Although alpha-thalassemia is probably present in Pakistan and Afghanistan, no data on population screens are yet available.

A-gamma to delta and beta genes, so that the majority of the hemoglobin found in the embryo are $\zeta_2\epsilon_2$ (hemoglobin Gower 1), $\zeta_2\gamma_2$ (hemoglobin Portland), and $\alpha_2\epsilon_2$ (hemoglobin Gower 2). In the fetus until birth the major hemoglobin is $\alpha_2\gamma_2$ (hemoglobin F). The gamma chains occur as a mixture of two types of chain differing only by one amino acid at position 136. G-gamma contains glycine, whereas A-gamma has alanine at that position. In the healthy adult, the majority (95 to 97 percent) of the hemoglobin is $\alpha_2\beta_2$ (hemoglobin A) and a minor fraction (about 2.5 percent) is $\alpha_2\delta_2$ (hemoglobin A_2). A small amount of hemoglobin F (always less than 2 percent) may also be found. Figure 12–2 demonstrates the relative amount of the different globin chains produced from embryonic stage to early childhood. Table 12–1 lists the different normal hemoglobins found throughout human development, as well as the abnormal hemoglobins found in patients with thalassemia. Figure 12–3 is a diagram of the location of the different globin genes on the human chromosomes. The zeta and alpha genes are found on chromosome 16. There are two closely linked alpha genes, both active and coding for identical alpha globin chains although at different levels of activity in the normal adult. The alpha 2 globin gene is expressed at two to three times the rate of the alpha 1 globin gene. On chromosome 11 are found the genes for the epsilon, G-gamma, A-gamma, delta, and beta

globins. Detailed mapping of the deoxyribonucleic acid (DNA) by restriction endonucleases shows great similarity between the two alpha genes, as well as the two gamma genes, the delta gene, and the beta gene. (For an explanation of the DNA analysis method, see the section on gene analysis.) It is tempting to speculate that multiple occurrences of these similar genes on the same chromosome were caused by duplication of an ancestral gene during evolution. Figure 12–4 illustrates the formation of the normal human hemoglobin from two identical globin chains coded by chromosome 11 and two identical globin chains coded by chromosome 16.

Figure 12–5 is a diagram of the biochemical progression from the original chromosomal DNA to the final globin chain polypeptide. The gene is represented by a length of chromosomal DNA, which consists of alternating coding and noncoding (or intervening) sequences. Only the coding sequences contain the information that will be finally translated into the polypeptide chain. The exact role of the intervening sequences is not clear at present, although it is thought that they may be involved in the initiation and the rate of progression of the synthetic process. The DNA is transcribed into a large ribonucleic acid (RNA) called heterogeneous nuclear RNA (hnRNA), which contains all the coding and noncoding sequences of the genes. This hnRNA is then processed into the messenger RNA (mRNA),

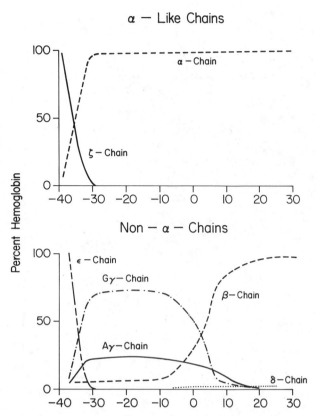

Figure 12–2. Relative production of the different globin chains from conception to 30 weeks after birth. (*Top*) zeta embryonic chain production has been almost totally replaced by alpha chain production around 12 weeks after conception. (*Bottom*) epsilon chain production runs in parallel with zeta chain production. The beta chain production stays at very low levels from 6 weeks after conception until it increases suddenly a few weeks before birth, while the gamma chain production suddenly decreases. The delta chain production starts a few weeks before birth and stays low. The Gγ chain to Aγ chain production ratio is 3 : 1 before birth and gradually reverses to 2 : 3 during the first few months of life.

Table 12–1. **COMPOSITION OF HEMOGLOBINS FOUND IN NORMAL HUMAN DEVELOPMENT AND ABNORMAL HEMOGLOBINS FOUND IN THALASSEMIA**

Globin Chains	Hemoglobin	State
$\alpha_2\beta_2$	A	Adult
$\alpha_2\delta_2$	A_2	
$\alpha_2{}^A\gamma_2$	F	Fetus
$\alpha_2{}^G\gamma_2$	F	
$\alpha_2\epsilon_2$	Gower 2	
$\zeta_2\epsilon_2$	Gower 1	Embryo
$\zeta_2\gamma_2$	Portland	
β_4	H	α-thalassemia
γ_4	Bart's	
α_2 precipitate	—	β-thalassemia

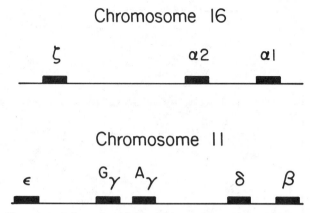

Figure 12–3. Location of the globin genes on chromosomes 16 and 11.

which contains only the coding sequences and which diffuses into the cytoplasm to be translated by the ribosomes into the final globin chain. Upstream of the coding portion of the gene (also called the 5′ direction) are promoter areas crucial to the level and accuracy of the gene expression.

PATHOPHYSIOLOGY OF THALASSEMIA

The genetic defect in thalassemia is the result of one of five processes:

1. A mutation in one of the noncoding intervening sequences of the original globin chain gene, producing inefficient splicing from hnRNA to mRNA, thereby decreasing the amount of mRNA produced.
2. A mutation in the promoter area decreasing the rate of expression of the gene.
3. The partial or total depletion of a globin gene, probably resulting from an unequal crossover.
4. A mutation at the termination of the gene which leads to the lengthening of the globin chain with additional amino acids, in which case the mRNA is unstable causing a reduction in globin synthesis.
5. A nonsense mutation leading to early termination of the globin chain synthesis

In all cases the final result is a decreased or absent production of one globin chain. There ensues a decrease in the amount of normal physiologic hemoglobin produced, resulting in a microcytic, hypochromic anemia. There will also be an excess of globin chains produced by the unaffected genes. In the case of α-thalassemia, the excess gamma chains and beta chains can form stable tetramers: hemoglobin Bart's (γ_4) and hemoglobin H (β_4), respectively. However, these hemoglobins are physiologically useless and will precipitate in older red cells, causing a shortened red cell lifespan. In the case of β-thalassemia, the excess alpha chains will form α_2 precipitates, which will cause hemolysis of the red cell precursors in the bone marrow, resulting in ineffective erythropoiesis. Recent studies suggest that

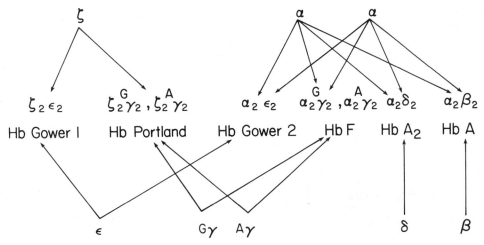

Figure 12-4. Formation of normal human hemoglobins.

unmatched globin chains interfere with the red blood cell membrane function causing defects that will result in hemolysis.

Beta-Thalassemia

In β-thalassemia the disease will not manifest itself until the switch from gamma chain to beta chain synthesis has been completed. This usually occurs several months after birth. Thus, the clinical presentation of a patient with this disease usually occurs during the first year of life. There often is a compensatory absolute or relative increase in production in gamma chains and delta chains, resulting in an increased level of hemoglobin F and hemoglobin A_2. The genetic background for β-thalassemia is very heterogeneous but may be broadly subdivided into β^0- and β^+-thalassemia.

β^0-Thalassemia

This gene results in complete absence of production of beta chains. This particular gene is commonly found in the Mediterranean area, particularly in Northern Italy, Greece, Algeria, and Saudi Arabia. It is also common in Southeast Asia. At the molecular level, there is heterogeneity in the basis for the genetic abnormality with at least eight genetic backgrounds described, each found in a specific geographic area.

β^+-Thalassemia

The β^+-thalassemia gene produces a reduced amount of beta chains. There is heterogeneity again in β^+-thalassemia, and at least three different genes have been described. The type 1 β^+-thalassemia gene produces the least amount of beta chains (about 10 percent of normal production) and is found throughout the Mediterranean region, the Middle East, the Indian subcontinent, and Southeast Asia. The type 2 β^+-thalassemia gene produces a greater amount of beta chains (about 50 percent of normal production) and is characteristically found in the blacks of West Africa and North America. The type 3 β^+-thalassemia gene produces an even greater amount of beta chains and causes a much milder form of β-thalassemia. It is found sporadically in Italy, Greece, and the Middle East.

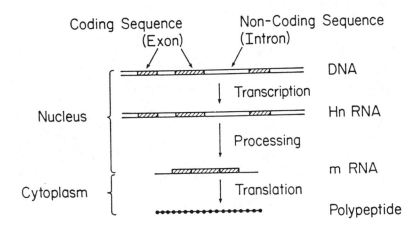

Figure 12-5. Diagram of the progression from gene to peptide.

Clinical Expression of the Different Gene Combinations

Homozygosity for the β^0- or β^+-thalassemia gene, or compound heterozygosity for the β^0 and β^+ genes, causes a severe form of thalassemia called thalassemia major. The only exception is perhaps the homozygous type 2 or type 3 β^+-thalassemia, which causes a milder form of thalassemia that has sometimes been called thalassemia intermedia. In thalassemia major a severe hypochromic, microcytic ane-

mia develops during the first year of life. The hemoglobin level is usually below 7 g/dl and consists mostly of hemoglobin F and hemoglobin A_2. This severe chronic anemia starting so early in life is a strong stimulus for erythropoiesis. This causes marked expansion of the marrow space and characteristic skeletal changes of the skull, long bones, and hand bones. The skull roentgenograms show widening of the diploid space and demonstrate characteristic radiating striations giving a typical hair-on-end appearance (Fig. 12–6). The marrow expansion

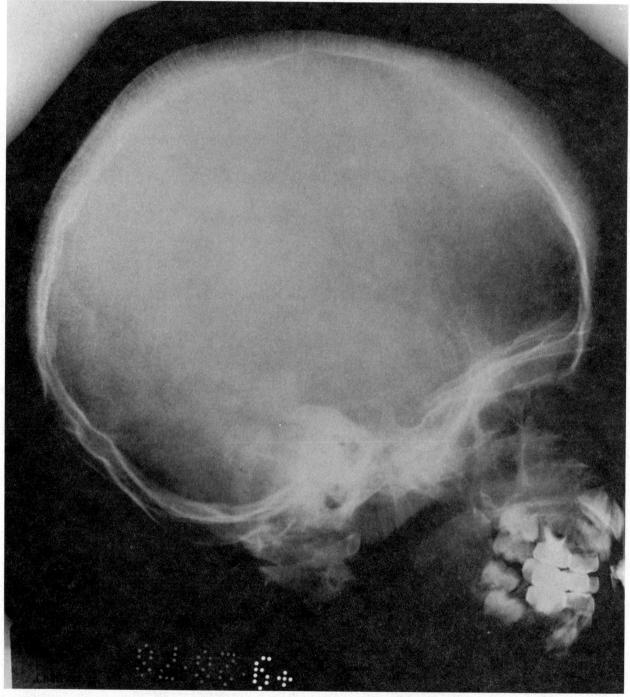

Figure 12–6. Skull roentgenogram of a 5-year-old child with homozygous beta-thalassemia. Note the dilatation of the diploic space and the typical "hair on end" appearance due to subperiostial bone growth in radiating striations.

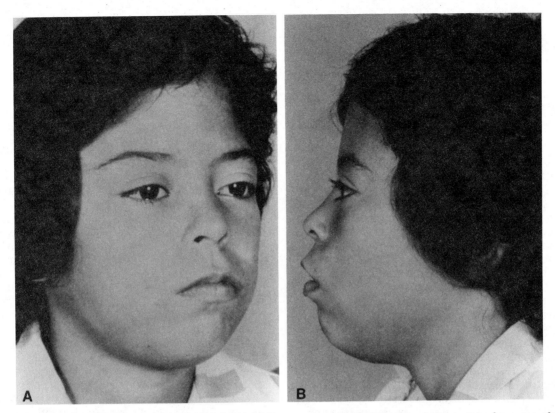

Figure 12–7. Face (A) and profile (B) of an 11-year-old child with homozygous beta-thalassemia who is receiving hypertransfusion. The characteristic facial changes are not as prominent as in an untransfused child but are still present. Note bossing of the skull, hypertrophy of the maxilla, with prominent malar eminences, depression of the bridge of the nose, and mongoloid slant of the eyes.

of the facial bones produces a characteristic facial appearance with hypertrophy of the maxilla causing forward protrusion of the upper teeth and overbite, a relatively sunken nose, widely spaced eyes, and prominent cheek bones resulting in a mongoloid facies (Fig. 12–7). The long bones of the hands and feet have cortical thinning with porosity of the medullary space. These changes are not a specific feature of thalassemia and are found in other severe chronic congenital anemias, but it may be in β-thalassemia major that these changes are most prominent. Without careful medical supervision and a therapeutic program including blood transfusions, iron chelation, and early treatment of infection, these children will have numerous complications such as massive hepatosplenomegaly, recurrent infections, spontaneous fractures, leg ulcers, dental and orthodontic problems, and compression syndromes due to tumor masses from extramedullary hematopoiesis. If the condition is left untreated, these children will usually die in early childhood.

Heterozygosity for the β^0- or β^+-thalassemia gene causes a mild form of chronic hypochromic, microcytic anemia that has been called thalassemia minor. While the degree of anemia is variable with hemoglobin levels from 10.5 to 13.9 g/dl, it is impossible to determine whether the patient has the β^0 or β^+ gene on clinical grounds alone. In general, the levels of hemoglobin F and hemoglobin A_2 are mildly elevated. The patients are usually completely asymptomatic, although symptoms may appear under stressful situations such as pregnancy. The patient with heterozygous β^+ type 3 thalassemia usually shows no clinical or laboratory evidence of anemia and has been called the silent carrier.

Alpha-Thalassemia

In contrast to β-thalassemia, α-thalassemia is usually manifested immediately at birth, and even in utero, as the alpha genes are activated early in fetal life. Another characteristic of α-thalassemia is that, because each chromosome 16 carries two alpha genes, the total normal complement of alpha genes is four. Thus, there will be a greater variety in severity of disease, as there may be one, two, three, or four alpha genes affected in a patient.

Owing to the wide variety of genetic backgrounds and the difficulty in defining the heterozygous carrier state, there has been much confusion in the classification and nomenclature of α-thalassemias. Much of this confusion is the result of the indiscriminate use of a phenotypic or genotypic classification without clear definition. We will use a genotypic classification that parallels the classification used for β-thalassemia.

Another characteristic of α-thalassemia is the fact that the decreased or absent alpha chain production will result in excess gamma chains during fetal life and at birth and in excess beta chains later on. This will cause the formation of stable tetramers, such as

γ_4 or hemoglobin Bart's and β_4 or hemoglobin H, that can be detected by hemoglobin electrophoresis. These stable, nonfunctional tetramers precipitate in older red cells, forming inclusion bodies and interfere with membrane function, which results in decreased red cell survival and may induce a hemolytic crisis during infectious episodes.

Alpha-Thalassemia 1 (α^0-Thalassemia)

Alpha-thalassemia 1 and α^0-thalassemia have been used synonymously in the past to describe a genetic determinant. However, because α-thalassemia 1 has been also used to describe the phenotypic or clinical expression of a disease, α^0-thalassemia is the preferred term for the description of the genetic determinant. This gene results in complete absence of production of alpha chains. This means that both alpha genes on chromosome 16 are nonfunctional. Studies by DNA hybridization techniques have shown that the α^0 determinant is the result of alpha gene deletions. In addition, they also demonstrated that there are at least five major haplotypes resulting in α^0-thalassemia, depending on the amount of DNA that has been deleted from the chromosome. Each haplotype appears to be characteristic of a certain population in the world. Genes for α^0-thalassemia are found frequently in Southeast Asia and less frequently in the Mediterranean area; they also occur sporadically in other parts of the world. These genes may possibly be recognized in adults through the detection of small amounts of zeta globin chain by radioimmunoassay.

Alpha-Thalassemia 2 (α^+-Thalassemia)

Again, α^+-thalassemia is the better term to describe the genetic determinant, as α-thalassemia 2 has been used to describe both the genetic determinant and a phenotypic expression. The α^+-thalassemia gene is characterized by a reduction in the output of alpha chains. This may be due to a deletion of a single alpha gene on chromosome 16, which leaves the other alpha gene intact and functional. Other types of α^+-thalassemia genes are due to nondeletion mutants that affect the regulation of the alpha chain synthesis. This is similar to the situation in the β-thalassemias. A third type of α^+-thalassemia genetic background is associated with alpha globin structural mutants, which may be a termination mutant such as hemoglobin Constant Spring (CS), hemoglobin Koya Dora (KD), hemoglobin Seal Rock (SR), or hemoglobin Icaria (Ic), or a single amino acid change such as hemoglobin Quong Sze (QS) or hemoglobin Swan Dok (SW). These structural mutants result in a decreased output of alpha chains due either to an instability of the corresponding mRNA or to a direct degradation of the abnormal alpha chain produced. Overall, a minimum of 12 major genetic defects resulting in the α^+-thalassemia gene have been defined using DNA hybridization techniques, sequencing analysis of the alpha genes as well as population studies. These different thalassemia genes result in different levels of alpha chain output. For example, the nondeletion regulatory type of defect, also called $\alpha\alpha^T$ and found in Saudi Arabia, is more severe than the single gene deletion type of defect, also called $-\alpha$ and commonly found throughout the Mediterranean area, Middle East area, Indian subcontinent, Southeast Asia, Africa, and Malaysia.

Clinical Expression of the Different Gene Combinations

Alpha-thalassemia can be divided into four clinical categories depending on the severity of the disease. The most severe expression of α-thalassemia is the hemoglobin Bart's hydrops fetalis syndrome, which is caused by homozygosity of the α^0-thalassemia gene. This is a lethal disease, and infants with hemoglobin Bart's hydrops fetalis die either in utero or soon after birth. They produce no alpha chain, and the only hemoglobins found are hemoglobin Bart's (γ_4) and hemoglobin Portland ($\zeta_2\gamma_2$). Because hemoglobin Bart's is useless as an oxygen carrier, survival of these fetuses into the third trimester or until birth is entirely due to the presence of hemoglobin Portland. At birth, these infants are severely anemic and edematous, demonstrating ascites, marked hepatomegaly, and splenomegaly. Significant morbidity and mortality can occur in the mothers owing to obstetric complications. This condition is quite common in Southeast Asia and is found sporadically in the Mediterranean area.

The second most severe clinical expression of α-thalassemia is hemoglobin H disease. In this entity only one alpha gene out of four is functioning. This is usually the result of a double heterozygosity of an α^0-thalassemia gene with an α^+-thalassemia gene but is also found in Saudi Arabia as the result of homozygosity of the more severe form of the α^+-thalassemia gene — the nondeleted $\alpha\alpha^T$ gene. Clinically, hemoglobin H disease is characterized by a variable degree of microcytic, hypochromic anemia, which is somewhat intermediate between the clinical pictures of thalassemia minor and thalassemia major and which has often been called thalassemia intermedia. These patients have mild to moder-and may develop the physical and bony characteristics of thalassemia major, as well as splenomegaly and hepatomegaly. They do, however, survive into adulthood without blood transfusion and do not usually suffer from severe iron overload. The anemia usually worsens with infections, pregnancy, and folic acid–deficiency states. Hemolytic crises may occur with infections. Adults with hemoglobin H disease have from 5 to 40 percent hemoglobin H, with the remainder being mostly hemoglobin A with a small amount of hemoglobin A_2 and hemoglobin Bart's. Infants who later develop hemoglobin H disease usually have between 19 and 27 percent hemoglobin Bart's at birth, with the remainder composed of hemoglobin F and hemoglobin A. Hemoglobin H and hemoglobin Bart's can easily be identified by hemoglobin electrophoresis, because they migrate anodally at pH 6.5 to 7.0. In addition, hemoglobin H shows a characteristic appearance of multiple ragged inclusions in

Table 12–2. **GENETIC BACKGROUND OF α-THALASSEMIA CLINICAL SYNDROMES (MATING COMBINATIONS)**

	CHROMOSOME				
	Normal	α^+			α^0
	GENES				
Genes	$\alpha\alpha$	$-\alpha$	$\alpha^{cs}\alpha$	$\alpha\alpha^T$	—
$\alpha\alpha$	N	αthal 2	αthal 2	αthal 2	αthal 1
$-\alpha$	αthal 2	αthal 1	αthal 1	αthal 1	H
$\alpha^{cs}\alpha$	αthal 2	αthal 1	αthal 1	αthal 1	H
$\alpha\alpha^T$	αthal 2	αthal 1	αthal 1	αthal 1	H
—	αthal 1	H	H	H	Bart's

$\alpha\alpha$ = normal haplotype; $-\alpha$ = deletion of one alpha gene; $\alpha^{cs}\alpha$ = Hb Constant Spring; $\alpha\alpha^T$ = nondeletion α-thalassemia gene; — = deletion of both alpha genes. (The clinical phenotype resulting from the combination of these haplotypes is found at the intersection of the corresponding column and row.) N = normal clinical phenotype; αthal 1 = α^0 trait, 5–15% Hb Bart's at birth, mild anemia; αthal 2 = α^+ trait, 0–2% Hb Bart's at birth, minimal hematologic changes; H = hemoglobin H disease; Bart's = hemoglobin Bart's hydrops fetalis.

many red cells after incubation with brilliant cresyl blue, the so-called golfball appearance.

The α^0-thalassemia trait, also called α-thalassemia 1 trait, is caused by the defect of two of the four alpha genes. This is usually the result of heterozygosity for the α^0-thalassemia gene but could also be the result of homozygosity for the α^+-thalassemia gene. The condition is characterized by the presence at birth of 5 to 15 percent hemoglobin Bart's, which disappears with development and is not replaced by hemoglobin H. There is a minimal amount of anemia with slight hypochromia and microcytosis present. After hemoglobin Bart's disappears, the hemoglobin electrophoretic pattern becomes normal.

The last category of α-thalassemia is the α^+-thalassemia trait, also called α-thalassemia 2 trait. This is the result of a defect in one of the four alpha globin genes and is characterized by the presence of a very small amount (up to 2 percent) of hemoglobin Bart's at birth; after the disappearance of hemoglobin Bart's during development, no recognizable hematologic abnormality is present.

Table 12–2 summarizes the different genetic backgrounds associated with the four different clinical expressions of α-thalassemia.

Delta-Beta Thalassemias and Hemoglobin Lepore Syndrome

Delta-beta ($\delta\beta$) thalassemias are a diverse group of thalassemias characterized by a combined defect in delta and beta chain synthesis. They can be described as demonstrating a normal level of hemoglobin A_2 and an unusually high level of hemoglobin F in the heterozygote, and absent hemoglobin A and A_2 in the homozygote. The delta-beta thalassemias can be subdivided into two groups according to the type of hemoglobin F produced. If both $^G\gamma$ and $^A\gamma$ chains are produced—that is, if both gamma genes are active—this variety is then called $^G\gamma^A\gamma\delta\beta$-

thalassemia. If only $^G\gamma$ chains are produced, which means that the A-gamma gene as well as the delta and the beta genes are inactive, this variety is then called $^G\gamma\delta\beta$-thalassemia. Another syndrome of delta-beta chain abnormality involves the production of an abnormal hemoglobin. This abnormal hemoglobin, called hemoglobin Lepore after the name of the family in which it was first found, has been shown to be a fusion of the delta and beta chains, which is the product of a fusion gene (hybrid) formed by an unequal crossover.

Figure 12–8 indicates diagrammatically the production of hemoglobin Lepore by this unequal crossover. At least three different hemoglobin Lepores have been described, varying in the exact location of the unequal crossover.

All delta-beta thalassemias studied thus far have been shown to be the result of a deletion. They can be described at the genetic level as three different entities, depending on the amount of DNA lost: hemoglobin Lepore syndrome results from a partial deletion of the delta and beta genes, $^G\gamma^A\gamma\delta\beta$-thalassemia from a complete deletion of the delta and beta genes, and $^G\gamma\delta\beta$-thalassemia from a deletion of the A-gamma gene in addition to the deletion of the delta and beta genes.

Delta-beta thalassemias are less common than β-thalassemias and have been found sporadically in Greeks, American blacks, Italians, and Arabs.

The gamma chain synthesis in delta-beta thalassemia is usually more efficient than in β-thalassemia, and in general the former results in a milder clinical disease than the latter. Patients with homozygous delta-beta thalassemia have a mild to moderate degree of anemia and rarely require blood transfusion, except occasionally during times of stress such as infection or pregnancy. The clinical course is usually described as thalassemia intermedia. This is also true of the double heterozygous delta-beta and β-thalassemia. However, the homozygous state for hemoglobin Lepore appears to be

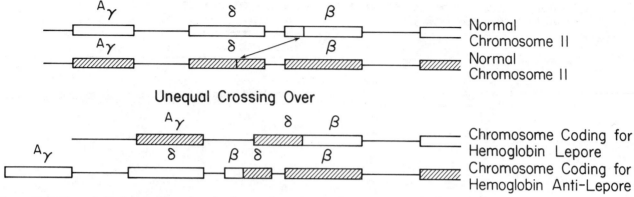

Figure 12–8. Hemoglobin Lepore formation. An abnormal crossing over between the beta and the delta genes gives rise to hemoglobin Lepore and to hemoglobin anti-Lepore.

somewhat more severe and closer to the clinical state of homozygous β-thalassemia. The majority of patients with homozygous hemoglobin Lepore are transfusion dependent. Double heterozygosity for β-thalassemia and hemoglobin Lepore also causes a clinical disorder similar to homozygous β-thalassemia.

Heterozygosity for delta-beta thalassemia and hemoglobin Lepore results in a mild form of anemia that is clinically described as thalassemia minor and is similar to the condition of patients with heterozygous β-thalassemia.

Hereditary Persistence of Fetal Hemoglobin

Hereditary persistence of fetal hemoglobin (HPFH) consists of a group of conditions characterized by the persistence of fetal hemoglobin synthesis into adult life. These conditions can be classified into two different categories according to the distribution of hemoglobin F among the red cells. Fetal hemoglobin is more resistant than adult hemoglobin to elution at acid pH and can be demonstrated on a peripheral blood smear by the acid elution test of Betke and Kleihauer **(see Color Plate 260)**. Using this stain, the hereditary persistence of fetal hemoglobin conditions can be divided into a pancellular form, in which hemoglobin F is uniformly distributed among the red cells, and a heterocellular form, in which hemoglobin F is found in a small percentage of the cells only. In the healthy adult, cells containing hemoglobin F can occasionally be found, but the amount is always less than 2 percent and is usually less than 1 percent. These cells are called F cells.

Heterocellular HPFH appears to be an inherited condition in which the number of F cells is increased without concurrent abnormalities in delta and beta chain production. Its most common form is the Swiss type, in which individuals have up to 3 percent hemoglobin F but are otherwise hematologically normal. At the DNA level, there appears to

be no gross abnormalities of the delta and beta genes.

On the other hand, pancellular HPFH appears to be a form of delta-beta thalassemia in which the gamma genes were not switched off and are able to compensate fully for the lack of delta and beta chain production. The most common form of pancellular HPFH is the Negro type, in which there is a deletion of the beta and delta globin genes that is associated with synthesis of $^G\gamma$ and $^A\gamma$ chains, which almost compensates for the lack of production of delta and beta chains. Hemoglobin F constitutes 100 percent of the hemoglobin in the homozygous state and 15 to 30 percent of the hemoglobin in the heterozygous state. The hemoglobin F is homogeneously distributed among the red cells and consists of a mixture of $^G\gamma$ and $^A\gamma$ chains. Clinically, the homozygotes will demonstrate features of thalassemia minor and the heterozygotes will be hematologically normal.

Another form of pancellular HPFH is the Greek type, in which about 15 percent hemoglobin F is present in the heterozygous state. This hemoglobin F is also found uniformly distributed among the red cells but is only of the A-gamma type. The homozygous state for this type of pancellular HPFH has not been described. In general, heterozygous or homozygous HPFH causes no significant clinical abnormalities.

Thalassemia Associated with Hemoglobin Variants

The molecular basis of the hemoglobinopathies can be broadly divided into two groups. In the first group the genetic defect involves the synthesis of the beta chain; this group includes β-thalassemia, hemoglobin S, hemoglobin C, and hemoglobin E. In the second group the genetic defect involves the alpha chain synthesis; the α-thalassemias are included in this group. Homozygosity or double heterozygosity for defective genes within the same group usually causes severe, often lethal disease. Double heterozygosity with one gene from one group and a second gene from the other group usually shows no interaction, and a defective gene in one group may even result in a clinical improvement of the condition of a patient who is homozygous for a defective gene in the other group. Although thalassemia has been described in association with a large number of hemoglobin structural variants, we will consider only the interactions with the more common hemoglobin variants (that is, β-thalassemia with hemoglobin S, hemoglobin C, and hemoglobin E, and α-thalassemia with hemoglobin S).

Beta-Thalassemia/Hemoglobin S

This condition was first recognized in individuals who had inherited a single hemoglobin S gene and who demonstrated about 65 percent hemoglobin S and 35 percent hemoglobin A, which is the reverse of the proportions found in patients with sickle-cell trait. This condition is the result of the inheritance of a hemoglobin S gene from one parent and the β-thalassemia gene from the other. Beta-thalassemia/hemoglobin S (also called the β-thalassemia sickle-cell syndrome) has been widely seen in Africa, the Mediterranean area, the Middle East, and the West Indies, as well as in North American blacks. There is great variety in the clinical severity of this syndrome, depending mostly on the type of β-thalassemia gene inherited. If the β-thalassemia gene is the β^0 type, no hemoglobin A will be produced and the clinical condition will be indistinguishable from classic sickle-cell anemia, characterized by severe anemia presenting in early childhood and recurrent sickling crises. If the β-thalassemia gene is β^+ type 1, a small amount of hemoglobin A will be produced, possibly representing up to 15 percent of the total hemoglobin. Patients in this group have severe anemia with a hemoglobin level in the 7 to 8 g/dl range and experience less frequent and less severe sickling crises than do those in the β^0 group. If the β-thalassemia gene is β^+ type 2, as is found in most American blacks, a greater amount of hemoglobin A will be produced, representing up to 30 percent of the total hemoglobin. Patients in this group have a very mild anemia with hemoglobin about 11 g/dl and are usually asymptomatic, the condition being diagnosed later in life or during a family study. These patients, as a rule, will not experience any sickling crisis, except under the most severe hypoxic conditions.

Beta-Thalassemia/Hemoglobin C

The β-thalassemia/hemoglobin C syndrome demonstrates great variability in clinical and hematologic manifestations, which is directly related to the type of β-thalassemia gene that interacts with the hemoglobin C gene; however, the great majority of patients with this syndrome are West African and North American blacks. In this racial group the more common β-thalassemia gene is β^+ type 2. In this case the β-thalassemia/hemoglobin C syndrome will be characterized by a mild degree of usually asymptomatic anemia, in which the clinical and hematologic findings are very similar to those found in heterozygous β-thalassemia.

Beta-Thalassemia/Hemoglobin E

Double heterozygosity for β-thalassemia and hemoglobin E is unusual in that it results in a clinical disorder that is much more severe than homozygous hemoglobin E disease. Patients with this syndrome are distributed widely throughout the Far East. The condition follows a clinical course very similar to that of homozygous β-thalassemia, with a very severe anemia occurring in early childhood and the development of the characteristic features of thalassemia major if the patient is not started on a regular blood transfusion program.

Alpha-Thalassemia with Sickle-Cell Anemia

The occurrence of α-thalassemia in conjunction with sickle-cell anemia has a positive influence on the clinical expression of the disease. Patients with such a genetic background have an increased percentage of hemoglobin F, which is thought to result in a decreased severity of the sickling process. Of interest is the fact that the amount of hemoglobin F present is roughly proportional to the number of alpha genes affected. Patients with the α^0-thalassemia trait have an average of 16 percent hemoglobin F, and those with the α^+-thalassemia trait have an average of 8 percent hemoglobin F.

CLINICAL COURSE AND THERAPY

The clinical course and therapy of patients with thalassemia can be broadly subdivided into three categories: thalassemia major, thalassemia intermedia, and thalassemia minor. A fourth category, thalassemia minima, is applied to healthy silent carriers who show no clinical symptoms and minimal to no hematologic abnormalities. Table 12–3 summarizes the different genetic backgrounds that result in each of these clinical outcomes.

Hemoglobin Bart's hydrops fetalis stands by itself as a single entity, in which the affected infants are either stillborn or die within a few days after birth. For this condition, no therapy is available. The clinical significance of this entity is related more to the obstetric problems that may arise in the affected infants' mothers. Pregnancy in these women is often complicated by toxemia, obstructed labor, and postpartum hemorrhage, which may result in severe morbidity and mortality. Clinical emphasis for this entity is on the prevention of the disease through early antenatal diagnosis, after which the pregnancy should be terminated for the protection of the mother's health.

Thalassemia major is the most severe clinical expression of thalassemia and characteristically occurs in patients with homozygous β^0 or β^+-thalassemia or with double heterozygous β^0- and β^+-thalassemia, as well as in patients with homozygous hemoglobin Lepore, double heterozygous β-

Table 12–3. **GENETIC BACKGROUND OF THE DIFFERENT CLINICAL COURSES OF THALASSEMIA**

Major	Intermedia	Minor	Minima
Homozygous β^0thal	Homozygous β^0 or β^+thal or double heterozygous β^0/β^+ thal in association with αthal	Heterozygous β^0thal	Heterozygous β^+thal (type 3)
Homozygous β^+thal (type 1)		Heterozygous β^+thal (type 1 or 2)	
Double heterozygous β^0/β^+thal	Homozygous β^+thal (type 2 or 3)	Heterozygous $\delta\beta$thal	
Homozygous Hb Lepore (some)	Homozygous Hb Lepore (some)	Heterozygous Hb Lepore	
Double heterozygous Hb Lepore/β^0 or β^+thal	Double heterozygous $\delta\beta$thal/βthal	Double heterozygous βthal/HPFH	Homozygous HPFH Heterozygous HPFH
Double heterozygous HbE/β^0 or β^+thal	Double heterozygous Hb Lepore/$\delta\beta$thal		
	Hemoglobin H disease	αthal 1	αthal 2

NOTE: Each column lists the genetic background associated with each category of thalassemia.

thalassemia/hemoglobin Lepore, and double heterozygous β-thalassemia/hemoglobin E.

Patients with untreated thalassemia major will usually present within the first year of life with failure to thrive, pallor, a variable degree of jaundice, and abdominal enlargement, with hemoglobin levels from 4 to 8 g/dl. All diagnostic work necessary to define exactly the type of thalassemia should be done at this time before blood transfusions are started.

It is now clear that a high transfusion program (hypertransfusion) that maintains the hemoglobin level at 11.5 g/dl on the average is better than an intermittent program that allows the hemoglobin level to drop to a point at which the child becomes severely symptomatic. Hypertransfusion allows for better development, suppresses ineffective erythropoiesis (thus preventing the serious bony deformities), and provides for an overall better quality of life. This, however, draws on considerable blood resources and may not be available in the very countries where thalassemia major is a serious public health concern.

In the presence of splenomegaly, splenectomy plays a clear role in decreasing the blood transfusion requirement. However, it should preferably not be performed until the child has reached at least 5 years of age, to decrease the risk of overwhelming infection, particularly that of pneumococcal origin.

With regular blood transfusion, these children survive but develop severe iron overload owing to increased iron absorption and to the loading of iron from the blood transfusions. This iron overload results in hemochromatosis, and these patients die in their second or third decade, usually of cardiac failure. In the meantime, they develop multiple organ damage, with lack of pubertal development probably due to iron toxicity to the pituitary gland, cirrhosis of the liver (which may be the result of either hemochromatosis or post-transfusion hepatitis), and diabetes due to iron toxicity to the pancreas.

This iron overload may be improved with the early introduction of iron chelation therapy. Recent assessment of iron chelation therapy with deferoxamine seems to indicate that an adequate iron balance can be achieved and that longer survival will be attained.

Alternate modes of therapy for thalassemia major in the future may be found in the areas of bone marrow transplantation, genetic engineering, and pharmacologic manipulations that may induce the "switching back on" of the gamma globin gene. The current optimal therapy for thalassemia major relies on intensive use of a fairly sophisticated level of health care that cannot be achieved in most of the countries where thalassemia major is a serious problem without shunting the major thrust of the health resources in that direction.

Another approach to this problem at the health planning level is to decrease the number of births of infants with thalassemia major. This has been successful in certain countries, particularly Cyprus, with the implementation of mass population screening for the detection of heterozygous carriers, genetic counseling, and antenatal diagnosis for couples at risk. Recent developments in antenatal diagnosis, using DNA hybridization techniques in association with chorionic villi sampling, enable physicians to make a diagnosis during the first trimester of pregnancy, thus making early termination of pregnancy much more widely available and acceptable.

Thalassemia intermedia covers a broad spectrum of clinical expression of thalassemia, bridging the gap between the severe, lethal form of thalassemia major and the mild, often asymptomatic anemia state of thalassemia minor. The definition of thalassemia intermedia is relative because the clinical state of patients in this group varies from a mild disability to severe incapacitation without transfusion. Thalassemia intermedia could be defined as a form of thalassemia in which patients have variable degrees of symptomatic anemia, jaundice, splenomegaly, and many of the complications of thalassemia major but will survive into adulthood without a large blood transfusion requirement.

The genetic background of thalassemia intermedia is also extremely varied. It includes patients with homozygosity for the less severe forms of the β-thalassemia gene (such as β^+ type 2 and β^+ type 3 thalassemia), homozygous delta-beta thalassemia, double heterozygous delta-beta thalassemia/β-thalassemia, and hemoglobin H disease, as well as patients who are homozygous for β-thalassemia but who have also inherited a gene for α-thalassemia or who have the ability to synthesize the gamma chains more efficiently. The exact definition of the genetic background of a patient with thalassemia intermedia requires a careful and extensive family study.

Patients with thalassemia intermedia usually present at a somewhat older age — usually after the age of 2 — and with a slightly higher level of hemoglobin (between 6 and 10 g/dl) than patients with thalassemia major. There is great overlap between the two conditions at presentation; however, it is very important to differentiate between them, as the only therapy for thalassemia major is regular blood transfusion in conjunction with iron chelation, whereas the management of thalassemia intermedia involves mostly supportive therapy with only occasional blood transfusion under special circumstances.

The serum bilirubin level is significantly more elevated in patients with thalassemia intermedia than in those with thalassemia major. Patients with thalassemia intermedia may develop the severe bony deformities and compression syndromes due to marrow hyperplasia and extramedullary erythropoiesis characteristic of thalassemia major. They are susceptible to frequent, sometimes severe, infections, and gallbladder problems due to the formation of gallstones. These children usually have an acceptable level of growth and development (although puberty may be delayed by a few years), and they reach adulthood if infections are controlled and if they enjoy good nutrition with particular emphasis on prevention of folic acid deficiency. They usually develop splenomegaly and may become transfusion dependent if severe hypersplenism occurs. This will usually require splenectomy. Children with thalassemia intermedia may develop iron overload as a result of increased gastrointestinal absorption, but this is a much slower process than that experienced by patients with thalassemia major, and the complications due to iron overload occur much later in life. Women with thalassemia intermedia who get pregnant require blood transfusions as well as folic acid supplementation throughout the pregnancy.

Thalassemia minor is a clinical entity in which the genetic defects of thalassemia are expressed as a mild microcytic, hypochromic anemia, usually in the 9 to 11 g/dl range, and is asymptomatic except during periods of stress such as pregnancy, infection, or folic acid deficiency. Most patients with thalassemia minor are heterozygous for the β^+-thalassemia gene, the β^0-thalassemia gene, or the α^0-thalassemia gene. The genetic background of thalassemia minor also includes heterozygosity for hemoglobin Lepore and for delta-beta thalassemia. Patients with thalassemia minor are usually diagnosed incidental to a family study of an index case with thalassemia major or by population screening. They usually require no therapy if they maintain good nutrition.

BLOOD TRANSFUSION IN THALASSEMIA

The three main concerns that need to be addressed regarding patients with thalassemia major who are on a regular blood transfusion program are (1) the development of iron overload, (2) the development of alloimmunization, and (3) the risk of transfusion-transmitted diseases. The problem of iron overload can be approached from one of two directions: by increasing the iron excretion or by decreasing the amount of iron transfused. This latter option can be performed by increasing the length of survival of the transfused red cells, which requires selection of the younger red cells (also called neocytes) for transfusion. Young red cells and reticulocytes have a lower specific gravity than old red cells, and by using a differential centrifugation technique the blood unit can be separated so that the upper layer of cells is collected. These red cells will have a much longer life expectancy and can decrease the transfusion requirement of a patient by lengthening the interval of the blood transfusion schedule.

Alloimmunization is a recurrent problem of all chronically transfused patients. These patients often develop antibodies to white cell as well as to red cell antigens. Antibodies to white cell antigens cause febrile nonhemolytic transfusion reactions that are unpleasant. These reactions can be avoided by routinely transfusing leukocyte-poor red cells. Alloimmunization to red cell antigens is a more serious problem, since this can cause acute or delayed hemolytic transfusion reactions and may seriously affect the availability of compatible blood. It is a good idea to obtain a complete phenotype of the patient's red cell before embarking on a regular transfusion program.

Transfusion-transmitted diseases are a common complication in multitransfused patients. Patients with thalassemia major often develop hepatitis, which is usually non-A, non-B hepatitis in countries where blood is routinely screened for the presence of the hepatitis B surface antigen (HBsAg). Hepatitis B as well as delta hepatitis can also be transmitted through blood transfusions and are the most common threat in certain parts of the world. Some patients may develop a chronic form of hepatitis that, in conjunction with the iron toxicity of iron overload, may damage the liver severely and result in cirrhosis of the liver.

LABORATORY DIAGNOSIS OF THALASSEMIA

The hallmark of thalassemia is the finding of a microcytic, hypochromic anemia. Although more sophisticated laboratory procedures are needed to define exactly the type of thalassemia, the original diagnosis of thalassemia can be made or strongly suspected on the basis of the results of routine hematology procedures.

Routine Hematology Procedures

Automated Blood Cell Analyzer

Modern electronic cell analyzers now routinely give the following parameters: red cell count (RBC), hemoglobin level (Hgb), hematocrit (Hct), mean corpuscular volume (MCV), mean cell hemoglobin (MCH), mean corpuscular hemoglobin concentration (MCHC), and red cell volume distribution width (RDW). The thalassemias in general are characterized by a decrease in Hgb, Hct, MCV, and MCH in conjunction with a normal to increased RBC, a normal to mildly decreased MCHC, and a normal RDW. The only exception is thalassemia major, in which the degree of anisocytosis is such that the RDW will be increased. The decrease in MCV is usually striking and disproportionate to the decrease in hemoglobin and hematocrit. This fact, in conjunction with the relatively high RBC and the normal RDW, offers a reliable discrimination index between heterozygous α- or β-thalassemia and iron deficiency. In iron deficiency, the RDW will be increased and the decrease in MCV less striking and only observed when the anemia is more severe. In heterozygous thalassemia, the MCH will usually be below 22 pg and the MCV below 70 fl, whereas the hemoglobin level will be in the 9 to 11 g/dl range.

Peripheral Blood Smear Examination

The careful examination of a well-prepared peripheral blood smear is essential to the diagnosis of thalassemia.

Wright's Stain. In homozygous β- and double heterozygous nonalpha-thalassemia, the peripheral blood smear demonstrates extreme anisocytosis and poikilocytosis with bizarre shapes, target cells, ovalocytes, and large number of nucleated red cells (**see Color Plate 98**). There is marked hypochromia and microcytosis. In heterozygous β-thalassemia, the cells are hypochromic and microcytic with a mild to moderate degree of anisocytosis and poikilocytosis. Target cells are frequent, and basophilic stippling is often seen (**see Color Plate 99**). The peripheral smear of a patient with the sickle-cell thalassemia syndrome can be differentiated from that of a patient with pure sickle-cell anemia by the presence of hypochromia, microcytosis, numerous target cells, and only an occasional sickled cell.

In hemoglobin H disease, the peripheral smear will demonstrate hypochromia with microcytosis, target cells, and mild to moderate anisopoikilocytosis. Patients with heterozygous α^0-thalassemia usually demonstrate a mild hypochromia and microcytosis, whereas those with heterozygous α^+-thalassemia usually have a perfectly normal peripheral smear.

Supravital Stains. The reticulocyte count is usually elevated up to 10 percent in hemoglobin H disease and up to 5 percent in homozygous β-thalassemia but is disproportionately low in relation to the degree of anemia in the latter condition.

In hemoglobin H disease, incubation of the red cells with brilliant cresyl blue stain will cause in vitro precipitation of hemoglobin H owing to the redox action of the dye. This will result in a characteristic appearance of the majority of the red cells, which will display multiple discrete inclusions, the appearance of which has often been compared to that of a golfball (**see Color Plate 100**). Occasionally, and after extensive searching, such cells containing hemoglobin H inclusions can be found in the α^0-thalassemia carrier.

In splenectomized patients with homozygous β-thalassemia or hemoglobin H disease, incubation of the blood with methyl violet stain can demonstrate Heinz body–like inclusions, which represent in vivo precipitation of the abnormal hemoglobin.

Acid Elution Stain. The acid elution technique originally described by Betke and Kleihauer is based on the fact that at an acid pH of about 3.3, hemoglobin A is eluted from an air-dried, alcohol-fixed blood smear, whereas hemoglobin F is resistant to elution. After such treatment and subsequent staining with eosin or erythrosin, normal adult red cells will appear as very faint ghosts. Red cells containing hemoglobin F will demonstrate a variable amount of stain, depending on the amount of hemoglobin F present. A controlled preparation containing a mixture of adult and cord cells must also be stained and examined in parallel to check the quality of the technique, as this technique is very sensitive to many variables.

This stain is very useful in demonstrating the distribution of hemoglobin F and can be used to differentiate between pancellular and heterocellular HPFH. It is also useful in differentiating heterozygous delta-beta thalassemia from heterozygous pancellular HPFH, as the former usually has a heterocellular distribution of hemoglobin F.

Osmotic Fragility

The red cells of patients with homozygous or heterozygous β-thalassemia, hemoglobin H disease, and α^0-thalassemia trait have a decreased osmotic fragility. This fact is not very useful for diagnostic purposes in a specific patient, but it is the basis of a simple, inexpensive method of screening for the thalassemia carrier state in large populations.

Hemoglobin Electrophoresis

Hemoglobin electrophoresis plays an important role in the diagnosis of thalassemia by allowing the detection of increased levels of hemoglobin A_2 and

Table 12–4. **HEMOGLOBINS A, A₂, AND F LEVELS IN THE DIFFERENT NONALPHA THALASSEMIAS**

	HbA (%)	HbA₂ (%)	HbF (%)
Homozygous β⁰thal	0	2–5	95–98
Homozygous β⁺ or double heterozygous β⁺/β⁰thal	5–35	2–5	60–95
Homozygous δβ thal	0	0	100
Homozygous Hb Lepore	0	0	75 (25% Hb Lepore)
Heterozygous β thal	90–95	3.5–7	2–5
Heterozygous δβ thal	80–92	1–2.5	5–20
Heterozygous Hb Lepore	75–85	2	1–6 (7–15% Hb Lepore)
Homozygous HPFH	0	0	100
Heterozygous HPFH (Negro type)	65–85	1–2.5	15–35
Heterozygous HPFH (Greek type)	75–85	1.5–2.5	15–25
Normal	97.5	2.5	0.2–1

hemoglobin F, as well as the presence of abnormal hemoglobins, such as hemoglobin H, hemoglobin Bart's, hemoglobin Lepore, hemoglobin Constant Spring, or other structurally abnormal hemoglobins that can be found in association with thalassemia (hemoglobin S, hemoglobin C, hemoglobin E). Table 12–4 contains a summary of the different patterns of the hemoglobins present in the nonalpha-thalassemia syndromes.

Routine hemoglobin electrophoresis to confirm the diagnosis of thalassemia is done at an alkaline pH around 8.4 on cellulose acetate or starch gel. At that pH the hemoglobins will migrate from the most cathodal to the most anodal in the following order: first hemoglobin Constant Spring, then hemoglobins A₂, C, and E migrate in the same band; next hemoglobins S and Lepore, again in the same band; next hemoglobin F, followed by hemoglobin A; then hemoglobin Bart's; and last hemoglobin H. The different patterns of migration of the different hemoglobins is illustrated in Figure 12–9. Cellulose acetate or starch gel electrophoresis can be done at low to neutral pH to easily detect hemoglobin H and hemoglobin Bart's, as they migrate anodally (that is, in a direction opposite that of other hemoglobins) at this pH.

Cellulose Acetate

Cellulose acetate electrophoresis is becoming more popular and has replaced starch gel electrophoresis in many laboratories, owing to its simple, rapid method. It uses a smaller sample than starch gel electrophoresis, however, possibly allowing minor components such as hemoglobin Constant Spring and small amounts of hemoglobin A₂ to be overlooked. Small amounts of hemoglobin A in the presence of mostly hemoglobin F also can be difficult to detect. Figure 12–10 demonstrates a strip of a cellulose acetate after electrophoresis of several hemoglobins.

Starch Gel

Starch gel electrophoresis is a little more cumbersome than cellulose acetate electrophoresis, because the starch gel must be prepared and poured and is more difficult to handle. The staining procedure is also more time consuming, with more difficult long-term storage. The results of the starch gel electrophoresis are similar to those of the cellulose acetate procedure. Electrophoresis with starch gel is

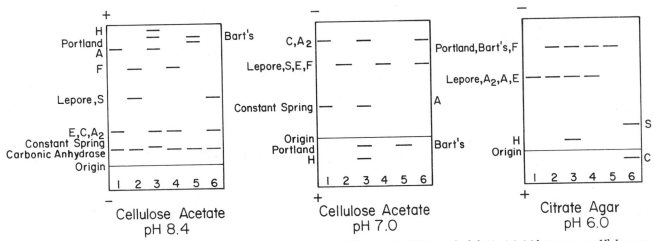

Figure 12–9. Diagram of the migration of the different hemoglobins at different pH. (1) Normal adult (A, A₂); (2) homozygous Hb Lepore (F, Lepore); (3) HbH/Constant Spring disease α^{cs}α/—(Constant Spring, A₂, A, Bart's, H); (4) double heterozygous HbE/beta-thalassemia (E,F); (5) Hb Bart's hydrops fetalis syndrome (Portland, Bart's); (6) HbS/C disease (S,C).

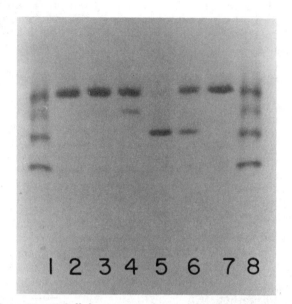

Figure 12–10. Cellulose acetate electrophoresis of the following samples: (1) AFSC control; (2 and 3) beta-thalassemia carriers (increased A₂ and F); (4) normal newborn; (5) HbS/beta-thalassemia (more hemoglobin S than A); (6) HbS heterozygote; (7) normal adult; (8) AFSC control.

better at defining the presence of hemoglobin Constant Spring and should always be used if such a variant is suspected.

Citrate Agar Gel

Citrate agar gel electrophoresis, which is performed at an acid pH between 5.9 and 6.2, has a minor role in the diagnosis of the thalassemias. It is mostly useful in defining structurally abnormal hemoglobins that are interacting with thalassemia because it allows the distinction between hemoglobin C and hemoglobin E and between hemoglobin S and hemoglobin Lepore.

Hemoglobin Quantitation

Although an experienced observer can detect an increased level in hemoglobin A_2 or hemoglobin F on cellulose acetate or starch gel electrophoresis, actual quantitation is necessary to truly establish the diagnosis of thalassemia.

Hemoglobin A₂ Quantitation

The elevation of hemoglobin A_2 is an excellent tool for the detection of a heterozygote carrier of β-thalassemia. It is characteristic of heterozygous β-thalassemia and specific with no overlap values between heterozygous carriers and healthy individuals. The level of hemoglobin A_2 ranges from 3.5 to 7 percent in heterozygous β-thalassemia, whereas normal values are always below 3.5 percent. A few rare variants of β-thalassemia with normal hemo-

globin A_2 do exist; this is called normal A_2 β-thalassemia and can only be distinguished in the carrier state from heterozygous α-thalassemia by globin chain synthesis. Also, in an iron-deficient patient with β-thalassemia minor, hemoglobin A_2 may be reduced to normal levels. The percent hemoglobin A_2 can be quantified either by elution following cellulose acetate electrophoresis or by microcolumn chromatography.

Hemoglobin F Quantitation

The hemoglobin F levels are useful in the definition of the type of thalassemia involved, and a summary of the levels of hemoglobin F corresponding to the different types of thalassemia can be found in Table 12–4. The hemoglobin F level is normally below 2 percent. Approximately half of the β-thalassemia carriers will have a mildly elevated level of hemoglobin F, usually below 5 percent. Quantitation of hemoglobin F can be done by an alkali denaturation method, in which hemoglobin A is denatured in the presence of an alkali solution while hemoglobin F is unaffected. Immunologic techniques using a specific antibody to hemoglobin F have been developed and are more accurate and practical. Prepared radioimmunodiffusion plates containing agarose with antisera to hemoglobin F are now available.

Routine Chemistry

The indirect bilirubin level is elevated in thalassemias major and intermedia, ranging from 1 to 6 mg/dl. It is characteristically more elevated in thalassemia intermedia than in thalassemia major.

The assessment of the iron status of the patient by the determination of the serum iron level, total iron-binding capacity (TIBC), and serum ferritin level is useful in the differentiation of a thalassemia carrier from a patient with iron-deficiency anemia, as well as in the assessment of the iron load in a patient with thalassemia major or intermedia. The serum iron and the serum ferritin will be low and the TIBC increased in patients with iron deficiency. These values are normal in patients with thalassemia minor unless they have concurrent iron deficiency. Patients with thalassemia major who have been transfused have increased levels of serum iron that will approach 100 percent saturation of the TIBC. The serum ferritin level will be elevated and will indicate the amount of iron deposited in the tissues.

Miscellaneous

Alpha/Beta Globin Chain Synthesis

The rate of synthesis of the globin chains can be measured in vitro by culturing reticulocytes from peripheral blood or nucleated red cells from the bone marrow in the presence of radioactively labeled leucine. The radioactive leucine is incorporated into the globin chains that are being synthesized. After the incubation is stopped, the red cells are lysed and the globin is precipitated and washed. The different globin chains are then separated by fractionation using CM-cellulose chromatography, and the radioactivity of each fraction is counted. In this way, a ratio of synthesis of alpha/beta globin chains can be determined. This is a very sophisticated technique that can be used on special occasions when it is vitally important to differentiate an α-thalassemia carrier from a normal A_2 β-thalassemia carrier, to identify a silent carrier of the β-thalassemia gene, or to unravel a complicated inheritance pattern of multiple types of thalassemia within a family.

Gene Analysis

This even more sophisticated technique using restriction endonucleases and hybridization with complementary DNA probes can study the genetic defects at the DNA level. The DNA is extracted from the nuclei of peripheral blood leukocytes and fragmented by enzymes called restriction endonucleases. These enzymes recognize specific sequences in the DNA and cleave the DNA at that particular point. Agarose gel electrophoresis is then performed on this fragmented DNA, which will separate the

fragments according to their molecular weight. The separated DNA fragments are then transferred on a nitrocellulose filter and fixed to this filter by baking. After a denaturation step to render the DNA single stranded, labeled complementary DNA (cDNA) probes that will recognize a specific globin gene are then incubated with the DNA fragments on the nitrocellulose filter. They will bind or hybridize to any DNA fragment whose sequence is complementary to theirs. In this way, one can demonstrate the specific globin gene that the cDNA probe recognizes. Its location on the nitrocellulose filter is dependent on the DNA fragment size containing the gene. This technique can detect complete deletion of a globin gene, partial deletion of a globin gene, and some minute mutations that may abolish a normal cleavage site or create a new cleavage site recognized by the specific restriction endonuclease used. These minute mutations that occur around the globin genes are inherited and have been found to be in linkage disequilibrium with specific defects of the globin gene complex. This type of analysis, called restriction fragment length polymorphism (RFLP), is now used in the antenatal diagnosis of thalassemia major. This method is illustrated in Figure 12–11.

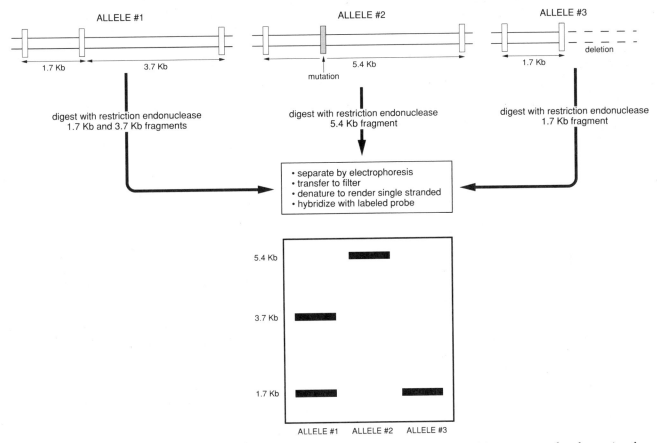

Figure 12–11. Diagram of principle of restriction fragment length polymorphism analysis: *Allele #1* is normal and contains three cleavage sites and yields two fragments 1.7 kb and 3.7 kb in length. *Allele #2* has a mutation at one cleavage site and only yields one fragment 5.4 kb in length. *Allele #3* has a deletion after the second cleavage site and yields one fragment 1.7 kb in length.

Table 12–5. **DIFFERENTIAL DIAGNOSIS OF MICROCYTIC HYPOCHROMIC ANEMIA**

	RDW	Serum Iron	TIBC	Serum Ferritin	FEP	A₂ Level
Iron deficiency	↑	↓	↑	↓	↑	nl
α-Thalassemia	nl	nl	nl	nl	nl	nl
β-Thalassemia	nl	nl	nl	nl	nl	nl
Hemoglobin E disease	nl	nl	nl	nl	nl	↑
Anemia of chronic disease	nl	↓	↓	↑	↑	nl
Sideroblastic anemia	↑	↑	nl	↑	↑	nl
Lead poisoning	nl	nl	nl	nl	↑	nl

RDW = red cell volume distribution width; TIBC = total iron-binding capacity; FEP = free erythrocyte protoporphyrin; nl = normal.

DIFFERENTIAL DIAGNOSIS OF MICROCYTIC HYPOCHROMIC ANEMIA

The differential diagnosis of microcytic hypochromic anemia includes iron deficiency, α-thalassemia, β-thalassemia, anemia of chronic disease, hemoglobin E disease, sideroblastic anemia, and lead poisoning. The evaluation of the clinical history, the hemoglobin level, and the red cell indices (in particular MCV and MCH) usually pinpoint the diagnosis. The sometimes difficult differential between the thalassemia carrier and the individual with iron deficiency can be done by evaluating the serum iron and ferritin levels and the TIBC. A markedly elevated free erythrocyte protoporphyrin (FEP) will identify a child with lead poisoning. Cellulose acetate electrophoresis will usually allow differentiation among a β-thalassemia carrier, an α-thalassemia carrier, and a person with hemoglobin E disease. The differentiation diagnosis of these diseases is summarized in Table 12–5.

CASE STUDY

A 25-year-old man of Chinese extraction is being evaluated because he was found to be anemic when he attempted to donate blood. He otherwise has no complaints; he is active in sports and feels healthy. A complete blood count gives the following results: RBC 5.76 million, Hgb 10.4 g/dl, Hct 35.9 percent, MCV 62 fl, MCH 18.1 pg, MCHC 29 percent, and RDW 13.5. The peripheral blood smear shows hypochromic, microcytic erythrocytes with a mild anisocytosis; occasional target cells but no basophilic stippling can be found.

The serum iron is 95 mg/dl (normal 60 to 150 mg/dl), the TIBC 305 mg/dl (normal 260 to 360 mg/dl), and the ferritin level 175 μg (normal 30 to 300 μg/dl). Cellulose acetate electrophoresis shows an increased amount of hemoglobins F and A₂, which are quantitated to 4.5 percent and 5 percent, respectively.

Questions

1. What are the diagnoses that you entertain at this time?

2. What laboratory tests do you think are most useful to diagnose the cause of his anemia?
3. What is your diagnosis now, and what is the significance of this diagnosis for this patient?

Answers

1. On clinical history alone, the possibilities of anemia of chronic disease and lead poisoning can be ruled out in a healthy young man. We are left with the possibility of iron deficiency, β-thalassemia carrier, α-thalassemia carrier, sideroblastic anemia, and hemoglobin E disease (which should be considered in a person of Chinese extraction).
2. A serum iron level, TIBC, serum ferritin level, and cellulose acetate electrophoresis are appropriate tests that may differentiate among these conditions.
3. Sideroblastic anemia and iron deficiency can be ruled out by the normal iron level, TIBC, and ferritin level. Although hemoglobin E migrates in the same area as hemoglobin A₂, on cellulose acetate electrophoresis, a patient with heterozygous or homozygous hemoglobin E would have a much larger amount of hemoglobin in that band; thus, hemoglobin E disease is ruled out. An α-thalassemia carrier would have a normal hemoglobin electrophoresis pattern; therefore, the diagnosis in this patient is heterozygous β-thalassemia.

Making the diagnosis of β-thalassemia heterozygosity in this patient is important for two reasons. First, the patient must be reassured that this level of hemoglobin and hematocrit is normal for him, and he should not be placed on iron therapy, which could be harmful. Second, the patient needs to be educated regarding the possibility of his having a child with a severe congenital anemia and its therapeutic implications, if he marries someone who is a carrier of β-thalassemia, hemoglobin E, or hemoglobin S. His spouse should be screened for the presence of these genes; genetic counseling such as antenatal diagnosis should be offered if in fact she is a carrier.

BIBLIOGRAPHY

Bank, A: Genetic defects in the thalassemias. Current Topics in Hematology 5:1, 1985.

Bunn, HF and Forget, BG: Hemoglobin: Molecular, Genetic and Clinical Aspects. WB Saunders, Philadelphia, 1986.

Higgs, DR and Weatherall, DS: Alpha thalassemia. Current Topics in Hematology 4:37, 1983.

Lehman, H and Huntsman, RG: Man's Hemoglobin. JP Lippincott, Philadelphia, 1974.

Liebhaber, SA and Manno, CS: Update on hemoglobinopathies. Diagn Med 29:1, 1983.

Lin-Fu, JS: Cooley's anemia, a medical review. US Department of Health and Human Services, Washington, DC, 1981.

Modell, B and Berdoukas, B: The Clinical Approach to Thalassemia. Grune & Stratton, New York, 1984.

Steinberg, MH: Review: Thalassemia: Molecular pathology and management. Am J Med Sci 296:308, 1988.

Weatherall, DJ (ed): The Thalassemias. Methods in Hematology. Churchill-Livingstone, New York, 1983.

Weatherall, DJ and Clegg, JB: The thalassemia syndromes. Blackwell Scientific, Boston, 1981.

WHO Working Group: Community control of hereditary anemias: Memorandum from a WHO meeting. Bull WHO 61:63, 1983.

WHO Working Group: Hereditary anemias: Genetic basis, clinical features, diagnosis and treatment. Bull WHO 60:643, 1982.

QUESTIONS

1. *What is the hemoglobin defect found in thalassemia syndromes?*
   a. Abnormal incorporation of iron molecule
   b. Defective production of the globin portion
   c. Excessive production of porphyrins
   d. Amino acid substitution

2. *What type of globin chains and hemoglobin are characteristics of α-thalassemia?*
   a. Two alpha chains and two beta chains (HbA)
   b. Two alpha chains and two delta chains (HbA₂)
   c. Four beta chains (HbH) or four gamma chains (HbBart's)
   d. Two alpha chains and two gamma chains (HbF)

3. *Which type of thalassemia has primarily hemoglobin Bart's and shows the following clinical expressions: infants die in utero or soon after birth; severe anemia, marked hepatomegaly and splenomegaly, and ascites?*
   a. Homozygous α-thalassemia
   b. Homozygous β-thalassemia
   c. Thalassemia minor
   d. Alpha-thalassemia trait

4. *What is the term for the clinical course of homozygous thalassemias due to defects in delta and beta chain synthesis?*
   a. Thalassemia minor
   b. Thalassemia major
   c. Thalassemia trait
   d. Thalassemia intermedia

5. *Hereditary persistence of fetal hemoglobin (HPFH) is characterized by the persistence of fetal hemoglobin into adult life. What are the clinical manifestations of this condition?*
   a. Chronic anemia with skeletal abnormalities due to excessive erythropoiesis
   b. Asymptomatic except during pregnancy or stressful situations
   c. Hydrops fetalis syndrome
   d. No significant abnormalities for heterozygous; minor symptoms for homozygous

6. *Which type of hemoglobin is commonly found in the β-thalassemia sickle-cell syndrome?*
   a. Hemoglobin S
   b. Hemoglobin C
   c. Hemoglobin E
   d. Hemoglobin F

7. *What is the clinical manifestation of α-thalassemia with sickle-cell anemia?*
   a. Severe, life-threatening anemia
   b. Relatively asymptomatic until placed in an oxygen-deprived environment
   c. Less severe than sickle-cell anemia alone
   d. Skeletal abnormality, but milder anemia than sickle-cell anemia

8. *What is the primary risk to thalassemia major patients who are on a high transfusion (hypertransfusion) program?*
   a. Hyperviscosity of the blood
   b. Iron overload
   c. Citrate toxicity
   d. Electrolyte imbalance

9. *What routine hematologic finding is indicative of thalassemia?*
   a. Microcytic, hypochromic anemia
   b. Macrocytic, hypochromic anemia
   c. Normocytic, normochromic anemia
   d. Macrocytic, normochromic anemia

10. *How can iron deficiency be distinguished from heterozygous α- or β-thalassemia?*
    a. RDW will be decreased in heterozygous thalassemia with increased MCH and MCV with Hgb in 10 to 14 g/dl range; iron deficiency with increased RDW, MCH, and MCV
    b. RDW normal in heterozygous thalassemia with decreased MCH and MCV with Hgb in 9 to 11 g/dl range; RDW increased in iron deficiency with decreased MCV and MCH only with severe anemia
    c. RDW increased in heterozygous thalassemia with decreased MCH and MCV with Hgb in 5 to 9 g/dl range; RDW normal in iron deficiency with normal MCV and MCH
    d. RDW, MCH, and MCV normal in heterozygous thalassemia; RDW, MCH, and MCV all increased in iron deficiency

11. *Which of the following cells might not be found in a patient with homozygous beta-thalassemia?*
    a. Target cells
    b. Ovalocytes
    c. Sickle cells
    d. Nucleated red cells

12. *Which test is useful in demonstrating the distribution of hemoglobin F and in differentiating pancellular HPFH, heterocellular HPFH, and heterozygous delta–beta-thalassemia?*
    a. Osmotic fragility
    b. Betke-Kleihauer acid elution test
    c. Serum ferritin level
    d. Complete blood count

13. *Which test is used as a screening method for detection of the thalassemia carrier state? (Use answer choices for question 12.)*

14. *Which electrophoresis media should be used if distinction is needed between hemoglobin C and hemoglobin E? (acid pH)*
    a. Cellulose acetate
    b. Starch gel
    c. Citrate agar
    d. Either cellulose acetate or starch gel

15. *How can hemoglobin H and hemoglobin Bart's be distinguished from other hemoglobins at low to neutral pH?*
    a. Speed of migration; faster than other hemoglobins
    b. Migrate in opposite direction of other hemoglobins
    c. Width of the band; wider than other hemoglobins
    d. Number of distinctive bands

16. *Which of the following findings would be indicative of heterozygous β-thalassemia?*
    a. Hemoglobin A_2 level 3.5 to 7%
    b. Hemoglobin F level below 2%
    c. Hemoglobin A level 65 to 85%
    d. Hemoglobin A_2 level below 3.5%

17. *Which of the following conditions would not show an elevated (above 2%) hemoglobin F?*
    a. Homozygous $β^0$ thalassemia
    b. Homozygous Hb Lepore
    c. Homozygous HPFH
    d. All conditions (a, b, and c) show elevated hemoglobin F

18. *What test results would help distinguish a thalassemia carrier from a patient with iron-deficiency anemia?*

a. Serum iron and serum ferritin will be low and TIBC will be increased in iron deficiency; normal in thalassemia minor
b. Serum iron and serum ferritin will be high and TIBC will be decreased in iron deficiency; only TIBC will be increased in thalassemia minor
c. Serum iron and serum ferritin will be normal and TIBC will be decreased in iron deficiency; serum iron and ferritin will be increased and TIBC will be decreased in thalassemia minor
d. Serum iron and serum ferritin will be increased and TIBC will be normal in iron deficiency; serum iron and ferritin will be decreased and TIBC will be increased in thalassemia minor

ANSWERS

1. b (p. 164)
2. c (p. 166)
3. a (p. 170)
4. d (p. 171)
5. d (p. 172)
6. a (p. 173)
7. c (p. 173)
8. b (p. 174)
9. a (p. 176)
10. b (p. 176)
11. c (p. 176)
12. b (p. 176)
13. a (p. 176)
14. c (p. 178)
15. b (p. 177)
16. a (p. 178)
17. d (p. 177)
18. a (p. 178)

CHAPTER 13

KATHRYN ANN GRENIER, M.T.(ASCP), C.L.S.(NCA)

Hemolytic Anemias: Intracorpuscular Defects

V. Paroxysmal Nocturnal Hemoglobinuria

OBJECTIVES

At the end of this chapter, the learner should be able to:
1. Define paroxysmal nocturnal hemoglobinuria.
2. Describe the red cell abnormality associated with paroxysmal nocturnal hemoglobinuria.
3. Describe the three types of paroxysmal nocturnal hemoglobinuria erythrocytes.
4. List clinical features of paroxysmal nocturnal hemoglobinuria.
5. List laboratory findings characteristic of paroxysmal nocturnal hemoglobinuria.
6. Describe the sugar water test (sucrose hemolysis test).
7. Describe Ham's test (acidified serum lysis test).
8. List therapies for treatment of paroxysmal nocturnal hemoglobinuria.

DEFINITION

Paroxysmal nocturnal hemoglobinuria (PNH) is an acquired hemolytic anemia with an insidious onset, resulting in a chronic hemolytic state. In this disorder, the red cell membrane is abnormal, causing the red cells to be highly sensitive to the hemolytic action of complement. This defect also affects leukocytes and platelets.[1] The membrane defect present in the blood cells is the result of an abnor-

mal clone of hematopoietic stem cells. Frequently associated with the chronic hemolysis are leukopenia, thrombocytopenia, hemosiderinuria, and hemoglobinuria.

HISTORY

In 1866, William Gull published the first case of PNH.[2] He described an anemic patient with "hematuria," which varied throughout the day but was the worst in the morning. He recognized that the urinary pigment was due to some breakdown product of the red cells. The second case of PNH was published in 1882 by Paul Strübing, a German physician.[3] He reported on a patient with "paroxysmal hemoglobinuria," and he too noted that this finding was most pronounced in the morning. Strübing related the hemolysis and hemoglobinuria to exercise and to the consumption of beer, and he hypothesized that the abnormality was a defect in the red cells and that hemolysis occurred when the abnormal red cells circulated through the kidney. Furthermore, he believed that an accumulation of carbon dioxide and lactic acid from the previous day's exertion caused the hemolysis. Subsequent to Strübing's report, several other descriptions of PNH appeared. In addition to the hemoglobinuria, Marchiafava[4] and Micheli[5] separately observed and described the presence of "perpetual hemosiderinuria." In 1911, Hijmas van den Bergh,[6] a Dutch physician, made the next significant observation by demonstrating that PNH red cells underwent lysis when the serum and cells were exposed to carbonic acid. This was the first acidified serum lysis test.

In 1930, Thomas H. Ham described in detail the acidified serum lysis test (Ham test).[7,8] He acidified serum to a pH of 6.4 and noted that when mixed with red cells from a patient with PNH, the cells lysed. Ham observed that these cells had an increased sensitivity to some serum hemolytic protein (complement) that caused the cells to lyse when acidified. Ham also demonstrated that some patients with PNH, presenting with chronic hemoly-

sis, had positive acidified serum lysis test results but did not have hemoglobinuria.

Although PNH is fairly rare, much progress and research have increased our understanding of the mechanism of hemolysis, the role of complement, and causes of the defects.

ETIOLOGY AND PATHOPHYSIOLOGY

Paroxysmal nocturnal hemoglobinuria is an acquired intracorpuscular defect due to an abnormality in hematopoietic cell membranes. This abnormality causes the cells, especially the erythrocytes, to be more sensitive than normal to lytic action of complement (Fig. 13-1). This defect is associated with an abnormal clone of hematopoietic stem cells, probably resulting from a mutagenic event that is passed on to its progeny.[9] This defect may occur during the course of bone marrow hypoplasia or recovery from an aplastic episode,[10] although it has also occurred without evidence of marrow hypoplasia.

The membrane defect is due to a deficiency of the complement regulatory proteins decay-accelerating factor (DAF) and homologous restriction factor (HRF).[11-13] Decay-accelerating factor is a membrane protein that accelerates the spontaneous decay of the C3 convertase enzyme for both complement activation pathways. The deficiency of DAF expression is the molecular explanation for the underlying clonal abnormality that affects granulocytes, monocytes, and platelets as well as the erythrocytes in patients with PNH.[11,12,14] Homologous restriction

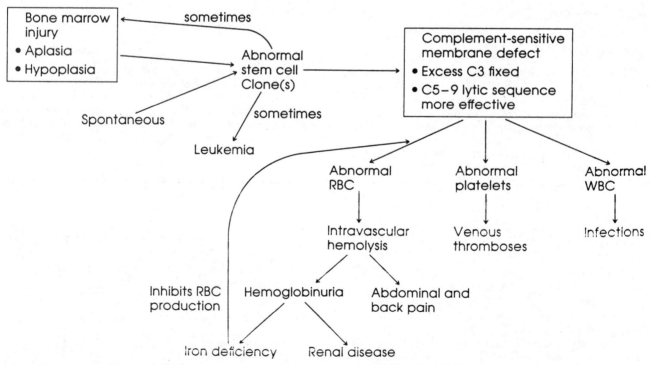

Figure 13-1. Pathophysiology of PNH. (From Beck, WS: Hematology, ed 3. MIT Press, Cambridge, MA, 1982, with permission.)

factor is a membrane regulatory protein that inhibits complement mediated lysis by the C5b-9 complex (membrane attack unit).[12,15] Studies on the affected erythrocytes also show the following abnormalities: decreased membrane acetylcholinesterase activity,[16,17] altered membrane lipids,[18] increased sensitivity to peroxidation,[19] and craters and pits of the erythrocyte membrane as demonstrated by electron microscopy.[20]

Complement has a major role in the pathogenesis of PNH and will be discussed in detail at the end of this chapter. The PNH erythrocytes have been classified into 3 categories based on their interaction with complement. In PNH, the erythrocytes react abnormally with complement components C3 and C5–C9. In PNH I, erythrocytes react normally with complement and are thought to represent residual normal cells because they are similar to normal erythrocytes in all respects.[21] The PNH II erythrocytes have moderate sensitivity to complement component C3 and are three to five times more sensitive to lysis by complement than are normal erythrocytes.[22] PNH II erythrocytes appear to be deficient in the complement regulatory protein DAF only.[11] PNH III erythrocytes are the cells most sensitive to complement, being 15 to 25 times more sensitive to complement component C3 than normal erythrocytes; in addition to binding increased amounts of C3, they also have increased sensitivity to the terminal complement component, C5-C9.[23] PNH III erythrocytes are deficient in both DAF and HRF membrane proteins.[11]

Patients with PNH usually have variable combinations of the three different types of PNH erythrocytes. Eighty percent of all patients with PNH have the combination of PNH I and PNH II cells, whereas the other 20 percent have variable combinations of PNH I, PNH II, and PNH III cells.[23] The degree of hemolysis depends on the proportion of abnormal cells and the severity of the cellular membrane defects. The proportion of abnormal cells varies from patient to patient, and the intensity of the clinical symptoms is related to the percentage of PNH III cells present.

CLINICAL FEATURES

Diverse clinical presentations of PNH are common. The disease most often occurs in middle-aged adults but occasionally occurs in children and the elderly. Both genders are equally affected. Most patients with PNH present with symptoms of anemia, which may be mild to severe and are due to the chronic hemolysis.

The classic presentation of hemoglobinuria, due to significant intravascular hemolysis, is most noticeable in the patient's first morning urine specimen. The cause of this sleep-induced hemolysis may be related to an increased retention of CO_2 and a slight drop in blood pH.[24] Up to 25 percent of patients present with this classic symptom;[23] however, irregular episodes of intravascular hemolysis with hemoglobinuria may be triggered by infections

(most commonly viruses), surgery, menstruation, administration of iron, and a variety of drugs.

In contrast to hemoglobinuria, hemosiderinuria is present in most patients. Recurrent hemolysis results in loss of body iron into the urine. This iron is derived from plasma hemoglobin that is absorbed and catabolized in the renal tubules. Iron-laden tubular cells appear in the urine and can be stained for hemosiderin. Prolonged loss of iron can lead to iron-deficiency anemia, which may mask the diagnosis of PNH.

Patients commonly present with infections, abdominal pain, headaches, and back pain – symptoms thought to be caused by intravascular thrombi. One of the major complications of PNH is the formation of venous thromboses of the portal, mesenteric, or hepatic veins. Formation of these thrombi may be attributed to the activation of complement sensitive platelets by the complement component C3.[10,25] Also, during the thrombotic episodes, features of disseminated intravascular coagulation (DIC) may appear (see Chapter 28).

Aplastic anemia may precede or coexist with PNH. In such cases, pancytopenia and marrow hypoplasia are present. Complement-sensitive erythrocytes occur transiently and in small numbers in certain patients with aplastic anemia. In a few patients complement-sensitive erythrocytes increase in number and persist, making these rare cases of aplastic anemia indistinguishable from PNH.

DIAGNOSIS OF PNH

The diagnosis of PNH depends on the detection of complement-sensitive erythrocytes in the peripheral blood.[10] The diagnosis is difficult if based solely on clinical features and evaluation of the bone marrow and peripheral blood smears. Paroxysmal nocturnal hemoglobinuria should be included in the differential diagnosis of patients with the following disorders: (1) hemolytic anemia of unknown etiology, (2) pancytopenia associated with a hypoplastic or aplastic bone marrow, (3) iron deficiency of unknown etiology, and (4) unexplained episodic hemoglobinuria.[26] It must also be differentiated from other causes of chronic hemolytic anemia (both inherited and acquired), congenital dyserythropoiesis type II, or hereditary erythroblast multinuclearity with positive acidified serum test (HEMPAS), and paroxysmal cold hemoglobinuria.[1]

LABORATORY EVALUATION

Characteristic laboratory findings in PNH are anemia, leukopenia, and thrombocytopenia.[27] The anemia may be mild to severe, depending on the number and type of PNH erythrocytes present. Hemoglobin levels may vary from normal to less than 6 mmol/liter. No characteristic red blood cell morphologic abnormalities are observed in the peripheral blood; in fact, patients most commonly present with normocytic, normochromic anemia. Slight macrocytosis and polychromasia, due to increased numbers of reticulocytes in the peripheral blood, may be seen (**see Color Plate 103.**). This reticulocytosis is a compensatory mechanism for the hemolytic process, and, although the reticulocyte count is usually elevated (5.0 to 10.0 percent), the absolute reticulocyte count may be low with respect to the degree of anemia present. This discrepancy is attributed to the presence of iron deficiency or to the bone marrow stem cell defect itself.[28] With associated iron deficiency, the erythrocytes appear microcytic and hypochromic. During an exacerbation of hemolysis, nucleated red blood cells may be seen in the peripheral blood smear. Spherocytes, although present in other types of hemolytic anemias, are generally not seen. Schistocytes or fragmented red blood cells are occasionally seen with acute hemolysis and may suggest the presence of an intravascular thrombosis.[23]

Also present in PNH erythrocytes is decreased membrane acetylcholinesterase, a finding that is most apparent in the reticulocytes.[10,16] The severity of the decrease in acetylcholinesterase activity parallels the severity of the disease.

Granulocytes, like the red cells, have the same membrane defects that render them more sensitive to the lytic action of complement and to antibodies.[29] When observed by light microscopy and with routine staining, however, they appear to have no characteristic morphologic abnormality. Leukopenia, primarily due to a decrease in granulocytes, is often observed. The granulocytes have decreased leukocyte alkaline phosphatase (LAP) activity ranging from zero to low normal (**see Color Plate 209**). The LAP score can aid in distinguishing PNH from aplastic anemia because in the latter the LAP score is normal to elevated (**see Color Plate 217**).

Platelet counts vary in PNH. Moderate thrombocytopenia is present, with counts ranging from 50 to 100×10^9 per liter. The platelets have the same membrane defect as the erythrocytes and granulocytes. Although decreased in number, the platelets have a normal function and lifespan.

Because almost all patients with PNH have hemosiderin in their urine, testing for urinary hemosiderin will aid in confirming the diagnosis. A random urine sample is centrifuged and the sediment stained with potassium ferrocyanide (Prussian blue), which will detect the presence of hemosiderin. If present, the hemosiderin granules will stain blue.

Hemoglobinuria, when present, must be differentiated from hematuria. This may be accomplished by performing a routine urinalysis with microscopic examination looking for the absence of intact red cells. Hemoglobinuria can lead to the formation of hemoglobin casts in the renal tubules and eventually may cause renal failure.

Other laboratory procedures that aid in diagnosing PNH are nonspecific tests of intravascular and extravascular hemolysis, including indirect bilirubin (increased), plasma hemoglobin (increased), haptoglobin (decreased but not very reliable), and Coombs' test (negative).

As expected, the bone marrow shows erythroid hyperplasia (**see Color Plate 104**). This is the result of increased erythropoiesis subsequent to chronic hemolysis. The increased erythropoiesis is usually normoblastic, although some megaloblastic change may be noted. Occasionally, a hypoplastic or even aplastic marrow is seen. The bone marrow usually reveals adequate numbers of myeloid and platelet precursors, except after an aplastic episode when the myeloid and platelet precursors are decreased. Bone marrow iron stains often reveal decreased iron stores.

DIAGNOSTIC TESTS

Sugar Water Test (Sucrose Hemolysis Test) (Color Plate 101)

The sugar water test is used as a screening procedure when the diagnosis of PNH is considered. The sucrose provides a medium of low ionic strength that promotes the binding of complement, especially C3, to the red cell membranes. The low ionic–strength solution used in the sugar water test activates complement via the classic or alternate pathway. The complement-sensitive PNH red cells are lysed, whereas normal cells will be unaffected.

To perform the sugar water test, the patient's cells are first washed, then mixed with ABO-Rh-compatible serum and sugar water. The tubes are incubated at room temperature for 30 minutes, after which time they are centrifuged. The percent hemolysis is then determined. Ten to 80 percent red cell lysis is seen in PNH (**see Color Plate 101**). Less than 5 percent red cell lysis is usually considered negative for PNH. A small amount of lysis (less than 5 percent) has been observed in patients with megaloblastic anemia, autoimmune hemolytic anemia, and leukemia. False-negative results occasionally occur if the serum lacks complement or if an unbuffered sucrose solution is used.

However, a definitive diagnosis of PNH depends on the results obtained with the Ham's test.

Ham's Test (Acidified Serum Lysis Test) (Color Plate 102)

The Ham's test, or acidified serum lysis test, is used to confirm the diagnosis of PNH. Serum is acidified, which activates complement via the alternate pathway and enhances the binding of C3 to the cell membrane. The PNH erythrocytes lyse because they are deficient in the membrane proteins DAF and HRF, rendering them more sensitive to lysis by complement. Normal erythrocytes will be unaffected. In order to confirm a positive Ham's test result, the following characteristics must be demonstrated: (1) hemolysis occurs with the patient's cells and not with control cells, and (2) hemolysis is enhanced by acidified serum and does not occur with the heat-inactivated serum[28] (heating serum to 56°C for 30 minutes inactivates complement activity). For an outline of the Ham's test procedure and

Table 13-1. **ACIDIFIED SERUM LYSIS TEST**

	1	2	3	4	5	6	7
Fresh normal serum	0.5 ml	0.5 ml			0.5 ml	0.5 ml	
Patient's serum			0.05 ml				
Heat-inactivated normal serum				0.5 ml			0.5 ml
0.2 N HCl		0.05 ml	0.05 ml	0.05 ml		0.05 ml	0.05 ml
50% patient's red cells	0.05 ml	0.05 ml	0.05 ml	0.05 ml			
50% normal red cells					0.05 ml	0.05 ml	0.05 ml
Pattern of lysis in positive test	Trace	+++	++	−	−	−	−

Source: Adapted from Dacie, JV and Lewis, SM: Practical Haematology, ed 4. Grune & Stratton, New York, 1968; from Henry, G: Clinical Diagnosis and Management by Laboratory Methods, ed 17. WB Saunders, Philadelphia, 1984, p 673.

results interpretation, refer to Table 13-1 (**see Color Plate 102**). This test is specific for PNH when it is shown that the patient's own serum is capable of lysing his or her own cells.[30]

A positive Ham's test result will be seen in the rare disorder congenital dyserythropoietic anemia (CDA) type II, or HEMPAS. In this disorder, lysis does not occur with the patient's own serum; lysis in this case is due to an unusual red cell antigen that reacts with IgM, a complement-activating antibody present in many normal sera.[27] The sugar water test for this disorder will also yield a negative result. Spherocytes also lyse in acidified serum due to the decreased pH; therefore, they will lyse in the tube containing the complement inactivated serum.[27]

THERAPY

No specific therapeutic regimen is employed in the treatment of PNH. Treatment is usually directed toward the complications that arise from infections, anemia, and thromboses. In uncomplicated mild cases, therapy is not needed.

In patients with severe iron-deficiency anemia, iron therapy is usually given, either orally or parenterally. However, patients may experience hemolytic episodes after iron therapy. Iron therapy causes an increase in the production of normal as well as abnormal erythrocytes. Oral administration of iron produces less hemolysis, but the iron loss as hemosiderin may be so great that the oral doses cannot compensate for the iron deficiency present.[31]

In the severely anemic patient, blood transfusions are required; however, stored whole blood or packed red cells may cause an exacerbation of hemolysis. This hemolysis is thought to be due to infusion of activated complement components; therefore, it is best to use washed or frozen deglycerolized red blood cells. Transfusions cause an increase in the red cell mass and hemoglobin level, while at the same time causing a temporary decrease in the production of the abnormal erythrocytes.

Hemolytic episodes associated with PNH may be controlled with the use of adrenocorticosteroids. Patients with any degree of bone marrow hypopla-

sia respond best to therapy with androgens. The androgens have a stimulatory effect on erythropoiesis and are thought to inhibit complement activation. Although androgens may be helpful, one must consider the possible side effects. Prednisone, a corticosteroid, has been used with success in suppression of hemolytic episodes. High doses of prednisone have proven the most beneficial but are associated with various side effects. However, moderate to high doses given on alternate days significantly decrease the side effects that may occur.[31]

Anticoagulant therapy is indicated in patients who are prone to the formation of venous thromboses or in whom a known life-threatening thrombosis exists. Heparin is the anticoagulant of choice in treating thromboses, but it can precipitate a hemolytic crisis. Administered in low doses, heparin can activate complement and thereby increase the probability of a hemolytic crisis.[32] However, when administered in high doses, heparin has been effective in the treatment of thromboses and has been shown to inactivate complement, thereby diminishing the chance of a hemolytic crisis.[32]

Certain patients with PNH have such severe bone marrow hypoplasia that a bone marrow transplant may be indicated; these transplants have been reported successful. After the transplant the abnormal clone of cells may be eliminated and replaced by a normal cell population.

CLINICAL COURSE AND PROGNOSIS

Paroxysmal nocturnal hemoglobinuria is a chronic disease. Patients have survived 20 to 43 years after diagnosis, although the average survival is 10 years.[27] The most common cause of death is thromboembolism. Patients with bone marrow hypoplasia often die of infections or hemorrhage.[23] In a minority of patients, the disease may decrease in severity or completely disappear with time. Some patients have complete clinical remissions with persisting laboratory abnormalities. Occasionally, acute myelogenous leukemia develops in patients with PNH.[33,34] When PNH transforms to acute leukemia, the abnormal complement-sensitive population of erythrocytes disappears.[27] Paroxysmal nocturnal hemoglobinuria has also been classified as a preleukemic or myelodysplastic syndrome.[35]

ROLE OF COMPLEMENT

Complement is a group of serum proteins that interact with each other to bring about, among other events, complement-dependent cell-mediated lysis. Complement can be activated by two different routes, the classic or the alternate (properdin pathway).

Classic Pathway

Activation of the classic pathway is initiated by immune complexes containing IgG (IgG1, IgG2, IgG3) or IgM. The first complement component, C1 consists of three subunits — C1q, C1r, C1s — as well as calcium (recognition unit). C1q initiates the complement cascade by interacting with the Fc (crystallizable fragment) portion of the immunoglobulin (Fig. 13–2). C1q then causes the activation of C1r, which then activates C1s. (A bar across the top of a

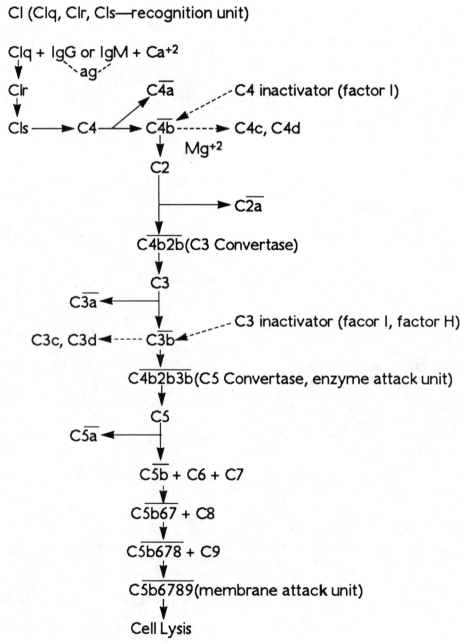

Figure 13–2. Classical pathway of complement activation.

complement component denotes its active form.) C4 is the second complement protein to be activated. This occurs when C1s cleaves C4 into its activated components, C4a, which remains in the plasma, and C4b, a small portion of which attaches to the cell membrane with the rest remaining in the plasma, inactivated. C2 attaches to C4b in the presence of magnesium and is then cleaved by C1s into the a and b subunits. C2b remains attached to C4b and forms the enzyme C3 convertase (C4b2b), and C2a is released into the plasma.

Amplification of complement activity occurs now with the action of C3 convertase on C3. This enzyme (C4b2b) cleaves C3 into its active components, C3a and C3b, and is able to cleave hundreds of C3 molecules. C3a is released into the plasma and acts as an

anaphylatoxin. C3b binds to the cell membrane and combines with C4b2b to form another enzyme, C5 convertase (C4b2b3b). Some of the C3b molecules attach to other sites on the cell, are inactivated (C3bi), or are cleaved by C3 inactivator to C3c, which is released into the plasma, and to C3d, an inactive subunit that remains attached to the cell. The components C4, C3, and C2 are referred to collectively as the enzyme activation unit.

C5 convertase (C4b2b3b) cleaves C5 into the components C5a, which is released into the plasma and acts as an anaphylatoxin and a chemotactic agent, and C5b, which binds C6 and C7 to the cell membrane. Membrane-bound C5b67 causes binding of C8, resulting in immediate ion flux into the cell. The C5b678 complex can bind up to six C9 mole-

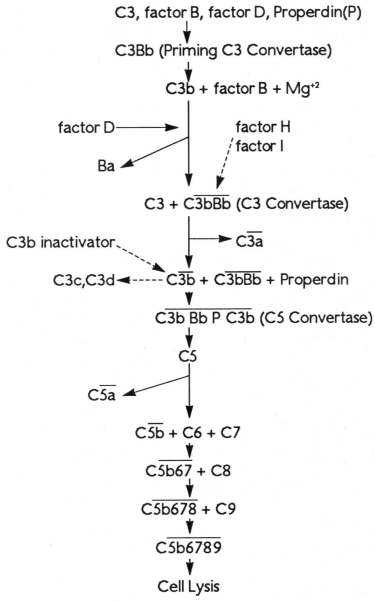

Figure 13-3. Alternate pathway of complement activation.

cules, together forming the membrane attack unit, C5b6789, which causes cell lysis and accelerated movement of ions into the cell. With binding of C9, cell lysis results (Fig. 13–2).

Complement activity is regulated by certain inhibitors (C1s inhibitor, C3b inactivator, and C4 inactivator) and by the instability of certain components (C4b2b, and C4b2b3b).[36]

Alternate (Properdin) Pathway

The alternate, or properdin, pathway of complement activation also results in cell lysis but by a different mechanism and group of proteins. The alternate pathway bypasses the complement components C1, C2, and C4 and enters at C3. This pathway consists of a distinct group of proteins: complement component C3; factor B, which is enzymatically cleaved into fragments Bb (biologically active) and Ba; factor D, which cleaves factor B; properidin (P), a serum protein that stabilizes the C3bBb complex; and factor H (C3b inactivator accelerator), which aids in controlling activation of the alternate pathway (Fig. 13–3).[37]

The alternate pathway may be triggered by certain microorganisms, polysaccharides, liposaccharides, aggregates of IgA, and cells or particles even in the absence of specific antibody. Present in the plasma are small amounts of a "priming" C3 convertase (C3Bb). The priming C3 convertase is produced continuously owing to spontaneous interaction of intact C3, factor B, factor D, and properdin, an event not requiring activating substances. This results in the formation of small amounts of C3b. C3b binds to the cell surface and, under appropriate conditions and in the presence of magnesium, causes the attachment of factor B. The bound factor B is cleaved by factor D, releasing the Ba fragment and uncovering the C3 cleaving site on the Bb fragment. The C3bBb complex can rapidly lose activity or disassociate unless properdin is present. Properdin binds to the C3b part of the complex and stabilizes it. The C3bBb fragment (C3 convertase) then cleaves more C3, resulting in C3a and C3b fragments. A complex of C3bBbPC3b (C5 convertase) forms and cleaves C5 to its fragments, C5a and C5b. C5b along with C6, C7, C8, and C9 form the membrane attack unit, the same way as in the classic pathway, which results in cell lysis (Fig. 13–3).

Control mechanisms also exist in the alternate pathway, just as they do in the classic pathway. Spontaneous dissolution of C3bBb may occur, or factor H with the factor I protein may compete with factor B, as may Bb for the C3b fragment, then blocking the formation of C3 convertase (C3bBb). Factor H may increase the susceptibility of C3b to be destroyed by C3b inactivator.[37]

CASE STUDY

A 43-year-old man presented to his physician with complaints of lower back pain, fatigue, easy bruising, and a sudden onset of dark urine upon arising in the morning. Laboratory studies and a bone marrow aspirate were then ordered by his physician, which disclosed the following:

1. Complete blood cell count (CBC)

Hct	28%
WBC	3.3×10^9/L
Platelet count	76.0×10^9/L
Reticulocytes	5.1%
Corrected reticulocytes	3.2%

   Differential:

Segmented neutrophils	34%
Lymphocytes	64%
Monocytes	2%
NRBC	1

   1+ Poikilocytosis
   2+ Anisocytosis
   2+ Polychromasia

   Color Plate 103 shows the peripheral blood smear from this patient.
2. The chemistry profile was normal except for an increased lactic dehydrogenase (LDH) value (780 IU/liter) and bilirubin (total 2.9 mg/dl, direct 0.4 mg/dl).
3. A urinalysis was performed and was positive for hemoglobin.
4. The bone marrow aspirate revealed a hypercellular marrow with relative erythroid hyperplasia. There were adequate numbers of myeloid and platelet precursors (**see Color Plate 104**).

Further studies were then performed after initial tests were finished.

5. Urinary hemosiderin: Positive
6. Sugar water test: Positive (12%)
7. Ham's test: Positive

Diagnosis: Paroxysmal nocturnal hemoglobinuria

REFERENCES

1. Williams, WJ, et al: Hematology, ed 2. McGraw-Hill, New York, 1977, p 560.
2. Gull, WP: A case of intermittent hematuria, with remarks. Guys Hospital Reports 12:381, 1866.
3. Strübing, P: Paroxysmale hamoglobinurie. Dtsch Med Wochenschr 8:1, 1882.
4. Marchiafava, E: Anemia emolitica con emosiderinuria perpitua. Policlinico (sez med) 18:241, 1931.
5. Micheli, F: Anemia (splenomegalia) emolitica con emoglobinuria-emosiderinuria tipo Marchiafava. Hematologica 12:101, 1931.
6. Hijmas, van den Bergh, AA: Ictere hemolytique avec crises hemoglubinuriques. Fragilite globulaire Rev Med 31:63, 1911.
7. Ham, TH and Dingle, JH: Studies on destruction of red blood cells—II. Chronic hemolytic anemia with paroxysmal nocturnal hemoglobinuria—Certain immunological aspects of the hemolytic mechanism with special reference to serum complement. J Clin Invest 18:657, 1939.
8. Ham, TH: Chronic hemolytic anemia with paroxysmal nocturnal hemoglobinuria—A study of the mechanism of hemolysis in relation to acid base equilibrium. N Engl J Med 217:915, 1937.
9. Rosse, WF: Phosphatidylinositol-linked proteins and paroxysmal nocturnal hemoglobinuria. Blood 75(8):1595, 1990.
10. Beck, WS: Hematology, ed 3. MIT Press, Cambridge, MA, 1982, p 211.
11. Nicholson-Weller, A, Spicer, DB, and Austen, KF: Deficiency

of the complement regulatory protein, 'decay accelerating factor' on membranes of granulocytes, monocytes and platelets in paroxysmal nocturnal hemoglobinuria. N Engl J Med 312:1091, 1985.

12. Rosse, WF: Paroxysmal nocturnal hemoglobinuria and decay accelerating factor. Annu Rev Med 41:431, 1990.
13. Zalman, LS, et al: Deficiency of the homologous factor in paroxysmal nocturnal hemoglobinuria. J Exp Med 165:572, 1987.
14. Eichner, ER, et al: Hematology—1989, Education program, American Society of Hematology, The Anemias; Paroxysmal Nocturnal Hemoglobinuria, Atlanta, 1989, pp 3–4.
15. Schonermark, S, et al: Homologous species restriction in lysis of human erythrocytes: a membrane derived protein with C8-binding capacity functions as an inhibitor. J Immunol 136:1772, 1986.
16. Chow, FL, Telen, MJ, and Rosse, WF: The acetylcholinesterase defect in paroxysmal nocturnal hemoglobinuria: Evidence that the enzyme is absent from the cell membrane. Blood 66:940, 1986.
17. Metz, J, et al: Acetylcholinesterase activity of the erythrocytes in paroxysmal nocturnal hemoglobinuria in relation to the severity of the disease. Br J Haematol 6:372, 1960.
18. Mengal, CE, et al: Studies of paroxysmal nocturnal hemoglobinuria erythrocytes: Increased lysis and lipid peroxide formation by hydrogen peroxide. J Clin Invest 46:1715, 1967.
19. Mengal, CE, et al: Biochemistry of PNH cells; nature of the membrane defect. Ser Haematol 5:88, 1972.
20. Lewis, SM, et al: Electron microscope study of PNH red cells and AET-treated normal cells (PNH-like), J Clin Pathol 24:667, 1971.
21. Rosse, WF and Adams, JP: The membrane abnormalities in paroxysmal nocturnal hemoglobinuria. Prog Clin Biol Res 30:457, 1979.
22. Dacie, JV: Paroxysmal nocturnal hemoglobinuria. Sangre 25:890, 1980.
23. Wintrobe, ME, et al: Clinical Hematology, ed 8. Lea & Febiger, Philadelphia, 1981, pp 312, 978.
24. Hemolytic anemia caused by intrinsic red-cell defects. In McKenzie SB: Textbook of Hematology. Lea & Febiger, 1988, pp 210–212.
25. Rosse, WF: Paroxysmal nocturnal hemoglobinuria in aplastic anemia. Clin Haematol 7(3):541, 1978.
26. Sun, NC: Hematology—An Atlas and Diagnostic Guide, ed 1. WB Saunders, Philadelphia, 1983, p 90.
27. Dacie, JV and Lewis, SM: Paroxysmal nocturnal hemoglobinuria, clinical manifestations, hematology and nature of the disease. Ser Haematol 5:3, 1972.
28. Kjeldsberg, C, et al: Hematologic Disease, Practical Diagnosis, ed 2. ASCP Press, Chicago, 1989, p 162.
29. Okuda, K, et al: Membrane expression of decay accelerating factor on neutrophils from normal individuals and patients with paroxysmal nocturnal hemoglobinuria. Blood 75(5):1186, 1990.
30. Hoffbrand, AV and Lewis, SM: Post Graduate Hematology, ed 2. Appleton-Century-Crofts, New York, 1981, p 232.
31. Rosse, WF: Treatment of paroxysmal nocturnal hemoglobinuria. Blood 60(1):20, 1982.
32. Logue, GL: Effects of heparin on complement activation and lysis of paroxysmal nocturnal hemoglobinuria red cells. Blood 50(20):239, 1977.
33. Cowell, DE, Pasquale, DN, and Dekker, P: Paroxysmal nocturnal hemoglobinuria terminating as acute leukemia. Cancer 43:1914, 1979.
34. Krause, JR: Paroxysmal nocturnal hemoglobinuria and acute nonlymphoblastic leukemia. Cancer 51:2078, 1983.
35. Rosse, WF: Paroxysmal nocturnal hemoglobinuria—present status and future prospects. West J Med 132(3):219, 1980.
36. Complement. In Muller, LE, et al: Manual of Laboratory Immunology, ed 2. Lea & Febiger, 1991, pp 120–141.
37. Fearson, DT and Austen, KF: The alternate pathway of complement—a system of host resistance to microbial infections. N Engl J Med 303:259, 1980.

BIBLIOGRAPHY

Dacie, JV and Lewis, SM: Paroxysmal nocturnal hemoglobinuria, clinical manifestations, hematology and nature of the disease. Ser Haematol 5:3, 1972.
Forman, K, et al: Paroxysmal nocturnal hemoglobinuria—a clinicopathological study of 26 cases. Acta Haematol 71:217, 1984.
Goetz, O and Muller-Eberhard, HJ: The alternate pathway of complement activation. Adv Immunol 24:1, 1976.
Hartman, RC and Jenkins, DE Jr: The "sugar water" test for paroxysmal nocturnal hemoglobinuria. N Engl J Med 275:155, 1966.
Hartman, RC, Jenkins, DE Jr, and Arnold, AB: Diagnostic specificity of sucrose hemolysis test for paroxysmal nocturnal hemoglobinuria. Blood 35:462, 1970.
Muller-Eberhard, HJ: Complement. Annu Rev Biochem 44:697, 1975.
Rosse, WF: Paroxysmal nocturnal hemoglobinuria—present status and future prospects. West J Med 132(3):219, 1980.

QUESTIONS

1. *Which statement best describes paroxysmal nocturnal hemoglobinuria?*
   a. Acquired hemolytic anemia associated with cellular membrane abnormalities
   b. Congenital hemolytic anemia associated with the inflammatory response
   c. Acquired or congenital hemolytic anemia associated with enzyme deficiencies
   d. Hemolytic anemia of unknown origin, associated with autoantibodies

2. *What causes the red cell defect of PNH?*
   a. Rare red cell antigens
   b. Deficiency of decay accelerating factor (DAF) and homologous restriction factor (HRF), complement regulatory proteins
   c. Excessive amounts of complement components C5–C9
   d. G6PD enzyme deficiency

3. *Which type of PNH erythrocyte is most sensitive to lysis by complement?*
   a. PNH I
   b. PNH II
   c. PNH III
   d. PNH I and II equally sensitive

4. *Which list is the most complete for clinical features of PNH?*
   a. Hemoglobinuria, hemosiderinuria, abdominal pain, headaches, and back pain
   b. Weakness, fatigue, hepatosplenomegaly, back pain
   c. Recurrent infections, skin ulcers, spontaneous fractures, dental problems
   d. Persistent bacterial infections, jaundice, kernicterus, and weight loss

5. *What nonspecific laboratory findings are characteristic for PNH?*
   a. Microcytic, hypochromic anemia; leukocytosis; thrombocytosis; decreased indirect bilirubin
   b. Macrocytic, hypochromic anemia; leukopenia with decreased lymphocytes; normal to

elevated LAP; thrombocytopenia; increased haptoglobin

c. Normocytic, hypochromic anemia; leukopenia with decreased neutrophils; thrombocytosis with giant platelets; decreased plasma hemoglobin

d. Normocytic, normochromic anemia; leukopenia with decreased granulocytes; low LAP; thrombocytopenia; urine hemosiderin

6. *Which of the following is a correct description of the sugar water test (sucrose hemolysis test)?*
   a. PNH cells are lysed by complement after exposure to low-ionic–strength sugar water.
   b. PNH cells are lysed by antibody and complement after heating to 56°C in sugar water solution (5%).
   c. Patient's serum is acidified to enhance complement binding and lysis of patient cells.
   d. Patient's serum is heat-inactivated and treated with HCl; complement is added; patient cell lysis occurs.

7. *What is a correct description of Ham's test (acidified serum lysis test)? (Use answer choices for question 6.)*

8. *Which of the following is not usually a treatment for PNH?*
   a. Anticoagulant therapy
   b. Blood transfusion/marrow transplant
   c. Adrenocorticosteroids
   d. Immunosuppressive therapy

ANSWERS

1. a (p. 183)
2. b (p. 184)
3. c (p. 185)
4. a (p. 185)
5. d (p. 185–186)
6. a (p. 186)
7. c (p. 186–187)
8. d (p. 187)

CHAPTER 14

DENISE M. HARMENING, Ph.D., M.T.(ASCP), C.L.S.(NCA)
RALPH L. B. GREEN, B.App.Sci.(MLS), F.A.I.M.L.S.

Hemolytic Anemias: Extracorpuscular Defects

VI. Immune and Nonimmune Hemolytic Anemia

OBJECTIVES

At the end of this chapter, the learner should be able to:

1. List mechanisms of immune hemolysis.
2. Define alloimmune hemolytic anemia.
3. Characterize immediate hemolytic transfusion reactions.
4. Characterize delayed hemolytic transfusion reactions.
5. Describe the causes of hemolytic disease of the newborn.
6. List hematologic findings for hemolytic disease of the newborn.
7. List treatments for hemolytic disease of the newborn.
8. Define autoimmune hemolytic anemia.
9. Characterize warm autoimmune hemolytic anemia.
10. List features of cold agglutinin syndrome.
11. Describe the principle of the Donath-Landsteiner test used for paroxysmal cold hemoglobinuria.
12. List mechanisms for drug-induced immune hemolytic anemia.
13. List classifications for nonimmune hemolytic anemias.
14. Describe the laboratory diagnosis for malarial infection.
15. Name other organisms associated with hemolytic anemia.

IMMUNE HEMOLYTIC ANEMIA

Immune hemolytic anemia is defined as a shortened red cell survival mediated through the immune response, specifically by humoral antibody. Immune-mediated hemolysis represents the results of an acquired extracorpuscular abnormality associated with demonstrable antibodies, as opposed to the inherited intracorpuscular defects described in Chapters 9 through 12, which represent intrinsic abnormalities of the patient's red cells.

Mechanisms of Immune Hemolysis

Immune hemolysis results from the premature removal from the circulation of red cells sensitized by antibody with or without complement. Removal is facilitated either by direct lysis or by phagocytosis of the cell.

Direct lysis usually occurs within the vascular system and results from activation of the classic complement pathway by IgG or IgM antibodies. The ability of IgG antibodies to activate complement is dependent on the IgG subclass. In order of efficiency IgG3 is greater than IgG1, which is greater than IgG2, whereas IgG4 is not capable of activating complement. The biologic properties of the IgG subclasses are summarized in Table 14–1. In addition, the concentration and distribution of IgG antibody on the red cell surface is also of importance, as it is necessary to have at least two antibody molecules in proximity, to allow crosslinking of at least two of the six receptors on C1q to start the activation process. The ability to get sufficient IgG molecules on the red cell surface in close relationship to one another is dependent as much on the number and distribution of red cell antigens as on the concentration and avidity of the antibody itself. Immunoglobulin M is a very efficient activator of complement, largely because of its pentameric structure. One molecule of IgM is theoretically capable of initiating complement activation by the classic pathway. Intravascular hemolysis requires the classic complement pathway going through to completion. This will occur only where the activation process is intense and overwhelms the natural regulatory steps in complement activation.

In recent years considerable interest has been shown in another mechanism of direct lysis of antibody-coated red cells. This mechanism is referred to as antibody-dependent cellular cytotoxicity (ADCC) and has been demonstrated in vitro; however, there is considerable conjecture as to whether the mechanism operates in vivo. Antibody-dependent cellular cytotoxicity results from IgG1- and/or IgG3-sensitized red cells interacting with effector cells having Fcγ1 and Fcγ3 receptors. Such cells include K cells, monocyte/macrophages, and granulocytes, specifically neutrophils. The process of hemolysis appears to result from the release of lytic enzymes from the effector cell, which act on the red cell membrane. The site of ADCC-mediated red cell destruction in the body is unknown.

Phagocytosis of red cells occurs extravascularly within either the spleen or the liver as a result of interaction with fixed phagocytic cells of the reticuloendothelial system (RES). Red cells sensitized with IgG1 or IgG3 antibodies are preferentially removed by splenic sequestration. As a result of its vascular structure, blood passing through the spleen becomes hemoconcentrated, which alters the ratio between free IgG in the plasma and cell-

Table 14–1. **BIOLOGIC PROPERTIES OF IgG ISOTYPES**

Characteristic	IgG1	IgG2	IgG3	IgG4
% Total serum IgG	65–70	23–28	4–7	3–4
Complement fixation (classic pathway)	Yes	Yes	Yes	No
Binding to macrophage Fc receptors	Yes	No	Yes	No
Placental transfer	Yes	Yes	Yes	Yes
Biologic half-life (days)	21	21	7–8	21

Source: Pittiglio, Baldwin, and Sohmer, 1983, p 66, with permission.

bound IgG. This permits the antibody-coated red cells to interact with the Fc receptors on the macrophages that line the splenic cords of the red pulp. This interaction may result in either complete or partial phagocytosis of the cell. In the latter case the cell membrane reforms to produce an irregularly shaped microspherocyte caused by alterations in the cell surface-to-volume ratio. These cells lack deformability and become physically trapped in the spleen; those that do escape from the spleen can be seen in the peripheral blood, and their presence is indicative of immune-mediated hemolysis (**see Color Plate 105**).

As previously mentioned, both IgG and IgM antibodies are capable of activating complement; however, the activation process does not always go to completion and in most cases will be stopped at the C3b stage owing to the action of factor I (FI), factor H (FH), and complement receptor 1 (CR1). Monocytes and macrophages have receptors for the breakdown products of C3. Complement receptor 1 interacts with the C3b molecule to produce immune adherence. In conjunction with FI, C3b is inactivated to iC3b, which is capable of interacting with CR1; however, iC3b is the only ligand for another complement receptor (that is, CR3), which is also found on monocytes and macrophages. Interaction of iC3b with CR3 results in phagocytosis of the target cell. As the active sites on C3b and iC3b are not exposed on native C3, the hemoconcentration of blood in the spleen does not contribute significantly to destruction of complement-coated cells in that organ. However, cells coated with both IgG and C3 are phago-

cytized more efficiently in the spleen than if they are sensitized by IgG alone.

The organ with the largest concentration of CR3-bearing macrophages is the liver; consequently this is the major site of destruction for cells coated with complement alone. There is little if any destruction of cells sensitized with IgG in the liver because of the high concentration of free IgG. Cells sensitized with IgG and C3 will be removed in both the spleen and the liver. Figure 14–1 summarizes the different mechanisms of immune hemolysis.

The presence and extent of immune hemolysis is the result of a number of interacting factors, which are summarized in Table 14–2.

Classification of Immune Hemolytic Anemias

Numerous classifications of immune hemolytic anemias have been proposed; however, three broad categories are usually used:
1. Alloimmune
2. Autoimmune
3. Drug-induced
In an alloimmune response, patients produce alloantibodies to foreign red cell antigens introduced into their circulation either through transfusion, pregnancy, or organ (such as bone marrow) transplantation. An autoimmune response occurs when patients produce autoantibodies directed against their own red cell antigens. A drug-induced immune hemolytic anemia is usually the result of a

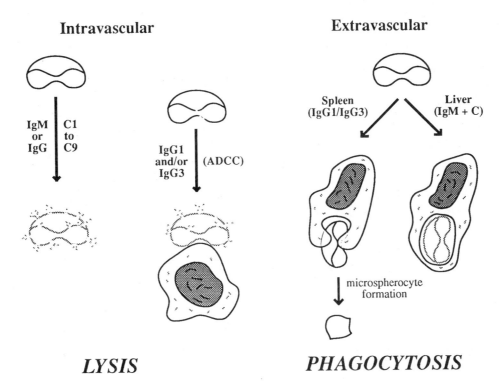

Figure 14–1. Mechanisms of immune hemolysis.

Table 14-2. **FACTORS INFLUENCING THE PRESENCE AND EXTENT OF IMMUNE HEMOLYSIS**

Antibody
Immunoglobulin class and subclass
Concentration
Avidity
Thermal reactivity (determined by the nature of the predominant noncovalent bonds formed at the time of the antigen antibody reaction)

Antigen
Number and density
Cellular distribution
Presence of soluble antigen

Complement
Concentration of complement factors
Concentration and activity of regulating factors

Reticuloendothelial System
Activity of phagocytic cells (influenced by underlying disease processes, generation and activity of lymphokines and interleukins, and any concurrent drug therapy)

Table 14-3. **CLINICAL FEATURES OF ACUTE HEMOLYTIC TRANSFUSION REACTION**

Fever	Hemoglobinuria
Chills	Shock
Chest pains	Generalized bleeding
Hypotension	Oliguria
Nausea	Anuria
Flushing	Back pain
Dyspnea	Pain at infusion site

patient's production of antibodies to a particular drug or drug complex, with subsequent damage to the patient's red cells.

ALLOIMMUNE HEMOLYTIC ANEMIA

Alloimmunization is the process in which the immune system of an individual is stimulated by foreign antigen with production of the corresponding antibody. The antibody produced by this immune response is termed an alloantibody. The antibody coats the foreign red cells introduced into the circulation, resulting in hemolysis. Alloantibody, or alloimmune hemolytic anemia may result from: (1) transfusion of blood (exposure to foreign donor red cell antigens) or (2) pregnancy (foreign antigens on fetal cells released into the mother's circulation). In recent years organ transplantation, particularly of bone marrow, has also been associated with the production of alloantibodies.

Transfusion Reactions

Hemolytic transfusion reactions may be classified as immediate (acute) or delayed. *Immediate hemolytic transfusion reactions* are characterized by acute intravascular hemolysis and are most commonly associated with ABO IgM isoantibodies, which activate complement.

Clinical features of an immediate transfusion reaction may be associated with a variety of signs and symptoms. Typical symptoms are fever, shaking, chills, pain at the infusion site, nausea, vomiting, lower back pain, hypotension, and chest pain (Table 14-3). In an anesthetized patient, the reaction may manifest itself as disseminated intravascular coagulation (DIC) with generalized bleeding and shock.

The reaction is termed "immediate" or "acute" because its manifestations occur within minutes to hours of transfusion of incompatible blood.

The process of hemolysis is initiated by the binding of the patient's alloantibody to the donor's (foreign) corresponding red cell antigen, which activates the complement cascade to completion, causing intravascular lysis of the transfused erythrocytes. (For a review of the process of intravascular hemolysis and the complement cascade, see Chapters 2 and 11 and the introductory section of this chapter.) The immediate type of transfusion reaction is most commonly associated with ABO incompatibilities. These reactions are severe because potent naturally occurring IgM and IgG anti-A or anti-B and, in the case of group O patients, anti-A,B are circulating in the patient's plasma at the time of transfusion.

The majority of other blood group antibodies destroy foreign red cells through extravascular hemolysis, since complement activation is only partial or is absent. However, in rare circumstances some IgG antibodies can bind complement and induce intravascular hemolysis. The most common offender is anti-Jk[a] (Kidd blood group system).

Laboratory findings include signs of a hemolytic process. Figure 14-2 charts the sequence of events that occur as a result of an intravascular hemolytic episode. Within hours plasma haptoglobin is depleted because as little as 5 ml of lysed red cells can bind all of the available haptoglobin. It is important to have a pretransfusion baseline level of haptoglobin for comparison with the post-transfusion level because it is an acute phase reactant protein and many factors affect its synthesis and could therefore lead to misinterpretation of results. Within 24 hours, the liver will synthesize new haptoglobin, returning the levels to normal.

Other laboratory findings include the presence of free plasma hemoglobin resulting in hemoglobinemia. The free hemoglobin is filtered through the kidneys, resulting in hemoglobinuria and hemosiderinuria. Hemoglobinuria may be confused with hematuria, especially when the urine is bright red. The urine in hemoglobinuria is clear, whereas in hematuria it is smoky. Analysis of the urinary sediment will usually distinguish the two quite readily, as intact red cells will be found in hematuria, provided that the osmolarity is not too low. Hemoglobinuria is always accompanied by hemoglobinemia.

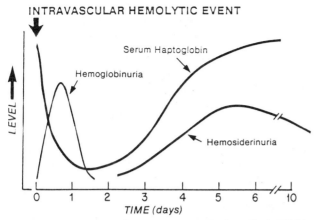

Figure 14–2. Indicators of acute intravascular hemolysis. Within a few hours of an acute hemolytic event, free hemoglobin is cleared from plasma and the serum haptoglobin falls to undetectable levels; hemoglobinuria ceases soon after. If no further hemolysis occurs, the serum haptoglobin level recovers, and methemalbumin disappears within several days. The urinary hemosiderin can provide more lasting evidence of the hemolytic event.

Other abnormal laboratory findings include elevated bilirubin (primarily indirect). Table 14–4 summarizes the laboratory findings of an acute, or immediate, hemolytic transfusion reaction. (For a review of the process of intravascular hemolysis and the laboratory parameters used to monitor the severity of the hemolysis, see Chapter 2.)

Treatment of an immediate hemolytic transfusion reaction focuses on prompt termination of the transfusion. Therapy is then directed toward maintaining diuresis, management of coagulopathy, promoting adequate renal blood flow, and treatment of hypotension.

The most common type of *delayed hemolytic transfusion reaction (DHTR)* results from an anamnestic or secondary response to transfused red cell antigens. This occurs in previously sensitized patients whose alloantibody level has dropped to the point of being undetectable, after initial stimulation. As a result, the initial antibody screen performed on the patient's pretransfusion serum sample yields a negative result. In most cases of DHTR, the antibodies implicated in the reactions are IgG immunoglobulins and are usually demonstrable in the patient's serum as early as 48 hours after transfusion. This type of reaction is termed "delayed" because it takes time for the patient to produce increasing levels of IgG antibodies that attack and destroy the transfused red cells. Characteristically the reaction may occur anywhere from 2 to 10 days following transfusion. The delay in the reaction and their generally mild nature means that many DHTRs may go undetected.

As with most hemolytic anemias, erythrocyte destruction is primarily extravascular, occurring within the cells of the reticuloendothelial system. As a result, spherocytes may be characteristically seen on the peripheral blood smear. (For a review of the process see Chapter 1 and also Mechanisms of Immune Hemolysis in this chapter.)

Hemoglobinemia and hemoglobinuria are not present as described in immediate hemolytic transfusion reactions. However, there are increases both in serum bilirubin (primarily indirect) and in urobilinogen in the urine and stools. Depending on when a patient is tested following transfusion, antibodies may be found coating the circulating transfused cells (positive direct antiglobin test result) and in the serum (positive antibody screen result).

Symptoms of a DHTR include fever, an unexpected fall in hemoglobin, mild jaundice, and anemia. Treatment is rarely necessary, and investigation focuses on accurately identifying the antibody to ensure that blood for future transfusions will be antigen negative for the patient's corresponding antibody. Table 14–5 lists the antibodies most commonly implicated in DHTR.

Hemolytic Disease of the Newborn

Hemolytic disease of the newborn (HDN) is an immune hemolytic disorder in which red cells of the fetus and newborn are destroyed by maternal IgG antibody. Generally, maternal antibodies provide the fetus with immune protection because the fetus is incapable of adequate immunoglobulin synthesis. The transport mechanism for maternal immunoglobulins is selective in that only IgG antibod-

Table 14–4. **LABORATORY FINDINGS IN AN IMMEDIATE (ACUTE) HEMOLYTIC TRANSFUSION REACTION**

Decreases in haptoglobin
Hemoglobinemia
Increase in lactic dehydrogenase (LDH)
Hemoglobinuria
Bilirubinemia (primarily indirect)
Methemalbuminemia (dependent on the severity of hemolysis)
Hemosiderinuria

Table 14–5. **ANTIBODIES MOST COMMONLY IMPLICATED IN DHTR**

Antibody	Blood Group System
Anti-Jk^a	Kidd
Anti-K	Kell
Anti-$\bar{c}$	Rh
Anti-E	Rh
Anti-Fy^a	Duffy
Anti-Jk^b	Kidd
Anti-C	Rh
Anti-e	Rh

ies can cross the placenta. When a mother is sensitized, either through a previous pregnancy or through transfusion, all maternal IgG antibodies (including the IgG blood group–specific antibodies) cross the placenta. If this antibody is specific for any antigen on the fetal red cells, destruction of these fetal red cells occurs, resulting in anemia. The term erythroblastosis fetalis is a synonym for HDN and describes the marked erythroblastic response to the immune hemolytic anemia present in the fetus.

The mother usually becomes immunized to foreign fetal red cell antigens during a larger fetal-maternal bleeds which may occur at the time of delivery. During the last half of pregnancy, small amounts of fetal red cells regularly enter the maternal circulation; however, this is rarely sufficient to induce sensitization. Even though the average bleed at the time of delivery is less than 1 ml of whole blood, it is estimated that at least 0.5 ml of fetal blood is necessary to promote alloimmunization.

Fetal red cells coated with maternal antibody are removed from the circulation by extravascular hemolysis. Responding to this increased red cell destruction, fetal hematopoietic tissue increases erythrocyte production. Because of the total commitment of the fetal bone marrow to hematopoiesis, extramedullary hematopoiesis occurs, resulting in liver and splenic enlargement. However, the fetus may not be able to compensate, and an anemia characterized by increased numbers of erythroblasts present during fetal development will then result. Hence, the term erythroblastosis fetalis has been used traditionally to describe HDN. The spectrum of clinical features ranges from mild anemia, jaundice, and hepatosplenomegaly to severe congestive cardiac failure with edema (hydrops fetalis).

The characteristic jaundice is a result of high levels of unconjugated bilirubin that have accumulated owing to increased red cell destruction. In utero, increased bilirubin crosses the placenta where it is conjugated and excreted by the maternal liver, as the fetal liver is not developed enough to handle this process. After birth, however, this maternal mechanism is no longer available and there is a buildup of the unconjugated bilirubin in the newborn. Because unconjugated bilirubin has a predilection for lipid tissue, a major potential consequence is the deposition of this bilirubin in the brain of the newborn, with the development of a condition known as kernicterus. This disorder occurs only in the newborn infant, as the liver enzyme, glucuronyl transferase, which is necessary to conjugate bilirubin, is poorly developed at that time. Table 14–6 summarizes the clinical features characteristic of HDN.

By far, the majority of the cases of HDN are caused by ABO and Rh incompatibility. The ABO incompatibility HDN, though more common, is generally much milder in severity than Rh hemolytic disease. The once-common Rh HDN is now a dying disease because the routine prophylactic use of Rh immune globulin (RhIg) has markedly decreased its inci-

Table 14–6. MAJOR CLINICAL FEATURES OF HDN

Anemia (erythroblastosis fetalis)
Jaundice (icterus gravis)
Severe edema (hydrops fetalis)
Hepatosplenomegaly

dence. However, even today occasional cases are still reported, which represent relatively severe forms of the disease. Table 14–7 lists the frequency of the various types of HDN.

Laboratory findings in patients with HDN include anemia, which may be mild (hemoglobin [Hgb] 130 g/liter) to severe (Hgb less than 80 g/liter) (normal hemoglobin for newborns is 140 to 200 g/liter); reticulocytosis; leukocytosis; numerous spherocytes (in ABO HDN); and nucleated red cells on the peripheral blood smear. As mentioned previously, bilirubinemia is present, and the result of the direct antiglobulin test on cord red cells is usually positive.

ABO HDN

ABO incompatibility, the most common form of HDN, rarely produces a clinical disease. The major clinical manifestation that occurs in approximately 10 to 20 percent of ABO-incompatible pregnancies is jaundice. This usually appears in the first 24 hours of life and is much milder than that associated with Rh HDN. Anemia is uncommon, and ABO HDN rarely causes stillbirths. Spherocytosis, however, is usually present on the peripheral blood smear. Group O mothers delivering group A or B infants usually account for most cases of this disorder, since O blood groups contain a significant amount of naturally occurring IgG anti-A,B. Therefore, ABO HDN characteristically can occur in the first-born child, as well as in subsequent pregnancies. Antenatal examination of the maternal serum is, however, unnecessary in almost all cases, as the serologic findings do not accurately predict or correlate with the incidence of ABO HDN. The direct antiglobulin test (Coombs' test) on cord blood usually yields a weakly positive result, but the results can vary from negative to moderately positive. The weak direct antiglobulin results have been explained by (a) the antigen density of A and B antigens on cord cells is approximately one-third that found on adult cells of the same group and (b) A and B antigens in the fetus can be found on cells other than red cells, especially if the fetus is a secretor and has soluble A or B antigen. The wide distribution of A and B antigen in the

Table 14–7. FREQUENCY OF TYPES OF HDN

ABO HDN	65%
Rh HDN	33%
Other	2%

fetus is also responsible for the mild clinical symptoms of ABO HDN. The offending maternal IgG anti-A,B is easily identified in the infant's serum and in eluates from the infant's red cells. Table 14-8 summarizes the main differences between ABO and Rh HDN.

Rh HDN

This disease results from primary sensitization of an Rh-negative mother with Rh-positive blood either by a previous pregnancy, blood transfusion, or abortion. The subsequent pregnancy of the Rh-negative mother carrying an Rh-positive fetus after initial sensitization results in HDN due to Rh incompatibility. Clinical manifestations include jaundice (appearing within 4 or 5 hours of birth), anemia, and hepatosplenomegaly. Hematologic laboratory results reflect the severity of the disease demonstrating decreased hemoglobin, increased reticulocyte count, and increased numbers of nucleated red cells in the peripheral blood smear. The previous discussion of erythroblastosis fetalis is characteristic of Rh HDN. Serologic findings include a positive antibody screen result and the identification of anti-D or other Rh antibodies in the serum of an Rh-negative mother, as well as a positive direct Coombs' test result on the Rh-positive cells of the infant. Antenatal diagnosis of Rh HDN is very important, and should be performed. Additionally, hemoglobin levels should be followed in a successfully delivered infant during the first month because of the risk of severe anemia developing during this time. Stillbirths and hydrops fetalis (previously described) are still major problems in Rh HDN. It is interesting to note that ABO incompatibility between mother and infant is protective for Rh HDN, because the fetal cells entering the mother's circulation will be destroyed by naturally occurring isoagglutinins, preventing Rh sensitization. (For comparison of Rh and ABO HDN, see Table 14-8.)

HDN due to Other Antibody Specificities

Approximately 2 percent of all cases of HDN are due to antibody specificities other than ABO or RhD. In most cases the pathology, investigation, and treatment parallel those for Rh HDN. Occasionally, however, an antibody to a high-frequency antigen is incriminated. Because of the difficulty of obtaining compatible blood, a number of in vitro techniques have been developed to assess the possible clinical significance of the antibody. Determination of IgG subclass and reactivity of the antibody in a monocyte/macrophage assay have been of limited success in giving useful information. Recently assays to determine the ability of an antibody to participate in ADCC have been introduced and early indications are that they may yield valuable information on clinical significance. Antibody-dependent cellular toxicity (ADCC) assays may be useful in any case of HDN in which a noninvasive procedure is required to determine clinical significance of antibodies. When antibodies to high-frequency antigens are incriminated in HDN and transfusion for the fetus or neonate is required, it may be necessary to look for antigen negative blood in siblings or ultimately from the mother herself.

Treatment

Treatment of HDN depends on the severity of the hemolysis and usually involves one of the following forms of therapy:

Table 14-8. **COMPARISON OF ABO AND Rh HDN**

	ABO	Rh
Severity	Mild	Severe
Child affected	First-born (40-50% of cases)	Usually second or subsequent births (first-born: 5% of cases)
Blood groups	Mother: O Child: A or B	Mother: Rh negative Child: Rh positive
Anemia	Uncommon/mild	Severe
Stillbirths/hydrops fetalis	Rare	Frequent
Jaundice	Mild	Severe
Spherocytes on peripheral blood smear	Usually present	None
Direct Coombs' test result	Negative or weakly positive	Positive
Maternal antibodies	Inconsistent/inconclusive	Always present
Antenatal diagnosis	Unnecessary	Necessary
Treatment (dependent on severity)	Phototherapy (common)	Exchange transfusion (common newborn treatment)
	Exchange transfusion (rare)	Intrauterine (common antenatal treatment)
Types of antibody	IgG (immune)	IgG (immune)
Prophylaxis	None	RhIG Antenatal RhIG

Antenatal treatment
  1. Intrauterine transfusion
  2. Umbilical vein transfusion
  3. Maternal plasmapheresis
  4. Intravenous immunoglobulin (IVIgG)
Treatment of newborn
  5. Exchange transfusion
  6. Phototherapy

The antenatal antibody screening of the mother's serum helps determine the severity of the disease, the need for aggressive monitoring, and a management strategy for the clinician. If anti-D antibodies are demonstrated in an Rh-negative mother, then Rh HDN will occur if the fetus is Rh positive. In the presence of a positive antibody screen result, the degree of alloimmunization should be determined by an antibody titer.

Using serial dilutions of the mother's serum, the strength of the antibody (titer) can be determined with corresponding RhD-positive cells. The value of the titer represents the lowest dilution with which the serum will react with the indicator cells. A titer of 1:2 represents very mild sensitization, whereas a titer of 1:512 represents severe immunization. It is important to note that following a secondary immune response, as a result of a subsequent pregnancy and continued transplacental hemorrhage immunizing the mother, the titer may be initially low and then increase to higher levels, with a significant risk of fetal death. Therefore, repeated serial titers (every 2 to 3 weeks) are particularly helpful in terms of the management of Rh HDN in immunized Rh-negative mothers.

If the titer remains below a determined critical level, then delivery can be performed at 38 weeks' gestation with a neonatal team present and blood available for an exchange transfusion if needed. The critical titer is determined by each institution (usually the titer is 1:16 or 1:32) and represents the maximum value at which there have been no stillbirths or severely affected infants. If the antibody titer reaches or exceeds the critical level, then amniocentesis and amniotic fluid analyses are performed to determine fetal condition. The practical spectrophotometric method of measuring amniotic fluid bilirubin developed by Liley provides a useful severity grading based on the gestational age and the relationship of amniotic fluid bilirubin levels. If intervention treatment is necessary and the fetus is too premature to deliver, then intrauterine transfusion remains the current therapy of choice. This procedure involves localization of the fetal peritoneal cavity with ultrasound waves and the injection of group O Rh-negative irradiated packed red cells into the fetal peritoneal cavity. The volumes used are determined according to the gestational age, and approximately 80 percent of the transfused red cells are eventually absorbed via lymphatic channels into fetal circulation. Once the transfusions are started, they should be repeated every 10 to 21 days until the infant is viable. The blood is routinely irradiated in this procedure to prevent the possible complication of graft-versus-host disease (GVHD).

In recent years improving technology has permitted percutaneous umbilical blood sampling (PUBS) to be performed using ultrasonic guidance. This procedure involves the insertion of a narrow (20 or 22) gauge spinal needle into the umbilical vein at a point adjacent to its junction with the placenta. The procedure can be performed as early as 17 weeks' gestation and allows direct testing to be performed on fetal cells. If blood can be sampled from the umbilical vein, it follows that it can also be transfused in a similar fashion. Umbilical vein transfusion (UVT) has been performed in a number of centers with varying degrees of success. With improvements in the technology it is likely that use of this form of therapy will increase in the future, particularly for severe forms of HDN.

Experimental maternal plasma exchange has been used when amniocentesis has indicated that the fetus is severely affected but too immature to be delivered. The objective of plasmapheresis in Rh HDN is the removal of the large quantities of circulating anti-D antibody in an attempt to reduce the amount of fetal red cell destruction. Plasma exchange is usually automated involving the use of cell-separating instruments and the routine removal of 2 to 3 liters of plasma, which is replaced with an albumin or plasma solution. The efficiency of this procedure has not yet been proved with any degree of certainty, and the reported clinical trials have not been controlled. Furthermore, this expensive procedure does not reduce the level of anti-D in the majority of cases and its overall value in preventing severe Rh HDN and fetal death has not been proved. One complication that has been reported with this procedure is a rebound phenomenon in which antibody levels are initially reduced but then return to very high levels a number of days afterward. In one report the procedure caused the mother to produce additional antibody specificities. The rebound phenomenon is thought to result from the removal of high-affinity antibody, which is acting as a positive feedback and regulating the level of antibody.

Another experimental approach to reduce the level of maternal antibody crossing the placenta, and hence affecting the fetal red cells, has been to give the mother high doses of intravenous immunoglobulin (IVIgG). The rationale for this approach is that the infused IgG causes feedback suppression of maternal antibody production while at the same time competing with maternal IgG for passage across the placenta. This procedure requires further study.

Exchange transfusion is the treatment of choice in affected infants requiring more than a single transfusion for correction of the anemia that is usually characteristic of Rh HDN. Serum bilirubin levels are generally used as the criteria for determining whether an exchange transfusion is necessary. Values vary, but bilirubin levels of greater than 10 to 12 mg/dl (171 to 205 μmol/liter) are strongly suggestive of the need for an exchange transfusion. However, the infant's entire clinical status must be considered before such a decision is made. An exchange transfusion attempts to accomplish four main objectives:

1. Remove antibody-coated fetal cells, reducing hemolysis
2. Lower bilirubin levels
3. Correct anemia by providing compatible red cells with adequate oxygen-carrying capacity
4. Decrease amount of circulating incompatible antibody

One major goal of exchange transfusion in Rh HDN is removal of bilirubin, not only in the initial exchange but also in subsequent exchanges. In Rh HDN, the blood selected for exchange transfusion should be Rh negative, ABO group-specific if the ABO group of the infant and mother are the same. If different ABO groups exist between the mother and infant, then group O blood should be used. For the first exchange transfusion, the selected blood is cross-matched against the mother's serum. Blood selected for subsequent exchange transfusions should be cross-matched with the mother's and infant's postexchange transfusion serum.

Treatment of patients with ABO HDN may require only phototherapy because the anemia in these patients is usually mild. If there is a need for exchange transfusion, which is rare, group O blood of the same Rh type as the infant's blood should be used, and this should be cross-matched with the mother's serum prior to transfusion.

Prophylaxis

Prevention of Rh HDN may be accomplished through the use of Rh immune globulin (RhIg), which is a passive form of anti-D, given within 72 hours of delivery to all Rh-negative mothers who have no detectable anti-D and who deliver a Rh-positive fetus. Postpartum testing to detect fetal-maternal hemorrhage (FMH) should be performed in all Rh-negative women at risk to determine if more than a single dose of RhIg is necessary. The Betke-Kleihauer acid elution procedure, or a modification thereof, is the most commonly used method for quantitating FMH. Using this stain, hemoglobin F (HbF) is resistant to acid elution and stains red with eosin dyes, whereas hemoglobin A (HbA) is eluted with acid and the red cells appear as colorless ghosts with the Betke-Kleihauer staining procedure (see Color Plate 259). The Betke-Kleihauer technique requires considerable expertise to obtain consistent results; accordingly, alternative techniques such as erythrocyte rosetting or enzyme-linked antiglobulin tests (ELATs) have been advocated. The rosetting procedure is quick but still involves considerable experience in its interpretation. Enzyme-linked antiglobulin test procedures are time consuming but can be semiautomated and the results, which are read by machine, can give consistent results. Irrespective of the method used to quantitate the degree of FMH, if it is greater than 30 ml of whole blood, then one dose of RhIg will not be sufficient to prevent alloimmunization.

Antenatal prophylactic RhIg is currently being routinely administered at 28 weeks' gestation (300 μg) to Rh-negative nonimmunized women to protect against FMH occurring during the third trimester. This type of prophylaxis eliminates the low failure rate (1 to 2 percent) of alloimmunization prevention that occurs when RhIg is administered only after delivery. The mother receiving this antenatal prophylactic dose of RhIg may demonstrate a positive antibody screen, owing to detectable levels of the passive anti-D in her serum. The weakly reacting passive anti-D may also cause a microscopically positive direct Coombs' test result in a Rh-positive newborn. Accurate records from the obstetrician and laboratory facilitates the blood bank's role in ascertaining whether the antibody was passively acquired or represents active alloimmunization. This confusion must be resolved, as postpartum RhIg must also be given to these women following delivery. If the cause of the maternal anti-D is still in doubt in an Rh-negative mother who has received antenatal doses, it must be assumed that it is a result of passive transfer, and the woman is still considered a candidate for RhIg at the time of delivery.

AUTOIMMUNE HEMOLYTIC ANEMIA

Autoimmune hemolytic anemia (AIHA) represents an abnormality within the immune system whereby the ability for self-recognition of an individual's own red cell antigens is lost. As a result, patients destroy their own red cells by producing autoantibodies, which bind to the patients' erythrocytes, inducing hemolysis. The majority of cases of AIHA can be divided broadly into warm or cold types. The warm type (WAIHA) is the most common, accounting for approximately 70 percent of all cases of autoimmune hemolytic anemia. This type involves autoantibodies whose serologic reactivity is optimal at 37°C. Cold AIHA involves autoantibodies whose optimal serologic reactivity occurs at 4°C but that also react at temperatures between 25 and 31°C. Two types of cold AIHA have been described: (1) cold agglutinin syndrome and (2) paroxysmal cold hemoglobinuria (PCH).

Drug-induced immune hemolytic anemia, which is sometimes difficult to distinguish from other cases of WAIHA, is the third type of AIHA, representing approximately 12 percent of the cases of AIHA in various studies.

Table 14–9 lists the frequency of the various types of AIHA.

Table 14–9. **PERCENTAGE OF REPORTED CASES OF AIHA**

Warm AIHA	70%
Cold agglutinin syndrome	16%
Paroxysmal cold hemoglobinuria	1–2%
Drug-induced	12%

Warm Autoimmune Hemolytic Anemia

Patients with WAIHA present a special problem to the blood bank. A significant percentage of cases suffer from an anemia severe enough to suggest the possible need for a transfusion. The degree of anemia is variable; however, hemoglobins less than 70 g/liter are frequently manifested. The onset of WAIHA is usually insidious and may be precipitated by a variety of factors such as infection, trauma, surgery, pregnancy, or psychologic stress. In other patients the onset is sudden.

Warm autoimmune hemolytic anemia may affect individuals of any racial background and of any age, including young children. The incidence of WAIHA in the community is estimated to be 1 in 80,000. There is a higher frequency of the disease in women than in men, which probably reflects the higher incidence of autoimmunity in women per se.

Warm autoimmune hemolytic anemia may be idiopathic, with no underlying disease process, or it may be secondary to a pathologic disorder. Table 14–10 lists the disorders reported to be associated with WAIHA. Signs and symptoms appear when a significant anemia has developed. Pallor, weakness, dizziness, dyspnea, jaundice, and unexplained fever occasionally are presenting complaints. Hemolysis is usually acute at onset and may stabilize or continue to accelerate at a variable rate.

The blood smear usually displays marked polychromasia, reflecting reticulocytosis, which is characteristic of a hemolytic anemia (**see Color Plate 105**). Spherocytosis and occasionally red cell fragmentation, indicating extravascular hemolysis, can be demonstrated along with nucleated red blood cells. An uncommon manifestation of WAIHA is reticulocytopenia. It is usually seen in the presence of a hyperplastic marrow, although it may also be associated with a hypoplastic marrow that is secondary to another underlying disease state. Because antigenic determinants on erythrocyte precursors can also react with the patient's red cell autoantibodies, reticulocytes can be destroyed as they are released from the bone marrow. Reticulocytopenia

Table 14–10. **DISORDERS REPORTED TO BE FREQUENTLY ASSOCIATED WITH WAIHA**

Reticuloendothelial neoplasms such as chronic lymphocytic leukemia, Hodgkin's disease, non-Hodgkin's lymphomas, thymomas

Collagen disease such as systemic lupus erythematosus, scleroderma, rheumatoid arthritis

Infectious diseases such as viral syndromes in childhood

Immunologic diseases such as hypogammaglobulinemia, dysglobulinemia, and other immune-deficiency syndromes

Gastrointestinal diseases such as ulcerative colitis

Benign tumors such as ovarian dermoid cysts

Source: Modified from Petz and Garratty, 1980, p 32.

at the time of intense hemolysis, therefore, is associated with a high patient mortality rate. Products of hemolysis such as bilirubin (particularly the unconjugated/indirect fraction) and urinary urobilinogen are increased. In severe cases, depleted serum haptoglobin, hemoglobinemia, hemoglobinuria, and increases in lactic dehydrogenase (LDH) may be demonstrated.

Hemolytic Process

In 80 percent of cases of WAIHA, the antibody causing the hemolysis is an IgG immunoglobulin, with IgG subclasses 1 and 3 associated with patients demonstrating clinical signs of hemolytic anemia. In the vast majority of cases hemolysis is extravascular and occurs predominantly in the spleen. It has been suggested that ADCC may be an important mechanism of hemolysis in WAIHA. (Refer to the introductory section of this chapter for a review of the mechanisms of immune hemolysis.)

Serologic Evaluation

Laboratory evaluation using a polyspecific antiglobulin reagent reveals a positive direct antiglobulin test (DAT) result. On further testing with monospecific antiglobulin reagents the DAT result is positive for both IgG and C3d in approximately two thirds of all cases. The remainder are positive with IgG (20 percent) or C3d (10 to 13 percent) alone. Occasionally the DAT result will be repeatedly negative in a patient who has clear evidence of hemolysis with no obvious cause. These patients represent a small group who are referred to as having DAT-negative AIHA. More sensitive techniques for the detection of IgG and/or C3d on red cells (such as ELAT) have shown that many of the patients have increased levels of either or both component on their cells, but this is below that normally detectable by a manual antiglobulin technique. Well-performed antiglobulin techniques can detect as few as 200 IgG molecules on the red cell surface. On the other hand, ELAT techniques are capable of detecting as few as 20 IgG molecules. In interpreting DAT results, it is important to remember that the test result, if positive, is not evidence that immune hemolysis is taking place, merely that if hemolysis is present or suspected it could be due to immune mechanisms. In a number of studies, it has been shown that the DAT result can be positive in up to 8 percent of hospitalized patients. In most of these the positivity is due to complement on the cells, probably as a result of the disease process from which the patient is suffering.

Tests on a patient's serum will usually show evidence of free autoantibody at low titer. On occasion it may be necessary to use an enzyme technique to detect the low levels of free antibody. The autoantibody can present several different problems in serologic testing. The serologic problems of WAIHA are twofold:

1. The patient's red cells are strongly coated with autoantibody, which interferes with phenotyping.

Table 14–11. **PRELIMINARY TESTING: SEROLOGIC PATTERN FROM A PATIENT WITH WAIHA**

Anti-A	Anti-B	Anti-A,B	A₁ Cells	B Cells	Anti-D	Rh Control
4+	neg	4+	neg	4+	3+	1+

Antibody Screen

	I.S.	37°C	AHG
I	neg	neg	2+
II	neg	neg	2+

PANEL RESULTS: 2+ reaction (AHG phase only) with all cells tested.

2. Autoantibody present in the serum may mask an underlying alloantibody.

A typical serologic pattern from a patient with WAIHA can be found in Table 14–11. As shown in the table there is often difficulty in obtaining accurate RhD results when using a potentiated typing reagent. This can be overcome by using a chemically modified reagent or one of the newer human monoclonal anti-D reagents.

Autoantibody Specificity

The autoantibodies producing WAIHA usually display broad specificity within the Rh system and react with all cells tested. Sometimes the autoantibody demonstrates a narrow specificity, the most common being anti-e. On rare occasions, other specificities have also been reported.

Treatment

The prognosis for patients with WAIHA is generally poor. Therapy is usually aimed at treating the underlying disease first, if one is present. Measures to support cardiovascular function are important in patients who are severely anemic. Transfusion is usually avoided, if possible, as this may only accelerate the hemolysis instead of ameliorating the anemia. However, transfusion is used in life-threatening situations.

As all donor blood will invariably be incompatible because of the broad reactivity of the autoantibody, it is general practice to use donor blood that is least reactive in the cross-match and that is antigen negative for any clinically significant alloantibodies that may also be present in the patient's serum. Blood is transfused slowly, in small volumes (100 ml), and the patient observed closely for any adverse reactions. Some hematologists advocate the use of phenotype-matched blood, irrespective of its degree of incompatibility in the cross-match for patients with WAIHA. The rationale for this approach is that patients with autoimmune antibodies are more likely to produce alloimmune antibodies, as immunologically they are considered to be "high responders." This in fact has not been shown to be the case and patients with autoantibodies have no greater incidence of alloantibodies than a normal patient.

The following three forms of treatment are generally used, depending on the severity of the disorder:

Corticosteroid Administration. This form of therapy involves the use of corticosteroids, such as prednisone. Initially, high doses of 100 to 200 mg of prednisone are maintained until the patient's hematocrit stabilizes. Patients who are not transfused respond to steroid therapy more rapidly than those who are transfused. Several mechanisms have been proposed for the action of prednisone, including (1) reduction of antibody synthesis, (2) altered antibody avidity and (3) alteration of macrophage receptors of IgG and C3, which reduces the clearance of antibody-coated red cells.

The dosage of prednisone should be reduced when the hematocrit begins to rise and the reticulocyte count drops. Finally, the steroids are withdrawn slowly over a period of 2 to 4 months. A beneficial response to the administration of prednisone is demonstrated in 50 to 65 percent of all cases of WAIHA. Recent reports on the use of the androgenic steroid Danazol 20 have also indicated some benefit in prednisone-resistant cases.

Splenectomy. If steroid treatment fails, or if a patient requires large steroid doses to control hemolysis, then splenectomy is usually recommended. The decision to perform a splenectomy requires clinical evaluation and judgment. However, there are three reasons for performing a splenectomy: (1) failure of steroid therapy; (2) need for continuous high steroid maintenance doses, and (3) complications of steroid therapy. Splenectomy decreases the production of antibody and removes a potent site of red cell damage and destruction. Patients who had a good initial response to steroids respond better with splenectomy than do those who failed steroid therapy initially.

It has been reported that as many as 60 percent of the patients with WAIHA benefit from splenectomy if steroid dosages greater than 15 mg/day are also used to maintain remission.

Immunosuppressive Drugs. This is usually the last approach used in the management of WAIHA. Azathioprine (Imuran) and cyclophosphamide are examples of cytotoxic immunosuppressive drugs that interfere with antibody synthesis by destroying dividing cells.

Experience in using this therapy is limited. The most detrimental side effect that threatens the common use of these drugs is the potential for neoplastic growth, as immunosuppressed patients have defective immune surveillance.

Cold Autoimmune Hemolytic Anemia (Cold AIHA)

Normal Cold Autoantibodies

Cold autoantibodies are present in all human sera to a greater or lesser degree. Cold autoantibodies found in the serum of normal, healthy individuals include anti-I, and anti-IH even though practically all adult red cells have the I and H antigens present on their red cells. Generally, most examples of anti-I, anti-H, and anti-IH have no clinical significance, and most of these autoantibodies are often too weak to be detected by routine serologic testing. This is primarily due to their low concentration in serum, failure to react at body temperature, and the fact that their optimal reactivity is at lower temperatures. Table 14–12 compares the characteristics of normal cold autoantibodies found in healthy adults with those of pathologic cold autoantibodies. These autoantibodies, termed autoagglutinins, differ in many ways from the pathologic cold autoagglutinins that produce cold AIHA.

Pathologic Cold Autoantibodies

Pathologic cold autoantibodies can be divided into (1) cold agglutinin syndrome (idiopathic cold AIHA); (2) secondary cold AIHA (cold autoantibodies related to infection); and (3) paroxysmal cold hemoglobinuria (PCH).

Cold Agglutinin Syndrome (Idiopathic Cold AIHA). Cold agglutinin syndrome, also called cold hemagglutinin disease (CHD) or idiopathic cold AIHA, represents approximately 16 percent of the cases of AIHA. A moderate chronic hemolytic anemia is produced by a cold autoantibody that optimally reacts at 4°C and also reacts between 25 and 31°C. The antibody is usually an IgM immunoglobulin, which quite efficiently activates complement.

Antibody specificity in this disorder is almost always anti-I, less commonly anti-i, and rarely anti-Pr.

Cold agglutinin syndrome occurs predominantly in older individuals, with a peak incidence after 50 years of age, and is found in all racial groups and affects both men and women. Although the disease is often called idiopathic, a careful evaluation of the patient may reveal the presence of a lymphoproliferative disorder. Because of this association it is prudent to investigate patients for possible malignancy when they present with a pathologic cold autoantibody and no obvious other cause (such as infection) exists.

Cold hemagglutinin disease is rarely severe and usually seasonal, as the winter cold months often precipitate the signs and symptoms of a chronic hemolytic anemia. Acrocyanosis of the hands, feet, ears, and nose is frequently the patient's main complaint, along with a sense of numbness in the extremities. Changes occur when the person is exposed to the cold because the cold autoantibody will precipitate autoagglutination of the individual's red cells in the skin capillaries causing local blood stasis. During cold weather, the temperature of an individual's skin and exposed extremities can fall to as low as 28°C, activating the cold autoantibody in these patients. This activated cold antibody agglutinates red cells and fixes complement as the erythrocytes flow through the capillaries of the skin, causing autoagglutination and signs of acrocyanosis. In addition, these patients may also experience hemoglobinuria, as complement fixation may result in intravascular hemolysis. However, this intravascular hemolytic episode is not associated with fever, chills, or acute renal insufficiency, which is characteristic of patients with PCH or severe WAIHA.

Patients usually display weakness, pallor, and weight loss, which are characteristic symptoms of chronic anemia. Cold hemagglutinin disease usually remains quite stable, and if it does progress in severity, it is insidious in intensity. Physical findings such as hepatosplenomegaly are infrequent owing to the mechanism of hemolysis. Other clinical features of cold hemagglutinin disease include

Table 14–12. **COMPARISON OF CHARACTERISTICS OF NORMAL AND PATHOLOGIC COLD AUTOANTIBODY**

Characteristic	Healthy	Pathologic
Thermal amplitude	<22°C	Broad: up to 32°C
Spontaneous autoagglutination	None	Significant degree which disperses on warming to 37°C
Titer	<64 at 4°C	>1000 at 4°C
Albumin enhancement	None	Reactivity enhanced
Clonality of antibody	Polyclonal	Idiopathic = monoclonal secondary to infection = polyclonal
Clinical significance	None	Causes cold AIHA
Usual antibody specificity	Anti-I	Anti-I
Direct antiglobulin test (DAT)	Negative or weak positive with polyspecific antiglobulin reagent	2 to 3+ with polyspecific antiglobulin reagent

jaundice and Raynaud's phenomenon (symptoms of cold intolerance, such as pain and a bluish tinge in the fingertips and toes, owing to vasospasm).

Laboratory findings in cold hemagglutinin disease include reticulocytosis and a positive DAT result (owing to complement coating only). It is suggested and recommended that a simple serum screening procedure be performed initially to test the ability of the patient's serum to agglutinate normal saline-suspended red cells at 20°C after a room temperature incubation. If this test result is positive, further steps must be taken to determine the titer and thermal amplitude of the cold autoantibody; if negative, the diagnosis of cold hemagglutinin disease is unlikely. The peripheral blood smear in patients with cold hemagglutinin disease may show rouleaux or autoagglutination, polychromasia, and a mild to moderate anisocytosis, and poikilocytosis (**see Color Plate 107**). Autoagglutination of anticoagulated whole blood samples is characteristic of cold hemagglutinin disease and occurs quickly as blood cools to room temperature, causing the binding of cold autoantibodies to the patient's red cells. As a result of this autoagglutination, performance of blood counts and preparation of blood smears are extremely difficult with blood samples from these patients. Leukocyte and platelet counts are usually normal.

The tendency for spontaneous autoagglutination of red cells in blood samples from patients with cold AIHA dictates that serum samples must be maintained and separated at 37°C if accurate results for the determination of antibody titer and thermal amplitude are to be obtained. Similarly, samples for the determination of DAT results must be collected into ethylenediamine tetracetic acid (EDTA) to inhibit any in vitro attachment of complement to the cells following collection. Table 14–13 summarizes the clinical criteria for diagnosis of cold hemagglutinin disease.

Secondary Cold AIHA (Cold Autoantibodies Related to Infection). Cold hemagglutinin disease can also occur as a transient disorder that is secondary to infections. Episodes of cold autoimmune hemolytic anemia often occur following upper respiratory infections. Approximately 50 percent of patients suffering from pneumonia due to *Mycoplasma pneumoniae* have elevated titers of cold autoagglutinins of greater than 64. In the second or third week of the patient's illness, cold hemagglutinin disease may occur in association with the infection, and a rapid onset of hemolysis as observed. Pallor and jaundice are characteristically present, and splenomegaly is usually found. Uncharacteristically, acrocyanosis and hemoglobinuria are unusual and are not consistently present. Resolution of the episode usually occurs in 2 to 3 weeks, as the hemolysis is self-limiting. The offending cold autoantibody is an IgM immunoglobulin with characteristic anti-I specificity. Very high titers of the cold autoagglutinin are seen almost exclusively in patients with mycoplasma pneumonia. It has been reported that the cold agglutinin produced in this infection is an immunologic response to the mycoplasmal antigens and this antibody cross-reacts with the red cell I antigen.

The antibodies produced in cold hemagglutinin disease and in the disorder secondary to mycoplasma pneumonia both have anti-I specificity. However, they differ in that the autoantibody in CHD is invariably monoclonal (IgM kappa light chain), whereas the autoantibody in the disease secondary to infection is polyclonal (IgM with both kappa and lambda light chain types). The monoclonality of the autoantibody in CHD suggests a possible underlying lymphoproliferative disorder. Red cells are sensitized with complement components owing to the cold autoantibody. If the complement cascade does not proceed to C9 (cell death by lysis), the macrophages of the RES system, particularly those within the liver, can still clear the sensitized red cells through their receptors for C3b fragments, thereby causing hemolysis. Red cells sensitized with C3b and iC3b and which escape the liver and to a lesser extent the spleen, become refractory to further hemolytic processes as the complement components are degraded to C3d for which there are no receptors on phagocytic cells. For this reason, the DAT result on the red cells of patients with cold AIHA has a positive result with monospecific anti-C3d antiglobulin reagents.

Infectious mononucleosis may also be associated with a hemolytic anemia due to a cold autoagglutinin. Although rather infrequent, it has been well documented that a high-titered IgM cold agglutinin with a wide thermal range anti-i specificity plays a major role in the hemolytic anemia associated with this viral infection. Acute illness with sore throat and high fever, followed by weakness, anemia, and jaundice are characteristic features of infectious mononucleosis.

Lymphadenopathy and hepatosplenomegaly are common findings. A larger percentage of patients with infectious mononucleosis have been reported to develop anti-i, but only a small number of these patients develop the antibody of sufficient titer and thermal amplitude to induce in vivo hemolysis. (For a review of infectious mononucleosis, see Chapter

Table 14–13. **CLINICAL CRITERIA FOR THE DIAGNOSIS OF COLD AGGLUTININ SYNDROME**

Clinical signs of an acquired hemolytic anemia, with a history (which may or may not be present) of acrocyanosis and hemoglobinuria upon exposure to cold

A positive DAT result using polyspecific antisera

A positive DAT result using monospecific C3 antisera

A negative DAT result using monospecific IgG antisera

The presence of reactivity in the patient's serum owing to a cold autoantibody

A cold agglutinin titer of 1000 or greater in saline at 4°C with visible autoagglutination of anticoagulated blood at room temperature

Table 14–14. **SECONDARY COLD AIHA**

Type of Infection	Cold Autoantibody Specificity
Mycoplasma pneumonia	Anti-I
Infectious mononucleosis	Anti-i
Lymphoproliferative disorder	Anti-i

18.) Table 14–14 lists the cold auto-antibody specificity most commonly found in the various infections that cause secondary cold hemagglutinin disease.

Treatment. The prognosis for patients with cold hemagglutinin disease is generally good. Most patients require no treatment and are instructed to avoid the cold, keep warm, or move to a milder climate. Patients with moderate anemia are given the same instructions, urging them to tolerate the symptoms rather than to use drugs on a therapeutic trial basis. There is some advantage to the use of plasma exchange in more severe cases, as IgM antibodies have a predominantly intravascular distribution. However, response to plasma exchange is still variable in this patient population. Corticosteroids have also been used but generally have had limited success. In some patients whose red cells are strongly sensitized with C3, successful results have been reported with corticosteroids. Some favorable responses have also been reported with the alkylating drug chlorambucil. Splenectomy is generally considered ineffective largely due to the fact that extravascular hemolysis predominantly occurs in the liver.

Transfusion is rarely required for these patients; however, if it is needed, blood should be ABO- and RhD-matched and lack any antigens for which the patient has an alloantibody. It should be warmed, preferably using a blood warmer and transfused slowly with constant monitoring of the patient for any adverse reactions.

Paroxysmal Cold Hemoglobinuria. PCH is the least common type of AIHA, with an incidence of only 1 to 2 percent. It is, however, more common in children in association with viral disorders such as measles, mumps, chickenpox, infectious mononucleosis, and the ill-defined flu syndrome.

Originally, PCH was described in association with syphilis, in which an autoantibody was formed in response to *Treponema pallidum* organism, the causative agent of the disease. However, with the discovery and use of antibodies to treat syphilis, PCH is no longer a commonly reported disorder related to syphilis.

Red cell destruction is due to a cold autoantibody termed an autohemolysin, which binds to the patient's red cells at low temperatures and fixes complement. Hemolysis occurs when the body temperature rises to 37°C and the sensitized cells undergo complement-mediated intravascular lysis. Uncharacteristically, this cold autoagglutinin is an IgG an-

tibody with biphasic activity; therefore, it is termed a biphasic hemolysin. The classic antibody produced in PCH is called the Donath-Landsteiner antibody, which characteristically is an IgG biphasic hemolysin with anti-P specificity.

In the Donath-Landsteiner test, two blood samples are drawn from the patient and maintained at different temperatures. One specimen is used as the control and kept at 37°C for 60 minutes. The other sample is cooled at 4°C for 30 minutes and then incubated at 37°C for another 30 minutes. Both samples are then centrifuged and observed for hemolysis. In a positive Donath-Landsteiner test result, hemolysis will be demonstrated in the sample placed at 4°C and then at 37°C, whereas no hemolysis is observed in the control sample. Table 14–15 summarizes the Donath-Landsteiner test. Determination of the specificity of the auto-antibody is indicated in all positive Donath-Landsteiner test results; however, this may be beyond the capacity of most blood banks owing to the need for red cells with rare phenotypes.

As the name of PCH implies, paroxysmal or intermittent episodes of hemoglobinuria occur upon exposure to the cold. These acute attacks are characterized by a sudden onset of fever, shaking chills, malaise, abdominal cramps, and back pains. All the signs of intravascular hemolysis are evident, along with hemoglobinemia, hemoglobinuria, and bilirubinemia depending on the severity and frequency of the attack (see Fig. 14–2). This results in a severe and rapidly progressive anemia with hemoglobin values frequently around 40 to 50 g/liter. Polychromasia, nucleated red blood cells, and poikilocytosis are demonstrated in the peripheral blood smear; these are consistent findings associated with a hemolytic anemia. These signs and symptoms, as well as hemoglobinuria, may resolve in a few hours or persist for days. Splenomegaly, hyperbilirubinemia, and renal insufficiency may also develop.

PCH is an acute hemolytic anemia occurring almost exclusively in children and young adults and almost always representing a transient disorder. Table 14–16 compares and contrasts PCH versus cold agglutinin syndrome.

Table 14–15. **DONATH-LANDSTEINER TEST**

	Whole Blood Sample 1 (Control)	Whole Blood Sample 2
Procedure		
1. 30 min	37°C	4°C
2. 30 min	37°C	37°C
3. Centrifuge and observe		
Results		
Positive	No hemolysis	Hemolysis
Negative	No hemolysis	No hemolysis
Inconclusive	Hemolysis	Hemolysis

Table 14-16. **COMPARISON OF PCH AND COLD AGGLUTININ SYNDROME**

	PCH	Cold Agglutinin Syndrome
Patient population	Children or young adults	Elderly or middle-aged
Pathogenesis	Following viral infection	Idiopathic/lymphoproliferative disorder/ following *Mycoplasma pneumoniae* infection
Clinical features	Hemoglobinuria: acute attacks upon exposure to cold (symptoms resolve in hours or days)	Acrocyanosis/autoagglutination of blood at room temperature
Severity of hemolysis	Acute and rapid	Chronic and rarely severe
Hemolysis	Intravascular	Extravascular/Intravascular
Autoantibody	IgG (anti-P specificity) (biphasic hemolysin)	IgM (anti-I/i) (monophasic)
DAT	3+ (polyspecific Coombs' sera)/neg IgG/3–4+ C3 monospecific Coombs' sera	3+ (polyspecific Coombs' sera)/neg IgG/3–4+ C3 monospecific Coombs' sera
Thermal range	Moderate (<20°C)	High (up to 30–31°C)
Titer (4°C)	Moderate (<64)	High (>1000)
Donath-Landsteiner test	Positive	Negative
Treatment	Supportive (disorder terminates when underlying illness resolves)	Avoid the cold

Treatment. For chronic forms of PCH, protection from cold exposure is the only useful therapy. Acute postinfection forms of PCH usually terminate spontaneously following resolution of the infectious process. Steroids and transfusions may be required, depending on the severity of the attacks. Table 14-17 reviews and compares characteristics of warm and cold autoimmune hemolytic anemias.

Mixed Autoimmune Hemolytic Anemia

In recent years a number of reports have drawn attention to the occurrence of mixed AIHA, in which patients exhibit autoantibodies having the characteristics of both warm and cold autoantibodies. This situation is not to be unexpected when one realizes that a number of the lymphoproliferative and collagen diseases may be associated with either form of autoantibody.

DRUG-INDUCED IMMUNE HEMOLYTIC ANEMIA

The administration of drugs may lead to the development of a wide variety of hematologic abnormalities, including immune hemolytic anemia.

Drug-induced immune hemolytic anemia, which is sometimes difficult to distinguish from other cases of WAIHA, represents approximately 12 percent of cases in various studies. However, drug-related immune hemolytic processes do not involve any known abnormality intrinsic to the red cell. Three recognizable mechanisms lead to the development of drug-related antibodies and drug-induced immune hemolytic anemia. One other mechanism can lead to positive DAT results; however, it has not been associated with the development of a hemolytic process.

Immune Complex Mechanism (Fig. 14-3)

The most common drugs involved in this response include quinidine and phenacetin. Table 14-18 lists other drugs involved in the immune complex mechanism. The patient responds to these drugs by producing an antidrug antibody, which forms an immune complex. The antibody drug complex then adsorbs onto the patient's red cells, which become innocent bystanders. Invariably complement is activated in this process.

Laboratory findings include evidence of intravascular hemolysis, with hemoglobinemia and hemo-

Table 14-17. **COMPARISON OF WARM AND COLD AUTOIMMUNE HEMOLYTIC ANEMIAS**

	WAIHA	Cold AIHA
Optimal reactivity	>32°C	<30°C
Immunoglobulin class	IgG	IgM (exception: PCH-IgG)
Complement activation	May bind complement	Binds complement
Hemolysis	Usually extravascular (no cell lysis)	Usually intravascular (cell lysis)
Frequency	70–75% of cases	16% of cases (PCH: 1–2%)
Specificity	Frequently Rh	Ii system (PCH: anti-P)

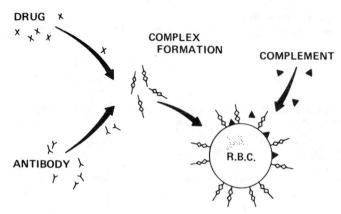

Figure 14–3. Immune complex mechanism. (From Petz, LD and Garraty, G (eds): Acquired Immune Hemolytic Anemias. Churchill Livingstone, New York, 1980, with permission.)

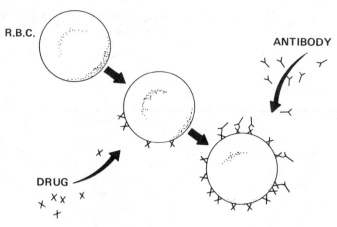

Figure 14–4. Drug absorption mechanism. (From Petz, LD and Garraty, G (eds): Acquired Immune Hemolytic Anemias. Churchill Livingstone, New York, 1980, with permission.)

globinuria being most notable. The antibody, which may be either IgM or IgG, is capable of activating complement. Only a small amount of the drug is necessary to produce an antibody response in a particular patient. The DAT result is positive, often only because of the presence of complement components on the red cell surface, since the immune complex has dissociated. In vitro agglutination reactions are generally observed during serologic testing only when the patient's serum, drug, and red cells are *all* incubated together. In addition, elution procedures often demonstrate nonreactive eluates.

Treatment is aimed at stopping the use of the drug. Although the production of antidrug antibodies is rare, when they are produced, hemolysis by this mechanism is common and onset is sudden and characterized by intravascular hemolysis and frequent renal failure. Therefore, immediate cessation of the drug is essential. Steroid treatment may also be given.

It is interesting to note that some of the drugs producing hemolysis by this mechanism (for example, quinidine) are also associated with the development of drug-induced immune thrombocytopenia (ITP). However, it is rare to find a patient with both hemolysis and thrombocytopenia being produced by antibodies to the one drug.

Table 14–18. **DRUGS IMPLICATED IN IMMUNE COMPLEX, OR "INNOCENT BYSTANDER," MECHANISM**

Quinidine	Insecticides
Quinine	Dipyrone
Phenacetin	Anhistine
Stibophen	Antazoline
P-Aminosalicylic acid	Chlorpromazine
Sulfonamides	Aminopyrine
Thiazide	Isoniazid

Drug Adsorption (Hapten) Mechanism (Fig. 14–4)

The drugs implicated in this response include the penicillins (which produce the second most common drug-induced hemolytic anemia) and rarely the cephalosporins and streptomycins. In this response, the drug is nonspecifically bound to the patient's red cells. It remains firmly adsorbed to the cells regardless of whether the patient develops an antibody to the drug. Hapten mechanism is also used to describe this response, because the drug's immunogenicity is determined by its ability to react chemically with serum proteins to form several haptenic groups. If the patient develops an antidrug antibody, it will react with the red cell–bound drug.

Laboratory findings include signs of extravascular hemolysis. Large doses of intravenous penicillin (10 million units daily) are needed to produce a response, although it should be noted that many patients who have received penicillins will have detectable IgM antipenicillin antibodies present at low titer. The onset is much less acute than that of the immune complex mechanism; the disorder developing over a period of 7 to 10 days. The DAT result is strongly positive owing to IgG sensitization, and a high titer of IgG antibody is present in the serum. Red blood cell eluates are nonreactive with red cell panels and react only with antibiotic-coated red cells. Treatment focuses on the discontinuation of the drug in the presence of an overt hemolytic anemia.

Membrane Modification Mechanism (Nonimmunologic Protein Adsorption) (Fig. 14–5)

As the name implies, the drug modifies the red cell membrane so that normal plasma proteins are adsorbed nonimmunologically. Cephalosporins are the drugs implicated in this response. Cephalothin-

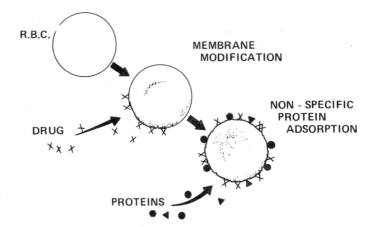

Figure 14-5. Membrane modification mechanism (From Petz, LD and Garraty, G (eds): Acquired Immune Hemolytic Anemias. Churchill Livingstone, New York, 1980, with permission.)

sensitized cells become coated with numerous plasma proteins such as albumin, fibrinogen, and globulins. Approximately 3 percent of patients receiving the drug develop a positive DAT result due to nonspecific protein adsorption by the red cells. However, hemolytic anemia has not been reported in association with this mechanism of drug-induced positive DAT results. Elution procedures result in nonreactive eluates. Hemolytic anemia associated with ingestion of these drugs has not been described in relation to red blood cell membrane modification.

Methyldopa-Induced Mechanism (Unknown Mechanism)

This represents the most common drug-induced immune hemolytic anemia, with an incidence of 0.8 percent. The drugs implicated in this response include methyldopa and related drugs (such as Aldomet, L-dopa), which are commonly prescribed for the treatment of hypertension. Drug-induced AIHA by this mechanism is difficult to diagnose because it mimics WAIHA. A positive DAT result develops in approximately 12 to 15 percent of the patients receiving Aldomet (alphamethyldopa), but AIHA develops only rarely in these patients (1 to 3 percent). Patients may continue to have a positive DAT result for up to 2 years after discontinuation of the drug. If anemia develops, it will do so gradually and depends on the dose of the drug. The antibodies produced by the patients suffering from this disorder are of the IgG immunoglobulin class, with specificities similar to those found in WAIHA. Most commonly the specificity of the antibody is anti-e–like, as it reacts more strongly with R_1R_1 and rr cells than with R_2R_2. Hemolysis is extravascular, and the DAT result is strongly positive owing to IgG sensitization. Atypically, the eluate yields a positive result, unlike all the other drug-induced positive DAT mechanisms in which the eluates are negative.

There are several hypotheses suggested for this drug-related hematologic problem; however, the exact mechanism is still unknown. Table 14-19 presents the four different theories proposed for the

Table 14-19. PROPOSED THEORIES FOR METHYLDOPA-INDUCED MECHANISM OF IMMUNE HEMOLYTIC ANEMIA

Normal RBC antigens are altered by the drug and are no longer recognized as "self," resulting in production of autoantibodies to these RBC antigens.

The drug acts as a hapten, resulting in the production of antibodies, which cross-react with normal RBC antigens.

The drug produces aberrations in the proliferation of normal lymphocytes, producing clones of abnormal immunologically competent cells, which produce antibodies against normal RBC antigens.

The drug affects the synthesis of IgG, exerting a direct effect on T lymphocytes, which results in a loss of suppressor function and subsequent proliferation of autoantibodies by B lymphocytes.

methyldopa-induced mechanism of immune hemolytic anemia.

Treatment

Discontinuation of the drug is the treatment of choice for patients with a drug-induced hemolytic anemia. The presence of a positive DAT result does not necessarily imply that the drug must be discontinued, if the effects of the drug are of therapeutic benefit. In general, however, other drugs should be substituted and the patient observed for resolution of the anemia to confirm a drug-induced hemolytic process. If the patient has a positive DAT result *without hemolysis*, continued administration of the drug is optional.

The classification used for the drug-induced immune hemolytic anemias provides a convenient mechanistic approach as to how drugs may be incriminated in immune hemolysis. Recent reports have drawn attention to the fact that some drugs may produce immune hemolysis by more than one mechanism.

Generally, the prognosis for patients with drug-induced hemolytic anemia is excellent. In Table

Table 14–20. **MECHANISMS LEADING TO DEVELOPMENT OF DRUG-RELATED ANTIBODIES**

Mechanism	Prototype Drugs	Immunoglobulin Class	DAT	Biologic Results	Frequency of Hemolysis
Immune complex formation (innocent bystander)	Quinidine Phenacetin	IgM or IgG	Positive (often to complement fragments only; however, IgG may be present)	Eluate often negative	Small doses of drug may cause acute intravascular hemolysis with hemoglobinemia and hemoglobinuria; renal failure is common
Drug adsorption (hapten)	Penicillins Cephalosporins Streptomycin	IgG	Positive (strongly) due to IgG sensitization	Eluate often negative	3–4% of patients on large doses (10 million units) daily of penicillin, which is one of the most common causes of drug induced immune hemolysis, usually extravascular in nature
Membrane modification (nonimmunologic protein adsorption)	Cephalosporins	Numerous plasma proteins (non-immunological sensitization)	Positive due to a variety of serum proteins	Eluate negative	No hemolysis; however, 3% of patients receiving the drug develop a +DAT
Methyldopa-induced (unknown)	Methyldopa (Aldomet)	IgG	Strongly positive (due to IgG sensitization)	Eluate positive (warm autoantibody identical to antibody found in WAIHA)	0.8% develop a hemolytic anemia that mimics a WAIHA (depends on the dose of the drug); 15% of patients receiving Aldomet develop a +DAT

14–20, the four recognized mechanisms leading to the development of drug-related antibodies are compared. Table 14–21 contrasts the antibody characteristics of the various types of autoimmune hemolytic anemias.

NONIMMUNE HEMOLYTIC ANEMIA

Classification

Acquired nonimmune hemolytic anemias represent a diverse group of conditions that lead to the shortened survival of red cells by various mechanisms. Often a number of mechanisms will be operative at the same time, e.g., malaria leads to mechanical destruction of red cells and in addition immunologic factors also play a role in the shortening of red cell survival. (See Fig. 14–5.) Classification may be made along either causative or mechanistic lines. Table 14–22 provides a classification incorporating both approaches.

Intracellular Infections

Malaria

Malaria is the most common protozoal infection in humans, and its high incidence in the tropical and subtropical regions of the world accounts for much of the anemia in the populations of those regions. It has been estimated that more than 400 million people suffer from the disease, resulting in the deaths of more than 1.5 million annually. Most fatalities occur in nonimmune children, whereas those who survive their childhood years invariably suffer from an ongoing debilitating disease. Over the last 20 years or so, many of the regions which had been subject to malaria control measures and in which the incidence of the disease had been significantly reduced, have seen a return of the disease in epidemic proportions. The increased incidence of infections has resulted from the organism becoming resistant to many of the antimalarial drugs, espe-

Table 14–21. **SUMMARY OF ANTIBODY CHARACTERISTICS IN AIHA**

	Warm Reactive Autoantibody	Cold Reactive Autoantibody	PCH	Drug-Related Autoantibody
Immunoglobulin characteristics	Polyclonal IgG, IgM, and IgA may also be present; rarely IgA alone	Polyclonal IgM-infection Monoclonal kappa chain IgM in cold agglutinin disease	Polyclonal IgG	Polyclonal IgG
Complement activation	Variable	Always	Always	Depends on mechanism of drug, antibody, and RBC interaction
Thermal reactivity	20°C–37°C; optimum 37°C	4°C–32°C occasionally to 37°C; optimum 4°C	4°C–20°C; biphasic hemolysin	20°C–37°C; optimum 37°C
Titer of free antibody	Low (<32) May only be detectable using enzyme treated cells	High (>512 at 4°C)	Moderate to low (<64)	Depends on mechanism of drug, antibody and RBC interaction
Reactivity of eluate with antibody screening cells	Usually panreactive	Nonreactive	Nonreactive	Panreactive with Aldomet type antibody. Nonreactive in all other circumstances
Most common specificity	Anti-Rh precursor -common Rh -LW -Enᵃ/Wrᵇ -U	-I -i -Pr	Anti-P	Anti-e–like: Aldomet, antidrug
Site of RBC destruction	Predominantly spleen with some liver involvement	Predominantly liver, rarely intravascular	Intravascular	Intravascular and spleen

cially chloroquine, while at the same time the mosquito vector has become resistant to insecticides, particularly DDT. Four species of malaria can normally infect humans: *Plasmodium vivax, P. falciparum, P. ovale,* and *P. malariae. P. vivax* and *P. falciparum* are responsible for most infections producing disease. In case of *P. falciparum* the disease can have a very rapid and often fatal course. *P. malariae* and *P. ovale* infections are uncommon and in the case of the latter are confined to areas of Africa.

The number of patients presenting with malaria is increasing in countries such as the United States, Europe, and Australia because of the increased travel by residents of these countries to tropical and subtropical regions in which the disease is endemic.

Life Cycle. The malarial parasite has a complex life cycle. The insect vector in its life cycle is the *Anopheles* mosquito, numerous species of which can transmit the parasite. Figure 14–6 illustrates the malarial life cycle. At the time of being bitten by an infected female mosquito, sporozoites within the mosquito saliva are injected into the victim's blood. They rapidly migrate to the liver where they invade the parenchymal cells and proceed to divide asexually to produce schizonts composed of thousands of merozoites. This process of exoerythrocytic schizogony occurs over 5 to 12 days, although it may be as long as 30 days with *P. malariae.* Rupture of the

schizont releases the merozoites which invade circulating erythrocytes. The number of merozoites released differs among the various species: in the case of *P. falciparum* it can be up to 40,000, whereas in *P. malariae* it may be only 2000 to 3000. Once in the erythrocyte they proceed to metabolize the hemoglobin and become the typical ring-form and/or ameboid trophozoite. After 2 to 3 days the parasite matures to an erythrocytic schizont composed of varying numbers of merozoites. The number of merozoites in an erythrocytic schizont, if detected in a peripheral blood smear, can be helpful in determining the species of parasite. On completion of erythrocytic schizogony the red cell ruptures to release the merozoites, which go on to infect other red cells. At the time of red cell destruction an infected patient will experience fever and chills. The periodicity between successive episodes of fever and chills is characteristic of the different malarial species. During these cycles of erythrocyte destruction and release of merozoites some of them may reinfect the liver, thereby producing a secondary, exoerythrocytic phase of infection. This process occurs for all species except *P. falciparum* and is responsible for the relapsing nature of malarial infections. After approximately 12 to 14 days some of the merozoites form male and female gametes. If an infected person is bitten by a mosquito at this stage,

Table 14–22. **CLASSIFICATION OF NONIMMUNE ACQUIRED HEMOLYTIC ANEMIAS**

Cause	Examples	Mechanisms
Infections		
Intracellular	Malaria	Physical disruption and immune
	Babesiosis	Physical disruption
Extracellular	Bartonella	Direct action on RBC membrane and RES sequestration
	Clostridia	Enzymatic action on RBC membrane
	Bacterial sepsis: meningococcal, pneumococcal	Physical disruption secondary to DIC
	Viral	?
Mechanical		
Macroangiopathic	Cardiac prosthesis	Physical disruption due to shear stress
	March hemoglobinuria	Physical disruption
Microangiopathic	Hemolytic uremic syndrome (HUS)	Physical disruption
	Thrombotic thrombocytopenic purpura (TTP)	Physical disruption
Chemicals and physical agents		
Oxidative agents	Dapsone at high dosage	Direct oxidation of RBC membrane components
Nonoxidative agents	Lead	Alteration of RBC membrane components
	Venoms	Possible direct effect on RBC membrane by enzymes
Osmotic effect	Water (drowning or water irrigation during surgery)	Osmotic lysis
	Burns	Localized dehydration
Acquired membrane disorders	Vitamin E deficiency; abetalipoproteinemia	RBC membrane oxidation; lack of membrane deformability
	Liver disease	Lipid abnormalities of RBC membrane lead to decrease in deformability
	Renal disease	Retained metabolic products cause membrane changes leading to a decrease in deformability
Hypersplenism		Sequestration of normal cells

the gametes will pass into the mosquitoes stomach where they will combine to produce an ookinete. The ookinete penetrates the stomach lining of the mosquito and produces an oocyst on the external wall. Sporozoites develop in the oocyst, which, upon rupturing, allows the sporozoites to pass through to the salivary gland, from which the life cycle begins once again.

Clinical Presentation. Typically patients seek medical alteration as a result of the often quite violent rigors, fever, and profuse sweating that accompany the periodic rupture of infected red cells. Early in the infection these episodes may not show classic periodicity, which, as mentioned, can be helpful in determining the species of parasite with which the patient is infected. In the case of *P. vivax, P. falciparum,* and *P. ovale* the interval between fevers is usually 48 hours and for *P. malariae* 72 hours. Periodicity may not be evident when a patient has multiple infections, which is not that uncommon. Nausea, vomiting, and diarrhea may be present. Patients frequently complain of headache, fatigue, and varying degrees of arthralgia and myalgia. Quite often these presenting symptoms are attributed to a viral infection, which, for a patient with *P. falciparum*

infection, can have fatal consequences. It is always advisable to inquire if the patient has been overseas and which countries have been visited.

Splenomegaly is present in 40 to 50 percent of patients with acute malaria. It is present in virtually all patients with chronic malaria, which accounts for the high incidence of splenomegaly in the tropics.

Infections with *P. vivax* and *P. ovale* show relatively benign courses if untreated. Relapses can occur for a number of years following initial infection resulting from secondary exoerythrocytic infection of the liver. In the case of *P. ovale,* relapses up to 20 years following initial infection have been reported.

P. malariae infections are generally quite mild; however, persistent infections are associated with the development of nephrotic syndrome, most probably due to the deposition of immune complexes involving parasitic antigen in the kidney. *P. falciparum* infection may be a rapidly progressive disease, and, unless accurately diagnosed and promptly treated, can prove fatal. Some patients may present with massive intravascular hemolysis evidenced by marked hemoglobinuria. Although

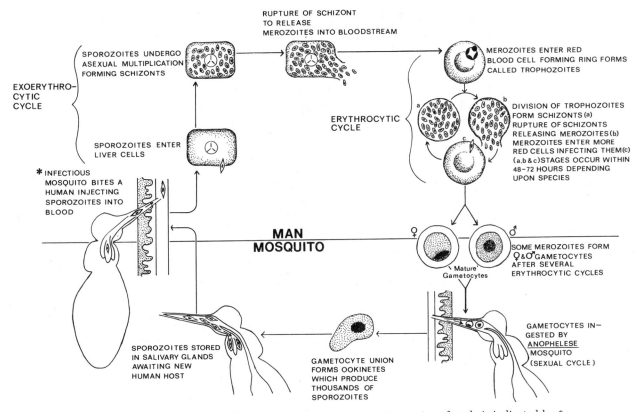

Figure 14-6. Malarial life cycle in humans and mosquitoes. Beginning of cycle is indicated by *.

this form of presentation is now relatively uncommon, it gave rise to the name "blackwater fever." The hemolysis is associated with jaundice and hypotension and quite often results in renal failure. Some patients will show evidence of DIC, which may be initiated by immune complexes and by the release of thromboplastic material when red cells rupture. Glomerulonephritis and nephrotic syndrome may also develop consequent to the presence of immune complexes and DIC.

In a small proportion of patients (2 to 3 percent), cerebral malaria may develop as a complication of the original disease. Evidence of cerebral malaria includes disturbances in consciousness ranging from lethargy to disturbances in movement, personality changes, and coma. Rare complications of falciparum malaria include respiratory and cardiac failure.

Pathogenesis. The ability of the malarial parasite to cause disease in humans is influenced by many factors, not all of which are well understood. The geographic distribution of the parasite corresponds very closely to a number of human genetic traits, and the associations have provided epidemiologists and population geneticists with an interesting source of data with which to study selective forces in evolution.

Susceptibility to Infection. The ability of the different species of malaria to infect and mature in red cells is controlled by several factors:

1. **Red cell maturity.** *P. vivax* and *P. ovale* selectively infect reticulocytes and young red cells. *P. falciparum* can infect red cells at any stage of development whilst *P. malariae* seems to infect senescent cells. The ability of *P. falciparum* to infect red cells at all stages of development contributes to the high parasitemia (up to 60 percent) seen in this infection compared to *P. vivax* (up to 10 percent).

2. **Blood group phenotype.** Recent studies have shown that merozoites of *P. vivax* and the simian malaria *P. knowlesi* must attach to specific receptors in the red cell surface to allow penetration of the cell. These receptors have been identified as the Duffy blood group antigen. Red cells that are genetically Fy(a − b−) or that have been enzymatically treated to remove the Duffy antigens are resistant to infection by the *P. vivax* merozoite. It is interesting to note that the frequency of the Fy(a − b−) phenotype in West African and American blacks is 68 percent compared with less than 1 percent in whites, which explains the well-known resistance of these populations to *P. vivax* infection. The red cell receptor for *P. falciparum* merozoites appears to be glycophorin A, as red cells from individuals with the rare En(a−) phenotype, which lacks this membrane glycoprotein, are resistant to infection.

3. **Membrane deformability.** Red cells from patients with hereditary pyropoikilocytosis (HPP) and Melanesian ovalocytosis are resist-

ant to invasion by malarial parasites, and this is thought to be due to their lack of deformability. The lack of deformability in these cells has been attributed to alterations in the red cell cytoskeleton.

4. **Hemoglobin variants.** Conflicting data exist on the association of different hemoglobin variants with resistance to maturation of the parasite in red cell. *P. falciparum* growth is retarded in cells with high hemoglobin F content. Contradictory reports exist for individuals with α- and β-thalassemia, those with hemoglobin E, and those heterozygous for hemoglobin S. On the other hand, individuals homozygous for hemoglobin C are resistant to malarial infection.

5. **Enzymopathies.** The only enzymopathy of interest is glucose-6-phosphate dehydrogenase (G6PD) deficiency. There are conflicting reports in G6PD deficiency and resistance to malaria. It is thought that resistance may be conferred only in areas where favism is present.

In general, the protection provided by abnormalities in hemoglobin and red cell enzymes is thought to be due to the red cell's high sensitivity to oxidant stress. Such sensitivity is well known for G6PD deficiency and was in fact first described in blacks who were being treated for malaria with the oxidant drug primaquine. The parasite itself contributes significantly to increases in oxidant stress within the red cell.

Development of Anemia. The anemia in malaria is largely due to the extravascular sequestration of infected cells in the spleen. The degree of anemia shows close, although not exact, correlation with the level of parasitemia in the peripheral blood; hence, anemia is most marked in *P. falciparum* infections and is quite mild with other species. Other factors contributing to the anemia include bone marrow suppression and immune hemolysis of opsonized uninfected red cells. In some patients with *P. falciparum* infection, it is possible to demonstrate a positive DAT result due to IgG.

As previously mentioned, some patients with *P. falciparum* infections may exhibit so-called blackwater fever. This was first demonstrated in whites who were being treated with quinine. The condition is not related to G6PD deficiency or to antibodies to quinine. The cause of blackwater fever is still unknown, but there is some evidence to show that it may be related to the level of parasitemia and the lack of immunity in the affected individual. Recent studies showing increases in oxidative stress produced by the parasite within the red cell, when combined with the ability of more than one *P. falciparum* merozoite to infect a cell and the concurrent administration of quinine, may stress the infected red cell sufficiently to produce intravascular lysis.

Cerebral, Pulmonary, and Renal Complications. *P. falciparum* is the only malarial infection in which these complications may arise. Each of them is due largely to the same mechanisms. First, the infected red cell undergoes a number of changes, including increases in permeability and glycolipid fluidity; at the same time it becomes less deformable. Second, *P. falciparum*–infected red cells acquire knoblike structures on the cell membrane. These knobs, which appear to contain malarial antigen, are responsible for cytoadherence and allow the infected cells to adhere to endothelial cells. This mechanism prevents the infected cells from being sequestered in the spleen; however, when combined with the lack of cell deformability, it contributes to sludging of the cells in small capillaries and, in many cases, physically blocks these capillaries. The result is that tissues and organs become anoxic and eventually their function is compromised.

Laboratory Diagnosis. Anemia associated with *P. falciparum* and, if present, with *P. vivax, P. malariae,* and *P. ovale,* is normochromic and normocytic. Leukopenia is present in many cases, as is thrombocytopenia — particularly in individuals with *P. falciparum* infections. Diagnosis of malaria is made by examination of a peripheral blood smear. Blood should be taken just prior to the onset of fever, as it is then that the parasitemia is greatest; however, this is only possible when periodicity of the infection is present. It is usual to examine an unfixed Giemsa- or Wright-stained thick blood smear to ascertain the presence of malarial parasites. Staining is usually performed at a pH of 7.2 to enhance the blue staining of the parasites' cytoplasm. Determination of the species of parasite may be made on this smear, particularly if schizonts or gametocytes are present; however, if only trophozoites are present it will be necessary to examine a stained thin blood smear. *P. falciparum* trophozoites are small, delicate ring structures that occasionally may appear to be adherent to the wall of the red cell. Often more than one parasite is present in a single cell **(see Color Plate 108).** *P. falciparum* gametocytes have a characteristic sausage or crescent shape, which assists immeasurably in identifying the type of infection. Occasionally it is possible to see irregular purple inclusions, called Maurer's dots, in the red cell cytoplasm, which are most probably breakdown products of hemoglobin. *P. vivax* trophozoites grow into characteristic band and ameboid forms that expand and distort the cell they infect. Bluish purple inclusions are often seen in red cells infected with *P. vivax* and *P. ovale* and are called Schüffner's dots **(see Color Plate 109).** Table 14–23 summarizes the features of the different malarial parasites infecting humans.

Immunoassays are being introduced to help screen large numbers of patients for the presence of infection. Flow cytometry has also been used with some success to show the presence of malarial parasites in red cells.

Treatment. Because of the potentially fatal nature of *P. falciparum* infections, it is advisable to treat all malarial infections as if they were caused by this organism. Therapy usually consists of administration of oral quinine sulfate 650 mg three times a day for 10 to 14 days. In severe infections the drug may be given intravenously. In addition oral

Table 14–23. **CHARACTERISTICS OF MALARIAL PARASITES INFECTING HUMANS**

	P. falciparum	*P. vivax*	*P. malariae*	*P. ovale*
Incubation period (days)	6–10	10–12	13–16	10–12
Asexual life cycle (hr)	48	48	72	48
RBCs infected	All	Reticulocytes	Senescent	Reticulocytes
Secondary exoerythrocytic development	No	Yes	Yes	Yes
Duration of relapses in untreated patients	Not applicable	3–5 yr	up to 40 yr	3–5 years
Level of parasitemia	50–60%	2–5%	2–3%	2–3%
Ring form	Small, delicate, may have two chromatin dots, often on edge of RBC Maurer's dots	Large irregular, poor outline One chromatin dot Schüffner's dots	Large thick, prominent chromatin dot	Large irregular, poor outline One chromatin dot Schüffner's dots
Schizonts	Rarely seen in peripheral blood 8–32 merozoites	Large, about same size as RBC 12–25 merozoites	Small "daisy-head" 6–16 merozoites	Irregular arrangement 4–16 merozoites
Gametocytes	Crescent or sausage shape	Round and expand RBC	Round, same size as RBC	

pyrimethamine 25 mg twice daily for 3 days and oral sulfadiazine 500 mg four times a day for 5 days are given. Patients with known *P. vivax*, *P. malariae*, and *P. ovale* infections can be treated with chloroquine phosphate to eliminate erythrocytic parasites and primaquine phosphate to clear hepatic parasites and prevent any future relapses of the infection.

In recent years considerable interest has been shown in the development of vaccine to combat malaria infection. The target for the vaccine has been the sporozoite, merozoite, or gametes, all of which, except the latter, represent the stages of development when the parasite is external to either parenchymal cells or the erythrocyte. Intracellular parasites are protected from the action of antibodies. Despite early promise, it now appears that a vaccine will be a long time in coming.

Babesiosis

Infection by this organism represents a zoonotic infection, as humans are not natural hosts for the parasite. The disease is carried by ticks (*Ixodes* species) and normally infects cattle, deer, and rodents. Infections tend to be self-limiting, although in splenectomized patients they can follow an acute course and be fatal. Patients usually present with a history of malaise, headache, and fever, sometimes associated with vomiting and diarrhea. In splenectomized patients this condition can progress to rigors, acute intravascular hemolysis with associated hemoglobinemia, hemoglobinuria, jaundice, and renal failure.

Diagnosis of the disease is made by examination of the peripheral blood, where parasites very similar to *P. falciparum* are seen in the red cells (**see Color Plate 110**). A history of possible exposure to ticks and a lack of recent travel to areas where malaria is endemic is helpful to correct diagnosis.

Treatment of babesiosis includes administration of quinine, chloroquine, and clindamycin. In severe forms of the disease, support for renal failure and possibly exchange transfusion may be necessary.

Extracellular Infections

Bartonellosis (Oroya Fever)

This disease is restricted to northern areas of South America including Peru, Ecuador, and Columbia. The name Oroya fever derives from the city of Oroya in the Peruvian Andes, where many railroad construction workers were affected by the disease in the late 1800s. It is also referred to as Carrión's disease, after the medical student who died as a result of a self-experiment designed to determine the nature of the infection.

Bartonellosis has a high fatality rate in nonimmune patients and is caused by the organism *Bartonella bacilliformis*. Infection is transmitted between affected individuals by the sand fly, and there does not appear to be any intermediate host. The organisms adhere to the red cell surface and appear as gram-negative rods in the acute phase of the disease. In the recovery phase they assume a coccoid appearance.

The disease has two clinical phases. The first is the hemolytic phase (Oroya fever), which may not occur in all patients. When it does occur, there is a rapid onset with marked intravascular hemolysis. Red cells are also sequestered in the spleen and liver. The anemia can be quite severe and blood smears show many nucleated red cells and a reticulocytosis. Antibiotic therapy including penicillin, streptomycin, and tetracyclines is effective in treating patients in this stage of the infection. The second stage of the disease (verucca peruviana) is nonhematologic and involves the development of verrucous nodes (warty tumors) over the patients face and extremities.

Clostridium perfringens (welchii)

This organism is responsible for the development of gas gangrene and is a gram-positive spore-forming bacillus. Infections in which it is involved are generally located in deep tissues where the anaerobic conditions required for the organism's survival exist. The organism is normally present in the environment and may infect tissues exposed by trauma and surgical procedures. There is a high incidence of the infection in septic abortions. The organism is responsible for extensive tissue damage due to the release of enzymes and toxins. Septicemia due to C. perfringens may produce an acute intravascular hemolytic process resulting from the release of an alpha toxin or lecithinase. This process, combined with phospholipases and possibly proteinases also produced by the organism, acts upon the red cell membrane to cause its destruction and subsequent lysis of the cell. Hemolysis is often severe, with marked hemoglobinemia and hemoglobinuria. Acute renal failure may develop quite rapidly, and prognosis is generally poor. Microspherocytes are a common finding in the peripheral blood smear. Leukocytosis with a shift to the left and thrombocytopenia is present in most cases.

Improvements in the maintenance of aseptic conditions during and following surgery and the decrease in criminal abortions have caused this form of presentation of hemolytic anemia to become quite uncommon.

Other Bacterial and Viral Infections

A wide variety of bacterial and viral agents are associated with infections in which hemolysis, to varying degrees, may be present. Many bacteria, through either the toxins that they produce or the formation of immune complexes involving soluble antigen of bacterial origin, may initiate DIC. This in turn may lead to microangiopathic hemolytic anemia (MAHA). Most often MAHA is associated with gram-negative bacteria producing septicemia. Microangiopathic hemolytic anemia is discussed in a later section of this chapter.

Some bacteria (such as Pseudomonas sp.) or their products (for example, deacetylases) may act on the red cell membrane to alter its antigenicity. This action, which is usually enzymatic, may lead to the exposure of crypt-antigens such as T, Tk, Th, and acquired B. These antigens are referred to as polyagglutination antigens because antibodies to them are present in the serum of most adults and the affected individual's cells will agglutinate when mixed with the serum of an ABO-matched person. For a short time the cells of the affected person are agglutinated by their own serum; however, production of the antibody stops as the immune system becomes exposed to this new self-antigen. Immune hemolysis is not a common occurrence in these cases.

Viruses may be associated with hemolytic anemia, primarily through their effects on the immune system. In many cases the infection will cause the production of autoantibodies which subsequently produce immune hemolysis of the red cells (see beginning of this chapter). Hemorrhagic fevers found in patients in the tropics have been associated with viral infections, but the mechanisms responsible for hemolysis are not well understood. Dengue and yellow fevers may show evidence of intravascular hemolysis.

Table 14–24 lists the organisms that have been associated with hemolytic anemia.

Mechanical Etiologies

The passage of red cells through the vascular system subjects the cell to a wide range of environmental conditions. As it travels around the body, shear forces on the cell are highly variable and are in-

Table 14–24. **ORGANISMS ASSOCIATED WITH HEMOLYTIC ANEMIA**

Bacteria	Viruses	Protozoa	Fungi
Bartonella bacilliformis	Coxsackie	Babesia microti	Aspergillus
Clostridium perfringens	Cytomegalovirus	Babesia divergens	
Escherichia coli	Epstein-Barr	Plasmodium falciparum	
Haemophilus influenzae	Herpes simplex	P. malariae	
Mycobacteria tuberculosis	Influenza A	P. ovale	
Mycoplasma pneumoniae	Rubeola	P. vivax	
Neisseria meningitidis	Varicella	Toxoplasma	
Salmonella sp.			
Shigella sp.			
Streptococcus sp.			
Vibrio cholera			
Yersinia enterocolitica			

fluenced by the size of the lumen of the vessel in which the cell is moving, the surface conditions of the vessel, the rate at which it is moving, and the number of other cells present at the same time. Other environmental conditions with which the cell must contend in its travels include changes in pH, in electrolytes, and in protein concentration. Factors that influence the shear forces on the cell may lead to mechanical disruption of the cell membrane with consequent hemolysis. Of the factors previously mentioned, the most important appears to be the surface conditions of the vessel with which the red cell interacts in its passage. Under normal conditions the endothelial cells lining the blood vessels provide an extremely smooth surface and do not impede the cell's passage, even when it must pass through a capillary with a diameter narrower than that of the cell itself. However, altered or abnormal surfaces may cause the cell to adhere momentarily to the surface, at which time the forces on it produced by the blood flow may cause it to stretch and rupture. Although red cells are normally quite deformable, they are not capable of being stretched to a great degree. The result of this mechanical rupturing of the cell membrane is to produce intravascular hemolysis accompanied by the presence of red cell fragments or schistocytes (**see Color Plate 119**).

Intravascular hemolysis accompanied by a significant number of schistocytes in the peripheral blood occurs in patients with a cardiac prosthesis, who suffer from the relative rare condition of march hemoglobinuria, or who have MAHA. The former two conditions may be referred to as macroangiopathic hemolytic anemias because larger blood vessels are involved in the hemolytic process.

Cardiac Prosthesis

Significant hemolysis following cardiac surgery is most common in patients who have received a plastic aortic valve, although all patients given an artificial valve or prosthetic patch will show evidence of some hemolysis. Hemolysis in patients receiving a homograft or xenograft is minimal. Artificial valves provide rough surfaces with which the red cells must interact in their passage through the heart. Once the implant is endothelialized, hemolysis is reduced.

The degree of anemia and fragmentation of red cells is highly variable. Usually the anemia is well compensated, leaving hemoglobin concentrations in the normal range. Occasionally a patient may have severe anemia and require transfusion. The peripheral blood smear shows many fragmented cells, including helmet cells. Occasionally microspherocytes are present. Leukocytes are usually normal, whereas platelets are often reduced owing to their interaction with the abnormal surface. Hemoglobinemia and hemoglobinuria are usually present, although the latter may be very mild. Hemosiderinuria is invariably present. Renal failure is rarely a complication in this type of hemolytic anemia. Haptoglobin levels are reduced.

Treatment of cardiac hemolysis can range from supportive therapy, which may include iron supplementation and transfusion if necessary, to reoperation to correct the faulty valve or vessel surface surgically.

March Hemoglobinuria

This form of hemolytic anemia was first described in the late 1800s in a young German soldier who presented with frank hemoglobinuria following a field marching exercise. The anemia has been described in joggers, marathon runners, and conga drum players. The cause of the anemia has been attributed to the direct physical disruption of the red cells as they flow through capillaries that are being subjected to intermittent but regular pressure. Patients who present with march hemoglobinuria following jogging may significantly reduce the incidence of episodes of hemoglobinuria if they wear cushion-sole shoes and jog on soft surfaces.

The blood picture of patients with march hemoglobinuria usually demonstrates a normal hemoglobin, although there may be an increase in the reticulocyte count. Hemoglobinemia and hemoglobinuria are episodic and present only following exercise. This obvious association with exercise is helpful in distinguishing the hemoglobinuria from other causes (such as PNH). Fragmented red cells are not a feature of the condition.

Microangiopathic Hemolytic Anemia

Hemolytic Processes. Microangiopathic hemolytic anemia is characterized by the presence in the peripheral blood of a large number of schistocytes and a low to low-normal platelet count. The extent of the anemia is variable but may be associated with the presence of a reticulocytosis. As the name implies, MAHA is associated with the presence of either localized or, less commonly, generalized abnormalities in the microcirculation. Most often the abnormalities in the microcirculation are due to the deposition of fibrin strands resulting from the intravascular activation of the coagulation system. Activation of the coagulation system in MAHA usually follows a chronic course in which the clinical condition is dominated by the hemolytic process. In contrast, DIC may present as an acute clinical condition in which excessive bleeding occurs with no evidence of hemolysis.

In MAHA the mechanical process leading to fragmentation of the red cells occurs as the blood flow forces the cells to negotiate a blood vessel whose lumen is restricted by fibrin strands. The red cells are physically torn as they are forced along a tortuous path within the narrow confines of the blood vessel. In addition to the intravascular hemolysis of the red cells, the fragments produced lack deformability, and there is an increase in extravascular hemolysis in the spleen.

Microangiopathic hemolytic anemia is associated with a wide range of conditions, but there are two in which it is a characteristic feature.

Hemolytic Uremic Syndrome. An acquired disorder found in infants and young children, hemolytic uremic syndrome (HUS) is characterized by intravascular hemolysis, renal failure, and thrombocytopenia.

Clinical Features. Hemolytic uremic syndrome is found predominantly in children under age 5, and the incidence decreases up to puberty; it is quite rare beyond that time. Generally, the syndrome becomes evident anywhere from 1 to 12 days following a systemic illness in which fever, diarrhea, and vomiting occur. Occasionally it may occur without any obvious preceding symptoms of disease. Quite often the illness and subsequent HUS occur in individuals who are in close relationship with each other (such as siblings and school children). This relationship indicates possible common precipitating factors, which may be environmental (such as infection) or genetic or both. The disease may show epidemic features and occur during certain seasons, most often autumn.

The onset of HUS is characterized by purpura or petechial hemorrhage, jaundice, hemoglobinuria, proteinuria, uremia, and hypertension. Involvement of the central nervous system is rare, although it may be evident in patients who exhibit severe hypertension.

This syndrome may develop rapidly as an acute disease, in which case it is important to institute early diagnosis and treatment. The mortality of the disease varies from 5 to 10 percent. Dialysis and the successful treatment of hypertension is critical to the eventual outcome of the disease. Blood transfusions and treatment of DIC, if a significant feature of the disease, is often necessary. Recent evidence has indicated that plasma exchange may be beneficial. Of those patients who survive the acute phase of the disease, approximately one third will recover completely, one third will develop chronic renal failure, and one third will develop persistent oliguric renal failure.

Laboratory Diagnosis. Peripheral blood smear examination reveals a decreased hemoglobin with an increased reticulocyte count indicating bone marrow compensation. This compensation may also result in normoblasts being present in the peripheral blood. The leukocyte count may be normal or raised, depending on the nature of the precipitating illness, and platelets are usually reduced. Coagulation studies for DIC may show normal results for the prothrombin time, activated partial thromboplastin time, and thrombin time. The fibrinogen level may be normal or increased. Tests for fibrin degradation products and D-dimer are usually raised with levels indicative of a chronic disease process. Examination of a peripheral blood smear will show the characteristic features of MAHA with many fragmented cells—schistocytes—and helmet cells. Polychromasia is increased and platelets are reduced. A differential leukocyte count may show neutrophilia. Biochemical studies reveal evidence of hemolysis (such as hyperbilirubinemia) and of renal failure (for example, raised urea and creatinine levels).

Thrombotic Thrombocytopenic Purpura. This disease bears many similarities to HUS, but there are also a number of distinctly different features. Thrombotic thrombocytopenic purpura (TTP) is a disease that presents mainly in adolescents and young adults of either gender, although there appears to be a slightly higher incidence in females. The disease is characterized by five predominant features: fever, anemia, thrombocytopenia, renal disease, and neurologic changes.

The exact etiology of the disease is unknown and it may occur secondary to infections and connective tissue disease. If it occurs in pregnant women, it must be differentiated from pre-eclampsia. The pathology of the disease does appear to result from the aggregation of platelets in small capillaries and their subsequent adherences to the vessel walls with consequent occlusion of the vessel by platelet plugs and fibrin. Some studies have shown that the vessel walls in affected patients lack the ability to synthesize prostacyclin, which functions as a platelet-antiaggregating agent.

Clinical Features. This condition is rare, but has a high fatality rate (greater than 50 percent); therefore, it is significant when it does occur. Onset of the condition is invariably sudden and patients usually present with fever and neurologic disturbances possibly including convulsions, hallucinations, coma, and paralysis. These signs may be accompanied by purpura and varying degrees of anemia. Occasionally the disease may present as an acute episode of bleeding usually into the gastrointestinal or genitourinary tracts. Purpura may be marked due to the accompanying decrease in the platelet count. In these cases the hemoglobin can fall very rapidly and the patient may be jaundiced and show evidence of hemoglobinuria. Bleeding episodes may be accompanied by concurrent hypertension. The time at which the features of the disease become evident can be quite variable and it may follow a fluctuating course. For example, neurologic disturbances may be the most obvious sign of a disease process and may lead to a patient being investigated over a period of time for a neuropsychiatric disorder. Renal failure is invariably present but it may be revealed only after laboratory investigation. Some patients show evidence of having possibly suffered from HUS in childhood.

Laboratory Diagnosis. Hematologic investigation of patients with TTP classically reveal a microangiopathic hemolytic anemia with thrombocytopenia (**see Color Plate 119**). The reticulocyte count is raised and occasionally nucleated red blood cells are present in the peripheral blood. There is often a neutrophilia with a shift to the left. Coagulation studies will often give a normal prothrombin time, activated partial thromboplastin time, and thrombin time. Tests for fibrin degradation products or D-dimer will often have elevated results, indicative of a chronic disease process. These test results may be quite abnormal if and when a patient is experiencing a bleeding episode, although the bleeding is mainly due to platelet consumption and not to consumption of coagulation factors. Biochemical studies often show raised lactic dehydrogenase levels as evidence of red cell hemolysis and hyperbilirubinemia. Creatinine levels may be increased when renal failure develops late in the disease process. Proteinuria is invariably present.

Treatment of patients with TTP requires aggressive therapy if they are to survive. This is usually done when both intensive care and renal dialysis facilities are on hand. Current treatment usually employs plasma exchange with infusion of fresh frozen plasma (FFP). Infusion of FFP alone may be sufficient to reverse the disease process. Not all patients will respond to FFP with or without plasma exchange. Such patients may benefit from the use of corticosteroids. Evidence of the possible role of prostacyclin in the disease has been the use of prostacyclin analogues or of drugs known to promote prostacyclin synthesis. Some patients benefit from splenectomy.

As infection is often thought to be a precipitating factor in the disease, the early use of broad-spectrum antibiotics, particularly in groups possibly at risk (such as pregnant women), may be advantageous.

Other Conditions. A wide range of disease processes may be accompanied by evidence of MAHA. Most often these are malignancies or infection. In the case of malignancies the red cell fragmentation occurs usually in the blood vessels of the developing tumor mass. The most common tumor associated with MAHA is mucoid-producing adenocarcinoma. Secondary tumors in the bone marrow will often show a MAHA picture accompanied by leukoerythroblastic changes in the peripheral blood. In most cases DIC is not a prominent feature of these conditions. Microangiopathic hemolytic anemia accompanied by DIC is a classic feature of promyelocytic leukemia (M3). In this condition the DIC is of more significance to the patient than is the MAHA.

Diseases in which changes to blood vessels occur (such as vasculitis), often owing to either infectious agents or immune processes, may show evidence of MAHA. Hence, MAHA may be seen in patients with acute glomerular nephritis and polyarteritis nodosa. Organ rejection often leads to deposition of fibrin in the microcirculation of the transplanted organ. While blood flow remains within the organ, evidence of MAHA may be seen. Septicemia due to meningococcal or pneumococcal infection often produces both MAHA and DIC. The DIC is usually the most significant pathology of the disease, and hemolysis may be only mild (see Chapter 28).

Chemicals and Physical Agents

Oxidative Hemolysis

As described in Chapter 10, the red cells of individuals who are congenitally deficient in a number of red cell enzymes may be hemolyzed following exposure to oxidative agents. However, the red cells of normal individuals may also be hemolyzed if the oxidative agent is sufficiently strong.

Oxidative stress on the red cell may affect the membrane of the hemoglobin molecule, with either the globin chains or the heme group being affected. Most oxidizing agents will influence the hemoglobin molecule, producing either Heinz body formation by denaturing globin chains or by oxidizing the heme group to produce methemoglobinemia.

Two drugs classically reported as producing hemolysis due to oxidative stress on normal red cells are dapsone and salazopyrine. Both drugs if taken in high enough doses will cause chemical damage to the red cell membrane and may lead to Heinz body formation. The red cells of affected patients will show characteristic "bite" formation in which a part of the cell appears to have been removed. Dapsone is employed for the treatment of patients with leprosy whereas salazopyrine is used for those with ulcerative colitis. In both groups of patients the hemolysis is usually well compensated. Hemolysis disappears once the drug is stopped, although cessation of the drug is usually not possible because of the disease being treated.

A wide range of chemicals may result in methemoglobinemia, particularly in young children. The most important of these are the nitrites, which can contaminate water or which may be present in high concentration in juices of some vegetables (such as spinach). Children are usually affected if their intake of these contaminated fluids is high and they have an impairment in their natural reducing mechanisms.

Combined analgesics such as aspirin, phenacetin, and codeine, when taken in sufficiently high doses, produced intravascular hemolysis characterized by the presence of methemoglobinemia and methemalbumin. Such drug combinations are generally no longer available over-the-counter, as they contributed to a high level of renal failure. This adverse effect is particularly evident in women who overuse the tablets.

Use of nitrates such as amyl or butyl nitrate have been associated with methemoglobinemia in patients who have indulged in excessive use of these compounds. Such chemicals constitute the recreational drugs known as "poppers."

Hemolysis has been produced in young infants by water-soluble vitamin K analogues. This hemolysis may be associated with methemoglobinemia, although it is not a consistent feature. The weed killer sodium chlorate may produce acute intravascular hemolysis if taken in large doses. Sufficiently large doses can be fatal, and the chemical is often implicated in cases of suicide.

Nonoxidative Hemolysis

Arsenic. Many industrial processes particularly those involving the action of acids and metals may give rise to the production of arsine gas. Continued exposure to the gas gives rise to intravascular hemolysis with anemia and hemoglobinuria. Marked methemalbumin formation causes the serum of affected patients to turn a characteristic brown and often to mask the presence of any red cells. Current concern for occupational health and safety requirements has seen that this hazard is being minimized in the workplace.

Lead. The affects of lead on hemoglobin synthesis have been known for a long time, and the anemia produced by lead exposure is usually caused by this process and not by direct hemolysis. The red cells of patients exposed to lead have a shortened red cell survival. Lead poisoning is usually a problem of young children who have been eating materials painted with lead-based paints. Children affected by lead poisoning may show a normocytic hypochromic blood picture, with classic punctate basophilic stippling. This is becoming much less a problem now, with legislation in most countries prohibiting toys and play equipment from being painted with lead-based paints. The other primary source of exposure is industrial activities. Prolonged exposure may lead to ringed sideroblasts evident in the bone marrow.

Copper. Very high levels of copper ions have been associated with intravascular hemolysis. These levels may occur as a result of suicide attempts in which copper sulphate solution is ingested or in Wilson's disease. The hemolytic process is unknown, although it has been shown that high levels of copper ions can affect a number of intracellular enzymes. The anemia may be associated with the presence of spherocytes.

Venoms. A number of venoms, particularly those from some spiders, contain potent enzymes capable of directly acting on the red cell membrane to produce lysis of the cell. Bee stings in some people may produce a hemolytic process. Snake venoms, although hemolytic in vitro, rarely cause hemolysis in vivo.

Osmotic Effects

Water. Patients in whom water irrigation has been used as part of a surgical process may show evidence of intravascular hemolysis. This is particularly so in men who may have had a transurethral resection for cancer of the prostate. Patients who have suffered from near drowning in fresh water may also show similar evidence. The peripheral blood picture in these patients generally shows many spherocytes.

Burns. Patients who have suffered severe burns to greater than 15 percent of their body will generally show evidence of intravascular hemolysis. The hemolytic process is thought to be due to the direct effect of the heat on the red cells in the affected area. Red cells that are heated to temperatures in excess of 49°C undergo changes including fragmentation, budding, and microspherocyte formation; blood collected within 24 hours of such heating will show evidence of these changes. Because the cells are osmotically and mechanically fragile, they are rapidly removed from the circulation, and blood collected after that time quite often is normal in appearance.

Acquired Membrane Disorders

A number of mechanisms can be implicated in producing changes to red cell membranes, which can result in the shortened lifespan of the cell. Any change that compromises the cell's deformability or its resistance to oxidative stress can potentially contribute to a hemolytic process.

Liver Disease

The red cells of patients with cirrhosis and acute hepatitis have a marginally reduced lifespan, which may give rise to an increased reticulocyte count; however, anemia in these patients is not common. The morphologic changes to the red cells seen in biliary obstruction are primarily due to the changes in cell-bound and free lipids which affect the shape of the red cell.

Zieve syndrome consists of mild hemolysis and acute abdominal pain associated with fatty liver and hyperglyceridemia. The syndrome, which is uncommon, occurs mainly in alcoholics. The blood picture may show the presence of spherocytes. The hemolytic anemia is usually self-limiting, and diagnosis of Zieve syndrome can be difficult because lipid changes may return to normal by the time of investigation.

Another condition that may be seen in liver disease is spur-cell anemia. In this condition the red cells assume a characteristic shape with a number of fine fingerlike spikes protruding from the cell **(see Color Plate 127)**. Some of these spikes may be surmounted by a knob. These cells are found in patients with alcoholic cirrhosis and probably result from increased cholesterol content in the red cell membrane. The cells lack deformability and are trapped within the microcirculation of the spleen.

Lipid Disorders

As seen in liver disease, acquired lipid disorders can affect the normal red cell morphology and lead to alterations in red cell deformability. A red cell abnormality due to a congenital form of lipid abnormality is seen in a β-lipoproteinemia. This rare condition is characterized by retinitis pigmentosa, steatorrhea, ataxia, and mental retardation. The red cells may contribute to the diagnosis of the condition as they assume the classic shape of acanthocytes **(see Color Plate 82)**. As with spur cells, acanthocytes lack the deformability to pass through the microvasculature of the spleen and become trapped, leading to a reduced red cell survival.

Vitamin E Deficiency

Vitamin E deficiency is rare in adults but may occur in infants who are fed a diet high in polyunsaturated fatty acids. The red cells of vitamin E–deficient infants are susceptible to oxidative stress and may lyse intravascularly.

Renal Disease

The anemia of renal disease is multifactorial, one part of which may be due to increased red cell destruction. In end-stage renal disease the accumulation of excretory products leads to unfavorable conditions for red cell survival. Many of the cells take on the appearance of burr cells, or echinocytes **(see Color Plate 124)**, which are round and have numerous small spines over their entire surface. Often, similar-looking cells are seen in a badly made blood smear; however, these cells are usually present only in certain areas of the smear, whereas in renal disease they occur uniformly throughout the smear. Other conditions in which echinocytes are seen include pyruvate kinase deficiency, where they are sometimes referred to as "thorny apple" cells, and in bleeding states associated with peptic ulcers. Generally these cells lack deformability and, besides being trapped in the spleen, become fragmented within the kidney where fibrin deposition often occurs. Dialysis removes the accumulated excretory products and the red cell morphology will often return to normal after a number of weeks.

Hypersplenism

This condition has been subject to a number of different interpretations over the years with respect to what it actually entails. It is now generally believed that hypersplenism is not itself a process but rather the result of a number of processes. The condition is one in which cells are selectively retained by the spleen and thus have a shortened cell survival. Interestingly, the spleen can be very selective regarding which cells it will retain: in idiopathic thrombocytopenic purpura only platelets are sequestered, whereas red cells have a normal survival.

The increased retention of cells is not always associated with splenomegaly, although in most cases splenomegaly is present. Similarly, the presence of splenomegaly does not necessarily mean that hypersplenism will be present.

Mechanisms that have been proposed to account for shortened red cell survival in patients with splenomegaly include the following: (1) increased

transit time in the spleen leads to metabolic stress on the cells due to the lower pH in the organ; and (2) increased transit time leads to a reduction in membrane lipids, which causes changes in the cells' surface-to-volume ratio, resulting in decreased cell deformability. Conditions associated with hypersplenism are listed in Table 14–25.

BIBLIOGRAPHY

Bowdler, AJ: Splenomegaly and hypersplenism. Clin Hematol 12:467, 1983.

Bowman, JM: Rh erythroblastosis fetalis. Semin Hematol 12:189, 1975.

Bowman, JM, et al: Rh iso-immunization during pregnancy: Antenatal prophylaxis. Can Med Assoc J 118:623, 1978.

Candle, MR and Scott, JR: The potential role of immunosuppression, plasmapheresis and desensitisation as treatment modalities for Rh immunisation. Clin Obstet Gynecol 25:313, 1982.

Carter, P, Koval, JJ, and Hobbs, JR: The relation of clinical and laboratory findings to the survival of patients with macroglobinaemia. Clin Exp Immunol 28:241, 1977.

Chaplin, H and Avioli, LV: Autoimmune hemolytic anemia. Arch Intern Med 137:346, 1977.

Chiu, D, Kuypers, F, and Lubin, B: Lipid peroxidation in human red cells. Semin Hematol 26:257, 1989

Cooper, RA: Haemolytic syndromes and red cell membrane abnormalities in liver disease. Semin Hematol 17:103, 1980.

Czuba, TL: Special problems in the mother and newborn. In Pierce, S and Wilson, JK (eds): Approaches to Serological Problems in the Hospital Transfusion Service. American Association of Blood Banks, Arlington, VA, pp 73–99, 1985.

Dacie, JV: Autoimmune hemolytic anemia. Arch Intern Med 135:1293, 1975.

Dike, AE: The role of plasma exchange in the management of hemolytic disease of the newborn: The Oxford Experience. Plasma Therapy and Transfusion Technology 5:23, 1984.

Frank, MM, Atkinson, JP, and Gadek, J: Cold agglutinins and cold agglutinin disease. Annu Rev Med 28:291, 1977.

Garratty, G: Drug-induced immune hemolytic anemia and/or positive direct antiglobulin tests. Immunohematology 2:1, 1985.

Garratty, G: Current viewpoints on mechanisms causing drug-induced immune hemolytic anemia and/or positive direct antiglobulin test. Immunohematology 5:97, 1989.

Garratty, G: Hemolytic Disease of the Newborn. American Association of Blood Banks, Arlington, VA, 1984.

Golbus, MS, et al: Rh isoimmunization following genetic amniocentesis. Prenat Diagn 2:49, 1982.

Gordon-Smith, EC: Drug induced oxidative haemolysis. Clin Haematol 9:557, 1980.

Hensleigh, PA: Preventing rhesus iso-immunization: Antepartum Rh immune globulin prophylaxis versus a sensitive test for risk identification. Am J Obstet Gynecol 146:749, 1983.

Karmali, MA, et al: The association between idiopathic haemolytic uraemic syndrome and infection by verotoxin-producing Escherichia coli. J Infect Dis 151:775, 1985.

Kwaan, HC: Clinicopathological features of thrombotic thrombocytopenic purpura. Semin Hematol 24:71, 1987.

Leddy, JP and Swisher, SN: Acquired immune hemolytic disorders (including drug-induced immune hemolytic anemia). In Samter, M (ed): Immunological Diseases, ed 3. Vol I. Little, Brown & Co, Boston, 1978, p 1187.

Marchand, A: Charting a course for hemolytic anemia. Diagn Med 19, 1981.

Marchand, A: Immune hemolytic anemia. Part I: Classification, manifestations and mechanism of destruction. Diagn Med 51, 1982.

Marchand, A: Immune hemolytic anemia. Part II: Test procedures and strategy. Diagn Med 25, 1983.

Mollison, PL: Blood Transfusion in Clinical Medicine, ed 6. Blackwell Scientific, Oxford, 1979, pp 693–709.

Table 14–25. **CONDITIONS ASSOCIATED WITH HYPERSPLENISM**

Idiopathic hypersplenism
Secondary hypersplenism associated with:
   Acute and chronic infections with splenomegaly: malaria, kala-azar, mononucleosis, brucellosis, viral hepatitis
   Infiltrating diseases: storage disorders, leukemia, lymphoma and cancer
   Inflammatory disorders: Felty's syndrome, systemic lupus erythematosus, sarcoidosis
   Congestive splenomegaly
   Chronic hemolytic diseases: hereditary spherocytosis, thalassemia, and so on

Murgo AJ: Thrombotic microangiopathy in the cancer patient including those induced by chemotherapeutic agents. Semin Hematol 24:161, 1987.

Petz, LD and Garratty, G: Acquired Immune Hemolytic Anemias. Churchill-Livingstone, New York, 1980.

Pittiglio, DH, Baldwin, AJ, and Sohmer, PR: Modern Blood Banking and Transfusion Practices. FA Davis, Philadelphia, 1983.

Queenan, JT: Current management of the Rh sensitised patient. Clin Obstet Gynecol 25:293, 1982.

Rote, NS: Pathophysiology of Rh iso-immunization. Clin Obstet Gynecol 25:243, 1982.

Sacher, RA and Lenes, BA: Exchanges transfusion. Clin Lab Med 1:265, 1981.

Scott, JR and Warenski, JC: Tests to detect and quantitate feto-maternal bleeding. Clin Obstet Gynecol 25:277, 1982.

Steiner, EA, et al: Percutaneous umbilical blood sampling and umbilical vein transfusions: rapid serological differentiation of fetal blood from maternal blood. Transfusion 30:104, 1990.

Tanowitz, HB, Robbins, N, and Leidlich, N: Hemolytic anemia: Associated with severe mycoplasma pneumoniae pneumonia. NY State J Med 78:2231, 1978.

Taswell, HF, Pineda, AA, and Moore, SB: Hemolytic transfusion reactions: Frequency and clinical laboratory aspects. American Association of Blood Banks 4:71, Arlington, VA, 1981.

Whitfield, CR: An obstetric overview of trends in the management of Rh hemolytic disease. Plasma Therapy Transfusion Technology 5:47, 1984.

QUESTIONS

1. *What are the mechanisms of immune hemolysis?*
   a. IgG or IgM antibodies that activate the classic complement pathway
   b. Antibody-dependent cellular cytotoxicity (ADCC) mediated by NK cells, monocytes/macrophages, and granulocytes
   c. Complement and phagocytic cells in a reaction of immune adherence
   d. All of the above

2. *What is the process in which the immune system produces antibodies to foreign red cell antigens introduced into their circulation through transfusion, pregnancy, or organ transplantation?*
   a. Alloimmune hemolytic anemia
   b. Autoimmune hemolytic anemia
   c. Drug-induced immune hemolytic anemia
   d. None of the above

3. *Which finding is not characteristic for immediate hemolytic transfusion reactions?*
   a. Acute intravascular hemolysis
   b. Most commonly caused by ABO IgM complement-activating antibodies
   c. Increase in plasma haptoglobin
   d. Hemoglobinemia, hemoglobinuria, and hemosiderinuria

4. *What is true concerning delayed hemolytic transfusion reactions?*
   a. Antibodies are not demonstrable in patient serum until 10 to 14 days after transfusion.
   b. Antibodies are usually IgG formed from a secondary response.
   c. Hemoglobinemia and hemoglobinuria are present.
   d. Findings include a negative direct antiglobulin test result and antibody screen.

5. *What causes HDN?*
   a. Maternal antibodies, formed as a result of a previous pregnancy, cross the placenta and attach to fetal cells.
   b. Fetal antibodies cross the placenta and attach to maternal red cells.
   c. Maternal antibodies attach to maternal red cells, which cross the placenta and enter fetal circulation.
   d. Fetal antibodies attach to fetal red cells and cross the placenta to enter the mother's circulation.

6. *Which of the following is not a hematologic finding for HDN?*
   a. Mild to severe anemia
   b. Microcytosis and hypochromia
   c. Reticulocytosis
   d. Spherocytes and nucleated RBCs

7. *Which of the following is a treatment for HDN?*
   a. Intrauterine or umbilical vein transfusion
   b. Maternal plasmapheresis
   c. Infant phototherapy
   d. All of the above

8. *What immune system abnormality results in the loss of self-recognition for an individual's own red cell antigens?*
   a. Alloimmune hemolytic anemia
   b. Autoimmune hemolytic anemia
   c. Drug-induced immune hemolytic anemia
   d. None of the above

9. *What is not a characteristic of warm autoimmune hemolytic anemia?*
   a. Variable anemia
   b. Reticulocytosis, spherocytosis, red cell fragmentation
   c. Positive result for Donath-Landsteiner test
   d. DAT result usually positive for both IgG and C3d

10. *What are features of cold agglutinin syndrome?*
    a. Usually an IgM antibody
    b. Reticulocytosis and positive DAT result
    c. Tendency for spontaneous autoagglutination of RBC samples
    d. All of the above

11. *What is the principle of the Donath-Landsteiner test?*
    a. Antibody binds red cells at 37°C and causes lysis at 4°C.
    b. Antibody binds red cells at 4°C and causes lysis at 37°C.
    c. Antibody binds red cells at 4°C or 37°C and causes immediate lysis.
    d. Antibody binds red cells at 4°C or 37°C but causes lysis only at 4°C.

12. *Which of the following is a mechanism for drug-induced immune hemolytic anemia?*
    a. Immune complex
    b. Drug adsorption (hapten)
    c. Membrane modification
    d. All of the above

13. *What are causes for nonimmune hemolytic anemia?*
    a. Infections
    b. Mechanical, chemical, and physical agents
    c. Acquired membrane disorders
    d. All of the above

14. *How is laboratory diagnosis made for malarial infection?*
    a. Examination of peripheral blood smear
    b. Recovery of the organism
    c. Measuring hepatic enzymes
    d. Skin testing

15. *Which of the following organisms are associated with hemolytic anemia?*
    a. *Mycoplasma pneumoniae*
    b. Epstein-Barr virus
    c. *Babesia microti*
    d. All of the above

ANSWERS

1. d (p. 194–195)
2. a (p. 195)
3. c (p. 196–197)
4. b (p. 197)
5. a (p. 197–198)
6. b (p. 198)
7. d (p. 199–200)
8. b (p. 201)
9. c (p. 202)
10. d (p. 204–205)
11. b (p. 206)
12. d (p. 207)
13. d (p. 212)
14. a (p. 214)
15. d (p. 216)

CHAPTER 15

SANDRA GWALTNEY-KRAUSE, M.A., M.T.(ASCP)

Anemia Associated with Other Disorders

OBJECTIVES

At the end of this chapter, the learner should be able to:
1. Define anemia associated with inflammation.
2. Identify laboratory findings characteristic of the anemia of inflammation.
3. List causes for anemia of inflammation.
4. Name the immune processes responsible for inducing the anemia of inflammation.
5. Describe the treatment for anemia of inflammation.

6. List causes for anemias not associated with the anemia of inflammation.
7. Describe the general laboratory findings associated with endocrine disease anemias.
8. Name the major cause of the anemia associated with renal failure.
9. Describe the typical appearance of red cells in anemia associated with liver disease.

At first glance, anyone skimming over the subjects for this chapter might very well wonder what anemia could possibly result from such a "mixed bag" of diseases. What do they have in common? These diseases are *systemic* diseases in which a variety of mechanisms may affect red cell production, survival, and integrity. All of these diseases are associated with an anemia that is secondary to the underlying disease state, and they are treated differ-

ently than other forms of anemia. Some of these diseases have something else in common: they are linked by ferrokinetics and the mechanism of inflammation. Anemia of chronic disorders (ACD) is the term that describes the anemia associated with chronic infections, inflammation, and malignancy. Anemia of chronic disorders is the hematologic consequence of the immune system during inflammation.

Recent research has demonstrated a mechanism involved in the inflammatory response to tissue injury that has rendered ACD obsolete. Most researchers will agree that ACD is misleading and has been retained only for lack of a better name. Anemia of inflammation (AOI) has been suggested as a more appropriate term because it describes the mechanism of the disorder and is therefore used throughout this chapter.

Anemias produced by inflammation and systemic diseases are perhaps the most common hematologic abnormalities encountered in the laboratory. It is important for the clinician and the medical technologist to recognize the characteristics of these anemias in patients with systemic diseases and to understand the basis of hematologic assays which can differentiate them from other causes of anemia. In some instances, anemia at the preliminary visit without other clinical symptoms may be the first indication of malignancy. A sudden change in the CBC of a patient who has been diagnosed with an inflammatory disease may indicate a new complication.

Patients with rheumatoid arthritis frequently develop anemia attributed to chronic inflammation. Those with chronic arthritis may later develop an iron-deficiency anemia due to chronic gastrointestinal blood loss from aspirin therapy. Not every systemic disease demonstrates anemia. Diabetes mellitus is not associated with anemia unless the patient has complications such as a chronic infection or develops renal failure. This chapter discusses the characteristic features of the anemia associated with inflammation (infection, inflammatory diseases, and malignancy) and the anemias seen in other systemic diseases (endocrine disorders, renal disease, and liver disease).

ANEMIA ASSOCIATED WITH INFLAMMATION

The exact mechanism for the anemia of inflammation is still evolving; recent research in this area has revealed that this anemia is a "cost paid" consequence to the host during the immune response to tissue injury. The anemia of inflammation is not a product of red cell antibody formation but rather a product of the host response to inflammation.

Characteristics of the Anemia of Inflammation

Anemia of inflammation is a hypoproliferative but mild anemia that is usually normocytic and normochromic but that may be microcytic or hypochromic if the disease increases in severity. Anemia of inflammation is characterized by low serum iron and a decreased total iron-binding capacity (TIBC), despite normal to increased iron stores in reticuloendothelial cells. The fact that iron stores can be elevated in bone marrow aspirates in AOI is helpful in differentiating this anemia from iron-deficiency anemia. Serum ferritin levels are usually

Table 15-1. **COMPARISON OF AOI WITH IRON-DEFICIENCY ANEMIA**

	Normal	AOI	IDA
Serum iron (μg/dl)	50-150	↓	↓
TIBC (μg/dl)	300-360	↓	↑
Ferritin (μg/dl)	20-250	↑	↓
Transferrin saturation (%)	20-45	↓	↓
FEPs (μg/dl of RBCs)	15-80	↑	↑
RE marrow iron deposits	2-3+	↑	↓
Sideroblasts (%)	40-60	↓	↓
Reticulocytes (%)	0.5-2.0	↓	↓

IDA = iron-deficiency anemia.

increased in AOI—another useful aid in differentiating it from iron-deficiency anemia (Table 15-1). Transferrin saturation generally falls between 5 and 16 percent. Free erythrocyte protoporphyrins (FEPs) are elevated.

Slight decreases can be seen in hematocrit (Hct), hemoglobin (Hgb), mean corpuscular volume (MCV), and mean corpuscular hemoglobin concentration (MCHC), with a corresponding increase in red cell distribution width (RDW).[1] The anemia can become fully developed within 1 to 2 months after the onset of illness and usually worsens if the underlying disease becomes aggravated and more severe.

Several other biochemical changes occur in patients with anemia of inflammation. Acute phase reactants appear in the serum, including fibrinogen, C-reactive protein, amyloid A protein, ceruloplasmin, haptoglobin, and C3. The increase in fibrinogen contributes to the accelerated erythrocyte sedimentation rate (ESR) seen in patients with cancer, infections, and rheumatoid arthritis.

Etiology and Pathophysiology

Despite current research in this area, evidence does not uphold one true etiology but rather several overlapping mechanisms, all induced by the inflammatory process. Possible etiologies for the AOI include (1) increased destruction of red blood cells (RBCs), (2) impaired iron metabolism due to faulty iron release from reticuloendothelial stores, (3) decreased erythropoietin levels, and (4) suppression of erythropoiesis by cytokines from activated macrophages and lymphocytes due to the underlying disease. Each of these possibilities is discussed farther on.

Shortened Red Cell Survival

Decreased lifespan of red cells is seen in patients with AOI. Mean survival of red cells in some cases is 90 days, compared with 120 days in healthy persons.[2] The mechanism for this decrease is unclear but may be due to the extracorpuscular effects of activated macrophage-monocytes of the reticuloendothelial system (RES). These cells have increased phagocytic capabilities in patients with inflammatory processes and may be responsible for the shortened erythrocyte survival. There are usually no demonstrable autoantibodies against red cell antigens responsible for this anemia.

Reticuloendothelial (RE) Iron Block

Anemia due to RE iron block is another possible contributor to AOI. Although there is a decrease in intestinal iron absorption and impaired iron reutilization by the hepatocytes in these patients, there is an abundance of iron transported to the RES stores. Macrophages of the RES demonstrate large coarse aggregates of iron despite the low serum iron. The iron appears trapped and unable to be fully utilized in erythropoiesis. This results in the paradoxic ferrokinetics typical of AOI. The resulting hypoferremia sets off a "domino effect" of decreased transferrin saturation, which limits the supply of iron to the marrow and increases the amount of FEP. Ferritin is increased because of the increased RES iron stores (see Chapter 6).

Decreased Erythropoietin Levels

One of the controversies regarding the anemia of inflammation is whether or not patients have an ineffective level of erythropoietin (EPO). The EPO levels in anemic patients with rheumatoid arthritis (RA), malignancy, and other chronic inflammatory disorders are elevated when compared with levels from patients with a normal hematocrit.[3] Still others have demonstrated that this response is blunted, relative to the anemia seen in control patients with uncomplicated iron-deficiency anemia.[4,5] From this information it appears that the patient attempts to counteract the anemia with increased EPO production by the kidneys but that the response is not adequate for compensation of the anemia.

Suppression of Erythropoiesis

The degree of anemia seen in patients with AOI correlates with the severity of the inflammatory disease. Inflammation is usually measured by ESR and the presence of other acute phase reactants. Serum from patients with RA, juvenile chronic arthritis (JCA), and systemic lupus erythematosus (SLE) inhibits erythropoiesis in cell culture and the inhibition correlates with the severity of the anemia and the inflammation.[6,7]

Role of the Inflammatory Response

In order to understand how AOI may develop, a brief discussion on the inflammatory response is necessary. Inflammation is one of the body's responses to tissue injury due to physical agents, foreign organisms, and immune reactions in the host. The inflammatory and hemostatic responses occur simultaneously to control damage at the injured area. Coagulation factors, and the complement, fibrinolytic, and kinin systems interact to modulate inflammation. When injury occurs, factor XII

(Hageman factor) is activated. Mast cells are also triggered to release histamine, which promotes vasodilation and increases vascular permeability. Factor XIIa activates factor XI and initiates intrinsic coagulation. Factor XIIa also activates kallikrein in the kinin system. Bradykinin is ultimately produced, which induces pain and increases blood flow to the site of injury. Kallikrein also activates the fibrinolytic system, and plasmin is produced. Plasmin splits fibrin into fibrin degradation products (FDPs), which increase vascular permeability. It also cleaves C3 into C3a, a potent anaphylatoxin and chemotaxin. During the inflammatory process, complement can be activated directly by microorganisms via the alternative pathway or via the antibody-induced classic pathway. The presence of C3a, C5a, and other chemotaxins attract phagocytes to the site of injury where they recognize and phagocytize foreign substances. Neutrophilic granulocytes, monocytes, and macrophages possess receptors for complement which can induce exocytosis of granules which contain proteolytic enzymes, free ion radicals, and other inflammatory metabolites.

Inflammation will persist as long as injury and damage persist. When the source of inflammation is persistent and the condition is chronic, mediators from the cell-mediated and humoral immune responses contribute to the onset of anemia.

Effect of the Cellular Immune Response (Tables 15–2 and 15–3)

The human host has two possible responses to the recognition of foreign antigens. Activation of the humoral immune system with antibody production from the B lymphocyte line is one response and is responsible for the immune hemolytic anemias. Another pathway is the cell-mediated immune response and the activation of T lymphocytes (Table 15–2), macrophages, and their cytokines. Humoral and cell-mediated immune responses are not entirely separate but rely on continuous interaction for effective immunity. Cytokines are responsible for a wide variety of activities (Table 15–3). The mechanism involved with these cellular reactions are complex and will vary with the source of the antigen.

Upon exposure to a specific antigen, antigen-processing cells (APCs) will take up, process, and present the antigens to T helper/inducer (CD4) cells that are specific for the antigen (Fig. 15–1). Antigen-processing cells are a type of macrophage-monocyte that possesses MHC–class II antigens. When the processed antigen is presented to a helper T cell, the monokine interleukin-1 (IL-1) is simultaneously produced in large quantities by the macrophage. This promotes T-cell proliferation and activation. These activated T cells secrete interleukin-2 (a lymphokine) which enhances the proliferation of helper/inducer (CD4) and suppressor/cytotoxic (CD8) T cells. Additional lymphokines are also secreted by activated T cells (Table 15–3).

Table 15–2. **THYMUS-DERIVED LYMPHOCYTES**

Helper (inducer) T cells
  Aid B-cell maturation in bone marrow
  Supply activating (permissive) signals to B cells
  Activate the generation of different antibody classes
  Activate effector T cells
Effector T cells
  Two types, producing delayed hypersensitivity and
      cytotoxic effects.
    Responsible for:
      1. Immunologic surveillance for malignant cells
      2. Eradication of established viral and fungal infection
      3. Eradication of intracellular bacterial infection
      4. Destruction of parasites
Suppressor (immunoregulatory) T cells
  Control inflammation produced by T cells
  Control antibody production
  Balance ratio of immunoglobulin classes
  Block activation of T- and B-cell clones reactive to "self"

Source: From Dwyer, JM: The Cell-Mediated Immune System. Cutter Biologicals, Emeryville, CA, 1982, p 3, with permission.

On their surfaces, macrophages have specific receptors that can bind the Fc portion of some immunoglobulins, C3 components of complement, and some lymphokines. Macrophages can have nonspecific receptors for antigen. The receptors for other immunologic products enable the cell to be phagocytic for microorganisms, tumor cells, and antigen-antibody complexes. During activation, macrophages change functionally and can synthesize and secrete oxygen metabolites, proteases (collagenase and plasminogen), tumor necrosis factor-alpha (TNF-α), and a variety of other substances that contribute to inflammation (Table 15–4).

Interleukin-1 is a monokine composed of two distinct proteins, IL-1α and IL-1β. The biologic activities of IL-1 include fever, neutrophilic leukocytosis, acute phase protein synthesis, lactoferrin release, production of lymphokines, and many other indicators of inflammation. Bacteria, fungi, bacterial toxins, immune complexes, and some tumor cells can induce IL-1 production by macrophages.

Interleukin-1 can induce neutrophilic leukocytosis, which is necessary for maintaining host defense at the site of tissue injury. With prolonged exposure to the stimulant, IL-1 will eventually lead to the production of colony-stimulating factor (CSF). Colony-stimulating factor is a family of hormones responsible for the growth of hematopoietic progenitor cells. Granulocyte macrophage-colony stimulating factor (GM-CSF) is one of these and acts specifically on colony forming unit-granulocyte/macrophage (CFU-GM) to stimulate the production of the granulocytic and monocytic series. Colony-stimulating factor is derived from activated monocytes-macrophages, activated T cells, and endothelial cells. It also programs the neutrophils for changes in movement and increases the expression of IgG and Fc receptors on neutrophils.[8] The production of IL-1, GM-CSF, and TNF-α also has a suppressive effect on erythrocytic precursor cells.

One of the consequences to this activated neutrophilic leukocytosis is the release of lactoferrin induced by IL-1.[9] Lactoferrin is an iron-binding protein, similar to transferrin, that is found in a variety of secretions. It is also found in the specific (secondary) granules of neutrophils and has a higher affinity for iron than serum transferrin. Lactoferrin does not transfer its iron to erythropoietic cells and it appears to be rapidly absorbed by macrophages.[10] During phagocytosis, IL-1 induces the release of lactoferrin into the phagolysosome and outside the cell, and is found in high concentrations at sites of inflammation. This mechanism of lactoferrin release and RE block may account for some of the hypoferremia seen in the anemia of inflammation.

What possible benefit to the host could result from an immune-mediated hypoferremia in response to an infection? The answer lies in the concept of nutritional immunity. Nutritional immunity is a mechanism wherein the host endeavors to starve the invading organism of nutrients needed for growth and pathogenesis. Iron is an essential nutrient for optimal growth of most organisms. Lactoferrin and transferrin inhibit bacterial growth by depriving the invader of iron by reducing the availability of free iron. Reducing the concentration of free iron in experimental systems will decrease the virulence of the organism and inhibit bacterial growth. Increased susceptibility to infection has been reported in conditions associated with hypoferremia such as hemochromatosis, in neonates receiving iron injections, in those receiving iron therapy for chronic pyelonephritis, and in patients with thalassemia. There is also an association between *Salmonella* infections and hemoglobinemia seen in patients with sickle-cell disease.[11]

The Role of Cytokines in the Suppression of Erythropoiesis

One of the newest keys to understanding anemia of inflammation is the suppressor/inhibitor effects on erythropoiesis by IL-1 and TNF-α. As stated previously, sera from patients with RA, SLE, and JCA have been shown to inhibit erythropoiesis in vitro. The inhibition of early erythrocytic progenitors, burst forming unit—erythroid (BFU-E) and colony forming unit—erythroid (CFU-E), corresponds with the severity of the anemia and indicators of inflammation such as the presence of acute phase reactants. Research now indicates that monokines may be the key signal regulating hematopoiesis in inflammatory disease states. Interleukin-1 and TNF are both products of macrophage activation and have received the greatest attention.[12]

Interleukin-1 has been examined for hematopoietic suppression because of its mediation of various facets of the acute phase reaction. There is also a close correlation between severity of anemia and inflammatory activity. Maury and colleagues[13] demonstrated that there was increased levels of

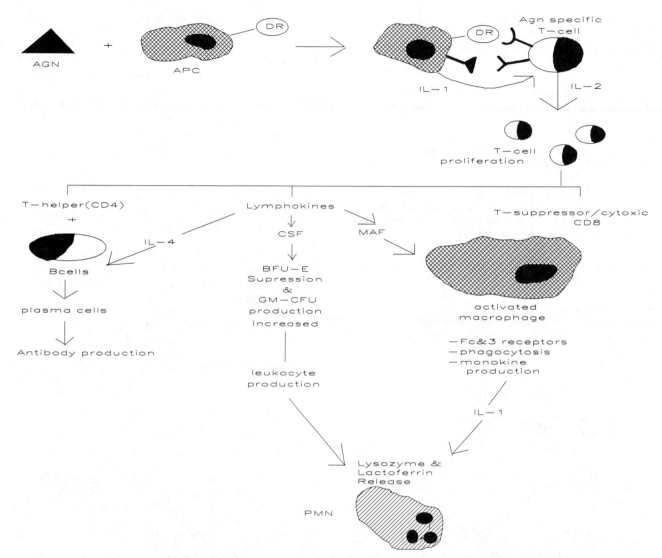

Figure 15 – 1. The mechanisms of cell-mediated immune response that lead to activation of T cells and macrophages we depicted. The monokines and lymphokines produced are mediators of the anemia of inflammation.

IL-1β in RA patients with anemia when compared with RA patients without anemia. This group also demonstrated that pure recombinant IL-1α and IL-1β, in concentrations similar to those found in arthritic patients, suppressed the colony formation of the erythroid, but not granulocyte-macrophage progenitor cells in normal bone marrow cultures.

Evidence also suggests that TNF, another monokine from activated macrophages, may be involved in the pathogenesis of AOI.[14] Very low concentrations of TNF were shown to inhibit erythroid progenitor growth in normal bone marrow cultures. This was demonstrated at concentrations similar to those found in affected patients. It has also been demonstrated that TNF mediates the hematopoietic colony-inhibiting activity of natural killer (NK) cells, showing a synergism with interferon gamma (INF-γ).[15]

It is becoming increasingly evident that what was originally regarded by early investigators as "simple

anemia" is far from being simple. The effect of monokines and lymphokines on hematopoietic, granulocyte, and macrophage progenitor cells appears to be responsible for AOI. Mechanisms responsible for host protection against infection and tissue injury indirectly become detrimental to the host. While the exact mechanism is still being researched, IL-1 and TNF-α (products of activated macrophages) have become key pathogenic factors. Theoretically, any disease that involves tissue injury and inflammation can, over a period of 1 to 2 months, result in anemia.

Treatment

The anemia seen with inflammatory processes is generally mild and usually does not require intervention. The degree of anemia correlates directly to the severity of the disease and the amount of inflammation. When the underlying disorder is

Table 15–3. **CYTOKINES THAT CONTRIBUTE TO INFLAMMATION**

Cytokine	Target Cell	Activity
IL-1	T cells, B cells, macrophages, and tissue cells	Lymphocyte activation, macrophage activation, acute phase reaction
IL-2	T lymphocytes	Stimulates proliferation of activated T cells
IL-3 (multilineage colony-stimulating factor)	Stem cells	Stimulates differentiation of bone marrow stem cells
IL-4 (B-cell growth factor)	B lymphocytes	B-cell proliferation
IL-5	B lymphocytes, eosinophils, precursor cells	B-cell growth and differentiation, eosinophil differentiation
IL-6	B lymphocytes, hepatocytes	Stimulates antibody production and acute phase reactants
Migration inhibition factor (MIF)	Macrophages	Inhibits migration
Macrophage activation factor (MAF)	Macrophages	Activates macrophages and enhances their functions
Leukocyte chemotaxis factor (LCF)	Phagocytes	Promotes chemotaxis to site of injury
Leukocyte inhibition factor (LIF)	Phagocytes	Inhibits migration
GM-CSF	Stem cells	Stimulates differentiation of granulocyte-monocyte precursor cells
M-CSF	Stem cells	Stimulates differentiation of monocytes
G-CSF	Stem cells	Stimulates differentiation of granulocytes
Interferon gamma (INF-γ)	Macrophages	Activates macrophages for cytotoxic functions; induces MHC II molecules on APCs
Tumor necrosis factor-alpha (TNF-α)	Macrophages, granulocytes	Activates macrophages, granulocytes, and cytotoxic cells

Table 15–4. **MACROPHAGE FUNCTIONS**

Production of IL-1
  Fever
  Neutrophil activation
  Release of acute phase reactants
  Lymphocyte activation and proliferation
    Lymphokine production
    Antibody production
Antigen Processing and Presentation
Tumor Destruction
  Production of TNF
  Cytotoxic action
  Toxic factors
Phagocytic Activities
  Fc and C3 receptors
  Microcidal and Bacteriostatic activities
  Protection from parasites
  Removal of particulate substances and damaged cells
  Lymphokine receptors (MAF, MIF)
Inflammation and Tissue Alterations
  Fibroblast activation
    Collagenase synthesis
  Synthesis and secretion of factors
    Lysozyme, plasminogen activators, elastase, complement components

treated, the hemogram results return to normal. If the inflammatory process is treated with long-term anti-inflammatory medications, acute phase reactants decrease, hemoglobin levels increase, and EPO levels decrease to normal levels.[3] When a disorder becomes exacerbated, or remains severe for a long time, the anemia is more severe and may necessitate treatment.

Despite the low serum iron levels, there is not a true iron deficiency. The treatment of this anemia with iron is ineffective and in some cases can actually be harmful. An excess of iron would increase the virulence of an infection and exacerbate an underlying infection. Depending on the hemoglobin and hematocrit levels, transfusion may be another possibility. In patients with severe anemia and no sign of remission in their disease, this may be a viable alternative, but only after a bone marrow evaluation of the iron stores.

In the past few years, recombinant human erythropoietin (rHuEpo) has offered a new alternative. Clinical trials have indicated that rHuEpo may improve erythropoiesis in most patients with anemia of renal failure.[16] More recently rHuEpo has been approved by the Food and Drug Administration (FDA) in treatment for the severe anemia in acquired immunodeficiency syndrome (AIDS) patients receiving azidothymidine (AZT) and in patients with RA. Although the anemia of inflammation in not entirely due to an EPO deficiency, high concentrations of this hormone were able to counteract the suppressive affects of IL-1.

Anemia Associated with Infection (Color Plates 111 to 113, 128 to 130)

Anemia is frequently seen with chronic infections. It can develop gradually in the first month of infection and will remain until the infection is successfully treated. Although most infections can now be treated effectively with antibiotic therapy, a number of chronic infections still remain that can produce anemia.

Bacterial

In general, any bacterium or fungus capable of persisting for more than 2 weeks can cause this type of anemia. The anemia seen in bacterial and fungal infections is the anemia of inflammation. The severity correlates with the intensity of fever and the presence of inflammatory products (acute phase reactants). Some examples of infections causing this form of anemia and the causative agents are listed in Table 15–5. All of these infections tend to be chronic and may result in weight loss and inflam-

Table 15–5. **EXAMPLES OF CHRONIC BACTERIAL AND FUNGAL INFECTIONS THAT COMMONLY CAUSE ANEMIA**

Infection	Common Etiologic Agents
Chronic meningitis	Mycobacterium tuberculosis, Cryptococcus neoformans, Coccidioides immitis
Malignant otitis externa	Pseudomonas aeruginosa
Empyema	Anaerobic bacteria, Staphylococcus aureus, aerobic gram-negative bacilli
Cavitary pulmonary disease	M. tuberculosis, Histoplasma capsulatum, Nocardia asteroides, Actinomyces israeli, anaerobic bacteria, Aspergillus niger, Blastomyces dermatidis, Pseudomonas pseudomallei
Endocarditis	Staphylococci and streptococci, Candida albicans
Intra-abdominal abscess (hepatic, splenic, renal, and so on)	Anaerobic bacteria, streptococci, aerobic gram-negative bacilli
Chronic peritonitis	M. tuberculosis
Chronic osteomyelitis	S. aureus, anaerobic bacteria, aerobic gram-negative bacilli, B. dermatidis
Chronic arthritis	M. tuberculosis

Source: From Strausbaugh, LJ: Hematologic Manifestations of Bacterial and Fungal Infections. In Bagby, GC (ed): Hematologic Aspects of Systemic Disease. Hematology/Oncology Clinics of North America, WB Saunders, Philadelphia, 1987, p 188, with permission.

mation. Other lingering infections such as leprosy, typhoid fever, tularemia, brucellosis, and Lyme disease can also produce this type of anemia.[13]

Anemia may also result from infection with organisms and various induced processes such as hemorrhage due to toxins and parasite invasion (see Chapter 14), virus-induced autoimmune hemolytic anemias (see Chapter 14), and virus-induced aplastic anemias (see Chapter 8).

Viral: Acquired Immunodeficiency Syndrome

Viral infections are usually not associated with AOI and are due to different mechanisms. One notable exception is the anemia associated with AIDS. Acquired immunodeficiency syndrome is a devastating condition caused by the destruction of CD4 T lymphocytes (helper/inducer cells) by the human immunodeficiency virus (HIV). The HIV renders the host immunocompromised and susceptible to several opportunistic pathogens. Most HIV-infected patients may develop pancytopenia or one or more of the cytopenias during the course of the disease. Anemia develops early and becomes more severe as the disease progresses. Approximately 75 percent of patients with AIDS are anemic.[17] Anemia has been noted in preliminary findings of HIV-infected individuals before secondary infections ensue and medications are started. Infections with Mycobacterium avium intracellulare, herpes simplex, Pneumocystis carinii, and cytomegalovirus (CMV) contribute to the state of chronic infection.

The hematologic picture seen in AIDS patients is a hypoproliferative anemia with a decreased reticulocyte count. Bone marrow aspirates demonstrate an increase in marrow reticulin and progressive aplasia. Decreased production of red cells can be attributed to several possible mechanisms:

1. There is a suppression of erythropoiesis due to an increase in cytokine production.
2. Bone marrow histiocytes have been observed phagocytizing red blood cells and white blood cells.
3. HIV antibodies circulate through the bone marrow and destroy altered precursor red blood cells.

Because of the already documented effects of IL-1 and TNF-α on erythropoiesis, current theory suggests that the inflammatory process is responsible for the anemia associated with AIDS.

Anemia in the AIDS patient is exacerbated by the use of zidovudine (AZT). Azidothymidine inhibits HIV replication and has helped to prolong life in many AIDS patients. Anemia and granulocytopenia are the major adverse effects associated with AZT.[18] Patients with less advanced AIDS at the initiation of AZT are less likely to develop severe anemia and granulocytopenia. When AZT therapy is stopped, increases in hematocrit and reticulocyte counts are observed. To treat this severe anemia, AZT therapy often must be discontinued or its dosage reduced. An even less attractive alternative is the transfusion of red blood cells. Recently the FDA has approved the use of rHuEpo to treat severe anemia in patients with AIDS. Recombinant human erythropoietin may reduce or eliminate the need for red cell transfusions in AIDS patients receiving AZT therapy.

Anemia Associated with Connective Tissue Disorders

All of the chronic systemic connective tissue diseases have the ability to produce AOI because they are by nature inflammatory diseases. Anemia is the most common hematologic abnormality seen in patients with RA, SLE, mixed connective tissue disease (MCTD), scleroderma, dermatomyositis, and Sjögren's syndrome.[19] These patients exhibit the laboratory features typical of AOI. Clinical symptoms of fever and inflammation are products of IL-1 and activation of macrophages. Macrophages, granulocytes, IL-1, TNF-α, lactoferrin, and other immune products are found in tissue fluids from these patients. Interleukin-1 has been demonstrated to stimulate the cellular responses that lead to the secretion of collagenase, protease, and lead to an increase in bone absorption and connective tissue destruction (see Table 15–2). There is a direct correlation between acute phase reactants, disease severity, and anemia.

Other factors may complicate the picture of this anemia. Iron-deficiency anemia may develop from gastrointestinal blood loss and peptic ulcer disease, either from the ingestion of aspirin or other anti-inflammatory drugs. Some collagen diseases (SLE, RA, and scleroderma) are also associated with the production of autoantibodies (see WAIHA, in Chapter 14). Renal disease is yet another complication of SLE, MCTD, and RA. The development of chronic renal disease, superimposed on the AOI, changes the hematologic picture (see under anemia of chronic renal failure).

The anemia of inflammation seen in connective tissue disorders is treated similarly to the other disorders in this group. If the underlying disease can be treated effectively to decrease the inflammatory process, the anemia will improve. Severe disease is associated with a more profound anemia. As stated previously, this anemia is refractory to iron therapy and transfusion may be necessary. In our present state of caution regarding the transfusion-transmitted viruses, the use of rHuEpo has become an attractive alternative to increase hematopoiesis in the anemic patient. Before undergoing elective joint repair surgery, the patient can donate an autologous unit of blood and decrease the risk of infection.[20]

Anemia Associated with Malignancy (Color Plate 122, 123)

Hematologic abnormalities are very common in patients with nonhematologic malignancies and depend on a multitude of factors (Table 15–6), which include the type of cancer, the site or sites involved in the body, the patient's therapy protocol,

Table 15–6. **MECHANISMS OF ANEMIA IN MALIGNANCY**

1. Direct Effects
   Replacement of marrow by malignant cells
      Primary hematologic malignancy
         Ineffective erythroid production
         Qualitative reduction in erythropoiesis
      Metastatic marrow infiltration
         Quantitative reduction in erythropoiesis
   Replacement of marrow by fibrosis
   Acute and chronic blood loss
2. Indirect Effects
   "Anemia of malignant disease"
   Anemia of associated organ failure (e.g., renal, hepatic)
   Malnutrition and vitamin deficiency
   Microangiopathic hemolytic anemia
   Immune hemolytic anemia
3. Treatment-Associated Anemia
   Immediate
      Chemotherapy
      Radiation therapy
   Late
      Secondary myelodysplasia/leukemia
      Idiopathic — ?Depleted marrow reserve
                  — Microangiopathic hemolytic anemia
                     (postmitomycin)

and whether the disease involves the hematopoietic tissues. Anemia is not an uncommon presenting symptom and can be due to decreased red cell production, increased destruction, and toxic effects of treatment.

Direct Effects

When the bone marrow is infiltrated by a malignant tumor (myelophthisis), it can lead to anemia (myelophthisic anemia). Leukoerythroblastosis (the presence of both immature white and red cells) can frequently be seen on the peripheral blood smear **(see Color Plate 213)** and is often a clue to marrow infiltration by the tumor. Marrow invasion can occur with solid tumors, particularly oat-cell carcinoma, carcinoma of the lung, breast carcinoma, prostate cancer, and in some instances lymphoma.[21] Extensive marrow invasion will eventually lead to pancytopenia. This anemia will usually improve when there is a response to treatment for the malignancy.

Primary hematologic malignancies such as the acute leukemias, definitely involve bone marrow infiltration with a proliferation of abnormal blast cells (see Chapter 18). Many of the chronic myeloproliferative diseases are associated with fibrosis of the bone marrow (see Chapter 21). The replacement of viable hematopoietic tissue in the marrow by pathologic, nonfunctioning fibrotic tissue results in pancytopenia.

Blood loss is another major cause of anemia in patients with malignancies. Chronic blood loss will result in a hypochromic anemia more consistent with iron-deficiency anemia than with AOI. Gastrointestinal tumors are associated with activation of the coagulation system, depletion of platelets and coagulation factors, and bleeding tendencies. Renal cell carcinoma can also produce significant blood loss through hematuria.[21]

Indirect Effects

Any malignant neoplasm that persists for more than a few weeks may result in the AOI. The anemia seen in malignancies is similar to other AOIs in that there is a correlation between the degree of anemia and the extent of the underlying disease. Severe anemia is usually seen in patients with metastatic cancer. The development of this anemia does not require or imply the invasion of the bone marrow by the tumor.

Malignant tumors elicit a chronic inflammatory response that is not related to necrosis or infection. The production and release of IL-1 and TNF-α by macrophages are responsible for the inflammatory process seen in malignancies. Most tumor destruction is cytolytic and cytostatic, involving activated macrophages, NK cells with INF-γ, and neutrophils. Destruction results predominantly from a nonphagocytic, contact-mediated event involving all three cell lines.[22] It is beyond the scope of this chapter to discuss the theories of tumor immunology, but the result of all these processes is the activation of macrophages and the chronic inflammatory process initiated by IL-1 and TNF-α. The consequence of the process is the alteration of normal red cell production resulting in anemia.

Anemia can be seen in patients with Hodgkin's disease. This anemia is usually related to AOI, but can also be due to a direct antiglobulin test (DAT)-positive hemolytic anemia.

Some cancers are associated with chronic liver or chronic renal disease. The resulting anemia is a reflection of those diseases or a combination of other etiologies. Advanced malignancies are also associated with malnutrition, especially in patients undergoing chemotherapy and/or radiation therapy. Anemia due to deficiency of vitamin B_{12}, folate, or iron may also develop. Microangiopathic hemolytic anemia is one of the more common sources of hemolytic anemia in widespread disseminated carcinoma. Activation of the coagulation system leads to fibrin deposition in small blood vessels causing mechanical shear-induced trauma to the red cells as they pass through the vessel (see Chapter 14). Schistocytes, fragmented cells, and helmet cells can be seen on the peripheral blood smear **(see Color Plate 122)**.

Treatment-Associated Anemia

Transient pancytopenia is expected in patients undergoing aggressive treatment in nonhematologic malignancies who do not have marrow invasion by tumor cells. Most combination chemotherapy protocols use one or more of the alkylating agents. When given frequently by intervals, they can cause a drastic decrease in the cell counts. One must remember that these drugs are designed to inhibit proliferating cancer cells and will also impair hematopoietic stem cells. The last cell line to show recovery from chemotherapy is the slower erythroid line. It will be interesting to see what the future holds for the use of rHuEpo in treated cancer patients to help accelerate erythropoiesis without reactivation of the cancer.

Summary

The anemia of inflammation is seen in chronic disease states such as infections, inflammatory diseases, and malignancies. Anemia of inflammation is hypoproliferative, normocytic, normochromic but can become microcytic, hypochromic if the disease increases in severity. Decreased serum iron and TIBC are seen despite increased iron stores in the bone marrow. Research indicates a suppressive effect on erythrocytic precursors in the presence of inflammatory mediators IL-1 and TNF-α. A blunted erythropoietin response has been noted in patients with severe inflammatory diseases. Hemogram results will return to normal once the underlying disorder has been treated.

ANEMIA ASSOCIATED WITH ENDOCRINE DISEASE

The spectrum of endocrine diseases and their effect on metabolism is wide. Many hormones are involved in the regulation of hematopoiesis and patients with endocrine disease can have disturbances in protein synthesis, energy metabolism, growth, and mineral metabolism. The resulting anemia is *not* due to the mechanisms involved in the anemia of inflammation. Diseases of the thyroid, gonad, pituitary, and adrenal glands are most often involved in the development of anemia.

Thyroid Disease

Thyroid hormones do affect erythropoiesis. Erythropoietin production by the kidney depends on the tissue oxygen tension, which is influenced by thyroid hormones. Thyroid dysfunction will either increase or decrease erythropoiesis by increasing (hyperthyroidism) or decreasing (hypothyroidism) the demand for oxygen. Hyperthyroidism may be associated with a mild erythrocytosis or no abnormal effect. Anemia is more common in hypothyroidism. The anemia picture is mixed. It is usually mild, normocytic, and normochromic when uncomplicated by nutritional deficiencies. Hemoglobin levels may be as low as 90 g/liter with a normal hematocrit.[23] The degree of anemia may not be reflected in bone marrow activity or hematocrit due to hypovolemia seen in these patients. In some patients, iron-deficiency anemia (hypochromic, microcytic) may develop as a result of menorrhagia, achlorhydria, or nutritional deficiency. Some hypothyroid patients develop a macrocytic anemia due to vitamin B_{12} or folate deficiency. Even patients who have normal vitamin B_{12} and folate levels frequently have macrocytosis with less ovalocytosis than nutritional deficiencies, but still exhibit an elevated MCV.

Hypogonadism

Androgens are other hormones that have an important role as stimulants of erythroid activity, both physiologically and therapeutically. The differences between hemoglobin concentrations in men and women are due to the effect of androgens. Healthy men have hemoglobin levels 10 to 20 g/liter higher than those of healthy women. Androgens seem to promote erythropoiesis in at least two ways: (1) by increasing the production of erythropoietin by the kidney; and (2) by directly stimulating the marrow in conjunction with erythropoietin. They are occasionally used pharmacologically to treat refractory anemias.

Men with hypogonadism, elderly men, and boys have hemoglobin levels similar to those in females. In the mature male with gonadal hypofunction, the decreased androgen levels result in a mild, normocytic, normochromic anemia and may be reversed with administration of androgens.

Pituitary Dysfunction

A mild, normocytic, normochromic anemia is seen in patients with hypopituitarism. The pituitary is responsible for the secretion of thyroid-stimulating hormone (TSH) and gonadotropins, which control the production of androgens. To correct this anemia, patients require not only the replacement of thyroid hormone and androgens but also the administration of steroids.

Adrenal Insufficiency

Adrenocortical insufficiency can result in a mild, normocytic, normochromic anemia. The anemia may not be evident because of the accompanying decrease in plasma volume. The etiology is unclear but may indicate erythropoietic activity by glucocorticoids.[23]

ANEMIA ASSOCIATED WITH RENAL DISEASE (Color Plates 120, 124, and 125)

Renal disease is associated with a wide variety of hematologic abnormalities including anemia, abnormal platelets, coagulopathy, and dysfunctional leukocytes. Anemia is a well-documented feature of acute and chronic renal failure. Patients with renal failure are anemic primarily because of blunted erythropoiesis due to an inadequate quantity of circulating erythropoietin and suppression of bone marrow response. In most causes it is a hypoproliferative, normocytic, and normochromic anemia but may evolve into other forms as a result of complications.

Pathophysiology

The major cause of the anemia associated with renal failure is decreased production of erythropoietin by damaged kidneys. The serum erythropoietin level in patients with renal failure is usually in the same range as normal nonanemic patients or slightly elevated, but is blunted when compared with anemic, nonuremic patients.[24] Some renal diseases (renal cell carcinoma, and polycystic kidney disease) are associated with erythrocytosis, but these patients may develop anemia (Table 15–7).

Inhibition of erythropoiesis has been demonstrated in the plasma of patients with chronic renal failure but identity of the inhibitor is unclear.[25] Parathyroid hormone and spermine have been investigated as uremic inhibitors with conflicting evidence as to their involvement in the development of this anemia. The possibility of IL-1 or TNF-α present as inhibitors in uremic plasma has not been thoroughly studied. Some forms of renal disease are products of immune complex disorders, infection, and other inflammatory diseases, so there is a possibility of some overlap between the etiologies of anemia of inflammation and the anemia of renal failure.

Mild hemolysis and decreased red cell survival also contribute to this anemia. Transfusion studies have shown that the hemolysis is caused by extracorpuscular factors and the defect is not intrinsic to the red cells. Hemolysis is due in part to acquired defects in the erythrocyte membrane sodium-potassium ATP-ase and pentose phosphate shunt. The latter defect leaves the cell susceptible to oxidants (sulfonamides and dialysis tap water) and can in-

Table 15–7. **MECHANISMS INVOLVED IN ANEMIA OF RENAL DISEASE**

Hypoproliferative Anemia
  ↓ Erythropoietin — ↓ Erythroid committed precursors
  Suppressive effects of uremic toxins on erythroid precursors
  Folate deficiency (hemodialysis)
Hemolytic Anemia
  Unfavorable chemical environment
  Uremic toxins
Dilutional Anemia
  Abnormal fluid retention
Blood Loss Anemia
  Gastrointestinal bleeding
  Blood drawn for laboratory tests
  Hemodialysis
  Chronic iron deficiency
Hypersplenism
  Chronic renal dialysis associated splenomegaly

duce Heinz body formation and hemolysis. Parathyroid hormone has been implicated as a source of hemolysis owing to its ability to increase osmotic fragility. Hypersplenism in patients on chronic hemodialysis also contributes to shortened red cell survival.

Coagulopathy develops in some patients with renal failure, and will demonstrate a microangiopathic picture on the peripheral blood smear.[25] Fibrin deposition in the capillary loops of the glomeruli contributes to the decreased survival (see Chapter 14).

Iron-deficiency anemia may develop in patients with renal failure because of blood loss during dialysis or occult gastrointestinal blood loss.

Treatment

Until the advent of rHuEpo there was no completely satisfactory treatment of the anemia associated with renal disease. Most patients treated with rHuEpo are able to become transfusion independent. Major side effects have included iron deficiency (treated with iron supplements) and an increase in blood pressure.[26] Erythropoietin levels increase with renal transplantation, but this drastic measure is reserved for patients with more severe problems than anemia. Hemodialysis will improve the anemia somewhat; however, the potential for the patient to develop anemia due to blood loss, iron or folate deficiency, or hemolysis is a calculated risk. Androgen therapy has been effective in increasing erythropoiesis, but it is not without side effects.

ANEMIA ASSOCIATED WITH LIVER DISEASE (Color Plates 126 and 127)

A wide array of hematologic disorders are encountered in patients with liver disease. Anemia associated with chronic liver disease is initially considered normocytic, normochromic but is often complicated by simultaneous effects such as iron deficiency (due to blood loss) or folate deficiency (due to poor dietary habits). Reticulocytosis, hypoferremia, increased TIBC, and increased ferritin levels are usually present. The morphology and degree of anemia, however, will differ somewhat depending on the nature of the liver disease. One of the most common forms of liver disease is due to chronic alcohol ingestion (Table 15–8).

Pathophysiology

Red cell shape, structure, and function are maintained by cholesterol and phospholipid levels, which are important factors in the deformability of the cell (see Chapter 3). Membrane lipids undergo change when the composition of plasma is altered. In liver disease, cholesterol and phospholipids are increased in plasma, which leads to alteration of the red cell.

Table 15–8. **MECHANISMS OF ANEMIA IN LIVER DISEASE**

Direct Effects
  Toxic effects of ethanol
    Vacuolization of marrow hematopoietic precursor cells
    Decreased marrow cellularity
    Megaloblastic changes unassociated with folate deficiency
  Acute and chronic blood loss
    Gastrointestinal bleeding (alcoholism)
    Liver disease–associated coagulopathies
  Viral suppression of erythropoiesis
Indirect Effects
  Dilutional anemia
  Hypersplenism, erythrocyte sequestration
  Hemolytic anemia
    Spur-cell anemia (acanthocytosis)
    RE macrophage activity
  Malnutrition
    Protein, folate, iron, and vitamin deficiencies
  Anemia of inflammation

In chronic liver disease the anemia may appear marked but does not correlate with the degree of hepatocellular failure or severity of disease. Target cells, macrocytes, and acanthocytes may be seen on the peripheral blood smear and are considered a consequence of altered lipid production **(see Color Plates 126 and 127**; see also Chapter 5). Hemolytic anemia may be present with macrocytes and spur cells (acanthocytes) because of the red cell membrane's rigidity or lack of permeability. A microcytic, hypochromic anemia may develop as a result of acute and chronic blood loss. Hypersplenism is found in 15 to 20 percent of patients with cirrhosis and advanced liver disease.[27] This complication can lead to decreased red cell survival.

Macrocytosis can also be seen in patients with cirrhosis, obstructive jaundice, and other types of liver disease. It is important to note that these macrocytes are round, with an increase in size but not in volume, and are not the macroovalocytes seen in megaloblastic anemia **(Color Plate 64)**. The MCV in liver disease is usually between 100 and 110 fl. Bone marrow examination shows macronormoblastic red cell precursors and no megaloblastic changes or hypersegmented neutrophils typical of a true megaloblastic marrow. The survival of these red cells is decreased owing to increased membrane lipids and lack of deformability. This type of macrocytosis does not respond to vitamin B_{12} or folate therapy, and usually resolves after improvement in liver function.

Megaloblastic macrocytes due to folate deficiency may be seen in fewer than 10 percent of patients with liver disease. Hemolytic anemia may be present in patients with chronic active hepatitis or other liver disease where splenomegaly is present. When the anemia is predominantly normocytic, normochromic it is attributed inflammation. The anemia of chronic liver failure is often complicated by portal hypertension, hypersplenism, and increased plasma volume seen in splenomegaly. These factors can yield a falsely decreased hematocrit and may cause difficulty in evaluating the anemia.

Anemia of Alcoholism

One of the widest array of hematologic abnormalities occurs in complications of acute and chronic alcoholism. Ethanol has direct toxic effects on precursor cells, marrow cellularity, and red cell morphology. Vacuolization of erythroblasts in the bone marrow can be observed in alcoholic patients. This phenomenon is also seen in chloramphenicol toxicity and results in red cell membrane damage.[28] Heavy, prolonged alcohol abuse will also result in decreased bone marrow cellularity. Macrocytosis is very common in chronic alcoholics and may not be due to megaloblastic anemia. In alcoholics who are not malnourished or have mild liver disease, there is still a macrocytosis that is not accompanied by neutrophilic hypersegmentation. The mechanism of macrocytosis in alcoholism is unknown. This change in cell size will remain until the patient stops consuming ethanol. The MCV remains elevated for 1 to 4 months afterward.[29]

Megaloblastic anemia is frequently seen in alcoholics who are admitted to a hospital. These patients suffer from folate deficiency due not only to malnutrition but also to the fact that ethanol itself interferes with folate metabolism. Iron deficiency due to chronic blood loss or poor nutrition may also be present with folate deficiency, demonstrating a dimorphic blood picture on the peripheral blood smear.

Hemolytic anemia can also be seen in alcoholics and is produced by several mechanisms. Hemolysis occurs in the spleen due to the activity of macrophages against the abnormal red cells which are high in cholesterol or phospholipid or both. Spurcell anemia (acanthocytosis) is mostly associated with severe alcoholic liver disease. Spur cells have an increase in cholesterol, which decreases the deformability of the cell as it passes through the spleen.

Anemia of inflammation is common in alcoholics and in patients with other liver diseases. It is rare to find a patient with liver disease in whom this is the only mechanism contributing to the anemia. The low serum iron seen in AOI may not be present but the increased reticuloendothelial iron may be seen on bone marrow examination.

Treatment

Treatment of the underlying liver disease is essential to the reversal of the anemia. Iron, vitamin B_{12}, and folate are not always effective in the treatment of the anemia unless the patient is deficient of iron or folate. If blood loss is a problem owing to gastrointestinal bleeding, transfusion may be necessary. Transfused red cells will acquire acanthocytosis as a result of the increased cholesterol deposition in the bilipid layer of the cell membrane. Their lifespan will become decreased, necessitating additional transfusions. Abstinence from alcohol will reverse the direct toxic effects on the bone marrow, and in a few months the MCV and red cell morphology should return to normal.

CASE STUDY

A 22-year-old woman was admitted for tests from the emergency department with fever, dysuria, and lower back pain. Immediate laboratory results revealed the following:

Urinalysis:	CBC:
4+ urine protein	WBC: 11.8×10^9/liter
1+ hemoglobin	RBC: 2.9×10^{12}/liter
Many bacteria	Hgb: 83 g/liter
Moderate blood	Hct: 0.25
Moderate WBCs	MCV: 88 fl
Casts: Few hyaline,	MCH: 29 pg
few granular	MCHC: 300 g/liter
Chemistry:	RDW: 14.7
	1+ aniso
	1+ poik
BUN: 113 mg/dl	1+ crenated RBCs
Creatinine: 7.7 mg/dl	

Blood cultures were drawn and eventually produced coagulase-negative *Staphylococcus*. Blood was still present in her urine after 2 days, and bleeding was noted from intravenous infusion sites. Coagulation tests were ordered before the patient was to go to surgery for kidney biopsy.

Platelet count: 296×10^9/liter
PT: 11.7 sec (control: 10.0–12.9)
APTT: 32 sec (control: 23–35)
Bleeding time: >20 sec
FDP: >40 μg/ml

This patient was suffering from bacterial sepsis and renal failure. The admitting CBC demonstrated a mild anemia with some crenated red cell morphology typical of renal disease. The patient had received several units of packed red cells with no noticeable difference in her hematocrit. The anemia could be the product of several mechanisms. First, there was blood loss from her abnormal platelets (see Chapter 26) and from the fact that she later developed DIC. Her presenting anemia was most likely due to the anemia of inflammation. Chronic and acute infections can produce this form of anemia. The anemia of renal disease was also present in this patient and was seen in conjunction with other etiologies of anemia.

REFERENCES

1. Baynes, RD, et al: Hematologic and iron-related measurements in rheumatoid arthritis. Am J Clin Pathol 87:196, 1987.
2. Lee, GR: The anemia of chronic disease. Semin Hematol 20:61, 1983.
3. Birgegård, G, Hällgren, R, and Caro, J: Serum erythropoietin

in rheumatoid arthritis and other inflammatory arthritides: Relationship to anaemia and the effect of anti-inflammatory treatment. Br J Haematol 65:479, 1987.

4. Baer, AN, et al: Blunted erythropoietin response to anaemia in rheumatoid arthritis. Br J Haematol 66:559, 1987.

5. Hochberg, MC, et al: Serum immunoreactive erythropoietin in rheumatoid arthritis: Impaired response to anemia. Arthritis Rheum 31:1318, 1988.

6. Dainiak, N, et al: Humoral suppression of erythropoiesis in systemic lupus erythematosus (SLE) and rheumatoid arthritis (RA). Am J Med 69:537, 1980.

7. Prouse, PJ, et al: Anaemia in juvenile chronic arthritis: Serum inhibition of normal erythropoiesis in vitro. Ann Rheum Dis 46:127, 1987.

8. Ogawa, M: Effects of hemopoietic growth factors on stem cells in vitro. In Golde, DW (ed): Hematopoietic Growth Factors. Hematology/Oncology Clinics of North America 3:454, WB Saunders, Philadelphia, 1989.

9. Klempner, MS, Dinarello, CA, and Gallin, JJ: Human leukocyte pyrogen induces release of specific granule contents from human neutrophils. J Clin Invest 61:1330, 1978.

10. Lee, GR: The anemia of chronic disease. Semin Hematol 20:61, 1983.

11. Strausbaugh, LJ: Hematologic abnormalities in patients with bacterial and fungal infection. In Bagby, GC (ed): Hematologic Aspects of Systemic Disease. Hematology/Oncology Clinics of North America 1:186, WB Saunders, Philadelphia, 1987.

12. Maury, CPJ: Anaemia in rheumatoid arthritis: role of cytokines. Scand J Rheumatol 18:3, 1989.

13. Maury, CPJ, et al: Mechanism of anaemia in rheumatoid arthritis: demonstration of raised interleukin 1β concentrations in anaemic patients and of interleukin 1 mediated suppression of normal erythropoiesis and proliferation of human erythroleukaemia (HEL) cells in vitro. Ann Rheum Dis 47:972, 1988.

14. Roodman, GD: Mechanisms of erythroid suppression in the anemia of chronic disease. Blood Cells 13:171, 1987.

15. Degliantoni, G, et al: Natural killer (NK) cell-derived hematopoietic colony-inhibiting activity and NK cytotoxic factor. Relationship with tumor necrosis factor and synergism with immune interferon. J Exp Med 162:1512, 1985.

16. Winearls, CG: Treatment of anaemia in haemodialysis patients with recombinant erythropoietin. Nephron 51(Suppl 1):26, 1989.

17. Spivak, JL, et al: Hematologic abnormalities in the acquired immune deficiency syndrome. Am J Med 77:224, 1984.

18. Fischl, MA, et al: Prolonged Zidovudine therapy in patients with AIDS and advanced AIDS-related complex. JAMA 262:2405, 1989.

19. Richert-Boe, KE: Hematologic complications of rheumatic disease. In Bagby, GC: Hematologic Aspects of Systemic Disease. Hematology/Oncology Clinics of North America 1:301, WB Saunders, Philadelphia, 1987.

20. Means, RT, et al: Treatment of the anemia of rheumatoid arthritis with recombinant human erythropoietin: Clinical and in vitro studies. Arthritis Rheum 32:638, 1989.

21. Dutcher, JP: Hematologic abnormalities in patients with nonhematologic malignancies. In Bagby, GC (ed): Hematologic Aspects of Systemic Disease. Hematology/Oncology Clinics of North America 1:281, WB Saunders, Philadelphia, 1987.

22. Roit, I, Brostoff, J, and Male, D: Immunology, ed 2. Gower Medical, London, 1989, p 18.11.

23. Orwoll, ES and Orwoll, RL: Hematologic abnormalities in patients with endocrine and metabolic disorders. In Bagby, GC (ed): Hematologic Aspects of Systemic Disease. Hematology/Oncology Clinics of North America 1:261, WB Saunders, Philadelphia, 1987.

24. Eschbach, JW and Adamson, JW: Anemia of end-stage renal disease (ESRD). Kidney Int 28:1, 1985.

25. Hocking, WG: Hematologic abnormalities in patients with renal diseases. In Bagby, GC (ed): Hematologic Aspects of Systemic Disease. Hematology/Oncology 1:231, WB Saunders, Philadelphia, 1987.

26. Johnson, CA and Chester, MI: Pathophysiology and treatment of the anemia of renal failure. Clin Pharm 7:117, 1988.

27. Phillips, DL and Keeffe, EB: Hematologic abnormalities associated with gastrointestinal disease. In Bagby, GC (ed): Hematologic Aspects of Systemic Disease. Hematology/Oncology Clinics of North America 1:207, WB Saunders, Philadelphia, 1987.

28. Girard, DE, Kumar, KL, and McAfee, JH: Hematologic effects of acute and chronic alcohol abuse. In Bagby, GC (ed): Hematologic Aspects of Systemic Disease. Hematology/Oncology Clinics of North America 1:321, WB Saunders, Philadelphia, 1987.

29. Lindenbaum, J: Hematologic complications of alcohol abuse. Semin Liver Dis 7:169, 1987.

BIBLIOGRAPHY

Chisholm, M: Haematologic disorders in liver disease. In Wright, R, et al: Liver and Biliary Disease. Pathophysiology, Diagnosis, Management. WB Saunders, Philadelphia, 1985, p 189.

Erslev, AJ: Anemia of Endocrine Disorders. In Williams, WJ (ed): Hematology, ed 3. McGraw-Hill, St. Louis, 1983, p 425.

Fantone, JC and Ward, PA: Mechanisms of Inflammation. In Cohen, AS and Bennett, JC (eds): Rheumatology and Immunology, ed 2. Harcourt Brace Jovanovich, New York, 1986, p 403.

Luksenburg, H: Anemia associated with other disorders: Infection, renal disease, liver disease, endocrine disease, connective tissue disease, and malignancies. In Pittiglio, DH and Sacher, RA (eds): Clinical Hematology and Fundamentals of Hemostasis. FA Davis, Philadelphia, 1987, p 172.

Savage, D and Lindenbaum, J: Anemia in alcoholics. Medicine 65:322, 1986.

Smith, HR and Chess, L: Cellular Basis of the immune response. In Cohen, AS and Bennett, JC (eds): Rheumatology and Immunology, ed 2. Harcourt Brace Jovanovich, New York, 1986, p 396.

Wiggins, RC, Fantone, J, Phan, SH: Mechanisms of Vascular Injury. In Tisher, CC and Brenner, BM (eds): Renal Pathology with Clinical and Functional Correlations. JB Lippincott, Philadelphia, 1989, p 975.

QUESTIONS

1. *What is anemia associated with inflammation?*
   a. Hematologic consequences of immune system during inflammation
   b. Diseases associated with an anemia primary to a secondary disease state
   c. Mechanism by which reduced erythropoiesis produces anemia
   d. Hemolytic processes initiated by antibody production

2. *Which of the following lists of laboratory findings would be most characteristic of the anemia of inflammation?*
   a. Normocytic, hypochromic; high serum iron; increased TIBC; decreased ferritin levels; decreases in hemoglobin hemocrit, and red cell indices
   b. Normocytic, normochromic; low serum iron; decreased TIBC; increased ferritin levels; decreases in hemoglobin, hemocrit, and red cell indices
   c. Microcytic, hypochromic; normal serum iron; decreased TIBC; normal ferritin levels; de-

creases in hemoglobin, hemocrit, and red cell indices
   d. Macrocytic, normochromic; low serum iron; decreased TIBC; decreased ferritin levels; decreases in hemoglobin and hemocrit; increases in red cell indices

3. Which of the following are causes for the anemia of inflammation?
   a. Increased destruction of red cells
   b. Impaired iron metabolism
   c. Suppression of erythropoiesis by cytokines
   d. All of the above are causes

4. What are the main immune processes responsible for reducing hematopoiesis and inducing nutritional immunity of anemia?
   a. Cytokines from macrophages and lymphocytes
   b. Antibodies from B lymphocytes
   c. Erythropoietin from kidney
   d. Hepatocellular factors from liver

5. What is the treatment for inflammatory anemia?
   a. Blood transfusion
   b. Iron therapy
   c. Treatment of the inflammation
   d. Human recombinant IL-1

6. What are causes for anemia not associated with inflammation?
   a. Malignancy and neoplastic processes
   b. Connective tissue diseases
   c. Bacterial and fungal infections
   d. Endocrine, kidney, and liver disease

7. What are the typical hematologic findings associated with anemia due to endocrine dysfunction?
   a. Mild, normocytic, normochromic anemia
   b. Anemia, abnormal platelets, and coagulopathy
   c. Target cells, macrocytes, and acanthocytes
   d. Marked anisocytosis and poikilocytosis, and dysfunctional leukocytes

8. What is the primary cause for anemia associated with renal disease?
   a. Blood loss from dialysis
   b. Decreased erythropoietin production
   c. Hemolytic processes
   d. Vitamin B_{12} and folate deficiencies

9. What is the typical appearance of anemia associated with liver disease?
   a. Normal red cell morphology with occasional ovalocytes
   b. Hypochromic microcytic
   c. Macrocytic normoblastic
   d. Megaloblastic

ANSWERS

1. a (p. 224–225)
2. b (p. 225)
3. d (p. 225)
4. a (p. 227)
5. c (p. 228–229)
6. d (p. 232–234)
7. a (p. 232)
8. b (p. 233)
9. c (p. 234)

PART THREE

WHITE BLOOD CELL DISORDERS

CHAPTER 16

RONALD G. STRAUSS, M.D.*

Cell Biology and Disorders of Neutrophils

CELL BIOLOGY OF NEUTROPHILS
PRODUCTION AND CIRCULATING KINETICS
NEUTROPHIL COUNTS IN BONE MARROW AND
  PERIPHERAL BLOOD
Marrow Counts
Blood Counts
Response to Infections
LOCOMOTION
PHAGOCYTOSIS AND PHAGOLYSOSOME FORMATION
BIOCHEMISTRY OF PHAGOCYTOSIS

DISORDERS OF NEUTROPHILS
NEUTROPENIA

Acquired Neutropenia
Congenital Neutropenia
QUALITATIVE DISORDERS
Chemotaxis
Cytoplasmic Granules
Biochemistry
Glycoproteins
Hyperimmunoglobulin E Syndrome
ABNORMAL MORPHOLOGY AND NORMAL FUNCTION

CASE STUDIES

OBJECTIVES

At the end of this chapter, the learner should be able to:
1. Name the three major types of leukocytes found in peripheral blood.
2. Describe the production and circulating kinetics of hematopoietic cells.
3. List normal values for various cell types found in the marrow.
4. List normal values for various cell types found in peripheral blood.
5. Characterize the changes in neutrophil count, morphology, and movement that occur in response to infections.
6. Describe the locomotion changes that occur in a neutrophil as a result of inflammatory reactions.
7. List the steps of phagocytosis and phagolysosome formation.
8. Name the biochemical mechanisms and products of phagocytosis.
9. Distinguish between quantitative and qualitative disorders of neutrophils.
10. List and define the two main classifications of neutropenia.
11. List and define four types of acquired neutropenia.
12. List conditions classified as congenital neutropenia.
13. Name conditions associated with a chemotaxis disorder.
14. Name conditions associated with a defect in cytoplasmic granules.
15. Name conditions associated with biochemical defects.
16. Describe neutrophil dysfunction associated with congenital deficiencies of neutrophil glycoproteins.
17. Describe disease characteristics associated with hyperimmunoglobulin E syndrome (Job's syndrome).
18. Name two conditions in which abnormal morphology and normal functions are found in neutrophils.

CELL BIOLOGY OF NEUTROPHILS

Three major types of leukocytes are found in blood: granulocytes, lymphocytes, and monocytes. Each major type is quite versatile. Granulocytes can be subdivided into three types (neutrophils, eosino-

phils, and basophils), based on morphology by light and electron microscopy and on the staining char-

*The author acknowledges receipt of Transfusion Medicine Academic Award K07 HL01426 and Research Career Development Award K04 HD00255 from the National Institutes of Health.

acteristics and contents of cytoplasmic granules. Likewise, lymphocytes can be subdivided into three broad categories designated T, B, and null lymphocytes. Monocytes become quite diverse when they enter tissues and differentiate into a variety of macrophages. Neutrophils are the most numerous leukocytes found in the blood, and the remainder of this chapter deals exclusively with this cell.

Production and Circulating Kinetics

All hematopoietic cells arise from a common, self-sustaining pool of pluripotent stem cells that become committed, as they mature, to a major cell line (granulocyte-monocyte, erythrocyte, or megakaryocyte). The clonal growth of committed granulocyte-monocyte stem cells in vitro is dependent on the presence of growth promoting substances called colony-stimulating factors (CSFs).[1,2] Although CSFs are found in increased quantities in the blood and urine of healthy individuals when there is an increased demand for neutrophils, CSF molecules produced locally within the bone marrow may have greater importance than those circulating in the bloodstream.[3] A major function of CSFs seems to be to amplify leukopoiesis (that is, to increase proliferation of previously committed cells) rather than to recruit new pluripotent stem cells into the granulocyte-monocyte differentiation pathway. Colony-stimulating factors also influence several functions of both neutrophils and monocytes, generally to enhance microbicidal activity. Many other factors interact with CSFs to influence leukocyte production and function, but the precise inter-relationships and relative biologic importance are incompletely defined.[4-6]

Once committed to the neutrophil cell line, the precursors progress in an orderly manner through stages of proliferation (myeloblast, promyelocyte, and myelocyte) and maturation (metamyelocyte and segmented polymorphonuclear neutrophils). Neutrophils can be stored in the marrow until their release into the peripheral blood. Once in the bloodstream, neutrophils are equally divided into marginating and circulating pools, between which there is a constant exchange of cells.[7] Marginating cells, which lie adjacent to the endothelial lining of blood vessels, can be mobilized into the flowing blood of the circulating pool during stress by epinephrine. Neutrophils leave the blood in a random fashion after a circulating half-life of approximately 7 hours and do not return to the blood from tissues.

Neutrophil Counts in Bone Marrow and Peripheral Blood

Alterations of the number and morphology of leukocytes in the bloodstream and bone marrow have long been used as clinical guides for the diagnosis of many diseases. These alterations may simply reflect the response of normal leukocytes to an underlying disease, or they may indicate a primary disorder of these cells, such as leukemia. Thus, a thorough knowledge of normal values is important so that deviations from normal can be readily recognized.

Marrow Counts

Although leukocytes are generally regarded to be residents of the blood, they use this fluid primarily as a route of transportation from sites of production in the bone marrow to sites of function in the tissues. Granulocytes, lymphocytes, and monocytes are formed in the marrow for release into the blood. In addition, lymphocytes proliferate in extramedullary lymphoid tissue. Values for the various cell types, as determined by differential cell counting of bone marrow samples from healthy individuals, are presented in Table 16-1.

Values are fairly constant except during infancy, when they vary according to age.[8] Erythrocyte precursors decrease shortly after birth and remain sparse until active erythropoiesis resumes during the second to third month of life. The percentage of granulocyte precursors (predominately neutrophils) falls precipitously during the first month of life due to a decrease in mature forms. Values are stable during infancy and increase during later childhood to adult levels. Lymphocyte numbers increase sharply during the first month of life, and this cell is the most numerous one in the marrow throughout infancy. Plasma cells are virtually absent until approximately 6 months of age. In older children and adults, mature granulocytes and granulocyte precursors outnumber erythroid about 3:1 with the postmitotic neutrophil forms (metamyelocytes and segmented polymorphonuclear neutrophils) predominating to form the storage pool. During bacterial infections the granulocyte-to-erythrocyte ratio can increase further owing to increased granulocyte production.

Blood Counts

Blood leukocyte counts are somewhat imprecise when clinical laboratories perform total and differential leukocyte counts manually. By using electronic, automated equipment, the margin of error can be reduced.[9] Blood leukocyte counts vary considerably with age; a broad range of acceptable normal counts is provided in Table 16-2. Generally, only mature, nondividing leukocytes are present in

Table 16-1. **PERCENTAGES OF PRECURSOR CELL TYPES IN THE BONE MARROW**

Cell Type	Birth	1 mo	3 mo	12 mo	Adult
Erythrocytes	7-21	3-12	8-19	4-12	18-30
Granulocytes	54-72	27-33	25-50	25-44	50-70
early:late	1:12	1:9	1:9	1:10	1:5
Lymphocytes	8-20	35-55	32-56	32-58	3-17
Plasma cells	0	0	0	0-1	0-2

Table 16–2. **RANGE OF BLOOD LEUKOCYTE COUNTS (ABSOLUTE NUMBER × 10³/μL)**

Cell Type	Birth	6 mo	4 yr	Adult
Total leukocytes	4–40	5–24	5–15	4–11
Neutrophils	2–20	0.5–10	1.5–7.5	1.5–7.5
Lymphocytes	1–9	1.5–22	1.5–8.5	1–4.5
Monocytes	0–2	0–2.5	0–1	0–1
Eosinophils	0–1.5	0–2.5	0–1	0–0.5
Basophils	0–0.3	0–0.4	0–0.2	0–0.2

the blood of healthy persons. However, if a large number of leukocytes are counted (for instance, in stained smears of a buffy coat preparation), immature myeloid cells, atypical lymphocytes, plasma cells, and even nuclear fragments of megakaryocytes can be found. Thus, unusual cells are occasionally found by chance, and a single strange or unexpected leukocyte should not be considered indicative of an abnormality unless other clinical or laboratory findings suggest the presence of disease.

A wide range of blood leukocyte counts exists at birth in healthy infants, and the neutrophil is the predominant cell.[10] Although not apparent on Table 16–2, significant changes in the differential white blood cell count occur during the first few days of life. At birth, the mean neutrophil count is about 8000/μl. This count rises rapidly to a peak value of about 13,000/μl at 12 hours of age but then drops to a mean of about 5000/μl by 72 hours of age. Thereafter, the neutrophil count slowly decreases so that the lymphocyte becomes the predominant cell by the age of 2 to 3 weeks (4000/μl). In addition, during the first few days of life, varying numbers of immature neutrophils such as myelocytes and metamyelocytes can be identified in the blood (so-called shift to the left). These immature neutrophils have been noted particularly in the blood of premature infants. Septicemia should be strongly suspected[11] when the left shift is carried to the extreme in the face of relatively low leukocyte counts (the absolute neutrophil count 3000/μl with 70 percent neutrophils being immature cells such as myelocytes and metamyelocytes). Finally, the monocyte count during the early days of life may transiently exceed values observed in older children and in adults.

The diurnal variation of neutrophil counts as observed in adults (significantly higher values in the afternoon than in the morning) has not been recognized in infants. No difference in normal values exists between boys and girls during childhood. However, in adults the total leukocyte count is higher in women than in men owing to a significantly higher neutrophil count,[12] a phenomenon apparently related to sex hormones.[13] The mean total leukocyte and neutrophil counts in normal black children more than 1 year old are lower than those in whites, although no racial differences are apparent in lymphocyte, monocyte, eosinophil, and basophil counts.[14]

Response to Infections

The characteristic response to bacterial infections is neutrophilia with an increased percentage of metamyelocytes (bands, stabs, and high-peroxidase cells), traditionally called a left shift. Many investigators have proposed criteria, based on total and differential leukocyte counts, in attempts to make an accurate distinction between bacterial infections and other disorders causing leukocytosis. Unfortunately, no method can predict the etiology of inflammation with complete accuracy—particularly to document whether or not a bacterial infection is present—and a number of reports have emphasized the lack of specificity and pitfalls of overinterpreting leukocyte counts.[15–17]

The kinetics of circulating neutrophils vary greatly depending on the type, duration, and intensity of the infection.[18] The immediate response to infection is transient neutropenia resulting from increased margination and accelerated delivery of neutrophils to the infected site. Within an hour, neutrophils are released from the bone marrow reserve into the bloodstream. In the early phases of infection, the circulating half-life of neutrophils is shortened and cell turnover is accelerated. Later, the circulating half-life becomes normal. Neutrophil production in the marrow increases by several mechanisms: (1) pluripotent stem cells are committed to the granulocyte differentiation pathway; (2) the generation (cell cycle) time of myelocytes is shortened; (3) myelocytes undergo an extra division (thus, the proliferative pool of precursors can be expanded independently of an increased input of pluripotent stem cells); and (4) transit time through the bone marrow is accelerated.

In addition to changes in the neutrophil blood count, neutrophil morphology can be altered by infection (**see Color Plates 128 to 130**). Cytoplasmic granules become prominent (toxic granulation), and large, bluish bodies (Döhle) may be seen. Döhle bodies consist of a few strands of rough endoplasmic reticulum that have aggregated.[19] They are similar, but not identical, to the inclusions found in the hereditary leukocyte and platelet disorder known as the May-Hegglin anomaly (see Chapter 26 for a description of the May-Hegglin anomaly) (**see Color Plate 134**). Finally, the cytoplasm may become vacuolated and, occasionally, contain ingested microorganisms. Although these features suggest the presence of infection, most of them can be seen with severe inflammation due to almost any etiology, including drug reactions.

The function of circulating neutrophils, as well as their number and appearance, can be affected by infection. Several functions have been studied during infections, and both enhanced and impaired functions have been reported when compared with normal values.[20,21] Although a number of exceptions exist, it is generally accepted that mild infections enhance neutrophil functions,[22,23] whereas neutrophil functions are impaired during severe infections. The role that these acquired functional abnormalities play in the course of infections is unknown. When investigating patients for qualitative neutrophil defects, remember that abnormalities of function may be the consequence, not necessarily the cause, of infections.

Locomotion

To participate in an inflammatory reaction in tissue, the neutrophil first slows its speed in the circulation and rolls along the walls of capillaries and venules. Eventually, the cell adheres to vascular endothelium and emigrates from the bloodstream by penetrating a narrow gap between endothelial cells. Neutrophils are briefly retained by the vascular basement membrane but then enter the tissues by passing through small openings in this membrane. This process is dependent on energy (adenosine triphosphate) production from glucose, requires calcium and magnesium, and is enhanced by the presence of chemotactic factors. A large number of substances generated by the inflammatory response have been demonstrated to be chemotactic factors.[24,25]

The first step in the process neutrophil locomotion is the binding of chemotactic factor molecules to specific receptors located on the plasma membrane of the neutrophil.[26] Depending on experimental conditions, chemotactic factor-receptor interaction can initiate a number of cellular functions in addition to chemotaxis. These functions include neutrophil aggregation (clumping), exocytosis (secretion) of the contents of cytoplasmic granules, and several biochemical changes including an increase in oxidative metabolism. A number of profound cellular effects follow binding of chemotactic factors to the neutrophil plasma membrane to mediate these functions.[24-26] Within seconds of chemotactic factor binding, the neutrophil membrane becomes more fluid, the concentration of cyclic adenosine monophosphate doubles, the electrical charge of the cell changes, and calcium is mobilized from the neutrophil membrane into the cytosol. Other findings that have been described within the first few minutes of chemotactic factor–neutrophil interaction include secretion of granular contents, movements of ions (potassium, sodium, and calcium), activation of enzymes, cellular swelling, and an increase in microtubule assembly. At present, most investigators consider the movements of calcium within the neutrophil to be a key event.

It is apparent that many humoral and cellular factors promote optimal chemotaxis. Similarly, several processes are involved in suppressing cell locomotion.[27-31] Controlled suppression of neutrophil locomotion is necessary to concentrate these cells at the inflammatory site by halting further migration. In addition, these suppressive mechanisms may protect normal tissues by limiting the inflammatory response. Neutrophils that have interacted with chemotactic factors become refractory or less responsive to subsequent exposure to chemotactic factors, a phenomenon called deactivation. An al-

most countless number of materials have been identified in normal plasma or serum and in inflammatory exudates and cellular extracts that suppress the chemotactic response in vitro.[30,31] These inhibitors can interact with chemotactic factors simply to inactivate them. Alternatively, some antagonists act directly on neutrophils to render them unresponsive to chemotaxins.

Phagocytosis and Phagolysosome Formation

Phagocytosis, the internalization of particles, is the first step in phagolysosome formation. Plasma proteins are necessary for the efficient phagocytosis of most pathologic microorganisms. These proteins, called opsonins, promote the interaction of the surfaces of microorganisms with receptors on the neutrophil plasma membrane.[32] Heat-stable opsonins are antibodies, most commonly of the IgG and IgM classes, with activity directed against antigens located on the surface of microorganisms. Generally, the opsonic activities of specific antibodies are enhanced via recruitment of the complement system.

The phagocytosis of particles bound to the neutrophil surface requires energy (adenosine triphosphate) that is generated via glucose phosphorylation by anaerobic glycolysis. Ingestion is a process of cell locomotion and shares many metabolic requirements with chemotaxis. For example, to ingest a particle that is attached to the neutrophil surface, pseudopods extend out and around the particle in cuplike fashion until they fuse. This movement requires energy, a functioning cytoskeleton, and calcium. Even before ingestion is complete, cytoplasmic granules approach the phagocytic vesicle, fuse with it, and discharge their contents into it (degranulate) to form a phagolysosome (Fig. 16–1). The molecular biology of degranulation and of granule secretion (exocytosis) is believed to be comparable. Secretion involves locomotion of cytoplasmic granules, and much of the molecular biology involved is similar to that pertaining to chemotaxis and phagocytosis.[33,34]

Information from in vitro studies suggests an orderly sequence of events for phagolysosome formation.[35-37] Discharge of secondary (specific) granules precedes that of the primary (azurophilic) ones. In rats and humans, the timing of degranulation has been coordinated with changes of intravesicular pH. The contents of secondary granules appear within the phagolysosome 30 seconds after ingestion, and the pH at this time ranges between 6.5 and 7.4. Myeloperoxidase, the marker for primary granules, is not detected until approximately 3 minutes after phagocytosis. The pH begins to fall at this time, and it reaches a level of about 4.0, 10 minutes after particle ingestion. The timing of sequential degranulation and pH changes seems well designed, as the contents of secondary granules function best at neutral pH and those of the primary ones function best in the acid range.

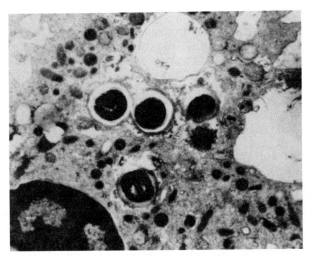 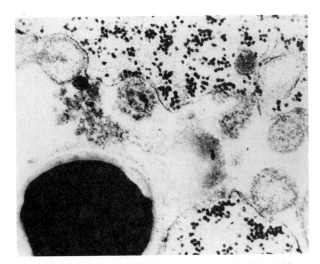

Figure 16-1. Electron microscopy of phagolysosome formation. (*Left*) staphylococci lie within phagocytic vesicles limited by sacs formed from inverted pieces of the neutrophil plasma membrane. Cytoplasmic granules are approaching the phagocytic vesicles. (*Right*) higher magnification that shows degranulation with the discharge of granule contents into the vicinity of the staphylococcus.

Biochemistry of Phagocytosis

Neutrophils consume glucose and oxygen during phagocytosis.[38-41] Glucose is metabolized via anaerobic glycolysis to provide adenosine triphosphate as energy for the ingestion of particles. A burst of oxidative metabolism accompanies phagocytosis and is characterized by an increase in oxygen consumption. The oxygen consumed is initially reduced to form superoxide anion and then is reduced further to hydrogen peroxide. Also, it has been demonstrated that human neutrophils produce a variety of reactive species of oxygen molecules such as hydroxyl radical (OH•) and singlet oxygen ($^1O_2$). A number of other biochemical reactions are associated with the postphagocytic oxidative burst, including the generation of chemiluminescence, reduction of tetrazolium dyes, oxidation and depletion of glutathione, iodination of proteins, production of lipoxygenase and cyclo-oxygenase products of arachidonic acid,[42] and cellular binding of estradiol.

Microorganisms within phagolysosomes are killed by a variety of oxygen-dependent mechanisms, the most important of which is the myeloperoxidase-hydrogen peroxide-halide system.[41] Myeloperoxidase is present in the primary granules and is delivered to the phagolysosomes by degranulation. Hydrogen peroxide is generated during the postphagocytic oxidative burst. Chloride ions are present within the cytosol and serve as the halide. Bacteria are killed by several reactive substances produced by this system.[41]

Lipid biochemistry is an area of postphagocytic metabolism that is currently being explored with great interest. Data are incomplete, but it appears certain that phospholipid metabolism, particularly that involving arachidonic acid, plays a crucial role in a number of neutrophil functions.[42] Neutrophils metabolize arachidonic acid to generate products of both the lipoxygenase (derivatives of hydroxyeicosatetraenoic acid) and cyclo-oxygenase (thromboxane and prostaglandins of the E and F series) pathways when activated by phagocytosis or surface-active agents such as chemotactic factors. Unstimulated (resting) neutrophils fail to produce these products or do so in much smaller quantities. These metabolites influence cellular function directly or by modulating the effects of other agents.

Neutrophils, like all aerobic cells, possess antioxidant protective mechanisms against self-inflicted damage (auto-oxidation).[43,44] Two isoenzymes of superoxide dismutase are present in human neutrophils. The majority of superoxide dismutase activity is present as the cytoplasmic copper-zinc enzyme, while the remainder is the manganese-containing enzyme found in mitochondria. Superoxide dismutase converts superoxide anion to hydrogen peroxide. The peroxide molecules are then metabolized to form water by glutathione peroxidase and catalase.

DISORDERS OF NEUTROPHILS

Neutropenia is a quantitative disease, defined as a mature blood neutrophil count of less than $1500/\mu l$. An increasing number of disorders are being reported with qualitative neutrophil abnormalities. In these disorders adequate numbers of neutrophils are usually present, but they function abnormally. Bacterial infections are the consequence of either severe neutropenia or neutrophil dysfunction. Effective neutrophils perform several processes that must interact in proper sequence to efficiently kill microorganisms. Multiple factors are involved in each of these processes, and neutrophil dysfunction may be the consequence of an abnormality in any one of them. The pathogenetic mechanisms responsible for the infectious complications and many of the principles of therapy are identical for both quantitative and qualitative neutrophil disorders. Accordingly, these disorders are considered together here.

Neutropenia

Neutropenia exists when the circulating blood contains less than 1500 mature neutrophils per μl (defined as segmented plus band forms). This traditional definition must be qualified, however, because the neutrophil count transiently decreases to less than 1500/μl during viral infection; maintains basal levels between 500 and 1500/μl in some normal blacks, Jordanian Arabs, and Yemenite Jews,[45] and occasionally is reported to be as low as 500/μl in healthy children under 4 years of age. Regarding the last, should counts of 1000 to 1500/μl be found in healthy children with normal hemoglobin and platelet values, no further studies are indicated except for periodic blood counts. If the neutrophil count is persistently less than 1000/μl, especially if the child has other evidence of disease, an explanation should be sought.

Recurrent, bacterial infections are the hallmark of persistent neutropenia,[46] and the clinical pattern is usually related to the neutrophil count. Generally, excess infections are not a problem if the neutrophil count is 1000 to 1500/μl, whereas life-threatening bacterial infections appear spontaneously in patients whose blood counts are less than 200/μl. Infections in patients with severe neutropenia are usually well controlled if the neutrophil count increases transiently in response to the stress of infection.

Neutropenia can be congenital or acquired, and it is produced by one or a combination of the following four general mechanisms: (1) decreased production by the bone marrow; (2) impaired release from the marrow into the blood; (3) increased destruction; or (4) maldistribution resulting in pseudoneutropenia. To demonstrate the mechanisms involved may require laboratory facilities that are generally not available, such as in vitro cultures to document the growth characteristics of bone marrow, radiolabeling to assess circulating kinetics, and immunologic techniques to detect neutrophil antibodies. However, a presumptive diagnosis can usually be made by a few simple studies in conjunction with the clinical findings. Marrow production can be estimated by examining smears of the marrow aspirate and sections of a needle biopsy specimen. Release of neutrophil from the marrow storage pool can be quantitated following adrenal corticosteroid stimulation, and the distribution of cells within the marginating and circulating pools of blood can be assessed by epinephrine.[47] It is also important regarding therapy, prognosis, and family counseling to determine whether the neutropenia is acquired or congenital.

Acquired Neutropenia

Most transient neutropenias in children are acquired rather than congenital, and *viral infections* are a frequent cause. Many children under 6 years old experience neutropenia with a relative lymphocytosis during viral infections. Bacterial infections can also be associated with neutropenia, sometimes due to endotoxemia. In these and in other nonviral infections, such as those due to *Mycobacterium tuberculosis* and *Histoplasma capsulatum*, the finding of an associated neutropenia (especially if accompanied by a marked left shift) is unusual and carries a poor prognosis. Newborns are particularly likely to develop severe neutropenia during bacterial infections due to depletion of the neutrophil storage pool in the bone marrow.[48] Acquired neutropenia as a component of pancytopenia occurs in patients who have *bone marrow failure* due to aplastic anemia, invasion with malignant cells, or toxic injury. The last can be either idiosyncratic or secondary to antitumor therapy. Anemia and thrombocytopenia are often associated, and the production failure is quickly identified by bone marrow examination.

Acquired immunoneutropenia can be idiopathic, can be related to drug ingestion, and can also be associated with diseases such as Sjögren's syndrome, systemic lupus erythematosus, rheumatoid arthritis, and infectious mononucleosis. Symptoms of the primary disease are usually present and immunohemolytic anemia and/or thrombocytopenia may coexist. Autoimmune neutropenia as an isolated feature in a child without an apparent underlying disease is an uncommon occurrence, although it is being recognized with increased frequency because of improved techniques in identifying neutrophil specific antibodies. Many instances of chronic benign neutropenia during childhood appear to be caused by antineutrophil antibodies.[49,50] Both clinical and laboratory findings are variable, and antibody in the patient's serum directed at antigens on autologous (patient) neutrophils must be demonstrated before an irrefutable pathogenic relationship is established. Adrenal corticosteroids may be helpful in some patients. Obviously, this therapy is not without risk in severely neutropenic patients and probably should be employed only when the diagnosis has been firmly made and when response to therapy can be monitored. Very high dose intravenous IgG has been used in immunoneutropenia with varying success.

Isoimmune (alloimmune) neonatal neutropenia that is analogous to isoimmune hemolytic anemia has been described in infants with severe, but transient, neutropenia.[51] Antibodies, demonstrated in both maternal and infant sera, react with infant and paternal neutrophils but not with maternal cells. Neutrophil specificity is demonstrated by adsorption of the antibody with neutrophils but not by other blood cells, and by the lack of interaction with other cells (for example, an absence of reactivity with lymphocytes). The mother becomes sensitized to neutrophil antigens shared by the infant and father. Once formed, antineutrophil antibodies cross the placenta. Of note, this mechanism does not occur with antileukocyte antibodies of broad specificity such as anti–human leukocyte antigen (anti-HLA). The latter are adsorbed and removed by the

HLA antigens of the placenta so that the fetus is not affected despite the frequent presence of leukoagglutinins (anti-HLA, but not antineutrophil) in many multiparous women. Isoimmune neonatal neutropenia is common in the first-born child. Severe neutropenia is present until 6 to 8 weeks of age and can be accompanied by skin and respiratory infections and even sepsis. Myeloid hyperplasia with depletion of the mature storage pool is generally seen in the bone marrow. Therapy is usually supportive and consists of antibiotics when infections occur. Intravenous IgG has been given to a few patients, but its efficacy has been difficult to prove.

Neutropenia associated with splenomegaly is rarely severe and, in itself, is usually not a cause for increased susceptibility to infections. Splenomegaly can result from portal hypertension, storage diseases (Gaucher's disease), work hypertrophy (hemoglobinopathies), autoimmune diseases (rheumatoid arthritis), myeloproliferative diseases, cancer, and various chronic infections. Pancytopenia is often present. Generally, the marrow is hypercellular with a depleted storage pool of mature neutrophil. The depletion of mature cells may give the false appearance of an arrest in maturation at the metamyelocyte stage. In contrast, a true maturation arrest, as seen in congenital agranulocytosis, occurs at the earlier promyelocyte-myelocyte stage. Because the degree of neutropenia seen is rarely of clinical significance, the blood count alone should not be used as an indication for splenectomy.

Congenital Neutropenia

Congenital agranulocytosis of the Kostmann type is characterized by a severe failure of neutrophil production with preservation of erythroid and megakaryocytic maturation in the marrow.[52] It is an autosomal recessive trait and is so rare that only about 30 patients were reported in the 20 years following the initial description of the disease.[52] Children with this condition are frequently seen during the first month of life with bacterial infections. The total white blood cell count may be normal, but a severe neutropenia (less than $200/\mu l$) will be present. The differential count may reveal increased monocytes and eosinophils. Neutrophil morphology is normal, but granulated monocytoid cells may be seen, presumably as circulating abortive forms of early neutrophil precursors. The marrow is cellular, and myeloid precursors are present. However, only rare neutrophil precursors mature beyond the promyelocyte or early myelocyte stages. Frequently, vacuoles and abnormally large granules are found in the cytoplasm of these cells.[53] In addition to the defect in maturation, proliferation of neutrophil precursors is decreased, and they die in the marrow.[54] Recently, a few patients have responded to experimental treatment with recombinant CSFs.[55]

The major condition to be distinguished from Kostmann's agranulocytosis is a heterogeneous group of disorders called *chronic benign neutropenia*.[49,50,56] Patients with this disorder have fairly persistent moderate to severe neutropenia with variable marrow findings. Marrow cellularity may be normal or decreased. True maturation arrest at the promyelocyte-myelocyte level is not seen, but the storage pool may be depleted to give the appearance of an arrest at the metamyelocyte level. Although the pathogenetic mechanisms may be multiple, an evaluation including anti-neutrophil antibodies should be done because this appears to be a frequent cause, particularly in children.[49,50] Bacterial infections may occur with increased frequency, but they are often well contained, as the blood neutrophil count may transiently increase in response to the stress of infection. The duration of neutropenia is unpredictable, but the disorder often improves over time, and the prognosis is generally good. The autosomal dominant, moderate neutropenia of blacks, Yemenite Jews, and Jordanians is sometimes included in this category.

A few patients have been described in whom neutropenia is related to an inability to release mature granulocytes into the blood—a disorder called *myelokathexis*.[57,58] At the time of bacterial infections, neutropenia is not present. Between infections, however, the neutrophil count decreases to extremely low values. Myeloid cells are present in the bone marrow, with an excessive number of mature neutrophils present. The nuclei of these cells are characterized by pyknotic lobes that are connected by thin, filamentous strands. Granulation frequently is absent, and vacuolization can be identified. Apparently, these cells become senescent and die in the bone marrow without being released into the blood. In one family, this disorder was judged to be inherited in autosomal recessive fashion.[58]

Organic acidemia with hyperglycinemia is a rare cause of neutropenia and pancytopenia. Patients with hyperglycinemia have developmental retardation, vomiting, lethargy, dehydration, and ketosis. They have repeated infections, and myeloid cells are decreased in the marrow. The diagnosis is established by the demonstration of hyperglycinemia and hyperglycinuria.

Cyclic neutropenia is associated with a variety of conditions and is the consequence of periodic marrow failure.[59,60] Experiments in gray collie dogs, a model of cyclic neutropenia, support the concept of a stem-cell defect because the disease is cured by marrow transplantation from healthy littermates. Moreover, the disease is produced in normal, healthy dogs transplanted with marrow from affected ones. The molecular defect of the stem cells is unknown. The clinical symptoms found at the nadir (that is, the lowest neutrophil count during the cycle) are mouth ulcers and skin or respiratory infections. Occasionally, bacterial infections can be more severe. In evaluating a patient with recurrent episodic periods of fever or infection, it may be necessary to do serial total and differential whole blood cell counts three times per week for at least 2 months to demonstrate the cyclic changes in blood neutrophils. Nadir points are reached about every 21 days. With increasing age, the cycles tend to dampen out; however, these patients, often have a persisting mild neutropenia.

Pancytopenia may occur in several congenital disorders in which neutropenia is a prominent feature. *Fanconi's anemia* is one such disorder; it is most likely inherited in autosomal recessive fashion. Marrow failure may not appear until the patient is 5 to 10 years of age.[61] Usually, anemia or thrombocytopenia is the early sign of disease, with neutropenia developing later. Evidence for congenital anomalies should be sought. These patients are frequently growth-retarded and may have areas of either hyperpigmentation or hypopigmentation of the skin. Approximately one third have an abnormality of the thumb; other skeletal anomalies are less frequently found. Renal anomalies are common. Fetal hemoglobin concentration is increased and can precede overt anemia — a fact that is useful in genetic counseling. Chromosomal breaks and recombination forms can be demonstrated in marrow cells, stimulated lymphocytes, and fibroblasts. The chromosomal abnormalities are probably related to the increased rate of cancer, particularly myeloid leukemia, observed in these patients. Androgenic hormones (sometimes combined with adrenal corticosteroids) are usually effective for treating the anemia, but neutrophils and platelet counts are less likely to respond. These patients seem particularly susceptible to the toxicities of irradiation and immunosuppressive therapy, and bone marrow transplantation carries an increased risk for them.

Another form of pancytopenia related to marrow failure is that associated with *dyskeratosis congenita*.[62] Patients with this disorder are frequently studied early in life because of failure to thrive. They have abnormalities of the epithelial surfaces, such as dyskeratosis and poor dental and nail formation. Progressive marrow failure usually occurs during the second half of the first decade. It is not associated with the chromosome abnormalities described in Fanconi's anemia, and it is not as responsible to androgen therapy.

Shwachman and co-workers described a rare form of congenital marrow failure that presents in early life as failure to thrive with evidence of malabsorption.[63] Patients have recurrent bacterial infections due to neutropenia. Some individuals also have impaired neutrophil locomotion. Anemia and thrombocytopenia may occur, as well. Initially the diagnosis may be obscured, particularly if a bacterial infection is present, because with the severe stress of infection the neutrophil count may be normal. As infection subsides, neutropenia becomes apparent. Thus, serial blood leukocyte counts may be necessary to document neutropenia. The bone marrow is usually hypocellular without indications of abnormal maturation, although maturation arrest can be seen. Pancreatic insufficiency is suggested by clinical features of malabsorption and can be documented by the absence of trypsin and other pancreatic enzymes in duodenal juices. The mechanism linking pancreatic insufficiency and marrow failure is unknown.

Additional rare causes of congenital neutropenia or pancytopenia are *reticular dysgenesis, cartilage-hair hypoplasia, transcobalamin II deficiency, osteopetrosis,* and *type IB glycogen storage disease.* The first three have associated immune defects. Additional diseases in which neutropenia and neutrophil dysfunction occur jointly, such as Chédiak-Higashi syndrome, are discussed later in this chapter.

Qualitative Disorders

Disorders of neutrophil function are characterized by bacterial infections that are due not to decreased numbers of neutrophils in the blood but to neutrophil dysfunction. These disorders will be grouped according to the major defect expressed, although it is recognized that multiple abnormalities (including neutropenia) can be detected in some patients.

Chemotaxis

Although these conditions are collectively referred to as chemotaxis disorders, it must be remembered that neutrophils are capable of three major types of locomotion: chemotactic factor–directed movement known as chemotaxis, nondirected random mobility, and chemotactic factor–stimulated random mobility known as chemokinesis. Detecting an abnormality in one type of movement will not guarantee defects in the other types. Moreover, in vitro assays of neutrophil movement may not correlate with each other or with in vivo studies. Finally, the basis for abnormal movement may lie with the neutrophil itself (intrinsic cellular defect) or with an imbalance of environmental agents promoting (chemotactic factors) and suppressing (cell- or chemotaxin-directed inhibitors) movement. Selected chemotaxis disorders are listed in Table 16–3. The listing is not intended to be all-inclusive as new conditions continue to be reported. Disorders are grouped according to the most acceptable pathogenetic mechanism, although it is realized that multiple mechanisms may be involved.

Cytoplasmic Granules

Myeloperoxidase (MPO) deficiency may be congenital or acquired.[64] Myeloperoxidase is present in the primary (azurophilic) granules of neutrophils, eosinophils, and monocytes-macrophages (located in different intracellular sites in these last cells, depending on their degree of differentiation). In congenital MPO deficiency, neutrophils and monocytes lack MPO but eosinophils are normal.[65,66] This usually is a mild disorder of autosomal recessive inheritance, but some patients may have severe *Candida* infections (**see Color Plate 111**). In vitro, MPO-deficient neutrophils are unable to kill certain types of *Candida*, but they eventually kill *Staphylococcus* and gram-negative enteric bacilli after prolonged incubation. Neutrophils that are MPO-deficient consume large amounts of oxygen after phagocytosis, and they exhibit prolonged stimulation of the

Table 16–3. **SELECTED DISORDERS OF NEUTROPHIL CHEMOTAXIS WITH SELECTED REFERENCES**

Intrinsic neutrophil defects

Lazy leukocyte syndrome	Lancet 1:665, 1971
Monosomy	Blood 54:401, 1979
Burns	Ann Surg 186:746, 1977
Congenital ichthyosis	J Lab Clin Med 82:1, 1973
Chédiak-Higashi disease	Medicine 51:247, 1972
Newborns	Pediatr Res 5:487, 1971
Actin dysfunction	N Engl J Med 291:1093, 1974
Glycoprotein deficiency	Blood 60:160, 1982
Immotile cilia syndrome	Lancet 2:893, 1978
Glycogenosis IB	J Infect Dis 143:447, 1981

Cell-directed inhibitors

Cancer	Clin Immunol Immunopathol 9:166, 1978
Surgical patients	Surgery 85:543, 1979

Chemotactic factor-directed inhibitors

Anergy (various causes)	J Immunol 113:189, 1974
Cytomegalovirus	J Pediatr 83:951, 1973
Liver cirrhosis	J Lab Clin Med 85:261, 1975
Acute lymphoblastic leukemia	Blood 54:412, 1979
Sepsis	J Surg Res 26:355, 1979

Undefined mechanisms

Influenza A virus	Scand J Immunol 6:897, 1977
Marrow transplant recipients	J Clin Invest 58:22, 1976
Hyperimmunoglobulin E	J Lab Clin Med 88:796, 1976
Uremia	J Lab Clin Med 88:536, 1976
Hemophilia	J Immunol 120:1181, 1978
Peridontitis	J Res 28:81s, 1980
Milk intolerance	Pediatrics 67:264, 1981

oxidative burst.[67] The diminished activity of MPO-dependent microbicidal activities seems to be partially offset by this generalized increase in oxidative metabolism. Myeloperoxidase deficiency can be recognized by either manual or automated histochemical techniques. Neutrophils that are recognized by automated counters using peroxidase staining will be reported as decreased in number, whereas unidentified leukocytes will appear to be increased. Wright-Giemsa staining, however, will reveal many of the large, unidentified cells to be neutrophils. Acquired MPO deficiency has been reported in patients with diabetes mellitus, leukemia, myeloproliferative disorders, megaloblastic anemia, and ceroid lipofuscinosis.

Chédiak-Higashi disease[68] is an autosomal recessive disorder characterized by partial oculocutaneous albinism, recurrent pyogenic infections, and the presence of giant lysosomes in most granule-containing cells, including all types of leukocytes (Fig. 16–2) (**see Color Plate 131**). Similar disorders have been described in whales, cattle, mink, and mice. A bleeding diathesis is due to both qualitative and quantitative abnormalities of platelet granules associated with reduced nucleotide and serotonin content. The susceptibility to infections is due to neutropenia, impaired chemotaxis, and delayed killing of ingested bacteria because of abnormal distribution and delivery of lysosomal enzymes. These patients usually die as a result of infection during childhood. Neutropenia is due to intramedullary destruction that is characterized by normal to increased numbers of precursors in the marrow, vacuolizations and inclusions in the precursors, poor release of neutrophils from marrow stores, normal half-life of circulating neutrophils, and increased serum concentrations of lysozyme. At times, splenic sequestration may contribute to the

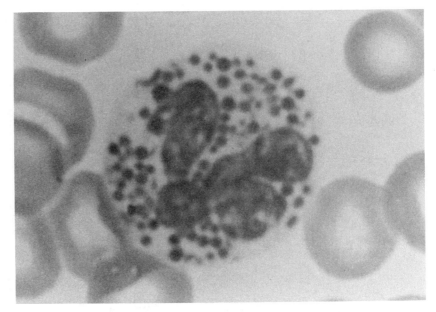

Figure 16–2. Neutrophil from a patient with Chédiak-Higashi syndrome. The cytoplasm is filled with strikingly large primary (azurophilic) granules.

neutropenia. Chemotaxis is impaired and may be related to a lack of cellular flexibility due to cytoskeletal abnormalities or to the presence of the giant cytoplasmic granules.[69] Microorganisms are ingested readily with normal to increased postphagocytic oxidative metabolism, but the delivery of peroxidase to the phagosome is delayed and there is delayed killing of most bacteria.

Abnormal neutrophil-specific granules with lactoferrin deficiency was first reported in a patient with recurrent staphylococcal skin and sinus infections but without serious deep tissue infections or sepsis.[70] Although rare, this disease has been recognized throughout the world, and it is important to remember it because it can be readily suspected by simple inspection of a stained blood smear. Neutrophils have bilobed nuclei with irregular, fingerlike projections (microlobes) and appear to be nearly devoid of cytoplasmic granules on Wright-Giemsa staining (Fig. 16–3). Primary granules are easily seen in neutrophils stained for MPO activity, but stains for secondary (specific) granules are negative (alkaline phosphatase was employed in the initial report). By electron microscopy, the azurophilic (primary) granules develop normally but the specific (secondary) granules are abnormal. They appear as flattened structures, limited by a trilaminar unit membrane that is in apposition centrally but is separated at the poles to form empty, bulbous enlargements. Neutrophils from the original patient contained less than 8 percent of the normal amounts of the specific-granule proteins lactoferrin and vitamin B transport protein.[71] Neutropenia is not a prominent feature, but has been noted occasionally. Neutrophil migration was impaired by both skin window and chemotaxis chamber techniques.[70] Neutrophils aggregated normally in response to chemotactic factors, but they tended to disaggregate unless additional lactoferrin was added to the reaction mixture.[71] Oxygen consumption and superoxide generation were elevated; however, hydroxyl radicals were produced at a significantly decreased rate (another defect probably related to lactoferrin deficiency). Giant abnormal phagolysosomes containing excessive numbers of bacteria were produced, and neutrophils appeared to disintegrate following phagocytosis, with release of viable organisms.[70] The basis for this disease is probably a congenital abnormality of specific granule formation with failure to deliver granule contents — particularly lactoferrin — to these granules. Malformation of specific granules has been reported also in bone marrow cultures of some patients with neutropenia, myeloproliferative diseases, and hairy-cell leukemia.

Biochemistry

It is logical to postulate that *deficiencies of glycolytic enzymes* (Embden-Meyerhof pathway), in a manner analogous to that seen in hemolytic anemias, might result in neutrophil dysfunction. However, clinically significant problems have not been reported; apparently, alternative metabolic pathways and microbicidal systems are available to compensate. As an example, phosphoglycerate kinase is an enzyme in the pathway that regulates one of the two adenosine triphosphate–generating steps. Congenital deficiency of this enzyme is inherited in an X-linked recessive manner and is characterized by hemolytic anemia and progressive central nervous system disease. Infections are not a major problem. Phagocytosis and killing of bacteria are normal because of a compensatory increase in mitochondrial oxidative metabolism.[72]

Neutrophils, monocytes, and eosinophils of children with *chronic granulomatous disease* are unable to kill certain microorganisms following normal engulfment. The characteristic clinical picture is of suppurative lymphadenitis, deep tissue infections (osteomyelitis, visceral abscess, perirectal abscess), recurrent pulmonary infections, hepatosplenomegaly, and infected eczematoid rash. The

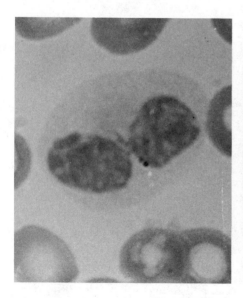
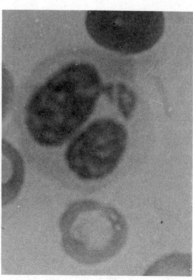

Figure 16–3. Neutrophils from a patient with the abnormal specific granule (absent lactoferrin) syndrome. Nuclear lobulation is decreased, and the cytoplasm seems to be devoid of granules.

basic abnormality is a complete inability to mount a postphagocytic oxidative burst. This disorder was originally described as an X-linked recessive disease of boys in whom severe bacterial infections appeared by 1 year of age, and most patients died of septicemia or chronic pulmonary disease in early childhood. However, much clinical experience has been gained since the description of this disease, and it is now clear that the disease can be much milder and may not be recognized until early adulthood. Moreover, it can occur in girls and, in these patients, is probably inherited in an autosomal recessive fashion. Pigment-containing macrophages are present throughout the reticuloendothelial system, in the lamina propria of the gastrointestinal tract, and adjacent to the inflammatory areas. Granuloma formation is the characteristic inflammatory lesion.

Neutropenia does not occur; neutrophilia is often present. A failure to reduce oxygen to reactive molecules is responsible for the microbicidal defect.[73-75] Several biochemical defects in the oxidase system have been reported in different patients, but variations in the activity of cytochrome b have permitted a classification of affected individuals.[76] Cytochrome b cannot be detected in the classic X-linked form or in a rare subset of autosomal recessive patients, whereas it is normal in most of the autosomal recessive patients. Engulfment of bacteria, glucose consumption and lactic acid production (anaerobic glycolysis), degranulation, and phagolysosome formation are normal. An increase in postphagocytic oxidative metabolism does not occur (that is, there is no increase in oxygen consumption, hexose monophosphate shunt activity, or superoxide anion and hydrogen peroxide production). The diagnosis is established by demonstrating a bactericidal defect due to the absence of the postphagocytic oxidative burst. The X-linked recessive inheritance can be confirmed by the presence of disease in male members of the maternal family and by the intermediate performance of neutrophils from the mothers and sisters of affected boys in certain oxidative assays (the histochemical slide test for nitroblue tetrazolium dye reduction). In most cases, these female relatives are clinically well, but occasionally an increased susceptibility to infections or a syndrome resembling systemic lupus erythematosus has been noted.

Other patients have been reported with clinical problems similar to chronic granulomatous disease. These disorders may have additional atypical features such as impaired chemotaxis, low serum concentration of IgA, progressive loss of cellular immunity, and bactericidal defects selective for only single bacteria. *Familial lipochrome pigmentation of histiocytes* is a similar disorder characterized by hypergammaglobulinemia, recurrent infections (particularly pulmonary), arthritis, splenomegaly, neutrophil metabolic abnormalities, and pigment-containing macrophages. *Glucose-6-phosphate dehydrogenase (G6PD)* is the enzyme regulating the flow of glucose into the hexose monophosphate shunt, and neutrophil function is abnormal only when enzyme activity is severely deficient. A syndrome similar to chronic granulomatous disease of childhood has been reported in both congenital and acquired G6PD deficiency.[77]

Glutathione peroxidase deficiency is considered by some[77a] to produce a variant of chronic granulomatous disease. *Glutathione reductase deficiency* is characterized by hemolysis and a variety of neutrophil defects that are not associated with clinical infections.[78] Chemotaxis, phagocytosis, lysosomal enzyme release, and results of studies of bacterial killing at a low bacteria-to-neutrophil ratio are normal. However, results of bacterial killing studies at a higher bacterial-to-neutrophil ratio are abnormal. The first few minutes of postphagocytic oxidative metabolism is normal, but the burst stops prematurely.[78] Intracellular levels of glutathione (GSH) drop rapidly, and neutrophils suffer oxidative damage (auto-oxidation). *Glutathione synthetase deficiency* has been described in a complex patient with oxoprolinuria, acidosis, hemolysis, and episodes of severe neutropenia.[79] Values for GSH in neutrophils were approximately 25 percent of normal, and hydrogen peroxide levels increased rapidly during phagocytosis. Although early postphagocytic events were normal, irreversible oxidative damage to the neutrophils (auto-oxidation) led to decreased killing of bacteria.

Information on *neutrophil dysfunction in infants* is conflicting and incomplete.[80] Abnormal neutrophil functions have been ascribed both to intrinsic cellular and to plasma defects. Chemotaxis is decreased, and the generation of chemotactic factors from infant serum is decreased. The responsible mechanisms remain undefined, although chemotactic factor binding by neonatal neutrophil seems to be normal.[81] Results of studies have been contradictory, and it is possible that some of this variability may be due to heterogeneity of neutrophil subpopulations.[82] In many studies, engulfment and killing of pathogenic bacteria was reported to be inefficient. Reports of oxidative metabolism are perplexing. Certain aspects such as oxygen consumption, hexose monophosphate shunt activity, nitroblue tetrazolium dye reduction, and superoxide anion generation seem to be increased, particularly when nonphagocytic (resting) neutrophils are studied. However, decreased oxidative metabolism has been reported when other aspects such as postphagocytic chemiluminescence and hydroxyl radical production have been assessed.[83,84] In addition, enzymes responsible for the detoxification of hydrogen peroxide (glutathione peroxidase and catalase) are decreased in neutrophils from newborns.[85] Glutathione levels in neonatal neutrophils are rapidly depleted by oxidant stress.[86] The increased production of reactive oxygen molecules such as superoxide anion and hydrogen peroxide on the one hand, and the decreased activity of oxygen detoxification enzymes on the other, suggest that neutrophils from infants may be prone to oxidant damage. Thus, it is suggested that auto-oxidation contributes, at least in part, to the effective functions of neonatal neutrophils. Other mechanisms undoubtedly are involved, however.

Glycoproteins

Several patients have been described with abnormal neutrophil functions that have been ascribed to congenital deficiencies of neutrophil glycoproteins.[87-92] These missing glycoproteins are believed to be associated with both the plasma membrane and cytoplasmic granules. Because abnormal function is a consequence of the diminished expression of these glycoproteins, they have been presumed to play crucial roles in normal neutrophil function. Many of the patients have had striking neutrophilia, delayed shedding of the umbilical cord, infection of the umbilical stump, impaired neutrophil adhesion, decreased chemotaxis, and diminished phagocytosis. Occasionally, abnormalities of other leukocytes (such as lymphocytes) have been demonstrated.[90] However, techniques of study have not been consistent among investigators. Patients with these disorders are being discovered with increasing frequency and will provide a focus of interest for quite some time.

Hyperimmunoglobulin E Syndrome

The combination of recurrent infections (typically with *Staphylococcus*) of skin and respiratory tract, decreased neutrophil chemotaxis, and high serum IgE has been called Job's syndrome.[93] Serum IgE is usually greater than 2000 IU/ml. Other manifestations of the disorder include coarse facies, eczema, mild eosinophilia, mucocutaneous *Candida* infections, depressed cell-mediated immunity, and the production of a chemotactic inhibitor by mononuclear cells. Many patients with variations of the syndrome have been reported, and the full spectrum of this disorder remains to be defined.

Abnormal Morphology and Normal Function

Several abnormalities of neutrophil morphology exist in patients without severe infections, involving neutrophil functions that are either normal or only slightly defective. Two conditions are characterized by abnormalities of the nucleus with regard to the number of nuclear lobes in mature neutrophil. In one of these conditions, *giant neutrophilic granulocytes with hypersegmentation* have been found to be inherited in a dominant fashion. In these patients 1 to 2 percent of neutrophils in the blood have five or more segments. A similar hypersegmentation of eosinophilic granulocytes has been described as being inherited in a dominant fashion.

At the other extreme (hyposegmentation) is the *Pelger-Huët anomaly*[94] (see Color Plate 132). When congenital, this anomaly is inherited as a dominant characteristic in which neutrophils are found to be bilobed or to have no lobulation whatsoever. The anomaly can be acquired as an idiosyncratic reaction to drugs and is recognized in some patients with leukemia, in which case the cells are often called pseudo–Pelger-Huët neutrophils. Clinically, there is no difficulty in distinguishing leukemia from the benign familial condition.

A number of abnormalities demonstrate an alteration of the morphology of neutrophil cytoplasm. Sometimes these findings can be of diagnostic significance. *Alder's anomaly* is the presence of dark-staining and coarse cytoplasmic granules in the cytoplasm of the three major leukocyte types (neutrophils, lymphocytes, and monocytes). In some patients only one cell line may be involved. This cytoplasmic anomaly, seen in association with the mucopolysaccharidoses, can also be found as an inherited anomaly without other demonstrable defects. On histochemical analysis the granules are found to contain mucopolysaccharide. Neutrophils in the *May-Hegglin anomaly* have blue-staining cytoplasmic inclusions that resemble Döhle bodies.[95] **(See Color Plates 133 and 134.)** On electron microscopy these neutrophils are shown to have large granule-free areas in the cytoplasm that contain fibrils of ribonucleic acid. In addition to the neutrophil finding, thrombocytopenia exists with the presence of platelets that tend to be large and poorly granulated.

CASE STUDIES

Case Study

History of Present Illness. A 3-year-old boy was admitted with a liver abscess. He had been ill with many infections since the age of 1 month. Types of infections included recurrent pyoderma, several episodes of pneumonia, perirectal abscess, osteomyelitis of the metacarpals, suppurative lymphadenitis, and mastoiditis. Organisms that were recovered from these sites of infection were *Staphylococcus*, *Serratia*, *Klebsiella*, and *Pseudomonas*. Despite these episodes of infection, he experienced normal growth and development. Immunization had been given without incident; in particular, he experienced no difficulties with live virus vaccines. The family medical history was remarkable in that an older brother and a cousin (a son of a maternal aunt) had suffered similar chronic infections, and one had died of chronic gram-positive pneumonia.

Physical Examination. He appeared to be generally well. The skin was covered with scattered areas of crusted scabs. Gram's stain of the moist base of a scab from the skin revealed gram-positive organisms (*Staphylococcus*). Lymph nodes in all areas were enlarged to 3 to 6 cm, and those in the neck were firm and tender. The tympanic membranes were scarred, and the right one was perforated. The lungs were normal. The liver was enlarged to 8 cm below the lower rib margin, and the spleen was so large that it extended into the pelvis.

Laboratory Data. The hemoglobin concentration was 9 g/dl, and the erythrocyte morphology was fairly normal except for slight hypochromia and variation in size. The total white blood cell count was 33,000/μl, with 28,000/μl neutrophils. The neutrophils contained toxic granules, Döhle bodies, and vacuoles. The platelet count was 427,000/μl. Concentrations of serum immunoglobulins and complement components were all increased moderately.

Neutrophilia was consistently found on several occasions when earlier laboratory data were reviewed. Neutropenia was never documented. Results of neutrophil migration studies were normal when assessed by both in vivo (skin window) and in vitro (chemotaxis chamber) techniques. Phagocytosis (ingestion) of *Staphylococcus*, yeast organisms, and latex particles was normal. The cytoplasm contained plentiful, prominent granules, and the degranulation process was intact. Oxidative metabolism in response to neutrophil stimulation was completely absent. Specifically, there was no postphagocytic increase in oxygen consumption, superoxide anion and hydrogen peroxide were not formed, and activity of the hexose monophosphate shunt was not increased. Finally, neutrophils were unable to oxidize and kill *Staphylococcus* that had been phagocytized. Neutrophils from the mother were studied and on some assays performed at about 50 percent of normal capacity.

Discussion. This patient exhibits characteristic features of the X-linked recessive form of chronic granulomatous disease of childhood, with severe and persistent infections caused by *Staphylococcus* and gram-negative organisms. Anemia and persistent neutrophilia are seen even when these patients are relatively free of infection. Neutrophils from these children are numerous, they migrate normally, they are capable of phagocytosis, and they form phagocytic vesicles. However, they are unable to kill the phagocytized microorganisms because they are unable to generate reactive forms of oxygen. In some families, the X-linked nature of the inheritance pattern can be established by finding disease in male members of the maternal family and by finding moderate defects in the mother. At present, treatment attempts to diminish the frequency of infections by giving long-term trimethoprim and sulfamethoxazole and promptly to treat established infections. Bone marrow transplantation is an experimental form of more definitive therapy.

Case Study

History of Present Illness. A 12-year-old girl was admitted with lobar pneumonia. She was perfectly well until 2 days before admission, when she began having fever and cough. Over the previous 48 hours, the temperature had remained at approximately 104°F, and the cough was increasing in intensity. On one occasion, the sputum contained a few flecks of blood. In the past, she had experienced only the usual number of minor respiratory infections, and she had never been this ill before. Approximately 6 hours prior to admission, she began to breathe rapidly and her lips became dusky.

Physical Examination. She was acutely ill and appeared short of breath. The temperature was 104°F, and she was listless and slightly cyanotic. The only other pertinent findings on the physical examination were confined to the right side of the chest. The

right upper chest was dull to percussion, and on auscultation there was very poor air exchange with many fine crackling rales.

Laboratory Data. The hemoglobin was 14 g/dl. The total white blood cell count was 35,000/μl, with 12,000 segmented neutrophils and 18,000 immature neutrophils (bands and stabs and myelocytes); the remainder were mononuclear leukocytes. The neutrophils were filled with toxic granulations and Döhle bodies, and vacuoles were quite abundant. A rare neutrophil contained tiny bodies that appeared to be gram-positive diplococci. The blood culture subsequently grew *Streptococcus pneumoniae*.

Discussion. This child with lobar pneumonia exhibits the typical picture of a neutrophilic, leukemoid reaction due to a bacterial infection. Both the absolute and relative neutrophil count were elevated with a marked increase in immature forms (bands, stabs, and myelocytes). Moreover, the alterations of neutrophil cytoplasm (toxic granules, Döhle bodies, and vacuoles) were characteristic of stress leukopoiesis. Obviously, the presence of intracellular microorganisms confirmed that this leukemoid reaction was due to a bacterial infection. However, none of the other features were specific for any single etiology. Other causes that must always be considered include other types of infections (such as *Staphylococcus*, other types of pyogenic bacteria, and leptospirosis), hypersensitivity drug reactions, burns, and other inflammatory diseases such as rheumatoid arthritis. It must also be remembered that during overwhelming infection, the leukocyte picture may actually be one of neutropenia, rather than neutrophilia. Even in this instance, however, the neutrophils that were present were frequently immature forms.

REFERENCES

1. Brennan, JK, et al: Chemical mediators of granulopoieses: A review. Exp Hematol 8:441, 1980.
2. Burgess, AW and Metcalf, D: The nature and action of granulocyte-macrophage colony stimulating factors. Blood 56:947, 1980.
3. Francis, GE, et al: Bone marrow endogenous colony stimulating factor(s): Relation to granulopoiesis in vivo. Exp Hematol 9:332, 1981.
4. Miller, AM, et al: Modulation of granulopoiesis: Opposing roles of prostaglandins F and E. J Lab Clin Med 92:983, 1978.
5. Verma, DS, et al: Human leukocyte interferon preparation blocks granulopoietic differentiation. Blood 54:1423, 1979.
6. Broxmeyer, HE, et al: Specificity and modulation of the action of lactoferrin, a negative feedback regulator of myelopoiesis. Blood 55:324, 1980.
7. Cartwright, GE, Athens, JW, and Wintrobe, MM: The kinetics of granulopoiesis in normal man. Blood 24:780, 1964.
8. Rosse, C, et al: Bone marrow cell populations of normal infants: The predominance of lymphocytes. J Lab Clin Med 89:1225, 1977.
9. Rosvoll, RV, et al: Visual and automated differential leukocyte counts. Am J Clin Pathol 71:695, 1979.
10. Manroe, BL, et al: The neonatal blood count in health and disease: I. Reference values for neutrophilic cells. J Pediatr 95:89, 1979.
11. Christensen, RD, Bradley, PP, and Rothstein, G: The leukocyte left shift in clinical and experimental neonatal sepsis. J Pediatr 98:101, 1981.
12. Bain, BJ and England, JM: Normal haematological values: Sex difference in neutrophil count. Br Med J 877:306, 1975.

13. Bain, BJ and England, JM: Variations in leucocyte count during menstrual cycle. Br Med J 2:473, 1975.

14. Caramihai, E, et al: Leukocyte count differences in healthy white and black children 1 to 4 years of age. Pediatrics 86:252, 1975.

15. Wright, PF, et al: Patterns of illness in the highly febrile young child: Epidemiologic, clinical and laboratory correlates. Pediatrics 67:694, 1981.

16. Morens, DM: WBC count and differential. Am J Dis Child 133:25, 1979.

17. Christensen, RD and Rothstein, G: Pitfalls in the interpretation of leukocyte counts of newborn infants. Am J Clin Pathol 72:608, 1979.

18. Walker, RI and Willemze, R: Neutrophil kinetics and the regulation of granulopoiesis. Rev Infect Dis 2:282, 1980.

19. Cawley, JC and Hayhoe, FGJ: The inclusions of the May-Hegglin anomaly and Döhle bodies in infection: An ultrastructural comparison. Br J Haematol 22:491, 1971.

20. McCall, C, et al: Functional characteristics of human toxic neutrophils. J Infect Dis 124:68, 1971.

21. McCall, CE, et al: Human toxic neutrophils: III. Metabolic characteristics. J Infect Dis 127:26, 1973.

22. Hill, HR, et al: Hyperactivity of neutrophil leukotactic responses during active bacterial infection. J Clin Invest 53:996, 1974.

23. van Epps, DE and Garcia, ML: Enhancement of neutrophil function as a result of prior exposure to chemotactic factor. J Clin Invest 66:167, 1980.

24. Becker, EL: Chemotaxis. J Allergy Clin Immunol 66:97, 1980.

25. O'Flaherty, JT and Ward, PA: Chemotactic factors and the neutrophil. Semin Hematol 16:163, 1979.

26. Schiffman, E: Leukocyte chemotaxis. Ann Rev Physiol 44:553, 1982.

27. Nelson, RD, et al: Chemotactic deactivation of human neutrophils: Possible relationship to stimulation of oxidative metabolism. Infect Immunol 23:283, 1979.

28. Gallin, JI and Wright, DG: Role of secretory events in modulating human neutrophil chemotaxis. J Clin Invest 62:1364, 1978.

29. Goetzl, EJ, et al: Specific inhibition of the polymorphonuclear leukocyte chemotactic response to hydroxy-fatty acid metabolites of arachidonic acid by methyl ester derivatives. J Clin Invest 63:1181, 1979.

30. Brozna, JP, et al: Chemotactic factor inactivators of human granulocytes. J Clin Invest 60:1280, 1977.

31. Ginsburg, I and Quie, PG: Modulation of human polymorphonuclear leukocyte chemotaxis by leukocyte extracts, bacterial products, inflammatory exudates, and polyelectrolytes. Inflammation 4:301, 1980.

32. Scribner, DJ and Farhney, D: Neutrophil receptors for IgG and complement: Their roles in the attachment and ingestion phases of phagocytosis. J Immunol 116:892, 1976.

33. Weissman, G, Smolen, JE, and Korchak, HM: Release of inflammatory mediators from stimulated neutrophils. N Engl J Med 303:27, 1980.

34. Ignarro, LJ, Lint TF, and George, WJ: Hormonal control of lysosomal enzyme release from human neutrophils. J Exp Med 139:1395, 1974.

35. Bainton, DF: Sequential degranulation of the two types of polymorphonuclear leukocyte granules during phagocytosis of microorganisms. J Cell Biol 58:249, 1973.

36. Jensen, MS and Bainton, DF: Temporal changes in pH within the phagocytic vacuole of the polymorphonuclear neutrophilic leukocyte. J Cell Biol 56:379, 1973.

37. Jacques, YV and Bainton, DF: Changes in pH within the phagocytic vacuoles of human neutrophils and monocytes. Lab Invest 39:179, 1978.

38. Weisdorf, DJ, Craddock, PR, and Jacob, HS: Glycogenolysis versus glucose transport in human granulocytes: Differential activation in phagocytosis and chemotaxis. Blood 60:888, 1982.

39. Badior, BM: Oxygen-dependent microbial killing by phagocytes. N Engl J Med 298:659, 1978.

40. DeChatelet, LR: Initiation of the respiratory burst in human polymorphonuclear neutrophils: A critical review. J Reticuloendothel Soc 24:73, 1978.

41. Klebanoff, SJ: Antimicrobial mechanisms in neutrophilic polymorphonuclear leukocytes. Semin Hematol 12:117, 1975.

42. Stenson, WF and Parker, CW: Metabolism of arachidonic acid in ionophore-stimulated neutrophils. J Clin Invest 64:1457, 1979.

43. Rister, M and Baehner RL: The alteration of superoxide dismutase, catalase, glutathione peroxidase and NAD(P)H cytochrome C reductase in guinea pig polymorphonuclear leukocytes and alveolar macrophages during hyperoxia. J Clin Invest 58:1174, 1976.

44. Higgins, CP, et al: Polymorphonuclear leukocyte species differs in the disposal of hydrogen peroxide (H_2O_2). Proc Soc Exp Biol Med 158:478, 1978.

45. Shoenfeld, Y, et al: The mechanism of benign hereditary neutropenia. Arch Int Med 142:797, 1982.

46. Howard, MW, Strauss, RG, and Johnston, RG, Jr: Infections in patients with neutropenia. Am J Dis Child 131:788, 1977.

47. Dale, DC, et al: Comparison of agents producing neutrophilic leukocytosis in man: Hydrocortisone, prednisone, endotoxin and etiocholanolone. J Clin Invest 56:808, 1975.

48. Christensen, RD, et al: Granulocyte transfusion in neonates with bacterial infection, neutropenia, and depletion of mature marrow neutrophils. Pediatrics 70:1, 1982.

49. Conway, LT, et al: Natural history of primary autoimmune neutropenia in infancy. Pediatrics 79:728, 1987.

50. Lalezari, P, Khorshid, M, and Petrosova, M: Autoimmune neutropenia of infancy. J Pediatr 109:764, 1986.

51. Lalezari, R and Radel, E: Neutrophil-specific antigens: Immunology and clinical significance. Semin Hematol 11:281, 1974.

52. Kostmann, R: Infantile genetic agranulocytosis. Acta Paediatr Scand 64:362, 1975.

53. Zucker-Franklin, D, L'Esperance, P, and Good, RA: Congenital neutropenia: An intrinsic cell defect demonstrated by electron microscopy of soft agar colonies. Blood 49:425, 1977.

54. Amato, D, Freedman, MH, and Saunders, EF: Granulopoiesis in severe congenital neutropenia. Blood 47:531, 1976.

55. Bonilla, MA, et al: Effects of recombinant colony-stimulating factor on neutropenia in patients with congenital agranulocytosis. N Engl J Med 320:1574, 1989.

56. Pincus, SH, Boxer, LA, and Stossel, TP: Chronic neutropenia in childhood: Analysis of 16 cases and a review of the literature. Am J Med 61:849, 1976.

57. Krill, CE Jr, Smith, HD, and Mauer, AM: Chronic idiopathic granulocytopenia. N Engl J Med 270:699, 1964.

58. Bohinjec, J: Myelokathexis: Chronic neutropenia with hyperplastic bone marrow and hypersegmented neutrophils in two siblings. Blut 42:191, 1980.

59. Andrews, RB, et al: Some immunological and haematological aspects of human cyclic neutropenia. Scand J Haematol 22:97, 1979.

60. Guerry, D, IV, et al: Periodic hematopoiesis in human cyclic neutropenia. J Clin Invest 52:3220, 1973.

61. Beard, MEJ, et al: Fanconi's anaemia. QJ Med 42:403, 1973.

62. Inoue, S, et al: Dyskeratosis congenita with pancytopenia (another constitutional anemia). Am J Dis Child 126:389, 1973.

63. Shwachman, H, et al: The syndrome of pancreatic insufficiency and bone marrow dysfunction. J Pediatr 65:645, 1965.

64. Cappelletti, P and Lippi, U: Hereditary myeloperoxidase deficiency: A rare condition? Diagnostic possibilities of a differential white cell autoanalyzer (Hemalog-D). Haematologica 68:736, 1983.

65. Nauseef, WM, Root, RK, and Malech, HL: Biochemical and immunologic analysis of hereditary myeloperoxidase deficiency. J Clin Invest 71:1297, 1983.

66. Kitahara, M, et al: Hereditary myeloperoxidase deficiency. Blood 57:888, 1981.
67. Rosen, H and Klebanoff, SJ: Chemiluminescence and superoxide production by myeloperoxidase-deficient leukocytes. J Clin Invest 58:50, 1976.
68. Root, RK, Rosenthal, AS, and Balestra, DJ: Abnormal bactericidal metabolic, and lysosomal functions of Chediak-Higashi syndrome leukocytes. J Clin Invest 51:649, 1972.
69. Oliver, JM: Cell biology of leukocyte abnormalities: Membrane and cytoskeletal function in normal and defective cells: A review. Am J Pathol 93:221, 1978.
70. Strauss, RG, et al: An anomaly of neutrophil morphology with impaired function. N Engl J Med 290:478, 1974.
71. Boxer, LA, et al: Lactoferrin deficiency associated with altered granulocyte function. N Engl J Med 307:403, 1982.
72. Strauss, G, McCarthy, DJ, and Mauer, AM: Neutrophil function in congenital phosphoglycerate kinase deficiency. J Pediatr 85:341, 1974.
73. Tauber, AI, et al: Chronic granulomatous disease: A syndrome of phagocyte oxidase deficiencies. Medicine 62:286, 1983.
74. Segal, AW: The electron transport chain of the microbial oxidase of phagocytic cells and its involvement in the molecular pathology of chronic granulomatosis disease. J Clin Invest 83:1785, 1989.
75. Galin, JI, et al: Recent advances in chronic granulomatous disease. Ann Int Med 99:657, 1983.
76. Parkos, CA, et al: Absence of both the 91KD and 22KD subunits of human neutrophil cytochrome b in two genetic forms of chronic granulomatous disease. Blood 73:1416, 1989.
77. Cooper, MR, et al: Complete deficiency of leukocyte glucose-6-phosphate dehydrogenase and defective bactericidal activity. J Clin Invest 51:769, 1972.
77a. Holmes, B, et al: Chronic granulomatous disease in females. A deficiency of leukocyte glutathione peroxidase. N Engl J Med 283:217, 1970.
78. Roos, D, et al: Protection of phagocytic leukocytes by endogenous glutathione: Studies in a family with glutathione reductase deficiency. Blood 53:851, 1979.
79. Oliver, JM, et al: Microtubule assembly and function in normal and glutathione synthetase-deficient polymorphonuclear leukocytes. J Immunol 120:1181, 1978.
80. Hill, HR: Biochemical, structural and functional abnormalities of polymorphonuclear leukocytes in the neonate. Pediatr Res 22:375, 1987.
81. Strauss, RG and Snyder, EL: Chemotactic peptide binding by intact neutrophils from human neonates. Pediatr Res 18:63, 1984.
82. Masuda, K, Kinoshita, Y, and Kobayashi, Y: Heterogeneity of Fc expression in chemotaxis and adherence of neonatal neutrophils. Pediatr Res 25:6, 1989.
83. Strauss, RG, Rosenberger, TG, and Wallace, PD: Neutrophil chemiluminescence during the first month of life. Acta Haematol 63:326, 1980.
84. Strauss, RG and Snyder, EL: Neutrophils from human infants exhibit decreased viability. Pediatr Res 15:794, 1981.
85. Strauss, RG, et al: Oxygen-detoxifying enzymes in neutrophils of infants and their mothers. J Lab Clin Med 95:897, 1980.
86. Strauss, RG and Snyder, EL: Glutathione in neutrophils from human infants. Acta Haematol 69:9, 1983.
87. Crowley, CA, et al: An inherited abnormality of neutrophil adhesion: its genetic transmission and its association with a missing protein. N Engl J Med 302:1163, 1980.
88. Buchanan, MR, et al: Studies on the interaction between GP-180-deficient neutrophils and vascular endothelium. Blood 60:160, 1982.
89. Arnaout, MA, et al: Deficiency of a granulocyte-membrane glycoprotein (gp 150) in a boy with recurrent bacterial infections. N Engl J Med 306:693, 1982.
90. Beatty, PG, et al: Absence of monoclonal-antibody-defined protein complex in a boy with abnormal leucocyte function. Lancet 1:535, 1984.
91. Andersen, DC, et al: The severe and moderate phenotypes of heritable Mac-1, LFA-1 deficiency: Their quantitative definition and relation to leukocyte dysfunction and clinical features. J Infect Dis 152:668, 1985.
92. Kobayashi, K, et al: An abnormality of neutrophil adhesion: Autosomal recessive inheritance associated with missing neutrophil glycoproteins. Pediatrics 73:606, 1984.
93. Donabedian, H and Gallen, JI: The hyperimmunoglobulin E recurrent-infection (Job's) syndrome. Medicine 62:195, 1983.
94. Johnson, CA, et al: Functional and metabolic studies of polymorphonuclear leukocytes in the congenital Pelger-Huet anomaly. Blood 55:466, 1980.
95. Cawley, JC and Hayhoe, FGJ: The inclusions of the May-Hegglin anomaly and Döhle bodies of infection: An ultrastructural comparison. Br J Haematol 22:491, 1972.

QUESTIONS

1. *Which of the following lists contains the three major types of leukocytes found in peripheral blood?*
   a. Myelocyte, myeloblast, and promyelocyte
   b. Neutrophil, eosinophil, and basophil
   c. Granulocyte, lymphocyte, and monocyte
   d. Erythrocyte, rubriblast, rubricyte

2. *What is the proper sequence of production and circulating kinetics of hematopoietic cells?*
   a. Amplification by CSF, proliferation, maturation, storage and/or release, removal
   b. Proliferation, maturation, amplification by CSF, storage and/or release, removal
   c. Maturation, proliferation, storage and/or release, amplification by CSF, removal
   d. Storage and/or release, proliferation, amplification by CSF, maturation, removal

3. *What are the normal percentages of precursor cell types in the bone marrow of adults? See a through d at the bottom of this page.*

4. *What is the predominant white cell type found in peripheral blood?*
   a. Monocyte
   b. Eosinophil
   c. Lymphocyte
   d. Neutrophil

	Erythrocytes	Granulocytes	Lymphocytes	Plasma Cells
a.	4–10	30–70	50–70	0–5
b.	18–30	50–70	3–17	0–2
c.	54–72	1–12	27–33	0
d.	0–10	50–70	30–50	0

5. *What happens to neutrophil count, morphology, and movement in response to infections?*
   a. Count decreases; morphology remains same; movement becomes increased
   b. Count increases; cytoplasmic granules become more prominent; movement is decreased
   c. Count decreases; Döhle bodies form; movement becomes increased
   d. Count increases; cytoplasmic granules become less prominent; movement remains same

6. *What changes occur in a neutrophil as a result of inflammatory reactions?*
   a. Binding of chemotactic factors; neutrophil aggregation; exocytosis; and increased metabolism
   b. Plasma membrane becomes rigid; penetration of chemotactic factors; and decreased metabolism
   c. Dispersion of neutrophils; increased endocytosis; decrease in chemotactic factors; no change in metabolism
   d. Deactivation of chemotactic factors; clumping of metabolic products from neutrophils; penetration of endothelium

7. *Which sequence is the CORRECT order for phagocytosis?*
   a. Release of cytoplasmic granules; binding of particle; ingestion; fusion to form phagolysosome
   b. Ingestion; binding of particle; fusion to form phagolysosome; release of cytoplasmic granules
   c. Binding of particle; ingestion; release of cytoplasmic granules; fusion to form phagolysosome
   d. Fusion to form phagolysosome; binding of particle; release of cytoplasmic granules; ingestion

8. *What are the two most important biochemical products manufactured by neutrophils that are involved in active phagocytosis?*
   a. Arachidonic acid and thromboxane
   b. Superoxide dismutase and catalase
   c. Glutathione peroxidase and copper-zinc enzymes
   d. Myeloperoxidase and hydrogen peroxide

9. *What is the difference between quantitative and qualitative disorders of neutrophils?*
   a. Quantitative refers to abnormal function of neutrophils; qualitative refers to abnormal number of neutrophils.
   b. Quantitative refers to abnormal number of neutrophils; qualitative refers to abnormal function of neutrophils.
   c. Both qualitative and quantitative are relative terms that refer to either abnormally high or low numbers of neutrophils.
   d. Qualitative and quantitative refer to the severity of abnormal functioning neutrophils.

10. *What are the two main classifications of neutropenia?*
    a. Isoimmune and autoimmune
    b. Alloimmune and autoimmune
    c. Acquired and congenital
    d. Organic and cyclic

11. *Which conditions are classified as acquired?*
    a. Viral infections, drug-related, or secondary to other conditions
    b. Lazy leukocyte syndrome, monosomy, glycoprotein deficiency
    c. Kostmann-type agranulocytosis, chronic benign neutropenia, myelokathexis, cyclic neutropenia
    d. Myeloperoxidase deficiency, Chédiak-Higashi disease
    e. Chronic granulomatous disease, G6PD deficiency, glutathione peroxidase deficiency

12. *Which conditions are classified as congenital? (Use answer choices for question 11.)*

13. *Which conditions have a chemotaxis defect? (Use answer choices for question 11.)*

14. *Which conditions are associated with a defect in cytoplasmic granules? (Use answer choices for question 11.)*

15. *Which conditions are associated with biochemical defects? (Use answer choices for question 11.)*

16. *What happens to neutrophils in the absence of certain glycoproteins?*
    a. No major changes in function
    b. Both structural and functional defects
    c. Primarily structural defects
    d. Primarily functional defects

17. *What is the major disease characteristic associated with Job's syndrome?*
    a. Recurrent staphylococcal infections of the skin and respiratory tract
    b. Recurrent viral infections
    c. Hyperpigmentation and swollen lymph nodes
    d. Lobar pneumonia

18. *What diseases are associated with abnormal neutrophil morphology?*
    a. Hyperimmunoglobulin E syndrome and Job's syndrome
    b. Chronic and acute lymphocytic leukemia
    c. Pelger-Huët anomaly and May-Hegglin anomaly
    d. Familial lipochrome pigmentation and G6PD deficiency

ANSWERS

1. c (p. 241)
2. a (p. 242)
3. b (p. 242)
4. d (p. 243)
5. b (p. 243)
6. a (p. 244)

7. c (p. 244)
8. d (p. 245)
9. b (p. 245–246)
10. c (p. 246)
11. a (p. 246–247)
12. c (p. 247–248)

13. b (p. 248)
14. d (p. 248–249)
15. e (p. 250)
16. b (p. 252)
17. a (p. 252)
18. c (p. 252)

CHAPTER 17

MICHELE L. BEST, B.S., M.T.(ASCP)

Infectious Mononucleosis and Reactive Lymphocytosis

HISTORY AND DEFINITIONS

MORPHOLOGY OF REACTIVE LYMPHOCYTES

CAUSES OF REACTIVE LYMPHOCYTOSIS

INFECTIOUS MONONUCLEOSIS
HISTORIC PERSPECTIVE

DISEASE DESCRIPTION AND ETIOLOGY
CLINICAL MANIFESTATIONS
TREATMENT
LABORATORY TESTS IN DIAGNOSIS

CASE STUDY

OBJECTIVES

At the end of this chapter, the learner should be able to:
1. Identify the distinguishing characteristics of reactive lymphocytes.
2. Name conditions that show reactive lymphocytes.
3. State a cause for heterophile-negative mononucleosis-like syndrome.

4. Describe clinical manifestations of EBV-associated infectious mononucleosis.
5. Discuss laboratory tests that are used to diagnose infectious mononucleosis.

HISTORY AND DEFINITIONS

The cell commonly described as the "atypical" lymphocyte has accumulated a rich history of observations and definitions from the time it was originally described in 1907 by Turk.[1] Since then, there have been as many new terms for this morphologic entity as observations. Turk initially described a deeply basophilic plasmacytelike cell, later referred to as a Turk cell, in the peripheral blood of a patient who was thought to have acute leukemia. Because the patient later recovered, this probably represents the first recorded case of infectious mononucleosis.

Downey and McKinlay[2] in 1923 described three separate morphologic types of abnormal cells seen in the blood of patients with infectious mononucleosis. The morphologic subtypes Downey I, II, and III were initiated. The Downey classification of atypical lymphocytes represents the first description of the diverse spectrum of morphologic observations seen when a T or B lymphocyte is stimulated by antigen. Although Downey's descriptions should be required reading for all students of hematology because of their historic and morphologic insights, the

separation of atypical lymphocytes into Downey subtypes has no practical value in today's laboratories.

Over the years, it became common practice to combine all lymphocytes that did not appear morphologically normal under the all-inclusive, vague heading of "atypical." The term atypical lymphocyte describes any abnormal lymphocyte morphology seen, regardless of whether the abnormality is benign or malignant. Atypical is still used in many laboratories in this way. It is also occasionally used to falsely describe normal variants because of the morphologic variation in normal lymphocyte populations.

A variety of other terms have cropped up since Downey's time to describe these same cell types. Virocyte, and immunoblast, as well as transformed, stimulated, and reactive lymphocytes, are among the more common terms used.

Elucidation of lymphocyte subtypes by advances in cellular immunology has led to a functional appreciation of the morphology of the atypical lymphocyte. These atypical cells represent T or B lymphocytes reacting to an antigenic stimulus and transforming into immune-responsive blast cells. These blast cells are called immunoblasts. All morphologic changes that occur during this transformation process are defined as reactive, transformed, or stimulated lymphocytes. The term *reactive lymphocyte* is preferred by many hematologists.

It is the author's opinion that the all-inclusive category of atypical lymphocytes should be replaced with the following more meaningful and specific categories of abnormal lymphocyte variants: (1) reactive, (2) abnormal, and (3) abnormal and immature. *Reactive* may be used to describe specific morphologic changes that are nonmalignant and elicited by a variety of antigens. *Abnormal* may be used to describe other morphologic abnormalities that do not appear reactive and that are probably due to lymphoid malignancy. If the cells also appear immature, they may be described as *abnormal and immature*. Malignant lymphocytic variants should also be described morphologically as cleaved, convoluted, or Burkitt's-like — whichever applies. Slides containing malignant or suspicious lymphocyte morphology must be reviewed by a pathologist, regardless of the number of such cells present. For the remainder of the text, reactive will be used to describe the atypical mononuclear cells seen in infectious mononucleosis and related syndromes.

MORPHOLOGY OF REACTIVE LYMPHOCYTES

A difficult morphologic challenge is the interpretation of a huge, deeply basophilic, immature-looking cell on a peripheral blood smear. The initial reflex is to regard the cell as malignant. Quite often these large, bizarre cells turn out to be reactive lymphocytes, which can achieve abnormal sizes (often greater than 30 μm) and can look quite ominous. These cells are commonly encountered on peripheral blood smears, and their recognition is essential.

Reactive lymphocytes range in size from that of a large normal lymphocyte to greater than 30 μm. Nuclear and cytoplasmic mass are both increased, contributing to the overall size increase. It is the nuclear and cytoplasmic morphology of the reactive lymphocyte that differentiates it from a normal, large lymphocyte or a monocyte. The contrasting morphology of a large normal lymphocyte, a monocyte, and several types of reactive lymphocytes is depicted in **Color Plates 135 through 139.**

The nucleus of a large lymphocyte has a densely stained, clumped chromatin with uneven streaks of parachromatin in the nucleus. Chromatin clumping is concentrated around the nuclear edges. The monocyte nucleus, in contrast, has a more lightly stained chromatin with a more even dispersion of chromatin clumps and parachromatin — the so-called lacy appearance. The clumps are smaller than those in the lymphocyte and tend to show less tendency to locate near the nuclear membrane. The nuclear chromatin of a reactive lymphocyte shows distinctive changes from the normal lymphocyte chromatin previously described. The chromatin is less intensely clumped, with more evidence of parachromatin in the nucleus and a more even pattern of clumping. Compared with that of a monocyte, the chromatin of a reactive lymphocyte is more densely stained and usually slightly more clumped. The chromatin density of a reactive lymphocyte is usually intermediate between those of a small lymphocyte and a monocyte. Nucleoli may or may not be visible in the reactive lymphocyte; when visible, they are generally multiple and small. Nucleoli may occasionally be larger and more prominent, but nucleoli in a reactive lymphocyte are hardly ever singular and prominent. Nuclear shape irregularities are common and often striking, varying from cleaved or convoluted to kidney bean–shaped or oblong. It must be emphasized that there is a wide range of reactive morphology from a very slight change in the nuclear chromatin clumping pattern to a very immature, blastlike nucleus with prominent nucleoli. These changes appear to reflect cells being "caught" in different stages of lymphocyte transformation.

Although nuclear abnormalities are important in the identification of reactive lymphocytes, cytoplasmic features are more striking and more differential. The cytoplasms of normal large lymphocytes and monocytes tend to be pale blue and gray, respectively, and possess an even staining quality, whereas the cytoplasm of a reactive lymphocyte is most notable for its increased degree of basophilia, which appears quite patchy (that is, the cytoplasm is unevenly stained). There are often linear or rodlike, clear, unstained areas in the cytoplasm adjacent to the nucleus. Often there is a perinuclear clearing or halo also. The cytoplasm of the reactive lymphocyte has traditionally been described as abundant and sprawled-looking with a scalloped, deeply basophilic cytoplasmic border that tends to be indented by the adjacent red cells.[8] These criteria are not as reliable as the cytoplasmic features cited earlier in recognizing reactive lymphocytes, because this scalloping effect will be seen only if the cytoplasm and the red cells are abundant. Prominent cytoplasmic granulation is present in some reactive lymphocytes, but it is neither a regular nor an identifying characteristic. Although frequently described in the literature, cytoplasmic vacuolation is not common in reactive lymphocytes.

A distinctive subtype of the reactive lymphocyte that bears special mention is the plasmacytoid lymphocyte (**see Color Plate 139**). These cells appear quite similar to plasma cells in the cytoplasm (that is, they are intensely basophilic with a developing perinuclear halo, or "hof"). However, the nuclear chromatin pattern is intermediate between that of a mature lymphocyte and that of a mature plasmacyte. Also, the nucleus-to-cytoplasm ratio is higher than that of a mature plasma cell. Plasmacytoid lymphocytes represent stimulated B lymphocytes maturing toward the plasma cell. When these cells are present in the peripheral blood, their immature precursor, the immunoblast, will often be seen also.

Immunoblasts have plasmacytoid intensely basophilic cytoplasms but possess immature blastic chromatin with nucleoli (**see Color Plate 138**). The mature end-product of B-cell maturation, the plasma cell, often accompanies plasmacytoid, reactive lymphocytes. The presence of plasma cells in the peripheral blood is more often reactive than malignant, especially when present with reactive lymphocytes.

When evaluating an abnormal lymphocyte population, the clinician must remember to look for heterogeneity or homogeneity of morphology. It is the heterogeneity of morphologic types in the patient's lymphocyte population that is most striking in infectious mononucleosis and other types of reactive lymphocytosis. The abnormal cell population should be evaluated as a group, and if quite heterogeneous, a reactive cause for the lymphocytosis should be searched for. In contrast, if the cells look abnormal and the population is homogeneous, malignant lymphoma should be ruled out.

CAUSES OF REACTIVE LYMPHOCYTOSIS

Reactive lymphocytes, as previously described, are present on peripheral blood smears in a wide variety of clinical conditions.

How many reactive lymphocytes, if any, are present on normal smears? This is a frequently asked question, and the answer largely depends on an individual laboratory's criteria for what constitutes "atypical." Sometimes a cell is called atypical because the technologist does not recognize the wide morphologic variation in normal lymphocyte populations. Therefore, lymphocytes that appear slightly different from normal are called atypical. If precise criteria are adhered to in the identification of truly atypical cells, the problem of overcalling atypical lymphocytes can be reduced. It is logical to assume that occasional lymphocytes reacting to antigen will be encountered in the blood of healthy individuals. Although it is rare to observe these lymphocytes while doing a 100-cell manual differential, the Technicon H-1 automated differential, which routinely counts a minimum of 10,000 cells, detects 1 to 3 percent large, unstained cells (LUCs) in normal, healthy individuals. These LUCs are usually identifiable as large lymphocytes or reactive lymphocytes, or both, on a low-power scan. Therefore, smears containing 1 to 2 percent reactive lymphocytes may be considered normal. Peripheral blood smears with greater than 5 percent atypical lymphocytes should be reviewed by a supervisor or pathologist.

Reactive lymphocytes are most striking in number and in morphology in infectious mononucleosis, cytomegalovirus infection, drug hypersensitivity, viral hepatitis, and toxoplasmosis, as well as after infusion of large amounts of blood during open heart surgery (postperfusion syndrome). Cells of similar morphology but fewer in number may be seen in any type of viral infection, including acquired immunodeficiency syndrome (AIDS), and in states of immunologic reactivity. Reactive lymphocytes with plasmacytoid features are often present on peripheral blood smears in drug hypersensitivity reactions, bacterial infections, and states of immunologic reactivity. It is common in the author's laboratory to see less than 10 percent plasmacytoid lymphocytes accompanying an elevated white blood count and a shift to the left in bacterial infection. Reactive lymphocytes should be interpreted as cells reactive to infection, but not necessarily to a viral infection because various bacterial infections and noninfectious conditions also are associated with the presence of reactive lymphocytes in peripheral blood.[9]

INFECTIOUS MONONUCLEOSIS
Historic Perspective

The clinical syndrome of mononucleosis was initially described by German physician Emil Pfeiffer[3] as "glandular fever." The symptomatology initially described of fever, sore throat, and lymphadenopathy closely correlates with the three most prominent symptoms of infectious mononucleosis. The syndrome was actually named "infectious mononucleosis" by Sprunt and Evans[4] in 1920, who were the first to associate the syndrome with atypical morphology of the white blood cells. Paul and Bunnell[5] in 1932 discovered a heterophile antibody in the serum of a patient with infectious mononucleosis. A heterophile antibody is an antibody that reacts with an antigen of an apparently unrelated animal species that is immunologically cross reactive. The heterophile antibody described by Paul and Bunnell[5] was found to agglutinate both horse and sheep erythrocytes.

Davidsohn and Walker[6] in 1935 described what is known today as the Davidsohn differential absorption test. They established that the key feature of the heterophile antibody in infectious mononucleosis is that it can be absorbed by beef erythrocytes but not by guinea pig kidney cells. This characteristic became the basic principle of the various rapid slide differential tests on the market today (Monospot, Monosticon, Monotest).

The causative agent of infectious mononucleosis remained a mystery until 1968 when Henle, Henle, and Diehl[7] described the association of infectious mononucleosis with rising titers of antibody to the Epstein-Barr virus.

Disease Description and Etiology

The term infectious mononucleosis is usually used to describe an acute, benign, febrile primary infection of lymphoid tissue by the Epstein-Barr virus (EBV), a herpes group deoxyribonucleic acid (DNA) virus. This virus infects both pharyngeal epithelial cells and B lymphocytes. The classic disease description includes (1) clinical manifestations of fever, sore throat, and cervical lymph node enlargement; (2) absolute lymphocytosis (greater than 4.5×10^9/liter) with at least 10 percent reactive lymphocytes (**see Color Plates 136 and 137**); and (3) a positive heterophile antibody test result. This combination of clinical, hematologic, and serologic evidence is considered essential for the diagnosis. The term chronic mononucleosis has been used to describe a chronic fatigue syndrome with symptoms resembling infectious mononucleosis. Most of these patients have not had prior documented infection with EBV, but some researchers have implicated EBV as the cause.

Over the years it became evident that the third criterion mentioned in the preceding paragraph is not present in all patients with infectious mononucleosis. Two categories of mononucleosis syndromes exist: (1) those that are heterophile antibody positive and (2) those that are heterophile antibody negative. Many cases of infectious mononucleosis, especially in children under age 10, fit into the second category because they lack a positive heterophile antibody test result. Children less than 3 years old are rarely heterophile antibody positive.[10] Until recently, these heterophile-negative cases have been a difficult diagnostic problem. This problem has been reduced with the advent of new specific and more sensitive tests for antibodies to EBV, the causative agent of infectious mononucleosis. The third criteria for diagnosis is now amended to a positive heterophile antibody test result or a positive EBV antibody titer.

Most cases of heterophile-negative mononucleosislike syndromes in adults are not caused by EBV at all, but by cytomegalovirus (CMV). This syndrome, called CMV mononucleosis, comprises about 65 percent of all heterophile-negative mononucleosis syndromes in patients 15 years of age or older.[11] Both CMV and EBV types of mononucleosis show identical hematologic morphology with numerous reactive lymphocytes and somewhat similar clinical symptoms; they can be differentiated only by specific viral antibody titers. Patients undergoing seroconversion to the human immunodeficiency virus (HIV) may also exhibit a mononucleosislike syndrome with atypical reactive lymphocytes in the peripheral blood. The remainder of this chapter deals with the more common type of infectious mononucleosis, that caused by the Epstein-Barr virus.

Strong evidence for the Epstein-Barr virus as the causative agent of the common type of infectious mononucleosis has been compiled and summarized by Henle and Henle.[12] The list includes the fact that only individuals who lack protective antibody to EBV get the disease. Also, individuals with classic heterophile-positive infectious mononucleosis demonstrate rising titers of EBV antibody during the course of the disease. The most compelling evidence is that continuous EBV-infected lymphoid cell lines can be developed using lymphocytes obtained from the blood of patients with infectious mononucleosis.

The virus is transmitted mainly via the exchange of oral secretions; hence the nickname "kissing disease." It afflicts mainly teenagers and college-aged adults 15 to 19 years of age who have somehow escaped previous infection by the EBV, which is ubiquitous in nature. Socioeconomic status seems to affect development of the immune status to this virus. In lower socioeconomic groups, 50 to 80 percent of children achieve immune status by the age of 4, whereas in more affluent children only 14 percent are immune by that age.[13] This appears to explain that fact that middle-class college students are particularly susceptible to this disease.

Clinical Manifestations

A combination of clinical and laboratory findings is required for the diagnosis of infectious mononucleosis. The clinical presentation of infectious mononucleosis is quite variable, depending on the age of the patient. In childhood, infections are often asymptomatic and remain undiagnosed because the typical symptoms and the heterophile antibody are absent. The teenager with infectious mononucleosis typically presents with a sore throat, fatigue, and transient cervical lymphadenopathy. Splenomegaly is present in 50 to 60 percent of cases. The clinical manifestations of infectious mononucleosis in teenagers and young adults are summarized in Table 17–1. Rare cases of infectious mononucleosis have been reported in older adults and the elderly. Liver involvement tends to be more striking than lymphadenopathy in older patients.[14] It should be remembered that CMV infection is more frequently encountered in this age group and that it tends to present with liver involvement also.

The usual case of infectious mononucleosis is uncomplicated and resolves in 2 or 3 weeks. Complications occur in 3 to 5 percent of cases. Common complications that occur include beta-hemolytic

Table 17–1. **CLINICAL MANIFESTATIONS OF INFECTIOUS MONONUCLEOSIS**

Common Manifestations (seen in >50% of patients)
Sore throat
Posterior cervical lymphadenopathy
Fatigue
Fever
Splenomegaly
Less Common Manifestations (seen in <50% of patients)
Hepatomegaly
Jaundice
Rash
Facial edema
Anorexia
Nausea and vomiting
Generalized lymphadenopathy

Source: Adapted from Schleupner and Overral.[15]

Streptococcus infection (group C or A) of the pharynx and a rash if the drug ampicillin is used to treat the sore throat. Rare complications including splenic rupture, pneumonia, immune thrombocytopenic purpura, Guillain-Barré syndrome, and hemolytic anemia have been reported.[15] Sporadic fatal cases of infectious mononucleosis do occur (about 1 in 3000 cases). Interestingly, all of these fatal cases showed splenomegaly and massive lymphoproliferation.

Treatment

Therapy for infectious mononucleosis depends on the severity of the symptoms. In most routine cases, no specific therapy is indicated other than bed rest and fluids. Steroids may be used to reduce pharyngeal inflammation, especially in cases of threatened airway obstruction.

Laboratory Tests in Diagnosis

Infectious mononucleosis is a disease state in which laboratory testing is essential to the diagnosis. The clinician presented with a patient in the suggestive clinical manifestations will most frequently order a complete blood count and a heterophile antibody test (often called a Monospot test).

The most important peripheral blood abnormality in infectious mononucleosis is the presence of more than 10 percent reactive lymphocytes (**see Color Plates 136 and 137**). These lymphocytes are not the EBV-infected B lymphocytes, but instead represent activated T lymphocytes responding to the infection. These activated cells often compose more than 50 percent of the circulating white blood cells and represent the earliest detectable laboratory abnormality in most patients. The morphology of reactive lymphocytes has been described in a previous section. In addition to the abnormality in morphology of the lymphocyte, there is an absolute increase in the number of total lymphocytes per cubic millimeter (greater than 4.5×10^9/liter for adults). The total white blood cell (WBC) count varies according to the clinical stage of infection. It is normal or decreased in the first week of illness and elevated with counts usually between 15 and 25×10^9/liter during the second and third weeks. Rarely, the WBC count may exceed 30×10^9/liter. The hemoglobin level and platelet count are usually normal; however, mild thrombocytopenia (100 to 150×10^9/liter) is seen in about one third of all cases. Spherocytosis, erythrophagocytosis, and cold autoagglutination may occasionally be seen as manifestations of an autoimmune hemolytic anemia, which may be severe in some cases. Cold agglutinins of anti-i specificity are present in 20 percent of patients with infectious mononucleosis.

The presence of absolute lymphocytosis with reactive lymphocytes on a patient's peripheral blood smear necessitates a logical scheme of laboratory testing for correct diagnosis (Fig. 17–1). The first test to be performed is a simple, inexpensive,

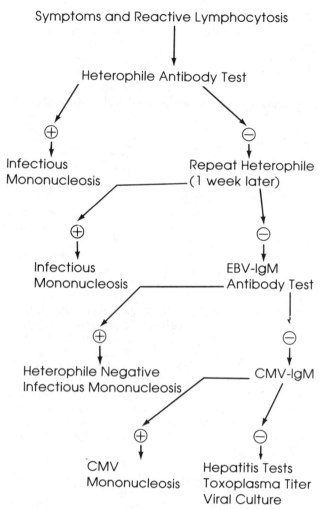

Figure 17–1. Laboratory diagnosis of reactive lymphocytosis.

rapid slide differential absorption test such as the Monospot test (Ortho Pharmaceuticals). This test detects the presence of the characteristic heterophile antibody by the ability of the antibody in the patient's serum to agglutinate horse red cells. It also tests for the differential absorption characteristic of the antibody in infectious mononucleosis by absorbing the serum with guinea pig kidney prior to adding horse red cells. The antibody in infectious mononucleosis is not absorbed by guinea pig kidney cells and thus, if present, agglutinates the horse red cells in the test system. The Monospot test using horse erythrocyte agglutination is a sensitive, rapid test for infectious mononucleosis. The Monosticon test (Organon) is another highly sensitive, rapid slide test for infectious mononucleosis. It tests for the differential absorption character of the heterophile antibody by using both beef erythrocytes and guinea pig kidney cells. This kit incorporates a combination horse-sheep erythrocyte stromal antigen instead of just horse erythrocytes to demonstrate the agglutination ability of the heterophile antibody.

It is important to remember that heterophile antibody titers are sometimes not elevated to detectable levels until the second or third week of the disease course. Therefore, it is possible to see greater than 10 percent reactive lymphocytes early in the course of infectious mononucleosis and to have a negative heterophile antibody test result. This test should be repeated in 7 to 10 days if the morphology is suggestive of infectious mononucleosis. If the repeat heterophile result is negative, other tests must be performed to determine the cause of the hematologic abnormality (Fig. 17–1).

The tests for antibody response to the EBV are highly specific and sensitive. A variety of tests for antibodies to Epstein-Barr viral antigens have been described (Table 17–2), including IgM and IgG antibody tests to viral capsid antigen (EBV-VCA), available at larger clinical laboratories and reference laboratories. These tests are not routinely performed in most hospital laboratories. A rise in the titer of IgM-EBV antibodies occurs initially and parallels the rise in titer of heterophile antibodies during the disease course. The IgM antibody is detectable in 82 percent of cases in the first week and in 100 percent by the third week.[16] Its presence constitutes conclusive evidence of current EBV infection especially in combination with a low titer of antibody to Epstein-Barr nuclear antigen (EBNA). IgG-EBV antibody is detectable early also; however, its presence indicates current or past infection. IgG antibody is present in detectable titer in 87 percent of cases during the first week of illness and in 100 percent by the third week.[16] A rise in titer must be shown to indicate a current infection. It is advisable to perform the IgG or IgM-EBV antibody titers on all heterophile-negative cases. It is prudent to order these tests immediately for children suspected of having infectious mononucleosis, as there is a high probability that the heterophile test result will be negative. If these specific test results are negative, other tests—particularly a CMV-IgM antibody titer—should be performed to determine the cause of the reactive lymphocytosis (Fig. 17–1 and Table 17–3). Viral culture may be helpful as an adjunct to the CMV-IgM titer for conclusive evidence of CMV infection.

Other laboratory tests with diagnostic significance in infectious mononucleosis are the liver enzyme tests such as the serum aspartate aminotransferase (AST), serum alanine transferase (ALT), and alkaline phosphatase tests. Eighty to 90 percent of patients with infectious mononucleosis demonstrate abnormal liver function with elevated levels of these enzymes yet rarely have jaundice as a clinical manifestation.

CASE STUDY

A 25-year-old white man was admitted to the hospital with symptoms of anorexia, fever, malaise, and headache. He had recently noted a darkening of his urine. He had been taking no prescribed medication.
Physical Examination: Slight splenomegaly, no lymphadenopathy.
Laboratory Data:

WBC	=	11×10^9/liter
RBC	=	4.72×10^{12}/liter
Hgb	=	14.0 g/dl

Table 17–3. **DIFFERENTIAL DIAGNOSIS OF LYMPHOCYTOSIS**

Viral
  Infectious mononucleosis
  Measles
  Mumps
  Chickenpox
  Infectious hepatitis
  CMV mononucleosis
Bacterial
  Tuberculosis
  Whooping cough
  Brucellosis
  Typhoid fever
  Paratyphoid fever
During recovery from acute infections (especially in children)
Neoplasms
  Lymphocytic leukemia
  Lymphoma
  Macroglobulinemia
Miscellaneous
  Rickets
  Syphilis
  Malnutrition
  Hyperthyroidism
  Acute infectious lymphocytosis
  Autoimmune diseases
  Allergic reactions

Table 17–2. **SUMMARY OF SPECIFIC ANTIBODY TESTS TO EBV ANTIGENS**

Test Name	Description	Clinical Significance
EBV-VCA (IgM)	IgM antibody to viral capsid antigen	Present at detectable levels in first week of infection; the best indicator of current infection
EBV-VCA (IgG)	IgG antibody to viral capsid antigen	Present at detectable levels about 7 days after exposure; indicates either current or past infection; a rise in titer must be demonstrated on acute and convalescent sera
EBNA	Antibody to EBV nuclear antigen	Appears late in first month of infection and persists indefinitely; indicates past infection
EBV-EA	Antibody to EBV early antigen complex	Seen in <5% of normal, healthy subjects; indicates EBV-carrier state

Hct	=	42%
MCV	=	89 fl
MCH	=	29.7 pg
MCHC	=	33%
Reticulocyte count	=	2%
Platelet count	=	252×10^9/liter
Coombs' test; direct antiglobulin test (DAT)	=	Negative
Differential	=	31% segmented neutrophils
	=	32% lymphocytes
	=	31% reactive lymphocytes
	=	6% monocytes
	=	Red cell morphology — normal
Serum bilirubin	=	1.4 mg/dl (0.2–1.0)
AST level	=	257 U/liter (0–41)
ALT level	=	85 U/liter (0–45)
Monospot test	=	Negative (initially and on repeat)
Hepatitis B antigen	=	Negative
Toxoplasma titer	=	Negative

Questions

1. What is the differential diagnosis?
2. What do the clinical symptoms suggest?
3. What do the laboratory test results indicate?
4. What further laboratory tests should be performed in this case?

Answers

1. The differential diagnosis in this case includes EBV infectious mononucleosis, CMV mononucleosis, viral hepatitis, and toxoplasmosis.
2. The clinical findings are fairly nonspecific and can be associated with all of these infections. A darkening of the urine could indicate the presence of increased amounts of urine urobilinogen, which would be present in hemolytic anemia or liver disease. Of particular interest is the fact that classic symptoms of EBV infectious mononucleosis—sore throat and cervical lymphadenopathy—were not present.
3. Laboratory findings show an absolute lymphocytosis with reactive lymphocyte morphology and evidence of hepatic dysfunction (elevated AAT, ALT, and slightly elevated serum bilirubin). Reactive lymphocytosis is seen in all of the aforementioned infections. Liver involvement, while most striking in hepatitis, is also seen in EBV and CMV mononucleosis.
4. Further tests indicated by the hematology and chemistry findings included a heterophile antibody test, hepatitis B antigen test, and toxoplasma titer. These tests were negative and rule out hepatitis B infection and toxoplasmosis. Therefore,

this case was interpreted as a heterophile-negative infectious mononucleosis syndrome. For accurate diagnosis, EBV and CMV antibody titers had to be performed. The EBV-IgG on this patient showed no change in titer between the acute and convalescent specimens; the CMV-IgM antibody titer was elevated at 1:256. CMV-IgM titers of greater than 1:32 are considered diagnostic of an active CMV infection.

This patient therefore had CMV mononucleosis, which when symptomatic, presents with nonspecific symptoms of fever, malaise, headache, and liver involvement in young adults (20 to 40 years). The blood picture is indistinguishable from that of the classic EBV infectious mononucleosis. This infection should be suspected when the heterophile test result is negative in a patient who lacks the typical symptoms of EBV infectious mononucleosis—sore throat and lymphadenopathy.

REFERENCES

1. Turk, W: Septische Erkranhungen bei Verkummerung des Granulozylensystems. Wien Klin Wochenschr 20:157, 1907.
2. Downey, H and McKinlay, CA: Acute lymphadenosis compared to acute leukemia. Arch Intern Med 32:82, 1923.
3. Pfeiffer, E: Drunsenfieber. Jarbuch Fur Kinderheilkunde 29:257, 1889.
4. Sprunt, TP and Evans, FA: Mononuclear leukocytosis in reaction to acute infection (infectious mononucleosis). Bull Johns Hopkins Hosp 31:410, 1920.
5. Paul, JR and Bunnell, WW: The presence of heterophile antibodies in infectious mononucleosis. Am J Med Sci 183:80, 1932.
6. Davidsohn, I and Walker, PH: Nature of heterophile antibodies in infectious mononucleosis. Am J Clin Pathol 5:455, 1953.
7. Henle, G, Henle, W, and Diehl, V: Relation of Burkitt's tumor-associated herpes-type virus to infectious mononucleosis. Proc Natl Acad Sci USA 59:94, 1968.
8. Kapff, C and Jandl, J: Blood Atlas and Sourcebook of Hematology. Little, Brown, Boston, 1981, p 122.
9. Miale, JB: Laboratory Medicine Hematology. CV Mosby, St Louis, 1982, p 166.
10. Karzon, DT: Infectious mononucleosis. Adv Pediatr 22:231, 1976.
11. Horwitz, CA, Henle, W, and Henle, G: Diagnostic aspects of cytomegalovirus mononucleosis syndrome in previously healthy persons. Post Grad Med 66:153, 1979.
12. Henle, W and Henle, G: Epstein-Barr virus and infectious mononucleosis. N Engl J Med 288:263, 1973.
13. Henle, G and Henle, W: Observations on childhood infections with the Epstein-Barr virus. J Infect Dis 121:303, 1970.
14. Horwitz, CA, et al: Clinical and laboratory evaluation of elderly patients with heterophile-antibody positive infectious mononucleosis: Report of seven patients ages 40 to 78. Am J Med 61:333, 1976.
15. Schleupner, C and Overral, J: Infectious mononucleosis and Epstein-Barr virus. Post Grad Med 65:83, 1979.
16. Evans, AS, et al: A prospective evaluation of heterophile and Epstein-Barr virus-specific IgM antibody tests in clinical and subclinical infectious mononucleosis: Specificity and sensitivity of the tests and persistence of the antibody. J Infect Dis 132:546, 1975.

QUESTIONS

1. *Which of the following is a distinguishing feature of the morphology of reactive lymphocytes?*
   a. Homogeneity of appearance
   b. Blastlike nucleus
   c. Unevenly stained basophilic cytoplasm
   d. Prominent singular nucleoli

2. *Which condition shows increased reactive lymphocytes on peripheral blood smears?*
   a. CMV infection
   b. EBV infection
   c. Drug hypersensitivity states
   d. All of the above

3. *What is the most frequent cause of a heterophile-negative mononucleosislike syndrome?*
   a. Human immunodeficiency virus
   b. Cytomegalovirus
   c. Hepatitis B
   d. *Toxoplasma gondii*

4. *Which of the following symptoms is not typical of EBV-associated infectious mononucleosis?*
   a. Urticaria
   b. Sore throat
   c. Fever
   d. Cervical lymphadenopathy

5. *Which of the following laboratory test results would not indicate a diagnosis of infectious mononucleosis?*
   a. More than 10 percent reactive lymphocytes
   b. Absolute increase in number of total lymphocytes
   c. Large, bizarre platelets
   d. Detection of heterophile antibody
   e. Cold agglutinins of anti-i specificity

ANSWERS

1. c (p. 259)
2. d (p. 260)
3. b (p. 261)
4. a (p. 261)
5. c (p. 262–263)

CHAPTER 18

MARY LORING PERKINS, M.S., M.T.(ASCP)S.H.

Introduction to Leukemia and the Acute Leukemias

INTRODUCTION TO LEUKEMIA
DEFINITION
HISTORIC PERSPECTIVE
CLASSIFICATION
ETIOLOGY AND RISK FACTORS
Host Factors
    Heredity
    Chromosome Abnormalities
    Immunodeficiency
    Chronic Marrow Dysfunction
Environmental Factors
    Ionizing Radiation
    Chemicals and Drugs
    Viruses
INCIDENCE
COMPARISON OF ACUTE AND CHRONIC LEUKEMIA

INTRODUCTION TO ACUTE LEUKEMIA
CLINICAL FEATURES
LABORATORY EVALUATION
Specimens
Evaluation of morphology
Cytochemistry
    Myeloperoxidase
    Sudan Black B
    Specific Esterase (Naphthol AS-D
      Chloroacetate)
    Nonspecific Esterase (Alpha-naphthyl Acetate
      or Butyrate)
    Periodic Acid–Schiff Reaction
Immunologic Marker Studies
    Surface Markers
    Cytoplasmic Immunoglobulin
    Terminal Deoxynucleotidyl Transferase

Cytogenetics
TREATMENT

ACUTE MYELOID LEUKEMIA
FAB CLASSIFICATION
SURFACE MARKER ANALYSIS
ACUTE MYELOBLASTIC LEUKEMIA WITHOUT
    DIFFERENTIATION (M1)
ACUTE MYELOBLASTIC LEUKEMIA WITH
    DIFFERENTIATION (M2)
ACUTE PROMYELOCYTIC LEUKEMIA (M3)
ACUTE MICROGRANULAR PROMYELOCYTIC LEUKEMIA
    (M3m)
ACUTE MYELOMONOCYTIC LEUKEMIA (M4)
ACUTE MYELOMONOCYTIC LEUKEMIA WITH
    EOSINOPHILIA (M4E)
ACUTE MONOCYTIC LEUKEMIA (M5)
ERYTHROLEUKEMIA (M6)
ACUTE MEGAKARYOBLASTIC LEUKEMIA (M7)

CASE STUDY

ACUTE LYMPHOBLASTIC LEUKEMIA
FAB CLASSIFICATION
IMMUNOLOGIC CLASSIFICATION
Lymphocyte Ontogeny
    B-Lymphocyte Development
    T-Lymphocyte Development
Immunologic Subtypes
CHILDHOOD VERSUS ADULT ALL
PRECURSOR B-CELL ALL
B-CELL ALL (BURKITT'S LYMPHOMA)
T-CELL ALL

CASE STUDY

OBJECTIVES

At the end of this chapter, the learner should be able to:
1. Define leukemia.
2. Describe the classification of leukemias.
3. Name risk factors for leukemia.
4. Differentiate between acute myeloid leukemia and acute lymphoblastic leukemia.
5. Distinguish among types M1 through M6 of acute myeloid leukemia.
6. Distinguish among types L1 through L3 of acute lymphoblastic leukemia.

INTRODUCTION TO LEUKEMIA

Definition

Leukemia is a malignant disease of hematopoietic tissue, characterized by replacement of normal bone marrow elements with abnormal (neoplastic) blood cells. These leukemic cells are frequently (but not always) present in the peripheral blood and commonly invade reticuloendothelial tissue including the spleen, liver, and lymph nodes. They may also invade other tissues, infiltrating any organ of the body. If left untreated, leukemia eventually causes death.

Historic Perspective

The discovery of leukemia as a clinical entity was made by John Bennett[1] in Scotland and Rudolf Virchow[2] in Germany, who independently published their findings in 1845. Several cases of leukemia were reported in the literature prior to this; however, it was Bennett and Virchow who recognized the significance of their observations and attempted to define this remarkable new disease.[3] They both made their discovery during the autopsy of victims of a progressive chronic disease of unknown origin. Here they discovered a huge spleen and purulent-appearing blood. The blood, when observed with a microscope, revealed an astounding increase in "colorless" corpuscles. The cause, however, was not clear. Bennett suggested that the marked increase in white blood cells was due to an inflammatory process; Virchow, however, chose to call it simply *Weisses Blut* (white blood), later translated into Greek as *leukemia*, and proposed that leukemia was caused by an overgrowth, or hyperplasia, of white cells. The argument between Bennett and Virchow ensued and continued for several years, but in time even Bennett rejected inflammation as the cause.

Virchow persisted in his study of the nature of leukemia and eventually published a summary of his studies, classifying the disease into two groups —one with primarily splenic involvement, the other with primarily lymph node involvement.[4] Today these are recognized respectively as chronic myelocytic leukemia and chronic lymphocytic leukemia.

In 1857 Friedrich gave a classic account of an acute form of leukemia characterized by a rapidly fatal course,[5] but not until 1889 was the term "acute" first used by Epstein to classify leukemia.[6] Further classification based on cell morphology was made possible in 1877 by Paul Ehrlich's discovery of a triacid stain that permitted the differentiation of blood cells. It was readily shown that acute leukemia was associated with primitive cells whereas chronic leukemia was associated with well-differentiated cells.

At the turn of the century Naegeli described the myeloblast and divided the acute leukemias into myeloblastic and lymphoblastic.[7] A decade later Schilling described a monoblastic variant. Thus, the main morphologic variants of acute and chronic leukemia were well established by 1930.[8] Since that time classification of leukemia has been refined, and clinically distinct subgroups have been recognized. Today the clinical laboratory plays an important role in the diagnosis and classification of leukemia. The standard morphologic classification of leukemia is now augmented by cytochemical, cytogenetic, and immunologic techniques. Together these methods are used to identify patients with different forms of leukemia who may benefit from different treatment protocols.

Certainly the most significant advance in our understanding of leukemia has been in the area of treatment. Complex therapy protocols using cytotoxic drugs, radiation, and, in some cases, bone marrow transplantation have improved the survival of many patients with leukemia—especially those with acute forms. This is most notable for children who have acute lymphoblastic leukemia (ALL). Before the 1960s, childhood ALL was universally fatal, but with current treatment programs more than half of children with ALL have the potential for cure.[9,10]

Classification

Leukemia is classified according to *cell type*, with regard to both cell maturity and cell lineage. *Cell maturity* is used to distinguish between acute and chronic forms of leukemia. When the malignant cells are immature (stem cells, blasts, or "pro" forms), the leukemia is classified as acute; when the cells are predominantly mature, it is classified as chronic. In general these two groups correspond to a rapid (acute) or slow (chronic) clinical course. Leukemias are further divided according to *cell lineage* into the lymphoid and myeloid groups. The term myeloid (*myelo*, Greek for marrow; *eidos*, form) includes granulocytic, monocytic, megakaryocytic, and erythrocytic leukemias. Thus, combining cell maturity and cell lineage, leukemia has four broad groups: acute lymphoblastic (ALL); acute myeloblastic (AML), also called acute nonlymphoblastic leukemia (ANLL); chronic lymphocytic (CLL); and chronic myelocytic (CML). These groups are further divided according to more specific cell types, as outlined in Table 18–1. For example, ALL is classified as either B or T lineage, and AML is subdivided into the groups of acute myeloblastic, promyelocytic, myelomonocytic, monocytic, erythrocytic, and megakaryoblastic.

Etiology and Risk Factors

Leukemia is a genetic disorder that is probably caused by a mutation and altered expression of oncogenes,[11] which are normal genes that regulate cell proliferation and differentiation, though this has not been totally proven. It is thought that an abnormal expression of these genes results in unregulated cell growth and possibly malignant transformation. Although the events that lead to this are not understood, a number of host factors and several environ-

Table 18–1. **CLASSIFICATION OF LEUKEMIA**

Type of Leukemia	Abbreviation	FAB*	Alternate Names
Acute Myeloid			Acute nonlymphocytic (ANLL)
Acute myeloblastic leukemia	AML		
Without maturation		M1	
With maturtion		M2	
Acute promyelocytic leukemia	APL	M3	Hypergranular promyelocytic
Acute myelomonocytic leukemia	AMML	M4	Naegeli-type leukemia
Acute monocytic leukemia	AMoL	M5	Schilling-type leukemia
Erythroleukemia	AEL	M6	Di Guglielmo's syndrome, erythremic myelosis
Acute megakaryoblastic leukemia	AMegL	M7	
Acute Lymphoid	ALL		
Early pre-B cell ALL		L1, L2	Common ALL
Pre-B–cell ALL		L1, L2	Common ALL
B-cell ALL		L3	Burkitt's leukemia
T-cell ALL		L1, L2	
Chronic Myeloid			
Chronic myelocytic leukemia	CML		Chronic granulocytic leukemia
Chronic eosinophilic leukemia	CEL		
Chronic basophilic leukemia	CBL		
Chronic Lymphoid			
Chronic lymphocytic leukemia	CLL		
B-cell			
T-cell			
Prolymphocytic leukemia	PLL		
Hairy-cell leukemia	HCL		Leukemic reticuloendotheliosis
Plasma-cell leukemia			Multiple myeloma, leukemic phase
Sézary syndrome			Mycosis fungoides, leukemic phase

*French-American-British classification of acute leukemia.

mental factors have been identified that are associated with an increased risk for leukemia.

Host Factors

Heredity. Leukemia does not appear to be inherited, although some individuals have an increased predisposition for acquiring it. An identical twin of a patient with acute leukemia has a markedly increased risk of developing leukemia. There is also an increased incidence of leukemia, although less dramatic, in other family members of the patient with leukemia.[12]

Chromosome Abnormalities. Leukemia occurs with increased frequency in patients with congenital disorders that have an inherited tendency for chromosomal fragility (such as Bloom's syndrome and Fanconi's anemia) or with an abnormality in the number of chromosomes (such as Down's syndrome, Klinefelter's syndrome, and Turner's syndrome). An 18- to 20-fold increased incidence of acute leukemia is seen in children with Down's syndrome.[13]

Immunodeficiency. An unusually high incidence of lymphoproliferative disease (lymphoid leukemia and lymphoma) has been noted in patients with hereditary immunodeficiency states including ataxia-telangiectasia and sex-linked agammaglobulinemia. It has recently been suggested that patients with ataxia-telangiectasia may have a defect that interferes with T- and B-lymphocyte gene rearrangements.[14]

Chronic Marrow Dysfunction. Patients with chronic marrow dysfunction abnormalities have an increased risk of their disorder transforming into acute myeloid leukemia. This includes patients with myelodysplastic syndromes, myeloproliferative syndromes, aplastic anemia, and paroxysmal nocturnal hemoglobinuria.

Environmental Factors

Ionizing Radiation. An increased incidence of leukemia is also associated with exposure to ionizing radiation. This fact is dramatically illustrated by data collected after the atomic bomb was exploded over Hiroshima and Nagasaki (Fig. 18–1). The occurrence of leukemia in survivors exposed to atomic radiation was many times that of individuals not exposed, and it was highest in those closest to the explosion.[15] Both acute and chronic forms of leukemia were reported, including AML, ALL, and CML.

Chemicals and Drugs. A variety of chemicals and drugs have been associated with development of leukemia. In humans, benzene is the most frequently documented chemical.[16] Other agents include chloramphenicol and phenylbutazone. Cer-

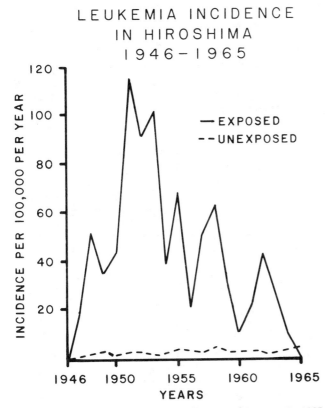

Figure 18–1. The leukemia incidence in Hiroshima, 1946–1965 in individuals exposed and those unexposed to atomic radiation. (From Gunz,[2] p. 528, with permission.)

tain cytotoxic chemotherapeutic agents, especially alkylating drugs, are also associated with leukemia development, and the risk in patients receiving alkylators is increased by the use of therapeutic radiation. This has been noted particularly in patients with Hodgkin's disease.

Viruses. The human T-cell leukemia/lymphoma virus-I (HTLV-I) has been implicated as the causative agent of adult T-cell leukemia/lymphoma (ATL). This rare form of chronic leukemia has a helper/inducer T-cell phenotype and is endemic to southwestern Japan, the Caribbean basin, Africa, and several other geographic regions.[17] Another, related virus, HTLV-II, has been isolated from patients with atypical hairy-cell leukemia (a chronic lymphoid leukemia).[18] Also, the Epstein-Barr virus has been closely associated with cases of African Burkitt's lymphoma.[19,20]

Incidence

The overall incidence of leukemia in the United States is 8 to 10 new cases per 100,000 individuals per year. In 1989 just over 27,000 new cases were reported, about half of them acute and half chronic.[21] Leukemia strikes more adults than children (10 : 1) and has a slightly increased incidence in men compared with women (1 to 2 : 1).

Acute leukemia occurs at all ages, but ALL (acute lymphoblastic) is more common in children and AML (acute myeloblastic) is more common in adults. Seventy-five percent of childhood leukemias are classified as ALL, whereas nearly 80 percent of all AMLs occur in adults.

Chronic leukemia is generally considered to be a disease of adults. Chronic lymphocytic leukemia is extremely rare in children and is unusual before the age of 40. Chronic myelocytic leukemia may be seen at any age, but its peak incidence is between 30 and 50 years of age; the disease is rare in children.

Comparison of Acute and Chronic Leukemia

The clinical and laboratory features of acute and chronic leukemia differ in a number of areas, as summarized in Table 18–2. Patients with acute leukemia usually have a sudden onset of symptoms, and, if untreated, the disease is rapidly fatal in 6 months or less. In contrast, patients with chronic leukemia tend to have an insidious (lacking symptoms) onset and a longer clinical course, usually lasting 2 to 6 years.

Patients with acute and chronic leukemia also show differences in their hematologic parameters. In general, bone marrow failure and its sequelae are much more prominent in patients who first present with acute leukemia than in those presenting with chronic forms. Anemia invariably occurs in the acute leukemia patient; it may be mild but can be quite severe. These patients tend to have a low-normal to decreased platelet count, and their white blood cell count is highly variable. The white blood cell count can be markedly elevated with numerous blasts, or it may be normal or, in some cases, even decreased. Typically the normal white blood cells are diminished in number. In chronic leukemia patients, anemia is often mild at presentation. The platelet count is usually normal, but it may actually be increased in cases of CML. Chronic leukemia patients almost always present with elevated white blood cell counts; often the increase is quite striking.

Patients with either acute or chronic leukemia can present with enlargement of the spleen, liver, or lymph nodes, but this is seen more consistently in patients with chronic leukemia whose organs may

Table 18–2. **COMPARISON OF ACUTE AND CHRONIC LEUKEMIAS**

	Acute	Chronic
Age	All ages	Adults
Clinical onset	Sudden	Insidious
Course (untreated)	<6 mo	2–6 yr
Leukemic cells	Immature	Mature
Anemia	Mild–severe	Mild
Thrombocytopenia	Mild–severe	Mild
WBC	Variable	Increased
Organomegaly	Mild	Prominent

be profoundly enlarged. Organomegaly is less prominent in patients with acute leukemia.

INTRODUCTION TO ACUTE LEUKEMIA
Clinical Features

The majority of patients who have acute leukemia present with a clinically abrupt onset of signs and symptoms lasting only a few weeks. Patients often seek medical attention because of weakness, bleeding abnormalities, or flulike symptoms. These abnormalities reflect the failure of the bone marrow to produce adequate numbers of normal cells and are caused by the proliferation and accumulation of leukemic cells in the marrow. Unless halted, this marrow involvement causes life-threatening complications including anemia, thrombocytopenia, granulocytopenia, and their sequelae. Anemia, the most consistent presenting feature, is associated with fatigue, malaise, and pallor. Bleeding abnormalities caused by thrombocytopenia and in some cases by disseminated intravascular coagulation (DIC) are also common. The hemorrhagic tendency may be mild and restricted to easy bruising, petechiae, and mucosal bleeding; or the bleeding may be more severe involving the gastrointestinal tract, genitourinary tract, or central nervous system. Infections occur frequently and result from severe granulocytopenia. Bacterial infections are common (for example, *Staphylococcus*, *Pseudomonas*, *Escherichia coli*, and *Klebsiella*) but fungal infections also occur (for example, *Candida* and *Aspergillus*). Viral infections are less common.[22]

Infiltration of other tissues, especially organs that play a role in fetal hematopoeisis, is common. Patients may present with an enlarged spleen, liver, or lymph nodes; these occur particularly often in acute lymphoblastic and acute monoblastic leukemia (AMoL), less often in the other acute nonlymphoblastic leukemias. A mediastinal mass due to thymic involvement is a hallmark of T-cell ALL. Gingival hypertrophy and oral lesions are primarily seen in AMoL. Bone or joint pain caused by pressure of the expanding leukemic cell population in the mar-

row cavity may accompany any of the acute leukemias. An ominous finding, infrequently seen when patients first present, is central nervous system disease. It is associated with symptoms of increased intracranial pressure (nausea, vomiting, headache, papilledema) or cranial nerve palsies. These clinical features and their relationship to pathophysiology are summarized in Table 18-3.

Five to 10 percent of cases of AML are preceded by a recognizable "preleukemic" (myelodysplastic) syndrome. The myelodysplastic syndromes (MDS) are more common in patients over 50 years old and are associated with unexplained and persistent anemia, leukopenia, thrombocytopenia, and monocytosis, alone or in combination. The myelodysplastic syndromes are discussed in more detail in Chapter 19.

Laboratory Evaluation

When acute leukemia is suspected, a series of laboratory tests is required to confirm the diagnosis and to classify the disease. The distinction between AML and ALL is particularly important; major differences between these two groups are outlined in Table 18-4.

Table 18-3. CLINICAL FEATURES OF ACUTE LEUKEMIA

Pathogenesis	Clinical Manifestation
Bone marrow failure	
Anemia	Fatigue, malaise, pallor
Thrombocytopenia	Bruising, bleeding
Granulocytopenia	Fever, infections
Organ Infiltration	
Marrow expansion	Bone or joint pain
Spleen	Splenomegaly
Liver	Hepatomegaly
Lymph nodes	Lymphadenopathy
CNS	Neurologic symptoms
Gums, mouth	Gingival hypertrophy, oral lesions

Table 18-4. COMPARISON OF ACUTE MYELOBLASTIC AND ACUTE LYMPHOBLASTIC LEUKEMIA

Factor	AML	ALL
Age	Common in adults, rare in children	Common in children, rare in adults
Blood	Anemia, neutropenia, thrombocytopenia; myeloblasts and promyelocytes	Anemia, neutropenia, thrombocytopenia; lymphoblasts and prolymphocytes
Morphology	Medium-to-large blasts, more cytoplasm than lymphoblasts, cytoplasmic granules, Auer rods; fine nuclear chromatin and distinct nucleoli	Small or medium blasts, scarce cytoplasm, no granules; fine nuclear chromatin and indistinct nucleoli
Cytochemistry	Positive peroxidase and Sudan black; negative TdT	Negative peroxidase and Sudan black; positive TdT
Extramedullary and focal disease	Common in spleen and liver; less common in lymph nodes and CNS	Common in lymph nodes, spleen, liver, CNS, and gonads

AML = acute myeloblastic leukemia; ALL = acute lymphoblastic leukemia; TdT = terminal deoxynucleotidyl transferase; CNS = central nervous system
Source: From Kjeldsberg, CR (ed): Practical Diagnois of Hematologic Disorders. ASCP Press, Chicago, 1989, p 349, with permission.

A preliminary work-up should include a complete blood count (CBC), platelet count, and white cell differential in order to assess the peripheral hematologic parameters. Anemia, which may be mild to severe and is usually normochromic, normocytic, is the most consistent finding. Typically the platelets are decreased although they may be normal in number. The white blood cell (WBC) count is variable, ranging from decreased to markedly elevated. The peripheral blood smear usually reveals blasts or other immature cells, but it is possible to find only a few (subleukemic) or no (aleukemic) blasts. Features associated with myelodysplastic syndromes are sometimes present, including pseudo–Pelger-Huët cells and hypogranular neutrophils. These features are more common in elderly patients with acute myeloid leukemia.

Once the preliminary hematology studies are complete, a bone marrow aspirate and biopsy should be obtained. Review of the marrow aspirate and biopsy is essential for establishing the extent of marrow involvement. The actual percentage of blasts necessary for the diagnosis is somewhat arbitrary; however, the most widely accepted classification system (French-American-British [FAB]) requires 30 percent.[23,24] The marrow aspirate is generally the specimen of choice for classification of leukemia by morphologic and cytochemical criteria.

It is helpful to follow a systematic approach in the evaluation of the leukemic cells starting with a review of their morphology, which provides important clues about the leukemic cell lineage and helps determine which other studies are required to make a definitive diagnosis. Review of the morphology should be followed by cytochemistry and immunologic cell marker studies. A battery of cytochemical stains that identify granulocytic and monocytic components is used to distinguish between ALL and AML. When results are positive, they exclude ALL and help subclassify AML. Another useful marker is the nuclear enzyme terminal deoxynucleotidyl transferase (TdT), which is present in most cases of ALL but not of AML. Immunologic cell marker studies are used to further characterize acute leukemia and are essential for immunophenotyping ALL.

Other laboratory studies used to evaluate acute leukemia include chromosome analysis and electron microscopy. Chromosome analysis is emerging as a valuable tool in identifying prognostically important subgroups of patients.[25] Occasionally, electron microscopy studies are necessary to make a definitive diagnosis of poorly differentiated leukemia or acute megakaryoblastic leukemia.

The purpose and principles of these laboratory methods is discussed below; detailed procedures are outlined in Chapter 30.

Specimens

Before any laboratory work is started, care must be taken to ensure that an adequate specimen is obtained and that it is properly handled. Lack of technical excellence may obscure or complicate an otherwise straightforward diagnosis; an inadequate or improperly handled specimen is the most common cause of an incorrect diagnosis.

Ideally evaluation of the peripheral blood cell morphology should be done using nonanticoagulated fingerstick smears. Anticoagulant ethylenediaminetetraacetic acid (EDTA) causes subtle morphologic artifacts of nucleated cells and platelets. A specimen left in EDTA for more than 30 minutes may show artifactual vacuolation of monocytes and neutrophils, nuclear shape changes and swelling, as well as degranulation of platelets.[26,27]

Before a bone marrow specimen is collected, arrangements for special studies including cytochemistry and immunophenotyping should be made and any special handling procedures noted. This is also true for cytogenetic or electron microscopy studies. During the bone marrow procedure the aspirate is collected first and smears made immediately to avoid problems with clotting. Properly pulled smears made on clean cover slips result in excellent thin aspirate smears. Although similar smears may also be made on glass slides, they tend to be somewhat thicker. As the aspirate smears are pulled, the presence of bone marrow spicules should be confirmed. If spicules are not present, another aspiration may be necessary. For immunophenotyping or cytogenetic studies the marrow aspirate is anticoagulated by aspirating directly into a syringe coated with heparin. After sufficient aspirate material is collected the biopsy is obtained. The biopsy should be used, before fixation, to make touch preps by gently touching or rolling the biopsy along a glass slide. Touch preps are especially important when the aspirate produces a dry tap. Further details of the bone marrow procedure are discussed in Chapter 2.

Evaluation of Morphology

The leukemic cell morphology is evaluated on a Romanowsky- (Wright-Giemsa) stained blood or bone marrow smear in carefully chosen areas in which cells are not distorted in shape or poorly stained by overcrowding. In the hands of an experienced morphologist the correct classification of cell type is often apparent; however, additional testing is always necessary to confirm the diagnosis.

Acute myeloblastic leukemia and acute lymphoblastic leukemia are classified into morphologic subgroups that are described later in this chapter. However, it is worth noting several cytologic features (Table 18–5) that are helpful in distinguishing between lymphoblasts and myeloblasts. These include the size of the blast, amount of cytoplasm, nuclear chromatin pattern, and the presence of nucleoli. The typical myeloblast (Fig. 18–2) is a large cell (15 to 20 μm in diameter) with a moderate amount of cytoplasm. Its nucleus has a fine reticulated chromatin pattern, and multiple distinct nucleoli are often present. The typical lymphoblast (Fig. 18–3) is a smaller cell with scant cytoplasm. The nuclear chromatin often appears more dense than in the myeloblast, and nucleoli are usually indistinct when present. (For a review of morphologic descriptions of the blast stage, see Chapter 1.)

Table 18–5. **MORPHOLOGIC FEATURES TO DIFFERENTIATE ACUTE MYELOBLASTIC LEUKEMIA FROM ACUTE LYMPHOBLASTIC LEUKEMIA**

	AML Myeloblast*	ALL Lymphoblast*
Blast size	Large	Small
Cytoplasm	Moderate	Scant
Chromatin	Fine, lacy	Dense
Nucleoli	Prominent (usually >2)	Indistinct (usually ≤2)
Auer rods	Present in 50–60%	Never present

*These are general features; morphology may vary considerably.
Source: From Kjeldsberg, CR (ed): Practical Diagnosis of Hematologic Disorders. ASCP Press, Chicago, 1989, p 374, with permission.

Granulocytic differentiation is suggested by the presence of azurophilic granules. An additional and very helpful morphologic feature is the Auer rod, whose presence rules out ALL. Auer rods are an abnormal fusion of primary granules and are pathognomonic for a myeloproliferative process— particularly, AML (and rarely chronic myelocytic leukemia or CML in myeloid blast crisis);[28] they have also been described in myelodysplastic syndromes.[29] On Romanowsky-stained smears, Auer rods appear as pink- or purple-staining rods or splinter-shaped inclusions (**see Color Plate 140**). They are present in up to 60 percent of patients with AML,[30] but it may take a long careful review of the blood or marrow smear to find them. In acute progranulocytic leukemia Auer rods are easy to find, some cells having bunches of cigar-shaped rods.

Cytochemistry

Special stains are used to identify chemical components of cells such as enzymes or lipids. These cytochemical stains are an important aid in the classification of acute leukemia because they identify cellular components that are associated with specific cell lines. For example, a positive myeloperoxidase or Sudan black B stain indicates myeloid differentiation, and a positive nonspecific esterase stain indicates monocytic differentiation. When these stains are positive, lymphoid origin is ruled out. Thus, the cytochemical stains help distinguish

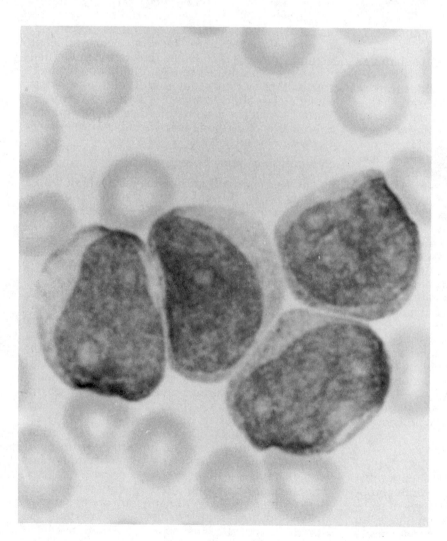

Figure 18–2. Myeloblasts.

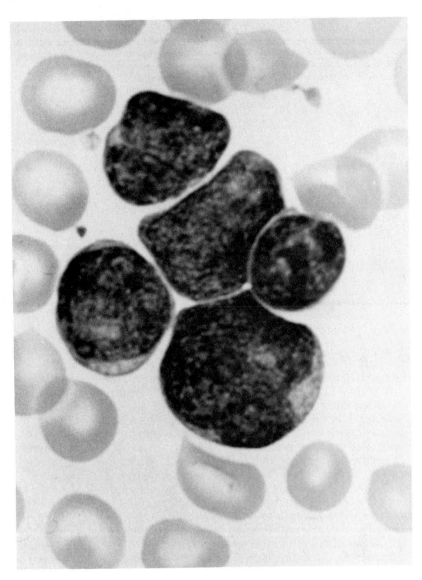

Figure 18-3. Lymphoblasts.

between ALL and AML. They are also used to help subclassify AML.

The cytochemical reactions are performed by applying staining techniques to peripheral blood smears, bone marrow smears, or touch preparations. Fresh preparations are preferred, especially for enzyme reactions. Control smears can be fixed in the appropriate fixative, allowed to air dry, and stored at − 20° for future staining. Caution should be taken when interpreting cytochemical stains. It is the leukemic cell population whose identity (cell lineage) is in question; therefore, a positive reaction is determined by finding positive staining in the leukemic blasts rather than in mature cells. Table 18-6 summarizes the cytochemical reactions that are useful in the classification of acute leukemia.

Myeloperoxidase (Color Plate 141). Peroxidase is present in the primary granules of myeloid cells. These granules first appear in the early promyelocyte (late blast) and persist through subsequent stages of cell maturation. Monocytes have variable staining with peroxidase and are most often only weakly positive. This enzyme is not present in lymphocytes or their precursors and is therefore useful in differentiating AML from ALL. It is more specific for granulocytic differentiation than the Sudan black B stain.

Smears are incubated in a buffered solution of hydrogen peroxide with an appropriate substrate such as 3-amino-9-ethylcarbazole (AEC). In the presence of the enzyme peroxidase, the hydrogen peroxide oxidizes the substrate, resulting in precipitation of a colored product at the site of enzyme activity. Effort should be made to use fresh smears when staining for peroxidase because the enzyme is labile.

Sudan Black B (Color Plate 142). Phospholipids, neutral fats, and sterols are stained by Sudan black B (SBB). This reaction is thought to be due to the solubility of the dye in the lipid particles. Phospholipids occur both in primary and secondary granules of granulocytic cells and to a lesser extent in monocytic lysozomal granules.

The SBB is the most sensitive stain for granulo-

Table 18–6. **SUMMARY OF CYTOCHEMICAL REACTIONS USEFUL IN DIAGNOSING ACUTE LEUKEMIA**

Special Stain	Site of Action	Cells Stained	Comment
Myeloperoxidase	Mainly primary granules; Auer rods	Late myeloblasts, granulocytes; monocytes less intensely	Valuable in that the primary granules are not always visible: separates AML (+) from ALL (−)
Sudan black B	Phospholipids: membrane of primary and secondary granules	Late myeloblasts, granulocytes; monocytes less intensely	Parallels peroxidase, but smears do not need to be fresh
Specific esterase (naphthol AS-D chloroacetate)	Cytoplasm	Neutrophilic granulocytes; mast cells	Parallels peroxidase, but less sensitive; useful on paraffin-embedded tissues
Nonspecific esterase (Alpha-naphthyl acetate (ANAE) and butyrate)	Cytoplasm	Monocytes; focal staining in T cells; ANAE also + in megakaryocytes	Useful for determining degree of monocytic differentiation; separates mono (+) from myelo (−) blasts
Periodic Acid–Schiff	Glycogen and related substances	Lymphocytes; granulocytes; megakaryocytes	Helpful in supporting diagnosis of erythroleukemia

cytic precursors with a staining pattern that generally parallels the myeloperoxidase stain. As with the peroxidase stain the SBB is used to differentiate AML from ALL. Positivity seldom occurs in lymphoid cells, but rare cases of SBB-positive ALL are observed.[31] The SBB stain, whose reactivity does not diminish with time, is particularly useful for specimens that are not fresh.

Specific Esterase (Naphthol AS-D Chloroacetate) (Color Plate 143). The specific esterase stain roughly parallels the peroxidase and Sudan black B stains, although it is not as sensitive and it is negative in eosinophils and monocytes. Its most important use is in demonstrating myeloid differentiation in paraffin-embedded tissue sections.

Smears or hydrated paraffin tissue sections are incubated in a buffered solution containing the substrate naphthol AS-D chloroacetate and a diazo salt (pararosaniline). The esterase enzyme within neutrophils, basophils, mast cells, and their precursors hydrolyzes the chloroacetate. This hydrolyzed substrate rapidly couples with the diazo salt, causing dye to precipitate at the site of enzymatic activity.

Nonspecific Esterase (Alpha-Naphthyl Acetate or Butyrate) (Color Plate 144). The nonspecific esterase (NSE) stain is used to identify monocytic cells. It is diffusely positive in these cells and negative in granulocytic cells. Lymphoid cells are negative except in T lymphocytes which can demonstrate a focal staining pattern.

Just as with the specific esterase stain, the NSE stain is performed by incubating fixed smears in a buffered solution containing a substrate and diazo salt. The difference in staining specificity lies in the naphthol derivative used for the substrate and in the pH and time of incubation. Different substrates are available for use in the NSE stain. Alpha-naphthyl butyrate is the most specific for monocyte differentiation, whereas alpha-naphthyl acetate is more sensitive. Both are positive in monocytes and

their precursors as well as in macrophages. The alpha-naphthyl acetate, but not the butyrate, is also positive in megakaryocytes and platelets. Another substrate, naphthol AS-D acetate (NASDA), is less specific and stains both monocytes and granulocytes. This substrate must be used in conjunction with a sodium fluoride inhibition step, which renders monocytic cells negative and thus differentiates them from granulocytic cells which remain positive. Although NASDA is no longer routinely used, its staining pattern gave the nonspecific esterase its name.

Periodic Acid–Schiff Reaction. The periodic acid–Schiff (PAS) reaction stains for glycogen and related compounds, including mucoproteins, glycoproteins, glycolipids, and polysaccharides. Periodic acid (HIO_4) oxidizes glycols to aldehydes. The resulting aldehydes react with Schiff's reagent (fuchsin-sulfurous acid) to form a magenta color. Lymphocytes, granulocytes, monocytes, and megakaryocytes may be positive, having a diffuse or sometimes a granular staining pattern. Normal erythroid precursors are negative.

The PAS reaction is not very useful for characterizing acute leukemia. The typical block positivity **(see Color Plate 145)** associated with lymphoblastic leukemia may also occur in acute myeloid leukemia, especially the acute monocytic type.[32,33] Burkitt's type ALL (L3) is negative. The PAS stain should not be used to distinguish AML from ALL.

The PAS reaction may sometimes be helpful in supporting the diagnosis of erythroleukemia, where strong PAS positivity may be present in normoblasts. When present, this feature is helpful for differentiating erythroleukemia from pernicious anemia in which the PAS reaction is negative except in rare cases. Normoblasts may also be positive in sideroblastic anemia, iron deficiency, thalassemia, severe hemolytic anemias, and some of the myelodysplastic syndromes.

Immunologic Marker Studies

A number of immunologic methods have proved indispensable in the diagnosis and classification of acute leukemia, especially of ALL. Antibodies are used to detect markers associated with cell lineage and maturation stage. Depending on the location of these cell markers (cell surface, cytoplasm, or nucleus) different methods are used to detect them. The following paragraphs briefly introduce the immunologic cell marker procedures. Their utility in the evaluation of acute leukemia is discussed in the individual sections on AML and ALL.

Surface Markers. Surface markers are proteins on the cell membrane that can be detected with immunologic reagents. Different proteins are expressed at different stages of maturation; some are present early in development while others do not appear until much later. Still other proteins may appear, then disappear, only to reappear at a later stage of development. This unique expression of proteins enables them to be used as markers of both cell lineage and maturation stage.

Whereas some surface markers can be detected with polyclonal antisera, many can only be detected with monoclonal antisera. Table 18–7 lists monoclonal antibodies that are used to evaluate leukemias and other lymphoproliferative and myeloproliferative disorders.

Surface marker studies, in cases of acute leukemia, are done using cell suspensions from either bone marrow aspirates or peripheral blood. It is important to have fresh specimens with viable cells; nonviable cells lead to nonspecific staining and, if severe, may make interpretation impossible. An immunofluorescent method (direct or indirect) is used to stain the cells, and a fluorescent microscope or a flow cytometer is used to analyze them. (See Chapter 30 for a review of flow cytometry.) **Color Plate 146** shows the surface staining pattern, as observed with a fluorescent microscope, that is typical of a strongly positive reaction.

Cytoplasmic Immunoglobulin. The only cytoplasmic marker that is routinely evaluated in the work-up of acute leukemia is cytoplasmic immunoglobulin (μ heavy chain) which is reserved for study of B lineage ALL. It is a marker of pre-B cells.

Cytoplasmic μ (Cμ) is usually detected by using a direct immunofluorescent procedure to stain cells on a glass slide. Fresh blood smears, bone marrow smears, touch preparations, or cytocentrifuged preparations (cytopreps) may be used; but cytopreps of washed cell suspensions are preferred because they tend to produce lower background staining. Slides are fixed in acid alcohol, incubated with a fluorescein-conjugated antihuman IgM, and washed with buffered saline. A fluorescent microscope is used to determine if cytoplasmic staining is present. Pre-B cells are weak to moderately positive.

Table 18–7. **MONOCLONAL ANTIBODIES USED FOR STUDY OF LEUKEMIA AND LYMPHOMA**

Cluster	Common Names	Cell Type	Major Hematopoietic Reactivity
CD1a	T6, Leu6	T	Thym and Langerhan's cells
CD2	T11, Leu5	T	E rosette forming T cells
CD3	T3, Leu4	T	Mature T cells
CD4	T4, Leu3	T	Helper/inducer T-cell subset
CD5	T1, Leu1	T	Pan-T and some B cells
CD7	Leu9	T	Pan-T, early thymocytes
CD8	T8, Leu2	T	Suppressor/cytotoxic T-cell subset
CD10	J5, CALLA	B	B-cell precursors, some thym, grans, and CALL
CD11b	Mo1, Leu15	M/G	Monos and grans C3bi receptor
CD11c	Leu M5	M/G	Monos, myeloid precursors, but not grans
CD13	MY7	G/M	Most grans, minority of monos, and other
CD14	MY4, Leu M3	M/G	Monos, minority of grans, and DRC
CD19	B4, Leu12	B	B cells, early B-cell precursors
CD20	B1, Leu16	B	B cells, midstage B-cell precursors
CD21	B2	B	C3d receptor on B cells, and DRC
CD22	Leu 14	B	B cells
CD25	IL-2R1, IL-2R	T	IL-2 receptor on T cells and other
CD33	MY9	G	Myeloid progenitors
CD41	J15	P	Plts and megakaryocytes (GPIIb/IIIa)
CD42b	AN51	P	Plts and megakaryocytes (GPIb)
CD45	T200, HLe, LCA	Broad	Leukocytes
—	Ia, HLA-DR	Broad	B cells, activated T cells, and monos

B cells (or B) = B lymphocytes; Broad = reactivity with many leukocyte populations; CALL = common ALL; CD = cluster designation; DRC = dendritic reticulum cells; Grans (or G) = granulocytes; IL = interleukin; Monos (or M) = monocytes; pan-T = antigen present on majority of T lymphocytes; Plts (or P) = platelets; RS = Reed-Sternberg cells; T cells (or T) = T lymphocytes; Thym = thymocytes.

Terminal Deoxynucleotidyl Transferase (Color Plate 147). Terminal deoxynucleotidyl transferase is a unique nuclear enzyme (DNA polymerase) present in early lymphoid cells.[34] High levels are found in the majority (90 percent) of the lymphoblastic leukemias including both B- and T-lineage ALL but not in most cases of AML. Thus, TdT is a useful marker for differentiating ALL from AML. Detectable levels of this enzyme have been noted in 5 to 10 percent of the cases of AML,[35] although the level is usually lower than in lymphoblasts. Terminal deoxynucleotidyl transferase is also present in most cases of lymphoblastic lymphoma and in approximately one third of cases of chronic myelocytic leukemia in blast crisis (CML-BC).[36] Its presence in cases of CML-BC is a predictor of the likelihood of a favorable response of the disease to treatment with vincristine and prednisone.[37]

Terminal deoxynucleotidyl transferase can be detected by immunologic techniques (immunocytochemical or immunofluorescent) using fresh smears, touch preparations, or cytopreps. When heparinized specimens are to be studied the sample must be washed to remove heparin, which causes false-negative staining. A positive reaction is indicated by a nuclear staining pattern (see Color Plate 147).

Cytogenetics

Cytogenetic analysis of leukemic cells can provide important information that augments the standard criteria (morphology, cytochemistry, and immunology) used to classify acute leukemia. Indeed, future classification schemes may include cytogenetic criteria to define clinically unique subgroups. At present a number of chromosome abnormalities associated with distinct forms of leukemia already exist. A classic example of this is the Philadelphia chromosome (t[9;22]) associated with CML. Because there are also a growing number of chromosome abnormalities associated with the acute leukemias, it is generally accepted that most patients presenting with acute leukemia should be evaluated for cytogenetic abnormalities. In addition it is recommended that cases of ALL should have flow cytometric analysis for deoxyribonucleic acid (DNA) ploidy status.[38]

Cytogenetic studies are done by evaluating chromosome metaphase preparations to detect numeric and structural karyotype (*karyon*, nucleus; *typos*, mark) abnormalities. Normal human cells have 46 chromosomes and are said to be diploid (*diplous*, double; *eidos*, form)—that is, they have two haploid sets of chromosomes. Numeric abnormalities include both polyploid (multiples of haploid) and aneuploid (irregular multiples of haploid) changes. An aneuploid population can be either hypodiploid or hyperdiploid.

Structural abnormalities include translocations, inversions, deletions, duplication, and isochromosomes. Of particular importance to the study of acute leukemia are the translocations that result from the movement of a DNA segment from one chromosome to another. Usually these result from a reciprocal interchange of portions of two nonhomologous chromosomes.

Chromosomal abnormalities (both numeric and structural) are found in the majority of patients with acute leukemia including more than 60 percent of patients with AML and more than 65 percent of those with ALL. The most common structural abnormalities are translocations. A number of these have been associated with distinct subgroups of AML or ALL and can be assigned to poor, intermediate, or favorable prognostic groups. For example, patients with acute myelomonocytic leukemia (AML, M4) who exhibit an inversion or deletion of the long arm of chromosome 16 (inv [16q] or del [16q]) have a longer median survival than those with other types of AML. Table 18–8 lists common cytogenetic abnormalities associated with acute leukemia.

Treatment

Treatment of leukemia has two main goals: to eradicate the leukemic cell mass and to give supportive care. Cures are infrequently realized except in children with common ALL; however, induction of a complete remission is a realistic goal for most patients with acute leukemia. Complete remission is defined as the absence of any leukemia-related signs and symptoms and return of marrow and blood granulocyte, platelet, and red cell values to within normal limits.

Table 18–8. **COMMON CHROMOSOME ABNORMALITIES ASSOCIATED WITH ACUTE LEUKEMIA**

Chromosome Abnormality	Associated Disorder
t(8;21)	AML with myelocytic maturation (M2)
t(15;17)	Unique to APL (M3 and M3m)
16q abnormalities: inv(16) and del(16)	AMML with abnormal eosinophilia (M4E)
t(9;11)	AMol, especially poorly differentiated (M5a); also in other types of AML (e.g., AMML (M4))
t(9;22)	Most common in CML; occasionally found in AML and ALL (early pre-B, pre-B–cell, and T-cell phenotypes)
t(4;11)	Biphenotypic leukemia with lymphoblastic (early pre-B) and monocytic features: common in infants
t(1;19)	ALL, pre-B–cell phenotype (30% incidence in this group)
t(8;14), t(2;8), and t(8;22)	ALL, B-cell phenotype (Burkitt's lymphoma): c-*myc* oncogene translocated to chromosome with Ig heavy or light-chain gene
t(11;14)	ALL, T-cell phenotype (common thymocyte)

Three general types of antileukemic therapy are commonly employed: cytotoxic chemotherapy, radiotherapy, and bone marrow transplantation. Chemotherapy is the mainstay of treatment, although bone marrow transplantation is being used more frequently. Radiotherapy is used as an adjunct to chemotherapy in patients who have localized tissue involvement that may be targeted with irradiation.

The treatment of patients is administered in different phases including an induction and postremission phase. Induction therapy is designed to obtain a complete remission of the leukemia; its success is the best predictor of long-term disease-free survival. The approach to postremission phase treatment differs depending on the type of leukemia being treated. In children with ALL postremission therapy includes intensification, central nervous system (CNS) consolidation, and maintenance therapy. In patients with AML postremission therapy is more controversial as it contributes less toward improving the survival time of these patients.[22]

A number of different cytotoxic chemotherapeutic agents are used to treat acute leukemia. Their modes of action differ but in general they poison dividing cells, usually by blocking DNA or ribonucleic acid (RNA) synthesis. Currently a combination of drugs, each with a different mode of action, is used. This approach helps to overcome leukemic cell drug resistance. Prednisone, vincristine, and asparaginase are used in most induction regimens for treatment of childhood ALL. Patients with AML are usually treated with a combination of cytarabine and daunorubicin plus other agents. The drugs are given in dosages that have substantial toxicity, particularly to the marrow. The most common complications in patients undergoing chemotherapy arise from marrow hypoplasia.

Bone marrow transplantation has emerged as an important treatment modality, especially for patients with AML. The patient's bone marrow is completely eradicated with intensive chemotherapy and total body radiation. This is followed by rescuing the patient with donor bone marrow cells collected from a human leukocyte antigen (HLA)–compatible donor (or from the leukemia patient when he or she is in complete remission) by repeated bone marrow aspirates. The donor cells are processed and then infused into the recipient intravenously. The infused cells travel to the recipient's "empty" marrow, where they begin to multiply and repopulate the patient's marrow with healthy hematopoietic tissue. It usually takes 3 to 4 weeks for engraftment and 2 to 3 months before hematologic values return to normal.[22] The complications surrounding bone marrow transplants—including infections, hemorrhage and graft-versus-host disease (GVHD)—are numerous and can be fatal; it is not suitable therapy for all patients who have leukemia. For some, however, it offers a chance for long-term survival and a potential cure.

ACUTE MYELOID LEUKEMIA
FAB Classification

The need for uniform nomenclature and classification of acute leukemia prompted a group of French, American, and British hematologists to propose a new system in 1976.[39] This system, designated FAB, has proven to be useful in standardizing the morphologic classification of both acute myeloid and lymphoid leukemias. In the years since it was first introduced, the FAB cooperative group has made several modifications, striving to make the classification as objective and unambiguous as possible.[24] Although there are still some areas of ambiguity, the FAB system has gained wide acceptance.

The acute myeloid leukemias are divided into the following groups:
- M1: Myeloblastic without differentiation
- M2: Myeloblastic with differentiation
- M3: Promyelocytic
- M4: Myelomonocytic
- M5: Monocytic (a) well and (b) poorly differentiated
- M6: Erythroid
- M7: Megakaryoblastic

These groups are defined according to the predominant cell type observed on Romanowsky- and cytochemically stained blood and bone marrow aspirate smears (Table 18–9). Additional specialized studies are required to confirm the diagnosis of M7 (acute megakaryocytic leukemia). A summary of the cytochemical reactions in each type of AML is found in Table 18–10.

Acute myeloblastic leukemia, especially M6 type (erythroleukemia), is sometimes difficult to distinguish from certain myelodysplastic syndromes (refractory anemia with excess blasts, or RAEB, in transformation). To address this problem, the FAB cooperative group proposed revised criteria for the classification of AML including a stepwise evaluation of the bone marrow aspirate (Fig. 18–4).[24] A differential is done of all nucleated cells (ANC) and of only nonerythroid cells (NEC). The ANC differential is used to determine the percentage of erythroblasts (all nucleated erythroid precursors): those cases with greater than 50 percent erythroblasts are further evaluated to differentiate between M6 (blasts 30 percent or more of NEC) and MDS (blasts less than 30 percent of NEC); those cases with less than 50 percent erythroblasts are evaluated to differentiate between AML, types M1 through M5 (blasts 30 percent or more of ANC), and MDS (blasts less than 30 percent of ANC). The final classification of AML (M1 through M5) is based on characterization of the NEC fraction. All of these FAB subgroups are discussed in more detail later in this chapter.

The FAB classification system has largely failed to define groups of patients with AML that have substantially different clinical outcomes. These patients generally have similar clinical courses, regardless of their FAB subtype. An exception to this

Table 18–9. **FAB CLASSIFICATION OF ACUTE MYELOBLASTIC LEUKEMIA**

Type	Characteristics
M1	*Myeloblastic without differentiation:* marrow leukemia cells are primarily myeloblasts with no azurophilic granules
M2	*Myeloblastic with differentiation:* leukemia cells show prominent maturation beyond myeloblast stage
M3	*Promyelocytic:* abnormal, hypergranular promyelocytes dominate; Auer rods easily found; increased incidence of DIC
M3m	*Microgranular variant of M3:* indistinct granules; nucleus often reniform or bilobed; increased incidence of DIC
M4	*Myelomonocytic:* both monocytic (monocytes and promonocytes) and myeloid differentiation (maturation beyond myeloblast stage)
M4E	*M4 with bone marrow eosinophilia:* similar to M4 with marrow eosinophilia (abnormal and immature); associated with abnormal 16q karyotype
M5a	*Monocytic, poorly differentiated:* monoblasts predominate, typically with abundant cytoplasm and single distinct nucleoli
M5b	*Monocytic, well differentiated:* predominantly promonocytes in marrow and more pronounced maturation in blood
M6	*Erythroleukemia:* dysplastic erythroblasts with multinucleation, cytoplasmic budding, vacuolation, and megaloblastoid changes
M7	*Megakaryoblastic:* wide range of morphology, cytoplasmic projections sometimes present; electron microscopy or immunocytochemical stains necessary for diagnosis

rule may include patients with AML showing monocytic differentiation (M4 and M5b) who tend to have a lower rate of complete remission and a lower rate of survival.[30] Another FAB group, acute promyelocytic leukemia (M3), is associated with a longer average survival.[40] Because of the failure of morphologic and cytochemical classification to predict other clinicopathologic subtypes of AML, immunologic and cytogenetic techniques are being used increasingly to augment the FAB classification; these methods provide additional data which are useful in determining appropriate patient management.[41]

Surface Marker Analysis

The availability of myeloid-specific monoclonal antibodies has lead to the increased use of surface marker analysis in cases of AML. These studies are based on the fact that AML is a clonal disorder derived from an aberrant myeloid stem cell, which generally expresses surface membrane antigens that correspond to pathways of normal myeloid differentiation.[42,43] A schematic representation of these pathways is shown in Figure 18–5.

Although surface marker analysis of cases of AML is not as important as it is in cases of ALL, it does provide useful information. These studies complement morphologic and cytochemical studies; they can be used to distinguish between cases of AML and ALL, especially when the leukemic cells are poorly differentiated with negative or equivocal cytochemical stains. There is also some evidence that certain antigens have prognostic significance. For example, Griffin and co-workers showed that patients with AML whose leukemic cells expressed either MY4 (CD13) or MY7 (CD33) antigens had a lower rate of complete remission than patients whose cells did not express either of these antigens.[44]

When surface marker analysis is done to distinguish between AML and ALL it is important to choose a panel of monoclonal antibodies that includes several myeloid-associated antibodies (such as MY4, MY7, MY9, and Mo1) as well as B- and T-lymphocyte–specific antibodies. More than one myeloid-associated antibody is necessary because no single antibody can detect all forms of AML.

The surface phenotypes expressed in cases of AML do not correlate well with the FAB subgroups. Although cases of AML with monocytic differentiation (M4 and M5) usually express monocyte-related surface markers and cases of acute promyelocytic leukemia (M3) tend to express a promyelocyte phenotype,[42] other AML subgroups have widely variable phenotypes. Occasionally cases of acute leukemia are found which express antigens of multiple lineage (both myeloid and lymphoid). These rare cases of biphenotypic leukemia may reflect the origin of the malignant cells from an early progenitor cell common to both myeloid and lymphoid development.

Acute Myeloblastic Leukemia without Differentiation (M1)

The leukemic cells seen in cases of AML, M1 subtype, are predominantly poorly differentiated myeloblasts (**see Color Plates 148 and 149**). The nucleus typically has a fine lacy chromatin pattern and distinct nucleoli. The amount of cytoplasm is usually moderate, though this varies. According to FAB criteria less than 10 percent of the leukemic

Table 18–10. **CYTOCHEMICAL REACTIONS IN ACUTE MYELOBLASTIC LEUKEMIA**

	FAB Classification					
	M1	M2	M3	M4	M5	M6
Peroxidase or Sudan black	>3%	>50%	Near 100%	20–80%	Variable	>3%
Nonspecific esterase	<20%	<20%	Variable	20–80%	>80%	Variable

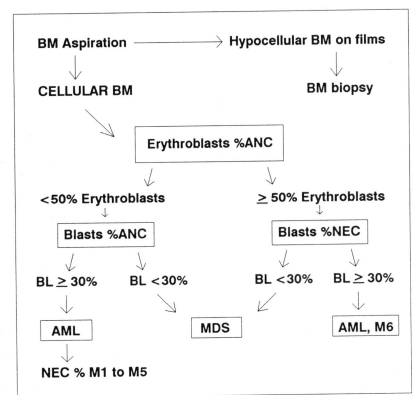

Figure 18–4. Suggested steps in the analysis of a bone marrow (BM) aspirate to reach a diagnosis of acute myeloid leukemia (AML) (M1 to M6) or myelodysplastic syndrome (MDS). BL = blast cells; ANC = all nucleated bone marrow cells; NEC = nonerythroid cells, bone marrow cells excluding erythroblasts. (From Bennett, et al,[24] with permission.)

cells have azurophilic granules (primary granules) when observed on a Romanowsky-stained smear. The peroxidase or Sudan black reactions must demonstrate at least 3 percent positivity (in the population of abnormal cells) to exclude lymphoblastic leukemia and less than 50 percent positivity to keep the leukemia within the M1 subgroup. The NSE reaction is positive in less than 20 percent of the cells. Auer rods, when present, are particularly helpful in distinguishing M1 from ALL (L2 variant).

Acute Myeloblastic Leukemia with Differentiation (M2)

In cases of AML, M2 subtype, the leukemic marrow infiltrate resembles M1 except evidence of maturation to or beyond the promyelocyte stage is present (**see Color Plates 150 and 151**). Romanowsky-stained bone marrow smears show that promyelocytes constitute greater than 10 percent of the immature cells. More than 50 percent of the leukemic cells are peroxidase or Sudan black posi-

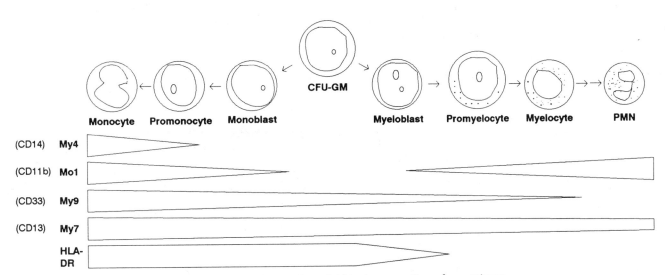

Figure 18–5. Distribution of myeloid and monocytic surface antigens.

tive (**see Color Plate 152**). The NSE activity does not exceed 20 percent.

The acute myeloblastic leukemias (M1 and M2 types combined) are the most common types of AML. Together, types M1 and M2 account for approximately 50 percent of cases of AML.[45] Aside from their morphology and cytochemistry they do not have unique features that set them apart from other myeloid subgroups. Although a translocation of chromosomes 8 and 12 (t[8;21]) has been identified in approximately 18 percent of patients with AML, type M2,[46] this chromosome abnormality has also been found, albeit less frequently, in other FAB groups of AML.

Acute Promyelocytic Leukemia (M3)

The FAB system defines acute promyelocytic leukemia (APL) solely by morphologic criteria. The leukemic infiltrate is composed of abnormal promyelocytes with heavy granulation, sometimes obscuring the nucleus, and often abundant cytoplasm (**see Color Plate 153**). Auer rods are frequently seen, and some cells may contain bundles or stacks of Auer rods (faggot cells; with faggot meaning a bundle of twigs or sticks). The nucleus varies in size and shape and is often reniform (kidney-shaped) or bilobed. These cells react strongly positive with the peroxidase stain or Sudan black and are usually negative with the NSE stain, but cases with positive NSE activity do occur (**see Color Plates 154 and 155**).[47,48]

Acute promyelocytic leukemia is associated with a high incidence of DIC. The abnormal promyelocytes are rich in thromboplastic substances that, if released, trigger DIC. The majority of patients with APL present with hemorrhagic manifestations including petechiae, small ecchymoses, hematuria, and bleeding from venipuncture and bone marrow sites.[49] These presenting signs and symptoms may precede the diagnosis by several weeks. The most consistent coagulation abnormalities include a prolonged prothrombin time and thrombin time, elevated fibrinogen degradation products, and decreased amounts of serum fibrinogen and factor V.[50] Thrombocytopenia, which tends to be more severe than in other types of AML, is almost universally present.[51] Schistocytes are sometimes evident on the peripheral blood smear. Because of the complications associated with DIC, it is important to distinguish APL from other forms of AML. Anticoagulant therapy (heparin) is usually indicated in these cases and is most successful when initiated prior to antileukemic therapy.[49]

A unique feature of APL is the occurrence of a translocation involving chromosomes 15 and 17 (t[15;17]). This abnormality has not been reported in any other type of leukemia.[46,52]

Acute Microgranular Promyelocytic Leukemia (M3m)

A second form of APL is the microgranular variant (M3m). The leukemic cells of M3m have primary granules that are not readily visible on Ro-

manowsky-stained smears (**see Color Plate 156**). These granules can, however, be demonstrated with peroxidase and Sudan black staining or by transmission electron microscopy.[53] The disease, like typical APL, has a high incidence of DIC, and it is therefore important to recognize it for therapeutic considerations. Patients with the microgranular variant tend to have a higher white cell count than those patients with typical APL, and they may have a shorter survival.[30]

Morphologically, microgranular APL can be mistaken for acute myelomonocytic or monocytic leukemia. The leukemic cells appear monocytoid with prominent nuclear folding and abundant cytoplasm. The nucleus of most cells in the peripheral blood is reniform or bilobed. Granulation of these cells is scant or absent, although occasional cells with heavy granulation are almost always present. The bone marrow aspirate may reveal a morphologic pattern which more closely resembles typical APL.[54]

The diagnosis of M3m can be confirmed with cytochemical studies including a peroxidase or Sudan black stain which are strongly positive. The NSE reaction is usually negative, but can be positive.[48] Cytogenetic studies of microgranular APL reveal the same abnormal karyotype [t(15;17)] that is found in the hypergranular form.

Acute Myelomonocytic Leukemia (M4)

Acute myelomonocytic leukemia (M4) is one of the most commonly diagnosed forms of AML, second only to the M2 group.[30] The leukemic cells of M4 are characterized by both granulocytic and monocytic differentiation (**see Color Plates 157 and 158**). On a Romanowsky-stained smear it is usually easy to find cells with primary granules (granulocytic differentiation) as well as cells with folded nuclei and moderate to abundant cytoplasm (monocytic differentiation). Both the peroxidase (or Sudan black) and NSE reactions are positive in 20 to 80 percent of the cells (**see Color Plates 159 to 162**). When morphologic and cytochemical similarities make the distinction between M4 and M2 difficult, the diagnosis of M4 can be supported by finding a serum lysozyme level exceeding three times the normal level and a peripheral blood monocyte count of greater than 5×10^9/liter.[24]

Acute Myelomonocytic Leukemia with Eosinophilia (M4E)

Some cases of M4 are associated with eosinophilia (usually 5 percent or more of the nonerythroid cells). The eosinophils appear immature and may have large basophilic staining granules. Unlike normal eosinophils, these cells stain positive with chloroacetate esterase (specific esterase) and with the PAS reaction.

This M4 variant (M4E)[24] is closely associated with an abnormal chromosome 16, including either a deletion[55] or inversion of the long arm (16q).[56] Patients with the 16q abnormality and bone marrow eosinophilia have a longer median survival than patients with typical M4.

Acute Monocytic Leukemia (M5)

The FAB classification system divides acute monocytic leukemia (M5) into two subtypes: poorly differentiated (M5a) and well differentiated (M5b). Subtype M5a is characterized by a predominance of monoblasts, which typically are large, with abundant cytoplasm and distinct nucleoli (see Color Plate 163). Subtype M5b is characterized by a spectrum of monocytic differentiation including promonocytes and monocytes. The peripheral blood usually contains more monocytes than the bone marrow, in which the predominant cell is the promonocyte. This cell has abundant cytoplasm, its nucleus shows delicate folding or lobulation, and nucleoli may be seen (see Color Plate 164). Both subtypes of M5 show greater than 80 percent positivity with the NSE stain. The peroxidase and Sudan black stains are negative or only weakly positive. Color Plates 165 and 166 contrast the staining of AMoL (M5b) with NASDA without sodium fluoride (NaFl) and with NaFl.

Acute monocytic leukemia has distinctive clinical manifestations associated with the monocyte's propensity to migrate to extramedullary sites. Skin and gum involvement (see Color Plate 167) is particularly characteristic. Lymphadenopathy frequently occurs, and sometimes the spleen and liver are markedly enlarged.[57] Central nervous system involvement also has an increased incidence in these patients.[58,59]

The white blood cell count is frequently elevated in patients with AMoL; the median value of 60×10^9/liter was reported in one study.[60] Markedly elevated leukocyte counts in AMoL patients have been shown to have a significant correlation with increased lysozyme levels, renal failure, and hypokalemia.[61] Disseminated intravascular coagulation is relatively common in patients with AMoL, especially following therapy, although hemorrhagic features are not as prominent as in patients with acute promyelocytic leukemia.

Serum and urine lysozyme levels (muramidase) are often elevated in cases of AML that have a significant monocytic component, including both AML types M4 and M5. Lysozyme is a hydrolytic enzyme found in mature monocytes and to a lesser extent in granulocytes. Serum and urine levels of this enzyme are elevated when there is rapid cell turnover. Such elevations are most striking in the monocytic leukemias and are directly proportional to the amount of monocytic differentiation;[62] they are more elevated in cases of M5b than of M5a. Those patients who have heavy urinary excretion of lysozyme may develop a renal tubular defect that results in hypokalemia, hypocalcemia, and azotemia.

Abnormalities involving the long arm of chromosome 11 (11q) have been found in about 35 percent of all M5 AMLs and in an even higher percentage of patients with M5a. The 11q abnormality appears to be particularly associated with children with M5a.[46]

Erythroleukemia (M6)

Acute erythroleukemia is characterized by an abnormal proliferation of erythroid and myeloid precursors. Patients with erythroleukemia have hypercellular bone marrows with marked erythroid hyperplasia (greater than 50 percent of ANC) associated with abnormal erythroid forms. Megaloblastoid changes can be seen in the erythroblasts along with other dysplastic features including bizarre multinucleation, markedly vacuolated cytoplasm of erythroblasts, and cytoplasmic budding (see Color Plates 168 and 169). Positive PAS staining of the erythroblasts is consistent with but not specific for the diagnosis of erythroleukemia; however, negative staining does not rule it out. Myeloblasts and promyelocytes are present in increased numbers (greater than 30 percent of nonerythroid cells), and Auer rods may be seen. Abnormal megakaryocytes may also be present.

Erythroleukemia has three sequential morphologically defined phases in which the size of the myeloid component varies. They are (1) erythremic myelosis, in which there is a preponderance of abnormal erythroblasts; (2) erythroleukemia, in which an increase in erythroblasts and in myeloblasts is seen; and (3) myeloblastic leukemia.[63] It is well recognized that many patients who are diagnosed with erythroleukemia will have their disease evolve into a leukemic stage indistinguishable from AML—M1, M2, or M4 type.[39]

Anemia is invariably present in patients with erythroleukemia, often more so than in patients with other types of AML. Lack of a significant increase in reticulocytes is common and is due to ineffective erythropoiesis. Frequently in the peripheral blood nucleated red blood cells (NRBCs) and myeloblasts are present, but it is possible to see patients who are anerythremic (no NRBCs) or aleukemic (no blasts), or both.

Caution must be taken when the diagnosis of erythroleukemia is considered. The possibility of megaloblastic anemia due to either vitamin B_{12} or folic acid deficiency and sideroblastic anemia must be excluded. These nonmalignant disorders may sometimes mimic erythroleukemia. Congenital dyserythropoietic anemias and the myelodysplastic syndromes must also be ruled out.

Acute Megakaryoblastic Leukemia (M7)

Acute megakaryoblastic leukemia (AMegL) is a relatively uncommon form of leukemia characterized by extensive proliferation of megakaryoblasts and atypical megakaryocytes. Increasing recognition of this entity has been largely aided by the use of platelet peroxidase (PPO) ultrastructural studies. Platelet peroxidase, which is distinct from myeloperoxidase, is specific for the megakaryocytic cell line.[64] This enzyme appears early in the differentiation of these cells and is localized in the nuclear membrane and endoplasmic reticulum.[65]

Acute megakaryoblastic leukemia was not initially included in the FAB classification of AML because it could not be identified by conventional morphologic and cytochemical studies; however, in 1985 its increased recognition prompted the FAB cooperative group to add AMegL to the acute myeloid leukemia list, as M7.[66]

The blasts observed in AMegL display a wide range of morphology, from small cells with scant cytoplasm and dense chromatin to large cells with a moderate amount of cytoplasm and a fine reticulated chromatin pattern. Cytoplasmic projections are sometimes present (**see Color Plate 170**), and in some cases azurophilic granules resembling early granular megakaryocytes can be seen.[67] The presence of megakaryocytic fragments in the peripheral blood is also suggestive of AMegL.

Conventional cytochemistry studies can help support the diagnosis of AMegL, but they are not diagnostic. The myeloperoxidase and Sudan black reactions are negative, whereas reactions to acid phosphatase, PAS, and alpha-naphthyl acetate esterase (ANAE) are usually positive. The combination of a positive ANAE and a negative alpha-naphthyl butyrate esterase rules out monocytic leukemia and is highly suggestive of megakaryoblastic lineage.[68]

Electron microscopy studies for platelet peroxidase are recommended when possible, but the diagnosis of AMegL can also be made by using an immunocytochemical method to demonstrate platelet-specific antigens. Antibodies against factor VIII–related antigen and against the surface glycoprotein IIb/IIIa (fibrinogen receptor, CD41) are the most sensitive and specific immunologic markers of AMegL. These antigens can be demonstrated using standard blood and marrow smears or paraffin-embedded bone marrow biopsy sections.

Acute megakaryoblastic leukemia may arise against a background of myelodysplasia or de novo. It has been observed as a transformation of existing hematologic disorders such as sideroblastic anemia, chronic myelocytic leukemia, and myeloid metaplasia. Acute megakaryoblastic leukemia has also been associated with acute myelofibrosis, which is a myeloproliferative syndrome characterized by diffuse marrow fibrosis and pancytopenia but which usually lacks the splenomegaly and characteristic red cell morphology changes of chronic myelofibrosis. It has been suggested that acute myelofibrosis may be synonymous with AMegL.[69]

CASE STUDY

K.L. is a 42-year-old woman who presented with a 2-month history of fatigue and weakness and a 2-week history of a sore throat. She reported a 15-pound weight loss over the last month or two. One week prior to admission she started antibiotics for her sore throat, but she reported little improvement; she subsequently developed a peritonsillar abscess. On admission to the hospital she was found to have an elevated white blood cell count with a large number of blasts.

Upon physical examination, the patient appeared to be an anxious, middle-aged woman whose vital signs were normal, aside from a slightly elevated temperature (37.6°C). Her right tonsil was enlarged and erythematous. She had no adenopathy, and her liver and spleen were not palpable.

Laboratory studies were ordered and the following results were reported: hematocrit 19.5 percent; hemoglobin 6.3 g/dl; platelets 64×10^9/liter; and WBC 79.2×10^9/liter. The differential included 80 percent blasts. The majority of these cells were relatively large (15 to 20 μm) with a moderate amount of cytoplasm. The nuclei varied in shape from round or oval and some were indented or folded; most had several distinct small nucleoli. An occasional blast had azurophilic granules, but this was the exception. A bone marrow aspirate and biopsy were obtained, which both showed virtually total replacement of normal elements with sheets of poorly differentiated cells (**see Color Plate 171**). The biopsy was hypercellular, approaching 100 percent cellularity in some areas. The morphology of the aspirated cells was similar to those seen in the peripheral blood except that fewer of the cells had folded nuclei, and in general, the nuclear to cytoplasmic ratio was higher. Most of these cells showed very little differentiation, though occasional cells with granulation were noted. Rare Auer rods were also observed. Cytochemical studies done on the aspirate smears were positive: the myeloperoxidase stain was positive in approximately 30 percent of the blasts and the NSE (alpha-naphthyl butyrate) was positive in occasional cells (less than 10 percent).

Diagnosis: Acute myeloblastic leukemia, type M1.

Follow-up: HLA matching was performed on the patient's brother and sister, but neither had a compatible tissue type. The possibility of a bone marrow transplantation was subsequently ruled out. The patient was placed on a therapy protocol for acute myeloid leukemia. During her induction chemotherapy she developed typical problems of anemia, thrombocytopenia, and leukopenia. She required platelets and packed red blood cell transfusions. She also required broad-spectrum antibiotics for fever due to neutropenia although no specific pathogen could be identified. Three weeks after her induction chemotherapy a repeat bone marrow showed no residual leukemia. She remained in complete remission for 11 months but then relapsed. Attempts to induce a second remission were unsuccessful. She developed progressive hepatomegaly, jaundice, and persistent neutropenia. She also developed multiple infections and was unable to recover.

This case illustrates a typical course of acute myeloid leukemia. Although the patient was not cured, she did achieve and maintain a complete remission for nearly a full year.

ACUTE LYMPHOBLASTIC LEUKEMIA
FAB Classification

The FAB classification system separates acute lymphoblastic leukemia (ALL) into three morphologic groups (Table 18–11):

Table 18–11. **FAB CLASSIFICATION OF ACUTE LYMPHOBLASTIC LEUKEMIA**

Cytologic Features	L1	L2	L3
Cell size	Predominantly small cells, homogeneous	Large, heterogeneous	Large, homogeneous
Nuclear chromatin	Homogeneous in any one case	Heterogeneous	Finely stippled, and homogeneous
Nuclear shape	Regular, occasional clefting	Irregular, clefting, and indentation common	Regular (round to oval)
Nucleoli*	Inconspicuous	One or more; often large	One or more, prominent
Cytoplasm*	Scanty	Variable; often moderately abundant	Moderately abundant, strongly basophilic
Cytoplasmic vacuolation	Variable	Variable	Prominent

Source: Adapted from Bennett et al.[39]
*The most useful cytologic features in separating L1 from L2 lymphoblasts are amount of cytoplasm and presence and prominence of nucleoli.

- L1: Small, uniform lymphoblasts
- L2: Large, pleomorphic lymphoblasts
- L3: Burkitt's type (vacuolated and deeply basophilic cytoplasm)

The morphology of these groups is evaluated on a bone marrow aspirate smear rather than peripheral blood. Cases of *L1 ALL* (Fig. 18–6 and **Color Plates 172 and 173**) have a predominantly uniform population of small blasts with scant cytoplasm, a homogeneous chromatin pattern in any one case, and indis-

tinct nucleoli. The nuclear shape is regular, but occasional clefting may be present. Cases of *L2 ALL* (Fig. 18–7 and **Color Plates 174 and 175**) are characterized by a heterogeneous group of cells. Some blasts may exhibit L1 features, whereas others are larger and have more abundant cytoplasm, a variable chromatin pattern, and prominent nucleoli. Nuclear clefting and indentation are common. This type may be difficult to distinguish morphologically from AML, type M1. Cases of *L3 ALL* (Fig. 18–8 and

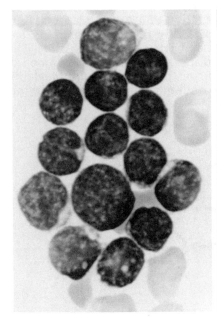 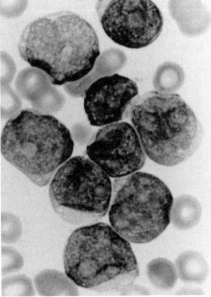 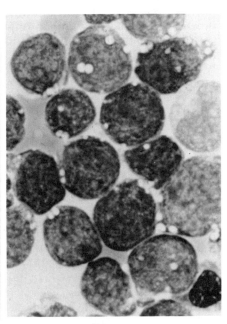

Figure 18–6. **Figure 18–7.** **Figure 18–8.**

Figure 18–6. Acute lymphoblastic leukemia—L1 morphology.
Figure 18–7. Acute lymphoblastic leukemia—L2 morphology.
Figure 18–8. Acute lymphoblastic leukemia—L3 morphology.

Color Plate 176) have a uniform population of blasts characterized by moderate to abundant cytoplasm that is deeply basophilic and has many vacuoles. The nucleus is round to oval without indentations. L3 ALL is referred to as Burkitt's type because its morphology is similar to that seen in Burkitt's lymphoma.

Because the distinction between L1 and L2 ALL is not always clear, the FAB cooperative group proposed a simple scoring system based on cytologic features.[70] Other groups have modified this system, assessing each case on a cell-by-cell basis to determine the percentage of L1 and L2 cells.[71,72] Individual L1 and L2 lymphoblasts can be differentiated most reliably by evaluating the nuclear to cytoplasmic ratio (high in L1, low in L2) and the absence (L1) or presence (L2) of nucleoli. Cases of pure L1 ALL (more than 90 percent L1 blasts) have the best prognosis, cases of pure L2 ALL (more than 50 percent L2 blasts) have a worse prognosis, and those cases with mixed cell types have an intermediate prognosis. The worst prognosis is seen in the L3 group.[73]

Immunologic Classification

In addition to morphologic criteria, ALL is also routinely classified by immunologic criteria. The lymphoblasts are phenotyped using traditional markers, including cytoplasmic immunoglobulin (μ heavy chain) and surface immunoglobulin (sIg), combined with surface markers detected with monoclonal antibodies (see Table 18–7). The nuclear enzyme TdT, found in immature lymphoid cells (both B and T lineage), is used to help distinguish between cases of ALL and AML.

To appreciate fully the immunologic classification of ALL and other lymphoproliferative disorders (such as CLL, lymphoma, and multiple myeloma) it is important to understand lymphocyte ontogeny. All of these neoplasias result from the uncontrolled proliferation of an abnormal clone of lymphoid cells — cells that have been "frozen" at a given stage of maturation retaining some features of their normal cell counterparts. In the case of ALL the malignant clone is arrested at an early stage of lymphocyte differentiation.

Lymphocyte Ontogeny

Lymphocytes originate from pluripotent stem cells (see Chapter 1, Fig. 1–2) that are present in the yolk sac, fetal liver, spleen, and bone marrow. At birth and into adulthood, the stem cells are normally found only in the bone marrow, where they respond to specific growth factors (hormonelike substances) that trigger their commitment toward B- or T-lymphocyte development. The microenvironment of these developing cells plays an important role in their maturation: B cells develop in the bone marrow (bursa-equivalent tissue), T cells in the thymus (from committed stem cells that have migrated there). Lymphocyte maturation in these organs is antigen-*independent*. After the lymphocytes have matured they migrate to the peripheral lymphoid organs including the lymph nodes, spleen, and other lymphoid tissues. In these organs the lymphocytes remain in a resting state until they are stimulated to undergo antigen-*dependent* development.

B-Lymphocyte Development. Early B-cell maturation (antigen-independent), which is particularly relevant to the classification of ALL, is divided into three stages: early pre-B cell, pre-B cell, and mature B cell (Fig. 18–9). These stages are identified by their expression of TdT, surface markers (HLA-DR, common ALL antigen [CALLA], CD19, CD20), and immunoglobulin (cytoplasmic or surface Ig). The *early-pre-B cell* is TdT positive and expresses HLA-DR, CD19, and usually CALLA (CD10). First HLA-DR, a histocompatibility-related antigen, is expressed, followed by CD19, and then CALLA. The most sensitive and specific surface marker for early B cells is CD19. During this stage the immunoglobulin genes begin to undergo rearrangements (see far-

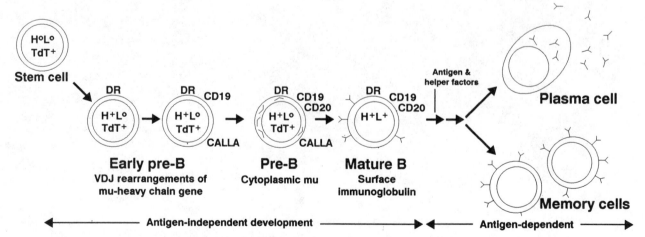

Figure 18–9. B-cell development; heavy chain (H) and light chain (L) are designated as H°, L° if in embryonic form and H+, L+ if rearranged.

ther on), followed by the production of cytoplasmic μ heavy chain. The presence of cytoplasmic μ distinguishes the *pre-B cell* from its predecessor, which otherwise has a similar phenotype. As the cell continues to mature, immunoglobulin light chains are produced and IgM is assembled and is inserted into the plasma membrane. This surface Ig (sIg) is the hallmark of the *mature B cell*, which no longer expresses TdT or CALLA. Each B cell expresses only one type of Ig light chain (kappa or lambda), a feature that is extremely helpful in identifying monoclonal proliferations of mature B cells.

Immunoglobulin genes are rearranged in a unique process that normally occurs only in cells committed toward B-cell differentiation. The Ig genes are composed of discontinuous segments of minigene families, which, when productively rearranged, encode for the heavy chain and the kappa or lambda light chains. The heavy chain gene (on chromosome 14) is composed of four minigene families including the variable (V_H), diversity (D_H), joining (J_H), and constant (C_H) regions. The C_H region has separate DNA sequences that encode for the different Ig isotypes including μ ($C\mu$), δ, γ, α, and ϵ. The V, D, and J regions are the first to undergo rearrangement forming a VDJ complex (Fig. 18–10). In this process intervening sequences (introns) are excised and the V, D, and J regions are spliced together. Messenger RNA (mRNA) is transcribed from this VDJ complex along with DNA sequences downstream from it, including an intron and the $C\mu$ region. The mRNA itself is then spliced to bring the VDJ complex adjacent to the $C\mu$ region, creating a template for cytoplasmic μ–heavy chain synthesis. This process is closely followed by a similar rearrangement of the kappa gene (on chromosome 2) which, if unsuccessful, is in turn followed by rearrangement of the lambda gene (on chromosome 22). As B-cell development continues, the heavy chain may undergo additional rearrangements in the C_H region, initiating an isotype switch from μ to δ. Both IgM and IgD are expressed on the surface of the majority of mature B cells.

After maturation in the bone marrow, B cells circulate through the blood to the peripheral lymphoid organs, where they remain in a resting state until stimulated by specific antigens to undergo further development. Activated B cells undergo clonal expansion, producing daughter cells that retain the same antibody idiotype (antigen-binding region).

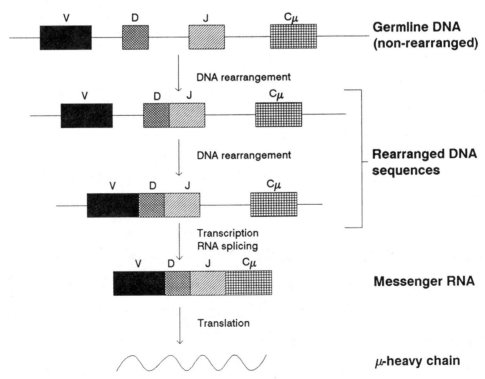

Figure 18–10. Schematic of immunoglobulin μ-heavy chain gene rearrangement. The variable (V), diversity (D), and joining (J) regions of germline DNA are linked through rearrangement and loss of intervening sequences. The VDJ complex, more intervening sequences, and a constant ($C\mu$) region are transcribed. The resulting RNA is spliced linking the VDJ and $C\mu$ regions and creating a template for the Ig μ-heavy chain.

Some daughter cells become memory cells and regain the small mature B-cell morphology and phenotype, whereas others continue development toward a short-lived antibody secreting cell, the plasma cell. During this final development, the Ig heavy chain may undergo another isotype switch, to IgG, IgA, or IgE. The plasma cell produces large quantities of Ig and is characterized by a high concentration of cytoplasmic Ig. It does not express sIg, CD19, or CD20, although other antigens, specific for plasma cells, are expressed (such as PCA-1 and PC-1).

T-Lymphocyte Development. In the past, T cells were identified by incubating lymphocytes with sheep red blood cells and observing for E-rosette formation (**see Color Plate 177**). Now, with the availability of monoclonal antibodies, T cells are identified and subclassified using immunologic reagents. T-cell development (antigen independent) in the thymus is divided into three main stages: stage I, early thymocyte; stage II, common thymocyte; and stage III, mature thymocyte. Stages I and II occur in the thymus cortex, and the last stage occurs in the thymus medulla. Like early B cells, thymo-

cytes express TdT and unique surface markers (Fig. 18–11). CD7, which is present on *early thymocytes*, is one of the earliest T-cell markers to be expressed; it is also the most sensitive marker for T-cell ALL.[74] Its expression is followed by that of CD2 and CD5. As the thymocytes move into stage II of thymic development they express CD1, a marker of *common thymocytes*, plus both CD4 and CD8. The next marker to be expressed is CD3; it is usually absent or only weakly expressed at stage II, but it is fully expressed in the *mature thymocyte* (stage III). At this stage CD1 and CD4 or CD8 are lost, giving the mature thymocyte a helper (CD4 +) or suppressor (CD8 +) phenotype.

During thymic maturation the T-cell synthesizes an antigen-receptor molecule called the T-cell receptor (TCR), which is closely associated with the CD3 molecule on the plasma membrane. Two TCR isotypes have been discovered, TCR-$\alpha\beta$ and TCR-$\gamma\delta$. The genes that encode for the α, β, γ, and δ polypeptides undergo rearrangement in a manner that parallels Ig gene rearrangements in the B cell. The TCR-β gene (on chromosome 7) rearrangements precede TCR-α gene (on chromosome 14) rear-

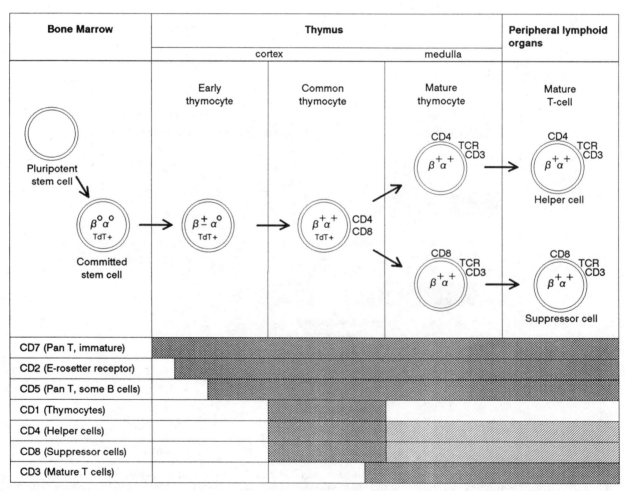

Figure 18–11. T-cell maturation. T-cell receptor (TCR) β and α chain genes are designated as $\beta°$, $\alpha°$ if in embryonic form and β^+, α^+ if rearranged.

rangements. Less is known about the γ and δ genes or about the function of the TCR-$\gamma\delta$, but it is clear that rearrangement of the γ gene precedes that of the α and β genes.[75] The majority of mature T cells express the TCR-$\alpha\beta$ isotype.

Immunologic Subtypes

The immunologic classification of ALL is based on the stages of lymphocyte development discussed above with four main groups whose phenotypes are summarized in Table 18-12. *Early pre-B-cell ALL* expresses HLA-DR and CD19. *Pre-B-cell ALL* has the same surface phenotype but also expresses cytoplasmic μ. Most of these precursor B-cell leukemias have CALLA (CD10) on their surface and are referred to as common ALL. Some of these, especially the pre-B-cell ALLs, also express CD20, a pan-B-cell marker that first appears during the midstage of B-cell development. *B-cell ALL*, which corresponds to the L3 morphology, is the only phenotype that can be reliably predicted based on morphology. It expresses sIg, CD19, CD20, and HLA-DR; it is TdT negative; and in most cases does not express CALLA. *T-cell ALL* is a heterogeneous group that expresses phenotypes that correspond to the different stages of thymocyte development; they are TdT positive and express CD7. A minority of these cases also express CALLA.

Before the availability of B-cell-specific monoclonal antisera (against CD19, CD20) many cases of ALL were classified as non-T, non-B because the lymphoblasts did not express the traditional markers of B or T lineage (cytoplasmic μ or sIg for B cells; or sheep E rosettes for T cells). The advent of CALLA antisera allowed many of the non-T, non-B ALLs to be classified as common ALL, yet there were still some patients, especially adults, whose cells did not react with CALLA. These cases were classified as *null-cell ALL*. It is now clear that the majority of these are derived from B-cell precursors, as confirmed by the leukemic cell's reactivity with CD19 antisera or the presence of Ig gene rearrangements.[76-78] Although gene rearrangement studies are rarely indicated in the work-up of acute leukemia, they can be performed in unusual cases where the standard cytochemical and immunologic methods fail to provide a specific diagnosis.

Childhood versus Adult ALL

The incidence of ALL differs markedly with age. For this reason and because of the generally poorer prognosis in adults, it is common to divide ALL into the broad groups of childhood and adult ALL. Generally the childhood groups consist of those patients who present with ALL at 15 years of age or younger.

The morphologic type L1 occurs most frequently in the pediatric age group, the L2 type in the adult age group. No significant differences occur in the incidence of L3 in children and adults.

B- and T-lineage ALLs occur at similar rates in children and adults, but differences in phenotypes are observed. For example, cases of childhood T-cell ALL rarely express HLA-DR, but this marker is expressed in a large percentage of adults with T-cell ALL.[79] Also, a higher proportion of adults with early pre-B-cell ALL do not express CALLA (what used to be classified as null-cell ALL).

Prognostic indicators are especially important in cases of childhood ALL. Most of these patients are able to achieve a complete remission, and many are potentially cured. Unfortunately some children relapse, and some of these eventually succumb to their disease. The therapy used to achieve a cure has potentially toxic effects which are a special concern in growing children. To help predict which children will have an optimal response to therapy, investigators have defined clinical prognostic factors. These allow the type and intensity of therapy to be more appropriately tailored to each child's prognosis.[80] Indicators of a poor prognosis include older age (over age 13 years), a high white blood cell count (greater than 20×10^9/liter), T-cell or mature B-cell phenotypes, L2 and L3 type morphology, and structural chromosome abnormalities. Children who have an early pre-B-cell phenotype, hyperdiploid lymphoblasts (greater than 50 chromosomes), and a low white blood cell count, and who lack a structural chromosome abnormality have a very good prognosis.[38,81]

Precursor B-Cell ALL

Precursor B-cell ALL, including both early pre-B-cell and pre-B-cell types, is the most frequently encountered form of lymphoblastic leukemia. It is

Table 18-12. IMMUNOLOGIC CLASSIFICATION OF ACUTE LYMPHOBLASTIC LEUKEMIA

	HLA-DR	CD19 (Pan-B)	CD10 (CALLA)	Cμ	sIg	CD7 (Pan-T)	TdT	FAB
Precursor B-cell ALL	+	+	−	−	−	−	+	L1, L2
Common ALL	+	+	+	−	−	−	+	L1, L2
Pre-B-cell ALL	+	+	+	+	−	−	+	L1, L2
B-cell ALL	+	+	−(+)	−	+	−	−	L3
T-cell ALL	−	−	−(+)	−	−	+	+	L1, L2
Null-cell ALL	+	−	−	−	−	−	+	L1, L2

*Immunoglobulin gene rearrangement studies have shown that most of these are precursor B-cell ALLs. CALLA = common ALL antigen: Cμ = cytoplasmic μ; sIg = surface immunoglobulin; TdT = terminal deoxynucleotidyl transferase; FAB = French-American-British classification; −(+) = majority negative, occasionally positive.

predominantly seen in the pediatric age group although it may occur at any age. Its peak incidence is between the ages of 3 and 5 years, and it is characterized in most childhood cases by L1 morphology. In adults L2 morphology is more common. The lymphoblasts frequently express CALLA, in which case the leukemia is called common ALL. Patients with common ALL usually present with disease predominantly localized in the blood and bone marrow. Prominent splenomegaly, hepatomegaly, and lymphadenopathy are infrequently seen at presentation. It is also uncommon for these patients to present with a markedly elevated white blood count (greater than 100×10^9/liter).

Pre-B–cell ALL (cytoplasmic μ present) is associated with a poorer outcome than cases of early pre-B–ALL (cytoplasmic μ absent). Both groups have a high rate of achieving complete remission; however, patients with pre-B–cell ALL appear to have a shorter duration of their remission.[82] Twenty to 30 percent of these patients have a translocation of chromosomes 1 and 19 (t[1;19]).[83] This abnormality is not generally found in cases of early pre-B–cell ALL.

B-Cell ALL (Burkitt's Lymphoma)

B-cell ALL is a homogeneous group that accounts for only a small portion (2 to 5 percent) of all cases of ALL. The majority of these patients have lymphoblasts with L3 morphology and a high concentration of surface immunoglobulin (usually sIgM). It is likely that these cells are derived from a transformed or stimulated B cell.[84] Virtually all cases have a characteristic translocation involving a rearrangement of the c-myc oncogene on chromosome 8 with the immunoglobulin heavy-chain gene on chromosome 14 or the light-chain genes on chromosomes 2 or 22 (t[8;14], t[2;8], or [t8;22]).[85,86]

The lymphoblasts found in cases of B-cell ALL are indistinguishable by cytologic, cytochemical, and immunologic criteria from tumor cells found in cases of Burkitt's lymphoma.[87] It is likely that patients with B-cell ALL are in a leukemic phase of Burkitt's lymphoma (non-African type).

The prognosis for patients with B-cell ALL is poor. They respond poorly to current chemotherapy regimens and rarely achieve remission.[88]

T-Cell ALL

T-cell markers are found in approximately 15 to 25 percent of all patients with ALL. Many of these cases can be classified into one of the three thymocyte stages of development.[89] CD7 is the most reliable marker of T-cell ALL, but CD2 and CD5 are also expressed in many cases. CD4 and CD8 are coexpressed in some cases and may be accompanied by the presence of CD3; approximately 10 percent express CALLA. The blasts of T-cell ALL are TdT positive and associated with both L1 and L2 morphology.

Patients with T-cell ALL often present with a me-

diastinal mass, a high white blood cell count (greater than 100×10^9/liter in 50 percent of cases), hepatosplenomegaly, and early meningeal involvement. Males are affected more often than females, and the disease occurs more often in older children. These patients generally have a poorer prognosis than those with common ALL. Efforts have been made to find prognostic factors that might help identify subgroups of patients within the T-cell ALL group who may benefit from different therapeutic protocols. Features that are most consistently correlated with a better response to therapy include a low white cell level, younger age (less than 15 years), and L1 morphology. There is also some evidence that certain surface markers may be associated with a better (CD5) or worse prognosis (CD3).[90,91]

When patients present with a mediastinal mass, it may be difficult to distinguish T-cell ALL from lymphoblastic lymphoma. The cytologic features of this type of lymphoma are similar to those of the leukemia although the lymphoma is generally associated with a more mature immunophenotype.[92] After a variable time patients with lymphoblastic lymphoma almost always develop bone marrow involvement, which renders their condition indistinguishable from that of patients who have T-cell ALL. The distinction between these disorders is generally based on clinical criteria. Patients who first present with prominent marrow and peripheral blood involvement are usually diagnosed with T-cell ALL.

CASE STUDY

T.J. was 4 years old when he was first brought to his family doctor with a 3-week history of fatigue, weakness, and a persistent sore throat. On physical examination he had a palpable spleen but no evidence of lymphadenopathy. He appeared pale and had multiple bruises over his lower extremities. A complete blood count (CBC), platelet count, and differential were done, with the following results:

CBC:

WBC	2.40×10^9/liter	MCV	87.0 fl
RCB	2.41×10^{12}/liter	MCH	29.0 pg
Hct	21.0 ml/dl	MCHC	33.3 g/dl
Hgb	7.0 g/dl	Platelets	6.7×10^9/liter

Differential:
3% Neutrophils
97% Blasts

A bone marrow examination was performed that revealed sheets of small blasts having scant cytoplasm and indistinct nuclei (**see Color Plate 178**).

Cytochemistry:
Peroxidase: Negative
NSE: Negative
TdT: Strongly positive
Surface Markers:

CD3	Negative	CD10	100%
CD5	Negative	CD19	98%
CD7	Negative	CD20	Negative

Cytoplasmic μ: Negative

Diagnosis: Acute lymphoblastic leukemia, common ALL (early pre-B; L1 type)

Follow-up: This patient started a treatment protocol for ALL, to which he responded very well. His physical examination 2 months after induction chemotherapy was unremarkable except for some hair loss. His CBC was entirely normal, although his white blood cell count was low-normal. A bone marrow examination at this time was also normal. He continued therapy, including one reintensification phase followed by maintenance therapy. Eight years later he is free of any signs of leukemia and is living a normal life.

REFERENCES

1. Bennett, JH: Two cases of disease and enlargement of the spleen in which death took place from the presence of purulent matter in the blood. Edinburgh Med Surg J 64:413, 1845.
2. Virchow, R: Weisses Blut. Froiep's Notien 36:151, 1845.
3. Gunz, FW: The dread leukemias and the lymphomas: Their nature and their prospects. In Wintrobe, MM (ed): Blood, Pure and Eloquent: A story of Discovery, of People, and of Ideas. McGraw-Hill, New York, 1980, p 511.
4. Virchow, R: Die farblosen Blutkorperchen. In Gesammelte Abhandlungen sur Wissen schaftlichen Medizin. Meidinger, Frankfurt, 1856.
5. Friedrich, N: Ein neuer fall von leukamie. Arch Pathol Anat 12:37, 1857.
6. Epstein, W: Ueber die acute Leukamia und Pseudoleukamie. Dtsch Arch Klin Med 44:343, 1889.
7. Naegeli, O:Über rothes Knockenmark und Myeloblasten. Dtsch Med Wochenschr 26:287, 1900.
8. Forkner, CE: Leukemia and Allied Disorder. Macmillan, New York, 1938, p 5.
9. Smithson, WA, Gilchrist, GS, and Burgert, EO: Childhood acute lymphocytic leukemia. CA-A Cancer Journal for Clinicians 30:158, 1980.
10. Pinkel, D: Curing children of leukemia. Cancer 60:1683, 1987.
11. Westin, EH, Wong-Staal, F, and Gallo, RC: Retroviruses and Onc genes in human leukemias and lymphomas. In Bloomfield, CD (ed): Chronic and Acute Leukemias in Adults. Martinus Nijhoff Publishers, Boston, 1985.
12. Gunz, FW, et al: Familial leukaemia: A study of 909 families. Scand J Haematol 15:117, 1975.
13. Evans, KIK and Stewart, JK: Down's syndrome and leukemia. Lancet 2:1322, 1972.
14. Carbonari, M, et al: Relative increase of T cells expressing the gamma/delta rather than the alpha-beta receptor in ataxia-telangiectasia. N Engl J Med 322:73, 1990.
15. Bizzozzero, OJ, Johnson, KG, and Cicco, A: Radiation-related leukemia in Hiroshima and Nagasaki, 1946–64. I. Distribution, incidence and appearance in time. N Engl J Med 274:1095, 1966.
16. Forni, A and Vigliani, EC: Chemical leukemogenesis in man. Ser Haematol 7:211, 1974.
17. Blattner, WA, et al: Epidemiology of human T-cell leukemia/lymphoma virus. J Infect Dis 147:406, 1983.
18. Rosenblatt, JD, Chen, ISY, and Golde, DW: HTLV-II and human lymphoproliferative disorders. Clin Lab Med 8:85, 1988.
19. de-The, G, et al: Epidemiological evidence for causal relationship between Epstein-Barr virus and Burkitt's lymphomas from Ugandan prospective study. Nature 274:756, 1978.
20. Geser, A, et al: Final case reporting from the Ugandan prospective study of the relationship between EBV and Burkitt's lymphoma. Int J Cancer 29:397, 1982.
21. Cancer Facts and Figures—1989. American Cancer Society, Atlanta, GA.
22. Gale, RP (ed): Leukemia Therapy. Blackwell Scientific, Boston, 1986.
23. Bennett, JM, et al: Proposals for the classification of myelodysplastic syndromes. Br J Haematol 51:189, 1982.
24. Bennett, JM, et al: Proposed revised criteria for the classification of acute myeloid leukemia. Ann Intern Med 103:626, 1985.
25. Yunis, JJ: Should refined chromosomal analysis be used routinely in acute leukemias and myelodysplastic syndrome? N Engl J Med 315:322, 1986.
26. Shafer, JA: Blood and marrow morphology in acute leukemia patients receiving chemotherapy: A photo-essay. Am J Med Technol 49:77, 1983.
27. Shafer, JA: Artifactual alterations in phagocytes in the blood smear. Am J Med Technol 48:507, 1982.
28. Wintrobe, MM (ed): Clinical Hematology, ed 8. Lea & Febiger, Philadelphia, 1981, p 1493.
29. Seigneurin, D and Audhuy, B: Auer rods in refractory anemia with excess blasts: Presence and significance. Am J Clin Pathol 80:359, 1983.
30. Stanley, M, et al: Classification of 358 cases AML by FAB criteria: Analysis of clinical and morphologic features. In Bloomfield CD (ed): Chronic and Acute Leukemias in Adults. Martinus Nijhoff Publishers, Boston, 1985, pp 147–178.
31. Stass, SA, et al: Sudan black B positive acute lymphoblastic leukemia. Br J Haematol 57:413, 1984.
32. Hayhoe, FGJ and Quaglino, D: Haematological Cytochemistry. Churchill Livingstone, Edinburgh, 1980, pp 130, 243, 265.
33. Bennett, JM and Reed, CE: Acute leukemia cytochemical profile: Diagnostic and clinical implications. Blood Cells 1:101. 1975.
34. Bearman, RM, et al: Terminal deoxynucleotidyl transferase activity in neoplastic and non-neoplastic hematopoietic cells. Am J Clin Pathol 75:794, 1981.
35. Casoli, C, Bonati, A, and Starcich, B: Ph¹-positive acute myelocytic leukemia with high TdT levels. Cancer 52:1210, 1983.
36. Kung, PC, et al: TdT in the diagnosis of leukemia and malignant lymphoma. Am J Med 64:788, 1978.
37. Marks, SM, Baltimore, D, and McCaffrey, R: Terminal transferase as a predictor of initial responsiveness to vincristine and prednisone in blastic chronic myelogenous leukemia. A cooperative study. N Engl J Med 298:812, 1978.
38. Look, AT: The emerging genetics of acute lymphoblastic leukemia: Clinical and biologic implications. Semin Oncol 12:92, 1985.
39. Bennett, JM, et al: Proposals for the classification of acute leukemia. Br J Haematol 33:451, 1976.
40. Cunningham, I, et al: Acute promyelocytic leukemia: Treatment results during a decade at Memorial Hospital. Blood 73:116, 1989.
41. Bloomfield, CD and Brunning, RD: FAB M7: Acute megakaryoblastic leukemia—beyond morphology (letter to editor). Ann Intern Med 103:451, 1985.
42. Griffin, JD, et al: Surface marker analysis of acute myeloblastic leukemia: Identification of differentiation-associated phenotypes. Blood 62:557, 1983.
43. Karen, DF (ed): Flow Cytometry in Clinical Diagnosis. ASCP Press, Chicago, 1989, pp 111, 114.
44. Griffin, JD, et al: Use of surface marker analysis to predict outcome of adult acute myeloblastic leukemia. Blood 68:1232, 1986.
45. Sultan, C, et al: Distribution of 250 cases of acute myeloid leukemia according to the FAB classification and response to therapy. Br J Haematol 47:545, 1981.
46. Bitter, MA, et al: Associations between morphology, karyotype, and clinical features in myeloid leukemias. Hum Pathol 18:211, 1987.
47. Liso, V, Troccoli, G, and Grande, M: Cytochemical study of acute promyelocytic leukemia. Blut 30:261, 1975.
48. Tomonaga, M, et al: Cytochemistry of acute promyelocytic leukemia (M3): Leukemic promyelocytes exhibit heterogeneous patterns in cellular differentiation. Blood 66:350, 1985.

49. Gralnick, HR and Sultan, C: Acute promyelocytic leukemia: Hemorrhagic manifestations and morphologic criteria. Br J Haematol 29:373, 1975.

50. Sultan, C, Surender, KJ, and Imbert, M: Variant form of hypergranular promyelocytic leukemia. ASCP Check Sample 25:4, 1983.

51. Jones, ME and Saleem, A: Acute promyelocytic leukemia. A review of the literature. Am J Med 65:673, 1978.

52. Rowley, JD, Golomb, HM, and Dougherty, C: 15/17 translocation. A consistent chromosomal change in acute promyelocytic leukaemia. Lancet 1:549, 1977.

53. Goulomb, HM, et al: "Microgranular" acute promyelocytic leukemia: A distinct clinical, ultrastructural, and cytogenetic entity. Blood 55:253, 1980.

54. Bennett, JM, et al: Correspondence: A variant form of hypergranular promyelocytic leukemia (M3). Br J Hematol 44:169, 1980.

55. Arthur, DC and Bloomfield, CD: Partial deletion of the long arm of chromosome 16 and bone marrow eosinophilia in acute nonlymphocytic leukemia: A new association. Blood 61:994, 1983.

56. LeBeau, MM, et al: association of an inversion of chromosome 16 with abnormal marrow eosinophils in acute myelomonocytic leukemia. N Engl J Med 309:630, 1983.

57. Rundles, RW: Monocytic leukemia. In Williams, WE, et al (eds): Hematology. McGraw-Hill, New York, 1972, p 896.

58. Meyer, RJ, et al: Central nervous system involvement at presentation in acute granulocytic leukemia: A prospective cytocentrifuge study. Am J Med 68:691, 1980.

59. Petersen, BA and Bloomfield, CD: Asymptomatic central nervous system leukemia in adults with ANLL in extended remission. Proc Am Soc Clin Oncol 18:341, 1977.

60. Tobelem, G, et al: Acute monoblastic leukemia: A clinical and biologic study of 74 cases. Blood 55:71, 1980.

61. Cuttner, J, et al: Association of monocytic leukemia in patients with extreme leukocytosis. Am J Med 60:555, 1980.

62. Catovsky, D, et al: Significance of cell differentiation in acute myeloid leukaemia. Blood Cells 1:201, 1975.

63. Pribilla, W: Erythramie und erythroleukamie. In Gross, R and Van de Loo, J (eds): Leukamie. Springer-Verlag, Berlin, 1972.

64. Breton-Gorius, J, et al: Megakaryoblastic acute leukemia: Identification by the ultrastructural demonstration of platelet peroxidase. Blood 51:45, 1978.

65. Breton-Gorius, J and Reyes, F: Ultrastructure of human bone marrow cell maturation. Int Rev Cytol 46:251, 1976.

66. Bennett, JM, et al: Criteria for the diagnosis of acute leukemia of megakaryocyte lineage (M7). Ann Intern Med 103:460, 1985.

67. Mirchandani, I and Palutke, M: Acute megakaryoblastic leukemia. Cancer 50:2866, 1983.

68. Koike, T: Megakaryoblastic leukemia: The characterization and identification of megakaryoblasts. Blood 64:683, 1984.

69. Bain, BJ, et al: Megakaryoblastic leukemia presenting as acute myelofibrosis: A study of four cases with the platelet-peroxidase reaction. Blood 58:206, 1981.

70. Bennett, JM, et al: The morphologic classification of acute lymphoblastic leukaemia: Concordance among observers and clinical correlations. Br J Haematol 47:533, 1981.

71. Miller, DR, Leikin, S, and Albo, V: Intensive therapy and prognostic factors in acute lymphoblastic leukemia of childhood: CCG 141. In Neth, R, Gallo, RC, and Graf, H (eds): Haematology and Blood Transfusion: Modern Trends in Human Leukemia IV. Springer-Verlag, Berlin, 1981.

72. Miller, DR, et al: Prognostic implications of blast cell morphology in childhood acute lymphoblastic leukemia: A report from the Children's Cancer Study Group. Cancer Treat Rep 69:1211, 1985.

73. Lilleyman, JS, et al: FAB morphological classification of childhood lymphoblastic leukemia and its clinical importance. J Clin Pathol 39:998, 1986.

74. Foon, KA and Todd, RF: Immunologic classification of leukemia and lymphoma. Blood 68:1, 1986.

75. Strominger, JL: Developmental biology of T cell receptors. Science 244:943, 1989.

76. Arnold, A, et al: Immunoglobulin-gene rearrangements as unique clonal markers in human lymphoid neoplasms. N Engl J Med 309:1593, 1983.

77. Korsmeyer, ST and Waldmann, TA: Immunoglobulin genes: Rearrangement and translocation in human lymphoid malignancy. J Clin Immunol 4:1, 1984.

78. Waldmann, TA, et al: Molecular genetic analysis of human lymphoid neoplasms. Ann Intern Med 102:497, 1985.

79. Sobol, RE, et al: Adult acute lymphoblastic leukemia phenotypes defined by monoclonal antibodies. Blood 65:730, 1985.

80. Weinberg, KI and Siegel, SE: Acute lymphoblastic leukemia in children. In Gale, RP (ed): Leukemia Therapy. Blackwell Scientific Publications, Boston, 1986, p 25.

81. Pui, CH, et al: Prognostic importance of structural chromosomal abnormalities in chldren with hyperdiploid (> 50 chromosomes) acute lymphoblastic leukemia. Blood 73: 1963, 1989.

82. Crist, W, et al: Prognostic importance of the pre-B-cell immunophenotype and other presenting features in B-lineage childhood acute lymphoblastic leukemia: A Pediatric Oncology Group study. Blood 74:1252, 1989.

83. Carroll, AJ, et al: Pre-B cell leukemia associated with chromosome translocation 1;19, Blood 63:721, 1984.

84. Brouet, JC and Seligmann, M: The immunologic classification of acute lymphoblastic leukemias. Cancer 42:817, 1978.

85. Taub, R, et al: Translocation of the c-myc gene into the immunoglobulin heavy chain locus in human Burkitt lymphoma and murine plasmacytoma cells. Proc Natl Acad Sci USA 79:7937, 1982.

86. Dalla-Favera, R, et al: Translocation and rearrangements of the c-myc oncogene locus in human undifferentiated B-cell lymphomas. Science 219:963, 1983.

87. Flandrin, G, et al: Acute leukemia with Burkitt's tumor cells: A study of six cases with special reference to lymphocyte surface markers. Blood 45:183, 1975.

88. Greaves, MF, et al: Immunologically defined subclasses of acute lymphoblastic leukaemia in children: Their relationship to presentation features and prognosis. Br J Haematol 48:179, 1981.

89. Reinherz, EL, et al: Discrete stages of human intrathymic differentiation. Analysis of normal thymocytes and leukemic lymphoblasts of T-cell lineage. Proc Natl Acad Sci USA 77:1588, 1980.

90. Pui, CH, et al: Heterogeneity of presenting features and their relation to treatment outcome in 120 children with T-cell acute lymphoblastic leukemia. Blood 75:174, 1990.

91. Shuster, JJ, et al: Prognostic factors in childhood T-cell acute lymphoblastic leukemia: A Pediatric Oncology Group study group. Blood 75:166, 1990.

92. Roper, M, et al: Monoclonal antibody characterization of surface antigens in childhood T-cell lymphoid malignancies. Blood 61:830, 1983.

QUESTIONS

1. *What is the best definition of leukemia?*
   a. WBC count $> 50 \times 10^9$/liter
   b. Replacement of normal bone marrow elements with neoplastic blood cells
   c. Fibrosis in the bone marrow and hematopoiesis in liver and spleen
   d. Leukocytosis with mixed cellularity with lymphoadenopathy and mediastinal masses

2. *What type of leukemia has immature malignant myeloid cells?*
   a. Chronic myelocytic leukemia
   b. Chronic myeloid leukemia

c. Acute myeloid leukemia
d. Acute type M6

3. *What are risk factors for the development of leukemia?*
   a. Chromosomal abnormalities
   b. Immunodeficiency
   c. Retroviruses
   d. All of the above

4. *What findings would be most useful for distinguishing AML from ALL?*
   a. Large blast cells with prominent nucleoli; Auer rods may be present; positive peroxidase and Sudan black; negative TdT
   b. Anemia, neutropenia, thrombocytopenia; numerous blast cells
   c. Small to medium blast cells with indistinct features; PAS and ANAE positive
   d. Blast cells with dense cytoplasm; negative peroxidase; positive Sudan black and TdT

5. *The WBC is 50 × 10⁹/liter with 80% blasts, 15% segs, and 5% lymphs. The bone marrow reveals sheets of immature cells. Cytochemical studies of these show that they are peroxidase positive (20%) and NSE negative. What is the diagnosis?*
   a. AML, M1 type
   b. AML, M3 type
   c. AML, M4 type
   d. AML, M5 type

6. *The WBC is 15 × 10⁹/liter with 90% blasts, 6% segs, and 4% monos. The blasts are relatively large and have abundant cytoplasm. More than 90% of them are positive with the NSE stain and an occasional blast is positive with Sudan black. What is the possible diagnosis? (Use answer choices for question 5.)*

7. *A 49-year-old woman, was admitted to the hospital for easy bruising and menorrhagia. She had evidence of DIC. Her WBC count is 3 × 10⁹/liter with 95% large atypical mononuclear cells. Many of these cells are packed with large purple-staining granules, some have multiple Auer rods, and all are strongly peroxidase positive. What type of leukemia is indicated? (Use answer choices for question 5.)*

8. *Cytochemical stains were performed on bone marrow smears from a patient with acute leukemia. All blasts were TdT negative. The majority of the blasts showed varying amounts of Sudan black positivity. Positive staining for NSE occurred in 50%. What type of leukemia is indicated?*
   a. Acute myeloblastic leukemia
   b. Acute lymphoblastic leukemia
   c. Acute myelomonocytic leukemia
   d. Acute erythroleukemia

9. *Bone marrow examination reveals a hypercellular marrow with lymphoblasts that react with antisera specific for CD7 and TdT; however, the lymphoblasts are negative for sIg and CD10 (CALLA). What is the diagnosis?*
   a. ALL, B-cell type
   b. ALL, early pre-B–cell type
   c. ALL, pre-B–cell type
   d. ALL, T-cell type

10. *A 4-year-old boy presents with bruising, fever, and coughing. His WBC is 15 × 10⁹/liter, Hct 23%, and platelets 53 × 10⁹/liter. A bone marrow aspirate is obtained and shows sheets of immature cells. Cytochemical studies for peroxidase and NSE are negative; the TdT is positive. Surface markers show the phenotype: HLA-DR +; CD19 +; CD10 +; cytoplasmic μ −; sIg −; CD7 −. What is the possible diagnosis? (Use answer choices for question 9.)*

11. *A 21-year-old patient's bone marrow is classified morphologically by the FAB system as an L3 acute lymphocytic leukemia. Which of the following results best supports this diagnosis?*
    a. Expression of CD19
    b. Presence of cytoplasmic μ
    c. Presence of surface immunoglobulin
    d. Nuclear TdT reactivity

ANSWERS

1. b (p 267)
2. c (p 267)
3. d (p 268)
4. a (p 270)
5. a (p 277–286)
6. d (p 277–286)
7. b (p 277–286)
8. c (p 277–286)
9. d (p 288)
10. b (p 287–288)
11. c (p 288)

CHAPTER 19

LLOYD A. SIMANDL, A.R.T. (CSLT)

Myelodysplastic Syndromes (MDSs)

OBJECTIVES

At the end of this chapter, the learner should be able to:
1. Name a leukemic trait shared by myelodysplastic syndromes.
2. List diagnostic criteria for myelodysplastic syndromes.
3. List characteristics for refractory anemia.
4. Identify features of refractory anemia with ringed sideroblasts (RARS).
5. Recognize the percentage of bone marrow blasts consistent with a diagnosis of refractory anemia with excess blasts (RAEB).
6. Name the terminating condition to refractory anemia with excess blasts in transformation (RAEB-T).
7. Identify the chromosome abnormality associated with myelodysplastic syndromes.
8. List factors used in the prognosis of myelodysplastic syndromes.
9. List diseases that may develop secondary to myelodysplastic syndromes.
10. Describe treatments for myelodysplastic syndromes.

Considering the diagnostic complexity of myelodysplastic syndromes (MDSs), it is not difficult to imagine the different names assigned over the years to this group of clinically diverse diseases. Preleukemias, preleukemic anemias, low-percentage leukemias, sideroblastic anemias, refractory anemias, smoldering leukemias, unresponsive anemias, subacute leukemias, dysmyelopoiesis, refractory cytopenias, chronic erythmic myelosis, oligoblastic leukemias, acute myeloproliferative syndromes, primary acquired panmyelopathy, and, finally, myelodysplasias or myelodysplastic syndromes are names applied throughout history to specify this group of hematopoietic disorders. Most of these definitions reflect specific interests of the various authors or are based on the outcome of the disease described, reflecting the key prognostic or diagnostic indicators. Subsequent to their designations, it has been found that some of these indicators were not accurate: some patients with "preleukemia," for example, did not progress to leukemia, whereas others, for example, with "refractory anemia," did. The issue becomes even more complicated with the attempts further to distinguish those disorders acquired as a primary condition from those acquired secondary to a treatment of a primary neoplasm or acquired by means of environmental factors.

Yet one thread of commonality emerged as early as 1949, when Hamilton-Paterson published a study of the likely transition of certain anemias into leukemia.[1] This thread continued ever since and was finally elaborated on by Bennett and associates,[2] with their original proposal for the classification and nomenclature of these disorders. This proposal was subsequently accepted by the French-American-British (FAB) Cooperative Group. Since then, this new classification has provided researchers and clinicians investigating these disorders with a common ground upon which to build a better understanding of these still mysterious diseases.

Today, although better classified and understood, myelodysplastic syndromes still remain a frustrating group of disorders ranging from mild anemias with little likelihood of evolving into acute leukemia to malignant diseases rapidly terminating as acute leukemia. In the same context, it is now known that the hematopoietic pluripotent stem cell is clearly involved in all types of MDS, yet this knowledge so far has failed to provide the patient with a satisfactory therapeutic regimen, with the possible exception of a bone marrow transplant.

ETIOLOGY OF MDS

The consensus held today is that all types of MDS are clonal abnormalities of hematopoietic pluripotent stem cell(s).[3-5] Such abnormal clonality is manifested by a spectrum of genetic alterations (see under Cytogenetics) resulting in a variable degree of impaired hematopoiesis, and in many cases a significant predisposition to the development of acute leukemia (see under Prognostic Criteria).[6] This theory is supported by the cytogenetic studies of Nowell[6] and the G6PD isoenzyme studies of Prchal, Abkowitz, and Raskind and their colleagues.[7-9] In some cases, a single clone producing the abnormal population undergoes successive mutations and steadily increases the number of affected cells yielding a frank leukemia picture. In other cases, multiple abnormal clones contribute to a faster transition into leukemia. In either category, the abnormal cell population effectively inhibits normal hematopoiesis and the leukemic cells displace normal bone marrow elements and enter into the peripheral blood circulation.

The exact mechanism causing the development of the initial abnormal clone of MDS is unknown, as the specific insult to the deoxyribonucleic acid (DNA) of an otherwise normal stem cell is not detectable by current methods of examination. However, certain assumptions can be made—namely, that a chemical, viral, and/or radiation insult is a prereq-

uisite to the development of MDS.[10-15] Also, some suggest a genetic predisposition to the development of MDS.[16] Whereas definitive proof of the primary insult is still elusive, there is common agreement that, after the alteration of the stem cell has taken place, this alteration is irreversible. The progression into a truly malignant transformation will then depend on the individual patient and/or on exposure to further insults to that individual's DNA.[17] It is this patient dependency and the degree and frequency of the DNA insult(s) that may explain why some patients progress to acute leukemia while others do not.

The mechanisms of these processes occurring within the hematopoietic system can so far only be suggested, as conclusive evidence of these events is still lacking. Some comparisons can be made, however, between the etiology of MDS and that of most myeloproliferative disorders (polycythemia rubra vera, myelofibrosis, essential thrombocythemia) and the relationship of both to leukemia. Leukemia is a clonal disturbance of hematopoietic cells inclusive of differentiation and proliferation. Diagnosis of leukemia is made when the cells of such a "disturbed" clone achieve hematopoietic dominance over all other hematopoietic cells. Myeloproliferative disorders, with their excessive proliferation, and MDSs, with their disturbed differentiation, thus share at least one of the three leukemic traits of differentiation, proliferation, and dominance. Diagnosis of leukemia, regardless of its prognostic outcome, allows the physician and patient a common ground of strategy. In MDS (and myeloproliferative disorders) this common ground is lacking, severely limiting the ability to influence the outcome. However, this limitation may prove valuable in the understanding of MDS etiology and pathogenesis, in that it allows researchers to observe the developmental mechanisms of leukemia, specifically with respect to the final step in such development: the establishment of leukemic cell dominance. Our current understanding of normal hematopoiesis is the result of more than two decades of investigative work using in vitro cultures.

It is clear that orderly hematopoiesis is a coupled process of proliferation and differentiation, with a stem cell pool carrying required genetic information to all progenitors. This is maintained by the process of self-renewal. Yet this coupled process of proliferation and differentiation may be controlled separately. Cell-to-cell interaction, growth factors, and random (stochastic) processes may affect any hematopoietic precursor individually.[18] Within these processes, a large body of evidence exists outlining the development of colony-forming units (CFUs) of individual (or mixed) precursors. It is also known that for proper growth CFUs require various colony-stimulating factors (CSFs). These CSFs appear to be for the most part glycoprotein hormones, produced in vivo by activated T cells, monocytes, endothelial, and stromal cells.[19-22] The genetic coding for the production of many of these CSFs or their receptors is on chromosome 5.[23-26] Coincidentally, chromosome 5 is the most frequent aberrant chromosome in all MDSs (except chronic myelomonocytic leukemia) (see under Cytogenetics). This aberration of chromosome 5 thus leads to refractory alteration in erythropoiesis and to similar changes in granulopoiesis and thrombopoiesis.

Therefore, a hypothesis may be put forward suggesting that in many cases of MDS a biologic event occurs, altering the genes of chromosome 5 (and possibly others) and resulting in the uncoupling of the two normal hematopoietic mechanisms— differentiation and proliferation. The resulting abnormal differentiation gives rise to MDS. A second biologic event, or an amplification of the first, results in increased proliferation, eventually culminating in leukemia. However, the recent developments in the study of oncogenes, growth factors, and the various cell cycle control mechanisms, along with the improvements in laboratory testing (such as in vitro cell cultures, purification of cell growth factors, improved cytogenetic techniques, and improved mapping of hematopoietic lineage with monoclonal antibody testing), will undoubtedly give us a better understanding of the etiology and pathogenesis of MDS as well as other hematologic malignancies in the future.

DIAGNOSTIC CRITERIA
Morphology — General Description

Once unexplained persistent anemia is established, diagnosis of MDS may be considered. This finding is frequently accompanied by neutropenia or monocytosis, or both. Bone marrow examination is essential for the diagnosis of MDS. The bone marrow should be normocellular to hypercellular and should present a variable degree of dyserythro-

poiesis, dysgranulopoiesis, and dysmegakaryocytopoiesis.[27,28] Generally, owing to the presence of anemia with impaired proliferation into peripheral blood, the bone marrow exhibits a decreased myeloid : erythroid (M : E) ratio (increased erythropoiesis). The peripheral blood absolute reticulocyte count will be decreased, and the mean corpuscular volume (MCV) will range from normal to elevated, depending on the degree of dyserythropoiesis present. Bone marrow iron deposits, myeloblast count, and other abnormalities will depend on subsequent classification of individual MDS. Qualitative and quantitative changes in granulocytes and thrombocytes (and their precursors) will also depend on the specific classification.

Morphology — Specific Features
Dyserythropoiesis (Figs. 19–1 and 19–2)

- Sideroblasts   type I   (1–5 granules)
            type II   (5–10 granules)
            type III   (numerous granules forming a ring around the nucleus)
- Multinuclearity
- Howell-Jolly bodies and nuclear fragments
- Cytoplasmic asymmetry
- Basophilic stippling
- Anisocytosis and poikilocytosis

Dysgranulocytopoiesis (Figs. 19–3 and 19–4)

- Hypogranulation
- Hyposegmentation with abnormal chromatin patterns (pseudo–Pelger-Huët)
- Hypersegmentation in bone marrow

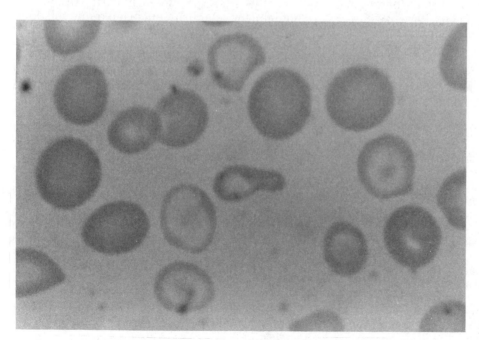

Figure 19–1. Refractory anemia (RA). (Peripheral blood 1000× magnification.) Note the dimorphism, anisocytosis, occasional target cells, and poikilocytosis.

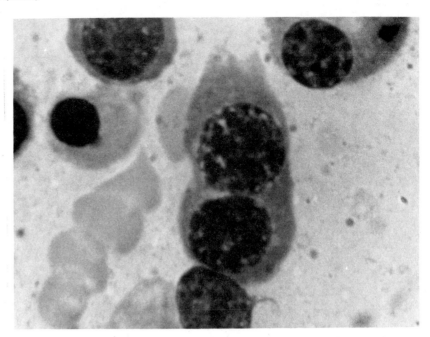

Figure 19–2. Refractory anemia. (Bone marrow 1000× magnification.) Note the large binuclear intermediate normoblast.

- Mixed eosinophilic and basophilic granules
- "Hybrid" myelomonocytes (confirmed by double esterase staining showing the presence of granulocyte specific chloroacetate esterase and monocyte specific alpha-naphthyl acetate esterase) (Fig. 19–5).

Dysmegakaryopoiesis (Figs. 19–6 and 19–7)

- Micromegakaryocytes
- Abnormal segmentation (hyposegmentation or hypersegmentation)
- Giant platelets

Figures 19–1 through 19–11 illustrate specific morphologic features of MDS, and Table 19–1 shows the relationships among MDS, myeloproliferative syndromes and acute nonlymphocytic leukemia.

CLASSIFICATION OF MDS

The FAB classification of the myelodysplastic syndromes includes the following types:

1. Refractory anemia (without ringed sideroblasts) (RA) (Figs. 19–1 and 19–2)

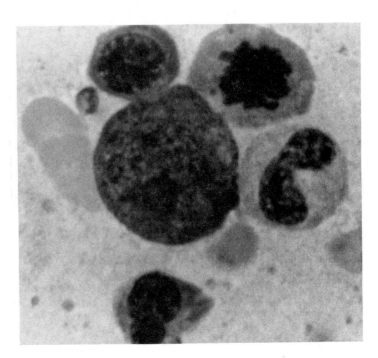

Figure 19–3. RA with excess blasts (RAEB). (Bone marrow 1000× magnification). (*Center*) Hypergranulated promyelocyte, (*center right*) "pelgeroid" band, (*upper right*) mitotic normoblast, (*center bottom*) binuclear normoblast.

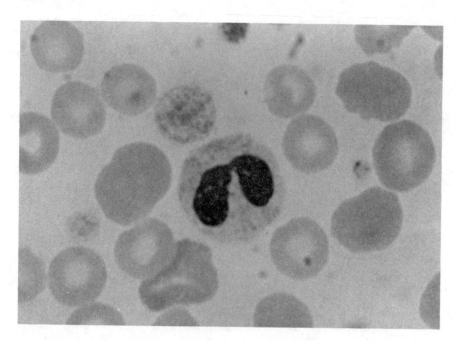

Figure 19-4. RAEB. (Peripheral blood 1000× magnification.) Note the pseudo Pelger-Huët band with abnormal chromatin.

2. Refractory anemia with ringed sideroblasts (RARS) or acquired idiopathic sideroblastic anemia (AISA) or primary acquired sideroblastic anemia (PASA)
3. Refractory anemia with excess blasts (RAEB) (see Figs. 19-3 and 19-4)
4. Refractory anemia with excess blasts in transformation (RAEB-T) (Figs. 19-7, 19-10, and 19-11)
5. Chronic myelomonocytic leukemia (CMML) (Fig. 19-6)

Refractory Anemia (RA) (Figs. 19-1 and 19-2)

This type of MDS is the mildest form of all, affording patients the longest survival. Most patients have a variable degree of cytopenias, with an average white blood cell (WBC) count of less than $3.9 \times 10^9/$ liter,[29] whereas the bone marrow shows increased erythropoiesis. Impaired release of erythrocytes results in variably decreased hemoglobin. Blast cells are rare in the peripheral blood (less than 1 percent)

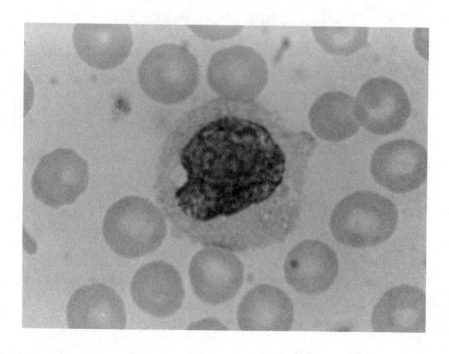

Figure 19-5. Chronic myelomonocytic leukemia (CMML). (Peripheral blood 1000× magnification.) Note the hybrid myelomonocyte.

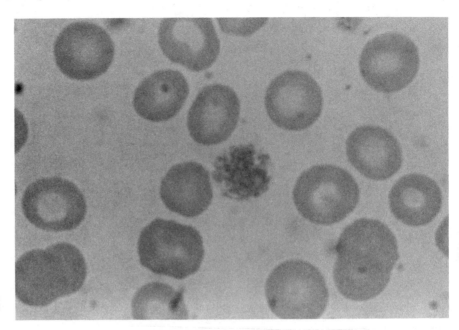

Figure 19–6. CMML. (Peripheral blood 1000× magnification.) Note the giant thrombocyte.

and found in normal numbers in the bone marrow (less than 5 percent). A significant criterion is the low number (or absence) of ringed sideroblasts not exceeding 15 percent of nucleated red blood cells. Bone marrow iron stores are inevitably elevated.

Refractory Anemia with Ringed Sideroblasts (RARS)

In many aspects similar to refractory anemia, RARS is distinct from RA mainly in its striking iron deposits encircling the nuclei of erythroid precur-

sors, thus forming ringed sideroblasts (**see Color Plate 56**). These are inevitably in excess of 15 percent of nucleated erythroid elements of the bone marrow, and frequently the percentage is much higher. The other distinct finding is that a comparatively low number of patients present with leukocytopenia or thrombocytopenia.[29] The elevated percentages of ringed sideroblasts with the accompanying failure of proper incorporation of iron into the hemoglobin molecule beside the production of normal erythroid precursors gives RARS another striking morphologic feature—erythroid dimorphism.

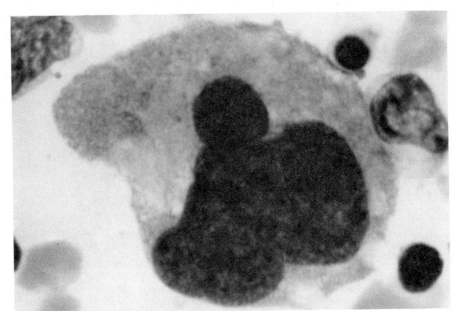

Figure 19–7. Refractory anemia with excess blasts in transformation (RAEB-T). (Bone marrow 1000× magnification.) Note the abnormal hyposegmented megakaryocyte.

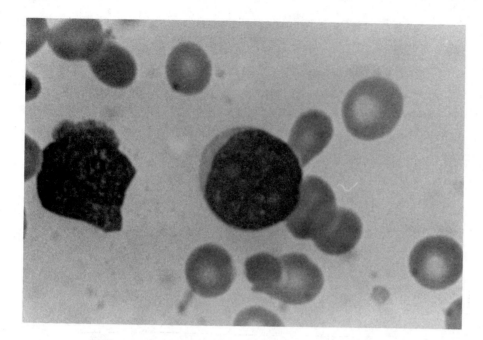

Figure 19–8. Acute myelocytic leukemia (M1, FAB classification). (Peripheral blood 1000× magnification.) Myeloblast.

Refractory Anemia with Excess Blasts (RAEB)

Refractory anemia with excess blasts represents the first overt classic relationship to ANLL—namely, elevated myeloblast count in bone marrow and myeloblasts circulating in the peripheral blood (see Figs. 19–3 and 19–4). Prior to the current definitions, "smoldering leukemia" applied to this condition. Its relationship to ANLL is also reflected in shortened survival as compared with survival in RA and RARS patients (see Prognostic Criteria). As with all other types of MDS, there is frequent dyserythropoiesis and dysmegakaryopoiesis resulting in cytopenia(s) and anemia with a variable degree of ringed sideroblasts. The most significant criterion applied to the MDS classified as RAEB is the total percentage of type I and type II myeloblasts in bone marrow of between 5 and 20 percent. The previously cited cytopenias and dyspoiesis morphologically separates RAEB from chronic granulocytic leukemia (CGL).

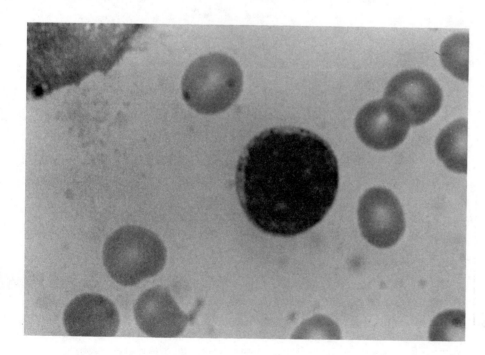

Figure 19–9. AML (M2). (Peripheral blood 1000× magnification.) Note the myeloblast.

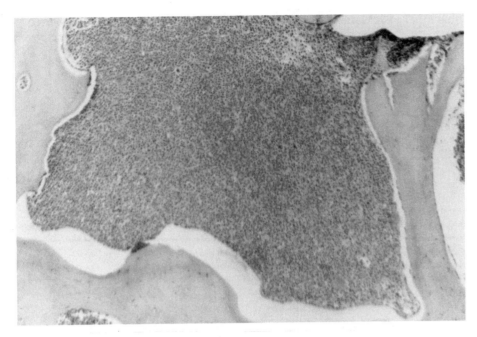

Figure 19–10. RAEB-T. (Bone marrow biopsy 40× magnification.) Note the increased cellularity.

Refractory Anemia with Excess Blasts in Transformation (RAEB-T) (Figs. 19–7, 19–10, and 19–11)

As the latest addition to the MDS family, RAEB-T became a recognized entity after the FAB reclassification of blasts into types I and II. The reclassification lowered RAEB criteria from a maximum of 30 percent blasts to a maximum of 20 percent blasts and deleted promyelocytes from the classification criteria. Because ANLL, to be so classified, must have at least 30 percent blast cells and RAEB must

not exceed 20 percent, the resulting gap needed to be filled; RAEB-T fills this gap. With its high blast count and increased peripheral blood blast circulation frequently above 5 percent, RAEB-T is the MDS with the highest conversion into ANLL and is also the MDS with the shortest survival.

Also, earlier criteria specified that the presence of Auer's rods always indicated ANLL, yet a number of cases exhibiting Auer's rods did not always appear to be full-fledged ANLL. This issue was further complicated when the FAB Group stipulated a 30 percent bone marrow blast count as a precondition

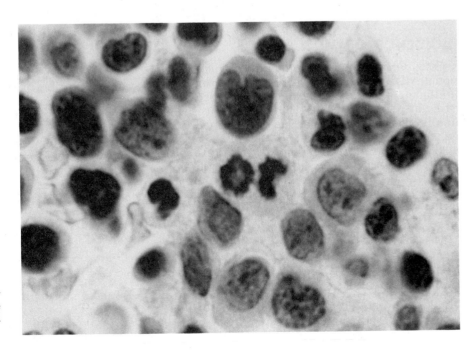

Figure 19–11. RAEB-T. (Bone marrow biopsy 400× magnification.) Note the increased cellularity, mitosis, and myeloid maturation.

Table 19–1. **RELATIONSHIP OF MDS, MYELOPROLIFERATIVE SYNDROMES, AND ANLL**

	BM Blasts	Cytopenia	Cytosis	Chrom	Dys	Other
RA	<5%	Yes	No	5q–	Yes	Ringed sideroblasts <15%
RARS	<5%	Yes	No	5q–	Yes	Dismorph, ringed sideroblasts >15%
RAEB	5–20%	Yes	No	5q–	Yes	Some with ringed sideroblasts
RAEB-T	20–30%	Yes	No	5q–	Yes	Some with ringed sideroblasts
CMML	<20%	No*	Yes	12q–	Yes	Monocytosis
CML	<30%	No*	Yes	Ph	No	Granulocytosis/thrombocytosis
PRV	<30%	No	Yes	N/A	No	Erythrocytosis
Myelofibrosis	<30%	No*	Yes	N/A	No	Granulocytosis/thrombocytosis/ tear drop cells/fibrosis in B.M.
Essential thrombocythemia	<30%	No*	Yes	N/A	No	Thrombocytosis/granulocytosis
ANLL (M1–M7)	>30%	No*	Yes	Many	No	Specific cell cytosis

*Except anemia due to bone marrow replacement.
Cytopenia = leukocytopenia (specific of general); Cytosis = leukocytosis (specific of general); Chrom = common cytogenetic aberration; Dys = dyserythropoiesis; N/A = not a key diagnostic determinant or not applicable due to lack of consensus.

to the diagnosis of ANLL. Again, this contradiction was eliminated by the introduction of RAEB-T. In other aspects, RAEB-T is similar to RAEB.

Chronic Myelomonocytic Leukemia (CMML) (Figs. 19–5 and 19–6)

It may be asked why CMML is included among the types of MDS. Its name even mentions leukemia. Indeed, there is little doubt that CMML is a frankly leukemic condition. Yet, if the monocytosis is excluded, what remains is a typical MDS, closely paralleling RAEB. The typical dyserythropoiesis, dysmyelopoiesis, and dysmegakaryopoiesis is always present, as is a similar blast distribution. In those cases (of CMML without prominent monocytosis) a diagnosis of RAEB may be made by mistake. It is only through careful analysis of chromosome abnormalities that the correct diagnosis can be made.

INCIDENCE OF MDS

Considering that the improvements in classification of MDS have been fairly recent, there are as yet limited data regarding the annual incidence of new cases of MDS. Between 1500 and 2000 cases annually in the United States can be estimated, based on earlier published data.[3] More information is available regarding age and sex distribution of MDS. The overall prevalence is in the older population of between 60 and 75 years of age.[31,32] The number of patients diagnosed for MDS under age 50 is described as being 3 to 30 percent, including rare pediatric cases.[33] There appears to be a higher frequency in males than in females.

OTHER DIAGNOSTIC CRITERIA

Cytogenetics

For more than 30 years, diagnosticians have relied on the assistance of chromosome analysis in the diagnosis of chronic myelogenous leukemia (CML) by mapping the presence of the Philadelphia chromosome (Ph). In the last decade specific chromosome aberrations were confirmed in most acute leukemias and myeloproliferative disorders. At the same time, such specific chromosomal abnormalities were also established in MDS. As in the case of the other hematologic malignancies, such specific aberrations are an important diagnostic tool in MDS, as well as an important prognosticator of the potential for leukemic transformation. Along with morphology and immunology, cytogenetics is an essential component of the diagnostic triangle.

On the whole, the incidence of nonrandom chromosomal abnormalities in MDS is likely to depend on the specific type of MDS. Also, the number of different abnormalities in each patient is closely related to the type of MDS. The frequency of a single chromosome being affected and/or multiple chromosomes being affected ranges from the lowest (in cases of RA) to the highest (in RAEB-T). The statistical analysis of these abnormalities tends to be somewhat inconsistent among various authors.[37–41] However, one specific abnormality, the deletion of a major portion of the long arm of chromosome 5, clearly emerges as the most common and consistent nonrandom chromosomal aberration in MDS. 5q– was present in more than 70 percent of patients with RA in Mitelman's 1985 study.[42] This association of RA with the frequency of 5q– is indeed so common that a number of authors describe the 5q– and RA relationship as being similar to that between CML and Ph.

Considerable evidence shows that if a single 5q– abnormality occurs in a patient with dyserythropoietic anemia, this inevitably will be RA with a predictable stable course, without a high probability of leukemic transition. However, the likelihood that a patient with MDS will only have one chromosomal abnormality is low. Even in RA the average number of chromosomal abnormalities is about 1.7, with the number of such abnormalities averaged across the whole group of MDS about 2.9. Attempts

Notes: RARS and Other Types of Sideroblastic Anemia

1. With respect to RARS it is important to note that it is a part of the MDS group of disorders. It is not related etiologically to congenital forms of sideroblastic anemias or to sideroblastic anemias acquired as secondary to other disorders.
2. Prior to the discussion of RAEB, the specific criteria applied to blasts and promyelocytes must be understood. These criteria are important to the classification of MDS and to the classification of acute nonlymphocytic leukemia (ANLL). Proposed by Bennett and co-workers[2,30] in 1982 and 1985, these criteria were subsequently accepted by the FAB Group. These criteria involve two items:
   a. Morphologic definition of myeloblasts (Figs. 19–8 and 19–9)
   b. Calculation of myeloblast percentage in bone marrow

MORPHOLOGIC DEFINITION OF MYELOBLASTS

Historically, the definition of a blast cell was fairly straightforward, fitting into the standard morphologic profile of size, chromatin pattern, nucleus-to-cytoplasm ratio, distinct basophilia, pattern of nuclear membrane, presence of nucleoli, and absence of any granulation (other than Auer's bodies in cases of acute leukemia). With the attempts of the FAB Group to establish criteria for MDS (and ANLL) this historic definition was no longer adequate. Therefore, the FAB Group established new criteria: type I blast and type II blast.

The historically distinct blast became the type I blast. A type II blast is slightly larger with a lower nucleus-to-cytoplasm ratio and always contains from one to six nonspecific azurophilic granule(s). All other morphologic findings are the same as for the type I blast. All more mature cells with a greater number of granules are classified as promyelocytes.

CALCULATION OF MYELOBLAST PERCENTAGE IN BONE MARROW

With the advent of the FAB Group classification criteria for ANLL (M1 to M7) and MDS, the determination of the myeloblast percentage became critical. Contrary to the reporting of peripheral blood, in which nucleated erythrocytic precursors are not part of the differential percentage, in bone marrow all nucleated cells (including erythrocytic precursors) are historically included. This created certain difficulties with the new FAB classification, especially in the distinction of FAB-M2, FAB-M6, RAEB, and RAEB-T. In order to eliminate those difficulties, FAB accepted the following standardization in reporting of blast counts. The calculation of the percentage of myeloblasts is achieved by excluding all erythroid nuclear precursors (E) from the count:

$$E = 65\% + \text{myeloblasts } 14\% + \text{others } 21\% = 100\%$$

The difference between 65 and 100 is 35; thus, 35 becomes 100 percent for such calculation. Therefore, myeloblasts are 14 of 35, or 40 percent.

Using this formula, the current proposal is:

>30% myeloblasts and the real % of E over 50% = M6
>30% myeloblasts and the real % of E under 50% = M2
20–30% myeloblasts and the real % of E under 50% = RAEB-T
5–20% myeloblasts and the real % of E under 50% = RAEB

to find another single type of chromosomal abnormality similar in consistency as RA and 5q— have not so far been successful; however, other significant data from this search emerged. These data demonstrated a frequency of other chromosomal abnormalities specific to ANLL as incidental to MDS. The proportion of such abnormalities and their frequency increases directly with the increase of the blast population in patients with MDS. Thus, RARS will have a greater proportion than RA, RAEB greater than RARS, and RAEB-T greater than RAEB. Some other common abnormalities are del(7q), −7, +8, trisomy 8, 11q−, and del(20). In general terms, these aberrations range from 1 to 2 percent in RA to more than 30 percent in RAEB-T. One notable MDS missing from the preceding chromosomal discussion is CMML. The reason for this omission is that the most frequent chromosomal abnormality, namely, the involvement of chromosome 5, does not occur in CMML. From this standpoint, CMML is

Notes: Nomenclature and Definition of Cytogenetic Terminology

Before continuing, the reader should be familiar with the following basic cytogenetic definitions:

1. Rearrangement symbols
   a. Translocation (t) = Transfer of chromosomal segment(s) from one chromosome to another
   b. Deletion (del) = Disappearance of a portion of a single chromosome
   c. Inversion (inv) = 180-degree rotation of a single chromosome
2. p = Short arm of a chromosome
3. q = Long arm of a chromosome
4. + or − symbol = Increase or decrease in length of the identified arm of a numbered chromosome (e.g., 5q− = shortened long arm of chromosome 5)
5. The specific chromosome affected is identified by its number followed by an arm designation in parentheses, preceded by a rearrangement symbol; e.g., del(5q)
6. Each arm of each chromosome contains specific regions. Several bands are found within each region. Both are numbered consecutively from the center of each chromosome outward. Consequently, in the case of a band designation (the smallest component of each chromosome) the following information is required:
   a. Chromosome number
   b. Arm designation
   c. Region number
   d. Band number in such region
   These are given in the aforementioned order without punctuation or spacing. For example, del(5)(q13q33) = bands 3 in regions 1 and 3 of the long arm of chromosome 5 are deleted.

These are not exhaustive rules and definitions of chromosome mapping. Special high-resolution chromosomal mapping techniques identify subbands and their specific breakpoints. Full discussion of these is beyond the scope of this text.[34-36]

clearly set apart from all other types of MDS. The data on frequencies of specific chromosomal abnormalities in CMML are varied. The 1986 French study[43] reported only 30 percent of 120 CMML cases with any chromosomal abnormalities, whereas a study by Heim and Mitelman[44] of 67 patients showed every patient having at least some abnormality across the entire chromosomal spectrum, the only exception being chromosome 14, which remained unaffected. A study by Yunis[45] also showed 79 percent of patients with MDS as having an abnormal chromosomal pattern. In CMML there appears to be only three abnormalities with a frequency of greater than 10 percent of cases: monosomy 7, trisomy 8, and deletion on the p arm of chromosome 12. Whereas the first two are also common to other MDS, the rearrangements of chromosome 12 appear to be unique to CMML in about 15 percent of cases. With the possible exception of abnormalities in chromosome 5 in cases of RA, the relationships of all other abnormalities to the various types of MDS or to the transition into leukemia at this time remain uncertain. Therefore, usage of these abnormalities in the determination of the pathogenesis of myelodysplasia must so far remain hypothetical. Setting aside the fact that the incidence and frequency of these aberrations is generally proportional to the likelihood of the development of leukemia, it is evident that only accurate cytogenetic characteriza-

tion and appropriate interpretation of subsequent findings may expand our knowledge of the associated pathogenesis of hematologic malignancies in general and of MDS in particular. Summarized in Figures 19–12 to 19–15 and in Table 19–2 is a comprehensive analysis of expected chromosomal aberrations by Heim and Mitelman.[44]

Immunology

Immunologic markers in all cases of acute lymphocytic leukemia (ALL) and other lymphoid malignancies are well established, and certain similar markers have been identified in many cases of ANLL. However, MDS, with respect to such markers, is still elusive. Although the findings are to date statistically inconclusive, some authors have reported different lymphoid abnormalities in a number of cases of MDS, including:

1. Clonal abnormality of lymphocytes alongside identical abnormality of myeloid precursors
2. Lymphocytopenia
3. Reduction of helper T cells
4. Deficiency of Epstein-Barr virus (EBV) receptors of B cells
5. Reduced number and/or impaired function of natural killer cells

Some patients with MDS were also observed with monoclonal gammopathy, whereas others had an

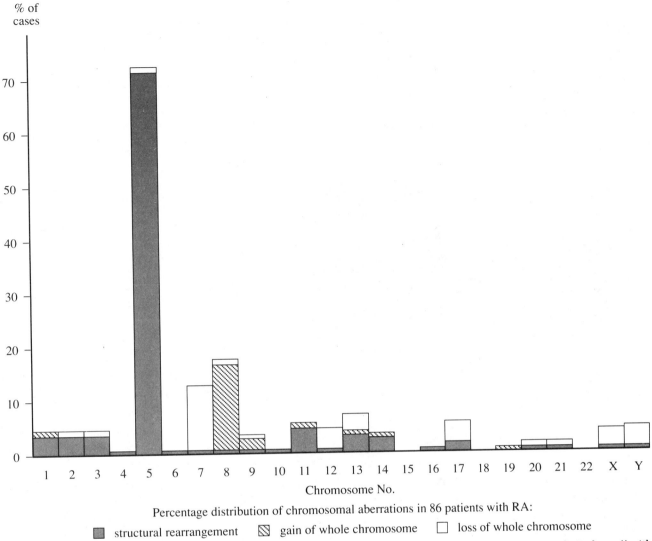

Percentage distribution of chromosomal aberrations in 86 patients with RA:

▨ structural rearrangement   ▧ gain of whole chromosome   ▢ loss of whole chromosome

Figure 19–12. Percentage distribution of chromosomal aberrations in eighty-six patients with RA. (From Heim and Mitelman,[44] with permission.)

increase or decrease of immunoglobulin levels. The latter was often observed in patients with CMML.

Whether these immunologic abnormalities are the result of lymphocytic (and/or plasmoid) abnormalities of the same stem cell clone involved in the specific MDS or whether they are caused by an interaction between normal lymphocytes and abnormal cells of the MDS clone is not known. Some also suggest that such lymphoid abnormalities may just coexist, unrelated to the MDS, and appear as a by-product of frequent infections in MDS patients or as a result of their old age. Today, the diagnostic value of immunologic markers is tentative. It appears, however, that a further accumulation of immunologic data may yield another reliable diagnostic tool in the future.

PROGNOSTIC CRITERIA

A number of investigators have published data outlining the prognostic criteria of MDS.[46–50] Although the consistency among the published data varies somewhat, certain prognostic criteria are clearly emerging, perhaps based on several individual factors that also may be combined in several scoring formulas. Factors frequently listed as having prognostic value are degree of cytopenia(s), degree of dysplasia, hemoglobin level, blast count in bone marrow and peripheral blood, presence or absence of abnormal chromosomes and the multiplicity of such abnormalities, and, last but not least, the specific type of MDS. Although all of these items are important, two types of scoring are currently in use and continue to be evaluated.

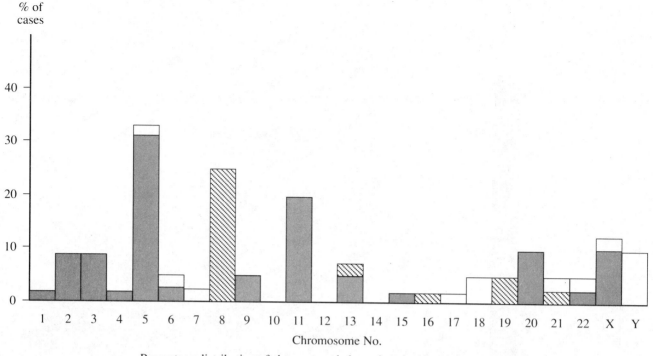

Percentage distribution of chromosomal aberrations in 40 patients with RARS:

■ structural rearrangement   ▨ gain of whole chromosome   □ loss of whole chromosome

Figure 19–13. Percentage distribution of chromosomal aberrations in forty patients with RARS. (From Heim and Mitelman,[44] with permission.)

The Bournemouth Score[51] and the FAB Score[28]

Based on standard hematologic criteria, the Bournemouth score assigns one point to each of the following:

$$Hgb < 100 \text{ g/liter } (10.0 \text{ g/dl})$$
$$\text{Neutrophil count} < 2.5 \times 10^9/\text{liter}$$
$$\text{Platelet count} < 100 \times 10^9/\text{liter}$$
$$\text{Bone marrow blast count} > 5\%$$

The resulting score is thus 0 to 4. Subsequently patients are divided into the following groups:

Group A = Score 0–1
Group B = Score 2–3
Group C = Score 4

Analysis of the scored group revealed a high statistical significance:

Group A = Median survival 62 months
Group B = Median survival 22 months
Group C = Median survival 8.5 months

The greatest survival variation was observed in group B patients. Further refinement of the group B problem may be provided by using good quality tre-phine biopsy to determine the presence of fine loci of immature precursors. The presence or absence of such either worsens or improves the prognosis, respectively.

Score based on more complex FAB criteria is consistent with the Bournemouth score.

This scoring system includes quantitative and qualitative parameters. The former include the levels of granulocytopenia, thrombocytopenia, and megakaryocytes in bone marrow. The latter consist of the proportion of dysgranulopoiesis and dysmegakaryopoiesis (dyserythropoiesis is not included in this scoring system). Therefore, two scoring tables are employed, a quantitative table and a qualitative one:

QUANTITATIVE

Score	Neutrophils	Score	Thrombocytes
0	$>3.0 \times 10^9/\text{liter}$	0	$>150 \times 10^9/\text{liter}$
1	1.0–$3.0 \times 10^9/\text{liter}$	1	100–$150 \times 10^9/\text{liter}$
2	0.5–$0.99 \times 10^9/\text{liter}$	2	50–$99.9 \times 10^9/\text{liter}$
3	$<0.5 \times 10^9/\text{liter}$	3	20–$49.9 \times 10^9/\text{liter}$
4	—	4	$<20 \times 10^9/\text{liter}$
2	Megakaryocytes $<1/1000$ nucleated B.M. cells		

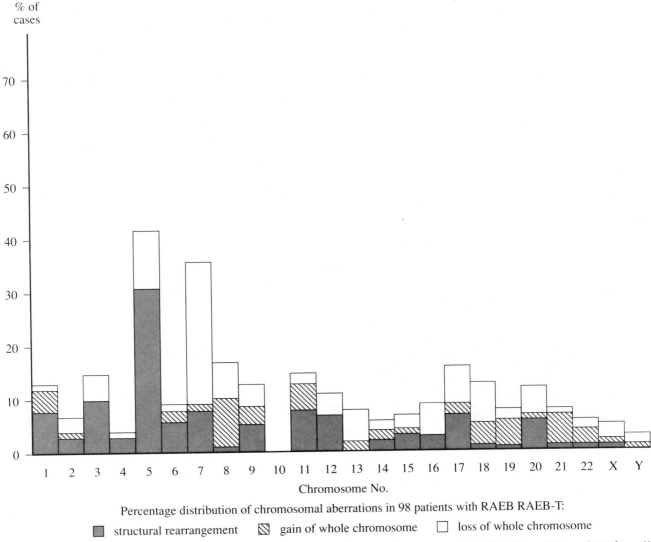

Percentage distribution of chromosomal aberrations in 98 patients with RAEB RAEB-T:

▨ structural rearrangement   ▨ gain of whole chromosome   ☐ loss of whole chromosome

Figure 19–14. Percentage distribution of chromosomal aberrations in ninety-eight patients with RAEB-T. (From Heim and Mitelman,[44] with permission.)

QUALITATIVE

Score	In Bone Marrow
2	Hypogranular cells >20%
2	Abnormal nuclei >20%
2	Micromegakaryocytes or large megakaryocytes or mononuclear megakaryocytes or megakaryocytes with multiple small nuclei >30%

By adding the various scoring points, the range is from 0 to 15, with the highest score being based on the maximum points assigned to each element:

Quantitative: Neutrophils   3
               Thrombocytes   4
               Megakaryocytes   2

Qualitative: Hypogranular   2
               Abnormal nuclei 2
               Megakaryocytes   2
                               ___
                                15

As stated earlier, the survival statistics are approximately correlated as follows:

FAB   0–1 = Bournemouth 0–1
FAB   2–5 = Bournemouth 2–3
FAB   6–15 = Bournemouth 4

Significant evidence is also being compiled regarding the prognostic value of specific chromosomal abnormalities. There are clear indications that patients with MDS who do not have detectable chromosomal abnormalities have the best prognosis, surviving generally longer than 3 years.

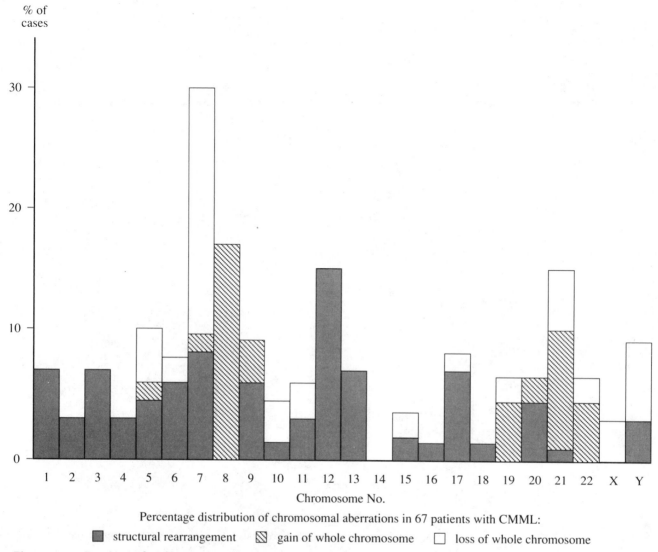

Percentage distribution of chromosomal aberrations in 67 patients with CMML:

▨ structural rearrangement   ▧ gain of whole chromosome   ▫ loss of whole chromosome

Figure 19–15. Percentage distribution of chromosomal aberrations in 67 patients with CMML. (From Heim and Mitelman,[44] with permission.)

Those with a single and stable chromosomal abnormality have a somewhat shorter survival, and those with more than three abnormalities have by far the worst prognosis.

There also is correlation between the individual type(s) of MDS and prognosis. This is of course related to the previously mentioned criteria, as RA, which shows the best prognosis, also has the least multiple chromosomal abnormalities, least blasts, least cytopenias, and so on. On the other hand,

Table 19–2. **SUMMARY OF THE PRINCIPAL CYTOGENETIC CHANGES (%) IN THE VARIOUS MDS SUBGROUPS**

	5q–	–5	–7	+8	del or +(11q)	del or +(12p)
RA	71	1	6	15	4	0
RARS	27	2	2	25	20	0
RAEB and RAEB-T	30	11	27	8	9	7
CMML	3	4	19	18	3	15

Source: Adapted from Heim and Mitelman.[44]

RAEB (or RAEB-T), having the worst prognosis, also possesses the most of the aforementioned negative prognosticators.

SECONDARY MDS

Successful treatment of a number of malignancies is sometimes complicated by the development of MDS (or leukemia) secondary to such treatment.[52-59] Also, the exposure to known toxins (such as industrial and environmental chemicals and contaminants) has been identified as a cause of secondary MDS.

As the etiology of the primary MDS is not fully understood, it may be possible that in the future there may be a fusion of at least some of the etiologies of primary and secondary MDS. Meanwhile, secondary MDS may be dealt with separately at least from one standpoint: a known cause. In all other aspects the distinction between primary and secondary MDS is insignificant.

With respect to the treatment of primary disease, a significant incidence of secondary MDS was identified subsequent to the treatment of the following:

- Hodgkin's disease
- Non-Hodgkin's lymphomas
- Multiple myeloma
- Ovarian cancer
- Lung cancer
- Breast cancer
- Testicular cancer
- Polycythemia rubra vera

Occasional incidence was described secondary to treatment of gastrointestinal and brain malignancies. Regardless of the frequency of such secondary MDS, there is little doubt that it is caused by the treatment of such diseases. In all cases, chemotherapeutic or radiation agents were identified. It is beyond the scope of this text to elaborate on the specific agents. In general, alkylating agents (such as nitrogen mustard and procarbazine busulfan) seem to be the second most frequently identified causes of secondary MDS, after irradiation. Whereas the causative agents are thus identified, the following questions remain to be answered:

- Is one agent more leukemogenic than another?
- Are the effects of a combination of these agents additive or synergistic?
- Does the method of delivery of these agents influence the incidence of secondary MDS?

Table 19–3. **PROGNOSTIC FACTORS IN MDS: SURVIVAL AND COMPLICATIONS FOR THE FIVE SUBGROUPS**

	Number of Patients	Survival (mo)	AML Death (%)	Death from Hemorrhage or Infections (%)	References
Refractory anemia (RA)	60	40	15	27	38
	53	32	11	36	46
	32	17	15	—	60
	30	52	20	57	61
	25	18	11*	59*	62
Refractory anemia with ringed sideroblasts (RARS)	20	52	20	15	38
	21	76	5	10	46
	15	13.9	7	—	60
	23	29	4	43	61
	12	31	11*	59*	62
Refractory anemia with excess blasts (RAEB)	97	10.6	44	37	38
	25	10.5	28	52	46
	21	14.3	38	—	60
	9	12	11	88	61
	14	11	56†	29†	62
Refractory anemia with excess blasts in transformation (RAEB-T)	—	—	—	—	38
	11	5	55	36	46
	21	3	47	—	60
	6	11	—	83	61
	23	4	56†	29†	62
Chronic myelomonocytic leukemia (CMML)	15	11.1	40	20	38
	31	22	13	13	46
	12	5	0/12	—	60
	1	2	—	100	61
	11	9.1	56†	29†	62

*RA and RARS.
†RAEB, RAEB-T, and CMML.
Source: Adapted from Spriggs, DR, Stone, RM, and Kufe, DW: The treatment of myelodysplastic syndromes. Clinics in Haematology, WB Saunders, London, p 1081, 1986.

- Is the duration or the amount of such treatment significant in the development of secondary MDS?
- Are the chemical agent(s) and the radiotherapy additive or synergistic?
- Is the radiotherapy alone significant?
- Are certain patients more susceptible than others?
- Are patients with a specific MDS more susceptible than other patients with a different MDS?

Once the answers to these questions are known and once corrective measures benefiting the patients are developed, secondary MDS, whether caused by therapy or by exposure to industrial factors, may be largely eliminated.

TREATMENT AND SURVIVAL

Refractory disease was first defined as a disease with a poor response to any treatment known at that time. Even today, most types of MDS remain refractory to all forms of treatment. In general, the treatment consists of prophylaxis against the effects of cytopenia(s), followed by the treatment of transitional leukemia. Table 19–3 indicates survival of patients with MDS and the predominant causes of death.

Therapy may be separated into three different groups, depending on the type of MDS and the age of the patient.

1. Older patients and those with RA and, in some cases, RARS. Supportive therapy for cytopenias includes transfusions of whole blood to treat anemia, transfusion of platelets to prevent hemorrhage, and transfusion of granulocytes as prophylaxis to infection. This may be supplemented by antibacterial and other antibiotic agents to treat opportunistic infections.
2. Younger patients and those with more advanced MDS (RAEB, RAEB-T, CMML). In addition to the aforementioned protocol, hormonal treatment with androgens, corticosteroids, and other myelostimulants and standard antileukemic treatment are used as needed to inhibit the abnormal clone proliferation.
3. The treatment of MDS with allogenic bone marrow transplant. Allogenic bone marrow transplantation is the only promising course of therapy for MDS.[63-65] The unfortunate limitation for bone marrow transplant candidates is the availability of suitable donor(s) and the required younger age. With the incidence of MDS being the highest in patients over age 50, the likelihood that a majority of patients can be so treated is low. In those patients receiving bone marrow transplants following complete body irradiation the survival statistics are steadily improving, with long-lasting remissions or cures reported in more than 50 percent of such patients.

In summary, with the exception of allogenic bone marrow transplantation, most patients with MDS respond poorly to all modes of treatment and succumb to opportunistic infections, bleeding complications, severe anemia, or some combination of these. Of those surviving these initial problems, most die after the transit into acute leukemia owing to the leukemic cell burden, and only a very few have a successful initial remission.

UNANSWERED QUESTIONS

Despite all the recent improvements in the diagnosis, classification, and treatment of MDS, many more questions have emerged. For example, when does MDS begin? This applies especially to RA and RARS, as in many cases the patient, feeling healthy, may not seek medical help. In such cases, how long does the patient truly suffer from this disease? Prior to diagnosis, when does the initial insult to the stem cell occur? And therefore, how valid is the statistical analysis of survival?

Even with the improved FAB classification the demarcation between the different MDS is, at best, arbitrary. It is therefore frequently difficult to assign a certain patient to a specific MDS, as the hematologic features may not be clearly defined. In many patients, the hematologic picture is altered from time to time, suggesting a revolving process rather than a strict transition from one type of MDS to another. Researchers hope that as more is learned about these disorders, more specific answers will allow a better understanding of why such apparently minor alterations in the cell differentiation can gradually evolve into a leukemic state. Because we are unable to detect the earliest changes in our stem cells, we cannot fully understand the development of MDS and of leukemia. It is therefore a hope for all that the key to the understanding of MDS will also open the door to the understanding of leukemogenesis.

CASE STUDY

An 80-year-old man was admitted to hospital complaining of general fatigue and shortness of breath, which he had experienced for the past 4 months. Otherwise, his previous medical history was uneventful. Upon examination he presented with pallor but had no hepatomegaly or splenomegaly.

Peripheral blood findings were:

WBC 1.9×10^9/liter
Hgb 87 g/liter (8.7 g/dl)
MCV 82 fl
Thrombocytes 109×10^9/liter
Marked anisocytosis
Moderate anisochromia
Occasional target cells
3% Blasts
Occasional pelgeroid cells

Bone marrow findings showed marked hypercellularity due to the increase in myeloid cells. Many of these were intermediate morphology with a moderate amount of cytoplasm, fine azurophilic granulation evenly distributed, and the occasional folded nucleus suggestive of monocytoid differentiation. Esterase stain failed to demonstrate a significant monocyte component. Because of the granulation pattern, the exact number of blast cells was difficult to attain and the count showing 24 percent is a conservative figure. Auer's rods were also present. Dysplasia of maturing myeloid and erythroid cells was evident.

Cytogenetic findings:

Monosomy 7

5q —

Diagnosis: Refractory anemia with excess of blast cells in transformation (RAEB-T).

Follow-up: Currently, the patient is undergoing a standard regimen, with transfusions to alleviate the effects of anemia and leukocytopenia.

ACKNOWLEDGMENTS

I wish to thank Judi London, R.T., for typing and assisting with the manuscript; Sharon Christensen, R.T., and George Zizka, respectively, for evaluation and searches for references; Vivian Tang, R.T., for selection of slides; and Sylvia Sinclair, R.T., for support and for many useful discussions.

REFERENCES

1. Hamilton-Paterson, JL: Preleukemia anaemia. Acta Haematol 2:309, 1949.
2. Bennett, JM, et al: Proposals for the classification of the myelodysplastic syndromes. Br J Haematol 51:189, 1982.
3. Mayer, RJ and Canellos, GP: Preleukaemic syndromes and other myeloproliferative disorders. Gunz, FW and Henderson, ES (eds): Leukaemia, ed 4. Grune & Stratton, New York, 1983.
4. Greenberg, PL: The smouldering myeloid leukaemic states: Clinical and biological features. Blood 61:1035, 1983.
5. Francis, GE and Hoffbrand, AV: The myelodysplastic syndromes and preleukaemia. In Hoffbrand, AV (ed): Recent Advances in Haematology. Vol 4. Churchill Livingstone, London, 1985, pp 239–267.
6. Nowell, PC: Cytogenetics of preleukaemia. Cancer Genetics and Cytogenetics 5:265, 1982.
7. Prchal, JT, Throckmorton, DW, and Carrol, AJ: A common progenitor for human myeloid and lymphoid cells. Nature 274:590, 1978.
8. Abkowitz, JL, et al: Pancytopenia as a clonal disorder of a multipotent haemopoietic stem cell. J Clin Invest 73:258, 1984.
9. Raskind, WH, et al: Evidence for a multistep pathogenesis as a myelodysplastic syndrome. Blood 63:1318, 1984.
10. Brandt, L, Milsson, PG, and Mitelman, F: Occupational exposure to petroleum products in men with acute non-lymphatic leukaemia. Br Med J 1:553, 1978.
11. Blair, A, Fraumeni, JF, and Mason, TJ: Geographic patterns of leukaemia in the United States. J Chron Dis 33:251, 1980.
12. Brandt, L: Environmental factors and leukaemia. Medical Oncology and Tumour Pharmacotherapy 2:7, 1985.
13. Marshall, CJ and Rigby, PWJ: Viral and cellular genes involved in oncogenesis. Cancer Surveys 3:183, 1984.
14. Wong-Staal, F and Gallo, RC: Human T-lymphotropic retroviruses (review). Nature 317:395, 1985.
15. Smith, PG: Current assessment of 'case clustering' of lymphomas and leukaemias. Cancer 42:1026, 1978.
16. Krontiris, TG, et al: Unique allelic restriction fragments of the human Ha-ras locus in leukocyte and tumour DNAs of cancer patients. Nature 313:369, 1985.
17. Jacobs, A and Clark, RE: Pathogenesis and clinical variations in the myelodysplastic syndromes. In Clinics in Haematology. WB Saunders, London, Vol 15, No 4, 1986, p 925.
18. Sachs, L: Constitutive uncoupling of pathways of gene expression that control growth and differentiation in myeloid leukemia: A model for the origin and progression of malignancy. Proc Natl Acad Sci USA 77:6152, 1980.
19. Broudy, VC, Zuckerman, KS, and Jetmalani, S: Monocytes stimulate fibroblastoid bone marrow stromal cells to produce multilineage hematopoietic growth factors. Blood 68:530, 1986.
20. Burgess, AW, Camakaris, J, and Metcalf, D: Purification and properties of colony-stimulation factor from mouse lung-conditioned medium. J Biol Chem 652:1998, 1977.
21. Nicola, NA, Metcalf, D, and Matsumot, M: Purification of a factor inducing differentiation in murine myelomonocytic leukemia cells. J Biol Chem 258:9017, 1983.
22. Stanley, ER and Heard, PM: Factors regulating macrophage production and growth: Purification and some properties of the colony stimulation factor from median conditioned by mouse L cells. J Biol Chem 252:4305, 1977.
23. LeBeau, MM, Westbrook, CA, and Diaz, MO: Evidence for the involvement of GM-CSF and FMS in the deletion (5q) in myeloid disorders. Science 31:985, 1986.
24. Pettenati, MJ, LeBeau, MM, and Lemmons, RS: Assignment of CSF-1 to 5q33.1: Evidence for clustering of genes regulating hematopoiesis and for their involvement in the deletion of the long arm of chromosome 5 in myeloid disorders. Proc Natl Acad Sci USA 84:2970, 1987.
25. Roussel, MF, Sherr, CJ, and Barker, PE: Molecular cloning of the c-fms locus and its assignment to human chromosome 5. J Virol 48:770, 1983.
26. Yarden, Y, Escobedo, JA, and Kuang, W-J: Structure of the receptor for platelet-derived growth factor helps define a family of closely related growth factor receptors. Nature 323:226, 1986.
27. Bennett, JM: Classification of the myelodysplastic syndromes. In Clinics in Haematology. WB Saunders, London, Vol 15, No 4, 1986, p 909.
28. Varela, BL, Chuang, C, and Woll, JE: Modifications in the classification of primary myelodysplastic syndrome: The addition of a scoring system. Haematol Oncol 3:55, 1985.
29. Beris, P, Graf, J, and Wiescher, PA: Primary acquired sideroblastic and primary acquired refractory anemia. Semin Hematol 20:101, 1983.
30. Bennett, JM, Catovsky, D, and Daniel, M-T: Proposed revised criteria for the classification of acute myeloid leukemia. Ann Intern Med 103:626, 1985.
31. Linman, JW and Bagby, GC: The preleukemic syndrome (hemopoietic dysplasia). Cancer 42:854, 1978.
32. Weber, RFA, et al: The preleukemic syndrome. I. Clinical and hematological findings. Acta Med Scand 207:391, 1980.
33. Bland, J and Lange, B: Preleukemia in children. J Pediatr 98:565, 1981.
34. First International Workshop on Chromosomes in Leukemia: Chromosomes in acute nonlymphocytic leukemia. Br J Haematol 39:311, 1978.
35. Rowley, JD: Mapping of human chromosomal regions related to neoplasia: Evidence from chromosomes 1 and 17. Proc Natl Acad Sci USA 74:5729, 1977.
36. Van Den Berghe, H, et al: Simultaneous occurrence of 5q— and 21q— in refractory anemia with thrombocytosis. Cancer Genet Cytogenet 1:63, 1979.
37. Billström, R, Nilsson, PG, and Mitelman, F: Cytogenetic analysis in 941 consecutive patients with haematologic disorders. Scand J Haematol 37:29, 1986.
38. Coiffier, B, Adeleine, P, and Viala, JJ: Dysmyelopoietic syndromes. A search for prognostic factors in 193 patients. Cancer 52:83, 1983.
39. Ker Khofs, H, Hagemeijer, A, and Leeksma, CHW: The 5q—

chromosome abnormality in haematological disorders: A collaborative study of 34 cases from the Netherlands. Br J Haematol 52:365, 1982.
40. Knapp, RH, Dewald, GW, and Pierre, RV: Cytogenetic studies in 174 consecutive patients with preleukemic of myelodysplastic syndromes. Mayo Clin Proc 60:507, 1985.
41. Rowley, JD: Non random chromosome changes in hematologic diseases. In Atlas of Blood Cells. Vol 2. Lea & Febiger, Philadelphia, 1981.
42. Mitelman, F: Catalog of Chromosome Aberrations in Cancer, ed 2. Alan R Liss, New York, 1985.
43. Groupe Français de Cytogénetique Hématologique: Cytogenetics of chronic myelomonocytic leukemia. Cancer Genetics and Cytogenetics 21:11, 1986.
44. Heim, S and Mitelman, F: Chromosome abnormalities in the myelodysplastic syndromes. In Clinics of Haematology. WB Saunders, London, Vol 15, no 4, 1986, p 1003.
45. Yunis, JJ: New chromosome techniques in the study of human neoplasia. Hum Pathol 12:540, 1981.
46. Mufti, GF, Stevens, JR, and Oscier, DG: Myelodysplastic syndromes: A scoring system with prognostic significance. Br J Haematol 59:425, 1985.
47. Varela, BL, et al: Modifications in the classifications of primary myelodysplastic syndromes: the addition of a scoring system. Haematol Oncol 3:55, 1885.
48. Todd, WM and Pierre, RV: Pre-leukaemia: A long term prospective study of 326 patients. Blood 62(Suppl 1):184a, 1983.
49. Todd, WM and Pierre, RV: Pre-leukaemia: A long term prospective study of 326 patients. Scand J Haematol 36(Suppl 45):114, 1986.
50. Groupe Français de Morphologie Hématologique: French registry of acute leukemia and myelodysplastic syndromes. Cancer 60:1385, 1987.
51. Mufti, GJ and Galton, DAG: Myelodysplastic syndromes: Natural history and features of prognostic importance. In Clinics in Haematology. WB Saunders, London, Vol 5, No 4, 1986, p 953.
52. Adamson, RH and Sieber, SM: Chemically induced leukemia in humans. Environmental health. Perspective 39:93, 1981.
53. Coleman, CN, et al: Secondary leukemia and non-Hodgkin's lymphoma in patients treated for Hodgkin's disease. In Rosenberg, SA and Kaplan, HS (eds): Malignant Lymphoma: Etiology, Immunology, Pathology, and Treatment. Academic Press, New York, p 259.
54. Pedersen-Bjergaard, J and Larsen, SO: Incidence of acute nonlymphocytic leukemia, preleukemia, and acute myeloproliferative syndrome up to 10 years after treatment of Hodgkin's disease. N Engl J Med 307:965, 1982.
55. Aisenberg, AC: Acute nonlymphocytic leukemia after treatment for Hodgkin's disease. Am J Med 75:449, 1983.
56. Boice, D, Jr, et al: Leukemia and preleukemia after adjuvant treatment of gastrointestinal cancer with semustine (methyl-CCNU). N Engl J Med 309:1079, 1983.
57. Papa, G, et al: Acute leukemia in patients treated for Hodgkin's disease. Br J Haematol 58:43, 1984.
58. Pedersen-Bjergaard, J, et al: Risk of acute nonlymphocytic leukemia and preleukemia in patients treated with cyclophosphamide for non-Hodgkin's lymphomas. Ann Intern Med 103:195, 1985a.
59. Pedersen-Bjergaard, J, et al: Acute nonlymphocytic leukemia, preleukemia, and solid tumors following intensive chemotherapy of small cell carcinoma of the lung. Blood 66:1393, 1985b.
60. Vallespi, T, et al: Myelodysplastic Syndromes: a study of 101 cases according to FAB classification. Br J Haematol 60:19, 1985.
61. Wiesdorf, DJ, et al: Chronic myelodysplastic syndrome: short survival with or without evolution to acute leukemia. Br J Haematol 55:691, 1983.
62. Tricot, F, et al: Prognostic factors in the myelodysplastic syndromes: importance of initial data on peripheral blood counts, bone marrow cytology, trephine biopsy and chromosomal analysis. Br J Haematol 60:19, 1985.
63. Guinan, EC, et al: Bone marrow transplantation for children with myelodysplastic syndromes. Blood 73 (2):619, 1989.
64. Appelbaum, FR, et al: Treatment of preleukemic syndromes with marrow transplantation. Blood 69:92, 1987.
65. Deeg, HJ: Marrow transplantation in preleukemia. J Nat Cancer Inst 76:1329, 1986.

QUESTIONS

1. *Which leukemic trait(s) is/are shared by MDS?*
   a. Excessive cell proliferation
   b. Disturbed cell differentiation
   c. Cell dominance
   d. Combination of two of the above traits

2. *Which of the following is not considered a diagnostic criterion of MDS?*
   a. Dysgranulopoiesis
   b. Bone marrow hypocellularity
   c. Granulocytopenia
   d. Ringed sideroblasts

3. *Which of the following is not a characteristic of refractory anemia?*
   a. Cytopenia
   b. Increased bone marrow iron stores
   c. Ringed sideroblasts >15% of nucleated RBCs
   d. Few blast cells in peripheral blood

4. *What is the most diagnostic criteria for RARS? (Use answer choices for question 3.)*

5. *Based on FAB classification, which of the following bone marrow blast percentages will be consistent with RAEB?*
   a. 5–20%
   b. 20–30%
   c. Over 30%
   d. Less than 5%

6. *What is the most likely terminating disease of RAEB-T?*
   a. CML
   b. CMML
   c. Hodgkin's lymphoma
   d. ANLL

7. *Which of the following chromosomes will be affected in MDS (except CMML)?*
   a. 5
   b. 9
   c. 11
   d. 14

8. *What will adversely affect the prognosis of MDS?*
   a. Lack of any chromosomal abnormality(ies)
   b. FAB score of 1 or 0
   c. Dysplasia(s)
   d. Age under 50

9. *Which of the following is usually not a primary disease that leads to development of secondary MDS?*
   a. Hodgkin's lymphoma
   b. Systemic lupus erythematosus
   c. Polycythemia vera
   d. Multiple myeloma

10. *Which treatment would be appropriate for a 40-year-old patient with RAEB?*
    a. Transplantation therapy and antibiotics
    b. Hormonal treatment, myelostimulants, and antileukemic treatment
    c. Bone marrow transplant
    d. All of the above

ANSWERS

1. b (p 293)
2. b (p 294)
3. c (p 295 – 296)
4. c (p 297)
5. a (p 298)
6. d (p 299)
7. a (p 300)
8. c (p 303)
9. b (p 307)
10. d (p 308)

CHAPTER 20

LAUREL KREWSON HOLMER, M.Ed., M.T.(ASCP) S.H.

Chronic Leukemias

OBJECTIVES

At the end of this chapter, the learner should be able to:
1. List general features of chronic lymphocytic leukemia.
2. Name laboratory methods used to study lymphocytes in lymphoproliferative disorders.
3. List diagnostic criteria of chronic lymphocytic leukemia.
4. Describe treatment for chronic lymphocytic leukemia.
5. Explain differential diagnostic criteria that are used to characterize lymphocytic leukemias, lymphomas, and lymphoproliferative disorders.
6. List general features of chronic myelogenous leukemia.
7. Name laboratory features characteristic of chronic myelogenous leukemia.
8. Describe treatment for chronic myelogenous leukemia.
9. Explain differential diagnostic criteria that are used to characterize chronic myelogenous leukemia.

CHRONIC LYMPHOCYTIC LEUKEMIA

Chronic lymphocytic leukemia (CLL) is included in a general category of conditions known as the lymphoproliferative disorders (Table 20–1). Unlike disorders causing a reactive lymphocytosis such as infectious mononucleosis and viral infections and some cases of large granular lymphocytosis, which generally have a benign clinical course, the other lymphoproliferative disorders are characterized by a monoclonal proliferation and accumulation of malignant lymphocytes. Chronic lymphocytic leukemia is the most common type of all the leukemias and is most frequently a neoplasm of B lymphocytes (B-CLL), although malignant proliferation of T lymphocytes (T-CLL) can also occur. A peripheral blood and bone marrow lymphocytosis dominates the he- matologic abnormalities of CLL. Morphologically, the lymphocytes have a relatively mature, well-dif- ferentiated appearance with a hypercondensed, al- most soccerball-like nuclear chromatin pattern. Bare nuclei called smudge cells are commonly seen (Fig. 20–1) (**see Color Plate 180**). The consequences of the accumulating lymphocyte mass include neu- tropenia, anemia, and thrombocytopenia. The nor- mal bone marrow elements literally get crowded out by the excessive lymphoid production and packing of the marrow space by malignant lympho- cytes. A variable degree of lymphadenopathy or splenomegaly or both may be present. Altered hu- moral immunity in patients with CLL results from suppression of all classes of immunoglobulin, lead- ing to hypogammaglobulinemia and an increased susceptibility to infections. Another important

Table 20–1. **THE LYMPHOPROLIFERATIVE DISORDERS**

Acute lymphoblastic leukemia (ALL)
Chronic lymphocytic leukemia (CLL)
Prolymphocytic leukemia
Non-Hodgkin's lymphomas
Hairy-cell leukemia
Sézary syndrome
T-gamma lymphocytosis (large granular lymphocytosis (LGL))
Reactive lymphocytosis

complication of altered immunity that can develop in the CLL patient is autoimmune disease. The production of autoantibodies may lead to idiopathic thrombocytopenic purpura (Chapter 26) and autoimmune hemolytic anemia (Chapter 14), thus further compromising the patient's hematologic status.

Patients with CLL are typically over 50 years of age at the time of diagnosis and frequently have a prolonged survival, quite often succumbing to an unrelated disorder associated with the elderly; however, some patients die within a few years of diagnosis. Generally 50 percent of CLL patients will be alive 5 years after diagnosis, whereas 30 percent of patients can expect a survival of at least 10 years.

Etiology and Pathophysiology

Although ribonucleic acid (RNA) tumor viruses (retroviruses) are a common cause of leukemia in animals, and exposure to certain agents such as radiation may lead to other chronic leukemias—namely chronic myelogenous leukemia (CML)—there is to date no specific etiologic agent or cause of CLL. A possible viral etiology continues to be investigated since the isolation of a type C retrovirus from the leukemic cells of patients with T-cell malignancies.[1-3] The finding of retroviruslike particles and reverse transcriptase activity in cultured cells

of patients with B-derived CLL[4] supports a viral etiology of CLL, but additional studies are needed. Infection with human T-cell lymphotropic virus type I (HTLV-I) has preceded the development of CLL in some patients.[5]

The pathophysiology of CLL is directly related to the accumulation of "long-lived," immunologically dysfunctional lymphocytes in the peripheral blood and bone marrow. Additional infiltration of the lymph nodes and spleen by the malignant lymphocytes occurs in 50 percent of patients, while cutaneous invasion occurs in 5 percent of patients.[6] As the bone marrow becomes more extensively infiltrated by the leukemic clone, marrow replacement results in anemia, thrombocytopenia, and neutropenia (**see Color Plates 181 and 182**). Organ infiltration can lead to massive adenopathy with splenomegaly, hypersplenism, and subsequent peripheral cytopenias. An increased tendency for hemorrhage further contributes to anemia and compromises hemostasis.

Patients with CLL have significantly impaired immunologic activity. Hypogammaglobulinemia is found in approximately 50 percent of patients with CLL. The deficiency in immunoglobulin leads to infections with a variety of agents. Bacterial infections, especially of the respiratory tract, urinary tract, and skin, as well as viral infections such as herpes zoster and herpes simplex, are common and dramatically contribute to patient morbidity and mortality (Fig. 20–2). Autoimmunity is a phenomenon frequently seen in CLL, with 15 to 35 percent of patients developing autoimmune hemolytic anemia at some time during the course of the disease.[6] Antibodies produced against red blood cells and detected with the direct antiglobulin (Coombs') test may precede, occur simultaneously with, or follow the development of CLL. Red cell aplasia is rare.[7] Autoantibodies to platelets and neutrophils may also develop and lead to immune thrombocytopenic purpura (ITP) and neutropenia. The production of autoantibodies coupled with marrow crowding and hypersplenism can lead to strikingly low peripheral platelet and neutrophil counts. The propensity to develop autoantibodies has not been traced to production by the malignant B-cell clone; however, interestingly, the relatives of patients with CLL have been shown to have an increased risk of autoimmune diseases.[8] Immunoparesis in some patients also includes the production of paraproteins. Bence Jones paraproteinemia has been reported in up to 20 percent of patients with CLL,[9] and heavy-chain paraproteins, either IgM or IgG, can be detected in these patients. Figure 20–3 summarizes the pathophysiology of CLL.

Immunologic Features and Methods for Studying Lymphocytes

In normal adult peripheral blood, 30 percent of the circulating lymphocytes have surface immunoglobulin (SIg) and are B cells, whereas 70 percent have no SIg and are T cells or null cells. Based on

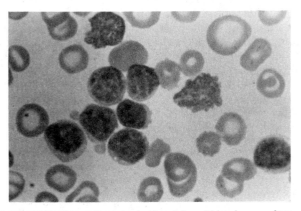

Figure 20–1. Photomicrograph of peripheral blood smear from a patient with CLL. Note the characteristic mature-appearing lymphocyte morphology with hypercondensed nuclear chromatin creating a soccer-ball pattern. Two smudge cells are also seen. Note the lack of platelets in this thrombocytopenic patient.

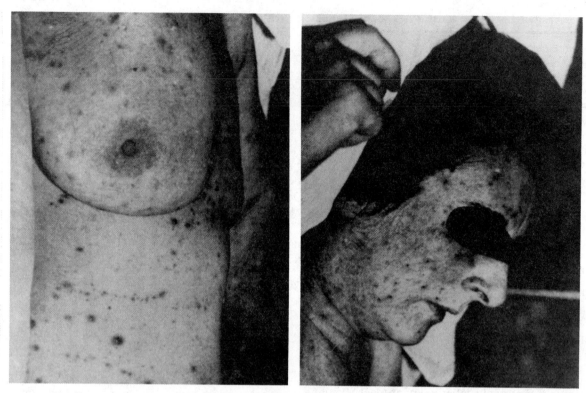

Figure 20–2. Severe generalized herpes zoster with a varicelliform rash in a patient with chronic lymphocytic leukemia. (From Henderson, ES: Diagnosis of Leukemia. In Gunz, FW and Henderson, ES [eds]: Leukemia, ed 4. Grune & Stratton, New York, 1983, p 409, with permission.)

morphologic features alone, it is not possible to distinguish B cells from T cells. When a lymphoproliferative process exists, it is important to be able to characterize the nature of the lymphocytes involved. A number of methods are available to study lymphocytes in lymphoproliferative disorders such as CLL, and these are listed in Table 20–2.

For the most part, the diagnosis of CLL can be done morphologically. Diagnosis is confirmed by a fairly straightforward immunologic characterization of the neoplasm as either B cell or T cell, using the large number of monoclonal antibodies available for detecting differentiation antigens (cluster differentiation [CD] antigens), as shown in Table 20–3. Monoclonal antibodies are homogeneous populations of antibody molecules generally produced by somatic cell hybrids (hybridomas) between activated normal B cells and a plasmacytoma cell line. A list of currently accepted CD designations and some basic information concerning the molecules defined by these antibodies has been established by the Fourth International Workshop and Conference on Human Leukocyte Differentiation Antigens.[9] Monoclonal antibody technology is possible because, as lymphocytes mature from pluripotent stem cells and migrate to lymphoid tissue, they acquire a variety of developmental markers that are helpful in identifying lymphocyte subpopulations. Expression of cell-surface membrane markers in B-cell maturation include SIg, multiple

B-cell antigens, Ia antigens, Fc receptor for IgG, and complement receptors. The malignant B lymphocytes of CLL do not progress normally to the final stages of B-cell development—the plasma cells—but rather appear to be developmentally arrested at an early to intermediate B-lymphocyte stage of differentiation, as seen in Figure 20–4. Studies have shown, however, that under certain in vitro conditions, such as stimulation with phorbol ester, typical CLL cells can undergo transformation to more mature levels of B-cell development.[10,11] In addition to low-density SIg with kappa or lambda light chain, the characteristic phenotype for B-CLL is expression of CD19, CD20 or CD24, and CD5. Of particular interest is the unique expression of CD5 in B-CLL, which has led to much speculation regarding its functional role and mechanisms of regulation. Additionally, high affinity for binding mouse erythrocytes (M rosettes) and low expression of B maturation antigens detected by CD22 typify B lymphocytes of CLL.

As mentioned earlier, T-CLL is rare, but it can be distinguished from B-CLL on the basis of differentiation antigens, as shown in Figure 20–5. The E-rosette receptor, a receptor for sheep red blood cells on T lymphocytes, is another important marker for T-cell identification.

The demonstration of SIg is the classic marker for B cells, while the detection of a predominance of *either* kappa or lambda light chains indicates mono-

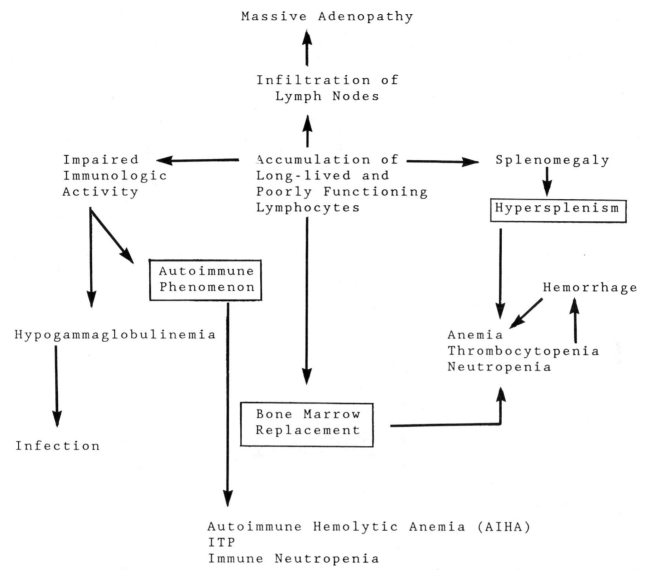

Figure 20-3. The pathophysiology of chronic lymphocytic leukemia. Three major processes typically interact: marrow replacement by long-lived lymphocytes, hypersplenism, and autoimmunity.

clonality.[12] When the conventional techniques fail to reveal the nature of the lymphoid neoplasm, molecular probe technology, using deoxyribonucleic acid (DNA) probes, can often contribute to the diagnosis and classification of malignancy by detecting gene rearrangements that occur in lymphocytes. On a molecular level, the rearrangement of heavy chain immunoglobulin genes, followed by rearrangement of light-chain genes proceeding from mu to kappa to lambda, is the earliest detectable commitment to B-cell development and a demonstration of monoclonality.[13] Monoclonality, rather than polyclonality (the presence of a mixture of kappa *and* lambda–bearing B lymphocytes) is a feature of many malignancies, including CLL; however, it is not, per se, indicative of malignancy. Analogous to immunoglobulin gene rearrangements in B cells is the ability of molecular probes to detect rearrange-

ment patterns of the genes coding for the T-cell receptor (TCR), the antigen-specific surface molecule characteristic of T cells.[14] With the use of Ig and TCR gene probes to detect gene rearrangements at the molecular level, the unusual case of CLL that cannot be diagnosed and classified by morphology and cell markers can now be characterized. It is extremely important that the final diagnosis of any lymphoproliferative disorder is made as a result of composite information from clinical data and from morphologic, histologic and immunologic analysis.

When the number of neoplastic cells is low, a technique for amplifying a specific segment of DNA called the polymerase chain reaction (PCR) can be applied to improve sensitivity. Polymerase chain reaction methodology involves denaturation, primer annealing, and polymerization and yields millions of copies of the originally scarce sequence of DNA.[15]

Table 20-2. **METHODS USED TO STUDY LYMPHOCYTES IN LYMPHOPROLIFERATIVE DISORDERS**

Method	Marker Detected or Feature Demonstrated
Cytochemistry	Absence of peroxidase, Sudan black B, and esterase positivity in lymphoblasts
	Tartrate-resistant isozyme 5 of acid phosphatase (TRAP) in hairy cells
	Localized alpha-naphthol acetate esterase (ANAE) positivity in Golgi area of T cells (i.e., T-ALL, Sézary cell, T-CLL)
Cytogenetics	Consistent chromosomal abnormalities such as t(8;14): B-cell ALL, Burkitt's lymphoma; t(14;18): follicular lymphoma; trisomy 12: CLL, WDLL; t(11;14): WDLL; t(4;11): ALL-FAB classification L_2
Electron microscopy	Nuclear and cytoplasmic ultrastructure such as nuclear whorls in Sézary cells and ribosomal lamellar cytoplasmic aggregates in hairy cells
Immunofluorescence	Surface and cytoplasmic immunoglobulin on B cells TdT on pre-B cells and immature T cells
Immunoperoxidase flow cytometry	Various differentiation antigens on B cells and/or T cells using monoclonal antibodies (see Table 20-3)
Molecular probes	Rearrangements of the B-cell Ig and TCR genes
Rosette formation	Sheep erythrocyte receptor on T cells

Table 20-3. **CLUSTER DIFFERENTIATION (CD) ANTIGENS USEFUL IN MARKING LYMPHOCYTES IN LYMPHOPROLIFERATIVE DISORDERS**

Markers (CD Designation)	Monoclonal Antibodies	Clinical Application
B Cells		
CD5	T1, T101, Leu1	B-CLL, some NHL, T lymphomas
CD9	BA-2 (p24)	Pre-B
CD10	J5, BA-3 (CALLA)	Lymph progenitor, CALL, some NHL
CD19	B4, Leu12	CALL, B-CLL B-PLL, HCL
CD20	B1, Leu16	CALL, B-CLL, B-PLL, HCL
CD24	BA-1	Most B cells
CD22	B3, Leu14	Late B cells, hairy cells
CD25	TAC (IL-2 receptor)	HCL
T Cells		
CD1	T6	Some T-CLL, T-PLL, T-ALL
CD2	T11, Leu5, 9.6 (E rosette)	T-CLL, T-PLL, Sézary cells, LGL, ATLL
CD3	T3, Leu4	T-CLL, T-PLL, Sézary cells, IM
CD4	T4, Leu3	T-PLL, Sézary cells, IM, ATLL
CD5	T1, Leu1, 10.2	T-CLL, T-PLL, Sézary cells, ATLL
CD7	3A1, Leu9	T-PLL
CD8	T8, Leu2	T-CLL, some LGL, IM
CD25	Tac (IL-2 receptor)	ATLL
CD57	Leu7 (HNK1)	LGL

B-CLL = B-lineage chronic lymphocytic leukemia; NHL = Non-Hodgkin's lymphoma; CALL = Common acute lymphocytic leukemia; B-PLL = B-lineage prolymphocytic leukemia; HCL = Hairy-cell leukemia.

T-ALL = T-lineage acute lymphoblastic leukemia; LGL = Large granular lymphocytosis (T-gamma lymphocytosis); ATLL = Adult T-cell leukemia/lymphoma; IM = Infectious mononucleosis; HNK = Human natural killer.

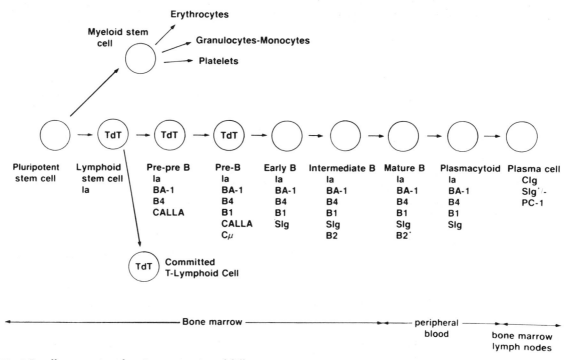

Figure 20–4. B-cell maturation showing expression of differentiation antigens using monoclonal antibodies. Very young B cells have only heavy chains of cytoplasmic IgM, but as the cells mature complete immunoglobulins are detected on the cytoplasmic membrane. Lymphocytes in CLL are developmentally at the early B/intermediate B stage. BA1 = CD24, B4 = CD19, B1 = CD20, B2 = CD21, SIg = surface immunoglobulin; CIg = cytoplasmic immunoglobulin. (From McKenzie, SB: Textbook of Hematology. Lea & Febiger, Philadelphia, 1988, p 72, with permission.)

This technique may be valuable for detecting minimal residual disease in patients who have previously been treated for leukemia or lymphoma but currently lack histopathologic evidence of relapse.[16,17] The purpose of using PCR is to identify as early as possible those patients who will subsequently relapse but who currently have only 1 to 5 percent malignant cells present or have gene rearrangements present in malignant clones that require amplification in order to be detected.

Clinical Features

Chronic lymphocytic leukemia occurs mainly in older adults, with 90 percent of all cases occurring in persons over age 50. In patients under 40 years of age CLL is rare; however, CLL in young adults has been described.[18] Like most other leukemias and myeloproliferative disorders, men are more likely to be affected than women, showing a 2:1 incidence. Unlike acute leukemia, the signs and symptoms of CLL develop gradually and the onset of the disease is difficult to pinpoint. In fact, it is not unusual for the disease to be accidentally discovered during the course of a routine visit to a physician. The duration of a relatively asymptomatic phase of CLL is extremely variable. Unexplained absolute and persistent lymphocytosis; cervical, supraclavicular, and/or axillary lymphadenopathy; and splenomegaly are the earliest signs of CLL. As the

disease progresses, chronic fatigue, recurrent or persistent infections, and easy bruising are consequences of anemia, neutropenia, B-cell immunologic dysfunction, and thrombocytopenia. Hepatomegaly may accompany splenomegaly. Dermatologic manifestations such as nodular and diffuse skin infiltrations, erythroderma, exfoliative dermatitis, and secondary skin infections may occur. Leukemic lymphocytes may invade unusual locations such as the scalp, orbits, subconjunctivae, gums, pharynx, pleura and lung parenchyma, gastrointestinal tract, prostate, and gonads.[19] Chronic lymphocytic leukemia has also been reported to occur simultaneously with acute myeloblastic leukemia (AML).[20]

Laboratory Features

The requirements for the diagnosis of CLL have undergone revision since earlier criteria were established by Rai and colleagues[21] in 1975 and by Binet and co-workers in 1981.[22,23] The most recent diagnostic criteria by the International Workshop on Chronic Lymphocytic Leukemia recommends a minimum peripheral blood B-cell lymphocytosis of $5000/\mu l$ (5×10^9 cells/liter) along with a 30 percent lymphocytosis of the bone marrow consisting of morphologically mature–appearing lymphocytes.[24] These guidelines are similar to an earlier set of criteria established by the National Cancer Institute—

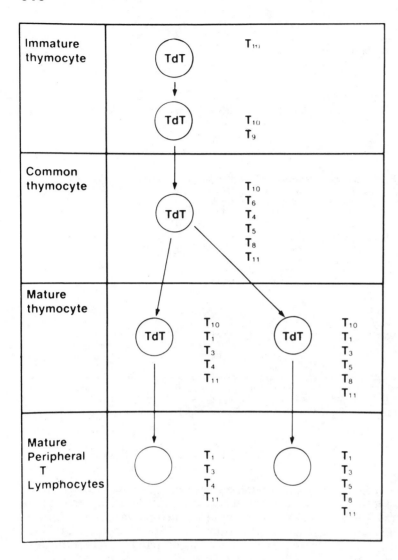

Figure 20–5. T-cell maturation showing immunologic maturation using monoclonal antibodies. Three intrathymic maturation stages precede release of mature T lymphocytes into the peripheral blood. T antigens refer to the antigens detected by OKT antibodies (produced by Ortho Pharmaceutical Corporation) and correlate with CD designation as follows T_1 = CD5, T_3 = CD3, T_4 = CD4, $T_{5,8}$ = CD8, T_6 = CD1, T_{11} = CD2. (From McKenzie, SB: Textbook of Hematology. Lea & Febiger, Philadelphia, 1988, p 70, with permission.)

sponsored working group to assist clinicians in clarifying a diagnosis when borderline disease features were encountered.[25] Anemia, when it occurs, is usually normochromic, normocytic, with a normal or low reticulocyte count. Autoimmune hemolytic anemia may precede, accompany, or follow the development of CLL and be characterized by a secondary reticulocytosis, positive direct antiglobulin test result, and an elevated indirect serum bilirubin level. A decreased platelet count is not uncommon in CLL and is related to bone marrow replacement by leukemic cells, hypersplenism, and/or platelet antibodies.

The lymphocytes of CLL may be morphologically indistinguishable from normal mature lymphocytes when examined with Wright's stain. Alternatively, the leukemic lymphocytes may have exaggerated nuclear chromatin clumping with numerous dark-staining chromatin aggregates separated by light-staining areas of parachromatin. The staining pattern that results from the contrast between the nuclear chromatin and parachromatin resembles the surface pattern of a soccerball, which may be a helpful image to recall in distinguishing the lymphocytes of CLL from those of other lymphoproliferative disorders. The morphology of peripheral blood lymphocytes in CLL is duplicated in the bone marrow aspiration and biopsy specimen (Fig. 20–6). The extent of marrow infiltration varies from patchy accumulations of lymphocytes to diffuse sheets that involve the entire marrow space.

Although the morphologic characteristics of the lymphocytes involved in most cases of CLL are quite distinctive, the membrane phenotype of the proliferating neoplastic cells needs to be determined for a definitive diagnosis. Immunologic features and methods used to characterize lymphocytes as B cells or T cells were discussed earlier under Immunologic Features and Methods for Studying Lymphocytes.

Immune dysfunction within the proliferating B cells is indicated by the presence of hypogammaglobulinemia or hypergammaglobulinemia and monoclonal gammapathy.

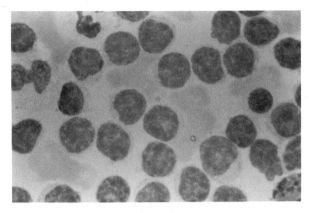

Figure 20-6. Photomicrograph of bone marrow aspirate smear from a patient with CLL. Note monotonous appearance of mature-appearing lymphocytes with condensed nuclear chromatin.

Chromosomal Abnormalities

The malignant lymphocytes of CLL have a low mitotic rate and respond poorly to in vitro stimulation; however, the use of various B-cell mitogens (such as pokeweed, lipopolysaccharide from *Escherichia coli*, Epstein-Barr virus, dextran sulfate, and protein A sepharose) enhances the growth of the leukemic B cells so that enough cells in mitosis can be obtained for chromosomal analysis.[26] The most common chromosomal abnormality in B-CLL is an extra chromosome 12, called trisomy 12, which may occur alone or together with other abnormalities. The placement of chromosomal segments in the 14q band (14q+) and structural alterations on chromosomes 6, 11, 12, or 13 are other common aberrations seen in CLL.[27] Interestingly, some of the sites of chromosomal abnormalities involve the chromosome bands that contain immunoglobulin genes. The site of the human heavy chain gene is 14q32; it is commonly involved in chromosomal translocations in B-lymphoid neoplasms. In fact, 14q32 universally shows up in a reciprocal translocation in Burkitt's lymphoma as t(8;14)(q24;q32) and is also seen in some cases of B-CLL as well as multiple myeloma and small-cell and diffuse large-cell lymphomas.[28] Additionally, oncogenes—the cellular genes which, when genetically altered, have the potential to cause or contribute to malignant expression—have been detected in certain chromosomal segments.[29] The aforementioned 8q24 is the c-*myc* oncogene that is translocated to the 14q chromosome, whereas the proto-oncogene c-k-*ras* is located on chromosome 12. The presence of additional chromosomes as well as multiple chromosomal abnormalities in B-CLL have been implicated as poor prognostic indicators.[30]

Frequently T-CLL is associated with the chromosomal inversion inv(14)(q11;32), an extra 8q, and structural abnormalities in chromosome 7. The site of the alpha TCR locus is 14q11 while the location of the beta TCR locus is 7q35. Rearrangement patterns in the alpha and beta TCR genes provide useful cell-specific markers to identify and study T-cell neoplasms.[31]

Clinical Course, Prognostic Factors, and Staging

The overall median survival for patients with CLL is currently 4 to 5 years. Chronic lymphocytic leukemia can be an indolent disease with an asymptomatic presentation and may not require any treatment until progressive lymphocytosis of the peripheral blood and marrow, lymphadenopathy, splenomegaly, anemia, neutropenia, thrombocytopenia, autoimmune phenomena, and infection develop. This may be as late as some 10 to 15 years from initial diagnosis. In contrast to an indolent course, approximately 20 percent of patients with CLL have a very aggressive clinical course that progresses rapidly from initial diagnosis and results in death within 1 to 2 years. The wide variation seen among patients is not fully understood, but clinical and physical data have been used to try to predict the CLL patient's prognosis and identify various stages and risk groups.

The Rai system,[21] the Binet system,[22] and the International Workshop on CLL system[23] are the three major staging systems developed for CLL; however, only the Rai system is widely used in the United States. The Rai and Binet staging systems, along with median survival for each system by stage, are shown in Table 20-4. The Binet and Rai systems are combined according to the International Workshop on CLL recommendations in the following manner: A(O), A(I), A(II); B(I), B(II); C(III), C(IV). Staging systems for CLL are not able to predict consistently whether a patient's clinical course is more likely to be indolent or progressive. The most reliable predicting factors for indolent CLL are blood lymphocyte doubling time (LDT) greater than 12 months[32] and a nondiffuse pattern of bone marrow lymphocyte infiltration,[33,34] along with a Rai stage of O, I, or II. A short LDT, a diffuse lymphocyte infiltration of the bone marrow, and a Rai staging of III or IV, are associated with a more progressive clinical course.

Three types of transformation in B-CLL have been described: (1) prolymphocytoid transformation, which is relatively low grade and slowly progressive; (2) Richter's syndrome (diffuse large-cell lymphoma); and (3) immunoblastic transformation, which is rapidly progressive and accounts for about 5 percent of all deaths due to CLL.[35] Transformation to acute leukemia is unusual in CLL, unlike the blast cell transformation that is responsible for almost all deaths in chronic myeloid leukemia. Most patients with CLL die without a major or recognizable morphologic change of the leukemic cell population and usually succumb to infection or a cause totally unrelated to their CLL, such as cardiovascular disease. When there is a proliferation of a new population of lymphoid cells—namely, larger cells with immature-appearing morphologic features, finer nuclear chromatin pattern, and a prominent nucleolus—the onset of the terminal transforma-

Table 20-4. **STAGING SYSTEMS FOR CHRONIC LYMPHOCYTIC LEUKEMIA**

STAGE			
Original Rai System	Modified Rai System	Clinical Features	Survival (yr)
0	Low	Lymphocytosis in PB and BM ($\geq 5 \times 10^9$ lymphs/liter in PB, $\geq 30\%$ lymphs in BM)	>12.5
I	Intermediate	Lymphocytosis + enlarged lymph nodes	8.5
II	Intermediate	Lymphocytosis, lymphadenopathy, adenopathy, splenomegaly, ± enlarged spleen	6
III	High	Lymphocytosis + anemia (Hgb < 11 g/dl)	1.5
IV	High	Lymphocytosis + thrombocytopenia (platelets <100 × 10⁹/liter)	1.5
Binet System			
A		2 or fewer node-bearing regions* >10 + no anemia or thrombocytopenia (Hgb ≥10 g/dl, platelets >100 × 10⁹/liter)	>10
B		3 or more node-bearing regions + no anemia or thrombocytopenia	5
C		Anemia and/or thrombocytopenia independent of regions involved	2

PB = Peripheral blood.
BM = Bone marrow.
*Cervical, axillary, inguinal, palpable spleen and liver.

tion of CLL is suggested. This morphologic transformation is often accompanied by the appearance of complex chromosomal changes not present earlier or in addition to the commonly present trisomy 12. The proliferation of a more malignant clone of cells is accompanied by an increasing resistance to therapy and an exceptionally poor prognosis. Because of the leukemogenic potential of agents used to treat CLL, it is likely that the exposure to therapeutic doses of radiation and chemotherapy plays a role in its transformation; however, the possibility of the transformation representing an end phase of the natural history of CLL cannot be ruled out. A variety of techniques are available to help determine whether the transformation represents a clonal evolution of the original CLL or an independent disease; these include cytogenetic analysis, immunoglobulin gene rearrangement by Southern blot analysis, and anti-idiotypic antibodies.[36]

Treatment

Some patients diagnosed with CLL do not require immediate treatment; however, when the signs and symptoms of progressive disease appear, it is time to begin therapeutic intervention. Major physical and clinical signs and symptoms identify advancing disease and are indications for treatment. These include progressive marrow failure with resulting anemia, thrombocytopenia, and neutropenia; progressive lymphocytosis; progressive lymphadenopathy; enlarging spleen; autoimmunity (autoimmune hemolytic anemia or idiopathic thrombocytopenic purpura); increased susceptibility to infection by bacteria, fungi, or viruses; and persistent constitutional symptoms such as night sweats, fever, and weight loss. There is currently no curative therapy for CLL, therefore, the goal of treatment is to reduce signs and symptoms of

disease with minimal discomfort or risk to the patient.

Conventional treatment for CLL is chemotherapy using the oral alkylating drugs chlorambucil (Leukeran), cyclophosphamide (Cytotoxan), and the corticosteroid prednisone. Combinations of chemotherapeutic agents are used for patients refractory to conventional therapy or those with advanced disease. These combination regimens include cyclophosphamide, vincristine (Oncovin), and prednisone (CVP);[37,38] cyclophosphamide, doxorubicin (Adriamycin), vincristine, and prednisone (CHOP);[39] and the Sloan Kettering M-2 protocol consisting of vincristine, cyclophosphamide, BCNU (carmustine), melphalan, and prednisone.[40] Because of the chronic, progressive nature of CLL and the marked variability in the pace of the clinical course, guidelines for patient management have been developed.[25] Table 20-5 summarizes the initial management of patients with CLL according to Rai staging groups.

Numerous chemotherapeutic programs using single agents or multiagent regimens are associated with partial control of disease, but survival is not necessarily prolonged.[41] Additionally, no chemotherapeutic agent can be used without potential side effects. For instance, although the cytoreductive drug chlorambucil is free of side effects such as alopecia or cystitis that result from many cytotoxic agents, it has a powerful cytotoxic effect on pluripotential hematopoietic stem cells. The bone marrow failure that may follow the use of chlorambucil can result in severe anemia and thrombocytopenia. Cyclophosphamide may be less toxic to platelets; however, severe cystitis is a formidable risk. As with the use of chlorambucil, prednisone has a preferentially lymphocytic activity that may result in excretion of large amounts of purine catabolites and the risk of renal insufficiency, due to urate nephropathy,

Table 20-5. MANAGEMENT RECOMMENDATIONS FOR CLL

Rai System Risk Group	Management Recommendation
Low (Stage 0)	Observation each 1-3 mo
Intermediate (Stages I and II)	Chlorambucil, cyclophosphamide, or radiation if symptomatic. Observation only if asymptomatic.
High (Stages III and IV)	Combination chemotherapy: prednisone with chlorambucil or cyclophosphamide *or* Intensive regimens: CHOP (cyclophosphamide, doxorubicin, Oncovin, prednisone), M-2 protocol (vincristine, carmustine (BCNU), cyclophosphamide, melphalan, prednisone)

mandating the administration of allopurinol. The use of aggressive multiagent regimens also presents potential hazards, in addition to presenting a financial burden that may not be justified, given the uncertain likelihood of response or prolonged survival.

Radiation therapy is an alternative or adjunctive approach in treating CLL. Leukemic lymphocytic masses in enlarged lymph nodes and in the spleen may respond to focused, local irradiation to relieve discomfort or eliminate obstruction. As with chemotherapy, irradiation also has its detrimental effects, especially in terms of causing life-threatening neutropenia. Total body or mediastinal irradiation is not commonly used to treat CLL; however, a more generalized remission has been reported using this approach.[42] Splenectomy is recommended in patients with massive splenomegaly and autoimmune hemolytic anemia or autoimmune thrombocytopenia resulting from splenic pooling uncontrolled by chemotherapy;[43] however, this surgery may have considerable risks depending on a number of variables such as patient age, cardiovascular status, and marrow function.[44] Leukopheresis and extracorporeal irradiation are two additional techniques that temporarily lower the white blood cell count but are time consuming and not cost effective compared with conventional chemotherapy.

In addition to chemotherapeutic intervention, the use of high-dose intravenous gammaglobulin therapy prevents major bacterial infections,[45,46] and the immunosuppressant cyclosporin, a fungal metabolite, helps to prevent or treat red cell aplasia — both of which can be management problems in the CLL patient. Experimental therapies are also being studied and include the adenosine deaminase inhibitor deoxycoformycin (Pentostatin),[47,48] fludara-

bine monophosphate,[49,50] 2-chlorodeoxyadenosine,[51] and the use of the monoclonal antibody anti-CD5.[52] Radioimmunoconjugates composed of a monoclonal antibody conjugated to a radioisotope such as ^{131}I and immunotoxins consisting of a monoclonal antibody such as CD19, coupled with a toxin such as the plant toxin ricin,[53] have been developed. Studies on the effectiveness of these types of agents for treating CLL are ongoing. The use of interferon alpha (IFN)-α to treat CLL has been widely studied[54-57] but has shown limited antitumor activity, unlike the highly successful responses seen with hairy-cell leukemia. The lymphoid growth factor, interleukin-2 (IL-2), as well as other biologic mediators of lymphoid activity, is also the target of investigation for clinical trials in the treatment of CLL.[58] Another agent, etoposide, has been used to treat patients with T-cell CLL and CD4 positivity who were refractory to standard CLL chemotherapy.[59]

Bone marrow transplantation (autologous and allogeneic) is being explored as a possible curative therapy for patients with aggressive CLL, especially in patients under age 50.[60]

Differential Diagnosis

As previously outlined in Table 20-1, CLL is a lymphoproliferative disorder that must be differentiated from other malignant or reactive lymphoid proliferations; namely, acute lymphoblastic leukemia (ALL); prolymphocytic leukemia (PL); non-Hodgkin's lymphomas, especially well-differentiated lymphocytic lymphoma (WDLL) and poorly differentiated lymphocytic lymphoma (PDLL); hairy-cell leukemia (HCL); Sézary syndrome; T-gamma lymphocytosis; and reactive lymphocytosis associated with viral infection such as infectious mononucleosis or infection with cytomegalovirus (CMV). The morphologic and immunologic characteristics of these lymphoproliferative disorders are shown in Table 20-6. In addition to these disorders, other hematologic malignancies may be confused with CLL. These include adult T-cell leukemia/lymphoma (ATLL)[61,62] and Waldenström's macroglobulinemia.[63]

The diagnosis of CLL is relatively straightforward and requires a sustained absolute lymphocytosis of mature-appearing lymphocytes in the absence of other causes. When the peripheral blood lymphocyte count is at least 10×10^9/liter (which is typically the case), the finding of either a lymphocyte infiltration of the bone marrow of greater than 30 percent lymphocytes of all nucleated cells or a B-cell phenotype of the circulating lymphocytes is consistent with a diagnosis of CLL. When lymphocyte counts are between 5 and 10×10^9/liter, both bone marrow infiltration of greater than 30 percent lymphocytes *and* B-cell phenotype are necessary for the diagnosis of CLL.

The distinction between CLL and ALL is easily made in most instances based on morphologic differences of the proliferating cell population (Fig.

Table 20–6. **MORPHOLOGIC AND IMMUNOLOGIC CHARACTERISTICS OF LYMPHOPROLIFERATIVE DISORDERS**

Identifying Characteristic	ALL	CLL	PL	PDLL	HCL	Sézary Syndrome	T-Gamma Lymphocytosis	Infectious Mononucleosis
						Disorder		
Predominating or significant cell type	Lymphoblast	"Mature" lymphocyte	Prolymphocyte	"Abnormal" lymphocyte	Hairy cell	Sézary cell	Large granular lymphocyte	Atypical lymphocyte
Nuclear chromatin pattern	Fine	Condensed; "soccerball"	Moderately condensed	Condensed	Fine to moderately condensed	Dark-staining	Condensed	Varies but generally less condensed than normal lymphocyte
Nuclear shape	Varies; round/oval	Regular	Regular	Irregular with cleffs, notches, folds	Regular to slightly irregular; may have some folding	Irregular; many folds	Regular	
Nucleoli prominent	Prominent	Not prominent	Prominent	Not prominent	Not prominent	Not prominent	Not prominent	May be prominent
Cytoplasm	Scanty	Scanty	Scanty to moderate	Scanty	Moderate with hairlike projections	Scanty	Moderately abundant with prominent vacuoles and/or azurophilic granules	Abundant; may have azurophilic granules and/or vacuoles
Cell size	Varies; generally homogeneous population with some variation in size and age	Varies; homogeneous population	Varies; heterogeneous population	Varies	Varies	Varies	Large	Large
Immunologic marker profile	**Common ALL** (early B) (70%) HLA-DR TdT CD19 CD10 (CALLA) CD20 **Early T-cell ALL** (15–20% of ALL is T-cell type)	**B-cell CLL (98%)** Weak SIg (IgM, IgD) HLA-DR CD5 CD19/20/24 CD22 **T-cell CLL (2%)** CD2 (E rosette) CD3 CD8	**B-cell PL (80%)** Strong SIg HLA-DR CD19/20/24 CD22 ±CD10 **T-cell PLL (20%)** CD2 (E rosette) CD3, CD4, CD5 CD7, ±CD8	**B-cell** Strong SIg HLA-DR CD19/20/24 ±CD10 (CALLA)	**B-cell Subset** Strong SIg HLA-DR CD19/20/24 CD22 CD25 (IL-2 Receptor, Tac)	**T-cell Lymphoma** E rosette CD2, CD3, CD4 CD5	**T-cell CLL (LGL)** Fc gamma receptor CD2 (E rosette) CD3 CD8 CD57 (HNK-1)	**Reactive T Cells** CD3 CD8 or CD4

ALL = Acute lymphoblastic leukemia; CLL = Chronic lymphocytic leukemia; PL = Prolymphocytic leukemia; PDLL = poorly differentiated lymphocytic lymphoma; HCL = Hairy-cell leukemia; HNK = Human natural killer cell.

20–7A,B) **(see Color Plates 172 to 174 and 182)**. The smoother nuclear chromatin pattern of the lymphoblast compared with the heavy condensation of nuclear chromatin in the CLL lymphocyte is readily appreciated when examining an appropriate monolayer area or featheredge of a well-stained blood smear. The age of the patient is also helpful when considering a diagnosis of lymphocytic leukemia. Chronic lymphocytic leukemia is typically seen in patients over 50 years of age and only rarely reported in children,[64] whereas ALL is the most common form of childhood leukemia. The dramatic prognostic and therapeutic implications of misdiagnosing a chronic leukemia for an acute leukemia or vice versa cannot be overstated.

Prolymphocytic leukemia (PL) is characterized by a predominance of circulating prolymphocytes (greater than 55 percent, usually greater than 70 percent). Prolymphocytes are larger, less mature-appearing cells than the typical lymphocytes seen in CLL, with moderately condensed nuclear chromatin and a prominent vesicular nucleolus (Fig. 20–C) **(see Color Plate 183)**. The clinical and laboratory features that make PL a distinct disorder include extreme leukocytosis (often more than 100×10^9/liter) and prominent splenomegaly without substantial lymphadenopathy.[65-67] As in all disorders accompanied by leukocytosis, morphologic detail of the predominating cell may not be appreciated unless appropriate areas of well-stained blood and bone marrow smears are examined. Prolymphocytes may be seen in patients with CLL but comprise less than 10 percent of the circulating cells (Fig. 20–7D) **(see Color Plate 184)**. When 11 to 55 percent prolymphocytes are present, a mixed-cell type of CLL, designated CLL/PL, is diagnosed.[68] This category includes patients with prolymphoid transformation.[69] Most cases of PL are B cell in nature (B-PL), as demonstrated by strong SIg (compared with weak SIg in CLL) and reactivity with the B-cell markers CD19, CD20, CD24, and CD22; but T-PL does exist. If four positive criteria for B-CLL are set—weak SIg, greater than 30 percent mouse erythrocyte binding (M rosettes), less than 50 percent CD5-positive cells and less than 30 percent CD22-positive cells—then a combination of three or four of these markers is seen in 80 percent of cases of typical CLL, in 65 percent of CLL/PL cases, and in none of B-PL cases.[70] Two cytochemical techniques that are helpful in distinguishing T cells from B cells are the alpha-naphthol acetate esterase (ANAE) stain and the acid phosphatase reaction.[71] The typical T-lymphocyte pattern with ANAE is one large, localized dot of reaction product positivity **(see Color Plate 185)**.

Well-differentiated lymphocytic lymphoma is a diffuse non-Hodgkin's lymphoma that is characterized by neoplastic transformation of B lymphocytes **(see Color Plate 186)**. When WDLL progresses to a leukemic phase, the circulating cells cannot be morphologically differentiated from those of CLL (Fig. 20–7E) **(see Color Plate 187)**;[72] however, the treatment and prognosis are often quite similar for both.

Poorly differentiated lymphocytic lymphoma, also a non-Hodgkin's lymphoma, consists of B lymphocytes that may be nodular (follicular) or diffuse in distribution[73] **(see Color Plate 188)** and can progress to a leukemic phase. The circulating cells of PDLL are morphologically characterized by nuclei that are irregular in shape and demonstrate irregular clefts, notches, or folds that may traverse the entire width of the nucleus (Fig. 20–7F) **(see Color Plate 189)**. These abnormal lymphocytes typically have very scanty cytoplasm and were formally called "lymphosarcoma cells."[74] As a result of more definitive means of classification, however, that term is no longer used. As compared with immunologic markers in B-CLL, PDLL shows strong SIg, low M-rosette positivity, positive CD22, usually negative CD5, and often positive CD10.

Another form of B lymphocyte–derived chronic leukemia is hairy-cell leukemia (HCL), so named because of the fine, hairlike, irregular cytoplasmic projections that typify the disease (Fig. 20–7G) **(see Color Plate 190)**. Pancytopenia is common in HCL, unlike the other lymphoid disorders discussed in this chapter, along with splenomegaly, marrow fibrosis, and responsiveness to interferon and pentostatin. Because a bone marrow aspirate is often difficult to obtain as a consequence of associated fibrosis (the so-called dry tap), a bone marrow biopsy section is essential for diagnosis and shows hairy cells surrounded by a clear zone that separates one cell from another, creating a "fried-egg" appearance **(see Color Plate 191)**. The most characteristic cytochemical feature of hairy cells is a strong acid phosphatase reaction that is not inhibited by tartaric acid, known as the tartrate-resistant acid phosphatase (TRAP) stain **(see Color Plate 192)**; this enzyme corresponds to the isoenzyme 5 demonstrable on polyacrylamide gel electrophoresis.[75] Immunologic markers that support the diagnosis of HCL are reactivity with CD19, CD20, CD24, and CD25, the monoclonal antibody that recognizes the IL-2 (Tac) receptor. An HCL variant with splenomegaly and a leukocytosis has been described,[76] as has a splenic form of non-Hodgkin's lymphoma that resembles HCL, called splenic lymphoma with villous lymphocytes (SLVL).[77]

The leukemic phase of the cutaneous T-cell lymphoma, mycosis fungoides, is called Sézary syndrome, and is hallmarked by abnormal circulating lymphocytes called Sézary cells.[78] A Sézary cell is typically the size of a small lymphocyte and has a dark-staining, hyperchromatic nuclear chromatin pattern with numerous folds and grooves described as cerebriform (Fig. 20–7H) **(see Color Plate 193)**. Nuclear folding is best appreciated at the ultrastructural level using electron microscopy. A less common large-cell variant of the Sézary cell is larger than a neutrophil and often larger than a monocyte but has the same grooved nuclear chromatin pattern as the smaller Sézary cell. The bone marrow is infrequently involved. The diagnosis of Sézary syndrome is dependent on the primary diagnosis of the cutaneous T-cell lymphoma mycosis fungoides in

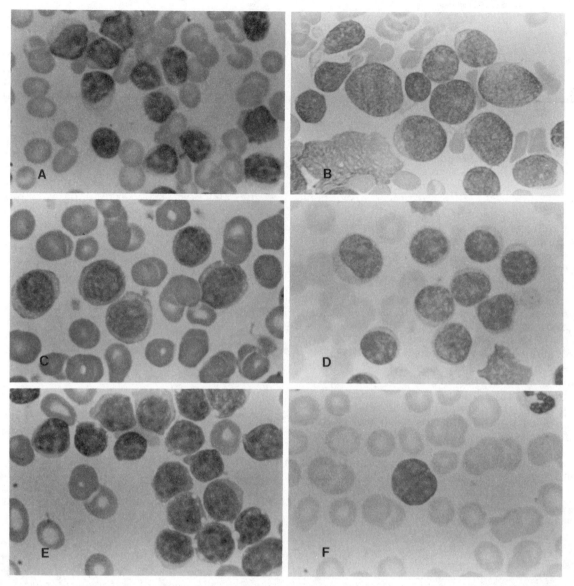

Figure 20–7. Peripheral blood smears of various lymphoproliferative disorders. *(A)* chronic lymphocytic leukemia (CLL), *(B)* acute lymphoblastic leukemia (ALL), *(C)* prolymphocytic leukemia (PL), *(D)*, CLL with occasional prolymphocyte, *(E)* well-differentiated lymphocytic lymphoma (WDLL) in leukemic phase, *(F)* poorly differentiated lymphocytic lymphoma (PDLL) in leukemia phase, *(G)* hairy cell leukemia (HCL), *(H)* Sézary syndrome, *(I)* adult T-cell leukemia/lymphoma, *(J)* T-gamma lymphocytosis with large granular lymphocytes (LGL), *(K)* infectious mononucleosis with atypical lymphocytes, and *(L)* plasma cell dyscrasia.

which a skin biopsy shows the typical pattern of infiltration in the upper dermis with accumulation of lymphocytes, histocytes, and Sézary cells within a vacuole forming structures called Pautrier microabscesses **(see Color Plate 194)**. The nuclear folding of a Sézary cell may, at first glance, suggest a monocytic cell line; however, a monocyte gives a diffuse pattern of cytoplasmic positivity with the nonspecific esterase stain ANAE mentioned earlier, compared with a localized dotlike positivity pattern that identifies T cells. Immunologic marker studies of Sézary cells show a mature T-lymphocyte phenotype with reactivity for CD2, CD3, and CD4, the monoclonal antibody that recognizes the helper/ inducer subset of T lymphocytes; CD8, the mono-

clonal antibody that recognizes the cytotoxic/suppressor subset, does not show reactivity.

Adult T-cell leukemia/lymphoma is more common in the Orient and the Caribbean and is characterized by high titers of the human type C retrovirus HTLV-I, lymphadenopathy, hypercalcemia, bone and skin lesions, and from 10 to 80 percent abnormal lymphoid cells in the blood and bone marrow. The most outstanding feature of these abnormal lymphocytes is the nuclear shape, which often is "cloverleafed" (Fig. 20–7I) **(see Color Plate 195)**. There is marked variation in cell size, ranging from that of a small lymphocyte to that of a large monocyte. Nucleoli are typically inconspicuous but, when present, may be prominent and cause confu-

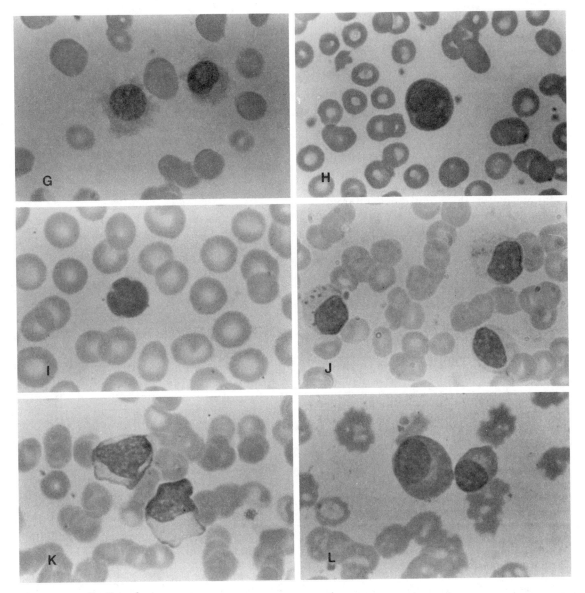

Figure 20–7. *Continued.*

sion with prolymphocytes. The clinical course of ATLL can be acute with a high white count and survival less than 1 year, chronic with a lower white count and survival of more than 1 year, or "smoldering" in which the white count is normal with low numbers of abnormal T lymphocytes. As in T-PL and Sézary syndrome, ATLL cells show reactivity with CD2, CD3, CD4, and CD5, and consistently express CD25, the monoclonal antibody that recognizes the receptor for IL-2.

Chronic T-gamma lymphoproliferative disease has the morphologic distinction of persistent circulating lymphocytes that have abundant cytoplasm that usually contain azurophilic granules (large granular lymphocytes, or LGLs) (Fig. 20–7J) (**see Color Plate 196**). These lymphocytes constitute 50 to 95% of the circulating white cells. This T lymphocytosis is often associated with cytopenias, usually neutropenia, and a chronic and stable clinical course. It is very likely synonymous with T-CLL when the absolute lymphocyte count is more than 5×10^9/liter for longer than 6 months.[79] Immunologic markers demonstrate a spectrum of antigenic profiles but most commonly show a membrane phenotype of CD3 and CD8 reactivity, although more aggressive forms of T-gamma lymphocytosis may show unusual phenotypes. As demonstrated by DNA analysis, the proliferation is clonal, unlike that in reactive T lymphocytosis.

Reactive lymphocytosis is self limiting, rarely exceeds 5×10^9/liter, and is most commonly caused by viral infection such as infectious mononucleosis, viral hepatitis, and infection with CMV in adults and *Bordetella pertussis* in children.[80] The atypical lymphocyte that characterizes the viremia is T cell in origin, has abundant cytoplasm that varies in degree of basophilia, is large with an often irregular nuclear outline resembling a monocyte, and has moderately coarse nuclear chromatin; cytoplasmic vacuolization may be present (Fig. 20–7K) (**see Color Plate 197**). Reactive B-cell lymphocytosis is rare.

The plasma cell dyscrasias—Waldenström's macroglobulinemia, multiple myeloma, and plasma cell leukemia—may be associated with the presence of abnormal circulating plasma cells (Fig. 20–7L) (**see Color Plate 198**). Plasma cells and plasmacytoid lymphocytes are characterized by abundant basophilic cytoplasm, an eccentric nucleus with clumped nuclear chromatin, and a prominent perinuclear clear zone. Plasma cells are end-stage B lymphocytes with the aforementioned characteristic morphology and distinctive immunologic markers—namely, the presence of monoclonal cytoplasmic immunoglobulin and expression of CD38.[80]

CASE STUDY

I.B. was a 74-year-old black woman with a medical history of chronic obstructive pulmonary disease (COPD), hypertension, renal insufficiency, sickle-cell trait, and CLL. Chronic lymphocytic leukemia had been diagnosed in 1973 and treated with chlorambucil and prednisone; an exacerbation of symptoms in 1984 required treatment with chlorambucil, vincristine, and bleomycin. Her last chemotherapy had been in May 1984. In June 1984 a bone marrow specimen showed no lymphoid infiltrates. The patient was doing well until approximately 2 weeks earlier, when she noted generalized fatigue. The day before seeking medical attention her nephew found her to be confused, minimally communicative, and quite weak. She had diarrhea at the time. She was admitted to the hospital after being found unable to speak and rubbing her stomach. In the emergency department the patient became gradually more unresponsive and appeared to be guarding her abdomen. She was intubated. Upon examination, blood was found rectally and in the nasogastric tube. She was also discovered to be markedly acidotic with a pH of 6.7. Her lactic acid was 15.8 mmol/L with no acetone or ketones present and her glucose less than 10 mg/dl. She was found to have DIC, with positive fibrinogen degradation products, a fibrinogen of 48 mg/dl, and prolonged PT and PTT. The patient was thought to be clinically septic and was given clindamycin, gentamicin, and ampicillin. She was treated with sodium bicarbonate for her acidosis, and the DIC was treated with platelets, fresh frozen plasma, and blood products. Blood pressure maintenance was difficult, and the patient became oliguric. A Swan-Ganz catheter was inserted, and supportive care with fluid, blood products, sodium bicarbonate, and pressor agents was continued, but the patient became progressively less responsive. She became edematous, particularly around the face. Blood and urine cultures were negative. Tracheal sputum showed gram-negative rods, and x-ray examination showed an abdominal ileus and increased congestion in the lungs with some left lower lobe atelectasis. The patient had an episode of bradycardia, and then expired.

Autopsy findings were remarkable for a monomorphic lymphocytic infiltrate of lymph nodes, liver, and spleen, which also showed the presence of sickled red blood cells (**see Color Plates 199 through 201**). The pyloric region of the stomach showed a large ulcer that contained necrotic tissue, chronic inflammation, adenocarcinoma, and colonization with nonseptate fungus resembling *Candida* (**see Color Plate 202**). Sections of the trachea showed multiple colonies of fungus with hyphae present along the tracheal epithelium and invading the tracheal mucosa; upon gomori methenemine silver (GMS) staining no septation and branching of the hyphae were shown to be present, consistent with *Candida* infection (**see Color Plate 203**).

This case illustrates how susceptibility to opportunistic infections and immunologic deficiency can contribute to morbidity and mortality in a patient with CLL. Although patients with CLL frequently have a prolonged survival and succumb to an unrelated disorder, the course of CLL varies widely in different patients.

CHRONIC MYELOGENOUS LEUKEMIA

Chronic myelogenous leukemia (CML), also known as chronic granulocytic leukemia (CGL) or chronic myeloid leukemia, is a clonal myeloproliferative disorder of the hematopoietic pluripotent stem cell that has undergone neoplastic transformation and is characterized by excessive production of granulocytes and their precursors.[81–84] Although CML was first described in 1845,[85–87] not until 1960 was it associated with a consistent chromosomal abnormality. This chromosome was called the Philadelphia chromosome (Ph), because it was first identified at the University of Pennsylvania School of Medicine in Philadelphia.[88] This was the first report of a chromosomal abnormality associated with a malignancy and was described as a small, deleted G group chromosome in the metaphases recovered from the bone marrow of patients with CML. Approximately 90 to 95 percent of patients with typical cases of CML carry the Ph chromosome in their leukemic cells;[89] consequently, its presence is virtually diagnostic of the disease. Another hallmark of CML is consistent molecular genetic aberrations involving two proto-oncogenes: c-*abl* and c-*sis*. In addition to the presence of the Ph chromosome, CML is characterized by marked leukocytosis with the presence of all stages of granulocytic maturation, organomegaly (especially splenomegaly), and low levels of leukocyte alkaline phosphatase (LAP). The clinical course may be characterized by three separate phases: (1) the chronic phase, which is generally controllable with chemotherapeutic agents and lasts 2 to 5 years; (2) the chemotherapy-resistant phase called the accelerated phase, which lasts approximately 6 to 18 months; and (3) the blastic acute leukemialike phase called blast crisis, which averages 3 to 4 months and is generally unresponsive to treatment, including those used for de novo acute leukemia,[81,90,91] or the course may be biphasic, in which case the chronic phase progresses directly to blast crisis.

Chronic myelogenous leukemia is primarily considered an adult leukemia because it usually occurs in individuals between 30 and 50 years old. However, the disease can strike any age group, including the elderly, infants, and toddlers. Although rare, when the disease is diagnosed in infants and toddlers, it is called juvenile CML and demonstrates marked hematopoietic, cytogenetic, and clinical differences from the adult form.[92,93] Chronic myelogenous leukemia accounts for approximately 20 to 25 percent of all leukemia cases and in Western countries is diagnosed in about 2 out of every 100,000 people annually, resulting in an estimated 5000 new cases each year.[94] There is a slight male predominance and the median survival is 3 to 4 years once the diagnosis of CML is made.

Etiology, Pathogenesis, and Pathophysiology

Chronic myelogenous leukemia is a clonal stem cell disorder. Although the majority of patients with CML have no history of excessive exposure to ionizing radiation or chemical leukemogens, the implication of causation or presumed role in leukemogenesis of a variety of agents is well documented. These include exposure to ionizing radiation,[95] as was seen in radiologists prior to the use of safety shielding techniques, in patients treated for ankylosing spondylitis, in survivors of nuclear explosions as in the atomic bomb explosions in Hiroshima and Nagasaki, and following the administration of cytotoxic drugs—especially alkylating agents and biologically active chemicals such as benzene.[96] The cause in more than 95 percent of CML cases is unknown. A viral etiology continues to be explored, using animal models.[97] Chronic myelogenous leukemia is not an inherited disease but appears to be acquired, as suggested by the rarity of familial aggregations of CML[98] and the failure of the second member of pairs of identical twins to have or develop the chronic leukemia.[99] The Ph chromosome is not present in nonhematopoietic tissues, nor is it found in parents or the offspring of patients.

The Ph chromosome has been found in neutrophil, monocyte, erythrocyte, platelet, and basophil precursors from CML patient's blood and bone marrow.[100] This unicellular stem cell origin helps to define the translocation that produces the Ph chromosome as a clonal abnormality and provides the subsequent progeny with a growth advantage over normal cells. Chromosomal banding analysis using Giemsa-trypsin (G bands) or quinacrine fluorescent (Q bands) shows that the Ph chromosome is derived from the G-group chromosome 22 rather than chromosome 21 as originally thought.[101-103] In accordance with the standardized system of nomenclature for human genetics established by the Paris conference,[104] the following symbolic designations are used to describe chromosome regions and their alterations: t stands for translocation; the + or − sign when placed before the chromosome number indicates additional or missing chromosomes, and when

placed after the chromosome number indicates an increase or decrease (deletion) in the length of that chromosome. The designation for the short arm of a chromosome is p (the portion above the centromere), and q represents the long arm of the chromosome (the portion below the centromere). The numbers listed immediately after the p and q designations represent the regions and bands along the p or q arm of the chromosome; subbands within a band are indicated by numbers following a decimal point. In CML the main portion of the long arm of chromosome 22 is deleted and translocated most often to the distal end of the long arm of chromosome 9 (or to another chromosome in variant translocations), resulting in an elongated chromosome 9 (9q+). A small part of chromosome 9 is reciprocally translocated to the broken end of the deleted chromosome 22 (22q−). The unequal exchange of chromosomal material results in the tiny or minute chromosome 22, which is smaller than any normal chromosome and is easily recognized as the Ph chromosome under the microscope following appropriate cell culture, harvesting, chromosome preparation, and staining (Fig. 20–8). Thus, the notation for the most common translocation in CML is t(9;22)(q34.1;q11.1), frequently simply referred to as the 9/22 translocation.

Approximately 5 percent of CML patients have the deleted portion of chromosome 22 translocated to other chromosomes[105]—t(4;22), t(12;22), and t(19;22)—called simple variant Ph translocations; other patients have complex variant Ph translocations involving more than one chromosome in addition to chromosome 22[106]—t(9;11;22). Additionally it has been found that on occasion the Ph chromosome may be masked by the presence of chromatin material translocated to the deleted chromosome 22 from one of the other chromosomes involved in the rearrangement.[107] Nonrandom chromosomal abnormalities such as duplication of the Ph chromosome, trisomy 8, and isochromosome 17 are detected in at least 50 percent of patients in accelerated phase of CML and in up to 80 percent of those who develop blastic phase.[108]

Changes at the gene level in proliferating leukemic cells appear to endow clonal advantage on the cell because of gene deregulation or because qualitatively altered gene products are produced. Some of the genes involved in chromosomal alterations

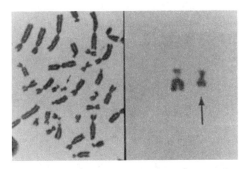

Figure 20–8. Philadelphia chromosome A *(left)* and B *(right).*

have been identified as cellular proto-oncogenes. A proto-oncogene is a normal cellular gene that, when activated by a molecular process such as mutation, deletion, and insertion of DNA sequences, can be converted to an oncogene, a gene that can cause malignant transformation. Human transforming DNA sequences have been found to be homologous to various viral oncogenes (v-onc) and are called cellular oncogenes (c-onc).[109] The proto-oncogene c-abl is the human counterpart to the Abelson murine leukemia virus (v-abl) and normally resides on chromosome 9 at band 9q34, the same location involved in the 9/22 translocation in CML. Since chromosome rearrangements have been shown to be associated with activated genes in appropriate cells,[110] it is possible that regulation of cell growth and differentiation may be expressed inappropriately as a result of chromosomal changes. Breakpoint cluster region (bcr) refers to the narrow 5.8 kilobase DNA fragment localized on chromosome 22 that defines the chromosomal break associated with the Ph chromosome abnormality and is based on restriction enzyme patterns of DNA probes from normal persons and those with CML.[111] In CML the balanced translocation between chromosomes 9 and 22 results in c-abl shifting from 9q34 to the bcr gene at 22q11. The subsequent formation of a bcr/abl hybrid gene product, a 210-kilodalton protein

possessing increased tyrosine kinase activity, provides an important mediator of oncogenesis that may have a potential in the pathophysiology of CML.[112] Most patients with CML have both the Ph chromosome as well as the rearrangement of the bcr/c-abl genes; however, some patients with clinically documented CML lack the Ph chromosome but have the bcr/c-abl gene rearrangement.[113] The gene rearrangement of the bcr region of chromosome 22 can be detected using DNA technology in Southern blots[114] or biotin-labeled gene probes.[115] The molecular basis of the Ph chromosome is summarized in Figure 20–9.

Another cellular oncogene, c-sis, the homologue of the transforming gene of simian sarcoma virus, has been mapped to chromosome 22. In CML, c-sis is translocated from chromosome 22 to a recipient chromosome, usually chromosome 9.[116] The oncogene c-sis encodes sequences for the B chain of platelet-derived growth factor (PDGF)[117] which may play a role in the myelofibrosis which accompanies some cases of CML. The involvement of the cellular proto-oncogenes c-abl and c-sis in the pathogenesis of CML continues to be studied.[118]

The category of Ph-negative CML has led to much discussion in the past.[119–121] Patients whose disease was once diagnosed as Ph-negative CML may be reassigned as a result of the development of criteria

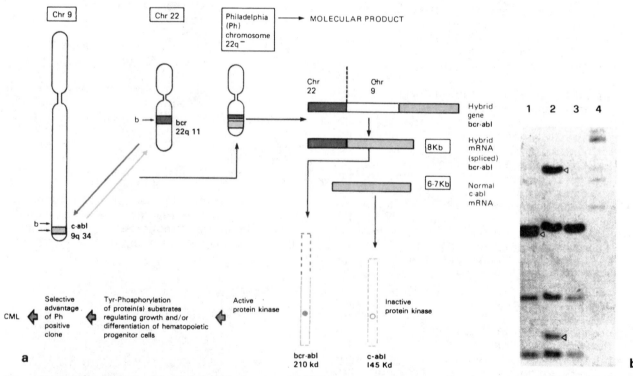

Figure 20–9. Molecular basis of the Philadelphia chromosome. (A) Sequence of molecular and biochemical events involved in generating the Ph-chromosome and its phenotypic consequences, (B) southern blot analysis of DNA from CML cells analyzed with a bcr probe to show clonal rearrangements in the bcr region. (Lane 1) Ph-positive CML DNA showing one rearranged band. (Lane 2) Ph-positive CML (as in Lane 1) but with different breakpoint in bcr region. (Lane 3) Ph-negative leukemic cell DNA showing no rearranged bcr. (Lane 4) molecular weight markers. (From Greaves, MF: Cellular Identification and Markers. In Zucker-Franklin, D, Greaves, MF, et al [eds]: Atlas of Blood Cells. Lea & Febiger, Philadelphia/E E edi-ermes, Milano, 1988, p 43, with permission.)

for the myelodysplastic syndromes (Chapter 19) and other myeloproliferative disorders (Chapter 21). The conditions that are characterized by the absence of the Ph chromosome and are readily distinguishable from CML on clinical and hematologic grounds include chronic neutrophilic leukemia,[122] the myelodysplastic syndrome chronic myelomonocytic leukemia (CMML),[123] and juvenile CML.[92] Rarely, true Ph-negative CML does exist and is diagnosed by the same clinical and hematologic parameters, other than the presence of Ph chromosome, as classic CML. However, in the majority of these patients the molecular defect, namely the juxtaposition of c-abl and bcr genes as seen in typical CML, can be demonstrated even though there is no cytogenetic evidence of the Ph chromosome. Occasionally patients are encountered who lack the Ph translocation, bcr rearrangement, and a bcr/abl gene product, but have a disease phenotype at the time of a diagnosis that is a morphologic facsimile of classic chronic phase CML. The disease in these individuals follows a clinical course that is not marked by increases in blast cells.[124]

Clinical Features

Patients with CML may be asymptomatic or symptomatic. Detecting CML in its early stages may be difficult, and it is not uncommon for the disease to be discovered accidentally during a routine physical examination or hematologic evaluation, analogous to the incidental discovery of CLL. When symptoms do appear, the most common complaints of patients are general malaise; complaints attributable to anemia such as weakness, fatigue, diminished exercise tolerance, dizziness, headache, fever, and irritability; complaints resulting from a hypermetabolic state such as excessive perspiration, night sweats, and weight loss; bone tenderness and aching due to marked marrow expansion; and fullness in the upper abdomen with accompanying easy satiation or loss of appetite resulting from hepatomegaly and splenomegaly. Excessive bleeding after a minor injury or surgical procedure; bleeding in the form of purpura, retinal hemorrhages, or hematuria due to quantitative or qualitative platelet defects; or abnormal or unexplained bruising may also occur. Although less common, patients may experience an increase in infections, attacks of gouty arthritis due to the accumulating uric acid from myeloid cell breakdown, ankle edema, menorrhagia, peripheral vascular insufficiency, and priapism. On rare occasion, the presenting sign of a patient with CML is an infiltrating skin tumor or chloroma, so named because of the characteristic green color of the tumorous mass. Table 20–7 summarizes the clinical signs and symptoms of CML.

Laboratory Features

The laboratory features of CML, like the clinical features, are predominantly caused by the increased body load of myeloid cells, which may be

Table 20–7. CLINICAL SIGNS AND SYMPTOMS OF CHRONIC MYELOCYTIC LEUKEMIA (CML)/CHRONIC GRANULOCYTIC LEUKEMIA (GCL)

1. **Symptoms Related to Hypermetabolism**
   Weight loss, anorexia, low-grade fever, warm moist skin, night sweats, sternal tenderness (characteristic sign present in ⅔ of patients)
2. **Splenomegaly** (present in >90% of patients and frequently massive)
   Associated discomfort, pain, and indigestion
3. **Symptoms Related to Anemia**
   Pallor, dyspnea, tachycardia
4. **Other Physical Signs or Symptoms**
   Bruising or ecchymoses over the extremities, epistaxis, retinal hemorrhages, menorrhagia in females or hemorrhage from other sites

increased greater than 100-fold. The bone marrow produces and releases large numbers of cells, resulting in extreme leukocytosis, often in excess of 100×10^9/liter. A spectrum of myeloid forms is seen in the peripheral blood ranging from blast forms to mature neutrophils (Fig. 20–10) **(see Color Plate 204)**; however, the segmented neutrophil and the myelocyte are the most numerous forms in the differential count. The immaturity seen in the granulocytic series is referred to as a left shift. Eosinophils, basophils, and platelets may be increased (Fig. 20–11), and pelgeroid granulocytes may also be present at any phase of CML **(see Color Plate 205)**. As in other myeloproliferative disorders, the blood smears of patients with CML may demonstrate giant platelets or megakaryocytic fragments or both (Fig. 20–12). A normocytic, normochromic anemia that varies in degree from patient to patient but is frequently associated with hemoglobin levels below 10 g/dl is typically present. Nucleated red blood cells may be present with varying degrees of anisocytosis, poikilocytosis, polychromasia, basophilic stippling, and reticulocytosis (Fig. 20–13). As the

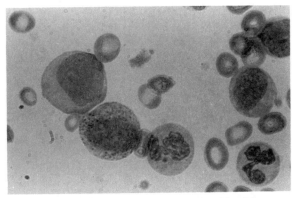

Figure 20–10. Photomicrograph of peripheral blood from a patient with CML showing a blast, promyelocyte, two segmented neutrophils, and a myelocyte.

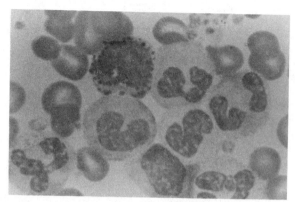

Figure 20–11. Photomicrograph of peripheral blood from a patient with CML showing various stages of myeloid maturation and a basophil.

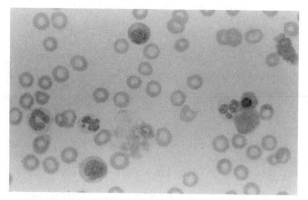

Figure 20–13. Photomicrograph of patient with a left shift in the granulocytic series, anemia, and a nucleated red blood cell consistent with a myeloproliferative disorder.

disease progresses, the degree of anemia may worsen, thrombocytopenia develops, and there may be a shift toward the younger myeloid forms with increasing numbers of blasts. Because CML is a clonal stem cell disorder, all cell lines in the peripheral blood may show quantitative and morphologic abnormalities.[125]

The bone marrow is hypercellular with a marked myeloid hyperplasia with a myeloid-to-erythroid (M:E) ratio of 10:1 instead of the normal M:E ratio of 3:1 (Fig. 20–14) (**see Color Plate 206**). A secondary myelofibrosis may accompany the CML and is diagnosed by examining the bone marrow biopsy specimen stained for reticulin or collagen fibers using a silver stain (**see Color Plate 207**). Sea-blue histocytosis, the appearance of storage cells with deep sea-blue pigmentation, may be seen scattered throughout the marrow of patients with CML. These contain accumulated glycolipids secondary to the expanded membrane turnover of the myeloid cell pool[126,127] (**see Color Plate 208**).

As mentioned earlier in 90 to 95 percent of CML patients, cytogenetic studies of the peripheral blood and bone marrow reveal the hallmark Philadelphia chromosome t(9;22)(q34;q11) resulting from the translocation of the c-*abl* proto-oncogene from chromosome 9 to the bcr gene of chromosome 22, and the reciprocal translocation of the c-*sis* proto-oncogene from chromosome 22 to chromosome 9.

Another characteristic laboratory finding in CML is low to absent levels of LAP, also called neutrophilic alkaline phosphatase (NAP) (**see Color Plates 209 and 210** to contrast absent LAP activity in CML with increased LAP activity in leukemoid reactions). During remission, LAP levels may increase as a reflection of enhanced maturation.[128] Although there is abnormal biochemical reactivity of LAP, not all bacteriocidal and phagocytic functions of the leukemic granulocytes are compromised; however, immunologic function such as adhesion to endothelial cells may be depressed.[129]

Other laboratory findings include elevated uric acid levels, elevated LDH, and increased levels of serum vitamin B_{12} —findings resulting from the increased catabolism of large numbers of granulocytes common to the myeloproliferative disorders.

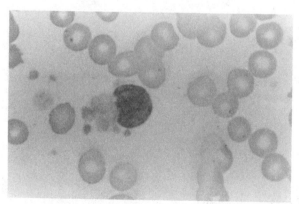

Figure 20–12. Photomicrograph of peripheral blood from demonstrating giant platelets and a megakaryocytic fragment.

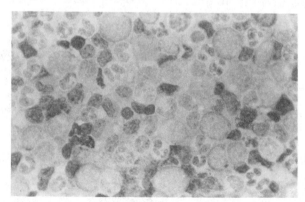

Figure 20–14. Photomicrograph of bone marrow aspirate from patient with CML. Note marked myeloid hyperplasia; 54× magnification.

Clinical Course and Prognostic Factors

As mentioned earlier, CML can be divided into two or three phases: Chronic, accelerated, and/or acute (blastic). The median survival from time of diagnosis is generally 3 to 4 years, and less than 30 percent of patients survive 5 years.[130] However, the chronic phase of CML is unstable and the transformation to the accelerated or blastic phase can occur at any time. In the majority of patients, transformation is associated with development of chromosomal abnormalities in addition to Ph. The blood picture changes from the spectrum of myeloid cells with neutrophils and myelocytes predominating to an increase in the number of blasts and promyelocytes. Systemic symptoms of fever, night sweats, or weight loss reappear or worsen, as does hepatosplenomegaly and extramedullary disease in the lymph nodes, bone, skin, and soft tissue.[131] The median time from development of extramedullary disease to blastic crisis is 4 months, and median survival is 5 months.

Acute blastic phase is the terminal event in CML and resembles acute leukemia in that the cells no longer differentiate to mature granulocytes and there are at least 30 percent blasts present in the bone marrow. The term maturation arrest refers to the absence of cellular differentiation beyond the blast or promyelocyte stage. The blasts of the blastic phase are usually myeloid as demonstrated by myeloperoxidase activity. However, approximately 25 percent of patients develop a lymphoid blast crisis as demonstrated by the immunologic markers terminal deoxynucleotidyl transferase (TdT) and common acute lymphoblastic leukemia antigen (CALLA). Less than 10 percent of patients develop megakaryocytic or erythroid blast crisis. Most patients die of complications arising during blast crisis, the most common of which are bleeding due to thrombocytopenia, infection, therapy-related marrow aplasia, or aplasia exacerbated by progressive myelofibrosis.

The prognosis in CML can be predicted by several factors present at the time of diagnosis which are associated with early transformation to blast crisis. These poor-risk factors include absence of the Ph chromosome or presence of other karyotypic abnormalities in addition to the Ph chromosome, large spleen or liver, thrombocytopenia (less than 150×10^9/liter) or thrombocytosis (greater than 500×10^9/liter), extreme leukocytosis (greater than 100×10^9/liter), peripheral blood blasts more than 1 percent, bone marrow blasts greater than 5 percent, and peripheral blood basophils over 15 percent.[132-135] Chronic myelogenous leukemia in myeloid blast crisis is also considered a poor-risk determinant, compared with lymphoid blast crisis, which traditionally is more responsive to chemotherapy. The morphologic, cytochemical, and immunologic characteristics of blast cells in CML have been widely studied.[136,137] In addition to the aforementioned prognostic factors, analysis at the molecular level in one study correlated the sublocation of bcr breakpoint with differences in the duration of the chronic phase.[114] The number and morphologic characteristics of megakaryocytes in bone marrow sections have also been used to identify histologic types of CML that may have prognostic significance.[138]

Treatment

The usual objective of therapy for the chronic phase of CML is to reduce the proliferating myeloid mass; relieve the symptoms of hyperleukocytosis, thrombocytosis, and splenomegaly; and maintain the patient in a symptom-free condition without causing therapy-related complications. This objective can be achieved by the conventional chemotherapeutic agents busulfan (Myleran) and hydroxyurea (Hydrea); however, neither cytotoxic drug postpones, prevents, or controls blast crisis. The only curative treatment for CML is bone marrow transplantation (BMT).[139]

Bone marrow transplantation can be syngeneic (donor is the patient's identical twin), allogeneic (donor is genetically compatible, most often human leukocyte antigen [HLA]–identical siblings), or autologous (patient's own chronic phase marrow or peripheral blood is transplanted). Syngeneic or HLA-identical allogeneic bone marrow transplantation following high-dose chemotherapy can eradicate the Ph chromosome-containing leukemic clone and is recommended within 1 year of diagnosis for patients in chronic phase under the age of 40 (under 55 at some centers)[140] and for any child with juvenile CML as soon as possible after diagnosis and identification of a suitable donor.[141] For patients without a suitable family donor, donor registries are being established to tally the names of volunteer unrelated allogeneic bone marrow donors. The importance of transplantation in the chronic phase rather than in the accelerated or blast phase is emphasized when considering the survival data. From 49 to 64 percent of patients receiving allogeneic transplants while in chronic phase enjoy long-term survival, compared with 15 to 30 percent for those transplanted in the accelerated phase and approximately 10 percent for those in the acute blastic phase.[142,143] Although transplantation gives CML patients hope for a cure, transplant-related mortality is high (20 to 30 percent), with graft-versus-host disease (GVHD) being a major cause of death. The incidence of acute GVHD can be reduced by depleting the donor marrow of the cells responsible for the GVHD reaction, namely T lymphocytes, by using various methods including T-cell monoclonal antibodies, E rosetting, and soybean lectin agglutination. Additionally, many transplant teams attempt to prevent GVHD by using methotrexate, cyclosporine, glucocorticoids, or a combination thereof. Unfortunately, the use of T depletion for GVHD prophylaxis significantly increases the incidence of leukemic relapse,[144-146] suggesting that the graft-versus-leukemia effect mediated by T lymphocytes is important in the successful cure of CML. Research is ongoing to retain the graft-versus-leukemia effect in spite of T-cell depletion.[147] The ability to determine the success of BMT in terms of detecting minimal residual disease has been dramatically enhanced by the DNA amplification technique called the PCR described briefly in the CLL section of this chapter (see under Immunologic Features and Methods for Studying Lymphocytes).[148-150]

The most popular chemotherapeutic agent used to palliatively treat CML is the oral alkylating agent busulfan (Myleran). Busulfan controls myelopoiesis and thrombopoiesis by acting on stem cells. This results in a slower but more prolonged control of disease than the other commonly used chemotherapeutic drug, the cell cycle–specific, antimetabolite hydroxyurea. Both busulfan and hydroxyurea are administered until there is a 50 percent reduction in the white cell count. As with most therapy, busulfan has side effects consisting mainly of life-threatening pancytopenia if dosage is not carefully monitored and rare, nonetheless severe, nonhematopoietic toxicity resulting in pulmonary fibrosis or a wasting syndrome resembling Addison's disease. Hydroxyurea is less toxic than busulfan and, because of its rapid cytoreductive capabilities, is invaluable in treating patients with leukostasis resulting from hyperleukocytosis syndrome. High-dose hydroxyurea is also being analyzed as a potential treatment to induce partial or complete restoration of Ph chromosome–negative hematopoiesis.[151] Other single chemotherapeutic agents used in CML include cyclophosphamide (cytoxan), 6-mercaptopurine, chlorambucil, thioguanine, melphalan, and dibromomannitol. Adjunctive or alternative measures for treating CML include leukopheresis, splenic irradiation or splenectomy, intensive combination chemotherapy, and immunotherapy; however, none of these approaches are guaranteed to prolong the duration of the chronic phase or improve overall survival. Cytogenetic responses have been reported with some combination regimens.[152]

The response to standard chemotherapeutic regimens is poor once the patient progresses to the accelerated or blast phase of CML. Standard AML therapy (cytosine arabinoside and thioguanine), when used in patients with myeloid blast crisis, rarely results in survival beyond 5 months, whereas patients with lymphoid blast crisis have a median survival of approximately 8 months when treated with standard ALL therapy (vincristine and prednisone). Chemotherapeutic agents for myeloid blast crisis in CML do not kill leukemic blasts in preference to normal hematopoietic blasts. It is the similarity in response of these cell populations to chemotherapy that constitutes the major obstacle to chemotherapeutic treatment of CML in myeloid blast crisis.

As mentioned earlier, interferons, naturally occurring proteins that exist in alpha, beta, and gamma forms, have antitumor activity and have

Table 20–8. DIFFERENTIAL DIAGNOSIS BETWEEN LEUKEMOID REACTION AND CML

	Leukemoid Reaction	CML
Toxic vacuoles	2–4+	0–1+
Toxic granules	2–4+	0–1+
Döhle bodies	Frequent	Rare
Eosinophilia	0	1–3+
Basophilia	0	1–3+
Pseudo-Pelger-Huët	0–1+	Occasional
Karyorrhexis	0–1+	1–2+
Giant bizarre nuclei	1–1+	1–3+
Leukemic hiatus	0	Occasional
LAP score	High	Low (most cases) Normal or high (rare)
Ph chromosome	—	+(85% of cases)

shown promise as a single component or as part of a combined modality to achieve hematologic remission.[153-156]

Differential Diagnosis

Chronic myelogenous leukemia is a myeloproliferative disorder and must be distinguished from the other hematologic disorders in this group, including polycythemia vera, essential thrombocythemia, and agnogenic myeloid metaplasia (Chapter 21). The presence of the Ph chromosome or bcr rearrangement, or both, and low to absent LAP activity are virtually pathognomonic for CML and clearly distinguish it from the other myeloproliferative disorders. Reactive granulocytic leukocytosis such as the leukemoid reaction or leukoerythroblastic blood picture that may accompany bacterial infection or acute hemolysis may be differentiated from CML mainly by their lack of the Ph chromosome and typical molecular aberrations of CML as well as their normal to high LAP levels. Table 20–8 summarizes the differential laboratory diagnosis between leukemoid reaction and CML.

CASE STUDY

E.P. is a 60-year-old white man who initially sought medical attention in March 1979 complaining of fatigue and fever. At that time, his white blood cell count was 45×10^9/liter with a left shift, hemoglobin 11.4 g/dl, hematocrit 35 percent, platelet count 500×10^9/liter, LAP score 0, and his spleen was palpable 8 cm below the left costal margin. The patient's history is significant for multiple exposures to a variety of herbicides and insecticides as a result of his occupation as a farmer. A bone marrow examination and cytogenetic studies revealed hypercellularity with marked granulocytic hyperplasia, an M:E ratio greater than 10:1 and the Philadelphia chromosome t(9q+;22q−). Treatment with the alkylating agent busulfan (Myleran) was started and continued at various intervals for the next 2 years. His white blood cell count began to drop within 2 weeks, and the symptoms of fatigue and fever subsided. The patient continued to do well until April 1983 when he again complained of chronic fatigue and was again found to have marked leukocytosis. He received hydroxyurea for the next 6 months with minimal improvement of his white blood cell count. He was admitted to the hospital 1 month later for further evaluation, which included another bone marrow examination and cytogenetic studies. This bone marrow showed hypercellularity with granulocytic hyperplasia, an M:E ratio of 8:1 with foci of blasts noted upon scanning the bone marrow aspirate and biopsy specimen. In addition to the Ph chromosome, an isochromosome of the long arm of chromosome number 17 (i[17q]) was present. A CBC at this time revealed a white blood cell count of 62×10^9/liter, hematocrit 38 percent, hemoglobin 12.8 g/dl, platelet count 269×10^9/liter, 36 segmented neutrophils, 5 bands, 1 metamyelocyte, 3 myelocytes, 13 promyelocytes, 21 blasts, 13 basophils, 3 lymphocytes, and 5 monocytes; pelgeroid granulocytes were also noted.

The patient was once again started on busulfan. More aggressive therapy was considered and discussed; however, the patient refused further treatment and discharged himself from the hospital against the advice of his physicians.

REFERENCES

1. Gallo, RC, et al: Association of type C retroviruses with a subset of adult T-cell cancers. Cancer Res 43:3892, 1983.
2. Popovic, RC, et al: Isolation and transmission of human retroviruses. Science 219:856, 1983.
3. Poisez, BJ, et al: Detection and isolation of type c-retrovirus particles from fresh and cultured lymphocytes with cutaneous T-cell lymphoma. Proc Natl Acad Sci USA, 77:7415, 1980.
4. Garver, FA, et al: Characterization of a human retrovirus from cultured chronic lymphocytic leukemia B-cells (abstr). Blood 64:202, 1984.
5. Mann, DL, et al: HTLV-I associated B-cell CLL: Indirect role for retrovirus in leukemogenesis. Science 236:1103, 1987.
6. Gale, PR and Foon, KA: Chronic lymphocytic leukemia — recent advances in biology and treatment. Ann Intern Med 103:101, 1985.
7. Chikkappa, G, Zarrala, MH, and Tsan, MF: Pure red cell aplasia in patients with chronic lymphocytic leukemia. Medicine 65:339, 1986.
8. Knapp, W, et al: CD antigens 1989. Blood 4:1448, 1989.
9. Patrick, CW: Chronic lymphocytic leukemia — a biologically diverse disease. Lymphocyte Workshop, University of Wisconsin, Milwaukee, 1985.
10. Conley, CL, et al: Genetic factors predisposing to chronic lymphocytic leukemia and to autoimmune disease. Medicine 5:323, 1980.
11. Caligaris-Cappio, F, et al: Lineage relationship of chronic lymphocytic leukemia and hairy cell leukemia with TPA. Leuk Res 8:567, 1984.
12. Knowles, DM: Lymphoid cell markers. Am J Clin Pathol 9:85, 1985.
13. Korsmeyer, SJ: Antigen receptor genes as molecular markers of lymphoid neoplasms. J Clin Invest 79:1291, 1987.
14. Foroni, L, et al: Rearrangement of the T-cell receptor delta genes in human T-cell leukemias. Blood 73:559, 1989.
15. Dimond, P: About PCR. Diagn Clin Testing 27:12, 1989.
16. Stevenson, MS, et al: Detection of occult follicular lymphoma by specific DNA amplification. Blood 72:1822, 1988.
17. Crescenzi, M, et al: Thermostable DNA polymerase chain amplification of t(14;18) chromosome breakpoints and de-

tection of minimal residual disease. Proc Natl Acad Sci USA 85:4869, 1988.
18. Spier, CM, et al: Chronic lymphocytic leukemia in young adults. Am J Clin Pathol 84:675, 1985.
19. Johnson, LE: Chronic lymphocytic leukemia. Am Fam Physician 38:167, 1988.
20. Conlan, MG and Mosher, DF: Concomitant chronic lymphocytic leukemia, acute myeloid leukemia, and thrombosis with protein C deficiency. Cancer 63:1398, 1989.
21. Rai, KR, et al: Clinical staging of chronic lymphocytic leukemia. Blood 46:216, 1975.
22. Binet, JL, et al: A clinical staging system for chronic lymphocytic leukemia. Cancer 48:198, 1981.
23. Binet, JL, et al: Chronic lymphocytic leukemia: proposals for a revised prognostic staging system. BRJ Haematol 48:365, 1981.
24. Binet, JL, et al: Chronic lymphocytic leukemia: recommendations for diagnosis, staging and response criteria: international workshop on CLL. Ann Intern Med 110:236, 1989.
25. Chenson, BD, et al: Guidelines for clinical protocols for CLL: Recommendations of the NCI-sponsored working group. Am J Hematol 29:152, 1988.
26. Rowley, JD and Testa, JR: Chromosomal abnormalities in malignant hematologic diseases. Adv Cancer Res 36:103, 1982.
27. Yunis, JJ: Chromosomal basis of human neoplasia. Science 221:227, 1983.
28. Gahrton, G, et al: Role of chromosomal abnormalities in chronic lymphocytic leukemia. Blood Review 1:183, 1987.
29. Croce, CM and Kloin, G: Chromosome translocations and human cancer. Science 3:54, 1985.
30. Whang-Peng, J and Knutsen, T: Cytogenetics: Methods and findings in hematologic disease. Laboratory Management 4:19, 1986.
31. Korsmeyer, SJ: Immunoglobulin and T-cell receptor genes reveal the clonality, lineage and translocations of lymphoid neoplasms. Important Advances in Oncology 3, 1987.
32. Montserrat, E, et al: Lymphocyte doubling time in chronic lymphocytic leukaemia: analysis of its prognostic significance. Br J Haematol 62:567, 1986.
33. Rozman, C and Montserrat, E: Bone marrow histologic pattern — the single best prognostic parameter in chronic lymphocytic leukemia: a multivariate survival analysis of 329 cases. Blood 64:642, 1984.
34. Rozman, C and Montserrat, E: Bone marrow biopsy in chronic lymphocytic leukemia. Nouv Rev Fr Hematol 30:369, 1988.
35. Galton, DA: Terminal transformation in B-cell chronic lymphocytic leukemia. Bone Marrow Transplant 4:156, 1989.
36. Foon, KA and Gale, RP: Clinical transformation of chronic lymphocytic leukemia. Nouv Rev Fr Hematol 30:385, 1988.
37. Liepman, M and Votaw, ML: The treatment of chronic lymphocytic leukemia with COP chemotherapy. Cancer 41:1664, 1978.
38. Oken, MM and Kaplan, ME: Combination chemotherapy with cyclophosphamide, vincristine and prednisone in the treatment of refractory chronic lymphocytic leukemia. Cancer Treat Rep 63:441, 1979.
39. Hansen, MM, et al: CHOP versus prednisolone + chlorambucil in chronic lymphocytic leukemia (CLL): Preliminary results of a randomized multicenter study. Nouv Rev Fr Hematol 3:433, 1988.
40. Kempin, S, et al: Combination chemotherapy of advanced chronic lymphocytic leukemia; the M-2 protocols (vincristine, BCNU, cyclophosphamide, melphalan, and prednisone). Blood 60:1110, 1982.
41. Cheson, BD: Current approaches to the chemotherapy of B-cell chronic lymphocytic leukemia: a review. Am J Hematol 32:72, 1989.
42. Richards, F, et al: The control of chronic lymphocytic leukemia with mediastinal irradiation. Am J Med 64:947, 1978.
43. Yam, LT and Crosby, WH: Early splenectomy in lymphoproliferative disorders. Arch Intern Med 133:270, 1974.

44. Spiers, ASD: Chronic lymphocytic leukemia. In Gunz, FW and Henderson, ES (eds): Leukemia, ed 4. Grune & Stratton, New York, 1983, p 709.

45. Cooperative Group for the Study of Immunoglobulin in CLL: Intravenous immunoglobulin for the prevention of infection in CLL. N Engl J Med 319:902, 1988.

46. Bunch, C: Immunoglobulin replacement in chronic lymphocytic leukemia. Nouv Rev Fr Hematol 30:419, 1988

47. Grever, MR, et al: Low dose deoxycoformycin in lymphoid malignancies. J Clin Oncol 9:1196, 1985.

48. O'Dwyer, PJ, et al: 2'-deoxycoformycin (pentostatin) for lymphoid malignancies. Ann Intern Med 108:733, 1988.

49. Grever, MR, et al: Fludarabine monophosphate: A potentially useful agent in chronic lymphocytic leukemia. Nouv Rev Fr Hematol 30:457, 1988.

50. Keating, MJ, et al: Fludarabine (FLU), prednisone (PRED): A safe effective combination in refractory chronic lymphocytic leukemia (CLL). Proc Am Soc Clin Oncol 780:201, 1989

51. Piro, LD, et al: 2-chlorodeoxyadenosine: an effective new agent for the treatment of chronic lymphocytic leukemia. Blood 72:1069, 1988.

52. Foon, KA, et al: Effects of monoclonal antibody therapy in patients with chronic lymphocytic leukemia. Blood 64:1085, 1984.

53. Nadler, L, et al: Anti-B4 blocked ricin immunotherapy for patients with B cell malignancies: Phase I trials of bolus infusions (abstr). Blood 74:121a, 1989.

54. Foon, KA, et al: Phase II trial of recombinant leukocyte A interferon in patients with advanced chronic lymphocytic leukemia. Am J Med 78:216, 1985.

55. O'Connell, MJ, et al: Clinical trial of recombinant leukocyte A interferon as initial therapy for favorable histology non-Hodgkin's lymphomas and chronic lymphocytic leukemia. J Clin Oncol 4:128, 1986.

56. Pangalis, GA and Griva, E: Recombinant alpha-2b-interferon therapy in untreated, stages A and B chronic lymphocytic leukemia. Cancer 61:869, 1988.

57. Rozman, C, et al: Recombinant a_2-interferon in the treatment of B chronic lymphocytic leukemia in early stages. Blood 71:1295, 1988.

58. Kay, NE, et al: Evidence for tumor reduction in refractory or relapsed B-CLL patients with infusional interleukin-2. Nouv Rev Fr Hematol 30:475, 1988.

59. Nierodzik, MJ, et al: Treatment of CD4 chronic lymphocytic leukemia (CLL) with etoposide (abstr). Blood 74:1039, 1989.

60. Michallot, M, et al: Allogenic bone marrow transplantation in CLL. Nouv Rev Fr Hematol 30:467, 1988.

61. Rai, KR, et al: Chronic lymphocytic leukemia. Med Clin North Am 68:697, 1984.

62. Uchiyama, T, et al: Adult T-cell leukemia: Clinical and hematologic features of 16 cases. Blood 50:481, 1977.

63. Krajny, M and Pruzanski, W: Waldenstrom's macroglobulinemia: Review of 45 cases. Can Med Assoc J 114:899, 1976.

64. Sonnier, JA, et al: Chromosomal translocation involving the immunoglobulin kappa-chain and heavy-chain loci in a child with chronic lymphocytic leukemia. N Engl J Med 309:590, 1983.

65. Galton, DAG, et al: Prolymphocytic leukemia. Br J Haematol 27:7, 1974.

66. Katayama, I, et al: B-lineage prolymphocytic leukemia as a distinct clinical pathological entity. Am J Pathol 99:399, 1980.

67. Lampert, I, et al: Histopathology of prolymphocytic leukemia with particular reference to the spleen: A comparison with chronic lymphocytic leukemia. Histopathology 4:3, 1980.

68. Melo, JV, et al: The relationship between chronic lymphocytic leukemia and prolymphocytic leukemia. I. Clinical and laboratory features of 300 patients and characterization of an intermediate group. Br J Haematol 63:377, 1986.

69. Enno, A, et al: "Prolymphocytoid" transformation of chronic lymphocytic leukemia. Br J Haematol 41:9, 1979.

70. Melo, JV, et al: The relationship between chronic lymphocytic leukemia and prolymphocytic leukemia. In Gale, RP and Rai, K (eds): Chronic Lymphocytic Leukemia: Recent Progress and Future Direction. Alan R Liss, New York, 1987, p 205.

71. Catovsky, D and Costello, C: Cytochemistry of normal and leukaemic lymphocytes: A review. Basic Appl Histochem 23:255, 1979.

72. Mann, RB, et al: Malignant lymphomas, conceptual understanding of morphologic diversity. Am J Pathol 94:105, 1979.

73. Aisenberg, AC: Cell lineage in lymphoproliferative disease. Am J Med 75:110, 1983.

74. Mintzer, DM and Hauptman, SP: Lymphosarcoma cell leukemia and other non-Hodgkin's lymphoma in leukemic phase. Am J Med 75:110, 1983.

75. Yam, LT, et al: Tartrate-resistant acid phosphatase isoenzyme in the reticulum cells of leukemic reticuloendotheliosis. N Engl J Med 284:357, 1971.

76. Catovsky, D, et al: Hairy cell leukemia (HCL) variant: An intermediate between HCL and B-prolymphocytic leukemia. Semin Oncol 11:362, 1984.

77. Melo, JV, et al: Splenic B cell lymphoma with circulating villous lymphocytes: Differential diagnosis of B cell leukemias with large spleens. J Clin Pathol 40:642, 1987.

78. Flandrin, G and Brouet, JC: The Sezary cell: Cytologic cytochemical and immunologic studies. Mayo Clin Proc 49:575, 1974.

79. Louhran, TP Jr, et al: Leukemia of large granular lymphocytes: Association with clonal chromosomal abnormalities and autoimmune neutropenia, thrombocytopenia and hemolytic anemia. Ann Intern Med 102:169, 1985.

80. Bennett, JM, et al: Proposals for the classification of chronic (mature) B and T lymphoid leukemias. J Clin Pathol 42:567, 1989.

81. Kantarjian, HM, et al: Chronic myelogenous leukemia—past, present, and future. Hematologic Pathology 2:91, 1988.

82. Champlin, RE: Chronic myelogenous leukemia. In Gale, R (ed): Leukemia Therapy. Blackwell Scientific, Boston, 1986, p 147.

83. Champlin, RE and Golde, DW: Chronic myelogenous leukemia: Recent advances. Blood 65:1039, 1985.

84. Koeffler, HP and Golde, DW: Chronic myelogenous leukemia—new concepts. N Engl J Med 304:1201, 1269, 1981.

85. Bennett, JH: Case of hypertrophy of the spleen and liver, in which death took place from suppuration of the blood. Edinburgh Med Surg J 64:413, 1845.

86. Craigie, D: Case of disease of the spleen in which death took place in consequence of the presence of purulent matter in the blood. Edinburgh Med Surg J 64:400, 1854.

87. Virchow, R: Weisses blut. Froiep Notizen 36:151, 1845.

88. Nowell, PC and Hungerford, DA: A minute chromosome in human chronic granulocytic leukemia. Science 132: 1497, 1960.

89. Rowley, JD: Ph[1]-positive leukemia, including chronic myelogenous leukemia. Clin Haematol 9:55, 1980.

90. Goldman, JM and Lu, Dao-Pei: New approaches in chronic granulocytic leukemia—origin, prognosis and treatment. Semin Hematol 19:241, 1982

91. Spiers, ASD: Chronic granulocytic leukemia. Med Clin North Am 68:713, 1984.

92. Glassy, EF and Sun, NCJ: Juvenile variant of chronic myelogenous leukemia. ASCP Check Sample H85-11, 1985.

93. Chi-Sing, NG, et al: Juvenile chronic myeloid leukemia. Am J Clin Pathol 90:575, 1988.

94. Bertino, JR, et al: Chronic myelogenous leukemia. Leukemia Society of America: Public education and information department booklet, New York, Jan 1988.

95. Gunz, FW: Ionizing radiation and human leukemia. In Gunz, FW and Henderson, ES (eds): Leukemia, ed 4. Grune & Stratton, New York, 1983, p 359.

96. Askoy, M, et al: Leukemia in shoeworkers exposed chronically to benzene. Blood 44:837, 1974.

97. Van Etten, RA, et al: A mouse model for chronic myelogenous leukemia (abstr). Blood 74:185, 1989.

98. Baikie, AG, et al: Cytogenetic studies in familial leukemias. Austral Ann Med 18:7, 1969.

99. Jacobs, EM, et al: Chromosome abnormalities in human cancer: Report of a patient with chronic myelocytic leukemia and his nonleukemic monozygotic twin. Cancer 19:869, 1966.

100. Sandberg, AA: The Chromosomes in Human Cancer and Leukemia. Elsevier, New York, 1980.

101. Whang-Peng, J and Knutsen, T: Cytogenetics: Methods and findings in hematologic disease. Laboratory Management 4:19, 1986.

102. Caspersson, T, et al: Identification of the Philadelphia chromosome on a number 22 by quinacrine mustard fluorescence analysis. Exp Cell Res 63:238, 1970.

103. Prieto, F, et al: Identification of the Philadelphia (Ph^1) chromosome. Blood 35:23, 1970.

104. Paris Conference: Standardization in human cytogenetics. Birth Defects 8:7, 1971.

105. Oshimura, M, et al: Variant Ph^1 translocations in CML and their incidence, including two cases with sequential lymphoid and myeloid crises. Cancer Genet Cytogenet 5:187, 1982.

106. Cork, A: Chromosomal abnormalities in leukemia. Am J Med Technol 49:703, 1983.

107. London, B, et al: A new translocation in chronic myeloid leukemia — t(4;9;22) — resulting in a masked Philadelphia chromosome. Cancer Genet Cytogenet 20:5, 1986.

108. Kantarjian, HM, et al: Characteristics of accelerated disease in chronic myelogenous leukemia. Cancer 61:1441, 1988.

109. Bishop, MJ: Cellular oncogenes and retroviruses. Annu Rev Biochem 52:301, 1984.

110. Hunter, T: Oncogenes and protooncogenes: How do they differ? J Natl Cancer Inst 73:773, 1984.

111. Groffen, J, et al: Philadelphia chromosomal breakpoints are clustered within a limited region, bcr, on chromosome 22. Cell 36:93, 1984.

112. Sandberg, AA, et al: The Philadelphia chromosome: A model of cancer and molecular cytogenetics. Cancer Genet Cytogenet 21:129, 1986.

113. Ganesan, TS, et al: Rearrangement of the bcr gene in Philadelphia chromosome-negative chronic myeloid leukemia. Blood 68:957, 1986.

114. Shtalrid, M, et al: Analysis of breakpoints within the bcr gene and their correlation with the clinical course of Philadelphia-positive chronic myelogenous leukemia. Blood 72:485, 1988.

115. Telzer, LL and Concepcion, EG: Detection of the gene rearrangement in chronic myelogenous leukemia with biotinylated gene probes. Am J Clin Pathol 91:464, 1989.

116. Groffen, J, et al: C-sis is translocated from chromosome 22 to chromosome 9 in chronic myelocytic leukemia. J Exp Med 158:9, 1983.

117. Doolittle, RF, et al: Simian sarcoma virus gene, v-sis is derived from the gene (or genes) encoding a platelet derived growth factor. Science 221:275, 1983.

118. Champlin, R: Chronic leukemia: Oncogenes, chromosomes and advances in therapy. Ann Intern Med 104:671, 1986.

119. Travis, LB, et al: Ph^1-negative chronic granulocytic leukemia: a nonentity. AJCP 85:186, 1986.

120. Fitzgerald, PH and Beard, MEJ: Ph-negative chronic myeloid leukemia. Br J Haematol 66:311, 1987.

121. Pugh, WC, et al: Philadelphia-negative chronic myelogenous leukemia: A morphological reassessment. Br J Haematol 60:457, 1985.

122. Krause, JR: Chronic neutrophilic leukemia. American Society of Clinical Pathology Tech Sample H-2, Chicago, 1989.

123. Bennet, JM, et al: The French-American-British (FAB) cooperative group. Proposals for the classification of the myelodysplastic syndromes. Br J Haematol 51:189, 1982.

124. Kurzrock, R, et al: Philadelphia-negative CML without bcr rearrangement: A chronic myeloid leukemia with a distinct clinical course (abstr). Blood 74:102, 1989.

125. Fialkow, PJ, et al: Chronic myelocytic leukemia: clonal origin in a stem cell common to the granulocyte, erythrocyte, platelet and monocyte/macrophage. Am J Med 63:125, 1977.

126. Brigden, ML and Preece, EV: An electrolyte abnormality in a case of chronic granulocytic leukemia. Lab Med 15: 761, 1984.

127. Ulirsch, R: Sea-blue histiocytosis in chronic myelocytic leukemia. American Society of Clinical Pathology Tech Sample H-4, Chicago, 1985.

128. Rosner, F, et al: Leukocyte alkaline phosphatase: Fluctuations with disease status in chronic granulocytic leukemia. Arch Intern Med 130:892, 1972.

129. Gordon, MY, et al: Adhesive defects in chronic myeloid leukemia. Curr Top Microbiol Immunol 149:151, 1989.

130. Sokal, JE: Evaluation of survival data for chronic myelocytic leukemia. Am J Hematol 1:493, 1976.

131. Terjanian, T, et al: Clinical and prognostic features of patients with Philadelphia chromosome positive chronic myelogenous leukemia and extramedullary disease. Cancer 59:297, 1987.

132. Gomez, GA, et al: Prognostic features at diagnosis of chronic myelocytic leukemia. Cancer 47:2470, 1981.

133. Tura, S, et al: Staging of chronic myeloid leukemia. Br J Haematol 47:105, 1981.

134. Sokal, JE, et al: Prognostic discrimination in "good-risk" chronic granulocytic leukemia. Blood 63:789, 1984.

135. Cervantes, F and Rozman, C: A multivariate analysis of prognostic factors in chronic myeloid leukemia. Blood 60:1298, 1982.

136. Polli, N, et al: Characterization of blast cells in chronic granulocytic leukaemia in transformation, acute myelofibrosis and undifferentiated leukaemia. I. Ultrastructural morphology and cytochemistry. Br J Haematol 59:277, 1985.

137. San Miguel, JF, et al: Characterization of blast cells in chronic granulocytic leukaemia in transformation, acute myelofibrosis and undifferentiated leukaemia. II. Studies with monoclonal antibodies and terminal transferase. Br J Haematol 59:297, 1985.

138. Lorand-Metze, I, et al: Histological and cytological heterogeneity of bone marrow in Philadelphia-positive chronic myelogenous leukaemia at diagnosis. Br J Haematol 67:45, 1987.

139. Alfan, NC: Therapeutic options in chronic myeloid leukemia. Blood Review 3:45, 1989.

140. Thomas, ED and Clift, RA: Indications for marrow transplantation in chronic myelogenous leukemia. Blood 73:861, 1989.

141. Sanders, JE, et al: Allogeneic marrow transplantation for children with juvenile chronic myelogenous leukemia. Blood 71:1144, 1988.

142. Goldman, JM, et al: Bone marrow transplantation for chronic myelogenous leukemia in chronic phase. Ann Intern Med 108:806, 1988.

143. McGlave, PB, et al: Therapy of chronic myelogenous leukemia with allogeneic bone marrow transplantation. J Clin Oncol 5:1033, 1987.

144. Santos, GW: Problems and strategies for bone marrow transplantation in acute leukemia and chronic myelogenous leukemia. Cancer Detect Prev 12:589, 1988.

145. Apperley, JF, et al: Bone marrow transplantation for chronic myeloid leukemia in first chronic phase: Importance of a graft-versus-leukaemia effect. Br J Haematol 69:239, 1988.

146. Goldman, JM: Allogeneic bone marrow transplantation: State of the art and future directions. Bone Marrow Transplant 4:131, 1989.

147. Champlin, R, et al: Selective CD8 depletion of donor marrow: retention of graft-versus-leukemia effect following bone marrow transplantation for chronic myelogenous leukemia (abstr). Blood 74:95, 1989.

148. Kohler, S, et al: Application of the polymerase chain reaction to the detection of minimal residual disease after bone marrow transplantation for patients with chronic myelogenous leukemia (abstr). Blood 74:96, 1989.

149. Synder, DS, et al: Definition of remission based on the expression of bcr-abl RNA following bone marrow transplant for chronic myelogenous leukemia in chronic phase (abstr). Blood 74:97, 1989.

150. Lee, M, et al: Clinical usage of polymerase chain reaction to analyze the bcr/abl splicing patterns and minimal residual disease in Philadelphia chromosome-positive chronic myelogenous leukemia (abstr). Blood 74:745, 1989.

151. Kolitz, JE, et al: Phase II trial of high-dose hydroxyurea in chronic myelogenous leukemia (abstr). Blood 74:577, 1989.

152. Kantarjian, H, et al: High doses of cyclophasphamide, BCNU and etoposide induce cytogenetic responses in most patients with advanced stages of Philadelphia chromosome-positive chronic myelogenous leukemia (abstr). Blood 74:1032, 1989.

153. Talpaz, M, et al: Chronic myelogenous leukemia: Hematologic remissions and cytogenetic improvements induced by recombinant alpha A interferon. N Engl J Med 314: 1065, 1986.

154. Niederle, N, et al: Interferon alpha-2B in the treatment of chronic myelogenous leukemia. Semin Oncol 16:29, 1987.

155. Higno, CS, et al: Alpha interferon induced cytogenetic remissions in patients who relapse with chronic myelogenous leukemia after allogenic bone marrow transplantation (abstr). Blood 74:307, 1989.

156. Talpaz, M, et al: Sustained complete cytogenetic responses among Philadelphia positive chronic myelogenous leukemia patients treated with alpha interferon (abstr). Blood 74:289, 1989.

QUESTIONS

1. Which features are characteristic of chronic lymphocytic leukemia (CLL):
   a. Most commonly a neoplasm of B lymphocytes; neutropenia; anemia; thrombocytopenia; hypogammaglobulinemia; autoimmune disease; may be caused by retroviruses
   b. Most commonly a neoplasm of T lymphocytes; lymphocytopenia; increased erythropoiesis; giant platelets; hypergammaglobulinemia; marked splenomegaly; may be caused by repeated bacterial infections
   c. Most commonly a neoplasm of plasma cells; leukopenia; hemolytic anemia; thrombocytosis; normal globulin levels; hemorrhagic disorders; may be caused by pre-existing autoimmune condition
   d. Most commonly a neoplasm of null cells; leukocytosis; normal RBC, hemoglobin, and platelets; hypergammaglobulinemia; marked lymphadenopathy; may be caused by neoplastic processes

2. Which of the following methods is not used for studying lymphocytes in lymphoproliferative disorders?
   a. Flow cytometry
   b. Cytochemical stains
   c. Molecular probes
   d. Chromatography

3. Which of the following diagnostic criteria is indicative of CLL?
   a. Minimum peripheral lymphocyte count of 50,000/mm³; 30% lymphoblastic infiltration of bone marrow; macrocytic, hypochromic anemia; increased mitogen response; usually no chromosomal abnormalities
   b. Minimum peripheral T-cell count of 7000/mm³; 50% lymphoblastic infiltration of bone marrow; microcytic, hypochromic anemia; normal mitogen response; presence of Philadelphia chromosome
   c. Minimum peripheral B-cell count of 5000/mm³; 30% lymphocytosis of bone marrow with mature-appearing lymphocytes; normocytic, normochromic anemia; decreased mitogen response; presence of trisomy 12
   d. Minimum peripheral leukocyte count of 150,000/mm³; 30% mature lymphocyte bone marrow infiltrate; normocytic, hypochromic anemia; normal mitogen response; presence of trisomy 14

4. What is the usual treatment for CLL?
   a. Primarily bone marrow transplant, followed by immunosuppressive therapy
   b. Chemotherapy, radiation therapy, radioimmunoconjugates, and biologic mediators
   c. Chemotherapy and bone marrow transplant
   d. Intravenous immunoglobulin therapy and immunosuppressive therapy

5. Which of the following indicates a diagnosis of CLL rather than other lymphoproliferative disorders?
   a. Absolute lymphocytosis of mature-appearing lymphocytes
   b. Predominance of circulating prolymphocytes
   c. Lymphocytes with irregular clefts or folds that show strong SIg, low M-rosette positivity, and CD22 positivity
   d. Hairy cells with strong TRAP reaction

6. Which feature is not characteristic of chronic myelogenous leukemia (CML):
   a. Presence of Philadelphia chromosome
   b. Consists primarily of a rapid cellular proliferation phase
   c. Excessive bleeding
   d. Weakness and increase in infections

7. Which list shows the primary laboratory features of CML?
   a. Leukocytosis with mature-appearing granulocytes; slightly decreased LAP; 1:3 M:E ratio; normocytic, hypochromic anemia
   b. Leukocytosis with blast forms; increased LAP; 3:1 M:E in bone marrow; microcytic, hypochromic anemia
   c. Leukocytosis with hypersegmented cells; normal LAP: 1:10 M:E ratio in bone marrow; macrocytic, hypochromic anemia
   d. Leukocytosis with all stages of granulocytic maturation; low to absent LAP; 10:1 M:E ratio in bone marrow; normocytic, normochromic anemia

8. What is the primary treatment for CML?
   a. Radiation and chemotherapy
   b. Chemotherapy and immunosuppressive agents

    c. Chemotherapy and bone marrow transplantation
    d. Biologic modifiers

9. *Which of the following indicates a leukemoid reaction rather than CML?*
    a. Absence of eosinophils and basophils in the peripheral blood
    b. Low LAP score with myeloblasts through segmented neutrophils in the peripheral blood
    c. Ph chromosome
    d. Blast crisis as the terminal phase of the disease

ANSWERS

1. a (p 312–313)
2. d (p 316)
3. c (p 317–319)
4. b (p 320–321)
5. a (p 321)
6. b (p 326–327)
7. d (p 329–330)
8. c (p 331)
9. a (p 332)

CHAPTER 21

BARBARA S. CALDWELL, M.T.(ASCP)S.H.

Myeloproliferative Disorders

OBJECTIVES

At the end of this chapter, the learner should be able to:
1. Describe the origin of myeloproliferative disorders.
2. List characteristics for chronic myeloproliferative disorders.
3. Identify the predominant abnormal erythrocyte morphology associated with idiopathic myelofibrosis.
4. Select features for myelofibrosis that distinguish it from chronic myelogenous leukemia.
5. List laboratory findings for polycythemia vera.
6. Select features for secondary polycythemia and relative erythrocytosis that distinguish them from polycythemia vera.
7. Describe the therapeutic control of polycythemia vera.
8. Name conditions that may cause an absolute erythrocytosis.
9. Recognize diagnostic criteria for essential thrombocythemia.

The term myeloproliferative disorders (MPDs) was proposed in 1951 by Dr. William Dameshek to describe a closely related group of acquired, malignant disorders that share several common clinical and hematologic features. He speculated on the presence of a common myelostimulatory factor that, under certain conditions, would cause prolif-eration of both hematopoietic cells and fibroblasts in the bone marrow. According to Dameshek, this factor also appeared to activate dormant embryonal hematopoietic tissue in the spleen and liver (extra-medullary hematopoiesis).[1] Myeloproliferative disorders classically embrace the clinical entities of chronic myelocytic leukemia, polycythemia vera, idiopathic myelofibrosis, and essential thrombocythemia. Although recent discoveries regarding hematopoiesis have necessitated certain modifications to the original hypothesis, the Dameshek concept of myeloproliferative syndrome has been widely accepted.

The MPDs may be divided into two groups, acute and chronic. The former include all the variants of acute nonlymphocytic leukemia (ANLL), which are morphologically designated according to the predominant cell type. The ANLL variants have been classified according to the French-American-British (FAB) system as M0 through M7 and all are characterized by excessive proliferation of immature cells (see Chapter 18 for complete discussion of these diseases). The chronic MPDs include chronic myelocytic leukemia (CML), polycythemia vera (PV), idiopathic myelofibrosis (IMF), and essential thrombocythemia (ET) (Table 21–1).

The evidence for the clonal and therefore neoplastic nature of the MPDs is derived from cytogenetic analysis isoenzyme studies of glucose-6-phosphate dehydrogenase (G6PD) and clonogenic assays.[2,3] These studies demonstrate that the hematopoietic abnormalities arise from a neoplastic transformation of a single multipotential stem cell; a progenitor cell that is committed to differentiation of myeloid cell lines (that is, granulocytes, monocytes, platelets, and erythrocytes).[4] Adams and coworkers[5] postulate that the increased sensitivity of the precursor granulocyte-macrophage, megakaryocytic, and erythroid progenitor cells to small amounts of growth factor accounts for the variably programmed predisposition of the affected stem cells to undergo transformation into abnormal blast-forming cells, as well as the subsequent deranged production of a spectrum of mature cells.

The specific entities within the myeloproliferative classification are designated according to the predominant cell type involved. Therefore, the most prominent features would be excessive production of granulocytes in CML, overproduction of erythrocytes in PV, and overproduction of platelets in ET. Idiopathic myelofibrosis is recognized by a prominence of marrow fibrosis and extramedullary hematopoiesis in the liver and spleen. The finding of a variable amount of fibrosis may complicate any of the chronic MPDs. Studies show, however, that the marrow fibroblasts do not share a common ancestry with the pluripotent hematopoietic precursor cell responsible for the hyperplasia and dysplasia that characterize each of the MPDs. Cell karyotypes and G6PD expression have both revealed the bone marrow fibroblasts to be polyclonally derived.[3,6] Therefore, fibrosis is thought to reflect a reactive rather than an intrinsic neoplastic process. (As mentioned earlier, the acute MPDs are discussed in Chapter 18 and the reader is referred to Chapter 20 for a discussion of chronic myelocytic leukemia).

There is a close qualitative and quantitative identity at the committed precursor cell level for IMF, PV, and ET, and, as such, these diseases will be discussed at length in this chapter. Cell culture studies by Adams and associates[5] suggest a progression of increasing abnormality in the stem cells, from the least abnormal in PV to the intermediate abnormality in ET to the most abnormal state in IMF. The pathophysiology, clinical, and laboratory findings, as well as therapy for each of these chronic MPD variants, are reviewed in detail.

COMMON CLINICAL AND HEMATOLOGIC FEATURES OF THE CHRONIC MYELOPROLIFERATIVE DISORDERS (MPDs)

All of the clinical variants of the chronic MPDs share, to varying extents, the following characteristics:

1. Predominantly affecting middle-aged and older groups
2. Insidious, sometimes asymptomatic onset
3. Panhyperplasia of bone marrow (granulocytic with or without monocytic, erythrocytic, and megakaryocytic elements)
4. Extramedullary hematopoiesis (myeloid metaplasia) manifested primarily in the spleen and less frequently in the liver
5. Bone marrow fibroblastic proliferation and reticulin/collagen formation
6. Transition often occurring between these disorders; overlapping manifestations possibly causing difficulty in classification (Fig. 21–1)
7. Increased propensity for terminating in acute leukemia
8. Bone marrow may demonstrate large numbers of megakaryocytes, sometimes atypical in appearance
9. Evidence of platelet dysfunction

Table 21–1. **MYELOPROLIFERATIVE DISORDERS (MPDs)**

Acute MPDs
Acute nonlymphocytic leukemia
  Acute myelogeneous leukemia
  Acute promyelocytic leukemia
  Acute myelomonocytic leukemia
  Acute monocytic leukemia
  Erythroleukemia
Unusual Variants
  Megakaryocytic leukemia
  Eosinophilic leukemia
  Basophilic leukemia
Chronic MPDs
  Chronic myelogeneous leukemia
  Idiopathic myelofibrosis/agnogenic myeloid metaplasia
  Polycythemia vera
  Essential or idiopathic thrombocythemia

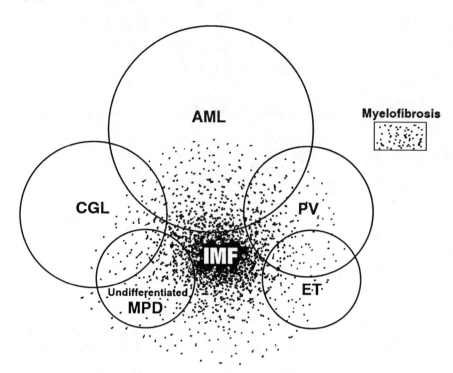

Figure 21–1. Myelofibrosis in the myelo-proliferative variants. Myelofibrosis occurs in a wide spectrum of myeloprolif-erative diseases, but is a predominant feature of idiopathic myelofibrosis (IMF). AML = acute myeloblastic leukemia, PV = polycythemia vera, ET = essential thrombocythemia, CGL = chronic gran-ulocytic leukemia (Adapted from Lewis,[19] p 17.)

10. Cytogenetic abnormalities, the most com-mon, in decreasing order of frequency, being 20q−, +8, +9, 13q−, and partial trisomy 1q7 (the Philadelphia chromosome +9;22 is present in about 90 percent of patients with CML)

A comparison of the amount of cellular prolifera-tions, leukocyte alkaline phosphatase (LAP), and cytogenetic findings in the MPDs is provided in Table 21–2.

SPECIFIC CHRONIC MPDs
Idiopathic Myelofibrosis

Definition and History

Within the family of myeloproliferative dis-orders, IMF is an important entity. The syndrome is characterized by the classic triad of findings of (1) fibrosis of the marrow, at first patchy and later widespread, which may or may not be accompanied by sclerosis; (2) extramedullary hematopoiesis or myeloid metaplasia of the spleen and liver; and (3) leukoerythroblastosis and teardrop poikilocy-tosis of the peripheral blood.

The first record of IMF was reported in 1879 by Heuck,[8] who described the case of a 24-year-old butcher who had been afflicted with severe fatigue for 1 year. Upon examination, severe anemia, leu-kocytosis with myeloid immaturity, and marked hepatosplenomegaly were noted. The patient sur-vived for only 2 years and, on autopsy, was demon-strated to have severe osteosclerosis and extrame-dullary hematopoiesis. Heuck[8] thus concluded, based on the unique features of the case, that mye-lofibrosis with myeloid metaplasia was distinct from leukemia.

Table 21–2. **DIFFERENTIAL CHARACTERISTICS OF THE CHRONIC MPDs**

	CML	Idiopathic Myelofibrosis	Polycythemia Vera	Essential Thrombocythemia
Erythrocytes	0−↓	0−↓	4+	0−1+
Granulocytes	4+	1−2+	1−2+	0−1+
Platelets	0−3+	0−3+	1−3+	4+
Fibroblasts	0−2+	2−4+	0−2+	0−2+
NRBCs	Rare	Common	Rare	Rare
LAP	↓↓	N−↑	Usually ↑	N
Bone marrow	Marked myeloid hyperplasia	Fibrosis, dry tap	Hypercellular, ↓ iron stores	Hypercellular, ↑↑↑ megakaryocytes
Special studies	Ph¹ chromosome	Marrow imaging	RBC mass ↑	—

According to Wintrobe, at least 37 synonyms have been assigned to this disease. Some of the most frequently used are agnogenic myeloid metaplasia, myelosclerosis, osteosclerosis, chronic erythroblastosis, aleukemic myelosis, and chronic or primary myelofibrosis. Recently the term idiopathic myelofibrosis with myeloid metaplasia (IMF/MM), or just idiopathic myelofibrosis for brevity, has been applied to this disorder, highlighting the essential features of fibrosis and extramedullary hematopoiesis.

Incidence, Epidemiology, and Etiology

There have been a limited number of epidemiologic studies on IMF. An overall annual incidence of 0.6 per 100,000 in western Australia was found by Woodliffe and Douigan[9]; the disease was stated to be one-quarter as common as chronic myelocytic leukemia in Denver by Ward and Block.[10] Male-to-female ratio is approximately 2:1. The age distribution is generally between 50 and 70; therefore, as with other MPDs, most IMF cases occur in middle-aged and elderly people. In the below 30 age group, fewer than 30 cases of this disorder have been reported.[11] Certain racial factors of interest have been studied. Idiopathic myelofibrosis is said to be rare in African and Spanish Americans[10] and is still occurring in the Japanese as a sequelae of the atomic bomb explosions there. It is generally more prevalent in white persons born in Europe, who have subsequently moved to Australia, than in other ethnic groups in that country.[9]

As the name implies, the etiology of the majority of patients with IMF is unknown. Exposure to ionizing radiation is most likely a factor in the development of some cases, as an increased incidence of IMF has been reported in survivors of the Hiroshima atomic bomb blast.[12] Myelofibrosis secondary to exposure to toxins such as benzene, toluene, arsenic, lead, and fluorine has been documented.[7,13] Conditions associated with abnormal immunologic mechanisms have been implicated in the genesis of IMF, as evidenced by its development in patients with systemic lupus erythematosus[14] and by the existence in a majority of IMF patients of a high proportion of peripheral leukocytes containing immune complexes.[15] Myelofibrosis has also occurred secondary to chronic infections, especially tuberculosis and histoplasmosis, and after myocardial infarction; however, the fibrosis seen in these disorders represents a secondary or reactive process.

In the setting of myeloproliferative disorders, a virtually identical syndrome develops in up to 20 percent of patients with polycythemia vera, as well as a small number of patients with essential thrombocythemia, and can be related to previous ^{32}P therapy.[16]

Pathogenesis

Stem Cell Defect. The hematopoietic abnormalities in idiopathic myelofibrosis arise from the mutation of a single multipotential stem cell, with bone marrow fibrosis occurring as a secondary, non-neoplastic process. As such, the pathogenesis of progenitor cell defect must be considered separately from that of the fibrosis.

The clonal proliferation of abnormal progenitor cells colony-forming unit-granulocyte/monocyte (CFU-GM) and colony-forming unit megakaryocyte (CFU-MK) has been well documented by isoenzyme and cytogenetic studies. Khan[17] and Jacobson[3] and their colleagues showed that in women heterozygous for G6PD isoenzymes A and B, the bone marrow fibroblasts express both isoenzymes but the blood cells express only one type. This finding, therefore, suggests that the blood cells are clonally derived, whereas the fibroblasts do not proliferate as a result of the malignant clone. Furthermore, Van Slyck and associates[18] showed that the blood cells from an IMF patient had a consistent chromosomal abnormality, in comparison to bone fibroblasts, which had normal karyotypes.

Marrow Fibrosis. The pathogenesis of fibro-osteosclerotic changes characterizing IMF is controversial. However, there is general agreement that the myelofibrosis is related to an increase in marrow collagen accumulation and that the source of collagen synthesis is in the fibroblasts. Hematopoietic cells, their products, or both, provide the provoking stimulus to activate the marrow collagen—producing cells, thus establishing the reactive nature of fibrosis.

A number of factors have been described that are capable of stimulating fibroblastic proliferation. There is current evidence that megakaryocytes are intimately involved in the pathway whereby increased collagen deposition takes place and as such are a prerequisite for osteosclerotic changes. One of the most fully characterized in terms of its biologic properties is platelet-derived growth factor (PDGF), which is released from abnormal megakaryocytes and platelets. An essential feature causally promoting the release of PDGF is ineffective megakaryopoiesis with intramedullary death of megakaryocytes.[7,20] Several reports postulate that immune complexes also interact with platelets to cause release of PDGF with subsequent activation of fibroblastic proliferation and collagen deposition. Furthermore, platelet factor 4, a cationic polypeptide synthesized by megakaryocytes and contained in platelet alpha granules, inhibits collagenase activity, thereby offsetting the natural balance between marrow collagen production and degradation. This action conversely leads to enhancement of myelofibrosis.[21]

Vitamin D appears to play a role in the regulation of collagen deposition in the marrow. Calcitriol (1,25-dihydroxyvitamin D_3), the active metabolite of vitamin D_3, inhibits collagen synthesis by suppressing megakaryocyte proliferation.[22] A deficiency of this factor would allow abnormal accumulation of marrow collagen hence leading to development of myelofibrosis (Fig. 21–2). The histologic course of IMF encompasses several phases.

In the so-called cellular phase of IMF the bone marrow displays panhyperplasia with a predominance of megakaryocytes. As the disease progresses there is deranged marrow architecture with an in-

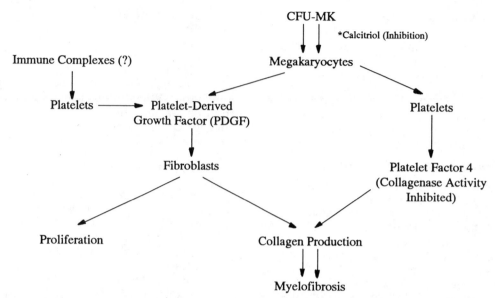

Figure 21–2. Schematic representation of possible relationships involved in collagen deposition in myelofibrosis.
*Calcitriol, 1, 15 $(OH)_2$ D_3 is the active metabolite of vitamin D_3.

crease in reticulin (or a neutral soluble collagen type III) and a progressive change to and deposition of the type I collagen, which is insoluble and cross linked. It is this type that occurs in IMF.[19] A marked increase in fibroblast and collagen proliferation, along with new bone formation are the hallmarks of the osteosclerotic phase.

The disturbance to the normal hematopoietic microenvironment is responsible for the hematologic abnormalities characteristic of IMF: increase in circulating stem cells, trilineage proliferation and dysplasia (particularly dysmegakaryocytopoiesis), and extramedullary hematopoiesis.[19]

Clinical Features

Myelofibrosis is a chronic progressive disorder with an insidious onset such that the patient may be symptom-free for many years. In about one third of cases, diagnosis is made following a routine physical examination and the incidental finding of unexplained splenomegaly and/or abnormal peripheral blood results. As the myeloid metaplasia gradually increases with eventual enlargement of the spleen and sometimes liver (see Color Plate 211), the patient will present with the customary sensations of splenomegaly; namely, left- or mid-abdominal fullness and distension and early satiety for food intake, resulting from decreased abdominal capacity due to splenic encroachment. With massive splenomegaly, urinary frequency and incontinence may be a problem. The splenomegaly in IMF is more pronounced than in almost any other disease.

Patients also present with the signs and symptoms of anemia, including weakness, pallor, lethargy, and dyspnea on exertion. Less than 10 percent of patients present with a serious bleeding diathesis,

but thrombocytopenia, qualitative platelet defects, and coagulation abnormalities may cause petechiae, ecchymoses, and gastrointestinal or urogenital bleeding. Bone pain is an occasional feature, usually occurring later in the disease process.

The metabolic consequences of myelofibrosis often result in the symptoms of night sweats, fever, itching, anorexia, and weight loss. Gout may be a complication stemming from hyperuricemia. Ward and Block[10] found gout in 16 percent of the patients with massive splenomegaly. Jaundice or ascites has been observed in a few patients, although the hepatomegaly is not generally excessive.

Extramedullary Hematopoiesis (Color Plate 212)

Splenomegaly is present to a varied degree in all patients. The spleen is mildly enlarged in one third of patients, palpable 5 cm below the left costal margin in another third, and massively enlarged in the remaining third.[23] The extraordinary splenic hyperplasia present in IMF is multifactorial in origin. The enlargement is due to a combination of extramedullary hematopoiesis and fibrosis, as well as congestion from increased blood flow through the celiac axis. The exaggeration of red cell pooling is so pronounced that up to two thirds of the red cell mass may be detained in transit through the splenic cords. Hematopoietic precursors evicted from the bone marrow find a hospitable surrogate microenvironment in the spleen and, to some extent, in the liver and lymph nodes. Stem cells capable of self-renewal give rise to neoplastic islands that may circulate via the splenic vein to other reticuloendothelial system organs. Extramedullary tumors may occasionally arise in the central nervous system, accounting for symptoms of speech impairment, semiblindness, partial paralysis, coma, and possibly death if the intracranial space has been invaded.[21]

Radiologic Features

Myelofibrosis is defined as an increase in fine fibers (reticular) in the marrow; myelosclerosis means an increase in coarse fibers (collagen), and osteomyelosclerosis refers to an additional new bone formation.[19] Approximately 40 to 50 percent of patients demonstrate radiologic osteosclerosis. The most readily recognizable pattern is diffuse increase in bone density in the long bones. In most cases this finding is readily visible on chest x-ray examinations.

Hematologic Findings

A normocytic, normochromic anemia is found in most patients at presentation and becomes more severe as the myelofibrosis progresses. The anemia results from a complex reaction of factors representing the additive effects of bone marrow failure, ineffective erythropoiesis, or dyserythropoiesis; pooling

of over 35 percent of the erythrocyte mass in the enlarged spleen (dilutional anemia); and an underlying hemolysis due to hypersplenism. In half of the anemic patients, there is shortened red cell survival due again to the ineffective erythropoiesis combined with hyperplasia. When severe hemolytic anemia occurs evidenced by marked reticulocytosis, it is generally antiglobulin (Coombs') test negative. However, in some cases of IMF, the erythrocytes are mildly Coombs' positive, resulting from deposition of IgG and IgM immune complexes and complement on the erythrocyte surfaces.[21]

Occasionally patients develop a hypochromic, microcytic anemia secondary to gastrointestinal bleeding or peptic ulcer, and sometimes the hyperproliferative state induces folate deficiency and a concomitant megaloblastic macrocytosis.

As the myelofibrosis progresses, the morphologic changes become increasingly abnormal and the classic leukoerythroblastic blood picture unfolds **(see Color Plate 213)**. The characteristic findings are the appearance of nucleated red cells, immature granulocytes, and teardrop poikilocytosis (Fig. 21–3). Improvement or even normalization of red cell

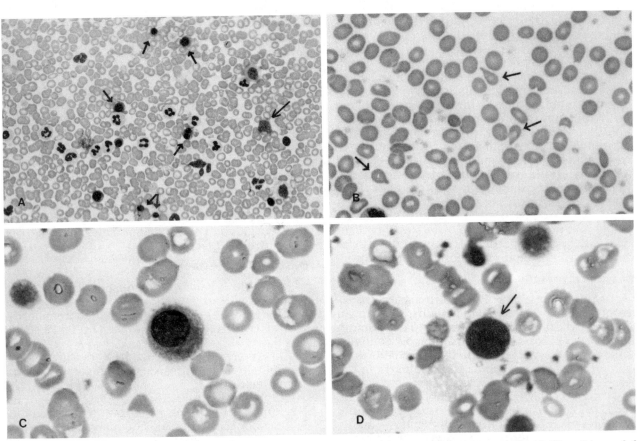

Figure 21–3. Leukoerythroblastosis, teardrop poikilocytosis, and abnormal platelet morphology associated with idiopathic myelofibrosis. (A) Leukoerythroblastosis. Note the myeloblast at the large arrow and the numerous nucleated red blood cells at the small arrows. (B) Teardrop poikilocytosis. (C) Dwarf megakaryocyte (or micromegakaryocyte). This pathologic alteration of a megakaryocyte may be found in any of the myeloproliferative disorders. Although often difficult to distinguish from cells of other lineages, observation of the marked cytoplasmic granularity and further comparison of this cytoplasm to that of other platelets present on the peripheral smear will aid in identification. (D) Dwarf megakaryocyte. The cell at the pointer displays cytoplasmic blebs or budding of platelets which is another characteristic of a micromegakaryocyte. Also note the giant platelets present on this peripheral blood smear.

morphology following splenectomy supports the concept of a causative relationship between splenic fibrosis and red cell changes.[24] Marrow fibrosis in conjunction with splenic fibrosis presumably accounts for teardrop formation, as the erythrocytes assume the teardrop shape (see Color Plate 214) upon passage through narrow, fibrotic sinusoids of the bone marrow and spleen.

The leukocyte count is variable in IMF. In about half of cases the white blood cell (WBC) count exceeds 10.0×10^9/liter; in approximately 35 percent the WBC count is normal; and in nearly 15 percent the WBC count is below normal.[10,25] As the disease evolves, the leukocyte level declines with an increase of immature myeloid cells dominating the peripheral blood picture, but not to the degree seen in acute myelocytic leukemia. In rare cases in which the WBC count exceeds 100×19^9/liter, the diagnosis of chronic myelocytic leukemia may be erroneously applied. The leukocyte alkaline phosphatase (LAP) score is typically normal or moderately increased. Serum levels of vitamin B_{12} are increased, but not to the degree found in untreated CML.

The platelet count may be normal, elevated, or decreased. In approximately 50 percent of IMF patients platelet counts are increased at time of diagnosis, and concentration may occasionally be in excess of 1000×10^9/liter. As the disease progresses, thrombocytopenia becomes increasingly prevalent. Giant dysplastic platelets are often conspicuous, and megakaryocytic fragments or even dwarf megakaryocytes may be present in the peripheral blood (Fig. 21–3). These findings attest to malignant platelet physiology and support the correlation of platelet dysfunction found in up to 50 percent of patients.[26] Platelet adhesiveness is often reduced and conversely spontaneous aggregation may occur, clinically resulting in increased risk of hemorrhage or thrombosis. According to one study by Silverstein,[23] the bleeding time (a measure of platelet number and function) was prolonged in 20 percent of patients, which is particularly important in relation to gastrointestinal or cerebral hemorrhage.

Bone Marrow Findings

Attempts at bone marrow aspirations are unsuccessful in nearly 90 percent of patients, resulting in the so-called dry tap of myelofibrosis. The reticulin and collagen fibrosis locks in the marrow contents, making a needle biopsy essential for a reliable diagnosis. Trilineage hyperplasia is found early in the disease, along with nonuniform fibrosis. At later stages, there are decreasing numbers of hematopoietic islands with residual foci consisting mainly of clumps of dysplastic megakaryocytes. Finally, marked hypocellularity is observed, and fibrotic features begin to predominate. In less than 10 percent of patients, osteosclerosis (new bone deposition) occurs (Table 21–3).

Coagulation Abnormalities

Platelet dysfunction (mentioned earlier) can cause troublesome hemostatic complications in

Table 21–3. **HISTOLOGIC COURSE OF IDIOPATHIC MYELOFIBROSIS**

1. Cellular Phase
   a. Diffusely hyperplastic; normal maturation of erythropoiesis and granulopoiesis
   b. Megakaryocytes may predominate; some immature forms
   c. Reticulin ± increase
2. Fibrotic Phase
   a. Megakaryocytes still predominant; decreasing numbers of other hematopoietic cells
   b. Altered sinus architecture
   c. Reticulin ++
   d. Collagen +
3. Sclerotic Phase
   a. Grossly disturbed architecture
   b. Markedly reduced hematopoiesis
   c. Megakaryocyte megakaryoblast clusters
   d. Fibroblasts +++
   e. Reticulin +++
   f. Collagen +++
4. Osteosclerotic Phase
   a. Fibroblasts +++
   b. Collagen +++
   c. Osteocyte proliferation with bone formation

Source: From Lewis, SM,[19] p 4, with permission.

IMF patients. In addition, patients in approximately half of the cases demonstrate prolonged prothrombin (PT) and thrombin times (TT), as well as elevated levels of fibrin degradation products and reduced levels of factors V and VIII. These features suggest occult disseminated intravascular coagulation (DIC). A normal euglobulin lysis time or a Fibrinosticon (Ortho Diagnostics) test may be useful in differentiating DIC from primary fibrinolysis.[4]

Hepatic dysfunction is found in many patients in the later stages of the disease, setting the scene for both coagulation factor deficiencies, chronic DIC, and fibrinolytic activation.

Differential Diagnosis

Idiopathic myelofibrosis must be distinguished from other diseases within the spectrum of the chronic MPDs, as well as differentiated from fibrosis secondary to infiltrative disorders (Tables 21–2 and 21–4).

The American Polycythemia Vera Study Group has defined myelofibrosis as encompassing the following features:
1. Splenomegaly
2. Fibrosis involving more than one third of the sectional area of an adequate bone marrow biopsy specimen
3. A leukoerythroblastic blood picture
4. Absence of increased red cell mass
5. Absence of Philadelphia (Ph) chromosome
6. Exclusion of systemic disorders
7. A diagnosis of osteomyelosclerosis requires the presence of sclerotic changes detected radiologically in axial skeleton long bones[7]

Table 21-4. **DIFFERENTIAL DIAGNOSIS OF MYELOFIBROSIS**

I. Idiopathic myelofibrosis/agnogenic myeloid metaplasia
II. Other chronic myeloproliferative disorders
  A. Chronic myelogeneous leukemia
  B. Polycythemia vera
  C. Essential thrombocythemia
  D. Transitional myeloproliferative disorders
III. Infiltrative disorders/secondary causes of myelofibrosis
  A. Metastatic carcinoma
  B. Granulomatous disorders
    1. Sarcoidosis
    2. Tuberculosis
    3. Histoplasmosis
  C. Hematologic malignancies involving bone marrow
    1. Acute leukemia
    2. Hairy-cell leukemia
    3. Myelodysplastic syndromes (preleukemia)
    4. Non-Hodgkin's lymphoma

Source: Adapted from Hoogstraten, B,[4] p 34, with permission.

Chronic myelogeneous leukemia is the disease considered most frequently in the differential diagnosis of IMF. In chronic cases of CML there is marked leukocytosis, whereas in IMF the WBC count is usually less than 30×10^9/liter. Red cell morphology in CML is generally normal or may show a slight amount of anisocytosis and poikilocytosis, compared with the significant teardrop poikilocytosis in IMF. The presence of the Ph[1] chromosome and the low LAP score are the strongest differentiating features that distinguish CML from IMF. Ordinarily, differentiation from CML is not difficult. However, in atypical cases such as Ph[1]-negative CML it may be virtually impossible to characterize CML as a separate entity from IMF with leukocytosis and minimal fibrosis (the cellular phase of IMF).

Approximately 15 to 20 percent of patients with known PV undergo a transition to terminal myelofibrosis with marked anemia, bone marrow fibrosis and hypofunction, and progressive splenomegaly. An intermediate or transitional myeloproliferative disease has been described as occurring in a group of patients with polycythemic peripheral blood counts and concomitant features of myelofibrosis, including myeloid metaplasia, leukoerythroblastic blood picture, and extensive reticulin/collagen fibrosis of the marrow. This subset of transitional patients seems to remain in a steady state for several years, whereas those patients in the terminal post-PV spent phase of myelofibrosis undergo a more aggressive course.

Idiopathic myelofibrosis must be differentiated from secondary causes of myelofibrosis. Metastatic carcinoma and granulomatous disorders such as tuberculosis, histoplasmosis, or sarcoidosis of the marrow can cause myelofibrosis. Certain hematologic diseases including acute leukemia, hairy-cell leukemia, myelodysplastic syndromes, and lym-phoreticular malignancies may induce secondary fibrosis (Table 21-4). The etiology of the infiltrative disorders can usually be established by careful scrutiny of the blood and bone marrow for evidence of abnormal cells that characterize the disease; by use of microbiologic cultures; and by other diagnostic tests such as chest x-ray examinations or skin tests. In certain situations (such as when a patient has acute leukemia) techniques of cytochemistry, immunologic surface markers, and electron microscopy studies may help define the nature of the malignancy.

Treatment

The primary aim of treatment in IMF is to improve the quality of life. Approximately 30 percent of patients will be asymptomatic at diagnosis, and, as there is no evidence that treatment increases survival time, these patients are best left untreated. Eventually, the majority of patients manifest symptoms due to anemia, splenic enlargement, bleeding, bone pain, or hypermetabolism. Treatment for these complications is palliative, and invasive procedures should be limited.

One of the major problems requiring therapy is anemia. An estimated 60 percent of IMF patients sooner or later will manifest signs of anemia during their clinical course.[23] Transfusion dependence develops as the anemia becomes more severe. In most cases, the anemia is normochomic, normocytic, whereas 5 percent of patients will develop iron deficiency anemia, and rare patients demonstrate folate or vitamin B_{12} deficiency. When nutritional deficiencies are suspected, patients are treated with iron, folate, or pyridoxine as appropriate. If inefficient erythropoiesis is the predominant mechanism, androgen therapy is indicated. Approximately 40 percent of anemic individuals respond to androgen therapy and should be given a trial of either oxymetholone (50 to 200 mg orally daily) or testosterone enanthate (400 mg intramuscularly every 3 to 4 weeks). Patients receiving oxymethalone require careful monitoring of liver function tests.[19] About 50 percent of patients respond to the combination of androgen and glucocorticoid therapy (prednisone, 30 mg daily), but long-term treatment may have annoying side effects, particularly fluid retention and hirsutism (excessive, unusual growth of hair, especially in women).[21]

The main aim of treatment in patients with progressive splenomegaly is to remove the spleen or reduce its size, thus relieving the severe pain due to pressure and ameliorating the constitutional symptoms of serious digestive disturbances, weight loss, and diarrhea. Chemotherapy is an alternative to splenectomy, reducing spleen size and controlling thrombocytosis, but it has little or no beneficial effect on the anemia. The alkylating agent busulfan (2 to 4 mg daily) or chlorambucil (4 to 6 mg daily), and more recently hydroxyurea,[28] have been used. This treatment must be strictly monitored by regular blood counts in order to avoid inducing dangerous cytopenias in the patient.

Radiation therapy is also considered in patients

with massive mechanical splenomegaly, although just as with the use of chemotherapy, the duration of the reduction in splenic size is usually measured in months. In patients having acute splenic infarction, ascites demonstrating prominent megakaryocytosis, or focal but severe bone pain, the use of radiation may produce gratifying effects.[23]

Although there is no general agreement on the indications and value of this invasive modality, splenectomy is important in the management of IMF patients with profoundly enlarged spleens. The main problem is that patients with symptoms that can be relieved by splenectomy are poor surgical risks, and "good risk patients seldom need palliative surgery."[29]

Four major life-threatening conditions have been espoused as situations warranting consideration of splenectomy:[30]

1. Painful splenic enlargement
2. Severe refractory hemolytic or dilutional anemia sufficient to cause cardiopulmonary symptoms
3. Severe, life-threatening thrombocytopenia
4. Portal hypertension with bleeding varices

Whenever splenectomy is contemplated, an extensive coagulation work-up is necessary, for bleeding is a major hazard.

As the spleen may become the major hematopoietic organ in patients whose marrow has been replaced by fibrosis, it is vital to ensure that splenectomy is considered only in patients in whom splenic hematopoiesis contributes a minor (less than 15 to 20 percent) proportion of total hematopoiesis. This can be quantified by bone imaging and measurement of transferrin-bound ^{52}Fe uptake. Mean survival following splenectomy is approximately 25 months. This procedure does not seem to alter the overall clinical course, and the mortality and morbidity are due mainly to bleeding, thromboembolism, and infection (the same causes as in patients who have not had splenectomy).

Allogeneic marrow transplantation following ablative chemotherapy/radiotherapy has been attempted in a few patients and offers a rational means for curing myelofibrosis. However, it is controversial whether or not the application of this rigorous therapy to a chronic disease, generally limited to the elderly, is judicious. Disappearance of fibrosis and regeneration of normal medullary hematopoiesis has been achieved in responsive patients, yet it is still to be ascertained whether the fibrosis found in IMF and the reactive fibrosis of other disorders is reversible and hence curable.

A significant new approach to the treatment of myelofibrosis is the use of antifibrosing agents such as penicillamine or colchicine. Biochemically, as myelofibrosis progresses, there is increasing conversion of soluble to insoluble collagen. Penicillamine interferes with the cross-linkage of collagen, and, therefore, with its use, a decrease in fibrous tissue occurs. Colchicine appears to cause its antifibrosing effect through two mechanisms: (1) it produces a decreased rate of procollagen and (2) it increases the secretion of collagenases.[19,31]

Prognosis

Patients with IMF comprise extremely heterogeneous populations and survival varies considerably. Median survival is approximately 5 years from the time of diagnosis; however, at least two major subpopulations have been identified. The first (low-risk) group is characterized by a benign or slowly progressive disease with a median survival of 10 years or longer and young age (under 45). The second, less fortunate (high-risk) group is distinguished by a short survival of 2 years and older age (over 45). Many patients in this subgroup die following acute blastic transformation.[32]

Beside age, a number of prognostic indicators have been identified, the most important with regard to long survival include the following:

1. Lack of symptoms
2. Effective erythropoiesis evidenced by hemoglobin level greater than 10 g/dl, reticulocyte count greater than 2 percent, bone marrow showing normal erythropoiesis
3. Platelet counts above 100×10^9/liter
4. Absence of significant hepatosplenomegaly

Conversely, patients with severe ineffective hematopoiesis and marrow failure, marked splenomegaly with plasma volume expansion and portal hypertension,[35] red cell mass reduction or excessive hemolysis fair poorly, having an average survival of only 1 to 2 years. The major causes of death are acute myocardial infarction, congestive heart failure, gastrointestinal and cerebral hemorrhage, and infection.

Between 5 and 20 percent of cases have a terminal transformation to leukemia, acute myelogenous leukemia in most instances, with a rapidly progressive, fatal cause. Rare patients die of liver or renal failure, and development of acute lymphocytic leukemia[33] and erythroleukemia[34] has been reported.

Major scientific advances and application of new knowledge have taken place in recent years. Relevant discoveries in the areas of collagen biochemistry and histochemistry, bone marrow ultrastructure, cell culture studies, and cell growth regulation have allowed a more in-depth understanding of the pathologic processes involved in the disease of myelofibrosis. As new, innovative strategies are applied to the treatment of this complex disease, it is hoped there will be a significant improvement in both the survival and quality of life of patients with IMF.

The Polycythemias

A number of diverse conditions may cause an elevation in the hematocrit (Hct). Initially these disorders can be separated into two groups based on the determination of the red cell mass (Table 21–5). In the absolute polycythemias, the red cell mass (or RC volume) is elevated, implying a true increase in the number of circulating erythrocytes. By contrast, in relative polycythemia, there is an increased Hct in the absence of an elevation in RC volume. This state is due to an increase in the ratio of RC mass to the plasma volume as would occur with dehydra-

Table 21–5. **CLASSIFICATION OF THE POLYCYTHEMIAS ACCORDING TO RED CELL VOLUME DETERMINATIONS**

Elevated Hematocrit (≥50 percent)

Absolute polycythemia (increased RC volume)
- Polycythemia Vera
- Secondary Polycythemia
- Idiopathic Erythrocytosis

Relative polycythemia (normal RC volume)
- Stress polycythemia (Gaisböck's syndrome)
- Dehydration

tion (wherein the plasma volume was contracted or decreased).

The absolute polycythemias may be further divided into three distinct groups: (1) the chronic myeloproliferative disorder, polycythemia vera, arising as a clonal hematologic malignancy of the bone marrow; (2) secondary polycythemias representing a physiologic response to abnormal stimulus (for example, tissue hypoxia and increased erythropoietic activity); or (3) an idiopathic group for which neither a myeloproliferative nor a secondary cause of sustained erythrocytosis can be implicated. An overall comparison of these three groups of polycythemia can be found in Table 21–6. Primary PV is discussed in length first.

Description, History, and Pathogenesis of Polycythemia Vera (Color Plates 215 and 216)

Polycythemia vera is a hematopoietic stem cell disorder predominantly characterized by accelerated erythropoiesis and to a varying degree by excessive proliferation of myeloid and megakaryocytic elements of the bone marrow. As mentioned earlier, the absolute increase in RC mass is the sine qua non for establishing the diagnosis of PV. In keeping with other myeloproliferative disorders, the manifestations of splenomegaly, myeloid metaplasia, and myelofibrosis are variably expressed at diagnosis and throughout the course of the disease.

Table 21–6. **FEATURES OF PV, SECONDARY (HYPOXIC) POLYCYTHEMIA, AND RELATIVE ERYTHROCYTOSIS**

Manifestations	Polycythemia Vera	Secondary Polycythemia	Relative Erythrocytosis
Clinical features			
Cyanosis (warm)	Absent	Present	May be present
Heart or lung disease	Absent	Present	Absent
Splenomegaly	Present in 75%	Absent	Absent
Hepatomegaly	Present in 35%	Absent	Absent
Laboratory features			
Arterial oxygen saturation	Normal	Decreased (rarely normal)	Normal
Red cell mass	Increased	Increased	Normal
Leukocyte	Increased in 80%	Normal	Normal
Platelet count	Increased in 50%	Normal	Normal
Nucleated red cells, poikilocytes	Often present	Absent	Absent
Leukocyte alkaline phosphatase (LAP)	Elevated	Normal	Normal
Bone marrow	Hypercellular; increased erythropoiesis and myelopoiesis; increased megakaryocytes; fibrosis	Increased erythropoiesis	Normal
Erythropoietin (EPO)	Decreased (rarely normal)	Increased (rarely normal)	Normal
Serum vitamin B_{12}	Elevated in 75%	Normal	Normal
Culture studies	Autonomous, erythroid proliferation	EPO dependent— colony formation	Not applicable

Most commonly, at the time of initial presentation, the degree of extramedullary hematopoiesis is usually mild and marrow fibrosis is most often minimal. However, 15 to 20 percent of cases transform to a spent phase, with progressive anemia and increasing splenomegaly; this development being virtually indistinguishable from idiopathic myelofibrosis.

The nature of this disease has been controversial over the years. Hippocrates recognized "plethora vera,"[35] and Von Haller in 1730[35a] associated thrombosis with the frequent occurrence of gangrene. Vasques, Cabot, and, in 1903, Olsen, first characterized the disease as autonomous erythrocytosis, additionally noting the concurrent feature of splenomegaly.[36] Turk[37] in 1904 described the leukoerythroblastic blood picture as well as documenting the finding of increased granulocytic and megakaryocytic activity. The replacement of normal marrow of fibrotic and sclerotic tissue was reported by Hirsch[38] in 1935; by 1938 Rosenthal and Bassen[39] had delineated the natural history and cause of the disease. The concept of the myeloproliferative diseases was originally proposed in the 1950s by Dameshek,[1] and since that time the body of knowledge encompassing polycythemia has greatly expanded.

It has now been clearly established that the cell of origin in PV is an abnormal pluripotent stem cell. This has been demonstrated by studies of black women with PV who were heterozygous for the two different G6PD isoenzymes. In these women only one of the isoenzymes was present in the progenitors and progeny of erythroid, granulocytic, monocytic, and megakaryocytic cell lines, whereas nonhematopoietic tissue displayed isoenzymes A and B.[2] In normal healthy women, equal amounts of isoenzyme types would be found in blood cells. These findings strongly suggest that the abnormal hematopoietic cells arise from a single malignant clone. Furthermore, some patients eventually develop marrow fibrosis and this occurrence appears to be a reactive process. Just as in myelofibrosis, the excessive fibroblastic proliferation is a result of the release of certain growth factors from abnormal megakaryocytes.[40]

When blood and bone marrow cells from patients with PV are cultured on semisolid media, erythroid colonies (colony-forming unit–erythroid [CFU-E], burst-forming unit–erythroid, [BFU-E]) will be formed without the addition of exogenous erythropoietin. This led to the original presumption that erythroid colonies grew spontaneously. It has now been suggested that the erythroid progenitors are extremely sensitive to low levels of erythropoietin supplied by the serum, which is inherently present in the basic culture medium. A small amount of normal stem cells are also formed in vitro, but it is likely that these residual normal stem cells are suppressed or inhibited in vivo by an unknown mechanism and that their numbers decline as the disease progresses.

Epidemiology

Polycythemia vera is a relatively rare disease, with an annual incidence of approximately 2 cases per 100,000 population. The median age at diagnosis is 60 years, but onset may occur from adolescence to old age. According to Danish and colleagues,[41] nine cases of childhood PV have been documented. Familial occurrences, although rare, have been reported. The disease has slightly higher incidence in men than in women. The etiology of PV remains unknown, as it is in other myeloproliferative diseases.

Clinical Features

Polycythemia vera has an insidious onset and is often discovered quite incidentally when, following a routine examination, an elevated hemoglobin (Hgb) or Hct is discovered. In other cases, development of characteristic symptoms related to increased red cell volume or hyperviscosity may herald the recognition of the disease (Fig. 21–4). Common complaints as a result of cerebral circulatory disturbances and transient ischemic attacks include headaches, dizziness, vertigo, visual phenomena (blurred vision, diplopia, scotomata), tinnitus, and rarely mild dementia. Vascular complications are manifested equally in arteries and veins. Thrombotic episodes such as phlebitis, myocardial infarction, erythromelalgia (painful, red extremities), paresthesias and burning sensation, particularly in the feet reflect impairment of blood flow to the peripheral circulation. Dawson and coworkers[42] proposed that the coexistent thrombocytosis acts in conjunction with the hyperviscosity and high blood volume to increase the incidence of thrombosis, thromboembolism, and hemorrhage in these patients. Incidence of morbidity and mortality from vessel wall disease is already high in this age group, and concomitant high Hct adversely influences the outcome of occlusive events.

Hemorrhagic diathesis is often seen in PV patients. Life-threatening hemorrhage may occur in association with trauma, surgery, or peptic ulcer. Spontaneous minor hemorrhages, in the form of epistaxis, gingival bleeding, and ecchymoses are common events almost certainly caused by qualitative platelet abnormalities.

The presence of splenomegaly in about 75 percent of patients is a finding of significant differential importance. The splenic enlargement is usually mild to moderate and is due to extramedullary hematopoiesis and not to the expanded blood volume per se (the spleen size does not diminish as blood volume is reduced by phlebotomy). Patients having moderate splenomegaly appear more likely to evolve to IMF at an early stage. Modest hepatomegaly is observed in one third of patients at the time of initial presentation (Table 21–6).

A common physical finding is ruddy cyanosis of the face, nose, ears, and lips. This facial plethora results from conjunctival and mucosal blood vessel congestion. Patients have stated that the appearance of their ruddy complexion has prompted friends to comment that they "look wonderful."[43]

Pruritus, occurring in about 30 percent of patients, is especially troublesome after a hot shower. The pathogenesis of the persistent itching and urticaria, occurring in 10 percent of patients, is related

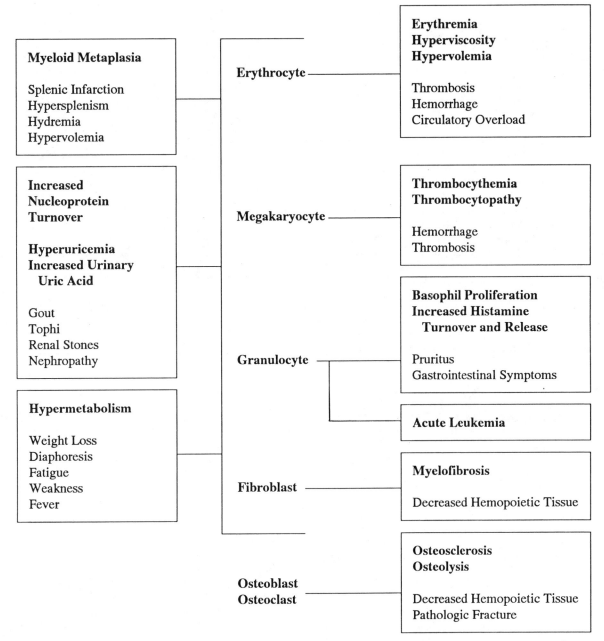

Figure 21–4. Physiologic complications of polycythemia vera. The clinical features of this disorder are attributable to the excessive proliferation of the three main hematopoietic cell lines and reactive proliferation of bone marrow fibroblasts. (From Gilbert,[27] p 359, with permission.)

to elevated levels of histamine produced by basophils and other granulocytes.

Fever, night (and day) sweats, and weight loss may occur resulting from the hypermetabolic state. Gout ascribed to increased nucleoprotein turnover occurs in 5 to 10 percent of patients. Uric acid calculi or urate nephropathy may arise from the increased uric acid excretion.

Laboratory Features

Elevation of the Hgb and Hct is the most important finding in PV; however, polycythemia may be masked if accompanying iron deficiency is present.

The diagnosis of PV requires the demonstration of an increase in red cell mass as part of the initial evaluation of a patient with erythrocytosis. The ^{51}Cr dilution technique is a simple, well-established method for direct measurement of total red cell mass. Absolute erythrocytosis is present in men with values at least 36 ml/kg and in women with at least 32 ml/kg. The plasma volume can be measured with human serum albumin labeled with ^{125}I or ^{131}I, and is normal or slightly reduced. A calculation of red cell mass from plasma volume gives unreliable results as a disproportionate increase in plasma volume occurs in pronounced splenomegaly due to red cell pooling.

Characteristically, at presentation there is increased red cell production at intramedullary sites. The erythrocytes are normochromic, normocytic, and have a normal lifespan. As the disease progresses, extramedullary ineffective hematopoiesis leads to an increasing anisocytosis and poikilocytosis, as well as a shortened red cell lifespan secondary to splenic sequestration.[44] Some patients demonstrate the microcytosis and hypochromia associated with iron deficiency (see Color Plate 215). This iron deficiency has been attributed to occult gastrointestinal blood loss and defective platelet function.[45] The reticulocyte count is usually normal, and only rarely will immature erythrocytes be found in the peripheral blood.

Relative and absolute granulocytosis occurs in two thirds of the patients. The elevation in total WBC count is usually moderate, with counts in the range of 12 to 25×10^9/liter. Occasionally basophilia and eosinophilia is apparent and few metamyelocytes, myelocytes, and even more immature cells may be seen on examination of the peripheral blood smear.

Thrombocytosis is present at the time of diagnosis in about one half of the patients with PV. The platelet count is most often moderately elevated, with counts between 450 and 800×10^9/liter, but in about 5 percent the platelet count exceeds 1000×10^9/liter. Morphologic alterations of platelets include the presence of giant platelets as well as deficient granulation. Studies show that most patients with PV form spontaneous megakaryocytic colonies analogous to the spontaneous erythroid colony formation seen in all MPDs.[46] Platelets from most patients demonstrate some abnormality in aggregation studies, but the results of these laboratory tests correlate poorly with clinical thrombotic and hemorrhagic episodes. Also of interest is the fact that in the majority of patients, even those with bleeding diathesis, the bleeding time, which is the best measurement of in vivo platelet function, is nearly always normal.[47]

When performing coagulation tests on PV patients, such as PT, activated partial thromboplastin time (APTT), and TT, the anticoagulant-to-blood ratio must be maintained at 1:9. Sodium citrate functions as an anticoagulant by binding calcium in plasma. In the case of erythrocytosis when plasma volume is decreased, citrate is left in excess in the vacutainer tube. This residual citrate will then be available to bind calcium in the test system, thus causing falsely prolonged clotting times. When the Hct is greater than 55 percent, the following adjustment for the volume of anticoagulant should be applied:

$$(0.00185) \ (V) \ (100 - Hct) = C$$
$$V = \text{Volume of whole blood}$$
$$C = \text{ml of anticoagulant}$$

The PT, APTT, TT, and fibrinogen levels are usually normal in patients with PV. The bone marrow is hypercellular with decreased fat content in nearly all cases. Panhyperplasia is evident to a varying extent, in contrast to the exclusive erythroid hyperplasia seen in secondary polycythemia (see Color Plate 216). Besides the striking increase in the number of megakaryocytes, they are often also increased in size. Marrow iron stores, demonstrated by Prussian blue staining, are reduced or absent. As previously mentioned, this apparently relates to chronic occult blood loss in addition to the increased utilization of iron in the process of excessive erythropoieses and the subsequent expansion of red cell mass. Early in the course of PV, fibrosis is a rare finding. If serial biopsies are performed, a progressive increase in reticulin deposits can often be demonstrated during the active phase of the disease and before the spent phase develops.[48] As the disease runs its course, cellularity usually decreases, although megakaryocytosis may persist. The transition to frank myelofibrosis occurs in 15 to 20 percent of patients.

The LAP activity is increased in 75 percent of patients with PV[7] (see Color Plate 217). The determination of the LAP may be inconsequential in differential diagnosis of erythrocytosis because some patients with PV have a normal LAP score, as do the majority of patients with secondary erythrocytosis (in the absence of inflammation, infection, or hormonal therapy).

Two of the three vitamin B_{12}–binding proteins, transcobalamin I and III, are frequently elevated in PV, as they are in other MPDs. Transcobalamin III is the binding protein most commonly elevated in PV, whereas transcobalamin I is predominantly increased in chronic myelogeneous leukemia.[49] These increased serum values are attributed to the excessive granulocyte turnover. Furthermore, the unsaturated vitamin B_{12}–binding capacity ($UB_{12}BC$) is increased in approximately 75 percent of patients.[50]

The arterial oxygen saturation is normal in most patients with PV; however, infrequently the oxygen saturation may be slightly lowered (88 to 92 percent). This feature is helpful in excluding erythrocytosis secondary to pulmonary and cardiac abnormalities, wherein the oxygen saturation is routinely decreased.

Hyperuricemia and uricosuria are present in 40 percent of PV patients at the time of presentation. This is a frequent finding in many hypoproliferative disorders where there is increased synthesis and degradation of cellular nucleotides. Most patients remain asymptomatic, but uncommonly clinical gout may develop.

Patients with PV have absent or reduced plasma and urine erythropoietin, which can now be measured by a very sensitive radioimmunoassay procedure. There is no significant rise in the levels of erythropoietin following phlebotomy and normalization of the Hgb and Hct. As mentioned previously, autonomous or spontaneous erythroid colonies may be grown in culture medium without the addition of exogenous erythropoietin. This finding is considered by many investigators to be of diagnostic value (Table 21–6).

Differential Diagnosis

The diagnostic criteria for evaluating a patient with erythrocytosis should encompass procedures that systematically exclude the various causes of secondary and relative polycythemia (Table 21–7). In 1968 the Polycythemia Vera Study Group (PVSG) developed a set of criteria that indicated, with a high degree of probability, the establishment of the diagnosis of PV (Table 21–8). Because of the sensitivity and specificity of these criteria, they have become the standard approach to this diagnostic problem worldwide.

As always, a careful history and physical should

Table 21–7. **CLASSIFICATION OF THE DISORDERS ASSOCIATED WITH POLYCYTHEMIA**

Primary Polycythemia
  Polycythemia vera
Secondary Polycythemia
  Physiologically appropriate increase in erythropoietin
    (hypoxic activation)
    High altitude
    Chronic pulmonary disease
    Cyanotic congenital heart disease
    Cirrhosis
    Alevolar hypoventilation (obesity/sleep apnea,
      pickwickian syndrome, intrinsic lung disease)
    Defective oxygen transport
      Smoking (carboxyhemoglobinemia)
      Methemoglobinemia
      High oxygen affinity hemoglobinopathies
    Defective oxidative metabolism (cobalt therapy)
  Physiologically inappropriate increase in erythropoietin
    Renal ischemia
      Renal tumors
      Renal cysts
      Renal transplant rejection
      Renal artery stenosis
      Hydronephrosis
    Neoplasms
      Uterine fibroids
      Hepatoma
      Cerebellar hemangioblastoma
    Endocrine disorders
      Pheochromocytoma
      Conn's syndrome
      Ovarian tumors (androgen secreting)
      Cushing's syndrome
    Miscellaneous causes
      Neonatal polycythemia
      Androgen therapy
      Hypertransfusion
Relative Polycythemia
  Stress polycythemia (Gaisböck's syndrome)
  Dehydration

Table 21–8. **PVSG CRITERIA FOR DIAGNOSIS OF PV***

Category A (Major Criteria)
  1. Elevated red cell mass
  2. Normal arterial oxygen saturation
  3. Splenomegaly
Category B (Minor Criteria)
  1. Leukocytosis
  2. Thrombocytosis
  3. Elevated leukocyte alkaline phosphatase score
  4. Increased serum vitamin B_{12} or vitamin B_{12}–binding
    proteins

*To establish a diagnosis of polycythemia vera, either all three diagnostic criteria from category A *or* an elevated red cell mass and normal arterial oxygen saturation *in addition to* two criteria from category B must be present.
Source: From Beck, WS: Hematology, ed 3. MIT Press, Cambridge, 1982, p 297, with permission.

preclude more extensive (and costly) diagnostic procedures. Of particular importance are such items as smoking, cardiopulmonary status, alcohol intake, family history, and examination for evidence of hepatosplenomegaly. It is imperative that the initial laboratory investigation include documentation of absolute increase in total red cell mass; this finding is associated with a variety of conditions causing absolute polycythemia.

Once it has been established that an increased red cell mass is present, other specific diagnostic studies are warranted to assist in the differential diagnosis of secondary polycythemia versus (primary) polycythemia vera (Fig. 21–5). Normal arterial O_2 and oxygen saturation (at least 92 percent), along with normal chest x-ray examinations, can help rule out chronic pulmonary or cardiac disease. Additionally, such patients have symptoms and other complications as a consequence of their primary, underlying disorder.

If evidence of tissue hypoxia is lacking, investigation for the presence of an occult erythropoietin-secreting tumor or other cause of inappropriate erythropoietin production should be undertaken. Common procedures at this level of evaluation include an intravenous pyelogram (IVP), renal ultrasound, abdominal and/or head computed tomography (CT) scan, and a liver scan. Carboxyhemoglobin levels should be measured in patients who smoke, as Hct levels higher than normal have been demonstrated in some of these patients.

Erythrocytosis in the absence of characteristic features of either polycythemia vera or cardiopulmonary secondary polycythemia should prompt consideration of the possibility of inherited hemoglobin abnormality (high oxygen affinity hemoglobin). Hemoglobin electrophoresis will be abnormal in the majority of these cases, but measurement of the oxygen affinity ($P_{50}O_2$) can help reveal those few cases in which the Hgb mutation is electrophoretically silent. Furthermore, family history can be very

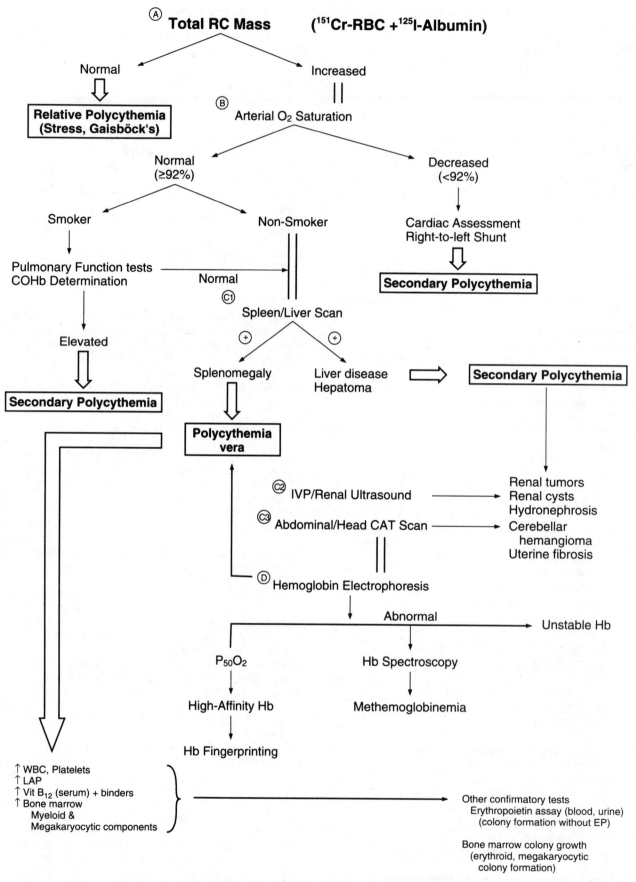

Figure 21–5. Diagnostic evaluation of polycythemia.

useful, as the inheritance mode of these disorders is autosomal dominant.

A serum erythropoietin assay may be helpful in distinguishing between primary and secondary polycythemia, although this determination is not always a reliable diagnostic feature. Most values in PV are decreased, but sometimes the result may be in the normal range. In difficult cases, culture studies of peripheral blood and/or bone marrow may identify autonomies producing erythroid colonies and hence verification of an MPD.

In summary, the most significant characteristic findings in PV are increased red cell mass, splenomegaly, pancytosis, and elevated LAP score. Occasionally a patient may present with a normal or near-normal Hgb, iron deficiency, splenomegaly, leukocytosis, and thrombocytosis, and the disease therefore may be difficult to distinguish from essential thrombocythemia. In this case the presumed blood loss and iron deficiency is masking the erythrocytosis of the underlying PV, and a trial of iron administration is warranted to establish a definitive diagnosis. In PV, the Hgb and Hct can be expected to rise to polycythemic levels, thus clarifying the diagnosis. Conversely, the combination of heavy smoking and excessive alcohol consumption has led to false-positive diagnoses of PV. In this setting the smoker's polycythemia and alcoholic liver disease, manifested by splenomegaly, elevated serum vitamin B_{12} levels, leukocytosis, and in some cases elevated LAP, have erroneously prompted diagnosis of PV.[51] Again, measurement of carboxyhemoglobin levels, bone marrow examination for presence of panhyperplasia, and erythropoietin assay (expected decrease) can help to rule in PV.

Treatment

Early descriptions indicated that the life expectancy of untreated PV patients averaged 6 to 36 months.[52,53] Over the years, therapeutic modalities have been complex and controversial. Today, however, these patients can enjoy a relatively normal lifespan if their disease is adequately controlled and monitored by their physician. No treatment at present can completely eradicate this disease.

The major complications of PV are thrombotic events due to hyperviscosity and complications due to transition to a MPD (myelofibrosis or leukemia or both). As such, PV therapy has two primary objectives: reduction of the total red cell mass and cytotoxic myelosuppression to control the malignant proliferative process. The treatment of the erythrocytic phase may be divided into induction and maintenance therapy.

Induction. Rapid reduction of the blood volume to normal can be accomplished by phlebotomy, thereby relieving the patient of the characteristic painful symptoms of hyperviscosity. This is a safe and relatively inexpensive method of controlling the erythrocytosis. Removal of 350 to 500 ml may be done every 2 to 3 days until the Hct is reduced to 40 to 45 percent. Recent studies have demonstrated the cerebral blood flow is significantly improved and

mental alertness heightened if the Hct can be maintained within this range.[54] Phlebotomies may then be performed bimonthly. In elderly patients or those with a history of cardiovascular disease, it is undesirable to remove more than 200 to 300 ml at a time. Surgery in an untreated patient is hazardous owing to the increased risk of thrombohemorrhagic complications. In such emergency situations, intensive phlebotomy accompanied by plasma infusion is advisable to maintain intravascular volume.

Because removal of every unit of blood causes a loss of approximately 250 mg of elemental iron, nearly all patients regularly treated by phlebotomy will develop iron deficiency with microcytic hypochromic red cell changes. Development of this iron deficiency and concomitant disruption of normal erythropoiesis allows maintenance of the Hct at acceptable levels with the decreased frequency of phlebotomies being required. Most patients do not show the classic symptoms of glossitis, dysphagia, cheilosis, weight loss, and so on generally associated with iron deficiency; however, some patients do have unexplained tiredness. Iron therapy is not usually required, but if iron is administered the Hct must be carefully monitored as it may rise quickly, necessitating more frequent phlebotomies. The microhematocrit method is preferred over the automated cell counter method, as the Hct may be overestimated by up to 10 percent at low mean corpuscular hemoglobin (MCH) and mean corpuscular hemoglobin concentration (MCHC) values.[7]

Management by phlebotomy alone is recommended for patients under 40, particularly for women in the childbearing years, unless specific thrombosis-associated risk factors are present (that is, high platelet counts, preexisting vascular disease). The major limitation of phlebotomy is that it has no suppressive effect on the abnormal bone marrow proliferation, particularly that of thrombocytosis. It does not alleviate pruritus or control any symptoms related to splenomegaly. As such, myelosuppression is often required to repress these manifestations.

Maintenance. Long-term control of the peripheral blood counts is essential to minimize the risk of thrombotic complications. Although phlebotomy relieves the burden of erythrocytosis, the reduction is short-term and many patients required additional myelosuppression, especially those with elevated platelet counts. Apparently no single therapy is optimal for patients of all ages and stages of this disease and therefore decisions as to the most effective approach must be based primarily on individual patient characteristics.

Extensive data on the management of PV by use of phlebotomy alone and/or in combination with the various myelosuppessive modalities are now available (PVSG). In this long-term study, 431 patients were randomized into three modes of treatment: phlebotomy alone, chlorambucil with phlebotomy as needed, and radioactive phosphorus ^{32}P and phlebotomy as needed. An additional study examined the results of long-term control of PV with a nonalkylating agent, hydroxyurea (HU). Patients treated with phlebotomy only exhibited an increased incidence of thrombotic complications, whereas significantly greater percentages of patients were regulated by either radioactive phosphorus or an alkylating agent that subsequently developed acute leukemia and other neoplasms. The comparison studies also show that HU, supplemented by phlebotomy, is *not* accompanied by excessive thrombotic complications and to date has *not* been shown to be leukemogenic.[55]

As a result of the PVSG's systematic study of prognostic indicators, complications, and effective therapeutic modalities, and because no form of treatment for PV is risk free, the PVSG suggests the following guidelines to provide the best control of the disease:

1. Because of the increased risk of vascular occlusion associated with age, patients over age 70 are most simply and effectively treated with radioactive phosphorus ^{32}P and phlebotomy as needed.
2. Patients under age 40 should be controlled with phlebotomy alone unless thrombosis-associated risk factors are demonstrated. If the requirement for phlebotomy is excessive or there is a history of a previous thrombotic episode, myelosuppression with HU is recommended even in this young age group.
3. As the role of myelosuppression is controversial in patients aged 40 to 70, phlebotomy alone can be used if no thrombosis-associated risks are present. If the aforementioned risk is identified, HU is again the current agent of choice.
4. Symptomatic hypersplenomegaly, resistant pruritus, bone pain, or poor veins may be other indications for the additive use of myelosuppression.[51,56]

Either chemotherapy or irradiation may be used to effect myelosuppression. Radioactive phosphorus ^{32}P is still probably the most convenient form of delivering myelosuppressive radiation and should be administered intravenously at a dosage of 2.3 to 5 mCi/m². In many cases, a single dose is sufficient to reduce spleen size and normalize the peripheral blood count. However, the response takes 2 to 3 months for maximal effect of chemotherapy. Sometimes a second small dose of 2 to 3 mCi/m² of ^{32}P is required after 3 to 4 months to arrest the disease completely. Satisfactory control of PV occurs in 75 to 85 percent of patients, and the duration of remission is typically 6 to 36 months. As there are very few side effects, this agent is particularly advantageous to patients who live lengthy distances from their physicians.[57] Although a low incidence of acute leukemia is a characteristic of the natural history of this disease, there is no doubt that there is a greatly increased risk for leukemic transformation in ^{32}P-treated patients. Approximately 10 to 15 percent of patients undergo a conversion to an acute, usually nonlymphocytic leukemia and, according to Williams,[30] this incidence is 20 to 40 times greater than that expected for a human population exposed to similar radiation doses and times at risk.

Because of its low mutagenic risk, HU has emerged as the preferred agent, particularly in the younger patients. The average dose of 1 g/day is sufficient to maintain a normal hematocrit and platelet count. Supplemental phlebotomies may be necessary. The initial response to HU treatment is positive, with between 80 and 90 percent achieving good control of the disease and more than 60 percent retaining long-term control after 5 years. In a high percentage of patients, HU also seems to have a beneficial effect on pruritus and splenomegaly.[58] Possible side effects include rashes, drug fever, and megaloblastoid changes.

Adjuvant therapy is often necessary to control hyperuricemia and hyperuricosuria. In addition to standard colchicine therapy, allopurinol (300 mg/day), an agent that blocks the formation of uric acid from its precursors, is used to prevent and/or control acute attacks of gout. In patients receiving myelosuppressive therapy, the need for allopurinol is diminished because of the decreased nucleic acid turnover effected by suppression of cellular proliferation.[30] Allopurinol may be continued indefinitely in patients treated by phlebotomy alone.

Severe pruritus is a distressing symptom in many cases. It is best managed by controlling the erythrocytosis; however, it may persist in some patients despite a normal Hct and physical examination. The antihistamine cyproheptadine and cimetidine may be of benefit. Cholestyramine, an anion exchange resin that functions by binding bile acids, has been reported to provide some relief of pruritus.

Course and Prognosis

The course of patients with PV is determined by the natural history of the disease and the development of complications that may or may not be related to the mode of therapy employed.

As previously mentioned, this disease progresses through several stages, each of variable duration. In the active erythrocytic phase, the red cell mass can be maintained at satisfactory levels with administration of treatment dictated by age and the presence of certain risk factors. Many patients eventually enter a period characterized by increasing anemia, and this spent phase is associated with transformation to frank myelofibrosis in 15 to 20 percent of cases. The progressive splenomegaly appears to be a manifestation of the natural course of the disease, but splenectomy carries a high incidence of morbidity and mortality in this group of patients. The treatment of this phase is predominantly supportive and may be very difficult. The cause of the anemia may be multifactorial, being due to one or more of the following factors: (1) iron, folic acid, or vitamin B_{12} deficiency; (2) inefficient hematopoiesis; or (3) splenic sequestration and destruction of erythrocytes, leukocytes, and platelets. As such, treatment of the anemia may involve appropriate nutritional replacement and/or administration of steroids to help control the ineffective erythropoiesis. Ongoing transfusion of packed red cells is often required. Despite possible splenic sequestration, thrombocytosis and leukocytosis may persist. Myelosuppressive therapy may be indicated to control the myelofibrotic proliferation. Prognosis is poor for this phase of the disease, and median survival is about 2 years.

Malignant transformation to acute leukemia, usually acute myeloblastic leukemia (AML), occurs in 10 to 15 percent of cases. This complication is almost universally fatal. As discussed earlier, the therapeutic modality affects the rate of leukemic transformation. In patients treated by phlebotomy alone, the incidence of transition to leukemia is only 1 to 2 percent, whereas those treated by chemotherapy have a risk approaching 15 percent. A few cases each have been documented of PV transforming into a myelodysplastic syndrome, myeloma, and also chronic lymphocytic leukemia.[7]

Reported survival rates in PV range from 8 to 15 years. Thrombohemorrhagic incidents account for 40 percent of deaths, and acute leukemia and myeloid metaplasia each account for 15 percent.[30] As the mean age of diagnosis is 60 years, many other patients die of additional unrelated reasons.

Continued research of the pathophysiologic abnormalities associated with this disease as well as the effects of various treatment modalities will undoubtedly lengthen the future life expectancy of patients with PV.

The Secondary Polycythemias

Absolute erythrocytosis may have a wide variety of causes (see Table 21–5). The secondary polycythemias differ from PV in that autonomous bone marrow proliferation occurs in PV. Increased secretion of erythropoietin has been implicated as the responsible stimulus for all cases of secondary erythrocytosis. These causes can be separated into three groups: those in which there is an appropriate, compensatory increase in erythropoietin; those resulting from an inappropriate or pathologic secretion of erythropoietin; and a miscellaneous category.

Appropriate Secondary Polycythemia

In this group of disorders, the underlying mechanism is release of erythropoietin as part of a compensatory effect to minimize impending tissue hypoxia. The most common causes of secondary polycythemia are cardiac or respiratory diseases that lead to significant arterial oxygen unsaturation. Of the lung diseases causing hypoxia and erythrocytosis, chronic obstructive pulmonary disease (COPD) is the most frequent offender. In COPD the release of erythropoietin appears to be appropriately responsive to the level of hypoxia; with the degree of increase in the Hct being inversely proportional to the arterial oxygen saturation. However, in some patients the erythrocytosis is not as marked as would be expected for the degree of oxygen unsaturation. The explanation for the erythropoietic unresponsiveness has not been fully explained. Other factors, such as carbon monoxide levels in smokers, shifting of the oxygen-dissociation curve, and the bone marrow suppressive effects of the underlying disease, may account for the con-

siderable individual variation in response to hypoxia. Other intrinsic lung diseases that may involve significant hypoxia are pulmonary fibrosis, pulmonary aneurysms, and hereditary hemorrhagic telangiectasia, when the lung is pathologically affected.

Right-to-left shunting in congenital heart disease is caused by a number of different anatomic defects and leads to profound arterial hypoxia and extreme erythrocytosis. Indeed, some of the highest hematocrits (75 to 80 percent) have been reported in some of these patients. The secondary polycythemia in these cardiac anomalies results from the shunting of poorly oxygenated venous blood into systemic circulations and necessitates surgical intervention. Only a few patients with inoperable conditions survive to adulthood. The issue of whether to reduce the elevated Hct of patients with inoperable lesions or those prior to cardiac surgery by phlebotomy is debatable. Although studies indicate that the increased red cell mass is of benefit in terms of tissue oxygenation,[59] there is high incidence of thrombosis related to raised blood viscosity. It is therefore recommended that the patients with particularly high hematocrits undergo phlebotomy to reduce the Hct to less than 65 percent. As there is much individual variation, no optimal target Hct for these patients has been endorsed.

Ascent to high altitudes causes tissue hypoxia due to the low atmospheric pressure. This leads to the release of erythropoietin with subsequent increase in red cell production. Although tolerance to high altitude varies, most healthy individuals experience no symptoms at altitudes of up to 7000 feet (2130 m). For the indigenous mountain inhabitants living higher than 16,440 feet (5000 m), hematocrits in the range of 60 to 70 percent are regularly seen. The physiologic adaptation of erythrocytosis allows most individuals to function normally, having lifespans equivalent to their counterparts at sea level.[60] The clinical and laboratory features of humans living at high altitudes include a ruddy cyanosis; venous and capillary engorgement of the conjunctiva, mucus membranes, and skin; emphysema; normocytic, normochromic erythrocytosis; increased reticulocyte count; and increased iron turnover.[61] The syndrome of acute mountain sickness occurs in nonacclimatized persons who rapidly ascend to high altitudes. The manifestations of cerebral hypoxia are headaches, dizziness, insomnia, weakness, nausea, and vomiting. Chronic mountain sickness was characterized by Monge in 1937. It is manifested by decreased exercise tolerance, marked cyanosis, plethora, and general emotional deterioration. The Hct values are comparatively higher than those seen in acclimatized individuals, due to even lower arterial oxygen saturation levels. Therapeutic phlebotomy provides relief of symptoms, but normalization of the Hct and disappearance of all signs of this disease involves a lengthy process after return to sea level.

The alveolar hypoventilation syndromes are characterized by impaired or inadequate ventilation. Intermittent alveolar hypoventilation has frequently been reported in healthy men during sleep[62] and if severe, can cause hypoxia, cyanosis, apnea, and secondary polycythemia. This condition may also be seen in neuromuscular disorders, in mechanical impairment of the chest wall, and in the colorful pickwickian syndrome (extreme obesity, somnolence, and associated erythrocytosis).

Heavy cigarette smoking (20 to 30 cigarettes per day) can result in carbon monoxide levels of up to 10 percent. When hemoglobin is bound to carbon monoxide, the resulting carboxyhemoglobin loses its capacity to carry oxygen. Tissue hypoxia results, the oxygen dissociation curve is shifted to the left, and, because of the reduced oxygen delivery, the erythropoietin level increases, causing a mild erythrocytosis. Environmental pollution from industrial sources and vehicle exhaust emissions have also been associated with increased levels of carboxyhemoglobin and mild erythrocytosis. As the increase in Hct is usually about 2 to 4 percent, the Hct may still fall within normal limits. Smokers with a concomitant lung disease or nocturnal hypoventilation most often have increased Hct levels.

Methemoglobinemia can result from a hereditary deficiency of the enzyme NADH-methemoglobin reductase, from ingestion of various drugs or toxic substance exposure, or from hemoglobin M disease. Methemoglobin is formed when heme iron is oxidized to the ferric state. In this oxidized form, the heme moiety is incapable of carrying oxygen and cyanosis is clinically observed. Interestingly enough, even alarming degrees of cyanosis may be seen with arterial oxygen saturation still being normal (92 percent or higher). Mild associated erythrocytosis is rare but, when present, is due mostly to a shift to the left of the oxygen-dissociation curve (increased oxygen affinity).

Cases of familial secondary polycythemia have been demonstrated wherein the hemoglobin molecule itself is abnormal. Amino acid substitutions in these variants may interfere with release of oxygen to the tissues by preventing normal conformational changes required for deoxygenation. This extraordinarily avid oxygen affinity leads to tissue hypoxia and increased erythropoietin production. A left-shifted oxygen-dissociation curve is characteristic, and a compensatory erythrocytosis ensues. Approximately 30 different high-affinity hemoglobin variants have been described, including hemoglobins Chesapeake, Rainier, Yakima, Hiroshima, Little Rock, and San Diego.

In many cases the aberrant hemoglobin is apparent on hemoglobin electrophoresis; however, in some patients the hemoglobin migrates along with hemoglobin A and is therefore undetectable. Determination of reduced oxygen affinity ($P_{50}O_2$) in patients with erythrocytosis of questionable origin is necessary to disclose these electrophoretically silent hemoglobins.

Inappropriate Secondary Polycythemia

A wide range of disorders have been associated with inappropriately increased erythropoietin pro-

duction and resultant erythrocytosis, in spite of the absence of generalized tissue hypoxia. This secondary polycythemia confers no physiologic advantage, and the underlying disease accounts for most of the clinical features observed in the patient. The Hct and red cell mass are increased, but classically there is no accompanying increase in WBC or platelet counts. Benign and malignant tumors may promote excessive secretion of erythropoietin. When these disorders are associated with thrombocytosis or granulocytosis, it may be difficult to establish a clear diagnosis. In this case, documentation of increased erythropoietin and the absence of splenomegaly can assist in ruling out primary PV.

A number of structural or functional renal disorders have been associated with an absolute polycythemia, apparently due to renal ischemia.[63] Renal tumors, solitary renal cysts, polycystic renal disease, renal artery stenosis, and hydronephrosis have all led to a varying degree of erythrocytosis. It has been determined that the erythrocytosis observed following renal transplantation is due to inappropriate production of erythropoietin by the native kidney rather than by the transplanted kidney.[64]

Certain neoplasms can evoke erythrocytosis due to inappropriate secretions of erythropoietically active substances. Hepatoma is common in the Far East and polycythemia occurs in approximately 12 percent of cases.[7] Erythrocytosis has been associated with the presence of large uterine fibroid tumors and ovarian carcinoma. Renal hypoxia and erythropoietin production may be caused by mechanical interference with blood supply to the kidneys, imposed by the large abdominal mass.[65] Cerebellar hemangioblastoma and various endocrine disorders account for less common causes of secondary polycythemia. In most cases, hematologic abnormalities remit when the tumor has been extirpated.

Neonatal polycythemia is designated when the Hct exceeds 70 percent. The causes are numerous and include placental transfusion, intrauterine hypoxia, endocrine disorders, and congenital anomalies. Possible manifestations of hyperviscosity include congestive heart failure, respiratory distress, and decreased renal function.[7] Phlebotomy with plasma replacement may be judiciously indicated in symptomatic babies.

A small number of families have been described with some members having idiopathic erythrocytosis. These patients may represent a heterogeneous group in which there has been inadequate investigation as to the causes of secondary polycythemia or in which absolute erythrocytosis is the only manifestation of PV. The precise mechanism responsible for this overproduction of erythropoietin has still not been elucidated.

Relative Polycythemia

Relative polycythemia may be seen in patients with an elevated Hct, normal red cell mass, and decreased plasma volume. Two groups can be clearly distinguished among patients with relative erythrocytosis. First, it is most often seen clinically in the group of patients having a depletion in circulating plasma volume caused by acute or subacute dehydration resulting from a number of conditions (such as burns). The second group of patients is characterized predominantly by asymptomatic middle-aged white men who are hypertensive, obese, and have a long history of heavy smoking. In 1905 Gaisböck[66] first described a condition of "polycythemia hypertonica" in several hypertensive patients who had increased red cell counts, plethora, but no accompanying splenomegaly. Today, this condition is variously termed Gaisböck's syndrome, stress or benign polycythemia, or pseudopolycythemia. It is well documented that excessive smoking causes mild to moderate erythrocytosis and a decreased plasma volume, hence the term smoker's polycythemia, as mentioned previously. Undoubtedly some patients with erythrocytosis merely represent the extreme physiologic range of Hct. The combined effect of a high-normal red cell mass and a low-normal plasma volume resulting in a so-called spurious erythrocytosis is not considered pathologic. Physical stress, extreme alcohol consumption, and diuretic therapy have also been documented as possible causes of plasma volume reduction.

This condition usually follows a benign course; however, a few patients may progress to an absolute polycythemia with an obvious underlying cause becoming apparent. There may be a few nonspecific symptoms reported in these patients such as headache, nausea, and dyspepsia. Hypertension, with possibly increased risk of thromboembolic complications, is seen in approximately one third of the patients. The Hct value is generally between 50 and 60 percent. Therapy indicated is in the form of encouragement of the cessation of smoking and/or alcohol intake, reduction of obesity, treatment of hypertension, stress counseling, and discontinuation of diuretic therapy when appropriate. On-going studies are investigating the efficacy of maintaining the Hct below 50 percent by phlebotomies. The risk of vascular occlusive episodes is presumably greatly decreased in this manner.

Essential Thrombocythemia

Essential thrombocythemia is a rare, chronic myeloproliferative disorder characterized by marked thrombocytosis associated with abnormal platelet function. Essential thrombocythemia was the last of the MPDs to be identified as a distinct entity, owing to the fact that extreme thrombocytosis is also frequently observed in CML, IMF, and PV. Sex-linked G6PD cell marker studies established ET as a clonal disorder involving the multipotential stem cell, which supported the placement of ET within the MPD classification.[67]

Diagnostic criteria that define ET were proposed by the PVSG in the mid 1970s. These guidelines

included (1) platelet count in excess of $600 \times 10^9/$ liter (and generally more than $1000 \times 10^9/$liter), (2) megakaryocytic hyperplasia in the marrow, (3) absence of identifiable causes of reactive thrombocytosis, (4) absence of the Ph[1] chromosome, (5) hemoglobin no higher than 13 g/dl or normal red cell mass, (6) absence of significant marrow fibrosis, and (7) presence of stainable iron in marrow or failure of iron trial.[68,69] Synonyms for this condition include idiopathic thrombocythemia, primary thrombocythemia, and primary hemorrhagic thrombocythemia.

Epidemiology

The mean age at time of diagnosis is approximately 60 years, the majority of patients being over age 50. This disease has occasionally been described in the 20- to 40-year age group, and very rarely in patients under age 20. Most studies do not demonstrate a statistical difference between frequency of males and females affected. The incidence of the disease has been estimated at seven per million population per year. The etiology of thrombocythemia remains unknown.

Clinical Features

Many patients are asymptomatic at diagnosis. With the introduction of automated instruments which routinely perform whole blood platelet counts, asymptomatic patients with coincidental high platelet counts are being discovered more frequently. Two thirds of patients in a recent study by Bellucci and colleagues[72] were found to be asymptomatic. Patients who are symptomatic present with hemorrhagic or vaso-occlusive symptoms, or both. In most instances bleeding is mild and manifestations are primarily mucocutaneous (epistaxis and ecchymoses); however, life-threatening hemorrhage may occur following accidental trauma or, rarely, following surgery. Gastrointestinal as well as esophageal variceal bleeding has also been reported. Hemorrhage has been attributed to several mechanisms: (1) platelet functional abnormalities; (2) thrombosis with infarction, ulceration of the infarction, and subsequent bleeding; (3) consumption of coagulation factors; and (4) increased numbers of circulating platelets causing excessive production of prostacyclin (PGI_2) by endothelial cells (increased PGI_2 suppresses platelet granule release and aggregation[45]).

Thrombosis, the other major manifestation of ET, is due to intravascular clumping of sludged, hyperaggregable platelets. Vascular occlusive symptoms are usually related to small vessel obstruction, although larger vessel occlusive events such as myocardial infarction and stroke may occur. Erythromelalgia of the toes, feet, and occasionally fingers (localized painful redness and burning) is a characteristic vaso-occlusive symptom and may progress to cyanosis and/or necrosis of the extremities. The toxic effect of the metabolites of platelet arachidonic acid appears to be responsible for the erythromelalgia, and this may be relieved by decreasing the platelet count or by use of anti-inflammatory agents.[70] Singh and Wetherly-Mein[71] suggest that thrombotic complications may be more common when the platelet count is greater than $2000 \times 10^9/$liter.

Neurologic manifestations are usually of a transient ischemic nature and include visual disturbances, headaches, paresthesias, dizziness, transient ischemic attacks, and rarely seizures. Complete stroke is an uncommon occurrence. In older patients, underlying degenerative vascular disease in combination with thrombocytosis and platelet functional defects all contribute to the thrombohemorrhagic complications.

Other signs and symptoms that have been observed in this disease are recurrent abortions and fetal growth retardation,[73] pruritus, gout, and priapism. Modest splenomegaly is present in approximately half of patients with ET. Splenic atrophy resulting from splenic vascular thrombosis and silent infarctions occurs in up to 20 percent of patients. According to Silverstein[80] patients with splenomegaly have a more favorable prognosis than do patients without splenomegaly. This is thought to be attributable to the beneficial effect of splenic sequestration of platelets.

Laboratory Features

The platelet count is always elevated, in the range of from 600 to $2500 \times 10^9/$liter. The peripheral blood smear reveals platelet anisocytosis, which correlates with an elevation of the platelet distribution width (PDW) as determined by automated instruments. Frequent abnormal morphologic findings include giant platelets (megathrombocytes) as well as microthrombocytes, platelet aggregates, abnormally granulated platelets, and megakaryocytic cytoplasmic fragments (Fig. 21–6) **(see Color Plate 218).**

A mild normocytic, normochromic anemia may be present in 15 to 20 percent of patients although the hemoglobin value is not usually less than 10 g/dl. When associated bleeding leads to iron-deficiency anemia, the MCV and MCHC will be decreased and a microcytic, hypochromic blood picture will be apparent upon examination of the peripheral blood smear. Erythrocyte morphologic findings reflective of hyposplenism, which occurs in the occasional patient with splenic infarction, and atrophy include the presence of Howell-Jolly bodies, Pappenheimer bodies (siderotic granules), target cells, and acanthocytes.

Leukocytosis is present in about one third of patients, with WBC counts rarely exceeding $50 \times 10^9/$liter. Neutrophilia is observed on the majority of patients with elevated WBC, but a mild eosinophilia and/or basophilia may occasionally be seen. Rarely, nucleated red cells and immature granulocytes may also be evident. The LAP score is variable but most commonly is normal.

The bone marrow in patients with ET demonstrates trilineage hyperplasia with a marked increase in the megakaryocytic component. The megakaryocytes are typically larger than normal and may be dysplastic in appearance **(see Color Plate 219)**. Stainable iron is present in most cases. Marrow karyotype is generally normal, but deletion of the long arm of chromosome number 21 (21q−) has been reported in some patients.[74] The PVSG, which has followed the largest series of strictly defined patients with ET, has been unable to confirm this finding.

Platelet function studies reveal a variety of abnormalities in most patients. Platelet aggregation is often decreased in response to epinephrine but a variable response to adenosine diphosphate (ADP) and collagen is seen. Studies have demonstrated both normal bleeding times (even in the case of pa-

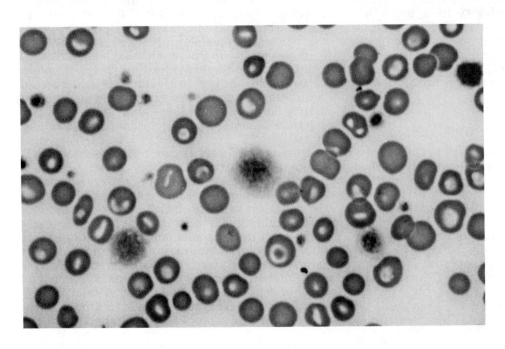

Figure 21–6. Peripheral blood smear in essential thrombocythemia. Note the presence of giant platelets (megathrombocytes).

tients with hemorrhagic tendencies[75]) and prolonged bleeding times. Reduced platelet factor 3, reduced platelet adhesion, low protein S levels,[76] and nucleotide storage pool defects have all been reported in association with ET. Despite all of these identified abnormalities, there is poor correlation with any of these findings and the incidence of clinical thrombohemorrhagic manifestations.

Differential Diagnosis

Essential thrombocythemia must be differentiated from the various cause of reactive thrombocytosis (Table 21–9), from other chronic MPDs with associated thrombocytosis, and from the myelodysplastic syndromes (MDSs) in which the platelet count is markedly elevated.

Most cases of extreme thrombocytosis represent incidental findings in patients with a wide variety of inflammatory and trauma–associated conditions. Reactive thrombocytosis, even when persistently present for weeks or months, is usually well tolerated in these patients and is not generally associated with thrombosis or hemorrhage. Bone marrow examination, virtually always performed in patients suspected of having MPD, is rarely done in instances of reactive thrombocytosis. The platelet count in secondary thrombocytosis seldom exceeds 1000×10^9/liter, commonly falling in the range of 500 to 750×10^9/liter. Platelet morphology and function is generally normal in chronic reactive states compared with the variety of abnormalities seen in MPDs.

When the platelet count is essentially greater than 600×10^9/liter and the bone marrow demonstrates predominant megakaryocytic hyperplasia, the diagnosis of ET should be investigated (Fig. 21–7). As there are no unique clinical, hematologic, or histopathologic findings in this disease, it is by nature a diagnosis of exclusion. At presentation, the hemoglobin should be less than 13 g/dl and the red cell mass normal in order to shift the diagnosis from PV with thrombocytosis (one third of PV cases) to ET. To ensure that masked PV has not been overlooked in those patients having a normal or decreased red cell mass due to iron deficiency, the establishment of the absence of marrow iron stores helps to exclude the diagnosis of ET. Additionally, if the clinical situation submits, a 1-month trial of iron therapy should be instituted. The response to iron therapy should be carefully monitored, and if a rise in the Hct and red cell volume is observed the patient should be evaluated for evidence of PV, evidence of blood loss, or both.

Chromosome analysis of the bone marrow should be performed to ensure that the Ph chromosome is not present, thereby excluding CML. In the approximately 15 percent of patients with CML and thrombocytosis that are Ph negative, the findings of profound myeloid metaplasia, low LAP score, and moderate to marked splenomegaly are important for supporting the diagnosis of CML.

Idiopathic myelofibrosis is often associated with extreme thrombocytosis. However, there is usually marked splenomegaly, a leukoerythroblastic blood picture, teardrop poikilocytosis, and the characteristic myelofibrotic involvement of the bone marrow (increased reticulin and collagen fibrosis). Additionally, the platelet morphology in ET has been described as nondysplastic, in comparison to the abundance of bizarre and atypical platelets seen in IMF.[77]

Myelodysplastic syndromes associated with thrombocytosis usually present with a more severe degree of anemia that is often macrocytic in appearance as compared with that seen in patients with ET. Additionally, the presence of either the 5q− syndrome or ringed sideroblasts in the bone marrow denotes a myelodysplastic syndrome as the cause of associated thrombocytosis rather than essential thrombocythemia.

Treatment

The therapeutic approach to ET depends upon a number of factors, including the patient's age and childbearing potential, the elevation of the platelet count, and, most important, the presence and duration of symptoms. Careful monitoring, without therapy specifically aimed at lowering the platelet count, is generally advocated for asymptomatic patients with extreme thrombocytosis. Young patients with few or no symptoms do not require treatment unless surgery is indicated or childbirth is imminent. In these cases plateletpheresis is useful in controlling the elevated platelet count. Additionally, a young patient with vaso-occlusive manifestations may respond to aspirin therapy alone.

In patients older than age 50 who are symptomatic, treatment is divided into the control of hemorrhage and manifestations of vascular occlusion, and the control of the progressive megakaryocyte proliferation. Acute hemorrhage and occlusive events indicate the necessity for immediate therapy. Plateletpheresis achieves a dramatic reduction in the platelet count in a matter of hours; however, this reduction is transient. Chemotherapy should be initiated whenever thrombohemorrhagic complications develop. A number of effective myelo-

Table 21–9. **CAUSES OF REACTIVE THROMBOCYTOSIS**

Acute hemorrhage
Splenectomy and hyposplenism
Postoperative
Malignancy
Chronic inflammatory disorders
Infection
Myelophthisic diseases
Hemolytic anemia
Iron deficiency
Drug-induced
Rebound recovery from thrombocytopenia
Exercise

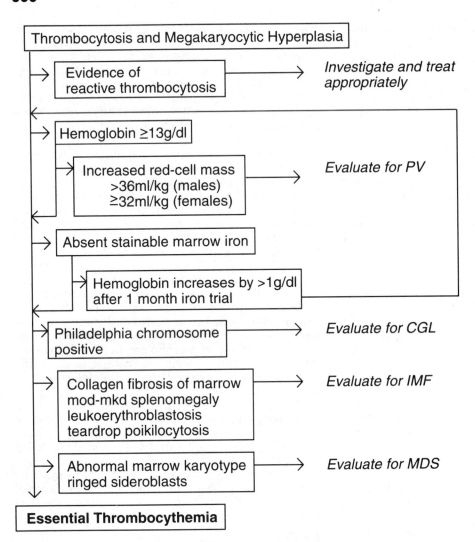

Figure 21–7. Differential criteria for diagnosis of essential thrombocythemia PV = polycythemia vera, CML = chronic myelogenous leukemia, IMV = idiopathic myelofibrosis, MDS = myelodysplastic syndrome. (Adapted from Iland,[82] p 167.)

suppressive agents have been used, but their use has been associated with an increased potential for induction of acute leukemia. Recently the antimetabolite hydroxyurea has emerged as the drug of choice because of its efficacy and low mutagenic risk. Hydroxyurea administration should be continued daily at a dosage of 15 mg/kg of body weight with adjustment according to response. In 90 percent of patients the platelet count will be decreased to less than 600×10^9/liter in 2 to 6 weeks.[70] A lower continuous dosage is required to maintain disease control, as once this treatment is halted the platelet count rises again. The only common side effects are dose-related, reversible leukopenia and macrocytic red cell changes.

Platelet antiaggregating agents, aspirin (300 mg daily) and dipyridamole (50 mg three times a day), have been shown to reverse incipient gangrene in patients with limb ischemia.[78] There is also some evidence that neurologic manifestations in ET are also improved through this therapy.[79] However, continuous use of aspirin once symptoms have abated or myelosuppression has controlled the platelet count, or both, is not advisable because of the significant risk of hemorrhage, particularly from the gastrointestinal tract.

Recent investigation of a new drug, anagrelide, for treatment of thrombocytosis has shown great promise.[80] Alpha interferon has also been advocated for treatment in ET.[81] This agent exerts an inhibitory effect on the growth of megakaryocyte progenitors which correlates clinically with a marked decrease in platelet count following treatment with interferon (IFN).

If surgery is indicated the platelet count should be controlled preoperatively by use of plateletpheresis or myelosuppression or both. Platelet concentrates may be needed to provide normal functional platelets.

Course and Prognosis

Recent follow-up studies by the PVSG and others suggest that survival time in ET is lengthy. Eighty percent will survive 5 years, with the prognosis particularly good for younger patients. Leukemic transformation can occur but seems to be an extremely rare event compared with the incidence of transitions found in other MPDs.

CASE STUDIES

Case 1

A 74-year-old man presented with complaints of increasing weakness, night sweats, shortness of breath, easy bruising, and a fever of 10 days' duration. The patient had lost about 10 lb over a 6-month period and noted early satiety. On physical examination he was found to appear pale and underweight and had a fever of 103°F. Massive splenomegaly, moderate hepatomegaly, and pulmonary congestion were noted. Purpuric lesions were present on the upper extremities.

Initial laboratory studies disclosed the following values.: WBC 30.5 × 10^9/liter, RBC 2.9 × 10^{12}/liter, Hgb 8.3 g/dl, Hct 25.8 percent, MCV 89 fl, MCH 28.6 pg, MCHC 32.2 percent, platelets (PLT) 650 × 10^9/liter. The differential count revealed 45 percent segmented neutrophils, 6 percent band neutrophils, 20 percent lymphocytes, 9 percent monocytes, 3 percent eosinophils, 3 percent basophils, 4 percent metamyelocytes, 3 percent myelocytes, 2 percent promyelocytes, and 5 percent "dwarf" megakaryocytes; and 15 nucleated red blood cells (NRBC)/100 WBC. Erythrocyte morphology demonstrated anisocytosis and poikilocytosis with prominent teardrop red cells, polychromasia, and basophilic stippling. Platelet number was increased and platelet morphology was abnormal, as evidenced by the presence of giant platelets and hyper and hypogranulated platelets and megakaryocytic fragments. Other laboratory tests included reticulocyte count 3.6 percent, LAP score 132 (normal 22 to 124), LDH 3054 μ/liter, uric acid 13.2 mg/dl, stool occult blood negative, Ph^1 chromosome negative, and direct antiglobulin test (DAT) negative. A bone marrow aspirate was attempted several times but was unsuccessful because of a dry tap. The bone marrow biopsy specimen revealed trilineage hyperplasia with many clumps of dysplastic atypical megakaryocytes. Extensive fibrosis was also noted. Bacterial and fungal bone marrow cell cultures were performed, and all results were negative.

Comment

The diagnosis of idiopathic myelofibrosis with myeloid metaplasia was made based on the classic findings of leukoerythroblastic anemia, marked splenomegaly, thrombocytosis with circulating megakaryocyte precursors, teardrop erythrocytes, and increased fibrosis of the bone marrow. Chronic myelogenous leukemia was excluded, as the majority of these patients have the Philadelphia chromosome, a low LAP, a higher proportion of myelocytes and myeloblasts, and a bone marrow showing predominantly granulocytic hyperplasia. Additionally the red cell morphologic changes—in particular teardrop red cells—are more prominent in myelofibrosis.

Fifteen to 20 percent of patients with known polycythemia vera undergo a transition to IMF; however, since there is no prior history of polycythemia (PV), this disease can be ruled out. Granulomatous disorders and acute leukemia can be excluded by careful scrutiny of the bone marrow and the negative microbiologic cultures. An increased platelet count and marked proliferation of bizarre megakaryocytes would be highly unusual in acute leukemia.

Another disorder involved in differential diagnosis is essential thrombocythemia. Again, these patients rarely show the red cell abnormalities associated with fibrosis in the marrow and splenic hematopoiesis, and the bone marrow is easily aspirated. The platelet count in ET is almost always greatly elevated, generally greater than 1000 × 10^9/liter, and immature granulocytes are rarely prominent.

Busulfan therapy was administered to this patient and continued over the course of 1 year. Blood transfusions were required every 3 to 4 weeks to counteract the impending anemia. Androgen therapy (danazol) was also initiated. The patient's condition gradually worsened, and it was evident that the chemotherapy was only mildly effective in decreasing splenic size. Splenectomy was performed in an attempt to ameliorate his anemia and relieve the constitutional symptoms of splenomegaly.

Four years after initial presentation this patient developed acute myelogenous leukemic and underwent a rapidly progressive fatal course. This case illustrates a typical course of myelofibrosis. The median survival is approximately 5 years and treatment has little effect in prolonging the survival.

Case 2

A 58-year-old man was admitted to the hospital with pain and swelling of the left arm suggestive of thrombophlebitis. He had presented to his physician 2 days earlier with complaints of pounding headaches, blurred vision, tinnitus, and generalized pruritus, especially after bathing. The patient had been treated for gout for the past 2 months. Family history is unremarkable for any hematologic disorders. The patient is a nonsmoker.

On physical examination, the patient's face appeared flushed and the retinal veins were engorged. Several ecchymoses were apparent on the legs. The spleen tip was palpable three fingerbreadths below the costal margin. No hepatomegaly or lymphadenopathy were observed.

Complete blood count revealed the following: WBC 20.3 × 10^9/liter, RBC 7.53 × 10^{12}/liter, Hgb 18.2 g/dl, Hct 58.0 percent, MCV 77 fl, MCH 24.2 pg, MCHC 31.4 percent, PLT 710 × 10^9/liter. The differential count demonstrated 80 percent segmented neutrophils, 8 percent band neutrophils, 9 percent lymphocytes, and 3 percent monocytes. Red cell morphology was consistent with a microcytic, hypochromic classification.

Subsequent investigations were undertaken as part of the diagnostic work-up of the erythrocytosis. Determination of the red cell mass (using the ^{51}Cr dilution method) was performed and found to be 41 ml/kg (normal, male, less than or equal to 36 ml/kg). The plasma volume was 40 ml/kg. Arterial oxygen saturation was 94 percent. The serum iron was 30 μg/dl (normal 50 to 150) and total iron-binding capacity (TIBC) 460 μg/dl (normal 250 to 450). Serum vitamin B_{12} was 925 pg/ml (normal 205 to 876) and vitamin B_{12} binding capacity was 2600 pg/ml (normal 1000 to 22). The LAP score was 198, and the uric acid determination was 10.3 mg/dl. A bone marrow examination revealed 95 percent cellularity with panhyperplasia and many large megakaryocytes. Iron stores were absent and the reticulin content was slightly increased.

Comment

Several findings in the history and physical examination suggest a presumptive diagnosis of PV. The nonspecific symptoms of headache and blurred vision are a result of cerebral circulatory disturbances due to hyperviscosity. Thrombotic episodes, such as the phlebitis recorded in this patient, are vascular manifestations resulting from the thrombocytosis in conjunction with the hyperviscosity and increased blood volume. The facial plethora and engorged retinal veins are findings associated with conjunctival and mucosal blood vessel congestion. Generalized pruritus occurs in 30 percent of patients with polycythemia and is related to hyperhistaminemia. The lack of cardiac or respiratory abnormalities, and the presence of normal arterial saturation is helpful in ruling out secondary polycythemia. The splenomegaly noted is a frequent finding in myeloproliferative disorders.

The most important clinical findings supportive of polycythemia are the elevation of the Hgb and Hct, increased red cell mass, and normal plasma volume. Furthermore, evidence of trilineage involvement, leukocytosis, and thrombocytosis, in addition to erythrocytosis and bone marrow panhyperplasia, strongly suggests a diagnosis of PV. Abnormal elevation of vitamin B_{12}, vitamin B_{12} binding proteins, uric acid, and LAP are all consistent with a myeloproliferative process and are helpful in establishing a diagnosis of PV. The low serum iron and absence of iron stores indicates concomitant iron deficiency. In most patients this is attributed to occult gastrointestinal blood loss and defective platelet function.

This patient fulfills all the diagnostic criteria for PV set forth by the PVSG. Since this 58-year-old patient has an elevated Hct and platelet count and is symptomatic (thrombophlebitis) both phlebotomy and myelosuppressive therapy were initiated. Colchicine and allopurinol were used to control the gout experienced by this patient. Pruritus was a persistent complaint despite the management of erythrocytosis by phlebotomy and hydroxyurea. Cyproheptadine was prescribed and found to be successful in controlling the pruritus.

Case 3

This 35-year-old white woman initially presented with thrombocytosis (platelet count 1200 × 10⁹/liter) discovered upon routine physical examination. Her WBC and Hgb were normal. The history was unremarkable except for occasional epistaxis and minor bruising. She was advised to have a routine follow-up examination and complete blood count (CBC) every 3 months and, despite a continually elevated platelet count, remained asymptomatic for 3 years. At that time she was seen by her physician with complaints of dizziness, visual disturbances, and erythromelalgia. She had also had recent dental surgery and experienced a major perioperative bleeding episode; mild splenomegaly was noted. Her platelet count was 2500 × 10⁹/liter, and PDW was increased. Other laboratory values were as follows: WBC 18.5 × 10⁹/liter, Hct 28.5 percent, prolonged bleeding time, reduced platelet adhesion, and defective platelet aggregation with epinephrine. Bone marrow biopsy demonstrated megakaryocytic hyperplasia with massive platelet clumping. Erythroid and myeloid hyperplasia, as well as a mild increase in reticulin content, were also observed.

Plateletpheresis was performed to rapidly reduce the marked thrombocytosis. The patient was treated with the myelosuppressive agent hydroxyurea in dosages varying from 1 g/day to 500 mg five times per week, depending on the platelet counts. The bleeding and vaso-occlusive symptoms were resolved and coagulation abnormalities corrected. Close follow-up is necessary for this patient to ensure continued beneficial clinical and laboratory response to all.

Comment

This case highlights the common findings in essential thrombocythemia: namely, marked increased platelet counts, thrombohemorrhagic events, splenomegaly, and bone marrow megakaryocytic hyperplasia. Although this is primarily a disease of upper middle-age (50 to 70) a second population of younger, predominantly female patients exists. Two thirds of patients are asymptomatic, as was this patient initially. With the advent of automated cell counters which routinely generate platelet counts, asymptomatic patients are being discovered more frequently.

The erythromelalgia noted in this patient represents one of the most characteristic vaso-occlusive manifestations. Prolonged bleeding after trauma or surgery is a common finding related to platelet dysfunction.

In an asymptomatic young patient it is advisable to withhold myelosuppressive therapy, as these patients do well for many years untreated. When patients requiring surgery present with preoperative findings of markedly increased platelet count and hemorrhagic complications, plateletpheresis will lower the platelet count dramatically. Additionally myelosuppression is necessary to control the hyperproliferative process.

Causes of reactive thrombocytosis, such as iron-deficiency anemia, malignancy, inflammatory disorders, splenectomy, and so on, are generally easy to exclude based upon the clinical and hematologic features of the individual patient. In order to reliably exclude the other chronic MPDs, the PVSG guidelines should be followed. To distinguish a patient with ET from an iron-deficient PV patient, a 1-month trial of oral iron should be instituted. The Hgb should not rise by more than 1 g/dl to support a diagnosis of ET. In patients with anemia, splenomegaly, and thrombocytosis, the presence of the Ph¹ chromosome conclusively rules out the diagnosis of ET.

The outlook for long-term survival in ET is encouraging as long as appropriate measures are taken to minimize thrombohemorrhagic complications. Many patients can tolerate markedly increased platelet counts for years without any complications. The introduction of plateletpheresis has allowed dramatic response in life-threatening or urgent surgical situations. Furthermore, the recent use of hydroxyurea has provided an effective chemotherapeutic agent that is associated with a lower mutagenic risk than that of traditional alkylating agents.

REFERENCES

1. Dameshek, W: Some speculations on the myeloproliferative syndrome. Blood 6:372, 1951.
2. Fialkow, PJ: The origin and development of human tumors studies with cell markers. N Engl J Med 291:26, 1974.
3. Jacobson, RJ, Solo, A, and Fialkow, PJ: Agnogenic myeloid metaplasia: A clonal proliferation of hemopoietic cells and secondary myelofibrosis. Blood 51:189, 1978.
4. Hoogstraten, B and Duiant, JR: Hematologic Malignancies. International Union Against Cancer, Current Treatment of Cancer. Springer-Verlag, Berlin/Heidelberg, 1986.
5. Adams, JA, Berrett, AJ, and Beard, J: Primary polycythemia, essential thrombocythemia and myelofibrosis—three facets of a single disease process? Acta Haematol (Basel) 79(1):33, 1988.
6. Greenberg, BR and Wilson, FD: Cytogenetics of fibroblastic colonies in Ph'-positive chronic myelogeneous leukemia. Blood 51:1039, 1978.
7. Hoffbrand, AV and Lewis, SM: Postgraduate Hematology, ed 3. Heineman Professional Publishing, Oxford, 1989.
8. Heuck, G: Zwei Falle von leukamia mit eigenthum lichem blut-resp knoch en markesbefund. Virchow Arch Pathol Anat 78:475, 1879.
9. Woodliffe, HJ and Douigan, L: Myelofibrosis: Incidence and prevalence in Western Australia. In Dahlem Workshop on Myelofibrosis-Osteosclerosis Syndrome. Pergamon Press, Oxford, 1974.
10. Ward, HP and Block, MH: The natural history of agnogenic myeloid metaplasia and a critical evaluation of its relationship with the myeloproliferative syndrome. Medicine 50: 357, 1971.
11. Boxer, LA, et al: Myelofibrosis-myeloid metaplasia in childhood. Pediatrics 55:861, 1975.
12. Anderson, RE, Hoshino, T, and Yamamoto, T: Myelofibrosis with myeloid metaplasia in survivors of the atomic bomb in Hiroshima. Ann Intern Med 60:1, 1964.
13. Bosch, W, et al: Toluene-associated myelofibrosis. Blut 58:219, 1989.
14. Rosen, PS, et al: Systemic lupus erythematosus (SLE) and myelofibrosis: A possible pathogenic relationship. Clin Res 21:565, 1973.
15. Lewis, CM and Pegrum, GD: Immune complexes in myelofibrosis: A possible guide to management. Br J Haematol 39:233, 1978.
16. Silverstein, MN: The evolution into and the treatment of late-stage polycythemia vera. Semin Hematol 3:79, 1976.
17. Khan, A, et al: A deficient G6PD variant with hemizygous expression in blood cells of a woman with primary myelofibrosis. Humangenetik 30:41, 1975.
18. Van Slyck, EJ, Weiss, L, and Dully, M: Chromosomal evidence for the secondary role of bone marrow fibroblast proliferation in acute myelofibrosis. Blood 36:729, 1970.
19. Lewis, SM: Myelofibrosis, Pathology and Clinical Management, Hematology. Vol 4. M. Dekker, New York, 1985.
20. Assoian, RK, et al: Cellular transformation by coordinated action of three peptide growth factors from human platelets. Nature 309:804, 1984

21. Jandl, JH: Blood, Textbook of Hematology. Little Brown, Boston, 1987.
22. McCarthy, DM: Fibrosis of the bone marrow: Content and causes. Br J Haematol 59:1, 1985.
23. Silverstein, MN: Agnogenic Myeloid Metaplasia. Publishing Science, Boston, 1975.
24. Manoharan, A, Hargrave, M, and Gordon, S: Effect of Chemotherapy on tear drop poikilocytes and other peripheral blood findings in myelofibrosis. Pathology 20:7, 1988.
25. Njoku, OS, et al: Anemia in myelofibrosis: Its value in prognosis. Br J Haematol 54:79, 1983.
26. Weinfield, A, Branehog, I, and Kutti, J: Platelets in the myeloproliferative syndromes. Clin Haematol 4:373, 1975.
27. Gilbert, HS: The spectrum of myeloproliferative disorders. Med Clin North Am 57:355, 393, 1973.
28. Laszlo, J, et al: The use of hydroxyurea in myelofibrosis. Minutes of Polycythemia Vera Study Group, November 1983.
29. Benbasset, J, et al: Splenectomy in patients with agnogenic myeloid metaplasia: An analysis of 321 published cases. Br J Haematol 42:207, 1979.
30. Williams, JW: Hematalogy, ed 3. McGraw-Hill, New York, 1983.
31. Rojkind, M: Anti-inflammatory and antifibrotic actions of colchicine. Myelofibrosis and the Biology of the Connective Tissue Symposium, New York, November 1982.
32. Barosi, G, et al: A prognostic classification of myeloid metaplasia. Br J Haematol 70:400, 1988.
33. Polliock, A, Prokocimer, M, and Matzner, Y: Lymphoblastic leukemia transformation (lymphoblastic crisis) in myelofibrosis and myeloid metaplasia. Am J Hematol 9:211, 1980.
34. Garcia, S, et al: Idiopathic myelofibrosis terminating in erythroleukemia. Am J Hematol 32:70, 1989.
35. Hippocrates: Dehumoribus. Chapter 1.
35a. Von Haller: Elementa physiologiae corporis humani. (Lausanne) 2:34, 1757.
36. Wasserman, LR: Polycythemia Vera Study Group: A Historical Perspective. Semin Hematol 23(3):183, 1986.
37. Turk, W: Beitrage zur Kenntnis des Symptomenbildes Polycythamie mit Milztumor und Zyanose. Wein Klin Wochenschr 17:153, 1904.
38. Hirsch, R: Generalized osteosclerosis with chronic polycythemia vera. Arch Pathol 19:91, 1935.
39. Rosenthal, N and Bassen, FA: Course of polycythemia. Arch Intern Med 62:903, 1938.
40. Castro-Malaspina, H, et al: Human megakaryocyte stimulation of proliferation of bone marrow fibroblasts. Blood 57: 781, 1981.
41. Danish, EH, Rasch, CA, and Harris, JW: Polycythemia vera in childhood: Case report and review of the literature. Am J Hematol 9:421, 1980.
42. Dawson, AA and Ogston, D: The influence of platelet counts on the incidence of thrombotic and hemorrhagic complications in polycythemia vera. Postgrad Med 46:76, 1970.
43. Rogers, BA: Want to live with Polycythemia vera for a few hours? Lab World 12:33, 1981.
44. Pollycove, M, Winchell, HS, and Lawrence, JH: Classification and evolution of patterns of erythropoiesis in polycythemia vera as studied by iron kinetics. Blood 28:807, 1966.
45. Reich, PR: Hematology, Physiopathologic Basis for Clinical Practice, ed 2. Little, Brown, Boston, 1984.
46. Juvonen, E: Megakaryocytic colony formation in polycythemia vera and secondary erythrocytosis. Br J Haematol 69:441, 1988.
47. Murphy, S, et al: Template bleeding time and clinical hemorrhage in myeloproliferative disease. Arch Intern Med 138:1251, 1978.
48. Ellis, JT, et al: Studies of bone marrow in polycythemia vera and the evolution of myelofibrosis and second hematologic malignancies. Semin Hematol 23(2):154, 1986.
49. Zittoun, G, et al: The three transcobalamins in myeloproliferative disorders and acute leukemia. Br J Haematol 31:287, 1975.

50. Gilbert, HS, et al: Serum vitamin B$_{12}$ content and unsaturated vitamin B$_{12}$–binding capacity in myeloproliferative disease. Ann Intern Med 71:719, 1969.

51. Berk, PD, et al: Therapeutic recommendations in polycythemia vera based on Polycythemia Vera Study Group Protocols. Semin Hematol 23(2):132, 1986.

52. Videbalk, A: Polycythemia vera, course and prognosis. Acta Med Scand 138:179, 1950.

53. Chievitz, E, and Thiede, T: Complications and causes of death in polycythemia vera. Acta Med Scand 172:513, 1962.

54. Thomas, DJ, et al: Cerebral blood flow in polycythemia. Lancet 2:161, 1977.

55. Kaplan, M, et al: Polycythemia vera: an update II, Semin Hematol 23(3):167, 1986.

56. Wasserman, LR: Polycythemia Vera Study Group: A historical perspective. Semin Hematol 23(3):183, 1986.

57. Donovan, PB: Progress in diagnosis and treatment of polycythemia vera. Lab World 12:25, 1981.

58. Sharon, R, Tatarsky, I, and Ben-arieh, Y: Treatment of polycythemia vera with hydroxyurea. Cancer 57:718, 1986.

59. Thorling, EB and Erslew, AJ: The "tissue" tension of oxygen and its relation to hematocrit and erythropoiesis. Blood 31:332, 1968.

60. Hurtado, A: Some clinical aspects of life at high altitudes. Ann Intern Med 53:247, 1960.

61. Eaton, JW, Skelton, TD, and Berger, E: Survival at extreme altitude: Protective effect of increased hemoglobin oxygen affinity. Science 183:743, 1974.

62. Block, AJ, et al: Sleep apnea, hypopnea and oxygen desaturation in normal subjects: A strong male predominance. N Engl J Med 300:513, 1979.

63. Balcerzak, SP and Bromberg, PA: Secondary polycythemia. Semin Hematol 12:353, 1976.

64. Dagher, FJ, et al: Are the native kidneys responsible for erythrocytosis in renal allorecipients? Transplantation 28:496, 1979.

65. Horwitz, A and McKelway, WP: Polycythemia associated with uterine myomas. JAMA 158:1360, 1955.

66. Gaisböck, F: Die Bedeutung des Blutdruckmessung fur die arztlichen Praxis. Dtsch Arch Klin Med 83:363, 1905.

67. Fialkow, PJ, et al: Evidence that essential thrombocythemia is a clonal disorder with origin in a multipotent stem cell. Blood 58:916, 1981.

68. Murphy, S, et al: Essential thrombocythemia: an interim report from the Polycythemia Vera Study Group. Semin Hematol 23(3):177, 1986.

69. Iland, HJ, et al: Differentiation between essential thrombocythemia and polycythemia vera with marked thrombocytosis. Am J Hematol 25:191, 1987.

70. Williams, WJ, et al: Hematology, ed 4. McGraw-Hill, New York, 1990.

71. Singh, AK and Wetherly-Mein, G: Microvascular occlusive lesions in primary thrombocythemia. Br J Haematol 36:553, 1977.

72. Bellucci, S, et al: Essential thrombocythemia, clinical evolutionary and biological data. Cancer 58:2440, 1986.

73. Falconer, J, et al: Essential thrombocythemia associated with recurrent abortions and fetal growth retardation. Am J Hematol 25:345, 1987.

74. Fuscaldo, KE, et al: Correlation of a specific chromosomal marker, 21q–, and retroviral indicators in patients with thrombocythemia. Cancer Lett 6:51, 1979.

75. Murphy, S, et al: Template bleeding time and clinical hemorrhage in myeloproliferative disease. Arch Intern Med 138:1251, 1978.

76. Conlon, M and Haire, W: Low protein S in essential thrombocythemia with thrombosis. Ann J Hematol 32:553, 1989.

77. Thiele, J, et al: Primary (essential) thrombocythemia versus initial (hyperplastic) stages of agnogenic myeloid metaplasia with thrombocytosis—a critical evaluation of clinical and histomorphological data. Acta Haematol 81:200, 1989.

78. Michiels, JJ, et al: Erythromelalgia caused by platelet mediated arteriolar inflammation and thrombosis in thrombocythemia. Ann Intern Med 102:466, 1985.

79. Jabaily, J, et al: Neurologic manifestations of essential thrombocythemia. Ann Intern Med 99:513, 1983.

80. Silverstein, MN, et al: Anagrelide: A new drug for treating thrombocytosis. N Engl J Med 318:20, 1988.

81. Gugliotta, L, et al: In vivo and in vitro inhibiting effect of alpha-interferon on megakaryocytic colony growth in essential thrombocythemia. Br J Haematol 71:177, 1989.

82. Iland, HJ, et al: Essential thrombocythemia: Clinical and laboratory characteristics at presentation. Trans Assoc Am Physicians 96:165, 1983.

QUESTIONS

1. *What is the origin of MPDs?*
   a. Fibroid infiltration of major organs
   b. Neoplastic transformation of multipotential stem cells
   c. Widespread deterioration of cellular functions
   d. Splenic sequestration of normal blood cells

2. *Which of the following is not a characteristic of chronic MPD?*
   a. Extramedullary hematopoiesis
   b. Possible termination in acute leukemia
   c. Cytogenetic abnormalities
   d. Hypoplasia of bone marrow

3. *What is the predominant abnormal erythrocyte morphology associated with idiopathic myelofibrosis?*
   a. Schistocytes
   b. Ovalocytes
   c. Teardrop cells
   d. Target cells

4. *Which features are the strongest characteristics of chronic myelogenous leukemia to distinguish it from myelofibrosis?*
   a. Presence of increased platelets and fibroblasts
   b. Decreased erythrocytes with abnormal morphology
   c. Increased leukocytes with hypercellular marrow
   d. Low LAP scores and presence of Ph^1 chromosome

5. *What are the laboratory findings in polycythemia vera?*
   a. Decreased hemoglobin and/or hematocrit; increased RBCs and granulocytes; decreased platelets
   b. Increased hemoglobin and/or hematocrit; increased RBCs, granulocytes, and platelets
   c. Normal hemoglobin and hematocrit; normal RBCs; increased granulocytes and platelets
   d. Increased hemoglobin and/or hematocrit; increased RBCs; decreased granulocytes and platelets

6. *Which features help to distinguish secondary polycythemia and relative erythrocytosis from polycythemia vera?*
   a. Absence of splenomegaly; normal leukocyte, platelet, and LAP levels
   b. Presence of splenomegaly; increased leukocyte, platelet, and LAP levels

    c. Presence of hepatomegaly; decreased leukocyte, platelet, and LAP levels

    d. Presence of both splenomegaly and hepatomegaly; increased leukocytes and platelets; decreased LAP score

7. *What is the safest and least expensive treatment for patients with polycythemia vera?*

    a. Chemotherapeutic agents

    b. Decrease of iron levels

    c. Therapeutic phlebotomy

    d. Decrease of erythropoietin levels

8. *Which condition will not cause an absolute erythrocytosis?*

    a. High altitude

    b. Chronic pulmonary disease

    c. Polycythemia vera

    d. Dehydration

9. *What condition is defined by a platelet count $> 1000 \times 10^9$/liter, megakaryocytic hyperplasia, absence of Ph chromosome, and hemoglobin ≤ 13 g/dl (or normal red cell mass)?*

    a. Essential thrombocythemia

    b. May-Hegglin anomaly

    c. Acute myelogenous leukemia

    d. Polycythemia vera

ANSWERS

1. b (p 339)
2. d (p 339)
3. c (p 340)
4. d (p 340)
5. b (p 349–350)
6. a (p 351–353)
7. c (p 353)
8. d (p 355–356)
9. a (p 357)

CHAPTER 22

JAMES M. LONG, M.D., Major, USAF, MC

Plasma Cell Disorders

OBJECTIVES

At the end of this chapter, the learner should be able to:
1. List laboratory tests for whole blood evaluation of immunoglobulin disorders.
2. Name laboratory tests and describe laboratory findings in serum evaluation of immunoglobulin disorders.
3. Name and describe laboratory tests for urine evaluation of immunoglobulin disorders.
4. List diagnostic criteria for multiple myeloma.
5. List diagnostic criteria for Waldenström's macroglobulinemia.
6. Describe heavy chain disease.

The plasma cell is the fully differentiated B lymphocyte (**see Color Plates 37 and 38**). Diseases of plasma cells are often a source of confusion to the novice but can be easily classified into a well-defined spectrum of disorders. Another name used in describing these disorders is monoclonal gammopathies. This denotes the clonal nature of the diseases and the excess production of immune globulins (also known as immunoglobulins or antibodies) seen in these illnesses. Clinical syndromes range from asymptomatic elevation of circulating globulins to rapidly debilitating, fatal illness. The value of the clinical laboratory in defining these disorders and providing the clinician with accurate data cannot be overemphasized.

To aid understanding of these illnesses, the development of lymphocytes and production of immune globulins is reviewed, followed by a discussion of the laboratory procedures used in their analysis. A brief overview of the individual diseases and the criteria for their differential diagnosis are then given, followed by more detailed clinical and laboratory descriptions of each in turn. The chapter ends with a series of illustrative case histories.

LYMPHOCYTE DEVELOPMENT

As discussed in the introductory chapters of this text, all subsets of lymphocytes develop from a common ancestor or progenitor cell. Through differentiation these cells become either B lymphocytes or T lymphocytes (Fig. 22–1). B lymphocytes produce antibody molecules under the influence of T lymphocytes. As T lymphocytes develop, they express one of two proteins, known as CD4 and CD8, on their surfaces. These antigens identify them as helper or suppressor cells, respectively. As their names imply, these T lymphocytes either stimulate or inhibit the antibody production of B lymphocytes. The complex interaction of antigen exposure with resulting antibody response by B lymphocytes under the modulation of helper and suppressor T lymphocytes results in an appropriate defense mechanism. When a B lymphocyte becomes autonomous, thus functioning irrespective of its controlling influences, it produces immunoglobulins (antibodies) in inappropriate amounts and in a functionally useless fashion. To allow a better understanding of these disorders, the next section briefly describes the structure and production of antibody molecules.

Fluorescent labeling studies have clarified the maturation sequence of B lymphocytes based on the location and type of immune globulins expressed. There are five classes of immune globulins, each possessing unique characteristics and function. These are named by the prefix Ig (denoting an immunoglobulin) followed by the class letter—IgG, IgA, IgD, IgM, IgE. Figure 22–2 demonstrates the evolution of an IgG-producing plasma cell. The pre-B lymphocyte has only IgM heavy chains in its cytoplasm. No surface immunoglobulins are found. With maturation IgM is first expressed on the surface; then IgG and IgD are expressed. In later stages of development, there is sequential loss of expression of surface IgM and IgD, leaving only surface IgG. In the final stage, the mature plasma cell, IgG, is produced only in the cytoplasm. Other immunoglobulin-producing cell lines follow a similar pattern of development. Depicted in Figure 22–3, deoxyribonucleic acid (DNA) is altered during the early stages of development, producing a progenitor for a clone of antibody-producing cells. The rearranged DNA in these cells is then translated via ri-

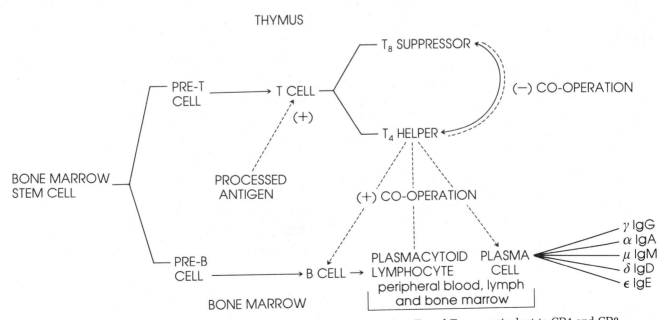

Figure 22–1. Development of T and B lymphocytes showing interaction. T_4 and T_8 are equivalent to CD4 and CD8.

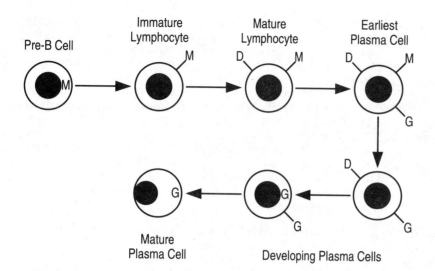

Figure 22–2. IgG-producing B-lymphocyte and plasma-cell development, showing location of immunoglobulins at different stages of development: M = IgM; D = IgD; G = IgG. (Adapted from Mellstedt, H, et al.)

bonucleic acid (RNA) into protein. This is followed by "packaging" in the Golgi apparatus, with later processing of the protein by addition of carbohydrates and disulfide bonds, to form the completed immunoglobulin molecule. The completed antibodies are then transferred to the cell surface where they are released by reverse pinocytosis.

IMMUNOGLOBULIN STRUCTURE AND FUNCTION

Immune globulins (antibodies) are proteins produced by B lymphocytes. Any substance that elicits an immune response is known as an antigen. Antibodies are unique in their ability to bind to an antigen with extreme specificity. Each immune globulin unit is composed of two identical heavy chains and two identical light chains (Fig. 22–4). Immune globulin units are often drawn stretched out into a Y configuration but in vivo are much more folded. There are five types of heavy chains corresponding to the five classes of immunoglobulins they define. They are named using the Greek letter equivalent of the immunoglobulin class: gamma for IgG, mu for IgM, alpha for IgA, delta for IgD, and epsilon for IgE. There are only two types of light chains: kappa and lambda. Only one type of light chain and one type of heavy chain are found in any one antibody molecule. An immune globulin molecule consisting of two gamma heavy chains and two kappa light chains would be designated IgG-κ, and so on.

The structure of an immunoglobulin unit is shown in Figure 22–4. A hinge zone of the heavy chains separates the molecule into two functional regions. One region of the molecule is formed by the amino-terminus of the two heavy chains. Each heavy chain is linked by disulfide bonds to a light chain. These form the antigen recognition sites. The opposite region of the molecule is composed of the carboxy ends of the two heavy chains and are linked at the hinge zone by disulfide bonds. This region determines whether the antibody can bind to complement or to neutrophils, or can activate some other effector mechanism.

The variable region of one light chain (V_L) and the variable region of one heavy chain (V_H) compose one binding site. Each immunoglobulin unit thus contains two antigen-binding sites. The variable regions of the light chains are not identical to those on the heavy chains, but the two make up a unique combination that determines the specificity or "idiotype" of the antibody molecule. These regions are called "variable" in that during development of the B lymphocytes, a rearrangement of the genetic material coding for this portion of the protein occurs. This results in each clone of cells having a unique sequence and antigen recognition capability. The remainder of the protein is designated the constant region; C_L in light chains, and C_H1, C_H2, and C_H3 in heavy chains. The peptide sequence for these regions is the same for all similar chains throughout the body. The gene sequences for the heavy chain are found on chromosome 14. The genes for the kappa and lambda light chains are found on chromosomes 2 and 22, respectively. Molecular weights and amino acid lengths are as noted in Table 22–1. IgM is found as a pentamer (composed of five immunoglobulin units). This gives it unique binding and physical properties. This is reflected in diseases caused by its overproduction, as will be seen later. IgA exists as a dimer (formed from two units), whereas IgG, IgD, and IgE are monomers.

There are subclasses of the immunoglobulins based on subtle differences in the heavy chains (Table 22–1). IgG3 causes some cases of hyperviscosity syndrome, discussed later.

LABORATORY EVALUATION OF IMMUNOGLOBULIN DISORDERS
Whole Blood

Complete Blood Count

The complete blood count (CBC) is performed by a standard automated cell counter, as described in Chapter 30. It measures the number of red cells, white cells, and platelets in the blood, which corre-

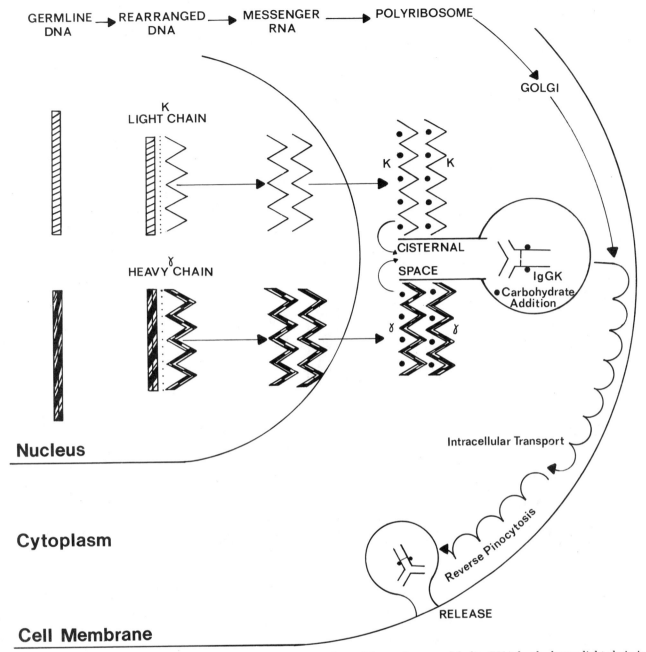

Figure 22–3. Illustration of the intracellular synthesis and export of an IgG-kappa immunoglobulin. DNA for the kappa light chain is found on chromosome 2; heavy chain DNA is found on chromosome 14. (Lambda light chain DNA sequence is on chromosome 22.)

lates well with bone marrow function. It is useful in the staging of plasma cell disorders, discussed later.

Peripheral Blood Smear

Wright's stains of peripheral blood smears from some patients with myeloma are bluish, which may be noted by experienced laboratory technologists and hematologists. This is due to increased background staining of the high levels of immunoglobulin in the plasma portion of the blood. Also seen is the "stacks of coins" arrangement of red blood cells on the smear, sometimes making it difficult to find a good area for examining red cell morphology. This

is caused by nonspecific antibody coating of red cells, causing them to adhere to each other in this fashion. Known as rouleaux formation, it is commonly seen in myeloma (**see Color Plate 225**). Although these clues can be the first evidence raising the suspicion of a plasma cell disorder, they are not diagnostic as they can be found in other inflammatory disorders as well.

Erythrocyte Sedimentation Rate

Erythrocyte sedimentation rate (ESR) is a measure of the rate at which red blood cells settle per hour. Rouleaux formation accounts for the high

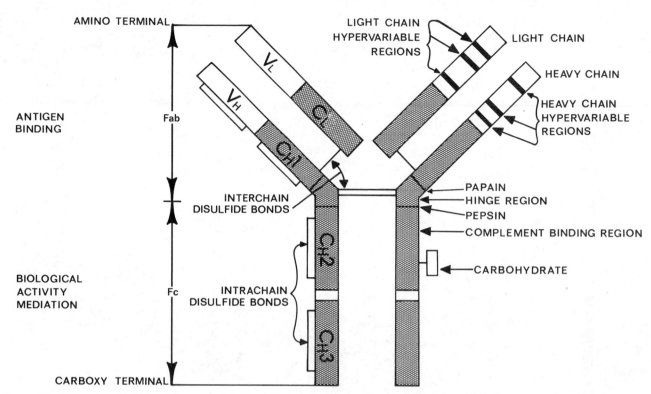

Figure 22–4. Structure of the basic immunoglobulin unit showing points of breakage by the proteolytic enzymes papain and pepsin. (See text for explanation.)

ESR seen in these diseases, in that stacked red cells have less surface area per red cell than they have individually. This causes less resistance to movement and a faster rate of descent. An otherwise unexplained elevation of ESR warrants serum protein electrophoresis to rule out multiple myeloma as a cause.

Serum

Serum Protein Electrophoresis

Serum protein electrophoresis (SPEP) is an analysis of the proteins present in the patient's serum based on size and electrical charge. A sample of serum is placed on a cellulose acetate support medium, which is saturated with a buffered electrostatic fluid. A continuous electrical current is then applied across the test field with resulting movement of the individual proteins. Those with the highest electrical charge will move fastest and therefore farthest. Heavier and less charged proteins will move more slowly and less far. Over time this results in a separation of the proteins on the cellulose acetate. The proteins are then stained. A densitometer may be used to determine the amount of protein present by the intensity of the stain. Several illustrative patterns are shown in Figure 22–5. The

Table 22–1. **IMMUNOGLOBULIN CLASSES: PHYSICAL AND BIOLOGIC PROPERTIES**

	IgG	IgA	IgM	IgD	IgE
Heavy chain class	γ	α	μ	δ	ϵ
Subclass	$\gamma^1\gamma^2\gamma^3\gamma^4$	$\alpha^1\alpha^2$	$\mu^1\mu^2$		
Molecular weights	150,000	160,000 (monomer) 400,000 (secretory)	900,000	180,000	196,000
Sedimentation coefficient	6.7	7–15	19	7	8
Serum concentration (mg/ml)	8–16	1.4–4.0	0.5–2.0	0–0.4	17–450 ng/ml
Biologic half-life (days)	23	6	5	2.8	2.4
Intravascular distribution (%)	45	42	76	75	51
Complement fixation	+ (variable)	—	++++	—	—
Placental transfer	+ ($\gamma^1\gamma^3$)	—	—	—	
Basophil/mast cell receptors	—	—	—	—	++++
Percent of total Ig	80	13	6	1	0.002

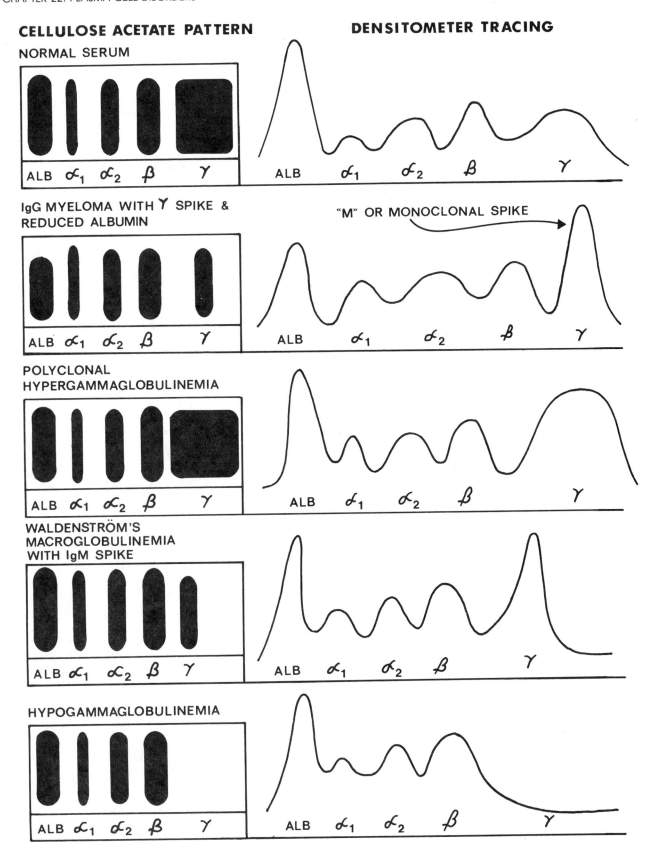

Figure 22–5. Patterns of serum protein electrophoresis showing characteristic patterns of normal serum, monoclonal M spike, polyclonal antibody production, IgM M spike, and the absence of antibody production seen in hypogammaglobulinemia.

first example shows an average-width band of normal immunoglobulin. When a disorder produces large amounts of identical immunoglobulin molecules, a narrow peak appears as shown in the second example. This occurs because their identical size and electrical charge cause them to move together in a narrow band. This is known as a monoclonal or M spike. Compare the M spike in the second example to the broad band caused by a high production of nonidentical immunoglobulins in the third example. This is commonly seen in infection or other immune reactions. IgM (five-unit pentamer) moves a shorter distance because of its heavier mass (fourth example in Figure 22–5), whereas IgA moves farther because of its higher electrical charge in comparison with IgG, IgD, and IgE. The last example shows the absence of a gamma peak seen in hypogammaglobulinemia.

The serum protein electrophoresis is thus a useful tool in determining whether or not a monoclonal protein is present. It is not reliable in defining to which immunoglobulin class a monoclonal protein belongs.

Immunoelectrophoresis

Following the finding of a monoclonal or M spike of immunoglobulin, immunoelectrophoresis (IEP) is used to define the antibody classes present in the serum sample. Agar is used as an electrophoresis medium with electrical separation performed, as for SPEP. Antisera (antibodies) to the immunoglobulins of the individual subclasses are then placed in troughs parallel to those containing the test serum. Specifically, anti-IgG, anti-IgM, and anti-IgA (for defining heavy chains), as well as antikappa and antilambda (for defining light chains), are used. The test serum and antisera are allowed to passively diffuse through the agar. When the antisera and the immunoglobulin meet in the agar between the troughs, they precipitate, forming visible bands. A normal serum sample is run for comparison. A thicker band in the test serum indicates an increased amount of immunoglobulin present. The antiserum causing the reaction then identifies the abnormal immunoglobulin. This test can be performed on serum or on concentrated urine samples.

A similar test is immunofixation in which a cellulose acetate strip impregnated with a monospecific antiserum is placed on the trough containing the electrophoresis-separated serum. It is then washed, with the antigen-antibody complexes remaining on the strip. Staining reveals the narrow bands consistent with a monoclonal gammopathy. This procedure is technically more difficult but is more sensitive. It may be used for evaluation of small amounts of monoclonal protein or when a false-negative IEP result is suspected. It should not be used as a standard screening procedure.

Immunoglobulin Quantitation

Evaluation of these diseases requires an accurate quantitation of the amount of monoclonal immunoglobulin present. The radial immunodiffusion method achieves this with an agar gel containing a known concentration of antisera to the immunoglobulin class being measured. The patient's serum or urine is placed into a small well cut into the agar and then allowed to diffuse. The interaction between the immunoglobulin and antiserum forms a visible precipitate in a ring pattern. The concentration of immune globulin in the sample is proportional to the diameter of the ring. Another method uses a nephalometer to measure the light scattering in a solution. The test serum and antiserum are placed in solution together. Antigen-antibody complexes produce turbidity and light scatter in proportion to the amount of antibody in the test sample. Its advantage is that it is not affected by the size of the individual antigens and accurately measures macromolecules such as IgM and polymerized IgA and IgG.

Urine

Urine Immunoelectrophoresis

Similar to the process described earlier, urine immunoelectrophoresis is used to distinguish between kappa and lambda light chains in urine. In disorders producing only light chains, urine is frequently positive while serum tests are negative.

Heat Precipitation Test

Urinary light chains (Bence Jones protein) have a unique identifying characteristic in that they are insoluble at 56°C. Slow heating results in visible precipitation of the proteins at this temperature, with solubility being regained at higher temperatures. Cooling from a temperature greater than 56°C results in a reversal of this process. Although 56°C is the quoted temperature, precipitation occurs over a range of temperatures from 45 to 60°C.

Sulfosalicylic Acid Test

The addition of sulfosalicylic acid to urine causes rapid precipitation of all urine protein and allows accurate quantitation of the total amount of protein in a 24-hour urine collection. The protein is then further evaluated as described earlier to establish the proportions of light chains, albumin, and so forth.

RADIOLOGIC EVALUATION OF PLASMA CELL DISORDERS
Radionuclide Skeletal Imaging

Multiple myeloma and related disorders evidence little or no osteoblastic activity, their predominant effect on bones being through osteoclast-activating factor (OAF). Because technetium phosphate bone scans show osteoblastic activity, they are generally not helpful in this group of disorders. They may be positive from secondary causes such as bone fractures.

Plain Film Radiographs

A standard survey of the skeleton for evaluation of plasma cell disorders includes films of the chest, skull, complete spine, the long bones of the extremities, and the pelvis. These areas are chosen because of the centralized location of red marrow in adults and because of the need to treat asymptomatic lesions in the weight-bearing bones that could lead to pathologic fractures from everyday activities.

The increased osteolytic activity results in punched-out lesions with sharply defined margins. Reactive osteoblastic activity evidenced by higher-density sclerotic bone is rare. Generalized loss of mineralization is common, especially in late cases of multiple myeloma. Vertebral compression fractures and pathologic fractures of ribs and weight-bearing bones frequently result.

Renal Imaging

Immunoglobulin can cause renal insufficiency by damaging renal tubules. Intravenous contrast used in imaging the kidneys is excreted in the urine. This can cause precipitation of urinary light chains and result in acute renal failure. For this reason, a screening SPEP and urine protein electrophoresis should be done as preliminary screens before using intravenous pyelography (IVP) to evaluate renal insufficiency. Radionuclide scans provide an effective means of evaluating renal function and retrograde pyelography can be substituted for evaluating possible obstruction in patients with known myeloma.

Spinal Cord Imaging

Plasmacytomas (tumors composed of plasma cells) can form in vertebrae and can cause spinal cord compression. When this occurs, prompt diagnosis and institution of therapy is required to preserve neurologic function. The "gold standard" for evaluating possible spinal cord compression is the myelogram. Only recently has its role been challenged by the noninvasive magnetic resonance imaging (MRI). This may provide equivalent data but at present is frequently not available on an emergency basis, except at major medical centers. Imaging of the entire canal is necessary to aid in irradiation and surgical treatment planning. Computed tomography (CT) is of limited use owing to the inability to perform longitudinal views of the skeletal axis. It can define cross-sectional anatomy in suspect areas.

EVALUATION OF SUSPECT PLASMA CELL DISORDERS

Patients with plasma cell disorders can present with a wide variety of symptoms or signs (Table 22–2). These problems include anemia, elevated serum calcium, renal failure, bone pain, lytic lesions on bone radiographs, elevated serum globulins incidentally found on chemistry panels, and

Table 22–2. **SIGNS AND SYMPTOMS OF PLASMA CELL DISORDERS**

Signs	Symptoms
Anemia	Tiredness
	Fatigue
	Shortness of breath
Hypercalcemia	Mental status changes
	Bone pain
	Kidney stones
	Constipation and abdominal pain
Renal failure	None (until late)
Bone lesions on radiograph	Bone pain
	Mass
	Pathologic fractures
Elevated serum globulins	Possible hyperviscosity syndrome
Serum hyperviscosity	Confusion
	Increased bleeding tendency
	Raynaud's phenomenon
	Visual complaints

symptoms possibly attributable to increased serum viscosity.

An appropriate evaluation of a suspect plasma cell disorder (Table 22–3) includes the following tests on serum: SPEP, calcium, phosphorus, blood

Table 22–3. **STANDARD EVALUATION OF PLASMA CELL DISORDERS**

Determine whether monoclonal protein is present
  Serum protein electrophoresis (SPEP)
  24-hour urine protein and protein electrophoresis (UPEP)
Characterize monoclonal protein
  Immunoelectrophoresis (IEP) of urine and serum
  Immunofixation electrophoresis if results are questionable
Evaluate bones with skeletal survey
Evaluate renal function
  Serum BUN
  Serum creatinine
  24-hour urine for creatinine clearance
Screening serum chemistry panel
  Calcium
  Total protein
  Albumin
  Uric acid
Evaluate bone marrow function
  CBC with reticulocyte count and WBC differential
  Bone marrow aspirate and biopsy
Evaluate for suppression of normal immunoglobulins
  Quantitative immunoglobulins
Serum viscosity
Miscellaneous
  Erythrocyte sedimentation rate (ESR)
  C-reactive protein
  Biopsy of mass or bone lesion if bone marrow is normal
  Beta-2 microglobulin if multiple myeloma diagnosed

urea nitrogen (BUN), creatinine. An M spike on SPEP should be evaluated further with IEP to define a specific immunoglobulin class. A CBC and an ESR are performed on whole blood. Urine is collected for 24 hours and assayed for total protein. The protein is then characterized by electrophoresis if present. A radiographic bone survey is done, which examines the skull, axial spine, and long bones of the extremities for lytic lesions. Intravenous iodine pyelography, used to evaluate renal anatomy and function, is scrupulously avoided when plasma cell disorders are being considered. Renal excretion of the contrast agent may cause precipitation of myeloma proteins in the renal tubules resulting in acute renal failure. If these tests support the suspicion of a plasma cell disorder, a bone marrow biopsy is usually done. Based on these studies a monoclonal gammopathy can be identified as being one of the diseases in Table 22–4, discussed individually later.

SOLITARY PLASMACYTOMA

The solitary plasmacytoma is a malignancy composed of a clone of plasma cells, which is localized to one area with no evidence of distant spread. It generally presents as pain or swelling in a bone (**see Color Plate 224**), although nonosseous soft tissue plasmacytomas are sometimes seen as well. Plain radiographs are often done first. Single, sharply circumscribed, lytic, punched-out lesions are the classic finding. These occur most commonly in the midshaft of one of the long bones of the extremities. There is usually evidence of swelling of the bone before the cortex is destroyed, but cortical destruction with an adjacent soft tissue mass is frequently seen. Complete evaluation is needed with the most common findings being a normal SPEP or a small M spike, with bone marrow, renal function, and radiologic bone survey as described earlier, all normal. Biopsy of the suspect lesion yields the diagnosis by demonstrating malignant plasma cells. With no other areas of involvement and with the criteria for multiple myeloma not met, these lesions are often treated with localized radiotherapy alone. Osseous plasmacytomas have a high tendency to develop into multiple myeloma (70 percent) or recur locally (15 percent) within 10 years of treatment. Extraosseous (soft tissue) plasmacytomas, on the other hand, are cured up to 70 percent of the time by surgical excision or by irradiation alone.

MULTIPLE MYELOMA

Description and Diagnosis

Multiple myeloma (MM) is a systemic disorder, meaning that malignant cells are not limited to any specific region of the body. It is not effectively treated with local measures such as surgery or radiotherapy. It is characterized by malignant plasma cells infiltrating the bone marrow (**see Color Plates 220 and 221**). There is often compromised marrow function and multiple lytic bone lesions (Figs. 22–6 and 22–7). High levels of circulating monoclonal immunoglobulin, excretion of light chains in the urine, renal insufficiency, hypercalcemia, and suppression of normal immunoglobulin production are commonly present. Criteria have been developed for the diagnosis of MM because there is variation in its clinical presentation. These criteria are outlined in Table 22–5. At least one major and one minor criterion must be met or three minor criteria with careful attention to the rules of combination given with the table. A bone marrow biopsy, radiologic bone survey, serum and urine protein electrophoresis and immunoelectrophoresis, as well as biopsy of suspicious masses (in the case of negative bone marrow findings) are required for complete evaluation.

Epidemiology

The overall incidence of this disease is three cases per 100,000, with a mean age of 63 years old. It is rarely seen in patients under 40 years of age (less

Table 22–4. **PLASMA CELL DISORDERS**

Solitary plasmacytoma
Multiple myeloma
  Smoldering myeloma
  Classic multiple myeloma
  Advanced myeloma
  Nonsecretory myeloma
Monoclonal gammopathy of undetermined significance
  (MGUS)
Waldenström's macroglobulinemia
Heavy chain disease (HCD)
  Gamma HCD
  Mu HCD
  Alpha HCD

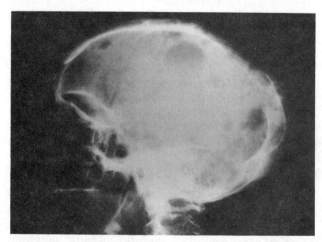

Figure 22–6. Skull radiograph showing discrete punched-out lesions characteristic of multiple myeloma (MM). This is due to production of osteoclast activating factor by clusters of malignant plasma cells.

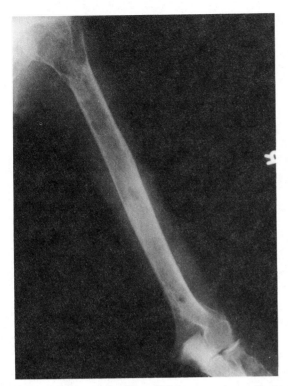

Figure 22-7. Radiographic film of left humerus in a patient with multiple myeloma. Areas with severe cortical bone destruction may fracture by everyday activities such as lifting or walking (pathologic fractures).

Table 22-5. **DIAGNOSTIC CRITERIA FOR MULTIPLE MYELOMA**

I. Biopsy proven plasmacytoma

II. >30% plasma cells in bone marrow

III. Monoclonal protein (M spike)

>3.5 g/dl of serum IgG or

>2.0 g/dl of serum IgA or

>1.0 g/24 hr of lambda or kappa urinary light chains (in absence of amyloidosis)

Minor Criteria

a. 10–30% plasma cells in bone marrow

b. M spike present but less than levels above

c. Multiple lytic bone lesions

d. Low normal immunoglobulins

IgM <50 mg/dl

IgA <100 mg/dl

IgG <600 mg/dl

Rules of Combination

A. One major and one minor criterion

1. I+b; I+c; I+d (not I+a)

2. II+b; II+c; II+d (not II+a)

3. III+a; III+c; III+d (not III+b)

B. Three minor criterion (must include a + b)

1. a + b + c

2. a + b + d

Source: Adapted from Durie, BGM and Salmon, SE: Staging kinetics and flow cytometry of multiple myeloma. In Wiernik, P, et al (eds): Neoplastic Diseases of the Blood. New York, Churchill Livingstone, 1985.

than 2 percent of cases). The rate of occurrence rises steadily with advancing age, to peak at 70 cases per 100,000 population at age 70. It has a well-defined male-to-female ratio of 1.6, and is twice as common in blacks as in whites.

Laboratory Findings

Rouleaux formation is common on peripheral blood smears. Accordingly, the Westergren ESR may be elevated to levels greater than 100 mm/hr (normal up to 13 mm/hr for men). Anemia and thrombocytopenia are seen with high tumor mass (see farther on). Bone marrow shows atypical plasma cells infiltrating the marrow with binucleate cells commonly seen (**see Color Plates 220 and 221**). Immunoglobulin may aggregate in the cytoplasm of some of these cells, staining red with Wright-Giemsa stain. These aggregates are called Russell bodies (**see Color Plate 220**). Flame cells are large, intensely staining multinucleated plasma cells that may be seen in myeloma (**see Color Plate 229**).

Elevated serum BUN and creatinine may indicate renal damage. Elevated serum calcium is frequently found and may be as high as 15 to 16 mg/dl (normal 8.5 to 10.5 mg/dl). This can cause an osmotic urine diuresis which compounds the hypercalcemia as well as the risk of renal failure. In advanced cases a high rate of cell turnover may cause an elevation of serum uric acid.

Pathophysiology

Multiple myeloma causes disease in four major ways (Fig. 22-8). First, malignant plasma cells produce OAF. This induces overactivity of osteoclasts with consequent bone reabsorption, leading to the characteristic lytic bone lesions with resultant pain and pathologic fractures, as well as elevation of serum calcium. Hypercalcemia can also induce pain, psychosis, kidney stones (nephrolithiasis), or frank renal failure. Intestinal dysmotility with constipation and abdominal pain are also seen ("bones, moans, stones, and groans").

Second, overproduction of immunoglobulin is one of the hallmarks of this disease. IgG is the most common, but IgA also accounts for 25 percent of cases. IgD, IgE, and IgM together account for less than 1 percent of cases (Table 22-6). There is often an excess of light chains formed, resulting in urinary excretion of the excess (Bence Jones proteins). Approximately 22 percent of cases exhibit light chain production only. These often have measurable proteins in the urine only. Less than 1 percent of cases will not produce any abnormal immunoglobulin.

Hyperviscosity syndromes may occur because of the high levels of immunoglobulins. This is more common with IgM (see discussion on Waldenström's macroglobulinemia later), although IgA and IgG3 may polymerize and cause similar problems. Myeloma proteins can also precipitate in the renal

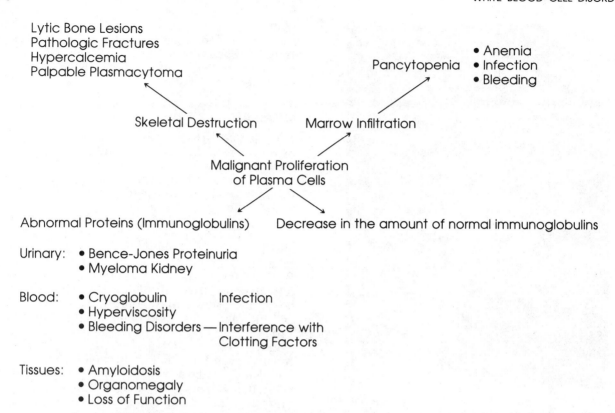

Figure 22–8. Mechanisms of disease in multiple myeloma. Skeletal destruction, abnormal immunoglobulin production, marrow failure, and decreased production of normal immunoglobulins all play a role.

tubules and result in renal failure. This can be precipitated (literally) by IVP with urinary excretion of the contrast medium.

Amyloid can form in many organ systems due to deposition of immunoglobulin light chains (**see Color Plate 227**). This can affect the kidneys, causing renal dysfunction and proteinuria. It can also affect the heart, causing conduction problems and heart failure. Carpal tunnel syndrome is not uncommon. Lambda light chains are most commonly found in patients with myeloma-related amyloidosis, yet kappa light chain deposition has been demonstrated as well.

Expanding cell mass is the third mechanism of disease. The proliferating myeloma cells can replace normal marrow (**see Color Plate 221**), result-

ing in decreased production of the formed blood elements (red cells, white cells, and platelets). This can cause symptoms of anemia, increased risk of infection, and prolonged bleeding. Expanding plasmacytomas may also impinge on adjacent structures, the most common and serious occurrence being spinal cord compression by a plasmacytoma arising from a vertebral body. Myeloma cells may diffusely infiltrate organs such as the liver, spleen, and kidneys, resulting in enlargement and dysfunction.

The fourth problem caused is the increased risk of bacterial infection due to lowered production of normal immunoglobulins (humoral immunity). Infection is the most common cause of death. Encapsulated bacteria, especially pneumococci, are the most dangerous organisms. They frequently cause multiple episodes of infection during the course of the disease. Cellular immunity is not affected, thus there is no increase in illness due to viruses, fungi, or acid fast organisms. All patients should receive pneumococcal vaccine on diagnosis. The benefits of prophylactic intravenous immunoglobulin in preventing infections are currently under study.

Staging and Prognosis

Untreated patients with MM have a median survival of 7 months. At present, there is no curative therapy. Most patients have been shown to have relatively slow-growing or indolent disease at time of

Table 22–6. **IMMUNOGLOBULIN CLASS FREQUENCIES FOUND IN MULTIPLE MYELOMA**

Class	Frequency (%)
IgG	52
IgA	25
Light chains only	22
IgD, IgE, or IgM	<1
Nonsecretory	<1

diagnosis. Rates of cell growth (as measured by labeling with tritiated thymidine) usually increase with the duration of disease. Survival is related to the mass of tumor cells present. This can be estimated from clinical parameters such as hemoglobin, serum calcium, serum and urine protein electrophoresis, and skeletal radiography, as shown in Table 22–7. Assignment to low tumor mass requires all the stage I criteria to be met. Any of the high mass stage III criteria is sufficient for inclusion in this poor prognostic group. Stage II, or intermediate mass, is assigned when one or more low mass criteria are not met, yet no high mass criteria are found. Median survival for the three groups are greater than 60 months for low mass, 41 months for intermediate mass, and 23 months for high mass. Renal function has also been shown to be highly prognostic for survival. The stage may be appended with an A or B, based on serum creatinine less than 2.0 mg/dl or 2.0 mg/dl or greater, respectively, indicating the influence of renal function on prognosis. Serum $\beta 2$ microglobulin is a nonspecific protein produced by a variety of tumors. Its serum level parallels tumor mass when corrected for degree of renal insufficiency. It is the most powerful single in-

Table 22–7. MYELOMA STAGING SYSTEM

Criteria	Median Survival
Stage I (low myeloma mass)	>60 months
(all criteria *must* be met)	
1. Hemoglobin >10 g/dl	
2. Corrected serum calcium <12 mg/dl	
3. Less than 2 lytic bone lesions	
4. Small M spike	
IgG <5 g/dl	
IgA <3 g/dl	
Urine light chains <4 g/24 hr	
Stage II (intermediate myeloma mass)	41 months
1. Does not meet *all* stage I criteria	
2. Does not meet *any* stage III criteria	
Stage III (high myeloma mass)	23 months
(any of the following criteria)	
1. Hemoglobin <8.5 g/dl	
2. Corrected serum calcium >12 mg/dl	
3. ≥2 lytic bone lesions	
4. Large M spike	
IgG >7 g/dl	
IgA >5 g/dl	
Urine light chains >12 g/24 hr	
Substaging	
A. Serum creatinine <2.0 mg/dl	
B. Serum creatinine >2.0 mg/dl	

Source: Adapted from Durie, BGM and Salmon, SE: Staging kinetics and flow cytometry of multiple myelomas. In Wiernik, P, et al (eds): Neoplastic Diseases of the Blood. New York, Churchill Livingstone, 1985.

Table 22–8. MYELOMA STAGING BASED ON $\beta 2$ MICROGLOBULIN AND SERUM ALBUMIN

Stage	$\beta 2$ Micro-globulin	Serum Albumin	Median Survival
I. Low Risk	<6 µg	>3.0 g/dl	55 months
II. Intermediate Risk	>6 µg	>3.0 g/dl	29 months
III. Poor Risk		<3.0 g/dl	4 months

Source: Adapted from Bataille, R, et al.

dicator of prognosis in MM. When used in conjunction with serum albumin, it may give the best stratification system for staging based on prognosis (Table 22–8). It may also be a useful marker for nonsecretory multiple myeloma as described later.

Clinical Course and Therapy

"Smoldering" Myeloma

Multiple myeloma often has a low rate of cell turnover at time of diagnosis. This is particularly true when an asymptomatic case is found on screening chemistry panels as an isolated elevated globulin level. Some patients have no findings necessitating treatment such as lytic bone lesions, hypercalcemia, or significant marrow or renal compromise. These patients can have a protracted period in which treatment may be withheld with close clinical and laboratory monitoring. Most cases will develop into the more classic, aggressive MM over a variable time ranging from months to years. As there is currently no curative therapy, they can be spared the toxicity of chemotherapy until such time as their disease requires it.

Classic Multiple Myeloma

Multiple myeloma most commonly presents with disease requiring treatment, be this elevated calcium, renal failure, lytic bone lesions, or low blood counts. Some cases of MM present with a problem requiring urgent treatment. When presenting with spinal cord compression, decompressing vertebral laminectomy with tissue biopsy is often indicated, followed by local radiotherapy while the myeloma work-up is pursued. A similar surgical approach is made if the patient presents with a pathologic fracture owing to extensive bone destruction from an expanding plasmacytoma. The surgical procedure allows for stabilization by internal fixation as well as tissue diagnosis. This is followed by radiotherapy as well.

Hypercalcemia is common and is treated acutely with saline hydration, furosemide (a loop diuretic), and glucocorticoids. Control sometimes requires calcitonin, etidronate, or mithramycin as well.

For nonemergent presentations, therapy is begun after a complete but rapid evaluation. Pain control is a major concern in patients with myeloma. Nonsteroidal anti-inflammatory agents are often useful, but narcotic analgesics are frequently required. Calcitonin is very useful in controlling the bone pain associated with myeloma, as well as in controlling the hypercalcemia. Although multiple chemotherapy regimens have been published, the standard regimen at present is oral melphalan and prednisone (MP). It is usually given for 4 consecutive days and repeated every 4 to 6 weeks. Progress is followed by monitoring the level of the monoclonal protein by SPEP and urine electrophoresis. Reported response rates range from 40 to 70 percent with this regimen. Invariably this treatment fails to control the disease at some point. When this happens, addition of other alkylators such as cyclophosphamide, anthracyclines, or nitrosourea class drugs may be of benefit, as is the vincristine, doxorubicin, and Decadron regimen noted later. High doses of glucocorticoids alone may have some benefit as a salvage regimen in patients with resistant disease. Trials of the clinical use of interferon-alfa in multiple myeloma are currently in progress. Isolated case reports of prolonged remission using allogeneic bone marrow transplantation can be found, but this therapy remains experimental because most individuals so treated have relapsed. This indicates that current therapies are inadequate to eradicate the disease.

Failure of chemotherapy to control the malignant clone eventually results in progressive multisystem failure. Pathologic fractures due to generalized demineralization of the bones commonly occur. Hypercalcemia as well as renal and bone marrow failure lead to death within weeks to months in resistant disease, most commonly from infection or renal insufficiency.

Myeloma patients treated with alkylator chemotherapy also have a significant risk of developing treatment-related acute myelogenous leukemia (AML). This risk may be as high as 20 percent in patients surviving 4 years after starting therapy. Prognosis for those affected is universally poor.

Late or Advanced Myeloma

Recent evidence suggests that the use of a more aggressive regimen for individuals with stage III, high-bulk disease may improve survival. The addition of cyclophosphamide and vincristine to standard melphalan and prednisone (VMCP), or regimens such as a 4-day continuous intravenous infusion of vincristine, doxorubicin, and oral dexamethasone (VAD), are often used, with response rates as high as 84 percent. Other regimens using various combinations of these drugs, as well as the nitrosoureas, have been published as well.

Plasma Cell Leukemia

The presence of plasma cells circulating in the blood (**see Color Plate 223**) is a late finding in advanced MM. Aggressive chemotherapy regimens such as VMCP, VAD, or others using nitrosoureas are frequently used in an attempt to reduce the tumor mass.

This should not be confused with primary plasma cell leukemia which differs from myeloma in that many immature plasma cells are found circulating in the blood, and severe compromise of the marrow is seen. The liver and spleen are usually quite enlarged. Hyperviscosity syndromes and bleeding due to platelet dysfunction are frequently seen. Bone involvement with resultant hypercalcemia is uncommon. Treatment is usually the same as for advanced myelomas with only 25 percent of affected individuals surviving longer than 1 year.

Nonsecretory Myeloma

A rare variant of MM, nonsecretory myeloma is a malignant clone of plasma cells too immature to secrete immunoglobulins. The predominant symptoms are of bone pain and hypercalcemia. Because of the lack of abnormal immunoglobulin production, less suppression of normal immunoglobulins is seen, resulting in a lower incidence of infection. There is a lower incidence of renal dysfunction as well, probably because of the absence of urinary light chain excretion and resultant kidney damage. This translates into an improved survival when compared with classic myeloma. Because there is no M spike to follow on electrophoretic studies, treatment decisions are more difficult. Beta-2 microglobulin may be useful as a tumor marker in this situation, as are serum calcium and periodic radiologic bone surveys.

MONOCLONAL GAMMOPATHY OF UNDETERMINED SIGNIFICANCE

Previously known as benign monoclonal gammopathy, monoclonal gammopathy of undetermined significance (MGUS) is a common finding in asymptomatic individuals in their sixth (1 percent of population) to eighth (3 percent of population) decades of life. It presents as an elevated globulin fraction on screening chemistry panels or as an M spike found on SPEP. By definition, there are no lytic bone lesions, an M spike less than 2 g, less than 10 percent plasma cells in the bone marrow, and normal levels of other immunoglobulins. Table 22–9 contains the criteria for diagnosis. Roughly 10

Table 22–9. **DIAGNOSTIC CRITERIA FOR MGUS**

I. M spike present
IgG <3.5 g/dl
IgA <2.0 g/dl
Urinary light chains <1.0 g/24 hr
II. <10% plasma cells in bone marrow
III. No bone lesions
IV. No symptoms
(all criteria must be met)

Source: Adapted from Durie, BGM and Salmon, SE: Staging kinetics and flow cytometry of multiple myeloma. In Wiernik, P, et al (eds): Neoplastic Diseases of the Blood. New York, Churchill Livingstone, 1985.

Table 22-10. **MGUS: 5-YEAR FOLLOW-UP**

Course of Illness	Fraction of Patients
No significant progression of M spike	57%
>50% increase in M spike	9%
Progression to malignant monoclonal gammopathy	11%
Death from unrelated cause	23%

percent of these individuals will progress to overt MM or other lymphocyte or plasma cell disorders at some time. The name has therefore been changed from benign monoclonal gammopathy to MGUS. Table 22-10 summarizes the outcome of patients with MGUS followed for 5 years. As there is no reliable means of predicting which patients will progress to other diseases, a second evaluation is performed 3 months after diagnosis, then every 6 months for life. No treatment is warranted.

WALDENSTRÖM'S MACROGLOBULINEMIA

Description and Clinical Characteristics

Macroglobulinemia refers to the overproduction of monoclonal IgM, a high molecular weight pentameric molecule. It is considered a low-grade malignancy with an insidious onset and a protracted clinical course. It is caused by the loss of regulation of a clone of cells which appear to be in an intermediate stage of development between the mature lymphocytes and the early plasma cells. Morphologically, these are commonly called plasmacytoid lymphocytes or "prolymphs" (**see Color Plate 226**). This is a disease most commonly seen in the seventh decade of life with no sex predilection. Life expectancy ranges from 8 months to 8 years.

The predominant early symptoms are vague weakness, fatigue, and weight loss. Later symptoms are caused by high levels of circulating IgM, abnormal bleeding, an enlarged liver and spleen, and, less frequently, enlarged lymph nodes. Table 22-11 compares the findings in MM and Waldenström's macroglobulinemia (WM). Diagnosis is made by the demonstration of plasmacytoid lymphocytes in the peripheral blood and bone marrow and an IgM M spike on SPEP.

Hyperviscosity Syndrome

Hyperviscosity occurs as a result of levels of monoclonal IgM as high as 10 g/dl. Viscous blood flows through small blood vessels more slowly than normal. This often causes altered neurologic function, with blurred vision, headache, and confusional episodes. This can progress to stuporous states and even frank coma. These mental changes are sometimes mistaken for psychiatric illness. Visual problems such as blurring and blind spots are common and can be caused by hyperviscosity alone. Damage to the retina caused by rouleaux formation within the retinal vessels (characteristic "sausage-link" pattern shown in **Color Plate 228**) may also play a role. The high level of protein also increases the serum oncotic pressure leading to an expanded intravascular volume. This can lead to congestive heart failure in some patients.

A cryoglobulin is a protein which precipitates on exposure to cold. In some cases of WM the IgM produced is a cryoglobulin. This can cause symptoms such as Raynaud's phenomenon (painful, cyanotic extremities on cold exposure), thrombosis of small arteries in exposed areas of the body, and renal damage (**see Color Plate 222** and Table 22-12).

Organ Involvement

Liver, spleen, and lymph node enlargement is present in less than half of affected patients. When present, the characteristic plasmacytoid lymphocytes can be found to be diffusely infiltrating these organs. Infiltration of neurologic structures is also seen in some cases. Nerve roots, meninges, as well as the brain itself can be affected and can present as a variety of neurologic complaints depending on the structures involved.

Hemostasis Problems

Bleeding problems are common in Waldenström's macroglobulinemia. Abnormalities of platelet function are demonstrated by a prolonged bleeding time despite normal numbers of circulating platelets. This is due to coating of the platelets with IgM molecules which impairs their adhesiveness

Table 22-11. **COMPARISON OF MULTIPLE MYELOMA AND WALDENSTRÖM'S MACROGLOBULINEMIA**

	Macroglobulinemia	Myeloma
Organomegaly	+++	+
Hyperviscosity	+++	+
Lytic bone lesions	+	+++
Renal failure	+	+++
Length of survival	++	+

Table 22-12. **CLINICAL FEATURES OF HYPERVISCOSITY SYNDROME**

Sign or Symptom	Fraction of Patients
Neurologic changes	20%
Retinopathy	35%
Hypervolemia/congestive heart failure	20%
Abnormal bleeding	20%
Enlarged liver and spleen	35%
Enlarged lymph nodes	45%

and aggregation. Coagulation time studies such as prothrombin time (PT) and APTT, which test the integrity of the coagulation cascade may also be affected. This and the ability to aggregate may be due to IgM interfering with normal interactions between fibrin monomers as well as with other coagulation factors. The compromise of both platelet and coagulation protein function makes bleeding problems frequent. Minor nose and gum bleeding are most common, but central nervous system and gastrointestinal bleeding are also seen.

Treatment and Prognosis

As is common with most low-grade malignancies, Waldenström's macroglobulinemia is not curable with current technology. The mainstay treatment for WM is with alkylator chemotherapy—most commonly, chlorambucil, cyclophosphamide, or melphalan. Anthracyclines such as doxorubicin can be used as well, especially when the disease becomes refractory to alkylators alone.

If severe symptoms such as loss of vision or neurologic function are present, IgM can be quickly removed from the circulation by plasmapheresis. Plasmapheresis replaces a portion of the patient's plasma with physiologic saline. This rapidly lowers the serum IgM levels, and thus viscosity, and relieves symptoms of impaired blood flow within hours. Chemotherapy should be started at the same time to provide long-term control.

Prognosis is estimated by the degree of marrow involvement. If more than 50 percent of the marrow is replaced by abnormal "plymphs," the median survival is approximately 8 months, while marrow with less than 20 percent involvement is associated with an average survival of 55 months.

HEAVY CHAIN DISEASE

Heavy chain disease (HCD) is very rare. This group of disorders is characterized by the excessive production of the heavy chain portion of the antibody subunit. These disorders represent a monoclonal process in which the cells have lost the ability to synthesize the light chain component of the immunoglobulin molecule. There are HCDs that correspond to each of the IgG, IgA, and IgM antibody classes. Each has a characteristic clinical presentation.

Gamma Heavy Chain Disease

Gamma HCD is a disease of the elderly. Lymphadenopathy, anemia, and fever are the most common presenting findings, often accompanied by malaise, weakness, and enlargement of the liver and spleen. Immunoelectrophoresis and SPEP reveal the presence of gamma heavy chains. Suppression of normal immunoglobulins is the rule. Bone marrow biopsy shows a mixed infiltrate of plasma cells, lymphocytes, eosinophils, and histiocytes. There are no lytic bone lesions. Survival varies from a few weeks to a few years. Chemotherapy has not been shown to be of benefit. Death is usually from infection or from progressive wasting and marrow replacement.

Alpha Heavy Chain Disease

This disease is frequently seen in, but not limited to, young Mediterranean individuals. For this reason, it is commonly known as Mediterranean lymphoma. Patients present with an abdominal mass. Bowel involvement with villous atrophy and malabsorption are hallmarks of the disease and may be related to the unusually high concentration of IgA-producing lymphocytes in the intestinal mucosa. This may occur due to chronic exposure to intestinal parasites, and responses to antibiotic therapy alone have been reported. Another variant is seen in which only respiratory tract mucosal involvement is found. Both show diffuse infiltration of involved areas with lymphocytes, plasma cells, and histiocytes. Alpha heavy chains circulating in the blood are required for the diagnosis. Chemotherapy regimens used to treat lymphomas have been used in this disease with generally poor results. Death usually occurs within months after diagnosis.

Mu Heavy Chain Disease

This disease is the rarest of the HCDs. Presenting symptoms most commonly include enlargement of the liver and spleen but not lymph nodes. Many circulating lymphocytes are present in a clinical setting of chronic lymphocytic leukemia (CLL). Mu heavy chains found in the blood make the diagnosis. Kappa light chains may sometimes be found in the urine of these patients. Bone marrow examination is significant for the presence of vacuolated plasma cells. Chemotherapy with alkylators such as chlorambucil are commonly used, as for common CLL.

CASE STUDIES

Case 1: Multiple Myeloma

A 71-year-old white man, a nonsmoker who used alcohol on holidays only, presented in January 1989 complaining of a constant aching pain in his chest and lower back. This had progressively worsened over the prior 3 months. He also had a 40-lb weight loss over the preceding 6-month period. His wife had noticed recent onset of increased somnolence during the day and occasional nonsensical statements. His only other medical problem was hypertension, which was adequately controlled with a beta blocker.

On examination, the patient was an elderly man, appearing his stated age, in mild discomfort. His temperature was 98.4°F; blood pressure standing 110/60 mmHg; supine 140/84 mmHg. Heart rate was 80 beats per min and did not change with position. He was unable to state the correct date or the current president but knew his name and current location. Further examination revealed generalized bony tenderness with a straightened lumbar curve. Cardiopulmonary examination was unremarkable. There were no enlarged lymph nodes. The prostate was normal.

Chest and spine radiographs were obtained, revealing generalized osteoporosis with compression fractures in the third and fourth lumbar vertebrae. Initial laboratory studies included a CBC with WBC count at 4500 cells/mm³ and a normal differential; hemoglobin was 10.5 g/dl; hematocrit was 32.2 percent. He had 220,000 platelets/mm³. The laboratory reported that the peripheral blood smear showed the presence of rouleaux formation. Electrolytes were unremarkable except serum calcium at 10.6 mg/dl (normal 8.5 to 10.5). Uric acid within normal limits at 7.5 mg/dl. Total protein was 8.2 g/dl, albumin was low at 2.6 g/dl, globulin fraction was elevated at 5.6 g/dl. Calcium corrected for low albumin was elevated at 11.7 mg/dl. Renal function appeared decreased with a serum creatinine of 1.7 mg/dl (normal up to 1.2) and BUN at 38 mg/dl (normal up to 28 mg/dl). Twenty-four–hour urine collection was negative for presence of protein.

The patient was hospitalized for management of hypercalcemia and to speed completion of evaluation. Serum calcium level was rapidly corrected with saline hydration, and the patient's mental status cleared over the following 3 days. Because of worsening back pain, a myelogram was performed, which showed no evidence of spinal cord compression. Serum creatinine and BUN normalized to 0.9 mg/dl and 23 mg/dl, respectively. A monoclonal gammopathy was revealed upon SPEP. Immunoelectrophoresis identified the M spike as IgG-λ. It was measured to be 4.7 g/dl. IgM level was 63 mg/dl, IgA was 120 mg/dl, and normal IgG was decreased to 350 mg/dl. Bone marrow biopsy specimen revealed 32 percent plasma cells in the bone marrow, many immature with binucleate forms. A bone survey was obtained, which demonstrated lytic lesions in his skull, pelvis, bilateral humeri, and multiple lytic lesions in both femurs with extensive osteoporosis in all areas (Figs. 22–9 and 22–10).

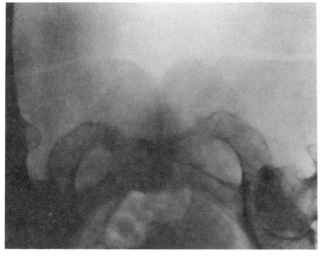

Figure 22–9. Pelvis radiograph of a patient with multiple myeloma showing the diffuse loss of bone seen in this disease.

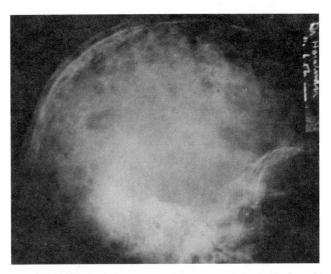

Figure 22–10. Extensive lytic skull lesions in a patient with multiple myeloma.

Questions

1. What features of the patient's illness confirm the diagnosis of multiple myeloma?
2. If the patient had only 15 percent plasma cells in the bone marrow, with everything else the same, would myeloma still be diagnosed?
3. What features of the patient's illness necessitate beginning treatment?
4. What stage disease does this patient have, and what are its implications for his treatment and survival?

Discussion

This unfortunate patient demonstrates many features of myeloma. He fulfills two major criteria for diagnosis: greater than 30 percent plasma cells in the bone marrow and IgG M spike greater than 3.5 g/dl. He also demonstrated two minor criteria—lytic bone lesions and decreased normal IgG. According to the rules of diagnosis, the presence of an IgG M spike above 3.5 g/dl with either decreased normal immunoglobulins or lytic bone lesions fulfills the diagnostic criteria. This is true even without an increase in marrow plasma cells.

Bone lesions, hypercalcemia, and anemia are all indications to begin therapy. The serum creatinine and BUN were elevated owing to dehydration on his initial presentation rather than renal failure. The patient does not fulfill all the requirements to be classed as a stage I myeloma. Since he has advanced lytic bone lesions, he fulfills one of the criteria for stage III disease. With a normal serum creatinine he would be classed as stage III A disease. Because high-bulk myeloma warrants more aggressive therapy, he was started on a four-drug regimen containing vincristine, melphalan, cyclophosphamide, and prednisone.

The patient has responded well to this treatment with a decrease in his M spike to 1.2 g/dl, which has been stable for 6 months. His femur lesions were too extensive for surgical stabilization and he has been confined to a wheelchair because of the high risk of femur fractures. Serum calcium has remained well controlled, and he has had no further weight loss. He was hospitalized most recently for pneumococcal pneumonia, recovering uneventfully on intravenous antibiotics. He has suffered two more vertebral compression fractures and, as a result, now shows some compromise of pulmonary function because of decreased chest volume. Pain control has been achieved with oral nonsteroidal agents with narcotic analgesics needed occasionally.

Patients with high-bulk, stage III disease have a median survival of 23 months. Pneumococcal pneumonia and other bacterial infections are the greatest risk. This is especially true when patients have pulmonary compromise, as in this case.

Case 2: MGUS

A 55-year-old white man was referred to the hematology clinic for evaluation of mild anemia (hematocrit 39 percent) found on routine health screening. He had no active medical problems and was taking no medications except a daily vitamin supplement. He had smoked one pack of cigarettes per day for 35 years and did not use alcohol.

Studies ordered by the referring physician included serum iron, total iron binding capacity, vitamin B_{12}, folate, thyroid panel, reticulocyte count, chemistry panel which included serum BUN and creatinine, and barium enema—all of which results were normal. A serum protein electrophoresis showed a monoclonal spike in the gamma region.

On evaluation in the hematology clinic, physical examination was entirely within normal limits. Laboratory evaluation demonstrated IgG-κ at 1.07 g/dl, with IgM at 144 mg/dl, IgA at 202 mg/dl, and IgG at 2430 mg/dl, all within normal limits. Sulfosalicylic acid test for protein on 24-hour urine collection was negative. A bone survey of the skull, spine, and pelvis was unremarkable. A bone marrow biopsy was performed, which showed normal cellularity, with a normal variety of cells present. Marrow plasma cells were not increased in number (3.2 percent). Some were noted to have nuclear maturation delay felt consistent with a monoclonal gammopathy.

Questions

1. What would you tell the patient about his prognosis?
2. What treatment would you offer now?
3. What follow-up should be instituted?

Discussion

The majority of patients who present with MGUS have a benign course and a normal lifespan. The cause of death is usually an unrelated event. This presentation is typical of most cases in which a screening SPEP for an unrelated problem demonstrates a small M spike with no other evidence of myeloma. No treatment is given, as there are no harmful effects arising from the small clone of cells producing the immunoglobulin. Because there is no indicator of which patients will progress to a more

malignant disorder, electrophoresis is repeated at 3 months and then every 6 months following. Any symptoms of persistent bone pain should be evaluated with appropriate radiologic studies.

This patient has had a benign course and is currently 3 years from diagnosis with the most recent SPEP showing a minimally changed M spike at 1.29 g/dl. Serial evaluations have showed variation from 0.85 g/dl to a high of 1.36 g/dl. One episode of bothersome low back pain prompted a repeat bone survey, the result of which was normal.

Case 3: Waldenström's Macroglobulinemia

A 59-year-old white man, editor of a local newspaper, was seen by his family physician for a check-up. He described an unintentional 35-lb weight loss over the preceding 18 months from his usual 200 pounds, as well as generalized loss of energy and libido. On questioning, he also admitted significant difficulty concentrating on his job and occasionally had episodes during which he was unable to understand what he was reading.

Past medical history was unremarkable. The patient exercised regularly and did not use alcohol or tobacco. His last health care evaluation had been 5 years earlier, and was normal. He was taking no medications.

Physical examination was normal except for a palpable spleen 3 cm below the left costal margin. Optic fundi were normal, lungs were clear, and there were no enlarged lymph nodes. Stool was negative for blood, and the prostate was normal.

Initial evaluation included a normal chest radiograph, a CBC that was abnormal with 10.5 g/dl of hemoglobin and a 30.2 percent hematocrit. His red cells were small but uniform in size; mean corpuscular volume (MCV) was 79 fl, and red blood cell distribution width (RDW) was 12.7 fl. He had 9700 WBCs with a normal differential and 298,000 platelets. Chemistry panel was normal except for a total protein at 8.7 g/dl and a low albumin level at 2.7 g/dl (serum calcium, BUN, and creatinine were all normal). Upon SPEP an M spike of 5.7 g/dl was revealed, with total IgM at 7.70 g/dl. A bone marrow biopsy specimen revealed increased cellularity with 23 percent plasmacytoid lymphocytes. A bone survey did not show any lytic lesions. Blood viscosity was moderately increased.

Questions

1. What findings are characteristic of Waldenström's macroglobulinemia?
2. What characteristics differentiate this presentation from the very rarely seen IgM multiple myeloma?
3. What condition(s) would require urgent plasmapheresis to remove IgM rapidly?
4. What is the patient's prognosis?

Discussion

The presentation is characteristic in that most patients with WM present with vague symptoms of weight loss and fatigue. This patient's spleen is mildly enlarged, and there are no other signs of extensive sludging on physical examination. In later stages, retinal vascular changes, enlarged liver, visual complaints, and more profound mental status changes could be expected to occur. Table 22–11 compares the findings of MM and those of WM. The lack of bone lesions and normal serum calcium are characteristic of WM. The lack of malignant plasma cells also supports the diagnosis. Neurologic dysfunction (somnolence, coma, or visual loss) is the primary indication for emergent plasmapheresis. Another reason would be tissue injury (ischemic necrosis) of skin or extremities, or any other manifestation of impending tissue damage due to high blood viscosity. This patient's expected survival is based on degree of marrow involvement with an expected survival of several years.

Treatment was begun with alkylator chemotherapy (chlorambucil), and the patient's symptoms resolved rapidly. His M spike rapidly decreased and remained decreased for 14 months. On progression, he was treated with cyclophosphamide, vincristine, and prednisone, and he again has remained stable for an additional 10 months. He has experienced only mild hair loss from his chemotherapy and is otherwise feeling well.

BIBLIOGRAPHY

Alexanian R, et al: High-dose glucocorticoid treatment of resistant myeloma. Ann Intern Med 105:8, 1983.
Bataille, R, et al: Prognostic factors and staging in multiple myeloma: A reappraisal. J Clin Oncol 4:80, 1986.
Buzaid, AC and Durie, BGM: Management of refractory myeloma: A review. J Clin Oncol 6:889, 1988.
Durie, BGM: Staging and kinetics of multiple myeloma. Semin Oncol 13:300, 1986.
Durie, BGM and Salmon, SE: A clinical staging system for multiple myeloma. Correlation of measured myeloma cell mass with presenting clinical features, response to treatment and survival. Cancer 36:1192, 1975.
Eisenberg, RL: Clinical immunology. In Diagnostic Imaging in Internal Medicine. McGraw-Hill, New York, 1985, pp 3–10.
Farhangi, M and Merlini G: The clinical implications of monoclonal immunoglobulins. Semin Oncol 13:366, 1986.
Gandara, DR, et al: Differential diagnosis of monoclonal gammopathy. Med Clin North Am 72:1155, 1988.
Jacobson, DR and Zolla-Pazner, S: Immunosuppression and infection in multiple myeloma. Semin Oncol 13:282, 1986.
Jandl, JH: Multiple myeloma and other differentiated B cell malignancies. In Blood: Textbook of Hematology. Little, Brown, Boston, 1987.
Kyle, RA and Garton, JP: Laboratory monitoring of myeloma proteins. Semin Oncol 13:310, 1986.
Kyle, RA and Garton, JP: The spectrum of IgM monoclonal gammopathy in 430 cases. Mayo Clin Proc 62:719, 1987.
Mellstedt, H, et al: Idiotype-bearing lymphoid cells in plasma cell neoplasia. Clin Haematol 11:65, 1982.
Rosen, SM, et al: The structure of immunoglobulins and their genes, DNA rearrangement and B cell differentiation, molecular anomalies of some monoclonal immunoglobulins. Semin Oncol 13:260, 1986.
Rota, S, et al: Multiple myeloma and severe renal failure: A clinicopathologic study of outcome and prognosis in 34 patients. Medicine 66:126, 1987.
Salmon, SE and Cassady, JR: Plasma cell neoplasms. In DeVita, VT, et al (eds): Cancer: Principles and Practice of Oncology. JB Lippincott, Philadelphia, 1989, pp 1853–1895.
Samson, D, et al: Infusion of vincristine and doxorubicin with oral dexamethasone as first-line therapy for multiple myeloma. Lancet 2:882, 1989.
Seligmann, M, et al: Heavy chain diseases: Current findings and concepts. Immunol Rev 48:145, 1979.
Woodruff, RK, et al: Solitary plasmacytoma. I. Extramedullary soft tissue plasmacytoma. Cancer 43:2340, 1979.

QUESTIONS

1. *Which laboratory test(s) for whole blood is/are used in the evaluation of plasma cell disorders?*
   a. CBC
   b. Peripheral blood smear
   c. ESR
   d. All of the above

2. *What laboratory serum tests are used for evaluation of plasma cell disorders, and how are they used?*
   a. First SPEP; if M spike is seen, then IEP or immunofixation to determine the specific antibody class
   b. Immunoelectrophoresis used to determine the antibody group and immunofixation or SPEP used to determine if light or heavy chain is increased
   c. First SPEP; if no abnormalities, then IEP or immunofixation used, as more sensitive indicators of increased antibody class(es)
   d. Either SPEP or IEP first; if M spike is seen, then immunofixation to determine the specific antibody class

3. *Which of the following tests can directly detect urinary light chains and is used to distinguish between kappa and lambda light chains?*
   a. Heat precipitation test
   b. Urine immunoelectrophoresis
   c. Sulfosalicylic acid test
   d. Both urine immunoelectrophoresis and sulfosalicyclic acid test

4. *Which list would contain diagnostic criteria for multiple myeloma?*
   a. Biopsy proven plasmacytoma and 10 to 30% plasma cells
   b. >30% plasma cells in bone marrow
   c. Biopsy-proven plasmacytoma and M spike present
   d. Monoclonal protein and M spike present

5. *Which of the following would be diagnostic criteria for Waldenström's macroglobinemia?*
   a. IgM M spike and hyperviscosity
   b. Lytic bone lesions and rouleaux
   c. Renal failure and >30% plasma cells
   d. M spike of IgM, IgG, or IgA; low-normal other immunoglobulins; inability to make light chains

6. *What are the characteristics of heavy chain disease? (Use answer choices for question 5.)*

ANSWERS

1. d (p. 368–370)
2. a (p. 372)
3. b (p. 372)
4. c (p. 374–375)
5. a (p. 379)
6. d (p. 380)

Dan M. Hyder, M.D.

The Lymphomas

OBJECTIVES

At the end of this chapter, the learner should be able to:
1. Name the cell characteristically found in Hodgkin's disease.
2. List distinguishing features for lymphocyte-predominance, mixed cellularity, lymphocyte-depletion, and nodular sclerosing Hodgkin's disease.
3. List distinguishing features for the four stages of Hodgkin's disease.
4. Describe the classification criteria for non-Hodgkin's lymphomas.
5. List some distinguishing features for various lymphomas.
6. Name tests that may be needed to provide a differential diagnosis for lymphomas.

The malignant lymphomas are a heterogeneous group of diseases that arise from cells of the lymphoid tissue (lymphocytes, histiocytes, and reticulum cells). They are broadly divided into the two major categories of Hodgkin's disease and the lymphocytic lymphomas. Although the vast majority of lymphomas within the second category are of lymphocytic origin, occasional cases do appear to arise from nonlymphoid cells. Consequently, the lymphocytic lymphomas are also frequently referred to as the non-Hodgkin's lymphomas (NHLs). This subdivision of the malignant lymphomas into two general categories has both biologic and therapeutic implications.

It is important for the student and clinician alike to be aware of the diagnostic difficulties often faced by the pathologist in evaluating lymphoid proliferations. Perhaps no area in pathology has produced as many subcategories of a basic disease process as the area of lymphoma diagnosis. The distinction between benign and malignant lymphoid proliferations, between Hodgkin's disease and non-Hodgkin's lymphoma, or among the subcategories of these two major types of lymphoma is frequently difficult, may require additional studies beyond light microscopy, and in some circumstances may be impossible to diagnose definitively.

HODGKIN'S DISEASE

Hodgkin's disease was the first of the lymphomas to be recognized. In 1832 Thomas Hodgkin described what he believed to be a primary yet benign disease of the lymphoid tissue.[1] Samuel Wilks in 1865 suggested that the disorder described by Hodgkin was a malignant process, and he was the first to apply the term Hodgkin's disease (HD) in honor of Hodgkin's original description of the process.[2] Sternberg[3] in 1898 and Reed[4] in 1902 described the distinct histologic features of Hodgkin's disease, including the peculiar cell that is the morphologic hallmark of Hodgkin's disease and that now bears their names: Reed-Sternberg cell (or Sternberg-Reed) (**see Color Plate 230**) (Fig. 23–1A).

Etiology and Pathogenesis

The continued usage of the term Hodgkin's disease rather than Hodgkin's lymphoma attests to the fact that the etiology and even the very nature of Hodgkin's disease (inflammatory/reactive versus malignant) remains uncertain. An intriguing possibility involves a viral etiology of Hodgkin's disease, with particular attention to certain ribonucleic acid (RNA) tumor viruses and Epstein-Barr virus. Conclusive experimental evidence, however, is lacking. Certain epidemiologic data such as the occasional occurrence of several cases of Hodgkin's disease within a small local and brief space of time (time-space clustering) would also suggest an infectious etiology. Other epidemiologic studies, however, have failed to support an infectious mode of transmission. The current view of Hodgkin's disease is that it is truly a malignant proliferation and that the malignant cells are the morphologically characteristic Reed-Sternberg cell and its variants (Fig. 23–1A through E). Despite the prevailing view that the Reed-Sternberg cell is the malignant cell of Hodgkin's disease, the origin of this cell remains an enigma. Kinship to almost every cell of the mononuclear phagocytic and lymphoreticular system has been proposed for the Reed-Sternberg cell. Functional, enzymatic, immunophenotypic, and genotypic data are conflicting, but the weight of the data strongly favors a heterogeneous rather than a single cellular origin for the Reed-Sternberg cell.

Pathology

A major success of 20th century medicine has been the development of a single, clinically useful classification scheme for Hodgkin's disease — namely, the Rye classification[5] (Table 23–1). The simplicity of the Rye classification, however, belies the histologic complexity of Hodgkin's disease. To those confronted with the challenge of making a histologic diagnosis of Hodgkin's disease, recourse to more complicated schemes such as the Lukes and Butler classification[6] (Table 23–2) is common practice. The student of Hodgkin's disease should be familiar with both.

The cytologic hallmark of Hodgkin's disease is the presence of an unusual giant cell, the Reed-Sternberg cell. The features of this cell include large size (up to 45 μm), abundant acidophilic cytoplasm, multinucleated or polylobated nucleus, and gigantic (greater than 5 μm) inclusionlike nucleoli (**see Color Plate 230**) (Fig. 23–1A). There is often clearing of the chromatin around the macronucleoli resulting in a distinct halo effect. It is necessary to identify at least one of these diagnostic Reed-Sternberg cells before a primary diagnosis of Hodgkin's disease can be made. The identification of Reed-Sternberg (or Reed-Sternberg–like) cells, however, is not a sufficient condition for the diagnosis of Hodgkin's disease. Reed-Sternberg–like cells are commonly seen in a variety of benign and malignant conditions other than Hodgkin's disease (Table 23–3). The diagnosis of Hodgkin's disease should be based on finding Reed-Sternberg cells in the proper cellular, stromal, and clinical setting. Many non-diagnostic variants of Reed-Sternberg cells have been described (Fig. 23–1). Observation of these cells is helpful in suggesting the possibility of Hodgkin's disease and in determining the subclassification of Hodgkin's disease.

The following discussion of the histologic subtypes of HD will follow the Rye classification scheme (Table 23–1). When appropriate, however, reference to the Lukes and Butler classification (Table 23–2) will be made.

Lymphocyte-Predominance Hodgkin's Disease

Lymphocyte-predominance (LP) Hodgkin's disease is a relatively uncommon variety of Hodgkin's disease. Its descriptive name is somewhat of a misnomer, as lymphocytes do not always predominate. Benign histiocytes, which are always a component of this disorder, may in fact predominate. The histologic importance of both lymphocytes and histiocytes in this subcategory of Hodgkin's disease is acknowledged in the Lukes and Butler designation for this disorder, lymphocytic and histiocytic (L and H) Hodgkin's disease. Although not distinguished by the Rye classification, both nodular and diffuse

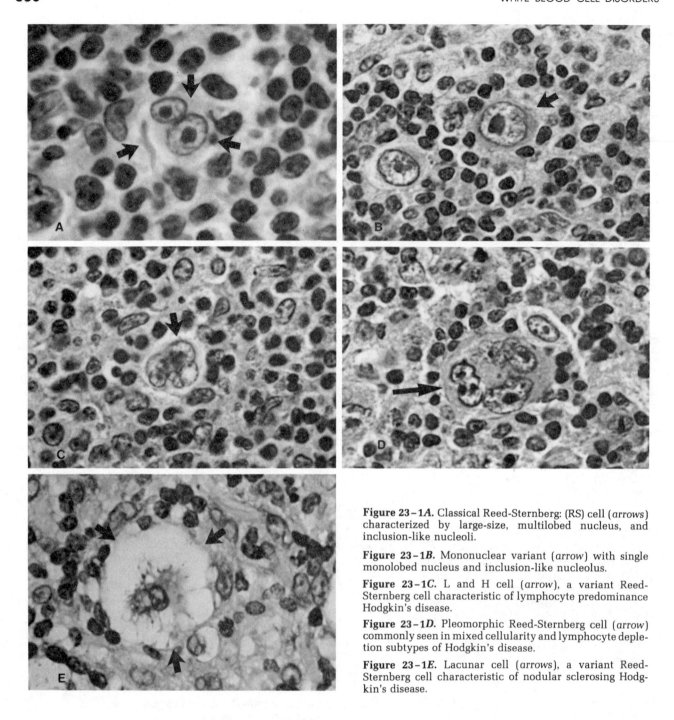

Figure 23–1A. Classical Reed-Sternberg: (RS) cell (*arrows*) characterized by large-size, multilobed nucleus, and inclusion-like nucleoli.

Figure 23–1B. Mononuclear variant (*arrow*) with single monolobed nucleus and inclusion-like nucleolus.

Figure 23–1C. L and H cell (*arrow*), a variant Reed-Sternberg cell characteristic of lymphocyte predominance Hodgkin's disease.

Figure 23–1D. Pleomorphic Reed-Sternberg cell (*arrow*) commonly seen in mixed cellularity and lymphocyte depletion subtypes of Hodgkin's disease.

Figure 23–1E. Lacunar cell (*arrows*), a variant Reed-Sternberg cell characteristic of nodular sclerosing Hodgkin's disease.

Table 23–1. **RYE CLASSIFICATION OF HODGKIN'S DISEASE[5]**

Nodular sclerosis
Lymphocyte predominance
Mixed cellularity
Lymphocyte depletion
Unclassified

forms of LP Hodgkin's disease are recognized in the Lukes and Butler classification.

The nodular variant is generally characterized by a vague nodularity, although in some cases nodularity may be well developed. The cellular milieu in both the diffuse and nodular varieties is composed of a mixture of small, normal-appearing lymphocytes; benign histiocytes; rare Reed-Sternberg cells; and variable numbers of a characteristic, though

Table 23–2. **LUKES AND BUTLER[6] CLASSIFICATION OF HODGKIN'S DISEASE**

Nodular sclerosis
Lymphocytic and histiocytic
   Nodular
   Diffuse
Mixed cellularity
Reticular
   Sarcomatous
   Nonsarcomatous
Diffuse fibrosis
Unclassified

Table 23–3. **DISEASES OF DISORDERS IN WHICH REED-STERNBERG–LIKE CELLS HAVE BEEN REPORTED**

Viral infection (eg, infectious mononucleosis)
Anticonvulsant-induced lymphadenopathy
Epithelial and stromal malignancies
Melanoma
Various lymphomas and leukemias
Myeloproliferative disorders

nondiagnostic, Reed-Sternberg variant referred to as an L and H cell (Fig. 23–1C). This cell has a variable amount of pale-staining cytoplasm, convoluted nucleus prosaically referred to as popcorn shaped, and an indistinct nucleolus. Plasma cells, eosinophils, fibrosis, and necrosis are usually absent. The paucity of Reed-Sternberg cells often makes definitive diagnosis difficult. Numerous histologic sections may need to be studied to find at least one classic Reed-Sternberg cell, which is a prerequisite for diagnosis. The histologic features of LP Hodgkin's disease must be distinguished from various reactive conditions such as infectious mononucleosis as well as from certain low-grade non-Hodgkin's lymphomas. Such differentiation may require special phenotypic and genotypic studies.

Mixed Cellularity Hodgkin's Disease

As its name implies, mixed cellularity (MC) Hodgkin's disease is characterized by a heterogeneous mixture of cells including lymphocytes, histiocytes, plasma cells, eosinophils, Reed-Sternberg

cells, and Reed-Sternberg variants (Fig. 23–2). Although the frequency of these cell types varies from case to case, the numbers of lymphocytes, Reed-Sternberg cells, and Reed-Sternberg variants are intermediate between the numbers found in LP Hodgkin's disease and those found in lymphocyte-depletion Hodgkin's disease. Specifically, the number of Reed-Sternberg cells and mononuclear Hodgkin's cells in mixed cellularity Hodgkin's disease has been defined as between 5 and 15 per high-power microscopic field.[7]

In addition to the cellular milieu there is usually an increase in the background stroma in the form of a disorderly, noncollagenous fibrosis distinct from that seen in nodular sclerosing Hodgkin's disease. Small areas of necrosis are commonly present. In some cases clusters of epithelioid histiocytes may be numerous, making distinction from Lennert's lymphoma (a T-cell lymphoma with high content of epithelioid histiocytes) difficult. The lymphocytes of Lennert's lymphoma are cytologically atypical, as opposed to the small, uniform features of the lymphocytes in all forms of Hodgkin's disease, including MC Hodgkin's disease. There is often only partial involvement of nodes in MC Hodgkin's disease. This is usually an interfollicular pattern that may be

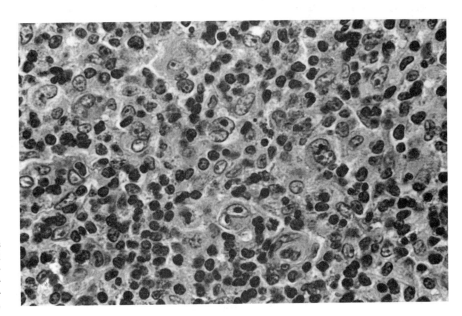

Figure 23–2. Mixed cellularity Hodgkin's disease. A polymorphous cellular milieu including small lymphocytes, eosinophils, plasma cells, and frequent Reed-Sternberg cells and their variants characterize this subtype of Hodgkin's disease.

missed on casual examination or confused with a reactive process.

Lymphocyte-Depletion Hodgkin's Disease

Lymphocyte-depletion (LD) Hodgkin's disease is at the opposite end of the cellular spectrum from LP Hodgkin's disease. Lymphocytes are sparse in this disorder, whereas Reed-Sternberg cells and Reed-Sternberg variants predominate. Other types of cells such as plasma cells, histiocytes, and eosinophils are infrequently found. In addition, irregular sclerosis is a major histologic component of LD Hodgkin's disease. This sclerosis ranges from a hypocellular reticular pattern of connective tissue to hypercellular proliferative fibrosis.

In the Lukes and Butler classification, two subtypes of LD Hodgkin's disease are recognized: the reticular and diffuse fibrosis types. The reticular subtype has been further divided into sarcomatous and nonsarcomatous variants. In the sarcomatous form of reticular LD Hodgkin's disease numerous bizarre, pleomorphic Reed-Sternberg variants (Fig. 23–1D) are present. The pattern of fibrosis and presence of bizarre Reed-Sternberg variants creates a pattern quite akin to that seen in pleomorphic sarcomas such as malignant fibrous histiocytoma. The nonsarcomatous form, on the other hand, is characterized by large numbers of classic Reed-Sternberg cells.

The diffuse fibrosis variant of LD Hodgkin's disease is truly cell-poor owing to the presence of abundant acellular, amorphous fibrillar connective tissue. Reed-Sternberg cells are less frequently found in this variant than in the reticular form of LD Hodgkin's disease.

There has been a marked decrease in the diagnosis of LD Hodgkin's disease during the past decade. This is not due to a decreased incidence of this form of Hodgkin's disease but to the recognition that many cases previously diagnosed as LD Hodgkin's disease are actually misdiagnosed cases of non-Hodgkin's lymphoma, particularly polymorphous T-cell lymphomas.[8] In fact, in some cases it may be impossible, even after detailed study including phenotypic and genotypic studies, to resolve the differential diagnosis between a pleomorphic NHL and LD Hodgkin's disease.

Nodular Sclerosing Hodgkin's Disease

The cardinal histologic features of nodular sclerosing (NS) Hodgkin's disease are birefringent collagenous sclerosis and the presence of classic Reed-Sternberg cells, as well as a distinctive Reed-Sternberg variant called a lacunar cell. The sclerosis observed in NS Hodgkin's disease differs from that seen in the other subtypes of Hodgkin's disease. In NS Hodgkin's disease, sclerosis is found in the form of well-organized bands of collagen that subdivide the tissue into distinct nodules (**see Color Plate 231**). Within the nodules is a variable mixture of lymphocytes, classic Reed-Sternberg cells, lacunar cells, plasma cells, eosinophils, and neutrophils. The lacunar cells often form distinct collections within the central region of the nodule (grouped lacunars) and these collections may be associated with focal necrosis. The lacunar cell is best identified in formalin-fixed tissue sections, where the artifact of formalin fixation produces a distinctive appearance of this Reed-Sternberg variant. The lacunar cell is separated from the surrounding cells by a large clear or pale-staining space (lacuna) (Fig. 23–1E). Wisps of cytoplasm may be seen in this space. The nucleus is large and often polylobated, and the nucleoli are small to intermediate size.

In some cases of Hodgkin's disease the characteristic cellular milieu of NS Hodgkin's disease may be seen, including the presence of large numbers of lacunar cells; however, the sclerotic bands are absent. These cases have been assigned by some authorities to a subcategory of NS Hodgkin's disease[9] (cellular phase of NS Hodgkin's disease). Others have assigned cases with this pattern to MC Hodgkin's disease.[10]

Sclerosis may be seen in many other lymphoid and nonlymphoid malignancies. For example, agnogenic myeloid metaplasia may produce a histologic pattern of fibrosis and cellular atypia virtually indistinguishable from NS Hodgkin's disease. Sclerosis alone, even when present as orderly bands of collagen, is not sufficient for a diagnosis of NS Hodgkin's disease.

Unclassified Hodgkin's Disease

A small percentage of cases of HD exhibit sufficient histologic features for a diagnosis of HD but insufficient features to be assigned to one of the aforementioned subcategories. These cases are assigned to the unclassified subcategory.

Histologic Progression

The concurrent evaluation of multiple sites of involvement with Hodgkin's disease usually demonstrates similar histology at each site. On the other hand, with the passage of time, reevaluation often reveals histologic progression in the sequence: LP Hodgkin's disease to MC Hodgkin's disease to LD Hodgkin's disease. Although it is often stated that NS Hodgkin's disease does not undergo such progression but remains NS Hodgkin's disease, there may be progression with time within the histologic spectrum of NS Hodgkin's disease. That is, cases of NS Hodgkin's disease initially rich in lymphocytes may undergo a progressive decrease in the number of lymphocytes with concomitant increase in the number of Reed-Sternberg cells and Reed-Sternberg variants equivalent to that seen in the non-NS types. Thus, NS Hodgkin's disease may pass through phases of LP to MC and LD. This progression, however, maintains the overall nodular sclerosing pattern of NS Hodgkin's disease. Eventually a stage of extreme cellular depletion may be reached, referred to as obliterative total sclerosis, in which few cellular elements, including Reed-Sternberg cells, are found.

Clinical Features

In the United States, Hodgkin's disease accounts for approximately one third of newly diagnosed cases of lymphoma. The incidence of Hodgkin's disease exhibits a bimodal distribution, with peaks between the ages of 15 and 35 and in the over-50 age group.

Most patients with Hodgkin's disease present with a complaint of painless lymph node swelling. Each subtype of Hodgkin's disease is associated with rather characteristic, but not totally specific, clinical features. Lymphocyte-predominant Hodgkin's disease occurs more often in males and is generally a disease of younger patients. The disease is usually localized at presentation to one peripheral node or node groups. Nodular sclerosing Hodgkin's disease, on the other hand, shows a female predominance and is usually associated with cervical, scalene, and/or supraclavicular adenopathy. An anterior mediastinal mass is often detected by chest radiograph. Most patients with NS Hodgkin's disease are asymptomatic on presentation. Mixed cellularity and lymphocyte-predominant Hodgkin's disease are most often seen in symptomatic patients with widely disseminated disease. Extranodal involvement is common in these two subcategories of Hodgkin's disease.

Diagnostic Evaluation and Staging

The diagnosis of Hodgkin's disease requires tissue biopsy and microscopic evaluation. Because of the complexities involved in accurate diagnosis and subclassification, adequate tissue should be obtained at the time of initial biopsy for routine light microscopic studies, as well as for ancillary studies such as immunophenotypic and genotypic analysis if these are deemed necessary.

Following a tissue diagnosis of Hodgkin's disease, the patient should be appropriately staged to determine the extent of disease and permit selection of appropriate therapy. The staging evaluation of Hodgkin's disease has become standardized and can be divided into clinical and pathologic staging. Clinical staging should be performed on all newly diagnosed patients with Hodgkin's disease. The elements of clinical staging are listed in Table 23–4. Pathologic staging requires exploratory laparotomy with multiple node samplings and splenectomy.

Table 23–4. **STAGING WORK-UP FOR HODGKIN'S DISEASE**

1. Initial tissue biopsy specimen demonstrating Hodgkin's disease
2. Careful history
3. Detailed physical examination
4. Laboratory studies (CBC; sedimentation rate; chemistry panel to include liver, kidney, and bone profiles)
5. Chest radiograph (anterior and lateral)
6. Bipedal lymphangiography

Table 23–5. **ANN ARBOR STAGING**[11]

Stage I	Involvement of single lymph node region or localized involvement of a single extralymphatic organ or site (I_e).
Stage II	Involvement of two or more lymph node regions on the same side of the diaphragm or localized involvement of a single associated extralymphatic organ or site and its regional lymph node(s) with or without involvement of other lymph node regions on the same side of the diaphragm (II_e)
Stage III	Involvement of lymph node regions on both sides of the diaphragm, which may also be accompanied by localized involvement of an associated extralymphatic organ site (III_e)
Stage IV	Disseminated (multifocal) involvement of one or more extralymphatic organs, with or without associated lymph node involvement, or isolated extralymphatic organ involvement with distant (nonregional) nodal involvement

Except at certain institutions, routine pathologic staging is not performed and is reserved for those cases where the results of pathologic staging would alter the therapy. The results of the staging evaluation are used to assign the patient to staging groups. The most widely used staging scheme is the Ann Arbor Classification (Table 23–5).[11] This scheme may be used with the data obtained from clinical or pathologic staging or both. In addition to the anatomic extent of the disease implicit in the staging categories, the disease is further classified according to the presence or absence of specific symptoms (Table 23–6). An A (asymptomatic) or a B (symptomatic) is then appended to the appropriate stage number.

The clinical utility of the Ann Arbor staging scheme stems from the predictable behavior of Hodgkin's disease. Hodgkin's disease is a lymph node–based disease and rarely, if ever, starts in extranodal sites. It spreads by the lymphatic route in an orderly and predictable pattern to contiguous lymph nodes. Only late in the disease course when hematogenous spread may occur does a more disorderly pattern of spread occur.

Treatment and Prognosis

Current modalities for the therapy of Hodgkin's disease are radiation, chemotherapy, or a combination of the two. The selection of therapy is directed by the results of the staging evaluation rather than

Table 23–6. **"B" SYMPTOMS**

1. Unexplained loss of more than 10% of body weight in the 6 months before admission
2. Unexplained fever with temperature above 38°C
3. Drenching night sweats

the specific histologic subtype. Regardless of the stage of the disease, therapy should be given with curative intent.

For stage I and II Hodgkin's disease, extended field or total nodal irradiation are the treatments of choice. The addition of chemotherapy or chemotherapy alone does not improve upon the results achieved by radiotherapy and subject the patient to the added risk of secondary malignancies (acute leukemia and non-Hodgkin's lymphoma) following chemotherapy. Long-term disease-free survival can be accomplished in approximately 75 percent of patients with early-stage Hodgkin's disease and recurrences after radiotherapy are generally responsive to chemotherapy. With appropriate therapy, the 10-year survival for stage I and II Hodgkin's disease now exceeds 80 percent. Ten-year survival for stage III and IV Hodgkin's disease has been successfully improved with aggressive chemotherapy, and now approaches 70 percent.[12]

NON-HODGKIN'S LYMPHOMA

Virchow in 1858[13] and Billroth in 1871[14] were the first to use the terms lymphoma and malignant lymphoma. The distinction between the two major categories of malignant lymphoma — the lymphocytic lymphomas and Hodgkin's disease — was suggested in 1893 by Dreschfield[15] and Kundrat.[16]

Etiology and Pathogenesis

Considerable insight into the mechanisms of lymphomagenesis has been achieved; however, there remain many gaps in our knowledge. It seems certain that a prerequisite for the development of lymphoma is damage to those regions of the genetic code that regulate the growth and reproduction of cells of the immune system. The inciting agents for this damage remain unknown, but it is believed that mutagenic factors such as chemicals, ionizing radiation, and certain viruses may play a role in initiating and promoting the damage. Although viruses such as the Epstein-Barr virus do not appear to be directly mutagenic, they may function via persistent antigenic stimulation as polyclonal mitogens that somehow favor the eventual selection of a single clone of non–growth-regulated (malignant) cells. This hypothesis is supported by the increased incidence of lymphomas in individuals with conditions associated with primary or acquired immunodeficiency (Table 23–7).

The genetic damage associated with the development of a lymphoma is often associated with numerical and/or structural alterations of chromosomes.[17] With high-resolution karyotyping techniques, nonrandom chromosomal abnormalities can be demonstrated in approximately 60 percent of cases of lymphoma. Certain types of lymphoma are highly correlated with specific chromosomal abnormalities—particularly translocations involving chromosomes 2, 8, 14, and 22. The pathogenic significance of these chromosomal

Table 23–7. CONDITIONS ASSOCIATED WITH INCREASED RISK OF DEVELOPING LYMPHOMA (NHL)

Sjögren's syndrome
Sarcoidosis
Systemic lupus erythematosus
Rheumatoid arthritis
Celiac disease
Dermatitis herpetiformis
Acquired immunodeficiency syndrome (AIDS)
Organ transplant recipients
Congenital immunodeficiency disorders

translocations relates to the function of the genetic material located at or near the site of these translocations. One of the breakpoints involved in B-cell lymphomas is at the site of the transcriptionally active immunoglobulin heavy or light chain (kappa and lambda) genes located on chromosomes 14, 2, and 22, respectively. For many T-cell lymphomas, a common breakpoint is in the region of one of the T-cell receptor genes. The other breakpoint is in the vicinity of a gene important in the regulation of cell growth and division. This growth-regulating gene, referred to as a proto-oncogene when it is normally located in the genome, is translocated to the region of one of the immunoglobulin genes (B-cell lymphomas) or T-cell receptor genes (T-cell lymphomas). In this new location, the growth-regulating gene functions abnormally and is now referred to as an oncogene. One of the best-studied examples of this process occurs in Burkitt's lymphoma, a B-cell lymphoma, in which the c-myc proto-oncogene located at region q24 on chromosome 8, is translocated to the immunoglobulin heavy chain locus at 14q32 (Fig. 23–3). This occurs in about 90 percent of patients with Burkitt's lymphoma. It is also found in about 40 percent of high-grade large cell lymphomas and therefore is not specific for Burkitt's lymphoma. The c-myc proto-oncogene normally functions in the nuclear signaling that switches cell proliferation on and off. The translocation of c-myc to the heavy chain locus deregulates the function of the c-myc gene resulting in uncontrolled cell proliferation. Chromosomal translocations represent only one mechanism for oncogene activation; other mechanisms include deletions, base pair mutations, and gene amplification. Oncogene activation-deregulation is believed to play a role in the development of most, if not all, lymphomas.

Pathology

Since the original suggestion by Dreschfield[15] that the lymphocytic lymphomas represent distinct histologic entities, a number of lymphoma classification schemes have been proposed. At least seven major classification schemes have been extensively used since the mid-1960s. Most of the classification

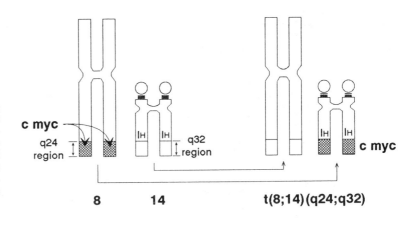

Figure 23-3. Reciprocal translocation t(8;14) (q24;q32) is seen in a majority of cases of Burkitt's lymphoma as well as some non-Burkitt's high-grade lymphomas. A reciprocal translocation of genetic material occurs between chromosomes 8 and 14. A distal portion of the long arm of chromosome 8, containing the c-myc proto-oncogene, is translocated to a site adjacent to the immunoglobulin heavy chain locus on chromosome 14.

schemes are based on the growth pattern — nodular or diffuse (Fig. 23-4A and B) — and on the cytologic features of the malignant cells. Other attributes of the cells such as immunophenotypic, genotypic, or functional capacity are not used in the common classification schemes. At present, the most widely used scheme in use by pathologists and clinicians in the United States is the modified Rappaport Classification[18] (Table 23-8) and in Europe the Kiel (Lennert's) Classification[19] (Table 23-9). To students, pathologists, and clinicians alike, this plethora of classification schemes, despite the intent to create order out of chaos, may result in considerable confusion. A critical analysis of these schemes conducted by the National Cancer Institute in the late 1970s revealed no significant differences in the various schemes with regard to their clinical utility. In acknowledgment of this fact, and in recognition of the confusion created by the lack of a standard classification scheme, the investigators in this multi-institutional study group proposed the Working Formulation for Clinical Usage[20] (Table 23-10).

In this classification scheme the lymphomas are broadly subdivided into the categories based on prognosis. These three groups are distinguished by survival data; that is, the group of patients with low-grade lymphomas experienced longer survival than

Table 23-8. **MODIFIED RAPPAPORT CLASSIFICATION[18]**

Nodular
    Lymphocytic, poorly differentiated
    Mixed lymphocytic-histiocytic
    Histiocytic
Diffuse
    Lymphocytic, well differentiated
    Lymphocytic, intermediate differentiated
    Lymphocytic, poorly differentiated
    Mixed, lymphocytic-histiocytic
    Undifferentiated, Burkitt's type
    Undifferentiated, non-Burkitt's type
    Histiocytic
    Lymphoblastic

the group with high-grade lymphomas. Survival in the intermediate-grade ranged between those of the two other groups. This scheme has now found wide acceptance in the United States, and it is hoped that it will become a common language throughout the world for categorizing the lymphocytic lymphomas. Use of a standard classification would greatly facilitate future clinical investigations.

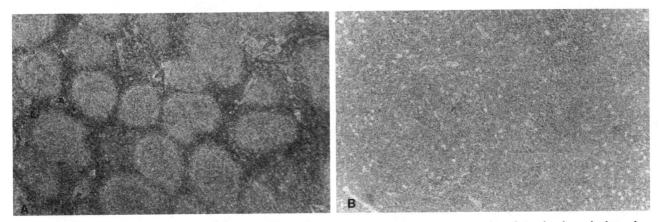

Figure 23-4. Growth patterns of the non-Hodgkin's lymphomas: (A) nodular (follicular) pattern resulting from closely packed neoplastic follicles without mantle zones. (B) diffuse pattern in which neoplastic cells are distributed as sheets of cells without follicular organization.

Table 23–9. **KIEL (LENNERT'S) CLASSIFICATION**[19]

Low-Grade
    Lymphocytic
    Lymphoplasmacytoid
    Centrocytic
    Centroblastic-centrocytic
        Follicular
        Follicular and diffuse
        Diffuse
High-Grade
    Centroblastic
    Lymphoblastic
        Burkitt's type
        Convoluted cell type
    Immunoblastic

Table 23–10. **WORKING FORMULATION FOR CLINICAL USAGE**

Low-Grade
  Malignant lymphoma, small lymphocytic
    Consistent with CLL
    Plasmacytoid
  Malignant lymphoma, follicular, predominantly small
    cleaved cell
    Diffuse areas
    Sclerosis
  Malignant lymphoma, follicular, mixed, small cleaved and
    large cell
    Diffuse areas
    Sclerosis
Intermediate-Grade
  Malignant lymphoma, follicular, predominantly large cell
    Diffuse areas
    Sclerosis
  Malignant lymphoma, diffuse, small cleaved cell
    Sclerosis
  Malignant lymphoma, diffuse, mixed, small and large cell
    Sclerosis
    Epithelioid cell component
  Malignant lymphoma, diffuse, large cell
    Cleaved cell
    Noncleaved cell
    Sclerosis
High-Grade
  Malignant lymphoma, large cell, immunoblastic
    Plasmacytoid
    Clear cell
    Polymorphous
    Epithelioid cell component
  Malignant lymphoma, lymphoblastic
    Convoluted cell
    Nonconvoluted cell
  Malignant lymphoma, small noncleaved cell
    Burkitt's
    Follicular areas

A conceptual understanding of the common classification schemes requires knowledge of the morphologic ontogeny of normal lymphocytes. Although it is customary to discuss the lymphomas with reference to one of the classification schemes, taking a more conceptual approach will facilitate understanding the relationship between the various classification schemes. If for no other reason than convenience, the lymphocytic lymphomas may be conceptualized as a malignant population of lymphocytes arrested at a particular stage (morphologic, genotypic, phenotypic, or functional) of lymphocyte maturation (see Chapter 18). Thus, we would expect to see lymphomas that express the attributes of cells found in each of the various normal lymph node compartments: the intrafollicular, mantle zone, and interfollicular compartments. As illustrated in Figures 23–5 and 23–6, each lymph node compartment is occupied by morphologically characteristic cells. Lymphomas morphologically resembling each of these normal lymphocytes, or mixtures of them, have been described. Table 23–11 illustrates the relationship between the Working Formulation and the various lymph node compartments.

Lymphomas Derived from Intrafollicular (Follicular Center) Lymphocytes

These lymphomas express a B-cell phenotype and may have a follicular (nodular) (see Fig. 23–4A), a diffuse (see Fig. 23–4B), or a mixed follicular and diffuse growth pattern. The four morphologically distinct lymphocyte cell types found in the normal follicle (Fig. 23–6) are the small cleaved, small noncleaved, large cleaved, and large noncleaved lymphocytes.

Lymphomas Composed of Small Cleaved Lymphocytes

The malignant cell in this lymphoma is the counterpart of the small cleaved follicular center cell. This cell is small (6 to 12 μm in diameter) with a small amount of cytoplasm, slightly to distinctly irregular nucleus (angulated, clefted), and indistinct nucleoli (Fig. 23–7). A predominantly follicular or mixed follicular and diffuse pattern is most commonly found. Pure diffuse lymphomas of this type are uncommon in the United States. This lymphoma is classified as low-grade (indolent) if follicular and intermediate-grade if diffuse.

Lymphomas Composed of Large Cleaved Lymphocytes

This lymphoma is composed predominantly (more than 75 percent) of large cleaved cells. These cells are from 15 to 20 μm in diameter and have modest amounts of cytoplasm, irregular vesicular nuclei, and indistinct nucleoli. A follicular, diffuse, or mixed pattern may be seen. This lymphoma is classified as intermediate-grade, regardless of pattern.

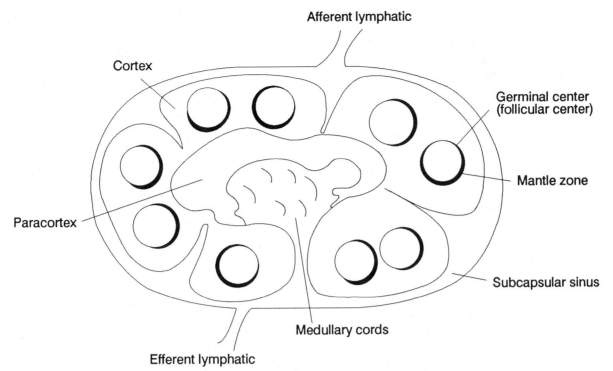

Figure 23-5. Anatomical compartments of the lymph nodes.

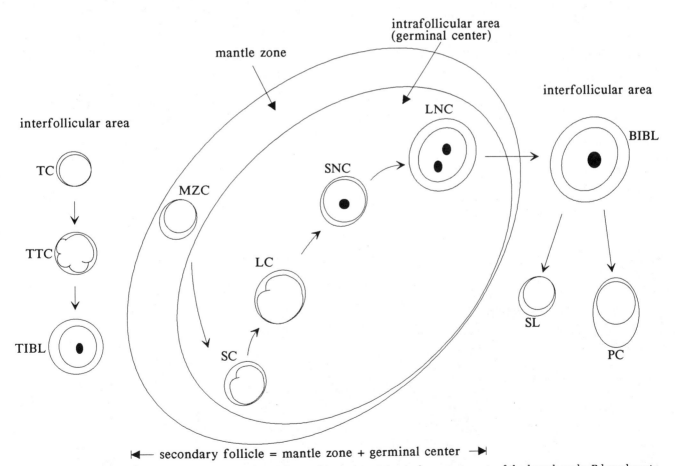

◄— secondary follicle = mantle zone + germinal center —►

Figure 23-6. Maturation of B and T lymphocytes in relationship to the anatomical compartments of the lymph node: B lymphocyte development occurs in all three of the compartments shown, whereas T lymphocyte transformation is confined to the interfollicular compartment. MZC, mantle zone cell; SC, small cleaved lymphocyte; LC, large cleaved lymphocyte; SNC, small noncleaved lymphocyte; LNC, large noncleaved lymphocyte; BIBL, B immunoblast; SL, small lymphocyte; PC, plasma cell; TC, T cell; TTC, transformed T cell; TIBL, T immunoblast.

393

Table 23–11. **LYMPHOMA CATEGORIES OF THE WORKING FORMULATION GROUPED BY ANATOMIC COMPARTMENTS OF THE LYMPH NODE**

Intrafollicular	Mantle Zone	Interfollicular
Small cleaved	Intermediate lymphocytic	Small lymphocyte
Large cleaved		Immunoblastic
Small noncleaved		True histiocytic
Mixed		Plasmacytoma

Lymphomas Composed of Large Noncleaved Lymphocytes

The majority of cells in this subcategory are 20 to 40 μm in diameter, have a modest amount of pyranophilic (RNA-rich) cytoplasm, round to oval vesicular nuclei, and small but distinct nucleoli. All three growth patterns (follicular, diffuse, or mixed) may be observed, and this group falls into the intermediate grade category.

Many large cell lymphomas are composed of a mixture of large cleaved and noncleaved cells and are so designated (Fig. 23–8).

Lymphomas Composed of Small and Large Lymphocytes (Cleaved and Noncleaved)

This subcategory is composed of a mixture of the cell types described earlier. The criteria for the diagnosis of mixed small and large cell vary with the different classification schemes and are largely subjective. Mann and Berard[21] have developed specific criteria for the follicular (nodular) variety of the follicular center cell lymphomas: between 5 and 15 large noncleaved cells per high-power field qualifies as mixed small and large cell, less than 5 per high-power field is considered small cleaved, and more than 15 per high-power field is large cell. Mixed small and large cell lymphoma is classified as low-grade if follicular and as intermediate-grade if diffuse.

Lymphomas Composed of Small Noncleaved Lymphocytes

The two recognized varieties of this subcategory are Burkitt's and non-Burkitt's types. A diffuse pattern is most commonly observed in both types, although a follicular pattern may occasionally be evident. In the Burkitt's form, a monomorphic pattern is observed, consisting of 15- to 20-μm cells with intense pyranophilic cytoplasm and uniform round nuclei with multiple distinct nucleoli (Fig. 23–9). Mitotic activity is very brisk. Numerous tingible-body macrophages (macrophages with phagocytized cellular debris) may be present and produce a "starry sky" pattern on low-power observation (**see Color Plate 232**). In the non-Burkitt's type the histologic features are similar to those of the Burkitt's variety, but there is greater nuclear size variation and nucleoli tend to be more prominent.

Lymphomas Derived from Mantle Zone Lymphocytes

In its early phase this lymphoma is characterized by broad expansions of the mantle zone of secondary follicles and in this phase is referred to as mantle zone lymphoma. This expansion is composed of a mixture of small uniform and small atypical lymphocytes that express the phenotype of mantle zone lymphocytes including monoclonal surface immunoglobulin. The residual germinal centers, however, are polyclonal. As the expansion progresses, a diffuse pattern supervenes (lymphocytic lymphoma of intermediate differentiation). In the mantle zone phase this lymphoma is classified as low-grade, whereas in the diffuse phase it is considered intermediate.

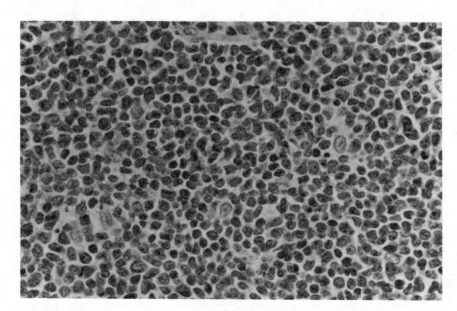

Figure 23–7. Malignant lymphoma, small cleaved cell is composed of small cells (6 to 12 μm in diameter) with scant cytoplasm and angulated or clefted nuclei with indistinct nucleoli.

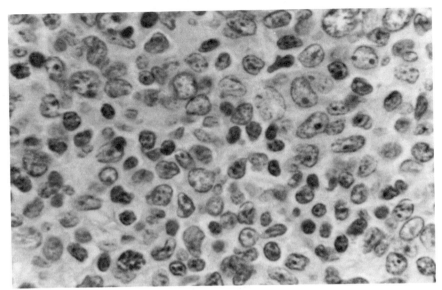

Figure 23-8. Malignant lymphoma, large diffuse cell composed of a mixture of large cleaved and noncleaved cells.

Lymphomas Derived from Interfollicular Lymphocytes

These lymphomas may express either a B- or a T-cell phenotype. Morphologic features alone are unreliable in assessing the B- or T-cell nature of these lymphomas.

Small Lymphocytic Lymphoma. This low-grade lymphoma is commonly referred to as well-differentiated lymphoma (Rappaport classification). It is the only low-grade lymphoma that does not have a follicular growth pattern. The growth pattern is diffuse, although a pseudofollicular pattern may be observed (Fig. 23-10A). These pseudofollicles, also called growth centers, do not have the cytologic or histologic features of true neoplastic follicles.[22] In the early phase of nodal involvement the neoplastic cells may be confined to the interfollicular areas with sparing of the normal follicles. Later, there is total effacement of lymph node architecture. The majority of the neoplastic cells are small, uniform lymphocytes with scant cytoplasm, round nucleus, clumped chromatin, and absent nucleoli; that is, they appear cytologically like normal lymphocytes (Fig. 23-10B). Admixed with these small lymphocytes are variable numbers of intermediate to large lymphocytes with large vesicular nuclei and distinct nucleoli. These cells are commonly found in increased numbers within the pseudofollicles. In approximately 40 percent of cases of small lymphocytic lymphoma a leukemic phase develops identical to that in chronic lymphocytic leukemia (CLL).

The vast majority of small lymphocytic lymphomas expresses a B-cell phenotype (98 percent in

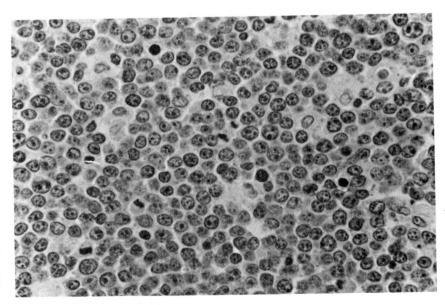

Figure 23-9. Malignant lymphoma, small noncleaved cell (Burkitt's lymphoma). The malignant cell of this subtype of lymphoma is characterized by relatively uniform cells 15 to 20 μm in diameter having a moderate amount of pyranophilic cytoplasm and round nuclei with multiple small distinct nucleoli.

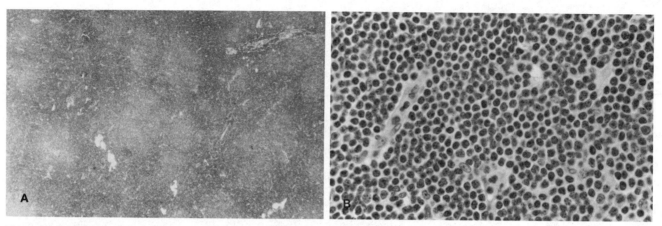

Figure 23-10. Malignant lymphoma, small lymphocytic (*A*) pseudofollicular growth pattern is evident due to the presence of numerous growth centers, (*B*) outside the growth centers this subtype of lymphoma is composed predominantly of sheets of small, mature-appearing lymphocytes.

Western countries). In addition to the expression of B-cell–associated antigens (CD19 through CD22; CD24), with sensitive techniques, low-density monoclonal surface immunoglobulin is detectable. The remaining 2 percent of these lymphomas express a mature T-cell phenotype, usually of the helper type [CD2(+)/CD3(+)/CD4(+)/CD5(+)/ CD7(+)/CD8(−)].

Small lymphocytic lymphomas may show evidence of plasmacytoid differentiation and are so designated. This subcategory of lymphoma represents the tissue expression of the clinical syndrome Waldenström's macroglobulinemia, although not all patients with plasmacytoid small lymphocytic lymphoma develop the clinical syndrome.

Immunoblastic Lymphomas. This category of high-grade lymphomas is associated with several distinctive cytologic patterns and may express either a B- or a T-cell phenotype. The correlation between cytologic features and phenotype is good but not absolute. Therefore, ancillary studies beyond light microscopy are required to determine the phenotype. The plasmacytoid subtype of immunoblastic lymphoma usually expresses a B-cell phenotype and is characterized by cells with moderate to abundant pyranophilic cytoplasm, large vesicular nucleus, and prominent nucleolus. Mitotic activity is brisk. The T-cell types of immunoblastic lymphoma most commonly have a clear cell, polymorphous, or epithelial pattern.

Lymphoblastic Lymphoma. The cells of lymphoblastic lymphoma are cytologically identical to the lymphoblasts of acute lymphoblastic leukemia. They have scant cytoplasm and nuclei with finely dispersed chromatin and absent or indistinct nucleoli. The nuclear contour may be either convoluted or nonconvoluted and mitotic activity is high. The cytologic and histologic features of this lymphoma may be confused with those of small, noncleaved lymphoma. Attention to nuclear features, as well as immunophenotypic and cytogenetic data,

can make the distinction between these two lymphoma types.

Approximately 70 percent of lymphoblastic lymphomas are of the T-cell type. Their phenotype is complex; however, most will test positive for terminal deoxynucleotidyl transferase (TdT) (see Chapter 18), which serves to distinguish them from other categories of lymphoma. The B-cell type of lymphoblastic lymphoma also shows a high frequency of expression of TdT.

Miscellaneous Lymphomas

A plethora of uncommon, unusual, and difficult-to-classify lymphomas has been described. Certain of these, although they do not fit neatly into the classification schemes, are distinct clinicopathologic entities worthy of discussion.

Cutaneous T-cell Lymphoma. This category includes a broad group of dysplastic and frankly malignant T-cell proliferations with a predilection for infiltration of the skin.[23] Disorders under this category include mycosis fungoides, Sézary syndrome, lymphomatoid papulosis, regressing atypical histiocytosis, and peripheral (post-thymic) T-cell lymphoma with skin involvement. B-cell lymphomas may occasionally secondarily involve the skin; however, this is seldom an isolated or presenting finding in B-cell lymphoma. Hodgkin's disease rarely involves the skin in the form of direct extension from adjacent involved lymph nodes.

Mycosis fungoides and Sézary syndrome, two related disorders, are characterized by infiltration of the dermis and epidermis by malignant T cells with a peculiar cerebriform nucleus. Thin sections of well-fixed paraffin-embedded material or plastic-embedded sections are required to appreciate this nuclear detail. In 90 percent of cases these cells exhibit a mature helper phenotype [pan-T(+), CD4(+), CD8(−)] and in 10 percent a mature suppressor phenotype [pan-T(+), CD4(−), CD8(+)]. In many cases, mycosis fungoides clinically progresses through three phases. In the premycotic phase, lasting from

6 months to 50 years, the T-cell infiltrate produces a nonspecific eczematous dermatosis that is difficult to differentiate from a benign inflammatory infiltrate. As the disease progresses, the infiltrate thickens to form distinct plaques and finally tumor nodules (**see Color Plate 233**). Systemic dissemination with lymph node, peripheral blood, and visceral organ involvement are more likely to develop in these later stages. In the related Sézary syndrome, the early erythroderma stage is associated with a leukemia of the characteristic cerebriform T cells (Sézary cells) (**see Color Plate 234**). Progression to the tumor stage is unusual in Sézary syndrome.

Angioimmunoblastic Lymphadenopathy with Dysproteinemia–like T-cell Lymphoma. In 1979 Shimoyama and co-workers[24] described a lymphoma with clinical and morphologic features similar to those of immunoblastic lymphadenopathy (IBL) and angioimmunoblastic lymphadenopathy with dysproteinemia (AILD).[24] These disorders are associated with evidence of hyperimmunity and often develop following exposure to certain drugs and infectious agents. There is a high frequency of evolution of these disorders to frank lymphoma. It is now generally recognized that the spectrum of clinicopathologic entities in this category range from benign (possibly premalignant) disorders to aggressive, rapidly fatal lymphomas.

Angiocentric T-cell Lymphomas. Angiocentric T-cell lymphoma[25] is the malignant member of a family of diseases that encompasses a variety of angiocentric and angiodestructive disorders (lymphocytic vasculitis, lymphomatoid granulomatosis, polymorphous reticulosis, and angiocentric T-cell lymphoma). The lymphoma is characterized by tissue nodules of atypical lymphoreticular cells centered about blood vessels, often resulting in their destruction. The lung is the most common site of involvement.

HTLV-I–Associated T-cell Lymphoma/Leukemia. This aggressive lymphoma is associated with the type C retrovirus HTLV-I and is most common in the endemic areas of Japan, Africa, and the southeastern United States.[26] It is often widely disseminated at presentation and clinically is characterized by lymphadenopathy, hepatosplenomegaly, involvement of the peripheral blood and cerebrospinal fluid (CSF), and hypercalcemia. Skin involvement mimics that of mycosis fungoides. In involved fluids such as peripheral blood or CSF the distinctive bizarre polypoid malignant cells are readily identified. These cells express a mature helper phenotype and also are positive for the T-cell growth factor receptor (IL-2 receptor).

True Histiocytic Lymphoma. Despite the common vernacular of the Rappaport classification, lymphomas of true histiocytes are uncommon. Morphologically they are indistinguishable from other large cell immunoblastic lymphomas; however, their enzyme and immunophenotypic profile is similar to that of histiocytes/monocytes.

Angiotropic Large Cell Lymphoma. This rare form of lymphoma (**see Color Plate 235**) was formerly referred to as malignant angioendotheliomatosis. When first described, this intravascular tumor was believed to be of endothelial origin.[27] Recent immunophenotypic and genotypic data, however, have demonstrated that the proliferation is lymphoid, expressing leukocyte common antigen (**see Color Plate 236**) and either T- or B-cell antigens.[28] Factor VIII antigen, present on endothelial cells, is absent on the tumor cells (**see Color Plate 237**). The tumor cells are confined to the lumens of blood vessels most commonly in the skin and central nervous system. This unusual form of lymphoma normally occurs in older adults; however, a few well-documented cases have been described in adolescents.[29] Prognosis is poor.

Clinical Features

Similar to Hodgkin's disease, patients with NHL most commonly present with painless lymph node swelling involving single or multiple sites. Different from Hodgkin's disease, up to one third of patients with NHL may present with involvement of lymphoid tissue other than lymph nodes (**see Color Plate 239**) such as gut and skin–associated lymphoid tissue, bone marrow, and tonsil. Neck nodes are the most frequently involved site.

The low-grade lymphomas are generally widespread at initial diagnosis with a high frequency of spleen, liver, and bone marrow involvement. The intermediate- and high-grade lymphomas are more often localized at presentation, with spleen, liver, and bone marrow occurring later in the clinical course. Extranodal (gut, CNS, skeletal, testicular) involvement is also common in the more aggressive grades of lymphoma. Peripheral blood involvement is uncommon in the NHLs except for small lymphocytic lymphoma (well-differentiated lymphocytic lymphoma) and lymphoblastic lymphoma. A CLL-like picture in the peripheral blood often develops during the course of small lymphocytic lymphoma. Frank acute lymphoblastic leukemia often supervenes in lymphoblastic lymphoma.

Except for lymphoblastic lymphoma, Burkitt's lymphoma, and some of the miscellaneous group of lymphomas, the NHLs are diseases of middle-aged and older adults. Approximately 40 percent of childhood lymphomas fall into the lymphoblastic category. In the United States, Burkitt's lymphoma accounts for about 30 percent of childhood non-Hodgkin's lymphomas (**see Color Plate 238**).

As a clinicopathologic entity Burkitt's lymphoma deserves special attention. This subtype of lymphoma was first described in 1958 by Dennis Burkitt. He noted the occurrence of a malignant tumor in children in East Africa that often presented as a destructive lesion of the jaw (Fig. 23–11). African (endemic) and nonendemic cases of Burkitt's lymphoma are now recognized. In younger children facial tumors are common, whereas in older children presentation with an abdominal tumor is more usual.

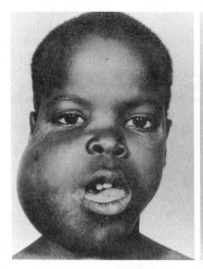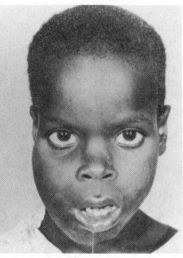

Figure 23–11. Burkitt's lymphoma before (*left*) and after treatment (*right*).

Diagnostic Evaluation and Staging

Tissue biopsy is required for the diagnosis and subcategorization of NHL. The mainstay of diagnosis is the histologic evaluation of well-stained tissue sections by an experienced pathologist. Ancillary studies, however, are often required and these include immunophenotypic studies, nucleic acid (DNA and RNA) content analysis, cytogenetics, gene rearrangement and functional studies (Table 23–12). The diagnostic difficulties fall into a relatively small number of categories; namely, differentiating (1) benign versus malignant lymphoproliferations, (2) lymphoma versus nonlymphoma, (3) T-cell versus B-cell lymphoma, and (4) non-Hodgkin's lymphoma versus Hodgkin's disease. One or more of the ancillary tests may be required to resolve the differential diagnostic dilemma, and rarely the dilemma may be unresolvable.

A word of caution: The reader should be aware that there are many technical and biologic pitfalls in the interpretation of these ancillary studies. These data must be interpreted in association with clinical and histologic findings.

Benign Versus Malignant

If light microscopic evaluation fails to distinguish a benign from a malignant lymphoproliferation, the demonstration of immunophenotypic or genotypic monoclonality would favor a malignant diagnosis. For B cells, immunophenotypic monoclonality is defined as restriction of immunoglobulin light chain production by a population of cells to a single light chain class, either kappa or lambda. Operationally, light chain monoclonality is present if the percentage of kappa-positive cells to lambda-positive cells (kappa-to-lambda ratio) falls outside of the expected ("normal") range or if "clonal excess" can be demonstrated by statistical comparison (Kolmogorov-Smirnov test)[30] of the kappa and lambda fluorescence intensity distributions. An example of monoclonality demonstrated by single

color flow cytometry is illustrated in Figure 23–12. For the interested reader, additional information is available regarding the detection of light chain clonality.[31–34] Unfortunately, at present, no practical method exists to define immunophenotypic T-cell clonality. Evidence for T-cell malignancy, however, may be suggested by immunophenotypically demonstrating an aberrant T-cell phenotype. Benign T-cell proliferations generally express a "normal" T-cell phenotype in which all pan-T–cell antigens (CD2, CD3, CD5, CD7) are expressed by the individual T cells. On the other hand, T-cell malignancies that might be confused with a benign T-cell proliferation often express an aberrant T-cell phenotype in which one or more of the pan-T–cell antigens are not expressed. Approximately 60 percent of peripheral T-cell lymphomas will express such an aberrant phenotype, with CD5 and CD7 being the most frequently absent antigens.[35]

A genotypic definition of both B- and T-cell clonality is possible. Clonal rearrangements of the T-cell receptor or immunoglobulin genes

Table 23–12. **ROUTINE AND ANCILLARY TESTS USEFUL IN THE EVALUATION OF LYMPH NODE BIOPSIES**

I. Fresh Tissue
  A. Bacterial/viral studies
  B. Cell suspension for surface marker, cytogenetic studies, and genotypic studies
  C. Frozen material for rapid diagnosis, histochemical and immunohistochemical stains

II. Fixed Tissue
  A. Paraffin-embedded for light microscopy and limited histochemical, immunohistochemical, and genotypic studies
  B. Resin (plastic)–embedded for electron microscopy and thin-section light microscopy

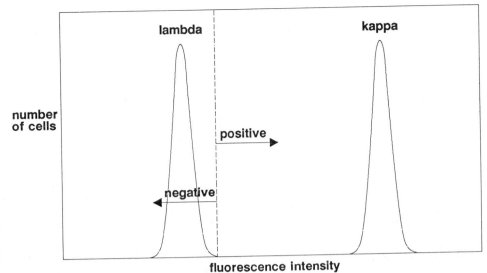

Figure 23-12. B-cell monoclonality detected by flow cytometry: overlay of single-parameter kappa and lambda fluorescence histograms demonstrating the presence of a monoclonal kappa population of cells.

(see Chapter 18) are detectable by the method of Southern analysis. Clonal rearrangement is present when bands other than germ-line bands are identified in the Southern blot (Fig. 23–13). The identification of a clonal rearrangement is indicative of a malignant proliferation. Although biphenotypic rearrangements (both T-cell receptor and immunoglobulin genes rearranged) may occur, the specific type of rearrangement is also useful in assigning lineage to the lymphoma—that is, a B-cell

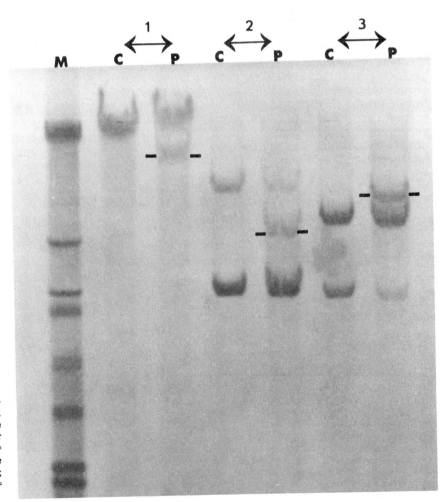

Figure 23-13. T-cell monoclonality demonstrated by Southern analysis: abnormal bands designated by small bars indicate clonal rearrangement of the T-cell receptor gene. M = molecular weight markers; C = control DNA to locate position of germ-line (nonrearranged) bands; P = patient DNA; 1 = Bam HI digest; 2 = Eco RI digest; 3 = Hind III digest.[36-38]

lymphoma if immunoglobulin gene rearrangement is found and a T-cell lymphoma if T-cell receptor gene rearrangement is found. (The interested reader is referred to other sources[36-38] for further details of the diagnostic utility of gene rearrangement studies.)

Although karyotypic analysis in a search for nonrandom chromosome abnormalities might be useful in distinguishing benign from malignant lymphoproliferations, the technical difficulties in performing this type of analysis have made cytogenetic studies an uncommon ancillary test in lymphoproliferation evaluation. The development of DNA probes for specific chromosomal alterations may obviate the necessity of performing karyograms in the cytogenetic evaluation of lymphoproliferations.

Lymphoma Versus Nonlymphoma

The differential diagnoses of large cell lymphoma and nonlymphoid malignancies such as amelanotic melanoma, poorly differentiated carcinoma, germ cell neoplasms, and round cell sarcomas is a frequently occurring problem in surgical pathology. A differential diagnosis is facilitated by determining the antigenic phenotype of the tumor cells. This is most commonly done by staining the cells by an immunoenzyme technique using a panel of antibodies directed against normal cellular differentiation antigens.[39] Although no single antibody is either 100 percent specific or sensitive for identifying the "cell of origin" of a tumor, with the aid of a panel of antibodies it is generally possible to define a phenotypic profile that permits identification of the type of tumor. From a therapeutic perspective it is most important to resolve the differential—carcinoma versus lymphoma versus sarcoma versus melanoma—which can usually be accomplished by a relatively small antibody panel (Table 23–13). Ad-

Table 23–13. **ANTIBODY PANEL FOR DISTINGUISHING AMONG THE FOUR MAJOR CATEGORIES OF CANCER**

Cancer Type	Antibody			
	Cytokeratin*	Vimentin†	LCA‡	S100§
Carcinoma	+	−	−	−
Sarcoma	−	+	−	−
Lymphoma	−	±	+	−
Melanoma	−	±	−	+

*Antibody directed against the cytokeratin group of intermediate filament proteins found in epithelial cells.
†Antibody directed against the 58-kilodalton intermediate filament protein found in mesenchymal cells.
‡Antibody directed against the 200-kilodalton leukocyte common antigen found in various hematopoietic and lymphoreticular cells.
§Antibody directed against the 25-kilodalton protein found in selected cells of the CNS, melanocytes, interdigitating reticulum cells, and so on. The antibody HMB-45 is more specifically restricted to melanocytes than anti-S100.

ditional refinement of the diagnosis, though it may not have therapeutic implications, may be possible with larger panels.

T-cell Versus B-cell Lymphoma

Although morphologic features may suggest a B- or T-cell phenotype, ancillary tests are required for specific distinction between B- and T-cell lymphoma. The immunophenotypic demonstration of light chain monoclonality and the expression of B lineage antigens (CD19 through CD22) or of an aberrant B-cell phenotype by the cells of a malignant lymphoma are indicative of a B-cell lymphoma.[30] Similarly, the expression of a normal or abnormal T-cell phenotype by the malignant cells is associated with T-cell malignancy.[35] Gene rearrangement studies appear to be more sensitive than immunophenotypic studies in distinguishing T-cell versus B-cell lymphoma; however, relatively few lymphomas require this technically more demanding procedure to make this distinction.

Hodgkin's Disease Versus Non-Hodgkin's Lymphoma

On morphologic grounds alone it is sometimes difficult, if not impossible, to distinguish Hodgkin's disease from non-Hodgkin's lymphoma. For this reason, and because of important therapeutic implications, there has been considerable interest in the utility of ancillary techniques to resolve this differential diagnosis. The literature is replete with contradictory studies concerning the significance of various tests in distinguishing Hodgkin's disease from NHL.[40] This state of affairs reflects defects in our understanding of the basic biologic differences between these disorders, as well as the nonspecificity of the tests. At present the only specific immunophenotypic distinction between these disorders is the presence of light chain monoclonality in B-cell NHLs and its absence in Hodgkin's disease.

Staging

The staging evaluation of the NHLs is similar to that for Hodgkin's disease. The Ann Arbor classification (see Table 23–5), the same staging scheme that was designed for Hodgkin's disease, is used also for non-Hodgkin's lymphomas. Because the natural history of Hodgkin's disease is different from that of NHL, there are certain problems with using the Ann Arbor classification in staging NHLs. Despite these drawbacks, the Ann Arbor scheme remains the staging scheme of choice. The major exception to this statement is Burkitt's lymphoma. In this lymphoma the bulk of tumor rather than sites of involvement, is a primary determinant of prognosis. Consequently, a different staging scheme is used for Burkitt's lymphoma (Table 23–14).

Treatment and Prognosis

For purposes of prognostic assessment and therapeutic selection, the NHLs can be grouped into two broad categories: the indolent lymphomas and the

Table 23-14. **STAGING CLASSIFICATION OF BURKITT'S LYMPHOMA**

Stage A	Single extra-abdominal site
Stage B	Multiple extra-abdominal sites
Stage C	Intra-abdominal tumor
Stage D	Intra-abdominal tumor with multiple extra-abdominal sites
Stage AR	Stage C disease with >90% of tumor surgically removed

diffuse aggressive lymphomas. The indolent lymphomas are the low-grade lymphomas of the Working Formulation (see Table 23-10). They are so designated because the median survival without therapy for this group of lymphomas is relatively long (7 to 9 years). The diffuse aggressive lymphomas encompass the intermediate- and high-grade lymphomas of the Working Formulation. Without treatment, these lymphomas are rapidly fatal (median survival is 6 to 12 months).

Therapy for the indolent lymphomas is controversial. Approximately 90 percent of these lymphomas are stage III or IV at presentation, and although sensitive to both radiation and chemotherapy, the disease is incurable. Current therapies are ineffective in prolonging survival in the low-grade lymphomas and a "watch and wait" approach has been adopted by many oncologists.[41] When symptoms warrant, or if the lymphoma progresses to a higher grade, therapy is instituted. In the small number of patients with stage I or II disease, involved or extended field radiation therapy may be useful.

Prior to the development of modern chemotherapeutic modalities, the indolent lymphomas were considered "favorable" lymphomas and the diffuse aggressive lymphomas "unfavorable." The situation is now reversed. The indolent lymphomas are recognized as clinically indolent but incurable with current therapies. On the other hand, the diffuse aggressive lymphomas are rapidly fatal if untreated but are potentially curable with aggressive chemotherapeutic strategies. The 10-year survival for the diffuse aggressive lymphomas treated aggressively with multiagent chemotherapy is now greater than for the indolent lymphomas. Long-term survival depends on achieving an initial complete remission. Therapy following relapse is usually ineffective. Patients who survive for 2 years without evidence of recurrence are considered cured, as relapses seldom occur after a 2-year disease-free interval. As survival is increased with aggressive therapy, the risk of secondary (chemotherapy-induced) acute nonlymphocytic leukemia is also increasing. Approximately 8 percent of patients develop acute nonlymphocytic leukemia within 10 years of chemotherapy for non-Hodgkin's lymphoma, and these leukemias are usually very resistant to therapy.

The therapeutic response of lymphoblastic lymphoma to aggressive chemotherapy has not been as impressive as with the other aggressive lymphomas. Adults older than 45 years tend to have longer survival than do younger patients; however, median survival is still short.[42]

REFERENCES

1. Hodgkin, T: On some morbid appearances of the absorbent glands and spleen. Medico-Chirurgicol Transactions 17:68, 1832.
2. Wilks, Sir S: Cases of enlargement of the lymphatic glands and spleen (or, Hodgkin's disease), with remarks. Guy's Hospital Reports 11:56, 1865.
3. Sternberg, C: Uber eine eigenartige unter dem Bilde der Pseudoleukamie verlaufende Tuberculose des lymphatischen Apparates. Zeitschrift für Heiltung 19:21, 1898.
4. Reed, DM: On the pathological changes in Hodgkin's disease, with special reference to its relation to tuberculosis. Johns Hopkins Hosp Rep 10:133, 1902.
5. Lukes, RJ, et al: Report of the Nomenclature Committee. Cancer Res 26:1311, 1966.
6. Lukes, RJ and Butler, JJ: The pathology and nomenclature of Hodgkin's disease. Cancer Res 26:1063, 1966.
7. Correa, P, et al: International comparability and reproducibility in histologic subclassification of Hodgkin's disease. J Natl Cancer Inst 50:1429, 1973.
8. Kant, JA, et al: A critical reappraisal of the pathologic and clinical heterogeneity of "lymphocyte depleted Hodgkin's disease." J Clin Oncol 4:284, 1986.
9. Kadin, ME, Glatstein, E, and Dorfman, RF: Clinicopathologic studies of 117 untreated patients subjected to laparotomy for the staging of Hodgkin's disease. Cancer 27:1277, 1971.
10. Lukes, RJ: Criteria for involvement of lymph node, bone marrow, spleen, and liver in Hodgkin's disease. Cancer Res 31:1755, 1971.
11. Carbone, PP, et al: Report of the Committee on Hodgkin's Staging Classification. Cancer Res 31:1860, 1971.
12. DeVita, VT, et al: Curability of advanced Hodgkin's disease with chemotherapy. Ann Intern Med 92:587, 1980.
13. Virchow, RLK: Die cellulare Pathologie in ihrer Begruendung auf physiologische und pathologische Gewebelehre. Hirschwald, Berlin, 1858.
14. Billroth, T: Multiple Lymphome: Erfolgreiche Behandlung mit Arsenik. Wien Med Wochenschr 21:1066, 1871.
15. Dreschfield, J: Ein Beitrag Zur Lehre von den Lymphosarkomen. Dtsch Med Wochenschr 17:1175, 1893.
16. Kundrat, H: Uber Lympho-sarkomatosis. Wien Klin Wochenschr 6:211, 234, 1893.
17. Heim, S and Mitelman, F: Cancer Cytogenetics. Alan R Liss, New York, 1989.
18. Berard, CW and Dorfman, RF: Histopathology of malignant lymphomas. Clin Hematol 3:39, 1974.
19. Lennert, K, et al: The histopathology of malignant lymphoma. Br J Haematol 31(Suppl):193, 1975.
20. Rosenberg, SA, et al: National Cancer Institute sponsored study of classification on non-Hodgkin's lymphomas: Summary and description of a working formulation for clinical usage. Cancer 49:2112, 1982.
21. Mann, RB and Berard, CW: Criteria for the cytologic subclassification of follicular lymphomas: A proposed alternative method. Hematol Oncol 1:187, 1983.
22. Nathwani, BN: Classifying non-Hodgkin's lymphomas. In Berard, CW, et al (eds): Malignant Lymphoma (IAP Monographs in Pathology; no 29). Williams & Wilkins, Baltimore, 1987.
23. Edelson, RL: Cutaneous T cell lymphoma. J Dermatol Surg Oncol 6:358, 1980.
24. Shimoyama, J, et al: Immunoblastic lymphadenopathy (IBL)-like T cell lymphoma. Jpn J Clin Oncol 9(Suppl):347, 1979.
25. Jaffe, ES: Postthymic lymphoid neoplasia. In Jaffe, ES and

Bennington, JL (ed): Surgical Pathology of the Lymph Nodes and Related Organs. WB Saunders, Philadelphia, 1985.

26. Gallo, RC: Human T cell leukemia/lymphoma virus and T cell malignancies in adults. Cancer Surv 3:113, 1984.

27. Drobacheff, C, et al: Malignant Angioendotheliomatosis: Re-classification as an angiotropic lymphoma. Int J Dermatol 28:454, 1989.

28. Ferry, JA, et al: Intravascular lymphomatosis (malignant an-giotheliomatosis): A B cell neoplasm expressing surface homing receptors. Mod Pathol 1:444, 1988.

29. Sangueza, O and Hyder, D: Intravascular lymphamatosis with T-cell phenotype in an adolescent. Archives of Derma-tology, in press.

30. Ault, KA: Detection of small numbers of monoclonal B lym-phocytes in blood of patients with lymphoma. N Engl J Med 300:1401, 1979.

31. Picker, LJ, et al: Immunophenotypic criteria for the diagnosis of non Hodgkin's lymphoma. Am J Pathol 128:181, 1987.

32. Tubbs, R, et al: Tissue immunomicroscopic evaluation of monoclonality of B cell lymphomas. Am J Clin Pathol 76:24, 1986.

33. Hsu, SM: The use of monoclonal antibodies and immunohis-tochemical techniques in lymphoma: Review and overlook. Hematol Pathol 2:183, 1988.

34. Little, JV, et al: Flow cytometric analysis of lymphomas and lymphoma-like disorders. Semin Diagn Pathol 6:37, 1989.

35. Weiss, FM, et al: Morphologic and immunologic character-ization of 50 peripheral T cell lymphoma. Am J Pathol 118:316, 1985.

36. Korsmeyer, SJ and Walkman, TA: Immunoglobulin Genes: rearrangement and translocation in human lymphoid malig-nancy. J Clin Immunol 4:1, 1984.

37. Bertness, VO, et al: T cell receptor gene rearrangements and clinical markers of human T cell lymphomas. N Engl J Med 313:534, 1985.

38. Cossman, J, et al: Molecular genetics and the diagnosis of lymphoma. Arch Pathol Lab Med 112:117, 1988.

39. Battifora, H: Recent progress in the immunohistochemistry of solid tumors. Semin Diagn Pathol 1:251, 1984.

40. Hyder, DM and Schnitzer, B: Analysis of hematopoietic/ lymphoreticular malignancies. In Keren, DF (ed): Flow Cyto-metry in Clinical Diagnosis. ASCP Press, Chicago, 1989.

41. Horning, SJ and Rosenberg, SA: The natural history of un-treated low grade non Hodgkin's lymphomas. N Engl J Med 311:1471, 1984.

42. Weinstein, JH, et al: Long term results of the APO protocol for treatment of mediastinal lymphoblastic lymphoma. J Clin Oncol 1:537, 1983.

QUESTIONS

1. What type of cell is characteristic for Hodgkin's disease?
   a. Reed-Sternberg cell
   b. Reactive histiocyte
   c. Convoluted cells
   d. Immunoblast

2. Which type of Hodgkin's disease shows benign lymphocytes, histiocytes, and L and H cells and rare Reed-Sternberg cells?
   a. Mixed cellularity
   b. Nodular sclerosing
   c. Lymphocyte predominance
   d. Lymphocyte depletion

3. Which stage of Hodgkin's disease shows involve-ment of two or more lymph nodes or extralym-phatic organs on the same side of the diaphragm?
   a. Type I
   b. Type II
   c. Type III
   d. Type IV

4. What disease classification schemes use criteria such as morphology, genotype, phenotype, or function of lymphocytes?
   a. Non-Hodgkin's lymphoma
   b. Hodgkin's disease
   c. Benign lymphoma
   d. Malignant lymphoma

5. Which lymphoma characteristically shows mac-rophages with phagocytized debris in a "starry sky" pattern?
   a. Immunoblastic lymphoma
   b. Burkitt's lymphoma
   c. HTLV-I–associated T-cell lymphoma/leuke-mia
   d. Small lymphocytic lymphoma

6. Which lymphoma shows an aggressive clinical course and is associated with a retrovirus? (Use answer choices for question 5.)

7. Which of the following tests would be least useful in providing differential diagnostic criteria?
   a. Cellular phenotyping
   b. Light microscopy
   c. Southern blot test
   d. Total lymphocyte counts

ANSWERS

1. a (p. 385)
2. c (p. 385–387)
3. b (p. 389)
4. a (p. 390)
5. b (p. 394)
6. c (p. 397)
7. d (p. 398–400)

CHAPTER **24**

CATHERINE M. SPIER, M.D.

Lipid (Lysosomal) Storage Diseases and Histiocytoses

LIPID (LYSOSOMAL) STORAGE DISEASES

GAUCHER'S DISEASE
CLINICAL FEATURES
Type I (Adult Gaucher's Disease)
Type II (Infantile, Acute, or Malignant Neuronopathic
 Gaucher's Disease)
Type III (Juvenile or Subacute Neuronopathic
 Gaucher's Disease)
LABORATORY DIAGNOSIS
PROGNOSIS

NIEMANN-PICK DISEASE
CLINICAL FEATURES
Type A
Type B
LABORATORY DIAGNOSIS
PROGNOSIS

TAY-SACHS DISEASE
CLINICAL FEATURES
LABORATORY DIAGNOSIS
PROGNOSIS

MUCOPOLYSACCHARIDOSES
CATEGORIES
CLINICAL FEATURES
LABORATORY DIAGNOSIS AND PROGNOSIS

HISTIOCYTOSES
SEA-BLUE HISTIOCYTE SYNDROME
OTHER HISTIOCYTIC DISORDERS (EOSINOPHILIC
 GRANULOMA, HAND-SCHÜLLER-CHRISTIAN DISEASE,
 LETTERER-SIWE DISEASE)

OBJECTIVES

At the end of this chapter, the learner should be able to:
 1. Describe the defect in lipid storage diseases.
 2. Name the enzyme deficiency of Gaucher's disease.
 3. List characteristics for type I, type II, and type III Gaucher's disease.
 4. Describe the appearance of Gaucher's cells.
 5. Name the enzyme deficiency of Niemann-Pick disease.
 6. List clinical features of Niemann-Pick disease.
 7. Describe the appearance of Niemann-Pick cells.
 8. Name the enzyme deficiency of Tay-Sachs disease.
 9. List clinical features of Tay-Sachs disease.
 10. List laboratory findings in Tay-Sachs disease.
 11. Describe clinical features of Hurler's syndrome, Hunter's syndrome, and other mucopolysaccharidoses.
 12. List laboratory findings in mucopolysaccharidosis disorders.
 13. Describe the characteristic cell of sea-blue histiocyte syndrome.
 14. Name other histiocytic disorders.

LIPID (LYSOSOMAL) STORAGE DISEASES

The lipid storage diseases, also known as lysosomal storage diseases because of the subcellular accumulation of unmetabolized material in lysosomes, are rare, autosomally inherited disorders. They are caused by various enzyme defects (inborn errors) in lipid metabolism (Fig. 24–1). Although many different types have been documented, the most widely known and well-established are those described subsequently. Certain ethnic groups, most notably the Ashkenazi Jews (those Jews who trace their origin to the Baltic Sea region), have an increased incidence of some lipid storage diseases, especially Gaucher's and Tay-Sachs, but all ethnic

A

GLOBOSIDE

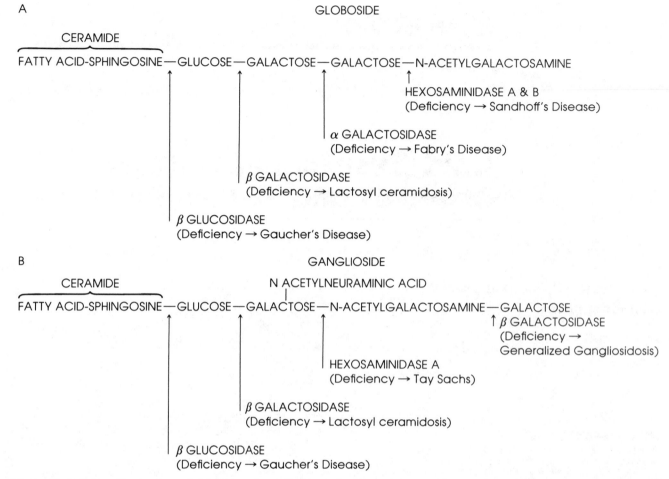

Figure 24–1. Schematic structure of globoside and ganglioside to show site of action of the several catabolic enzymes, which, when defective, result in one of the storage diseases. (From Wintrobe,[3] p 1341, with permission.)

groups are known to be affected. This group of disorders has wide clinical expression, ranging from essentially asymptomatic to severe and incapacitating with early death. None has an effective therapy. The aim of control in these disorders has been directed at prenatal detection. However, newer techniques such as enzyme replacement and gene manipulation are now being attempted. The results of these manipulations have shown variable degrees of success, and continued research is in progress. This chapter is devoted to a description of the clinical and pathologic features, as well as the prognosis and treatment, of the lipid storage diseases.

GAUCHER'S DISEASE

This disorder was first described in 1882 by Philippe C. Gaucher in a 32-year-old woman with an enlarged spleen. Gaucher believed the abnormal cells found in her spleen at autopsy were part of a primary splenic tumor. His observations were studied further and the entity we call Gaucher's disease was coined at the turn of the century by Dr. Nathan E. Brill of New York.[1]

Gaucher's disease has three clinically recogniz-

able types, but all are due to a deficiency of the enzyme β-glucocerebrosidase with an accumulation of the unmetabolized glucocerebroside in cells, especially of the reticuloendothelial system. The three types are the adult, or non-neuronopathic form (type I); the infantile, acute, or malignant neuronopathic form (type II); and the juvenile or subacute neuronopathic form (type III). All have in common the triad of hepatosplenomegaly (**see Color Plate 240**), Gaucher's cells in the bone marrow, and an increase in serum acid phosphatase. The severity of the disease and the patient's age when the disease is first manifested are related to the magnitude of the enzyme deficiency. Each type is described in detail later. Table 24–1 briefly summarizes the features of each type.

Clinical Features

Type I (Adult Gaucher's Disease)

This is the most common type of Gaucher's and is also the most common of the lipidoses.[2] It is seen most frequently in Ashkenazi Jews. The clinical onset of the disease is variable, being discovered in

Table 24–1. **GAUCHER'S DISEASE — CLINICAL SUBTYPES**

Clinical Features	Type I: Non-neuronopathic	Type II: Acute Neuronopathic	Type III: Subacute Neuronopathic
Clinical onset	Childhood Adulthood	Infancy	Childhood
Hepatosplenomegaly	+	+	+
Hematologic complications secondary to hypersplenism	+	+	+
Skeletal deterioration	+	–	+
Neurodegenerative course	–	+++	++
Death	Variable	By 2 yr	2nd–4th decade
Ethnic predilection	Ashkenazi Jews	Panethnic	Swedish

Source: From Desnick,[1] p 445, with permission.

most patients in childhood or early adulthood. It is not unheard of, however, for the diagnosis to be made in an older adult who comes to medical attention for other reasons and is incidentally noted to have splenomegaly, anemia, or thrombocytopenia. On physical examination, these patients are often noted to have a yellow to yellow-brown pigmentation of the skin and pinguecula, a yellowish discoloration near the sclerocoroneal junction of the eye. Enlargement of the spleen, usually accompanied by an enlarged liver, is almost always present and is due to the accumulation of Gaucher's cells. Lymphadenopathy, however, is uncommon. Bleeding episodes, most frequently of the nose or gums, are often described; normocytic anemia is common. Neurologic manifestations are rarely seen. Bony changes, noted especially in the femur, occur in from 50 to 75 percent of patients[3,4] and are due to the accumulation of Gaucher's cells in the marrow cavity, which expands and thins the overlying bone. This gives rise to the so-called flask-shaped deformity of the distal femur often seen on roentgenogram. Bone pain is common.[5] Survival of these patients is variable, and many have normal lifespans.

Type II (Infantile, Acute, or Malignant Neuronopathic Gaucher's Disease)

This form of Gaucher's disease is not common and is seen in all ethnic groups, although uncommonly in Jews. Familial intermarriage is frequently found in the infant's family history. The onset of multiple neurologic signs including difficulty swallowing, opisthotonos (extreme arching of the spine), and other manifestations of brain stem involvement are noted early in infancy. Enlargement of the liver and spleen is also present. The infant has great difficulty in feeding and fails to grow. Usually death intervenes before the age of 2 years.

Type III (Juvenile or Subacute Neuronopathic Gaucher's Disease)

This type of Gaucher's disease is characterized by physical findings and survival ranging between those of types I and II. It has been noted especially in a group of 12 children from northern Sweden, the offspring of several related intermarriages.[2] These children have neurologic disease, with the onset between 6 months and 1 year of age. Their clinical course is more prolonged than in type II disease, with survival to late childhood or adolescence. The more severe the neurologic disease, the shorter the survival.

Laboratory Diagnosis

Peripheral blood, bone marrow, and spleen are the sites most frequently examined in patients with Gaucher's disease. The peripheral blood nearly always demonstrates a moderate normocytic anemia without active signs of replacement, such as polychromatophilic cells or nucleated red blood cells. There is pooling of blood in the enlarged spleen and some degree of ineffective erythropoiesis, with decreased incorporation of iron in erythroid precursors in the bone marrow. Leukocytes are commonly decreased in number. Platelets are also usually decreased in number as a result of splenic sequestration. These patients may have a bleeding tendency, with nosebleeds especially common. Gaucher's cells are noted only rarely in the peripheral blood.

Bone marrow aspirates are often the first tissue in which Gaucher's cells are detected; these cells are required for the diagnosis (**see Color Plate 240**). They are histiocytes, 20 to 80 μm in diameter, found in moderate numbers and as clumps of cells in the thickest areas of the smear. One or more round to oval nuclei are present in each cell. The cytoplasm is faintly blue with Wright's stain and has a "crumpled tissue paper" or finely folded appearance. Electron microscopy has demonstrated that this appearance is due to lamellar bodies stacked inside secondary phagolysosomes.[5] These cells stain positive with periodic acid–Schiff (PAS), acid phosphatase, Giemsa, iron, Sudan black B, and oil red O, all because of the accumulation of the unmetabolized glucocerebroside.

The spleen is variably enlarged, owing to the accumulation of masses of Gaucher's cells. This enlargement is commonly up to 10 times normal splenic weight and can cause considerable discomfort to the patient.

Other organs and systems commonly affected include the liver and, in type II, the nervous system, pituitary gland, kidneys, lung, and ovaries.[6] All contain massive deposits of Gaucher's cells.

The serum acid phosphatase is increased, but proper detection requires the use of the substrate phenyl phosphate.[2] The isozyme measurement of this enzyme has shown that the tartrate-resistant fraction is what is increased in patients with Gaucher's disease.

With the advance of molecular techniques in the diagnosis of disease, much has been learned regarding Gaucher's disease. A review of polymerase chain reaction (PCR) techniques is available elsewhere.[7,8] Recently it has been shown through the use of PCR that the severity of disease in type I Gaucher's disease could be predicted based on the type of genetic mutation within the glucocerebrosidase gene that was detected using this type of deoxyribonucleic acid (DNA) analysis.[9] In this study, the single amino acid substitution of adenine for guanine was the most common finding in patients with type I Gaucher's disease. These types of advances are rapidly expanding the ability to diagnose Gaucher's disease, predict its severity, and perhaps even aid in its treatment.

Although the Gaucher's cell is pathognomonic of the disease in the proper clinical setting, so-called pseudo-Gaucher's cells have also been described. They are seen in disease states with increased cellular turnover, especially chronic myelogenous leukemia, in which the phenomenon was first described. In theory, the increased cell turnover presents so much glycosyl ceramide to the reticuloendothelial system (RES) that its enzyme system is overwhelmed and cannot adequately metabolize all of the material. The excess is therefore stored in histiocytes, with their end morphologic expression identical to that of true Gaucher's cells. This phenomenon is also seen in a variety of other disorders, including acute myelocytic leukemia, chronic lymphocytic leukemia, plasma cell myeloma, aplastic anemia, idiopathic thrombocytopenic purpura (ITP), thalassemia major, and rheumatoid arthritis.[6] The presence of Gaucher–like cells in patients with these diseases has no known prognostic significance. It should be emphasized that in each of these diseases there is no deficiency of the β-glucocerebrosidase, as there is in Gaucher's disease, but rather an overtaxation of a normal system.

Prognosis

As previously stated, the length of survival in patients affected with Gaucher's disease is variable and depends on the type. The adult form has the longest survival, with patients surviving commonly into adulthood. Survival beyond 2 years of age in the infantile form is rare. As with its clinical features, the survival in the juvenile form is intermediate between those of the first two, and these individuals usually live into adolescence.

NIEMANN-PICK DISEASE

Niemann-Pick disease is caused by a deficiency of the enzyme sphingomyelinase with a secondary accumulation of the unmetabolized lipid sphingomyelin as well as cholesterol. Sphingomyelin is a common constituent of cell membranes as well as cellular organelles; thus, a deficiency of sphingomyelinase is most serious. There is an increased incidence of Niemann-Pick disease in Jews, especially in consanguinous populations. Because of the very different clinical manifestations the disease may take, it has been divided into five types, A through E. Only the first two types will be described, as they account for more than 85 percent of all cases.[10]

Clinical Features

Type A

This form is also known as infantile or classic Niemann-Pick disease. This is the most common form of Niemann-Pick disease, accounting for up to 85 percent of all cases.[3,10] The onset is in early infancy and is associated with failure to thrive, difficulty feeding, and retarded physical and mental development. The skin has a waxy consistency. There is often jaundice at birth and usually hepatosplenomegaly, with a distended abdomen. The lymph nodes are enlarged as well. A cherry-red spot in the macula of the eye is found in approximately one half of the affected infants.[10] The neurologic symptoms are more pronounced in this type of Niemann-Pick disease than in any of the others. Deterioration is relentless, and survival past the age of 1 or 2 years is rare.

Type B

Also called the chronic, or adult, form, this type of Niemann-Pick disease is seen much less frequently than type A, with only 13 reported cases in the literature.[2] Clinical onset consisting of hepatosplenomegaly is usually found in infancy, but the central nervous system is not involved. Individuals with this type of disease may live longer than those with type A, but they do not survive beyond childhood or early adolescence.

Laboratory Diagnosis

There is a distinct pattern to the histiocytes in Niemann-Pick disease. These cells are most commonly seen in bone marrow and spleen, although they accumulate throughout the body and in the nervous system in patients with type A. They are large cells, 20 to 90 μm in diameter, with an inconspicuous nucleus. The cytoplasm is filled with and distended by round, uniformly sized droplets of accumulated lipid, turning the cell a very pale or light blue when Wright-stained (see Color Plate 241). Stains producing a positive reaction with Niemann-Pick cells are the lipid stains oil red O, Sudan black, and luxol fast blue; and acid phosphatase and nonspecific esterase. The PAS staining is weak, and the myeloperoxidase is negative.

Some adult patients with certain varieties of Niemann-Pick disease contain, in the bone marrow, a mixture of Niemann-Pick cells and sea-blue histiocytes, which are histiocytes distended with blue-staining ceroid on Wright's stain. It is believed that the sphingomyelin is gradually metabolized to the ceroid, thus generating the sea-blue histiocytes.[6] A marrow specimen with these findings would then need to be distinguished from the entity of sea-blue histiocytosis (see farther on).

Other disorders that may cause Niemann-Pick–like cells to be contained in the bone marrow are GM_1 gangliosidosis, lactosyl ceramidosis, and Fabry's disease.[6]

The peripheral blood is most remarkable for the vacuoles that may be found in lymphocytes and monocytes of a routine peripheral blood smear. These vacuoles are round, and from 2 to 20 may be found within one cell.[3] Anemia and leukopenia may be present but do not usually pose any threat to the patient. Serum lipids are not usually increased.[3]

Prognosis

There may be a slightly longer survival in patients with the other types of Niemann-Pick disease, but those with type A have a very short life expectancy. Survival past the age of 2 years is uncommon. Type E, which is very rare, has been found only in adults and is characterized by a mild chronic course and a lack of neurologic manifestations.[2]

TAY-SACHS DISEASE

Also known as amaurotic infantile idiocy or GM_2 gangliosidosis, Tay-Sachs disease was first described in 1881 by the British ophthalmologist Warren Tay and in 1886 by the New York neurologist Bernard Sachs. Its incidence in the Ashkenazi Jewish population is 100 times greater than that in the non-Jewish population.[11] It is estimated that this high-risk group has a 1 in 30 carrier rate.[12] This autosomal recessive sphingolipidosis is due to a deficiency of the enzyme hexosaminidase A, with an increase of the other isoenzyme, hexosaminidase B. The unmetabolized GM_2 ganglioside accumulates in almost all tissues and has its most devastating effects within the central nervous system and eye.

Clinical Features

Although affected infants appear normal at birth, by 6 months of age both physical and mental deterioration are notable. They have an exaggerated physical response to noise (the startle reflex). In addition, a cherry-red spot in the macula of each eye is found. The infants eventually go blind. Along with the continual deterioration, there is enlargement of the head (macrocephaly), seizures, and paralysis. The neurons are greatly enlarged by accumulation of the unmetabolized ganglioside in vacuoles in the cytoplasm. In contrast to many other lipid storage diseases, the spleen, liver, and lymph nodes are not enlarged.[2] Feeding is poor, and death eventuates by 4 years of age.

Variant forms of GM_2 gangliosidoses are known.[13] Though less common than infantile Tay-Sachs, they still occur most frequently among Ashkenazi Jews. These forms are commonly referred to as juvenile and adult (chronic) onset. These patients have physical disabilities related to the cerebellum and neurons controlling motor functions; functions of intelligence vary, and may be less severely affected in the adult form. Survival is quite variable.

Laboratory Diagnosis

The major site of pathology is in the central nervous system, and examination of other tissues is less instructive. The peripheral blood contains vacuolated lymphocytes. The number and size of the vacuoles are related to the duration of the disease; it is postulated, but not definitely proven, that they contain the unmetabolized lipid (**see Color Plate 242**).[14] Vacuolated lymphocytes, however, are not pathognomonic for Tay-Sachs disease, as they are also seen in Niemann-Pick disease and in certain types of leukemias. Foam cells, or vacuolated histiocytes, are found in the bone marrow. Presence of these cells too is helpful but not diagnostic.

Because of the high frequency of disease in certain populations, prenatal detection has taken on greater importance. Culture of fetal fibroblasts from the amniotic fluid can be undertaken to detect hexosaminidase A levels in the fetus. Mass screening programs of adults at possible risk for transmitting the disease have been undertaken, with variable success.[11]

The ability to examine the messenger ribonucleic acid (mRNA) and DNA in patients with noninfantile forms of Tay-Sachs, using the molecular techniques of RNAase protection assays and PCR, has pinpointed the defect to an amino acid substitution in the α- subunit of the β-hexosaminidase.[13] These results will undoubtedly be incorporated into genetic counseling for families.

Prognosis

The infantile form of Tay-Sachs disease is uniformly fatal before age 4. Enzyme replacement is now being attempted, and the final results of the potential therapy are not yet known. Patients with the juvenile and adult forms of Tay-Sachs disease have longer survival than those with the infantile form, although it is quite variable.

MUCOPOLYSACCHARIDOSES

The original description of children affected with different forms of the mucopolysaccharidoses (MPSs) was published within a relatively short time span at the turn of the century. Dr. John Thompson first described three young brothers with the characteristics, now called Hurler's syndrome, in London in 1900; Gertrud Hurler elaborated on his description, describing two unrelated boys in Munich in 1919 with very similar characteristics. In 1917, Hunter described two brothers with a constellation of abnormalities now recognized as Hunter's syndrome.

Like the previously described disorders, the MPSs show accumulations of unmetabolized material within lysosomes (see Color Plate 243). However, it is mucopolysaccharides, not sphingolipids, that accumulate. The clinical severity of these disorders varies widely. Products are found in the reticuloendothelial system (spleen, bone marrow, liver), lymph nodes, blood vessels, brain, heart, connective tissue, and urine.

Categories

The mucopolysaccharidoses have been arranged into seven types (Table 24–2 gives an abbreviated classification scheme), but there are only four possible unmetabolized products: keratan sulfate, dermatan sulfate, heparan sulfate, or chondroitin sulfate. With the exception of Hunter's syndrome, which is X-linked recessive, these disorders have an autosomal recessive mode of inheritance. There does not appear to be a significant increase of affected individuals within any one ethnic group. The final classification of MPS is still somewhat unclear because of the interrelationships with cystic fibrosis and glycolipid storage diseases.[4]

Clinical Features

Many clinical abnormalities are found within each type of MPS, and there are seven types of MPS; therefore, a detailed description of each is not possible here. The findings in Hurler's syndrome will be given in the most detail, because it is considered the prototype of the mucopolysaccharidoses.

In patients with Hurler's syndrome (MPS I), there may be a short period of apparently normal development, but this is only temporary. These individuals are abnormally short and have coarse facial features, with a broad, flat nose, widely spaced eyes, and thickened tongue and lips. Some authors have described their appearance as similar to that of a gargoyle (the carved heads sometimes found on older European churches). The amount of body hair is increased, dark, and especially prominent on the forehead. The skin is thickened. Patients are mentally retarded. Clouding of the corneas of the eyes is present. These individuals may have hearing loss or be completely deaf. The heart is damaged, owing to the accumulation of mucopolysaccharide in the valves and blood vessels. There is a humpback and prominent abdomen, with enlarged liver and spleen. The arms and legs are abnormal, with contractures of many joints. In addition, the hands are very wide and the fingers shortened.

In Hunter's syndrome (MPS II), the changes are similar, although not as severe. Corneal clouding is much less common. Patients affected with Sanfilippo's syndrome (MPS III) have a more normal stat-

ure but unfortunately many more severe neurologic problems and decreased survival. Compared with Hurler's syndrome, patients with Scheie's syndrome (MPS I S) have more prominent corneal clouding but less abnormality in stature, facial appearance, and mental development. Patients with Maroteaux-Lamy syndrome (MPS VI) have growth and skeletal abnormalities but no mental retardation. In Morquio's syndrome (MPS IV) patients have numerous skeletal changes, giving a markedly abnormal physical appearance; there is no mental retardation, however.

Laboratory Diagnosis and Prognosis

In contrast to the other lysosomal storage diseases, nonmetabolized products may be detected in the urine of patients with MPS. Using the toluidine blue spot test or the turbidity test to detect acid mucopolysaccharides is the initial screening test. The spot test may be unreliable, however, with up to 32 percent false-negative test results in patients with Hurler's syndrome reported.[15] Also of note is that the urine of normal healthy newborn infants may give false-positive results, a phenomenon that disappears by 2 weeks of age.[15] Any positive screening test result should be confirmed by column chromatography.

An interesting but somewhat inconsistent finding in the MPS in the peripheral blood is the presence of large granules in leukocytes, especially lymphocytes. These are known as Alder-Reilly bodies (see Color Plate 133). In polymorphonuclear leukocytes, this needs to be distinguished from toxic granulation, but the large size of the granules in MPS usually leaves little doubt. A metachromatic stain, such as toluidine blue, will aid in confirmation. These granules are found with much greater regularity, however, in histiocytes and lymphocytes in the bone marrow.[3]

The prognosis of the MPS varies somewhat with the type. Patients with Hurler's syndrome may live into their teens, whereas those affected with Hunter's syndrome may live into their 20s. Individuals who have Sanfilippo's syndrome do not usually survive to their teens. The theoretical aid of enzyme replacement therapy has yet to be translated into practical results.

HISTIOCYTOSES
Sea-Blue Histiocyte Syndrome

Although initially described in isolated case reports of young adults with an enlarged spleen, the syndrome of the sea-blue histiocyte is a genetic disorder with a benign course. The striking blue color of the histiocytes after staining with Wright's or May-Grünwald-Giemsa stain gives the syndrome its name.

The mode of transmission has not been clearly established, but autosomal recessive inheritance, with a variable degree of expression, appears most

Table 24–2. **MUCOPOLYSACCHARIDOSES (MPS)**

Name	Genetics	Accumulated Product	Enzyme Deficiency	Life Expectancy	Intelligence	Clinical Features
MPS I H (Hurler's)	AR	Heparan sulfate Dermatan sulfate	α-L-iduronidase	6–10 yr	Retarded	1. Onset 6–8 mo 2. Dwarfism 3. Large, long head 4. Flat, broad nose with upturned nostrils 5. Corneal clouding 6. Hepatosplenomegaly 7. Valvular lesions 8. Coronary artery lesions 9. Skeletal deformities 10. Joint stiffness
MPS I S (Scheie's)	AR	Heparan sulfate Dermatan sulfate	α-L-iduronidase	Normal	Normal	1. Onset after 5 yr 2. Near normal height 3. Corneal clouding 4. Valvular lesion 5. Coronary artery lesions 6. Finger stiffness
MPS I H-S (Hurler-Scheie)	AR	Heparan sulfate Dermatan sulfate	α-L-iduronidase	3rd decade	Mild retardation (may be normal)	1. Onset infancy 2. Dwarfism 3. Facial and bony lesions of Hurler's syndrome 4. Cardiac lesions

MPS II (Hunter) (wide range of severity)	X–R	Heparan sulfate
		Dermatan sulfate
			L-iduronosulfate sulfatase	2nd decade to normal	Mild retardation to normal	1. Similar to Hurler's syndrome, *but*
						  a. No corneal clouding
						  b. Retinal degeneration
						  c. Deafness
						  d. Nodular skin infiltrates

MPS III (Sanfilippo's A) (Sanfilippo's B) (Sanfilippo's C) (range of severity)	AR	Heparan sulfate Heparan sulfate Heparan sulfate	Sulfaminidase α-N-acetylglu-cosaminidase α-Glucos-aminidase	2nd–3rd decade	Retarded	1. Onset after 3 yr 2. Normal growth 3. Hurler facies 4. No corneal clouding 5. No heart disease 6. No hepatosplenomegaly 7. Mild skeletal changes
MPS IV (Morquio's) (wide range of severity)	AR	Keratan sulfate Chondroitin sulfate	N-acetylhexos-aminidase Sulfatase	3rd–6th decade	Normal	1. Dwarfism 2. Thoracolumbar gibbus 3. Kyphoscoliosis 4. Facies similar to Hurler's syndrome 5. Corneal clouding 6. Valvular and coronary artery lesions 7. Joint hypermobility 8. Genu valgum

MPS VI (Maroteaux-Lamy)	AR	Dermatan sulfate	N-acetylhexos-aminidase
			4-SO₄ sulfatase
				2nd decade	Normal	1. Similar to Hurler's syndrome, *but*
						  a. Preservation of intelligence
						  b. Longer survival

MPS VII (Glucuronidase deficiency disease)	AR	Dermatan sulfate Heparan sulfate Chondroitin sulfate	β-Glucuronidase	(?) Some restriction	(?) Retarded	Variable

AR = Autosomal recessive; X–R = X-linked recessive.
Source: From Robbins and Cotran,[12] p 250, with permission.

likely. Most patients are diagnosed before they reach 40 years of age. The earlier in life the disease is found, the more severe it is likely to be. Major findings on physical examination are splenomegaly and usually hepatomegaly. Also described, but occurring less consistently, are abnormalities of the eye, skin, and nervous system. Involvement of the lung may be noted on roentgenographic examination. Involvement of the lymph nodes is not seen.

Significant laboratory findings are usually confined to the blood. In the peripheral blood, thrombocytopenia is found with great frequency. Consequently, clinical manifestations such as epistaxis, gastrointestinal tract bleeding, and purpura may be expected. However, there is no correlation of the degree of thrombocytopenia with the size of the spleen.[16] Blood lipid levels are normal. Abnormal liver function study results are only rarely seen.

The bone marrow aspirate is usually the site of diagnosis. Histiocytes of variable size (20 to 60 μm) are present in greatly increased numbers. They contain the blue- to green-staining granules that vary in size, shape, and ability to take up the stain (**see Color Plate 244**). Thus, not all cells will have the same staining intensity. It is not currently known why the granules stain blue with these stains. The cells will also react with the PAS, Sudan black B, and acid fast stains, but not with toluidine blue or iron stains.[16,17] Tissue sections stained with hematoxylin and eosin show some of the cells with pale-yellow pigmentation but without cytoplasmic staining. Both histochemical stains and tissue lipid analysis have shown the cells to contain largely glycolipid, phospholipid, and sphingolipid.

The great majority of patients with this syndrome do well and have normal lifespans. Splenectomy is not inevitable; many patients never require removal of the spleen. As previously mentioned, manifestations of the disease at an early age may imply more severe symptomatology.

Acquired, or secondary, sea-blue histiocyte syndrome is briefly mentioned here. Cells identical in appearance to those in the primary disorder are found but in lesser numbers than in the primary syndrome. They are present in both the spleen and the bone marrow of patients with other, unrelated disorders. These disorders include ITP, chronic myelogenous leukemia (CML), sickle-cell anemia, thalassemia, polycythemia vera, sarcoidosis, and many other diseases.[3,17] The finding of these cells has led to the consideration that they may occur in individuals with a partial enzyme deficiency who are under stress from another disease.[16]

Other Histiocytic Disorders (Eosinophilic Granuloma, Hand-Schüller-Christian Disease, Letterer-Siwe Disease)

The group of "histiocytic" disorders described here may be thought of as an abnormal proliferation and accumulation of mature histiocytes, or Langerhans' cells. Langerhans' cells are large but inconspicuous cells in the skin, whose function is to process and present antigen to other cells in the area, including lymphocytes. These cells, as well as histiocytes, are normally found in small numbers in the skin and RES. Most patients are either children or young adults. A favorable outcome may be expected in most cases, with the exception of Letterer-Siwe disease, which may be fatal. These disorders may actually represent a continuum, from the unifocal and benign eosinophilic granuloma to the generalized and sometimes fatal Letterer-Siwe disease.[12] The term histiocytosis X is used generally to describe these disorders. Table 24–3 summarizes their major findings. The malignant histiocytic disorders are discussed elsewhere in this book.

The clinical presentation of these disorders may consist of a myriad of findings, a solitary lesion, or

Table 24–3. **MAJOR FINDINGS IN HISTIOCYTIC DISORDERS**

Disease	Age at Onset	Main Site(s) of Involvement	Course and Prognosis
Eosinophilic granuloma	Especially in males Children and young adults Often no symptoms until bone fracture	Unifocal — skull, rib, femur most common	Rare spontaneous healing; most require surgical removal; occasional patients develop recurrence later
Hand-Schüller-Christian disease	Usually <5 yr old	Multifocal — bones, skin, lymphoid tissue; triad of pituitary, eye, and skull involvement is characteristic but uncommon	50%: spontaneous recovery 50%: recovery with chemotherapy
Letterer-Siwe disease	Usually <3 yr old	Generalized — skin, lymphoid tissue, bones, +/− bone marrow; more severe and extensive than Hand-Schüller-Christian disease	Chemotherapy has improved prognosis, which was previously considered poor

anything between these two extremes. Removal of tissue for pathologic examination is necessary for the diagnosis. Microscopically, the different entities all have in common an accumulation of histiocytes with a distinctive appearance and a variable admixture of eosinophils, neutrophils, lymphocytes, plasma cells, giant cells, and foam cells in a fibrotic background. These cells also have characteristic organelles termed Birbeck or Langerhans' granules. Their shape has been likened to that of a tennis racket, and represents the internalized membrane of this antigen-presenting cell. They are visible only with the aid of the electron microscope.

There are no diagnostic findings on examination of the peripheral blood. In Letterer-Siwe disease, however, the coexistence of anemia or thrombocytopenia has been associated with a poor prognosis. This usually reflects involvement of the bone marrow by the disease.

REFERENCES

1. Desnick, RJ: Gaucher disease (1882–1982): Centennial perspectives on the most prevalent Jewish genetic disease. Mt Sinai J Med 49:443, 1982.
2. Kolodny, EH: Clinical and biochemical genetics of the lipidoses. Semin Hematol 9:251, 1972.
3. Wintrobe, MM: Clinical Hematology. Lea & Febiger, Philadelphia, 1981.
4. Stanbury, JB, Wyngaarden, JB, and Frederickson, DS: The Metabolic Basis of Inherited Disease. McGraw-Hill, New York, 1972.
5. Lee, RE: The pathology of Gaucher disease. In Desnick, RJ, Gatt, S, and Grabowski, GA (eds): Gaucher Disease: A Century of Delineation and Research. Progress in Clinical and Biological Research. Vol 95. Alan R Liss, New York, 1982, p 193.
6. Savage, RA: Specific and not-so-specific histiocytes in bone marrow. Lab Med 15:467, 1984.
7. Bell, J: The polymerase chain reaction. Immunol Today 10:351, 1989.
8. Erlich, HA (ed): PCR Technology. Principles and Applications for DNA Amplification. Stockton Press, New York, 1989.
9. Zimran, A, et al: Prediction of severity of Gaucher's disease by identification of mutations at DNA level. Lancet 2:349, 1989.
10. Volk, BW, Adachi, M, and Schneck, L: The pathology of sphingolipidoses. Semin Hematol 9:317, 1972.
11. Goodman, MJ and Goodman, LE: The overselling of genetic anxiety. Hastings Cent Rep 12:20, 1982.
12. Robbins, SL and Cotran, RS: Pathologic Basis of Disease. WB Saunders, Philadelphia, 1979.
13. Paw, BH, Kaback, MM, and Neufeld, EF: Molecular basis of adult-onset and chronic G_{M2} gangliosidoses in patients of Ashkenazi Jewish origin: Substitution of serine for glycine at position 269 of the α-subunit of β-hexosaminidase. Proc Natl Acad Sci USA 86:2413, 1989.
14. Brunning, RD: Morphologic alterations in nucleated blood and marrow cells in genetic disorders. Hum Pathol 1:99, 1970.
15. Henry, JB: Clinical Diagnosis and Management by Laboratory Methods. WB Saunders, Philadelphia, 1984, p 454.
16. Sawitsky, A, Rosner, F, and Chodsky, S: The sea-blue histiocyte syndrome, a review: Genetic and biochemical studies. Semin Hematol 9:285, 1972.
17. Silverstein, MN and Ellefson, RD: The syndrome of the sea-blue histiocyte. Semin Hematol 9:299, 1972.

QUESTIONS

1. *What defect is found in lipid storage diseases?*
   a. Subcellular accumulation of unmetabolized material in lysosomes
   b. Cellular accumulation of metabolites in cytoplasm
   c. Protein accumulation in cellular mitochondria
   d. Abnormal sequestration of minerals and trace elements in cellular nuclear organelles

2. *What is the enzyme deficiency of Gaucher's disease?*
   a. Sphingomyelinase
   b. Hexosaminidase A
   c. β-glucocerebrosidase
   d. α-galactosidase

3. *Which description best characterizes type I Gaucher's disease?*
   a. Found in any ethnic group; multiple neurologic signs including difficulty in swallowing and manifestations involving brain stem; enlargement of liver and spleen
   b. Found primarily in Ashkenazi Jews; yellow pigmentation of skin and eyes; bleeding episodes; bone changes; enlargement of liver and spleen
   c. Found in northern Sweden; neurologic disorders; bone disorders; skin pigment changes
   d. Found in Mediterranean; hypermetabolic manifestations; fever, lethargy, poor musculature, bone deformities

4. *What are the characteristics of Gaucher's cells?*
   a. Atypical lymphocytes with foamy cytoplasm
   b. Hypersegmented neutrophils with Auer's rods
   c. Large, multilobed monocytes with prominent red granules
   d. Histiocytes with blue, folded cytoplasm

5. *What is the enzyme deficiency of Niemann-Pick disease?*
   a. Sphingomyelinase
   b. Hexosaminidase A
   c. β-glucocerebrosidase
   d. α-galactosidase

6. *What are the clinical features of Niemann-Pick disease?*
   a. Waxy, jaundiced skin; retarded physical and mental development; cherry-red spot in macula of eye
   b. Startle reflex; blindness; macrocephaly; no enlargement of liver, spleen, or lymph nodes
   c. Abnormal facial features; deafness; increased body hair; mental retardation; heart damage; structural deformities
   d. Splenomegaly; hepatomegaly; eye, skin, nervous system, and lung abnormalities

7. *What are the characteristics of Niemann-Pick cells?*
   a. Atypical lymphocytes with large vacuoles

b. Cytoplasm filled with lipid droplets; inconspicuous nucleus
c. Vacuolated histiocytes or foam cells
d. Lymphocytes with Alder-Reilly bodies

8. *What is the enzyme deficiency of Tay-Sachs disease?*
a. Sphingomyelinase
b. Hexosaminidase A
c. β-glucocerebrosidase
d. α-galactosidase

9. *What are the clinical features of Tay-Sachs disease?*
a. Waxy, jaundiced skin; retarded physical and mental development; cherry-red spot in macula of eye
b. Startle reflex; blindness; macrocephaly; no enlargement of liver, spleen, or lymph nodes
c. Abnormal facial features; deafness; increased body hair; mental retardation; heart damage; structural deformities
d. Splenomegaly; hepatomegaly; eye, skin, nervous system, and lung abnormalities

10. *Which cell is found in Tay-Sachs disease, but is not considered diagnostic?*
a. Atypical lymphocytes with large vacuoles
b. Cytoplasm filled with lipid droplets; inconspicuous nucleus
c. Vacuolated histiocytes or foam cells
d. Lymphocytes with Alder-Reilly bodies

11. *What are clinical features of Hunter's and Hurler's syndromes?*
a. Waxy, jaundiced skin; retarded physical and mental development; cherry-red spot in macula of eye
b. Startle reflex; blindness; macrocephaly; no enlargement of liver, spleen, or lymph nodes
c. Abnormal facial features; deafness; increased body hair; mental retardation; heart damage; structural deformities
d. Splenomegaly; hepatomegaly; eye, skin, nervous system, and lung abnormalities

12. *Which cell may be found in MPS disorders?*
a. Large, foamy histiocytes with blue or green granules
b. Neutrophils with toxic granulation
c. Neutrophils with Döhle bodies
d. Lymphocytes with Alder-Reilly bodies

13. *What is the characteristic cell of sea-blue histiocyte syndrome? (Use answer choices for question 12.)*

14. *How are eosinophilic granuloma, Hand-Schüller-Christian disease, and Letterer-Siwe disease classified?*
a. Malignant lymphoproliferative disorders
b. Histiocytic disorders
c. Myeloproliferative disorders
d. Nonmalignant leukocyte disorders

ANSWERS

1. a (p. 403)
2. c (p. 404)
3. b (p. 404–405)
4. d (p. 405)
5. a (p. 406)
6. a (p. 406)
7. b (p. 406)
8. b (p. 407)
9. b (p. 407)
10. c (p. 407)
11. c (p. 408)
12. d (p. 408)
13. a (p. 408)
14. b (p. 410)

PART **FOUR**

HEMOSTASIS AND INTRODUCTION TO THROMBOSIS

CHAPTER 25

DENISE M. HARMENING, Ph.D., M.T.(ASCP), C.L.S.(NCA)

Introduction to Hemostasis: An Overview of Hemostatic Mechanism, Platelet Structure and Function, and Extrinsic and Intrinsic Systems

OBJECTIVES

At the end of this chapter, the learner should be able to:
1. List the functions of the vascular system.
2. Describe the major functions of the endothelium.
3. Name the three structural zones of platelets.
4. Describe the composition and functions of the peripheral zone.
5. Describe the composition and functions of the sol-gel zone.
6. Describe the composition and functions of the organelle zone.
7. Explain the role of platelets in the hemostatic process.
8. List steps in platelet plug formation.
9. Name essential elements for the process of platelet adhesion.
10. Describe the process of platelet aggregation.
11. Name the product responsible for stabilization of the hemostatic plug.
12. List characteristics for the contact coagulation proteins.
13. List characteristics for the prothrombin proteins.
14. List characteristics for the fibrinogen group.
15. Name factors unique to the extrinsic system.
16. Summarize the activity of the extrinsic system.
17. Name factors unique to the intrinsic system.
18. List the correct sequence of events in the intrinsic pathway that lead to the common pathway.
19. Name factors found in the common pathway.
20. List functions of thrombin.
21. Name substances that activate plasminogen to plasmin.
22. List functions of plasmin.
23. Explain the role of the kinin system in coagulation.
24. Name protease inhibitors.
25. List functions for C3a, C3b, C5a, and C1 inhibitor.
26. Describe the use of the prothrombin time test in monitoring hemostasis.
27. Describe the use of the activated partial thromboplastin time test in monitoring hemostasis.

PLATELETS AND HEMOSTATIC MECHANISMS

Hemostasis is the process by which the body spontaneously stops bleeding and maintains blood in the fluid state within the vascular compartment. Four major systems are involved in maintaining hemostasis:

1. Vascular system
2. Platelets
3. Fibrin-forming (coagulation) system
4. Fibrin-lysing (fibrinolytic) system

Three additional minor systems are also related to hemostasis:

1. Kinin system
2. Serine protease inhibitors
3. Complement system

The hemostatic mechanisms are designed rapidly to repair any vascular breaks and maintain blood flow within the vessels. However, there are potential risks associated with this rapid localized hemostasis: imbalance in one direction leads to excessive bleeding and in the other to thrombosis. There are also limits to the degree of vascular injury that may be controlled, as the process of hemostasis involves consumption of platelets and coagulation factors. The relative importance of the hemostatic mechanisms varies with vessel size. For example, breaks in capillaries seal directly and immediately with little dependence on hemostasis. However, arterioles and venules, once ruptured, become quickly occluded with a mass of fused platelets. Hemostasis in veins depends on vascular contraction as well as on perivascular and intravascular activation of hemostatic factors, as these vessles rupture easily with increased hydrostatic pressure due to trauma. Arterial hemorrhage is the most severe test of hemostasis, even though arteries are the most resistant of all vessels to bleeding because of their thick muscular walls. The process of vasoconstriction is crucial to successful thrombus formation in arteries. Generally, the larger the area of bleeding the larger the vessel involved.

Bleeding from arterioles and venules results in pinpoint petechial hemorrhages. Hemorrhaging from veins results in large, ill-defined, soft tissue bleeding termed ecchymoses. Bleeding from arteries manifests in rapidly expanding "blowout" hemorrhage. Each major and minor hemostatic system will be considered separately and then interrelated into the entire sequence of events in the maintenance of hemostasis.

Vascular System

The vascular system acts to prevent bleeding by (1) contraction of vessels (vasoconstriction) and reflex stimulation of adjacent vessels, (2) diversion of blood flow around damaged vasculature, (3) initiation of contact-activation of platelets with subsequent aggregation, and (4) contact-activation of the coagulation system (both extrinsic and intrinsic) leading to fibrin formation. Vascular integrity, which is influenced by vitamin C intake, is important in maintaining the fluidity of the blood. The blood vessel with its smooth and continuous endothelial lining and fibrous coat is designed to facilitate blood flow as well as participate in the process of hemostasis. The endothelial surface of the blood vessel is usually inert to coagulation factors and platelets. It is termed a nonwettable surface in that the physical and chemical characteristics of the endothelium allow a minimum of interaction between blood and the endothelial surface. However, when the endothelial lining is disrupted, underlying collagen and basement membrane are exposed, activating platelets and the plasma coagulation factors. This break in endothelium leads to platelet adhesion and thrombus formation, because the endothelial cells contain adenosine diphosphate (ADP), which is important in inducing aggregation of platelets. In addition, released tissue thromboplastin initiates fibrin formation through the extrinsic pathway of the coagulation system. The vascular response involved in the hemostatic mechanism usually lasts less than 1 minute.

Metabolic Functions of the Endothelium

One of the most important functions of the endothelial surface is its multiple antithrombotic properties. Glycocalyx, a mucopolysaccharide, coats the luminal surface of the endothelium and possesses the ability to stimulate weakly the physiologic anticoagulant antithrombin III (AT-III) through one of its constituents known as heparan sulfate. In addition, the vascular endothelial membrane also contains thrombin receptor sites, termed thrombomodulin, that neutralize the active enzyme thrombin, which is necessary in producing a fibrin clot with the coagulation cascade (see section on fibrin-forming system). This thrombomodulin-thrombin complex activates another important plasma protein called protein C, which is a potent and specific anticoagulant as well as an effective fibrinolytic agent important in maintaining the endothelium in a nonthrombogenic state (see section on protease inhibitors).

Other nonthrombogenic properties of the vascular endothelium include the enzyme ADPase, which degrades ADP, and synthesis of prostacyclin (PGI_2), which functions as a potent vasodilator and inhibitor of the platelet response. The endothelium is also rich in an activator of fibrinolysis called tissue plasminogen activator (TPA). With an appropriate stimulus, this substance is released and activates the plasma protein plasminogen to the enzyme plasmin, which ensures rapid lysis of the forming fibrin clot.

The endothelium plays a major role in the delicate balance between halting the bleeding (procoagulant activity, formation of a clot) and prevention of excessive pathologic thrombus formation by initiation of fibrinolysis and release of anticoagulant factors. The endothelium is also intimately involved in the metabolism and clearance of several small molecules such as angiotensin, serotonin, and bradykinin. These substances affect the regulation of blood pressure, the egress of fluid across the endothelium, and inflammation.

The vascular endothelial cells also synthesize a number of substances such as type IV collagen and fibronectin (a noncollagen glycoprotein) that are important for normal hemostasis and vascular integrity. Von Willebrand's factor, a part of the plasma factor VIII molecule, is also produced by the vascular endothelial cells as well as by megakaryocytes. A glycoprotein receptor for this factor is present on the surface of activated platelets and mediates platelet adhesion to a foreign surface such as collagen (see next section).

PLATELET STRUCTURE AND FUNCTION

Platelets are intimately involved in primary hemostasis, which is the interaction of platelets and the vascular endothelium in halting bleeding following vascular injury. As discussed in Chapter 1, platelets are cellular fragments derived from the cytoplasm of megakaryocytes present in the bone marrow. Platelets are released and circulate approximately 9 to 12 days as small, disc-shaped cells with an average diameter of 2 to 4 μm. On a Wright-stained peripheral blood smear, platelets appear as round or oval granular purple dots. The platelet's typical stained morphology consists of a clear zone of cytoplasm, termed hyalomere, which surrounds

a highly stained granulomere (Fig. 25–1). The normal platelet count ranges from 150,000 to 350,000, depending on the methodology employed. In the peripheral blood, approximately 30 percent of the platelets are sequestered in the microvasculature or spleen as functional reserves after their release from the bone marrow. Aged or nonviable platelets are removed by both spleen and liver. These anuclear cytoplasmic fragments (platelets) contain a number of interesting organelles, which are listed in Figure 25–2.

Structure

The platelet structure is quite distinct, leading to the subdivision into three defined zones that possess unique functional capabilities. These include (1) the peripheral zone (the stimulus receptor/transmitter region), (2) the sol-gel zone (the cytoskeletal/contractile region), and (3) the organelle zone (the metabolic/organella region). Table 25–1 summarizes the three described zones and their contents. These zones are prominently delineated by the circumferential band of microtubules found in the platelet (Fig. 25–3).

Peripheral Zone

The peripheral zone is a complex region of the platelet consisting of the glycocalyx (an amorphous exterior coat), plasma membrane, numerous deeply

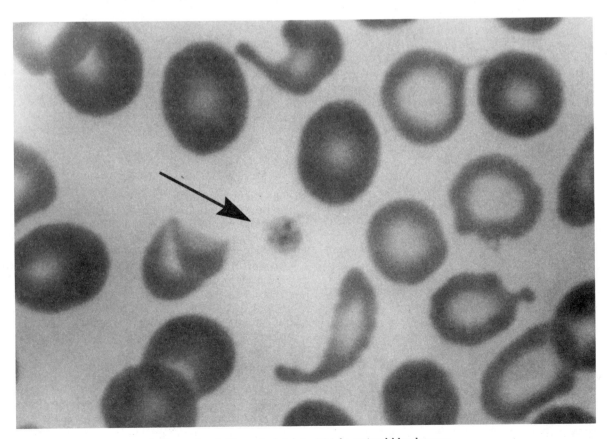

Figure 25–1. Normal platelets; Wright-stained blood smear.

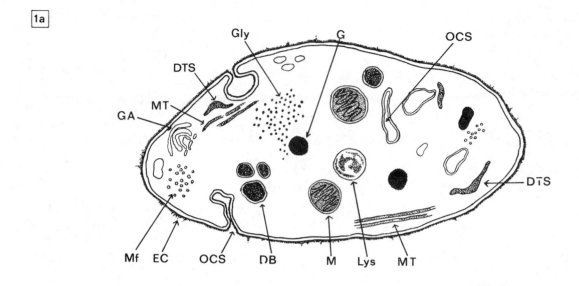

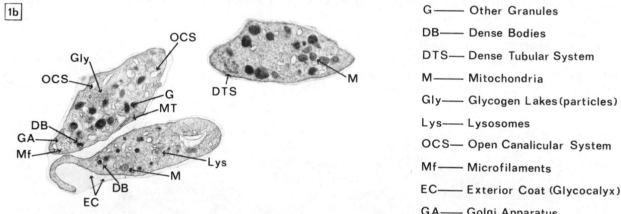

MT —— Microtubules

G —— Other Granules

DB —— Dense Bodies

DTS —— Dense Tubular System

M —— Mitochondria

Gly —— Glycogen Lakes (particles)

Lys —— Lysosomes

OCS —— Open Canalicular System

Mf —— Microfilaments

EC —— Exterior Coat (Glycocalyx)

GA —— Golgi Apparatus

Figure 25–2. Discoid platelets; (1a) summary diagram of the platelet organelles, (1b) transmission electron micrograph (TEM) of cross-sectioned platelets illustrating basic ultrastructure.

Table 25–1. **PLATELET ULTRASTRUCTURAL ZONES**

I. Peripheral Zone (Stimulus Receptor/Transmitter Region)
  A. Glycocalyx
  B. Plasma membrane
  C. Open canalicular system
  D. Submembranous region
II. Sol-Gel Zone (Cytoskeletal/Contractile Region)
  A. Circumferential microtubules
  B. Microfilaments
III. Organelle Zone (Metabolic/Organellar Region)
  A. Granules
    1. Alpha granules
    2. Dense granules
    3. Lysosomes
    4. Glycogen granules
  B. Mitochondria
  C. Dense tubular system
  D. Peroxisomes

penetrating surface-connecting channels known as the open canalicular system (OCS), and a submembranous area of specialized microfilaments.

The glycocalyx intimately surrounds the platelet and is considered an important component of the platelet membrane. A number of glycoproteins present in this area are responsible for blood group specificity (ABO), tissue compatibility (human leukocyte antigen [HLA]), and platelet antigenicity. Platelet membrane glycoproteins serve as receptors and facilitate transmission of stimuli across the platelet membrane. Platelet membrane glycoprotein Ib appears to be the receptor for plasma von Willebrand factor, which serves to mediate the adhesion of platelets to subendothelium. Glycoproteins IIb and IIIa function as receptors for fibrinogen, fibronectin and von Willebrand factor, thereby mediating platelet aggregation. In addition to these, the platelet membrane includes receptors for ADP, thrombin, epinephrine, and serotonin. Various en-

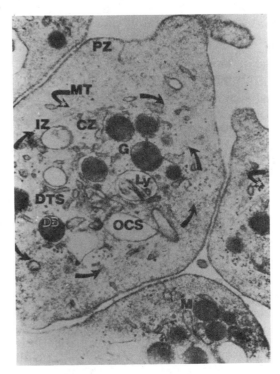

Figure 25 – 3. Internal anatomy of a stimulated platelet. Circumferential band of microtubules (MT) leads to reorganization of the internal structure of the platelet into three zones. The peripheral zone (PZ) is the region external to a circumferential band of microtubules (MT with * on *curved arrows*). The intermediate zone (IZ) (*encircling arrows*) includes the microtubules and the closely adjacent cytoplasmic material. The central zone (CZ) is internal to the microtubule band and contains many organelles such as granules (G), dense bodies (DB), dense tubular system (DTS), lysosomes (Ly), mitochondria (M), and many profiles of the open canalicular system (OCS). Magnification ×49,700. (From Barnhart, MI: Platelet responses in health and disease. Mol Cell Biochem 22:115, 1978, with permission.)

zymes have also been isolated in the plasma membrane of platelets.

The platelet membrane, similar to other plasma membranes, represents a fluid lipid bilayer composed of glycoproteins, glycolipids, and lipoproteins. The membrane phospholipid portion of the activated platelet serves as a surface for the interaction of the plasma proteins involved in blood coagulation, which assemble in complexes on the platelet's surface. Coagulation factors V and VIII also are present on the surface of the platelet membrane, as are various platelet factors (PFs) that participate in the formation of fibrin (that is, PF 3, PF 4). In addition to containing receptors for various stimuli, the peripheral zone of the platelet also contains the mechanism for the development of stickiness, which is essential for the adhesion and aggregation.

The membranous surface-connecting system referred to as the OCS consists of tubular invaginations of the plasma membrane that articulate throughout the platelet even though it is part of the peripheral zone. Platelet-stored products are released to the exterior through the OCS. The OCS

also facilitates collection of plasma procoagulants that aid in fibrin formation by providing increased surface absorptive area.

Sol-Gel Zone

The term cytoskeleton is often used to describe this zone. Within the matrix of the platelet are found microtubules, microfilaments, and submembranous filaments. Submembranous filaments are found within the peripheral zone and have been previously discussed. Microtubules and microfilaments are found within the sol-gel zone. The most numerous of the three fibers is the circumferential band of microtubules.

In the stimulated platelet (Fig. 25 – 3) contraction of the circumferential band of microtubules appears to be responsible for the centripetal movement and reorganization of organelles, which facilitates the secretory process. Microtubules appear to monitor the internal contraction of platelets, preventing secretion in response to only minimal stimulation, thereby regulating the degree of platelet response.

Microfilaments are interwoven throughout the cytoplasm of the platelet and are composed of actin and myosin-like contractile proteins. Actin is the major contractile protein in the platelet cytosol accounting for 20 to 30 percent of the total platelet protein, whereas myosin composes 2 to 5 percent of the total platelet protein (a sizable percentage for a nonmuscle cell). Microfilaments can convert from an unorganized gelatinous state to organized parallel filaments capable of contraction within seconds as the platelet's shape changes.

Organelle Zone

The organelle region is responsible for the metabolic activities of the platelet. Generally, the most numerous organelles are the platelet granules, which are heterogeneous in size, electron density, and chemical contents. Platelets contain three morphologically distinct types of storage granules: dense granules, alpha granules, and lysosomes containing acid hydrolases. Earlier studies reported the alpha granules as containing acid hydrolases. The alpha granules are more numerous (20 to 200 per platelet) and contain several different proteins, summarized in Table 25 – 2. The physiologic role of these proteins present in the alpha granules of platelets has not been clearly defined; however, it is

Table 25 – 2. **PROTEINS PRESENT IN PLATELET'S ALPHA GRANULES**

Platelet-Specific Proteins	Plasma Proteins
1. PF 4	1. Fibrinogen
2. β-thromboglobulin (β-TG)	2. vWF
3. Platelet-derived growth factor	3. V
4. Thrombospondin (TSP)	4. Albumin
5. Chemotactic factor	5. Fibronectin
6. Permeability factor	
7. Bactericidal factor	

Table 25-3. **CONTENTS OF PLATELET DENSE BODY GRANULES**

ADP	ATP
Calcium	Serotonin
Catecholamines (epinephrine, norepinephrine)	Pyrophosphate
	Magnesium

known that PF 4 neutralizes the anticoagulant heparin.

Dense bodies are fewer in number (2 to 10 per platelet) and represent densely opaque granules in transmission electron microscope (TEM) preparations. Table 25-3 lists the contents of the dense body granules in the platelet. The intragranular concentration of ADP and adenosine triphosphate (ATP) found in the dense bodies of the platelets is called the storage pool of adenine nucleotides. This contrasts with the metabolic pool of ATP and ADP that is found in the platelet cytoplasm. Physiologically, ADP is the most important substance secreted by the dense granules.

Acid hydrolases are enzymes active at a low pH and are contained within vesicles known as lysosomes. These lysosomes function to digest materials brought into the cell by endocytosis.

Many of the substances found in the storage granules of platelets are also substances normally found in plasma. Platelet agonists such as collagen, thrombin, and the cationophore A-23187 induce secretion from all three storage granules. Thromboxane A_2 (TXA$_2$), ADP, and epinephrine induce both dense and alpha granule secretion. Acid hydrolase secretion, in which the substances within the lysosomes are not completely secreted, differs from dense or alpha granule secretion in which virtually the entire granule content is secreted. The secretory processes depend on cellular ATP availability and are associated with increases in cytoplasmic Ca^{2+} levels.

The contents of both the alpha granules and dense bodies are released during the process called the release reaction, which is energy dependent. As a result of ADP released from dense bodies during the release reaction, additional platelets are drawn to the site of the vascular injury resulting in the formation of platelet aggregates. Both acquired and hereditary disorders have been described, resulting in decreased storage pool adenine nucleotides. Acquired abnormalities of platelet alpha or dense granules have been reported in patients who have undergone coronary bypass surgery. Patients with antibodies to platelets that induce platelet release in conditions of compensated autoimmune thrombocytopenia represent one type of acquired storage pool disease. Congenital abnormalities of alpha granules have also been reported, such as the gray platelet syndrome (see Chapter 26). These patients usually experience a mild clinical bleeding. A group of rare heterogeneous hereditary storage pool disorders also exists that includes Chédiak-Higashi syndrome, Hermansky-Pudlak syndrome, and Wiskott-Aldrich syndrome (see Chapter 26 for more details on these disorders). Other granules that can be found in the platelet as well as in other cells include lysosomes, peroxisomes, and glycogen granules.

The dense tubular system (DTS) is another important structure present in the cytoplasm of the organelle zone of platelets. This complex of dense tubules is analogous to the sarcotubules in skeletal muscle. It is derived from the smooth endoplasmic reticulum (ER) of immature megakaryocytes. The DTS is the site of prostaglandin synthesis and sequestration of calcium. It is primarily the release of calcium from the DTS that triggers platelet contraction and subsequent internal activation of platelets. It is also postulated that the DTS is involved in limited protein synthesis and serves as a reservoir for microtubular elements as well as submembranous and other microfilaments. Platelet activation is an energy-dependent process that relies on the metabolic function of mitochondria. Approximately 10 to 60 mitochondria per platelet are present that require glycogen as their source of energy for metabolism. It is estimated in the resting platelet that ATP (energy) production is generated by 50 percent glycolysis and 50 percent oxidative Krebs cycle. In the activated state, 50 percent of the ATP production in platelets occurs through the glycolytic pathway.

Function

Platelets have specific roles in the hemostatic process that are critically dependent on an adequate number of circulating platelets as well as on normal platelet function. The function of platelets in hemostasis include (1) maintenance of vascular integrity, (2) initial arrest of bleeding by platelet plug formation, and (3) stabilization of the hemostatic plug by contributing to the process of fibrin formation.

Numerous stimuli can trigger a platelet response termed activation, which may be transient, reversible, or irreversible. Activation refers to several separate responses of platelet function that include stickiness, adhesion, shape change, aggregation, and secretion release. Platelets respond in a graded fashion depending on the strength and duration of the stimuli, as well as the physiologic or pathologic state of the platelet.

Before proceeding, the reader should review the structure of the platelet, in order to visualize and understand subsequent events that occur in the platelet at the ultrastructural level during hemostasis (see Fig. 25-2).

Maintenance of Vascular Integrity

Platelets are involved in the nurturing of endothelial cells lining the vascular system. When a platelet adheres to the endothelial cell, the amount of cytoplasm between platelet and cell is reduced, and the platelet may eventually become incorporated into the endothelial cell. This process has an effect of nurturing or feeding the tissue cells by releasing endothelial growth factor. Through the

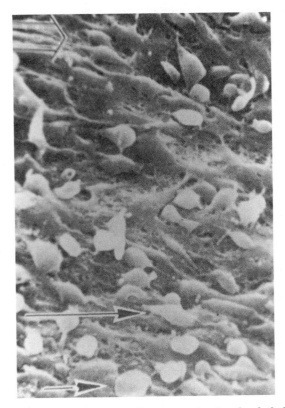

Figure 25-4. SEM of platelet adherence at the site of endothelial loss. *Short arrow* points to a discoid intact platelet with a single pseudopod, *long arrow* points to an elongated adherent platelet *double arrow* marks densely adherent platelets appearing as elongated humps fused to the subendothelial layer. (From Cotran, E: Robbins Pathologic Basis of Disease, ed 1, WB Saunders, Philadelphia, 1979, p 120, with permission.)

release of this mitogen (platelet-derived growth factor), vascular healing is also promoted by stimulating endothelial cell migration and medial smooth muscle cell migration in the vessel wall. Figure 25-4 shows a scanning electron micrograph (SEM) demonstrating platelet adherence at the site of endothelial loss compared with the normal smooth contour of the endothelial cell. In the absence of platelets, a large number of red cells migrate through the vessel wall, enter the lymphatic drainage, and appear as petechiae or purpura in the skin or mucous membranes. The process of maintenance of normal vascular integrity, involving nourishment of the endothelium by the platelet, or actual incorporation of platelets into the vessel wall, utilizes less than 10 percent of the platelets in the circulation but is nevertheless an important function.

Platelet Plug Formation

Various steps or processes are involved in the initial formation of a platelet plug: platelet adhesion, platelet aggregation, and platelet release reaction.

Adhesion. Exposure to subendothelial connective tissue, such as collagen fibers, initiates platelet adhesion. Adhesion is a reversible process whereby platelets stick to foreign surfaces. This process of

platelet adhesion involves the interaction of platelet surface glycoproteins with the connective tissue elements of the subendothelium.

Adhesion of platelets to subendothelial fibers is dependent on a plasma protein called von Willebrand factor (vWF), denoting that this factor is a component of the factor VIII complex (see section on coagulation system). Evidence indicates that vWF is synthesized by endothelial cells and megakaryocytes (precursors of platelets). Absorption of vWF occurs both on exposed subendothelial fibers and on the surface of circulating platelets as it attaches to the appropriate membrane surface glycoprotein Ib. In certain hereditary disorders, no platelet adhesion occurs and abnormal bleeding results because of the absence either of this plasma factor (von Willebrand's disease) or of the appropriate platelet membrane glycoprotein Ib (Bernard-Soulier syndrome). Platelets thus adhere to the area of injury at the endothelial lining or to each other when injured, acting to arrest the initial episode of bleeding. In Figure 25-5, a TEM demonstrates platelet adherence to subendothelial connective tissue at the focus of endothelial loss. A decrease in platelet number, therefore, leads to failure to block the site of injury, resulting in increased bleeding. Other platelets may adhere to the original contact platelets (adhering to the site of injury), producing the phenomenon of aggregation and resulting in thrombus formation in order to stop bleeding. It is interesting to note that platelet adhesion consumes little energy as measured by ATP use.

Aggregation. During platelet aggregation, the injured platelet changes shape from discoid to spherical with pseudopod formation (Fig. 25-6). Initial aggregation of platelets is caused by ADP, which is released from adherent platelets or endothelial

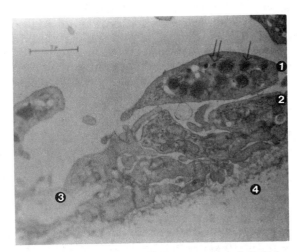

Figure 25-5. TEM of platelet adherence to subendothelial connective tissue at the focus of endothelial loss. (1) Intact platelet with pseudopod (*thin arrow* indicates alpha granule; *thick arrow* indicates dense body), (2) partially degranulated platelet, (3) degranulated platelet "ghost," (4) internal elastic lamina. (From Cotran, E: Robbins Pathologic Basis of Disease, ed 1. WB Saunders, Philadelphia, 1979, p 116, with permission.)

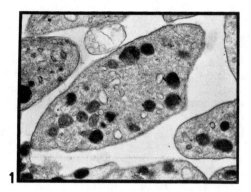

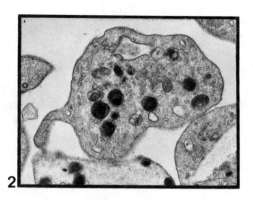

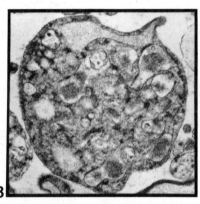

Figure 25–6. TEM showing disk-to-sphere transformation of an activated platelet. Note progression from (1) disk shape to (2) pseudopod formation to (3) degranulated ballooned sphere.

cells. A potent initiator of aggregation, ADP causes ambient discoid platelets to transform themselves into reactive spiny spheres. These spheres react with one another to form a mass of aggregated platelets (see Fig. 25–5). By binding specific membrane receptors, ADP induces further shape change of nearby circulating platelets, promoting additional aggregation. Both calcium and the plasma protein fibrinogen (coagulation factor I) are necessary for platelet aggregation. The interaction of ADP with its platelet membrane receptor mobilizes specific fibrinogen-binding sites consisting of two membrane glycoproteins.

The platelet-to-platelet interaction (initial aggregation) is a process of Ca^{2+}-dependent ligand formation between membrane-bound fibrinogen molecules. Fibrinogen is believed to bind to the calcium complex of platelet membrane glycoproteins IIb-IIIa (GPIIb-IIIa). Once fibrinogen binds to this complex, extracellular calcium-dependent fibrinogen bridges form between adjacent platelets, thereby promoting platelet aggregation. Aggregation does not occur in Glanzmann's thrombasthenia, an inherited condition in which platelets lack GPIIb and GPIIIa. Platelets will not aggregate in the absence of membrane glycoprotein, fibrinogen-binding sites, fibrinogen, or calcium. Binding of ADP to the platelet membrane activates phospholipase, an enzyme that cleaves the phospholipids present in the plate-

let membrane, freeing such fatty acids as arachidonic acid. Released arachidonic acid is converted in the cytoplasm of the platelet into the cyclic endoperoxides PGG_2 and PGH_2 by prostaglandin synthetase. This enzyme is commonly known as cyclooxygenase, and PGG_2 and PGH_2 are unstable compounds that are converted to TXA_2 by the enzyme thromboxane synthetase (Fig. 25–7). Thromboxane A_2, a potent aggregating agent of platelets, mediates the platelet release reaction as well as vasoconstriction. With its in vivo half-life of 30 seconds, thromboxane A_2 activity is limited in time, because it hydrolyzes spontaneously within the platelet to an inactive form (TXB_2). As TXA_2 is generated with subsequent aggregating effects on platelets, calcium, sequestered in the dense tubular system of the platelet, is extruded in the sol-gel zone. This process activates the Ca^{2+}-dependent actin-myosin–like contractile protein of the microfilament. Activation of the microfilaments results in a contractile wave centralizing organelles, which leads to the release of dense granules and activation of PF 3. Receptor sites of PF 3 then become exposed on the surface of the platelet membrane. Platelet factor 3 facilitates thrombin formation by the intrinsic coagulation system (see section on fibrin formation). Thrombin, also a potent platelet aggregator, can induce secretion of all types of granules (dense, alpha, and lysosomes).

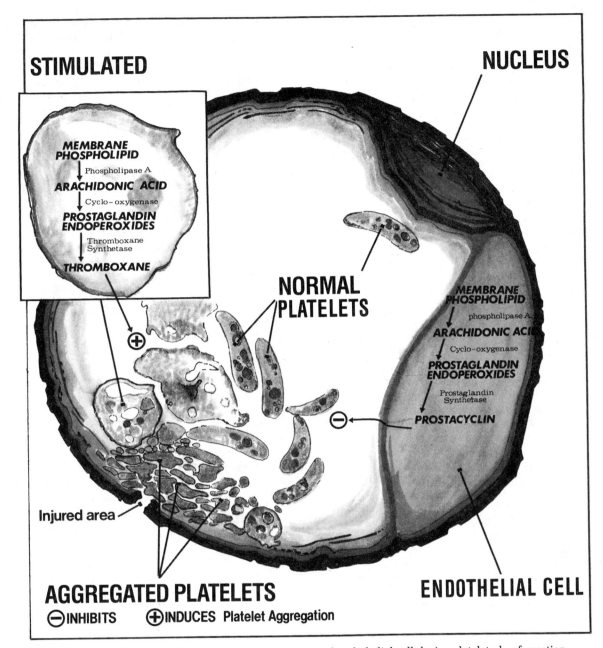

Figure 25–7. Synthesis of prostaglandins in platelets and endothelial cell during platelet plug formation.

In vitro platelet aggregation can be initiated by a variety of agents listed in Table 25–4. In vitro aggregation may be visualized as a two-phase process that may be reversible or irreversible, depending on the strength of the activation stimulus. Early aggregation, the primary (initial or first) wave of aggregation, involves contraction of the circumferential microtubules and reorganization and centralization of platelet organelles. Platelet aggregation results in decreased absorbance as measured by a platelet aggregometer. (For a review of the laboratory procedure for aggregation, see Chapter 30.) This first wave of aggregation is a reversible process as plate-

Table 25–4. **IN VITRO PLATELET AGGREGATORS**

ADP Collagen Epinephrine Thrombin Ristocetin	Common laboratory aggregating reagents
Arachidonic acid Immune products Snake venoms	Other aggregators

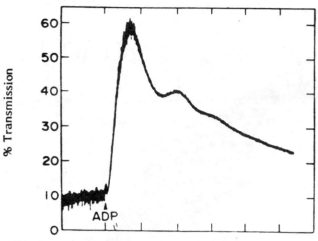

Figure 25-8. A typical biphasic response of in vitro platelet aggregation to ADP, as recorded by an aggregometer.

lets form loosely attached aggregates under such conditions as low concentrations of aggregating reagents or pathologically diminished platelet response.

The secondary wave of aggregation is dependent on the activation stimulus being strong enough to evoke the secretion of platelet granules as a consequence of stronger more complete contraction. Ultrastructurally, the internal reorganization of organelles is more severe, and degranulation is evident by the lack of density of the granules with TEM (see Fig. 25-6). Biochemical studies have confirmed the release of substances such as ADP serotonin and epinephrine; these are responsible for the secondary wave of aggregation, which is usually irreversible. Figure 25-8 depicts a typical biphasic response of in vitro platelet aggregation to ADP, as recorded by an aggregometer. It should be noted that aggregation is an energy-dependent process that greatly exhausts the platelet energy resources.

Secretion (Release Reaction). The release reaction from dense granules involves the secretion of ADP, serotonin (a vasoactive amine), and calcium. Responsible for further aggregation of more platelets, ADP serves to amplify the process previously described. Elevation of intracellular Ca^{2+} further amplifies the process by activating more calcium-sensitive phospholipases, which leads to further formation of TXA_2, as previously described. Amplification of the initial aggregation of platelets (a reversible phenomenon) results in secondary aggregation of many other platelets into an irreversible aggregation of a mass of degenerative platelet material without membranes. This mass is termed viscous metamorphosis (Fig. 25-9). Different substances are released at different rates, suggesting a heterogenicity of granules. The release of substances such as fibrinogen and B thromboglobulin confirms the degranulation of alpha granules. Secretion is an energy-dependent process that occurs only after internal reorganization and transformation have occurred, given a sufficiently strong platelet stimulus that results in an irreversible process (Fig. 25-10).

Effect of Aspirin on Platelet Plug Formation

Aspirin induces irreversible acetylation and inactivation of platelet cyclo-oxygenase, leading to the inhibition of endoperoxide and TXA_2 synthesis, thus preventing aggregation. Because platelets cannot synthesize cyclo-oxygenase, TXA_2 synthesis is inhibited for the entire lifespan of the platelet. Megakaryocytes are capable of synthesizing cyclo-oxygenase; therefore newly released platelets will show enzyme activity. Prostaglandins are present in many different tissues including endothelium. In endothelium, there is a pathway similar to the one described in platelets (see Fig. 25-7). Arachidonic acid in endothelium is converted to PGG_2 by cyclo-oxygenase but thromboxane is not formed. Instead prostacyclin PGI_2 is formed from the cyclic endo-

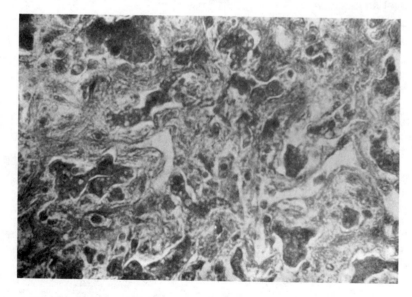

Figure 25-9. TEM of viscous metamorphosis.

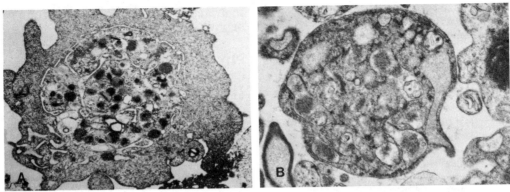

Figure 25-10. TEM of an activated and a degranulated platelet. (A) Early aggregation of activated platelet (the primary wave of aggregation, a reversible process). (B) Degranulated platelet (the secondary wave of aggregation, an irreversible process). (From Barnhardt, MI: Platelet responses in health and disease. Mol Cell Biochem 22:117, 1978, with permission.)

peroxides by the enzyme prostacyclin synthetase. PGI_2, produced in the endothelium, has an effect opposite to that of thromboxane on the platelet. Prostacyclin PGI_2 is a potent inhibitor of platelet aggregation and a vasodilator. Therefore, as long as the endothelium is intact and PGI_2 is made and secreted, platelet aggregation is limited in time. Aspirin also inhibits cyclo-oxygenase produced by the endothelial cells. Endothelial cells, however, possess the organelles necessary to synthesize cyclo-oxygenase, thereby regenerating enzyme activity as the level of circulating aspirin decreases. However, if very high doses of aspirin are ingested, both the endothelial and platelet cyclo-oxygenase will be affected and the effect will cancel out. Thus, a potential for thrombosis may occur.

Stabilization of Hemostatic Plug

The last stage involved in arresting bleeding after vessel damage is the formation of a stable platelet plug. This stabilization is achieved through the formation and deposition of fibrin, the end product of coagulation. Fibrin is formed as a result of a series of reactions that involve not only platelets but also various blood proteins, lipids, and ions (see section on fibrin-forming system).

As mentioned previously, platelets provide an optimal environment for fibrin formation by exposing certain phospholipids (PF 3) on the platelet membrane surface during aggregation. These membrane phospholipids provide a catalytic surface for the activation of various clotting enzymes or factors, such as factor X. In addition, certain coagulation factors (V and VIII) are present on the platelet membrane. All of these factors, in addition to others, are involved in the coagulation system, which leads to the generation of large quantities of thrombin on the aggregated platelet's surface. Thrombin then converts fibrinogen to fibrin (see section on fibrin-forming system). This allows stabilization of both adherent and aggregating platelets by the fibrin strands that form around them. These fibrin strands trap and enmesh all the activated platelets, resulting in the formation of a stable hemostatic plug. Figure 25-11 provides a review of the sequence of

events involved in platelet plug formation and the approximate time involved in each stage.

FIBRIN-FORMING (COAGULATION) SYSTEM

This system is mediated by many coagulation proteins normally present in the blood in an inactive state (coagulation factors). Secondary hemosta-

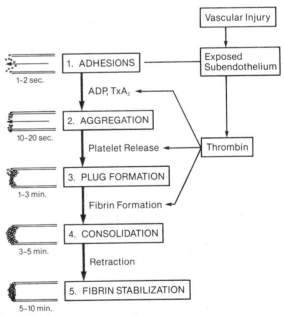

Figure 25-11. Sequence of events in hemostatic plug formation. (1) Platelet adhesion to exposed subendothelial connective tissue structures. (2) Platelet aggregation by ADP, thromboxane A_2, and thrombin recruitment through transformation of discoid platelets into reactive spiny spheres that interact with one another through calcium-dependent fibrinogen bridges. (3) Contribution of platelet coagulant activity to the coagulation process, which stabilizes the plug with a fibrin mesh. (4) Retraction of the platelet mass to provide a dense thrombus. (5) Fibrin polymerization and fibrin stabilization factor XIII. (From Thompson, AR and Harker, LA: Manual of Hemostasis and Thrombosis, ed 3. FA Davis, Philadelphia, 1983, with permission.)

Table 25-5. **NOMENCLATURE OF COAGULATION FACTORS**

Factor I	Fibrinogen
Factor II	Prothrombin
Factor III	Tissue thromboplastin (tissue factor)
Factor IV	Calcium
Factor V	Labile factor (proaccelerin)
Factor VI	Not assigned
Factor VII	Stable factor (serum prothrombin conversion accelerator, or SPCA)
Factor VIII	Antihemophilic factor (AHF)
Factor IX	Christmas factor (plasma thromboplastin component, or PTC)
Factor X	Stuart-Prower factor
Factor XI	Plasma thromboplastin antecedent (PTA)
Factor XII	Hageman factor (contact factor)
Factor XIII	Fibrin-stabilizing factor (FSF)
Fitzgerald factor	High molecular weight kininogen (HMWK)
Fletcher factor	Prekallikrein

sis is used to define the coagulation factor's role in the hemostatic mechanism (see Tables 25-5 and 25-8 for a review of the appropriate nomenclature and characteristics of these factors).

The coagulation factors are designated by Roman numerals. The numerical system adopted assigns the number to the factors according to the sequence of discovery and not to the point of interaction in the cascade. Table 25-5 lists the coagulation factors and their most commonly used designations. All the coagulation proteins are produced in the liver, with the possible exception of factor VIII.

Hemostatic Function

In terms of hemostatic function, the coagulation factors can be divided into three categories: substrate, cofactors, and enzymes. Factor I, fibrinogen, is regarded as the substrate of the blood coagulation system, because the formation of a fibrin clot from fibrinogen is the ultimate goal. Cofactors are proteins that accelerate the enzymatic reactions involved in the coagulation process. Factors III (tissue factor), V (labile factor), and VIII (antihemophilic factor, or AHF) and Fitzgerald factor (high molecular weight kininogen, or HMWK) are the cofactors of the blood coagulation system. All the rest of the coagulation factors are categorized as enzymes. These enzymes involved in coagulation can be divided into two groups: serine proteases and a transamidase. Factor XIII (fibrin-stabilizing factor) is the only transamidase of the coagulation proteins that functions to create covalent bonds between the fibrin monomers formed during the coagulation process to produce a stable fibrin clot. All the other factors that function as enzymes in coagulation are serine proteases. These proteases have serine as a portion of their active enzymatic site and function to cleave peptide bonds.

Physical Properties

On the basis of their physical properties, the coagulation proteins may also be conveniently divided into three other groups: (1) the contact proteins, (2) the prothrombin proteins, and (3) the fibrinogen or thrombin-sensitive proteins.

The contact group includes factors XII (Hageman factor) and XI, prekallikrein (Fletcher factor), and high molecular weight kininogen (Fitzgerald factor). This group is involved in the initial phase of the intrinsic activation of coagulation; its factors are not consumed during coagulation and therefore are present in both plasma and serum. The contact group of coagulation factors is fairly stable, is not absorbed by the reagent barium sulfate ($BaSO_4$), and is not dependent on vitamin K for synthesis. Although deficiencies of these coagulation proteins are associated with markedly abnormal laboratory tests, an isolated factor XI deficiency is associated with a mild bleeding disorder. Problems with thrombosis have been reported in patients with factor XII and Fletcher factor deficiencies.

The prothrombin proteins are generally low molecular weight proteins that include factors II, VII, IX, and X. This group is also known as the vitamin K-dependent coagulation proteins. Each member of this group contains a unique amino acid—gamma carboxyglutamic acid—that is necessary for attraction of these coagulation factors to the surface of activated platelets, where the formation of a fibrin clot occurs. The active participation of these proteins in blood coagulation is dependent on vitamin K, which is necessary for the conversion of glutamic acid to gamma carboxyglutamic acid. Drugs that act as antagonists to vitamin K inhibit this vitamin K-dependent reaction, which is required for functionally active coagulation factors of the prothrombin group. Patients who are vitamin K deficient exhibit decreased production of functional prothrombin proteins. Acquired deficiencies of the vitamin K-dependent coagulation factors are relatively common, as the body does not contain appreciable stores of vitamin K. Characteristic prototypes for developing a vitamin K deficiency include patients who have just had surgery and are receiving parenteral feeding, patients who are receiving high doses of intravenous antibiotics, and patients suffering from liver disease. The factors of the prothrombin group, except for factor II (prothrombin), are not consumed during coagulation. These factors are absorbed by the reagent $BaSO_4$ and are therefore not present in adsorbed plasma. However, they are present in fresh and stored plasma as well as in serum.

The fibrinogen group consists generally of high molecular weight proteins that include factors I (fibrinogen), V (labile factor), VIII (AHF), and XIII (fibrin-stabilizing factor). During coagulation, generated thrombin acts on all the factors in the fibrinogen group. Thrombin enhances the activity of factors V and VIII by converting these proteins to active cofactors, which are involved in the assembly of macromolecular complexes on the surface of activated platelets. Thrombin also activates factor XIII and converts fibrinogen (factor I) to fibrin. The fibrinogen group of coagulation factors is consumed during the coagulation process; therefore these factors are not present in serum. These factors are not absorbed by the reagent $BaSO_4$ and are present in adsorbed plasma. Factors V and VIII are the least stable factors, since their activity is relatively labile to degradation and denaturation. These factors are therefore not present in stored plasma. In addition to the presence of the fibrinogen group in plasma, these factors are also found within platelets. The fibrinogen group of coagulation factors have been reported to increase during conditions of inflammation both in pregnancy and with the use of oral contraceptives.

Blood Coagulation: The "Cascade" Theory

The process of blood coagulation involves a series of biochemical reactions that transforms circulating blood into an insoluble gel through conversion of soluble fibrinogen to fibrin. This process requires plasma proteins (coagulation factors) as well as phospholipids and calcium.

Blood coagulation leading to fibrin formation can be separated into two pathways, the extrinsic and intrinsic, both of which share specific common coagulation factors with the common pathway (Fig. 25–12). Both pathways require initiation, which leads to subsequent activation of various coagulation factors in a cascading, waterfall, or domino effect. According to the cascade theory, each coagulation factor is converted to its active form by the preceding factor in a series of biochemical chain reactions. Each reaction is promoted by the preceding

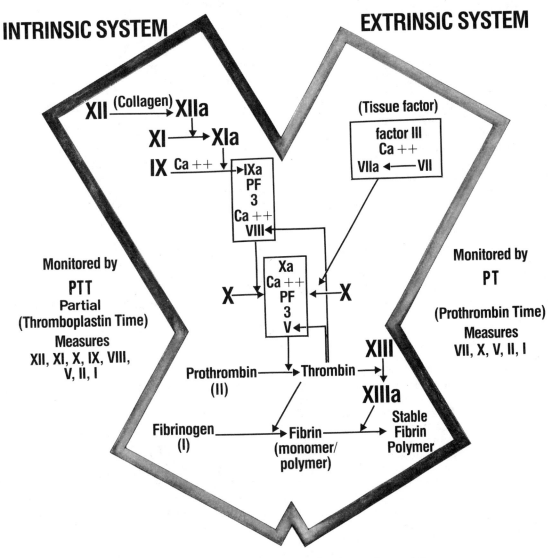

Figure 25–12. Formation of the "cascade" theory of coagulation.

reaction, and if there is a deficiency of any one of the factors, the following consequences result:

1. Coagulation cannot proceed at a normal rate.
2. Initiation of the next subsequent reaction is delayed.
3. The time required for the clot to form is prolonged.
4. Bleeding from the injured vessel continues for a longer time.

Eventually, both the extrinsic and intrinsic systems lead to generation of the enzyme thrombin, which converts fibrinogen to fibrin (Fig. 25–12).

The term extrinsic is used because this pathway is initiated when factor III (tissue thromboplastin), a substance not found in blood, enters the vascular system. The tissue factor includes a phospholipid component that is the source of required phospholipid in the extrinsic system. Phospholipid provides a surface for interaction of various factors. The phospholipids required in the intrinsic pathway are provided by the platelet membrane. In the intrinsic pathway, all the factors necessary for clot formation are intrinsic to the vascular compartment, as they are all found within the circulating blood (Fig. 25–12).

Extrinsic Pathway

In the extrinsic pathway, factor VII is activated to factor VIIa in the presence of calcium (factor IV) and the tissue factor (factor III), which is released from the injured vessel wall. In the extrinsic coagulation system, it is important to realize that this pathway bypasses the activation of factors XII, XI, IX, and VIII, requiring only activated factors VII, IV (Ca^{2+}), and III (a lipoprotein) to activate factor X to Xa. In Figure 25–12, one can see that the extrinsic pathway provides a means for quickly producing small amounts of thrombin leading to fibrin formation. In addition, the thrombin generated by this pathway can accelerate the intrinsic pathway by enhancing the activity of factors V and VIII. In the laboratory, the prothrombin time (PT) test is used to monitor the extrinsic pathway (for a review of the procedure see Chapter 30).

Intrinsic Pathway

Following exposure to foreign substances such as subendothelial collagen, activation of factor XII to XIIa initiates clotting through the intrinsic pathway. It should be noted that factor XII is only partially activated by this contact with a foreign substance. Fletcher and Fitzgerald factors are additionally needed to enhance or amplify the contact factors involved in the intrinsic system (Fig. 25–13). The activation of factor XII acts as the common link between many aspects of the hemostatic mechanism, including the fibrinolytic system, the kinin system, and the complement system (Fig. 25–13; also see section on fibrin lysing). Contact activation occurs in the absence of calcium and also refers to the activation of factor XI to factor XIa by factor XIIa.

The next reaction in the intrinsic pathway is the activation of factor IX to factor IXa by factor XIa, in the presence of calcium. Activated factor IX (IXa) participates along with the essential cofactor VIII in the presence of calcium and PF 3, a source of phospholipid, to activate factor X, which leads to the generation of thrombin and formation of fibrin. The macromolecular complex of IXa, VIII, X, and Ca^{2+} assembles on the surface of the activated platelet during the intrinsic pathway of blood coagulation. This surface provides a protective environment that facilitates the enzymatic reactions of the coagulation cascade without interference fom the physiologic anticoagulants normally present in plasma.

In regard to the intrinsic pathway, it is also important to be familiar with the properties of the factor VIII complex (Table 25–6). Factor VIII, which consists of several components, is the largest protein involved in the clotting cascade. The major portion of this protein is considered to be the carrier protein called von Willebrand factor (vWF). A smaller subunit or protein that is tightly associated is responsible for the clotting or procoagulant activity. Two other subunits have also been defined (Table 25–6). It should be noted that factor VIII requires enhancement by the generated enzyme thrombin to amplify its activity. In the laboratory, the activated partial thromboplastin time (APTT) test is used to evaluate the intrinsic pathway (for a review of this procedure see Chapter 30).

Common Pathway

The common pathway begins with the activation of factor X either by factor VIIa in the presence of cofactor, tissue thromboplastin (factor III), and calcium, or by factor IXa in the presence of the cofactor, factor VIII, calcium, and PF 3 (Fig. 25–14). After the formation of factor Xa, this activated factor along with cofactor V, in the presence of calcium and PF 3, converts factor II, prothrombin, to the active enzyme thrombin. This additional macromolecular complex of factors Xa, V, IV (Ca^{2+}), and II also assembles on the surface of activated platelets.

Activation of thrombin is slow, but once generated it further amplifies coagulation. Thrombin functions to do the following:

1. Convert fibrinogen to fibrin
2. Activate factor XIII
3. Enhance factor V and VIII activity
4. Aggregate more platelets

Thrombin acts on fibrinogen to form fibrin monomers. Fibrinogen is composed of three pairs of polypeptide chains (two alpha, two beta, and two gamma). Thrombin cleaves a portion of each of the alpha and beta polypeptides to form fibrinopeptides A and B. After this cleavage, the fibrinogen molecule is converted to a fibrin monomer (Fig. 25–15). Fibrin monomers quickly polymerize to form fibrin. Weak hydrogen bonding holds together fibrin in this initial clot, which can be dissolved by certain substances such as mild acid and urea. Activated factor XIII (XIIIa), a transamidase, with calcium induces cross-linking of the fibrin polymer. Covalent peptide bonds form between lysine and glutamic

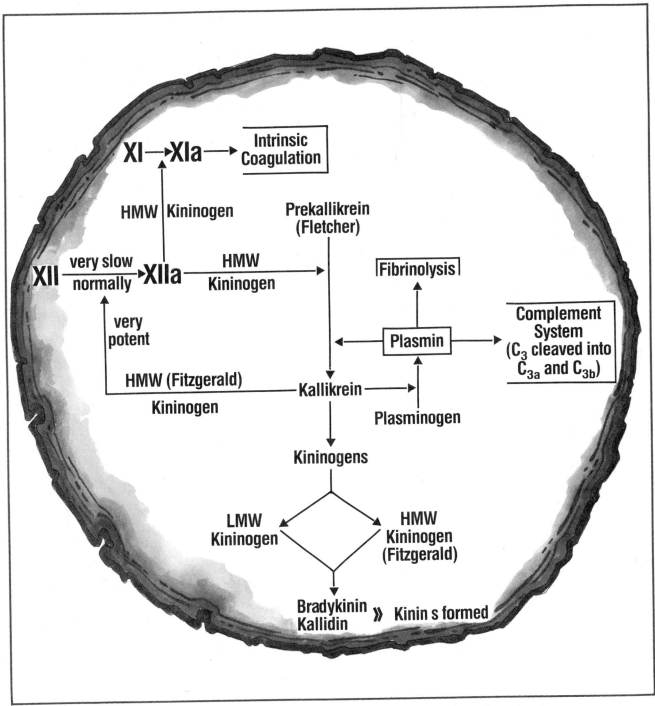

Figure 25–13. Interrelationship of coagulation, fibrinolytic, kinin, and complement systems.

acid moieties. The two gamma chains cross-link in a rapid fashion forming gamma dimers. The alpha chains cross-link slowly with two other alpha chains thereby forming a polymer meshwork. Fibrin contains approximately 100 photofibrils linked by a random fashion of branching.

By using the PT and partial thromboplastin time (PTT) test results in the laboratory, one can identify defects or deficiencies as occurring in the intrinsic, extrinsic, or common pathways of blood coagulation. Using Table 25–7 the reader can practice interpretation of these tests in identifying possible factor deficiencies. Table 25–8 summarizes the properties of the coagulation factors.

Table 25–6. **FACTOR VIII COMPLEX**

I. Smaller Protein Subunit
   Nomenclature
   VIII: (the factor VIII procoagulant protein) or VIII : C or
   VIII : AHF (the antihemophilic factor)
      Components
      a. VIII : Ag—antigen determinant of VIII, measured by
         immunoassays with human antibodies to VIII
      b. VIII—procoagulant property of normal plasma
         measured in the APTT test as procoagulant activity
   Characteristics
   1. Inherited recessive, sex-linked
   2. Acts as a cofactor in a complex with factor IXa, Ca²⁺,
      and PF 3 to activate X to Xa.

II. Major Protein Portion
   Nomenclature
   VIII : vWF (von Willebrand factor) or
   VIII : R (factor VIII–related protein)
      Components
      a. vWF : Ag—antigen determinant on VIII-related protein
         which is detected by using the heterologous
         antibodies to von Willebrand's factor
      b. Ristocetin cofactor (VIIIR : RC₀) or (VIIIR : vWF)—the
         property of normal plasma VIIIR that supports
         ristocetin-induced agglutination of washed normal
         platelets
   Characteristics
   1. Inherited autosomal dominant
   2. Responsible for platelet adhesion
   3. Responsible for ristocetin-induced aggregation of
      platelets
   4. Plays a role in regulating VIII : C synthesis; therefore,
      affects the plasma concentration of VIII : C as well as
      release of VIII from the site of production into circulation
   5. Stabilizes VIII : C when bound to VIII : R during
      circulation, and functions in prevention or protection
      of VIII : C from inactivation

Current Concepts of the Coagulation System

Division of the coagulation process into strictly defined extrinsic and intrinsic pathways has been abandoned, because the cascade theory has been extensively modified. It has been reported that factor VIIa of the extrinsic pathway can directly activate factor IX of the intrinsic pathway (Fig. 25–16). Additionally, it is reported that factor VII can be activated by factors XIIa, IXa, and Xa, and thrombin. It has therefore been hypothesized that factor VII may be the key regulatory protein that initiates blood coagulation. Until more information is generated, and for the simplicity of presentation, the reader should still be able to assimilate the classic cascade presentation of fibrin formation.

FIBRIN-LYSING (FIBRINOLYTIC) SYSTEM

The fibrin-forming and fibrin-lysing systems are intimately related. Activation of coagulation also activates fibrin lysis. Fibrinolysis, the physiologic process of removing unwanted fibrin deposits, represents a gradual progressive enzymatic cleavage of fibrin to soluble fragments. These fragments are then removed from the circulation by the fixed macrophages of the reticuloendothelial system (RES). This action of the fibrinolytic system reestablishes blood flow in vessels occluded by a thrombus and facilitates the healing process following injury. The fibrinolytic system is mediated mainly by the enzyme plasmin, which acts primarily on fibrin to produce lysis of the clot. Plasmin is generated from the circulating inactive zymogen called plasminogen. Plasminogen is activated to plasmin by various substances:

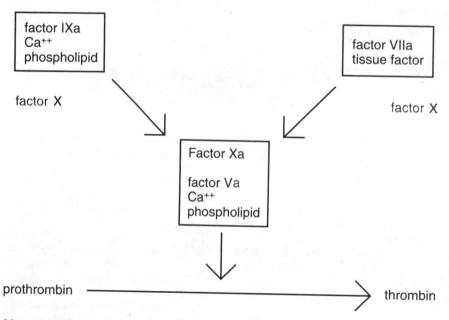

Figure 25–14. Role of factor X in blood coagulation. (Modified from MacGillivray, RTA and Fung, MR: Molecular biology of factor X. Clin Haematol 2:897, Oct 1989, with permission.)

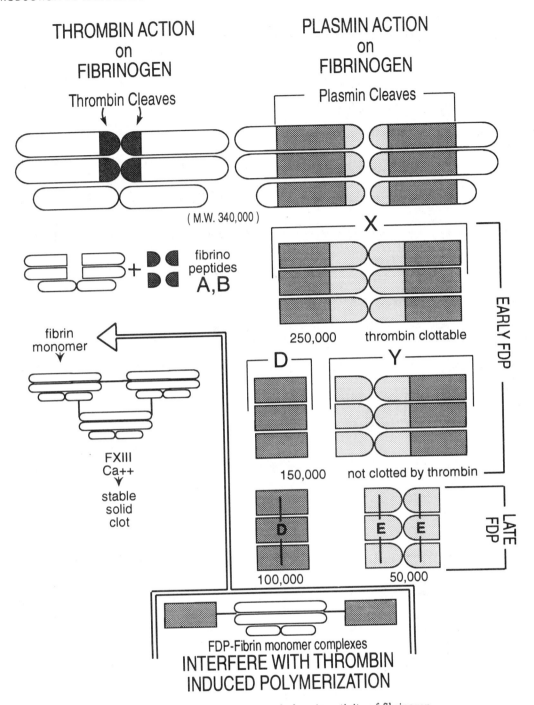

THROMBIN ACTION on FIBRINOGEN

Thrombin Cleaves

(M.W. 340,000)

+ fibrino peptides **A,B**

fibrin monomer

FXIII
Ca++

stable
solid
clot

PLASMIN ACTION on FIBRINOGEN

Plasmin Cleaves

X

250,000   thrombin clottable

D   **Y**

150,000   not clotted by thrombin

100,000   50,000

EARLY FDP

LATE FDP

FDP-Fibrin monomer complexes
INTERFERE WITH THROMBIN INDUCED POLYMERIZATION

Figure 25–15. Comparison of thrombin and plasmin activity of fibrinogen.

1. TPA (tissue kinase released from injured tissue or endothelium)
2. Kallikrein
3. Other substances: urokinase, streptokinase, and staphylokinase

In addition to plasmin, plasminogen, and plasminogen activators, inhibitors of plasmin are also a part of the fibrinolytic system.

It is important to realize that some of the same substances that initiate or enhance clot formation also initiate clot degradation. For example, in tissue, both tissue thromboplastin (initiator of extrinsic pathway of fibrin formation) and TPA (which activates plasminogen) are released with endothelial damage. Tissue plasminogen activator is produced by vascular endothelial cells and selectively binds to fibrin as it activates fibrin-bound plasminogen. Because circulating plasminogen is not activated by TPA, this biologic substance is efficient in dissolving a clot without causing systemic fibrinolysis and serves as an ideal therapeutic fibrinolytic agent. Biologic TPA has been successfully produced by recombinant deoxyribonucleic acid (DNA) technology and is currently in clinical trials. It is also

Table 25–7. **USE OF PT AND PTT FOR IDENTIFICATION OF FACTOR DEFICIENCIES IN COAGULATION STUDIES**

		CORRECTION STUDIES					
		PT		PTT			
Patient PT	Results PTT	Adsorbed Plasma Reagent	Serum Reagent	Adsorbed Plasma Reagent	Serum Reagent	Deficiency
N	Ab	—	—	C	NC	VIII
N	Ab	—	—	C	C	XI, XII*
N	Ab	—	—	NC	C	IX
Ab	Ab	C	NC	C	NC	V
Ab	Ab	NC	C	NC	C	X
Ab	Ab	NC	NC	NC	NC	II
Ab	N	NC	C	—	—	VII

N = normal time; Ab = abnormal time; C = time corrected to normal; — = not applicable; NC = time not corrected to normal.
*No associated bleeding occurs in this deficiency.

Table 25–8. **COAGULATION FACTOR NOMENCLATURE AT A GLANCE**

Factor	Synonym	Clotting Pathway	Molecular Weight	Site of Production
I	Fibrinogen	Both intrinsic, extrinsic, common pathway	340,000	Liver
II	Prothrombin	Both intrinsic, extrinsic, common pathway	70,000	Liver — Vitamin K-dependent
III	Tissue thromboplastin	Extrinsic system only	45,000	Thromboplastic activity present in most tissues
V	Labile factor proaccelerin	Both intrinsic, extrinsic, common pathway	330,000	Liver
VII	Stable factor proconvertin	Extrinsic system only	55,000	Liver — Vitamin K-dependent
VIII	Antihemophilic factor (AHF)/von Willebrand factor	Intrinsic system only	1–2 million	Possibly endothelial cells and megakaryocytes
IX	Christmas factor, plasma thromboplastin component (PTC)	Intrinsic only	57,000	Liver — Vitamin K-dependent
X	Stuart-Prower factor	Both intrinsic, extrinsic, common pathway	59,000	Liver — Vitamin K-dependent
XI	Plasma thromboplastin antecedent (PTA)	Intrinsic only	160,000	Liver
XII	Hageman factor/ contract factor	Intrinsic only	80,000	Liver
XIII	Fibrin-stabilizing factor (FSF)	Both intrinsic, extrinsic, common pathway	300,000	Liver or platelets
Prekallikrein	Fletcher factor	Intrinsic only	80,000	Liver
High molecular weight kininogen	Fitzgerald factor	Intrinsic only	120,000	Liver

(continued)

Note: Although not a coagulation protein or factor, calcium is sometimes denoted as factor IV.

important to note that thrombin generates fibrin and plasmin formation. In addition, prekallikrein (Fletcher factor) and HMWK (Fitzgerald factor) indirectly initiate clotting (via factor XIIa) as well as plasmin formation (see Fig. 25–13).

Action of Plasmin

Plasmin is a broad-spectrum endopeptidase (proteolytic enzyme) that acts nonspecifically, with a strong affinity for fibrin. Plasmin, however, cannot distinguish between the protein fibrin and fibrinogen. The action of plasmin begins by splitting off pieces of each of the alpha and beta polypeptides (a larger portion than that cleaved by thrombin) and a smaller piece of each of the two gamma polypeptides from fibrinogen. The remaining molecule is called the X monomer (which is still thrombin clottable). As plasmin continues its action, it further

splits the X monomer into a Y fragment (not clottable by thrombin) and a smaller D fragment. Further action of plasmin cleaves the Y fragment into D and E fragments. Therefore, the final fibrin-split products are 2D and 1E fragments generated from one molecule of fibrinogen (see Fig. 25–15). These products are collectively known as either fibrin degradation products (FDPs) or fibrin-split products (FSPs). Early FDPs include X monomer and Y fragments; late FDPs include D and E fragments. These fragments are important clinically because they can increase vascular permeability and interfere with thrombin-induced fibrin formation. In patients with certain disease conditions, when plasmin is activated, FDPs are measured.

In addition to its action on fibrin and fibrinogen, plasmin also destroys factors V, VIII, and other coagulation factors. Thus, plasmin acts to:

1. Destroy fibrin and fibrinogen

Table 25–8. **COAGULATION FACTOR NOMENCLATURE AT A GLANCE (*Continued*)**

Plasma Concentration (μg/ml)	Half-life Disappearance (hr)	Minimum Hemostatic Level	Storage Stability	Active Form	Other Characteristics (all factors are present in normal fresh plasma)
2500 (250 mg%)	120	50–100 mg%	Stable	Protein	Activity destroyed during coagulation process/present in absorbed plasma
100	100	40% concentration	Stable	Serine protease	Consumed during coagulation process
0				Cofactor	
5–12	25	5–10% concentration	Labile	Cofactor	Activity destroyed during coagulation process/present in absorbed plasma
1	5	5–10% concentration	Stable	Glycoprotein	Present in serum
7	10	30% concentration	Labile	Cofactor	Activity destroyed during coagulation process/present in absorbed plasma
4	20	30% concentration	Stable	Serine protease	Present in serum
5	65	8–10% concentration	Stable	Serine protease	Present in serum
4	65	20–30% concentration	Stable	Serine protease	Present in serum and absorbed plasma
29	60	0%	Stable	Serine protease	Present in serum and absorbed plasma
10	150	1% concentration	Stable	Transglutaminase	Actively destroyed during coagulation process/present in absorbed plasma
50	?	?	? Stable	Serine protease	
70	?	?	? Stable	Cofactor	

Note: Although not a coagulation protein or factor, calcium is sometimes denoted as factor IV.

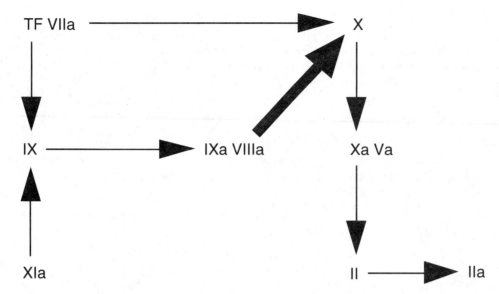

Figure 25–16. Simplified model for the initiation of the coagulation cascade. In this model the primary stimulus results from exposure of cell-bound tissue factor (*TF*) to circulating factor VII (FVII). This cofactor/zymogen complex cleaves FX to Xa and IX to Xa. The additive effect of FVIIIa in the conversion of X to Xa by FIXa is indicated by the *larger arrow*. FVIIIa increases the rate of this reaction by four orders of magnitude. Positive and negative feedback loops are not shown. (From O'Brien, DP: The molecular biology and biochemistry of tissue factor. Clin Haematol 2:803, Oct 1989, with permission.)

2. Produce FDP, which increases vascular permeability and interferes with thrombin-induced fibrin formation (Fig. 25–16)
3. Destroy factors V, VIII, and other coagulation factors
4. Indirectly enhance or amplify factor XII to XIIa (see Fig. 25–13)
5. Enhance or amplify prekallikrein conversion to kallikrein, liberating kinins from kininogen
6. Cleave C3 into fragments (see section on the complement system)

Enhanced fibrinolysis may be observed not only in patients with various coagulopathies but also in those with traumatic injuries, liver cirrhosis, and other pathologic states, and following major surgery.

KININ SYSTEM

The kinin system, important in inflammation, vascular permeability, and chemotaxis, is activated by both the coagulation and fibrinolytic systems. In this system, prekallikrein (Fletcher factor) is activated to kallikrein by factor XIIa (Hageman factor) and plasmin. Kallikrein is an enzyme that can act on kininogens—low molecular weight (LMW) and high molecular weight (HMW, or Fitzgerald factor) —and converts them to kinins. The kinins generated may include kallidin and bradykinin. Bradykinin functions to:

1. Increase vascular permeability
2. Contract smooth muscle
3. Dilate small blood vessels
4. Induce inflammation and pain
5. Release prostaglandins from tissues

The kinin system is also involved in the contact activation phase of the intrinsic pathway of coagula-

tion. Activation of factor XII to XIIa does not occur without kallikrein or HMWK. Kallikrein amplifies the generation of factor XII; and HMWK is an essential factor in the activation of factor XI to XIa. Fitzgerald factor (HMWK) is necessary in both the fibrin-forming and fibrin-lysing systems (see Fig. 25–13).

PROTEASE INHIBITORS

Because the fibrinolytic system is activated when coagulation is activated, extra fibrin is degraded and eliminated along with some of the coagulation factors. However, enzymes such as plasmin and kallikrein still circulate until they are eliminated by (1) liver hepatocytes (which have an affinity for activated enzymes), (2) RES (which picks up particulate matter), or (3) serine protease inhibitors present in plasma. Serine protease inhibitors attach to various enzymes and inactivate them. Important serine protease inhibitors include AT-III, $\alpha2$ macroglobulin, $\alpha2$ antiplasmin, $\alpha2$ antitrypsin, C1 esterase inhibitor, protein C and protein S inhibitors, and activated protein C inhibitor.

Antithrombin III, also termed heparin cofactor or factor Xa inhibitor, is the major inactivator of thrombin and Xa. It is considered the most important physiologic anticoagulant, as 80 percent of the antithrombin activity of normal human plasma is due to AT-III. In addition, AT-III inhibits factors XIIa, XIa, IXa, and VIIIa. Antithrombin III is also capable of inhibiting kallikrein and plasmin. In its natural state, AT-III is a slow progressive inhibitor. However, in the presence of heparin it becomes a very potent inhibitor of coagulation. Therefore, the efficacy of heparin therapy depends on the level of AT-III. Individuals who lack this inhibitor fail to respond to heparin therapy. Heparin forms a complex with AT-III. This combination exposes further sites on the AT-III molecule, increasing its ability to combine with sites on either thrombin or Xa, rendering the factor inactive. This complex is 100 times more potent as an anticoagulant than AT-III alone. The hemostatic result is an increase in the coagulation time. (Deficiency of AT-III, also known as hereditary thrombophilia, is an autosomal dominant disorder in which there is an increased tendency toward thrombosis. This inherited reduction in AT-III may account for as many as 2 percent of the cases of clinical pulmonary thromboembolism.)

Alpha-2 macroglobulin is a nonspecific inhibitor that works on many coagulation factors. The major blood inhibitor of plasmin is $\alpha2$ antiplasmin. Alpha-1 antitrypsin inhibits coagulation factors as well as fibrinolysis. C1 esterase inhibitor inhibits plasmin, kallikrein, and thrombin.

All of these protease inhibitors have broad spectrums of inhibition, even though specificity for one factor or more may be exhibited. Both kallikrein and plasmin are inhibited by all of these serine protease inhibitors.

Also included in this group is a vitamin K–dependent protein inhibitor known as protein C (autoprothrombin II-A). Protein C is a serine protease that acts as an anticoagulant by (1) proteolytically cleaving factors V and VIII, (2) competitively inhibiting factor Xa by the platelet-bound factor V mechanism, and (3) promoting fibrinolysis by stimulating the release of TPA from endothelial cells.

Another vitamin K–dependent protein, protein S, is a necessary cofactor for activated protein C in its role of inactivation of factor V. Deficiencies of protein C are associated with a predisposition for thrombosis.

Finally, it should be mentioned that the generation of activated protein C is regulated by its own specific inhibitor. Activated protein C (APC) inhibitor, along with AT-III and heparin cofactor III (HC-III), is the third heparin-sensitive protease inhibitor. Originally it was postulated that a deficiency of APC inhibitor was responsible for a combined deficiency of factors V and VIII. Recent studies indicate that this inhibitor appears to regulate protein C activation in vivo during coagulation as evidenced by a decrease in plasma concentration of the inhibitor proportional to the increase in FDPs as seen in disseminated intravascular coagulation (DIC).

COMPLEMENT SYSTEM

The complement system is composed of approximately 22 serum proteins, which, working together with antibodies and clotting factors, play an important role as a mediator of both the immune and allergic reactions. The reactions in which complement participates take place in the blood or in other body fluids. The most important biologic role of complement is the production of cell membrane lysis of antibody-coated target cells. Two independent pathways of activation of the complement cascade may occur along with a common cytolytic pathway. These are designated the classic and the alternate pathways of complement activation (see Chapter 13 for a review of the complement system).

Both the coagulation system and the fibrinolytic system are interrelated with complement. Plasmin is an important activator of complement, possessing the ability to cleave directly C3 into C3a and C3b. C3a is an anaphylotoxin causing increased vascular permeability via degranulation of mast cells releasing histamine. C3b is an opsonin causing immune adherence. C5a is not only an anaphylotoxin but is also a potent aggregator of platelets and a chemotactic agent for white blood cells. In addition, C1 esterase inhibitor is an inactivator of the complement sequence as well as inhibiting thrombin and plasmin.

The interrelationship of the coagulation, complement, and fibrinolytic systems is clinically demonstrated in the condition known as hereditary angioneurotic edema. In this disease, there is no inhibition of C1 enzyme activity. The allergic-type symptoms are increased in stressful conditions. Stress results in increased blood levels of plasmin and therefore complement activation. In the absence of adequate C1 inactivation, the body cannot rid itself of the complement products.

LABORATORY EVALUATION OF HEMOSTASIS

The diagnosis of any hemostatic disorder is made by the systematic evaluation of information obtained in the history and physical examination, along with the appropriate laboratory testing. Diagnostically, the most valuable data from a patient's history include:

1. Documentation of the physical appearance, site, severity, and frequency of bleeding episodes
2. A family history of bleeding disorders
3. An accurate drug history
4. Other contributing or underlying illnesses

Bleeding disorders present themselves differently depending on the causative problem. Patients with platelet disorders usually exhibit petechiae and mucous membrane bleeding. Patients with coagulation defects usually develop deep spreading hematomas and bleeding into the joints with evident hematuria.

Alteration of any aspect of the hemostatic mechanism may cause abnormal bleeding in a wide variety of familial and acquired clinical disorders. These defects may be classified into three broad categories that can be diagnostically approached by a systematic laboratory evaluation. These include (1) vascular and platelet disorders, (2) coagulation factor deficiencies, and (3) fibrinolytic disorders.

Although many laboratories differ in their approach to a bleeding disorder, a general profile of laboratory tests is usually established. This profile can often be used as a means of differentiation of various hemostatic problems. Laboratory screening tests routinely ordered usually include platelet count and peripheral blood smear examination, PT,

Table 25–9. **INTERPRETATION OF COAGULATION TEST RESULTS**

Test	Test Result		Possible Defect(s)
APTT and PT	Abnormal	Multiple:	1. Vitamin K defect
Thrombin time (TT)	Normal		2. Liver disease
			3. Inhibitor present
			4. Factors in common pathway (II, V, X)
APTT	Abnormal	Factor:	1. VIII, IX, XI, XII, Fletcher, Fitzgerald
PT	Normal		2. Lupus anticoagulant
PT	Abnormal	Factor:	1. VII
APTT	Normal		
APTT, PT, TT	Abnormal	Multiple:	1. Factor deficiencies (1)
			2. Severe liver disease
			3. DIC
			4. Potent inhibitor
			5. Hypofibrinogenemia or dysfibrinogenemia

PTT, and template bleeding time (TBT). Several laboratories also include the thrombin time as part of their initial coagulation workup.

As mentioned previously, the PT test measures the factors of the extrinsic pathway of coagulation (factors VII, X, V, II, and I). Factor VII is the only factor listed that is restricted to the extrinsic system, as factors X, V, II, and I are part of the common pathway (see Fig. 25–12). The PT test is ideally used to detect early vitamin K deficiencies, as factor VII has the shortest half-life of the coagulation factors and is vitamin K dependent. The PT test is also used to monitor oral anticoagulant therapy. Any abnormalities of these factors, a vitamin K defect, liver disease, or the presence of inhibitors will result in an abnormally prolonged PT.

The APTT, or PTT, test measures factors of the intrinsic pathway of blood coagulation (XII, Fletcher, Fitzgerald, XI, IX, VIII, X, V, II, and I). It should be noted that factors XII, XI, IX, VIII, Fletcher, and Fitzgerald are limited to the intrinsic system. Deficiencies or inhibitors of any of these factors will result in an abnormally prolonged APTT. Both the PT and APTT tests will show prolonged results with an abnormality of the shared factors of the common pathway (X, V, II, and I). A factor abnormality refers to a deficiency of that fac-

tor in plasma owing to any one of the following reasons:

1. Decreased synthesis
2. Synthesis of an abnormal functioning factor molecule
3. Excessive destruction of factors through acquired disorders
4. Inactivation of factors through circulating inhibitors

Table 25–9 summarizes the interpretation of the PT and APTT test results.

The thrombin time is a measure of the ability of thrombin to convert fibrinogen to fibrin and is particularly useful in the evaluation of circulating anticoagulants (pathologic inhibitors). The thrombin time is prolonged in the following conditions:

1. Hypofibrinogenemia and dysfibrinogenemia
2. Treatment with heparin
3. Circulating FDPs
4. Pathologic circulating inhibitors

Table 25–10 may be used as a general guide toward categorizing bleeding disorders into the groups previously listed, using the suggested screening tests. Additional laboratory testing is designed to narrow down the abnormality to one of these specific areas. As a result, laboratory testing can be divided into the following categories:

Table 25–10. **CLASSIFICATION OF BLEEDING DISORDERS BY SCREENING TESTS**

Test	Vascular Disorder	Quantitative Platelet Disorder	Qualitative Platelet Disorder	Factor Deficiency	Fibrinolytic Disorder (Acquired)
Platelet count	N	AbN	N	N	AbN
PT	N	N	N	AbN*	AbN
PTT	N	N	N	AbN*	AbN
TBT	AbN	AbN	AbN	N	AbN

N = normal; Ab = abnormal; PTT = partial thromboplastin time; TBT = template bleeding time.
*Dependent on the factor deficiency

1. Screening tests for vascular or platelet dysfunction (such as platelet aggregation, PF 3 assay)
2. Tests for coagulation (such as factor assays)
3. Special tests (for example, for fibrinolytic disorders: such as tests for determination of FDPs and protamine sulfate and ethanol gel tests for detection of fibrin monomers)

The reader may refer to subsequent chapters for a detailed discussion of the previously listed hemostatic disorders.

BIBLIOGRAPHY

Barnhart, MI: Platelet responses in health and disease. Mol Cell Biochem 22:113, 1978.
Baruch, D, et al: Von Willebrand factor and platelet function. Clin Haematol 2:627, 1989.
Berndt, MC, Fournier, DJ, and Castaldi, PA: Bernard-Soulier syndrome. Clin Haematol 2:585, 1989.
Caen, JP: Glanzmann's thrombasthenia. Clin Haematol 2:609, 1989.
Daniel, L and Tuszynski, P: Platelet contractile proteins. In Coleman, RW, et al: Hemostasis and Thrombosis. JB Lippincott, Philadelphia, 1987, pp 644, 649.
Decary, F and Rock, G: Platelet membrane in transfusion medicine. S Karger AG, Basel, Switzerland, 1988.
Dolan, G, Ball, J, and Preston, FE: Protein C and protein S. Clin Haematol 2:999, 1989.
Evans, VJ: Looking at platelets. J Med Tech 1:9, 1984.
Evans, VJ: Platelet morphology and the blood smear. J Med Tech 1:9, 1984.
Giannelli, F: Factor IX. Clin Haematol 2:821, 1989.
Glassman, B: Platelet abnormalities in hepatobiliary diseases. Ann Clin Lab Sci 20:119, 1990.
Hardisty, RM: Disorders of platelet secretion. Clin Haematol 2:673, 1989.
Hovig, T: Megakaryocyte and platelet morphology. Clin Haematol 2:503, 1989.
Jenny, RJ and Mann, KG: Factor V: A prototype pro-cofactor for vitamin K–dependent enzyme complexes in blood clotting. Clin Haematol 2:919, 1989.
Kaplan-Gouet, C and Salmon, Ch: Platelet Immunology. S Karger AG, Basel, Switzerland, 1988.
Kuast, TVD, et al: Localization of VIII CAg using different monoclonal antibodies against VIII C. Thromb Haemost 50:17, 1983.
Kwan, HC and Samana, MM (eds): Clinical thrombosis. CRC Press, Boca Raton, FL, 1989.
La Croix, KA and Davis, GL: A review of protein C and its role in hemostasis. J Med Tech 2:2, 1985.
Lane, DA and Caso, R: Antithrombin: Structure, genomic organization, function and inherited deficiency. Clin Haematol 2:961, 1989.
MacGillivray, RTA and Fung, MR: Molecular biology of factor X. Clin Haematol 2:897, 1989.
Mason, RG, et al: The endothelium: Roles in thrombosis and hemostasis. Arch Pathol Lab Med 101:61, 1977.
McGann, MA and Triplett, DA: Laboratory evaluation of the fibrinolytic system. Lab Med 14:18, 1983.
Menitove, JE and McCarthy, LJ: Hemostatic Disorders and the Blood Bank. American Association of Blood Banks, Arlington, VA, 1984.
O'Brien, DP: The molecular biology and biochemistry of tissue factor. Clin Haematol 2:801, 1989.
Pati, HP, Gupta, MK, and Saraya, AK: Screening tests for platelet function defect: Evaluation and recommendation. Hem Rev Comm 4:1, 1990.
Pennica, D, et al: Cloning and expression of human tissue-type plasminogen activator with DNA in E. coli. Nature 301:214, 1983.
Tuddenham, EGD: Factor VIII and haemophilia A. Clin Haematol 2:849, 1989.
Vermylen, J and Blockmans, D: Acquired disorders of platelet function. Clin Haematol 2:729, 1989.
Von Dem Borne, AEGK and Ouwehand, WH: Immunology of platelet disorders. Clin Haematol 2:749, 1989.
Walker, FJ: Protein C deficiency in liver disease. Ann Clin Lab Sci 20:106, 1990.

QUESTIONS

1. *How does the vascular system prevent bleeding?*
   a. Vasoconstriction
   b. Diversion of blood flow around damaged vasculature
   c. Initiation of platelet aggregation and fibrin formation
   d. All of the above

2. *Which of the following is not a function of the endothelium?*
   a. Clot formation
   b. Prevention of anticoagulant activity
   c. Prevention of excessive thrombus formation
   d. Initiation of fibrinolysis

3. *Which of the following are structural zones of platelets?*
   a. Peripheral zone
   b. Sol-gel zone
   c. Organelle zone
   d. All of the above

4. *What is not true concerning the peripheral zone?*
   a. Glycocalyx contains platelet antigens such as ABO and HLA
   b. Membrane phospholipid portions serve as the interaction surface for coagulation
   c. Microtubules and microfilaments found here are responsible for the structure and movement
   d. Factors V and VIII and PF 3 and PF 4 are present in this zone

5. *What zone regulates platelet response for section and shape change?*
   a. Peripheral zone
   b. Sol-gel zone
   c. Organelle zone

6. *Which of the following is not true concerning the organelle zone?*
   a. Responsible for metabolic activities of the platelet
   b. Contains dense granules, alpha granules, and lysosomes
   c. Contains the dense tubular system which is the site of prostaglandin synthesis and sequestration of calcium
   d. Contains the OCS to deliver stored products to the platelet surface

7. *What is not a role of platelets in the hemostatic process?*
   a. Induce fibrinolysis by activating plasmin
   b. Maintain vascular integrity

c. Cause initial arrest of bleeding by platelet plug formation
d. Stabilize platelet plug by fibrin formation

8. *What step(s) is (are) involved in the formation of a platelet plug?*
   a. Adhesion
   b. Aggregation
   c. Release action
   d. All of the above

9. *What plasma protein is necessary for the adhesion of platelets to subendothelial fibers?*
   a. Glycoprotein IIb
   b. vWF (von Willebrand factor)
   c. PF 3
   d. Factor X

10. *Which phase is a biphasic response in which ADP, a Ca^{2+} fibrinogen glycoprotein complex, phospholipase, cyclo-oxygenase, and thromboxane synthetase result in a contractive wave and eventual release of platelet granules and thrombin formation?*
    a. Platelet aggregation
    b. Platelet release action
    c. Stabilization of hemostatic plug
    d. Secondary hemostasis

11. *What product is responsible for stabilization of the hemostatic plug?*
    a. Thromboxane A_2
    b. PF 3
    c. Fibrin
    d. GPIIb

12. *Which of the following is not a characteristic of the contact coagulation proteins?*
    a. Group includes factors XII (Hageman factor) and XI, prekallikrein (Fletcher factor), and HMWK (Fitzgerald factor)
    b. Factors are present in both plasma and serum
    c. Dependent on vitamin K for synthesis
    d. Not absorbed by $BaSO_4$

13. *Which of the following is not a characteristic of the prothrombin proteins?*
    a. Consists of factors II, VII, IX, and X
    b. Factors are present in both plasma and serum
    c. Dependent on vitamin K for synthesis
    d. Present in absorbed plasma

14. *Which of the following is not a characteristic of the fibrinogen group?*
    a. Consists of factors I, V, VIII, and XIII
    b. Factors not present in serum; factors V and VIII not present in stored plasma
    c. Found in plasma, but not within platelets
    d. Not absorbed by $BaSO_4$

15. *Which factors are unique to the extrinsic system?*
    a. XII, XI, X, IV, VIII, V, II, I
    b. III, VII
    c. VII, X, V, II, I
    d. XII, XI, IV, PF 3, VIII

16. *What events do not take place in the extrinsic system?*
    a. Activation of factor X to Xa
    b. Acceleration of intrinsic pathway by enhancement of the activity of factors V and VIII
    c. Activation of factor XII to XIIa to initiate clotting
    d. Activation of factor VII to VIIa in the presence of Ca^{2+} and factor III

17. *What factors are unique to the intrinsic system? (Use answer choices for question 15.)*

18. *What is the proper clotting sequence for the intrinsic system that leads to the common pathway?*
    a. XII to XIIa; XI to XIa; IX to IXa; IXa + PF 3 + Ca^{2+} + VIII to X
    b. III + Ca^{2+} + VII to VIIa; X to Xa; Xa + Ca^{2+} + PF 3 + V to Va
    c. II to thrombin; V to X; Xa + IXa + PF 3 to fibrin
    d. XIII to XIIIa; IX to IXa; X to VIII

19. *What factor is not found in the common pathway?*
    a. Factor X
    b. Factor V
    c. PF 3
    d. Factor XIII

20. *Which of the following is not a function of thrombin?*
    a. Conversion of fibrinogen to fibrin
    b. Activation of factor XIII to stabilize fibrin
    c. Conversion of factor VII to VIIa
    d. Enhancement of factor V and VIII activity

21. *Which substance(s) activate(s) plasminogen to plasmin?*
    a. TPA
    b. Kallikrein
    c. Urokinase, streptokinase, and staphylokinase
    d. All of the above

22. *Which of the following is not a function of plasmin?*
    a. Destruction of fibrin, fibrinogen, factors V and VIII, and so on
    b. Conversion of XII to XIIa and prekallikrein to kallikrein
    c. Inhibition of XIIa, XIa, IXa, and VIIIa
    d. Cleavage of C3

23. *What system functions in inflammation, vascular permeability, and chemotaxis?*
    a. Kinin system
    b. Coagulation system
    c. Fibrinolytic system
    d. None of the above

24. *Which of the following are protease inhibitors?*
    a. Antithrombin III
    b. Alpha-2 macroglobulin
    c. Proteins C and S
    d. All of the above

25. *What component of the complement system is a potent aggregator of platelets and a chemotactic agent for WBCs?*
   a. C3a
   b. C3b
   c. C5a
   d. C1-INH

26. *What is the purpose of the PT test in monitoring hemostasis?*
   a. Measures factors of the extrinsic pathway
   b. Detects vitamin K defects
   c. Detects presence of inhibitors
   d. All of the above

27. *What is the purpose of the APTT test in monitoring hemostasis?*
   a. Measures factors of the intrinsic pathway
   b. Detects deficiency of factors for both intrinsic and extrinsic pathways
   c. Measures circulating FDPs
   d. Detects platelet dysfunction

ANSWERS

1. d (p. 416)
2. b (p. 416)
3. d (p. 417)
4. c (pp. 418–419)
5. b (p. 419)
6. d (pp. 419–420)
7. a (p. 420)
8. d (pp. 421–422)
9. b (p. 421)
10. a (pp. 421–422)
11. c (p. 425)
12. c (p. 426)
13. d (p. 426)
14. c (pp. 426–427)
15. b (pp. 427–428)
16. c (pp. 427–428)
17. d (pp. 427–428)
18. a (pp. 427–428)
19. d (pp. 427–429)
20. c (pp. 428–429)
21. d (pp. 430–431)
22. c (pp. 433–434)
23. a (p. 434)
24. d (p. 434)
25. c (p. 435)
26. d (p. 436)
27. a (p. 436)

CHAPTER 26

JANIS WYRICK-GLATZEL, M.S., M.T.(ASCP)

Quantitative and Qualitative Vascular and Platelet Disorders, Both Congenital and Acquired

OBJECTIVES

At the end of this chapter, the learner should be able to:
1. List factor decreases characteristic of von Willebrand's disease.
2. Characterize Bernard-Soulier syndrome.
3. Characterize Glanzmann's thrombasthenia.
4. List differential laboratory findings for congenital disorders of platelet function.
5. Record abnormal laboratory findings associated with disorders of platelet secretion.

6. List diseases that may show acquired qualitative platelet disorders.
7. Name causes for thrombocytopenia.
8. Name conditions classified as nonimmunologic causes for thrombocytopenia.

9. List conditions responsible for immunologic thrombocytopenia.
10. Describe disorders associated with thrombocytosis.
11. List conditions that show inherited vascular defects.
12. List conditions that show acquired vascular defects.

Hemostasis is a complex physiologic interaction of processes. Injury to the vascular system initiates the formation of a fibrin clot, which requires both cellular and molecular components of the vasculature and blood. Platelets play an essential role in maintaining hemostasis through the processes of adhesion, aggregation, secretion, and acceleration of blood coagulation resulting in fibrin formation. Abnormalities in any of the cellular or molecular components of hemostasis or in the interaction of these processes can result in hemorrhagic or thrombotic complications.

Numerous clinical conditions are associated with platelet dysfunction. Hemorrhagic manifestations of the skin and mucous membranes are commonly seen in platelet defects. Thromboembolic episodes occur less frequently. The most common symptoms associated with platelet defects include easy bruising, epistaxis, petechiae, prolonged bleeding from minor cuts, spontaneous gingival bleeds, menorrhagia, and gastrointestinal hemorrhage. Hemarthroses and the formation of deep hematomas after trauma generally do not occur; these clinical symptoms are distinguishing features of patients with coagulation abnormalities such as hemophilia. The hemorrhagic diathesis seen in patients with platelet defects is quite variable, depending on the specific platelet disorder and the individual patient.

The platelet count and bleeding time are common screening tests used to assess the platelets role in hemostasis. The platelet count is used to detect quantitative platelet disorders. The bleeding time detects quantitative and qualitative disorders as well as vascular abnormalities. In addition to the platelet count and the bleeding time, platelet aggregation, adhesion/retention, secretion, and platelet morphology are valuable laboratory tests used to diagnosis platelet abnormalities.

This chapter discusses the etiology, pathophysiology, clinical manifestations, and laboratory tests used to diagnosis the various qualitative and quantitative platelet abnormalities.

QUALITATIVE PLATELET DISORDERS
Congenital Disorders of Platelet Function

Congenital disorders of platelet function, known as thrombocytopathies, can be classified based on the platelet function or response that is abnormal. This classification currently includes defects of mechanisms involving (1) platelet adhesion, (2) platelet aggregation, (3) platelet storage or secretion, (4) platelet-coagulant protein interaction, and (5) platelet-agonist interaction. Table 26–1 lists the various congenital disorders as they relate to abnormal platelet function.

Disorders of Adhesion

Von Willebrand's Disease. In 1926, Dr. E.A. von Willebrand documented the investigation of a 5-year-old girl with a history of severe bleeding. After studying the family members, of whom approximately one third had a positive history for bleeding, he noted three clinical manifestations that separated this bleeding disorder from hemophilia—mucocutaneous bleeds, an autosomal dominant inheritance, and a prolonged bleeding time.

Early studies in patients with von Willebrand's disease (vWD) showed reduced levels of factor VIII. The prolonged bleeding time and low factor VIII levels were corrected after plasma infusion. Even infusion of hemophiliac plasma resulted in a prolonged increase in VIII levels. It is now known that as factor VIII levels rise, vWF:Ag levels decrease.

Von Willebrand's disease is a relatively common heterogeneous disorder. The heterogeneity of this disorder is seen in a variety of clinical manifestations including epistaxis, menorrhagia, easy bruisability, and bleeding following tooth extraction. Severe cases are characterized by recurrent potentially life-threatening bleeds, whereas mild cases may go undetected. Classic vWD is characterized by decreases in factors VIII, vWF, vWF:Ag, and ristocetin cofactor activity. An autosomal dominant pat-

Table 26–1. **CONGENITAL DISORDERS OF PLATELET FUNCTION**

Disorders of adhesion
  Von Willebrand's disease
  Bernard-Soulier syndrome
Disorders of aggregation
  Glanzmann's thrombasthenia
  Congenital afibrinogenemia
Disorders of secretion
  Storage pool deficiency
  Aspirinlike defects
  Miscellaneous congenital disorders
    May-Hegglin anomaly
    Hermansky-Pudlak syndrome
    TAR baby syndrome
    Wiskott-Aldrich syndrome
    Chédiak-Higashi syndrome

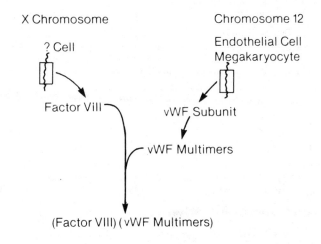

The Factor VIII/vWF Complex in Plasma

Figure 26–1. Factor VIII vWF complex in plasma.

tern of inheritance is most typical for vWD. Several studies also suggest an autosomal recessive mode of transmission with clinical manifestations similar to those found in hemophilia, with joint, muscle, and mucocutaneous bleeding less common. Variants of vWD exist, allowing subdivision into types.

The relationship between vWF and VIII activity of the factor VIII complex has been intensively studied (Figs. 26–1 and 26–2). Certain functions of the molecules are known. Von Willebrand Factor and VIII are believed to be individual molecules of different molecular weights capable of separation by gel filtration. Immunologic evidence seems to support this. Von Willebrand factor binds to VIII, forming a stable complex serving as a carrier for VIII and perhaps serving to stabilize the VIII molecule and increase its concentration at the site of tissue injury. The genes that code for vWD are autosomal, those that code for hemophilia are sex-linked. Endothelial cells and megakaryocytes are known to synthesize vWF. It is believed that vWF stimulates the production of the VIII molecule. Infusion of normal or hemophiliac plasma will result in a gradual increase in VIII levels followed by a decline and rather short-lived increase in vWF levels. Von Willebrand factor is an important molecule that interacts with the vessels and blood platelets and can be isolated in the plasma, platelets, and endothelial cells. The role that vWF plays in hemostasis is quite important as seen from the bleeding manifestation in patients with vWD. A deficiency of vWF results in abnormal platelet adhesion and abnormal coagulation.

The laboratory tests used in the diagnosis of vWD include the bleeding time, platelet retention-adhesion, activated partial thromboplastin time (APTT), factor VIII levels, vWF:Ag levels, platelet aggregation in response to ristocetin, and ristocetin cofactor activity. Crossed immunoelectrophoresis of the vWF:Ag and multimeric analysis of vWF:Ag by agarose gel electrophoresis are a few of the tests used to differentiate the types of vWD.

In vWD, the platelets are intrinsically normal. Platelet adhesion is dependent upon subendothelium, platelet membrane glycoprotein Ib (GPIb), and vWF. The platelet membrane receptor for vWF is thought to be GPIb. In vWD, characterized by the lack of vWF, and in Bernard-Soulier syndrome,

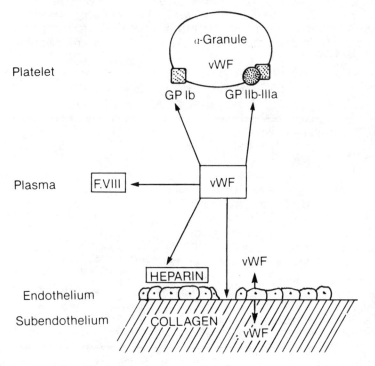

Figure 26–2. Schematic representation of the interactions between vWF, platelets and collagen of the subendothelium; vWF synthesized by endothelial cells is released in plasma and in the subendothelium; vWF is stored in the alpha granules of platelets and can be released after stimulation; vWF mediates platelet adhesion through binding to collagen and to platelet GPIb in the presence of ristocetin, as well as to platelet GP IIb-IIIa in the presence of physiologic agonists (thrombin, collagen, ADP); vWF also binds to F.VIII and to heparin.

characterized by the lack of GPIb, prolonged bleeding times and abnormal platelet adhesion are observed. This is by no means a detailed review of von Willebrand's disease; for a more complete discussion, see Chapter 27.

Bernard-Soulier Syndrome. Bernard-Soulier syndrome was first described in 1948 as a familial bleeding disorder characterized by a prolonged bleeding time and unusually large platelets. Today, it is known that Bernard-Soulier syndrome is a rare autosomal trait associated with decreased concentrations of the platelet surface GPIb as well as glycoprotein V (GPV) and glycoprotein IX (GPIX), causing decreased platelet adhesion to subendothelium.[1] Glycoprotein Ib is the platelet receptor for plasma vWF, one of at least six extracellular components involved in platelet-subendothelium interaction.[2] Glycoprotein V is believed to function in the platelets' response to thrombin; the function of glycoprotein IX is as yet uncertain.

Heterogeneity among the glycoprotein abnormalities in Bernard-Soulier indicates that there are multiple genetic defects. The presence of heterozygotes coincides with recognizable abnormalities such as occasional large platelets on the peripheral blood smear and a history of bleeding but few clinical problems. Homozygotes present with abnormal platelet function and morphology,[3] thrombocytopenia, and hemorrhagic disease. The binding of plasma vWF is necessary for platelet adhesion to other cells and vascular endothelium.[4] Lack of the receptor site, GPIb, impairs hemostasis.

Because so many possible molecular defects exist in Bernard-Soulier syndrome, it is anticipated that the disorder will become more complex. Certain criteria for the diagnosis of this bleeding syndrome have been established. These criteria are as follows:

1. An autosomal trait with clinical manifestations expressed in homozygotes (or double heterozygotes with two combined genetic abnormalities of GPIb, GPV, and GPIX)
2. Moderate thrombocytopenia (despite a normal number of marrow megakaryocytes)
3. A significant number of giant or large platelets present on peripheral blood smear; prolonged bleeding time—too prolonged for degree of thrombocytopenia
4. Absent platelet agglutination in response to bovine vWF or to human vWF plus ristocetin
5. Normal platelet aggregation in response to adenosine diphosphate (ADP), collagen, and epinephrine

Demonstration of an abnormality in platelet membrane GPIb is confirmatory for Bernard-Soulier syndrome. Abnormal laboratory results are presented in Table 26–2.

Bernard-Soulier syndrome must be differentially diagnosed from other congenital disorders of thrombocytopenia associated with giant platelets such as May-Hegglin anomaly or Gray platelet syndrome. Patients with May-Hegglin anomaly, a rare disorder, do not present with bleeding episodes in spite of moderate thrombocytopenia; their platelet membrane glycoprotein and platelet function are normal. Gray platelet syndrome, a very rare disorder, is characterized by mild bleeding episodes, thrombocytopenia, large platelets, and decreased content of the alpha granules; however, membrane glycoproteins are normal.

The nature of the bleeding episodes in patients

Table 26–2. **COMPARISON OF CLINICAL AND LABORATORY FINDINGS IN GLANZMANN'S THROMBASTHENIA AND BERNARD-SOULIER SYNDROME**

Laboratory Findings	Glanzmann's Thrombasthenia	Bernard-Soulier Syndrome
Platelet count	Normal	Decreased
Platelet morphology	Normal	Giant platelets
Bleeding time	Prolonged	Prolonged
Platelet adhesion	Normal	Abnormal
Platelet aggregation		
ADP	Abnormal	Normal
Thrombin	Abnormal	Abnormal
Collagen	Abnormal	Normal
Epinephrine	Abnormal	Normal
Platelet agglutination		
Ristocetin	Normal	Abnormal
vWF	Normal	Abnormal
Clot retraction	Abnormal	Normal
Platelet membrane		
Glycoprotein abnormality	GPIIb–IIIa	GPIb
Inheritance	Autosomal recessive	Autosomal
Bleeding manifestations	Menorrhagia, purpura, easy bruising, mild or severe mucocutaneous bleeds	Severe hemorrhage in homozygotes

with Bernard-Soulier syndrome is similar to that described for Glanzmann's thrombasthenia. Hemorrhagic episodes are treated with transfusions of platelet concentrates, often unsatisfactorily.

Disorders of Aggregation

Glanzmann's Thrombasthenia. Glanzmann's thrombasthenia was first described in 1918 by Glanzmann as "hereditary hemorrhagic thrombasthenia."[5] Early observations in patients with this disorder showed heterogeneity of the disease.

Glanzmann's thrombasthenia is a rare autosomal recessive disorder of platelet function associated with an abnormality of membrane glycoproteins IIb and IIIa, thereby causing decreased platelet aggregation.

The defect stems from the lack of fibrinogen binding to platelet surface membranes or binding in such reduced amounts as to result in the platelets' inability to bind to one another during reactions that normally result in aggregation.[5] The GPIIb-GPIIIa complex is the binding site on platelets for fibrinogen and other contact-promoting proteins.

The exact nature of the genetic defect remains unknown. It is believed, however, that GPIIb and GPIIIa are products of separate genes and messenger ribonucleic acid (mRNA) and that both proteins must associate or complex to provide a stable platelet membrane.[6] The complex GPIIb-GPIIIa is present on myeloid, lymphoid, and endothelial cells, where it is speculated to function in intracellular adhesion.[7]

Platelets in Glanzmann's thrombasthenia show the disc-to-sphere transformation[8] as a result of stimulation by aggregating agents and can undergo the release reaction. They do not aggregate, however, and therefore cannot form normal hemostatic plugs.[9]

Clinical manifestations are quite variable, ranging from minor bruising to severe and potentially fatal hemorrhages, with the severity of bleeds consistent within single families. The most common bleeding symptoms include easy bruisability, epistaxis, spontaneous gingival bleeding, prolonged bleeding from minor cuts, and menorrhagia. Gastrointestinal hemorrhages are less common. The formation of deep hematomas and recurrent hemarthrosis after trauma do not occur in Glanzmann's thrombasthenia, although this is a classic feature of hemophilia. Certain criteria for diagnosing Glanzmann's thrombasthenia have been proposed:

1. A wide variation in hemorrhagic symptoms, ranging from minor bruising to severe mucocutaneous bleeds, beginning during infancy
2. An autosomal recessive trait with clinical manifestations expressed in homozygotes only
3. Prolonged bleeding time
4. Normal platelet count; normal platelet morphology
5. Absent platelet aggregation to ADP, thrombin, collagen, and epinephrine; normal platelet agglutination to ristocetin and bovine vWF

Laboratory findings which are hallmarks of this disorder, include a normal platelet count, prolonged bleeding time, absent aggregation to ADP, collagen, thrombin and epinephrine and absent clot retraction (Table 26–2).

Glanzmann's thrombasthenia is differentially diagnosed from disorders of platelet function associated with a normal platelet count. Von Willebrand's disease, a more common disease than Glanzmann's thrombasthenia, presents with mucocutaneous bleeds similar to patients with thrombasthenia; however, vWD is ruled out by the absence of platelet aggregation to ADP and thrombin. Platelet agglutination by ristocetin, which may be absent in vWD, is normal in Glanzmann's thrombasthenia. Storage pool deficiencies show abnormal rather than absent platelet aggregation and normal clot retraction. In congenital afibrinogenemia, the bleeding time may be prolonged, plasma coagulation tests are abnormal, and clot retraction may occur if the blood clots.

Patients with Glanzmann's thrombasthenia who present with severe bleeding episodes require platelet transfusions. Supportive therapy should be used judiciously, as patients may develop alloantibodies to normal platelet GPIIb and GPIIIa, as well as anti–human leukocyte antigen (HLA) antibodies, and thus become refractory to supportive therapy.[10]

Disorders of Platelet Secretion

Storage Pool Deficiencies. Platelet secretion is a process that involves the release of contents from both alpha granules, including lysosomes and dense granules.

In platelets, ADP and adenosine triphosphate (ATP) are stored in two pools—the metabolically active pool within the cytoplasm and the nonmetabolic storage pool in the electron-dense granules. Upon platelet stimulation, the electron-dense granules are released. Inherited storage pool deficiencies are associated with abnormal platelet function and bleeding manifestations.

This heterogeneous group of inherited platelet disorders is characterized by defects in platelet secretion. They may be classified based on impaired ADP secretion due to decreased stores of ADP and ATP in electron-dense granules (storage pool deficiencies) or defects in the release mechanism (aspirinlike defects).

Clinically bleeding manifestations are generally mild to moderate. Common features include easy bruising, postoperative bleeding, menorrhagia, and epistaxis.

Abnormal laboratory findings associated with these disorders include a prolonged bleeding time, absent or diminished secondary aggregation in response to ADP and epinephrine, decreased aggregation to collagen, decreased platelet retention to glass beads, and impaired platelet factor (PF) 3 availability. The platelet count and platelet morphology are most often normal. The use of electron microscopy is helpful in classifying the disorder as either storage pool deficiency or impaired release mechanism.

Decreases in substances within the electron-dense granules is characteristic of storage pool deficiencies; however, rare documented cases of alpha granules have been reported.[11] Weiss and associates[12] have suggested a system for classification based on morphologic evaluation of platelet granules by electron microscopy and analysis of granule substances.

Congenital Defects. In many patients, reference has been made to storage pool deficiencies associated with other congenital conditions. In the Hermansky-Pudlak syndrome, oculocutaneous albinism with increased ceroid of the reticuloendothelium, a platelet deficiency of nonmetabolic ADP is noted. In patients with Chédiak-Higashi syndrome, characterized by partial oculocutaneous albinism and increased susceptibility to pyogenic infections, an associated storage pool defect is seen. In the syndrome of thrombocytopenia with absent radius (TAR baby syndrome), there are multiple skeletal and cardiac abnormalities with a storage pool defect. A storage pool defect has been shown in patients with Wiskott-Aldrich syndrome, characterized by immunologic alteration, recurrent pyogenic infections, and eczema. Thrombocytopenia results from qualitative defects and shortened platelet survival. Ehlers-Danlos and osteogenesis imperfecta, inherited connective tissue disorders, have been associated with defects of platelet aggregation and adhesion (see inherited vascular disorders). May-Hegglin anomaly, an autosomal dominant trait, is characterized by thrombocytopenia, giant platelets, and Döhle bodies. Most patients are asymptomatic. Platelet function abnormalities are not a consistent finding in patients with this anomaly. Alport's syndrome, an inherited disorder, characterized by deafness and nephritis is associated with giant platelets and thrombocytopenia. Bleeding is most often mild and presents as epistaxis. Laboratory findings in this disorder may include abnormal platelet aggregation in response to collagen and ADP, impaired PF 3 availability, and an abnormal bleeding time.

Abnormal platelet aggregation and PF 3 activity is seen in glycogen storage disease type I (glucose-6-phosphate dehydrogenase, or G6PD, deficiency). The mild clinical bleeds and the abnormal platelet function tests improve upon treatment for the enzyme deficiency. The platelet defects are thought to be secondary to the metabolic defect.

Afibrinogenemia, an extremely rare inherited disorder, is associated with abnormal platelet function. Fibrinogen is essential for aggregation with ADP. Abnormal platelet aggregation in response to ADP, decreased platelet retention, impaired PF 3 activity, and a prolonged bleeding time have been reported in patients with afibrinogenemia. Aggregation studies with ADP are restored to normal upon addition of fibrinogen. The treatment of choice for bleeding in these patients is administration of platelet concentrates. In patients who have very mild bleeding, the syndrome may not be detected.

Acquired Qualitative Platelet Disorders

Renal Disease — Uremia

Bleeding has long been recognized as a common, yet sometimes severe, complication of uremia. Patients with acute and chronic renal failure hemorrhage predominantly from mucous membranes. Petechiae, purpura, epistaxis, ecchymoses, and gastrointestinal bleeds are common.[13] Severe hemorrhages within serous cavities and muscles may also occur.

A number of different laboratory findings and clinical symptoms suggest that platelet dysfunction with abnormal platelet–vessel wall interaction is the major cause of hemorrhage. Decreased PF 3 availability was the first recognized platelet defect.[14] Other rather consistent platelet abnormalities seen in uremia are reduced platelet retention to glass bead columns;[15] abnormal platelet aggregation in response to ADP, epinephrine, and collagen;[16] and prolonged bleeding times. The bleeding time and reduced platelet retention is used as means to assess the hemorrhagic tendency of patients with uremia.[17] However, no correlation exists among serum levels of creatinine, uric acid, or urea with prolonged bleeding times or reduced platelet retention.[18]

Metabolic abnormalities of platelets have been seen in uremia and include abnormal GPIb or a block in binding of vWF to GPIb, abnormal prostaglandin synthesis, abnormal platelet serotonin and ADP storage pool defects, abnormal β-thromboglobulin (β-TG), and elevated intracellular calcium levels. A correlation of the metabolic changes with functional defects has not yet been established.

Various studies have been conducted to determine which of the metabolites is responsible for the qualitative platelet abnormalities seen in patients with renal failure. The cause remains unknown.

Hemodialysis or peritoneal dialysis, or both, is the treatment of choice to correct the hemostatic defect in uremia; however, platelet function abnormalities may remain. Administration of cryoprecipitate to patients unresponsive to dialysis has also been used as a means of therapy.[19] The use of the vasoactive peptide, 1-Deamino-8-D-arginine-vasopressin (DDAVP) in uremic patients has prevented clinical bleeds in patients following surgical procedures and has shortened the bleeding time temporarily.[20]

Paraproteinemias

Coagulation abnormalities, acquired circulating anticoagulants, and platelet dysfunction are associated with the malignant paraproteins. Bleeding is a common clinical manifestation of the various paraproteinemias. There is, however, a greater frequency of bleeding and platelet dysfunction seen in Waldenström's macroglobulinemia and in IgA multiple myeloma as compared to IgG multiple myelomas.[21] The occurrence of bleeding correlates with the findings of abnormal platelet function.

Platelet abnormalities are demonstrated by reduced PF 3 availability, reduced platelet retention, abnormal aggregation, and prolonged bleeding time. Abnormal fibrin polymerization, thrombocytopenia, and hyperviscosity are often seen in patients with dysproteinemias, and may contribute to the hemorrhagic episodes.[21]

The exact mechanisms by which these abnormalities occur have not been well defined. Binding of the paraprotein to the platelet membrane may interfere with the function of the membrane.[21] Coating of the collagen fibers by the abnormal protein has also been reported.[22]

Myeloproliferative Disorders

The myeloproliferative disorders (MPDs) include polycythemia vera (PV), agnogenic myeloid metaplasia, chronic myelocytic leukemia (CML), and essential thrombocythemia (ET). This group of disorders has many clinical and hematologic features in common; however, the platelet defects in each appear to differ. Concomitant hemorrhage and thromboembolic episodes are frequent in patients with myeloproliferative disorders. The hemorrhagic manifestations include ecchymoses, epistaxis, and mucocutaneous bleeds of the gastrointestinal and genitourinary tracts. Thrombosis occurs in both the arterial and venous circulation and includes deep vein thrombosis, stroke, pulmonary emboli, and thrombosis of the hepatic, portal, splenic, and mesenteric veins. The exact mechanism of platelet dysfunction and hemostatic defect is uncertain. In many cases, the degree of thrombocytosis is a contributing factor to the complications seen in the MPDs (see Color Plate 251).

Thrombosis rather than hemorrhage is a major complication in PV, as a result of hyperviscosity, increased red cell mass, thrombocytosis, intravascular coagulation, and qualitative platelet defects. It has been suggested that hyperviscosity and increased red cell mass lead to thrombosis, creating problems in the cerebral, retinal, and pulmonary circulation, thus contributing to the clinical manifestations in PV. Thrombocytosis is generally moderate, in the range of 500,000 to 1,000,000/μl and is seen in approximately 50 to 60 percent of cases.[23] Platelet defects are thought to be responsible for much of the hemostatic problems found.

Abnormal platelet aggregation in response to epinephrine, ADP, and collagen has been reported.[24] Evidence of in vivo platelet activation and intravascular coagulation, as evidenced by increased plasma levels of β-TG and low platelet serotonin levels,[25] as well as abnormal levels of fibrinogen and prothrombin,[26] have also been reported in cases of PV.

Bleeding and thrombosis are seen in patients with CML; however, thrombosis occurs much less frequently than bleeding. When a bleeding diathesis does occur, mucocutaneous bleeds, retinal hemorrhages, and hematuria may occur. It is thought that the acquired platelet defects seen in CML result from dysplastic platelet production.

Decreased or absent platelet aggregation in response to ADP, epinephrine, and collagen have been reported in cases of CML.[27] A prolonged bleeding time is often seen in patients with CML in remission as well as in those in blast crisis.[27] A factor V deficiency has been reported in some cases of CML.[28] Increases in platelet vWF have also been noted.[29]

Patients with agnogenic myeloid metaplasia may experience bleeding such as ecchymoses and urogenital bleeds. Thromboembolic complications, with the exception of hepatic and portal vein thrombosis, occur rather infrequently. It has been suggested that of all the MPDs, agnogenic myeloid metaplasia is associated with the greatest degree of platelet defects.[27]

Decreased platelet adhesion and prolonged bleeding time are relatively common findings in patients with agnogenic myeloid metaplasia.[27] Storage pool deficiencies and impaired platelet aggregation have also been reported.[30]

Essential thrombocythemia, characterized by platelet counts of 1,000,000/μl or greater, is associated with both bleeding and thrombosis, although bleeding episodes occur more often. Evidence suggests that thrombocytosis alone does not account for the bleeding and thrombotic episodes seen in ET,[31] but the combination of thrombocytosis and abnormal platelet function determine the hemostatic defects in ET.

Decreased platelet aggregation in response to epinephrine[32] as well as decreased platelet retention[27] are consistent findings in patients with ET. Impaired PF 3 availability and platelet hyperactivity[33] have been reported in patients with thrombosis in ET. Several platelet defects have been described in ET, but what predisposes patients to bleeding or thrombotic manifestations is still uncertain.

Management of patients with MPDs aims at reducing the risk of hemorrhage and thrombotic complications. Myelosuppressive and cytotoxic therapy is often used. In patients with the MPDs and thrombocytosis, the syndromes of cerebral ischemia are often therapeutically treated by plateletpheresis and chemotherapy. The use of antiplatelet drugs such as aspirin is controversial.

Acute Leukemias and Myelodysplastic Syndromes

Thrombocytopenia and platelet defects have been associated with manifestations of clinical bleeding in the acute leukemias and the myelodysplastic syndromes. Morphologic changes in megakaryocytes may contribute to the qualitative platelet defects seen in these diseases.

Acquired von Willebrand's Disease

Acquired vWD is a bleeding disorder that has been found in patients with myeloproliferative disorders, lymphoproliferative diseases, monoclonal gammopathies, and collagen vascular diseases.

Most patients are 40 years old or older, with no previous history of bleeding. Bleeding presents with an insidious onset and manifests as mucocutaneous or post-traumatic hemorrhage.

Laboratory findings seen in acquired vWD include a prolonged bleeding time (variable); decreases in plasma levels of factor VIII, vWF : Ag, and ristocetin cofactor; and variable decreases in vWF multimers. Platelet vWF is generally normal. Following infusion of plasma or cryoprecipitate, there is an absence in the rise in plasma factor VIII levels observed in most patients with classic vWD.

Spontaneous remission and remission after therapy for the underlying disease is often seen. Therapeutic use of DDAVP has been observed to correct the bleeding time and increase the level of vWF. A response to the use of corticosteroid therapy has been documented.

Cardiopulmonary Bypass

Alterations in hemostasis and the potential for life-threatening hemorrhage have been well documented in patients undergoing cardiac surgery and cardiopulmonary bypass (CPB). Various hemostatic abnormalities have been implicated in the development of the hemorrhagic manifestations of CPB surgery. They include coagulation factor deficiencies, increased fibrinolytic activity, thrombocytopenia, disseminated intravascular coagulation (DIC), and inadequate heparin neutralization or protamine excess.[34] The development of thrombocytopenia during surgery is thought to be due to hemodilution, formation of intravascular platelet thrombi, platelet utilization in the pump, and peripheral destruction as a result of DIC.[34] Platelet defects such as decreased platelet adhesion, abnormal platelet aggregation, increased plasma levels of β-thromboglobulin, and PF 4 (signs of platelet activation) and membrane damage have all been seen. During CPB, a prolonged bleeding time in the face of a platelet count of $100,000/\mu l$ is often seen. It has been suggested that platelet activation and platelet dysfunction account for the majority of hemostatic alterations seen during this procedure.[35] Platelet concentrates are administered to stop the bleeding, and antiplatelet drugs are used to control platelet activation during the CPB procedure.

Liver Disease

Chronic liver disease is often associated with a significant hemorrhagic diathesis as a result of multiple alterations in hemostasis. These alterations include decreased synthesis of blood coagulation factors and their inhibitors, increased fibrinolytic activity, evidence of intravascular coagulation, thrombocytopenia, and platelet defects.

Mild to moderate thrombocytopenia is seen in approximately one third of patients with chronic liver disease as a result of splenic sequestration secondary to congestive splenomegaly associated with portal hypertension.[34] Abnormal platelet function tests found in patients with chronic liver disease include reduced platelet adhesion; abnormal platelet aggregation to ADP, epinephrine, and thrombin; and abnormal PF 3 availability. An acquired storage pool deficiency has also been suggested.[35] The exact mechanism responsible for the platelet defects seen in patients with chronic liver disease is not known.

In patients with alcoholic cirrhosis, thrombocytopenia and platelet abnormalities may result from the direct toxic effects of alcohol on bone marrow megakaryocytes, leading to an ineffective thrombopoiesis.

Transfusion with platelet concentrates may ameliorate the bleeding and thrombocytopenia associated with chronic liver disease. The rise in platelet count following transfusion may not be as expected if splenic sequestration occurs.

Acquired Storage Pool Deficiencies

Acquired storage pool deficiencies have been reported in patients with systemic lupus erythematosus (SLE), idiopathic thrombocytopenic purpura (ITP), thrombotic thrombocytopenic purpura (TTP), DIC, hemolytic uremic syndrome (HUS), MPDs, hairy-cell leukemia, and acute nonlymphocytic leukemia, as well as in CPD. The platelet defect is most likely due to the underlying disease process.

Disseminated Intravascular Coagulation

This consumptive coagulopathy is associated with thrombocytopenia and platelet defects. The bleeding diathesis seen in this disorder results from the consumption of platelets, coagulation factors, and increased fibrinolytic activity. Qualitative platelet defects such as impaired platelet aggregation,[36] acquired storage pool deficiencies,[37] and a prolonged bleeding time[37] have been described in DIC (see Chapter 28 for a detailed discussion of DIC).

Drug Therapy

A large variety of pharmacologic drugs has been shown to inhibit platelet function, thereby increasing the risk of bleeding. Occasionally, as with heparin therapy, the risk of thrombosis is increased. Individual susceptibility to the effects of these drugs varies greatly. The use of antiplatelet drugs in patients with hemostatic abnormalities often predisposes them to severe complications.

The use of aspirin has been well documented to inhibit platelet aggregation and platelet secretion in response to ADP, epinephrine, and low concentrations of collagen. Prolonged bleeding times are associated with the use of aspirin. The effect of aspirin on the bleeding time is generally dose dependent, but extremely prolonged bleeding times at lower dosages have been reported. Aspirin inhibits prostaglandin synthesis by irreversible acetylation and inactivation of cyclo-oxygenase, thereby inhibiting endoperoxide and thromboxane A_2 synthesis — important mediators of platelet release. The inhibitory effect of aspirin on thromboxane A_2 synthesis will remain for the lifespan of the platelet. Patients with hemophilia, vWD, or major underlying hemostatic defects may develop significant or spontaneous bleeds upon aspirin ingestion and therefore should not use aspirin or aspirin-containing compounds.

Nonsteroidal anti-inflammatory agents, such as indomethacin, ibuprofen, phenylbutazone, and sulfinpyrazone inhibit cyclo-oxygenase. The effect of these drugs on platelets is short-lived and reversible.

Cyclic AMP (cAMP) plays a major role in mediating platelet activity. Platelet response is inhibited when intracellular levels of cAMP are raised. Drugs such as dipyridamole inhibit phosphodiesterase, an enzyme capable of inactivating cAMP. Dipyridamole has a rather minor effect on platelet function. When administered with aspirin, it exerts an antiplatelet effect. Dipyridamole does not prolong the bleeding time.

Sulfinpyrazone is a competitive inhibitor of platelet cyclo-oxygenase. Bleeding times are not prolonged, and platelet aggregation is generally normal. Its mechanism of action as an antiplatelet agent is not well understood.

Antimicrobial drugs such as penicillin, ampicillin, and carbenicillin may inhibit platelet function.[38] When administered in high doses, bleeding may occur. Cephalosporins may also inhibit platelet function. These drugs affect platelet aggregation, platelet secretion, and platelet adhesion.[39]

Dextran infusion is also known to prolong the bleeding time. Platelet function tests such as aggregation, PF 3 availability, and platelet retention have all been shown to be abnormal with the use of dextran.[40] It is believed that dextran interferes with the platelet's surface membrane.

Heparin is known to cause thrombocytopenia with an increased risk for thrombosis (see section on nonimmune thrombocytopenia).

Several drugs inhibit platelet function by mechanisms still unknown. The list of such drugs includes vasodilators, chemotherapeutic drugs, antihistamines, ethanol, local anesthesia, radiographic dyes, and foods such as garlic, ginger, and onions.

Numerous other conditions have been associated with an acquired platelet defect. These include paroxysmal nocturnal hemoglobinuria (PNH), infectious mononucleosis, severe vitamin B_{12} deficiency, diabetes, hyperbetalipoproteinemia, congenital heart defects, and hypothyroidism. The pathogenesis of these various disorders is uncertain.

Platelet Antibodies

Disorders such as ITP, SLE, and Graves' disease have been reported in association with increased platelet-associated antibodies.[40] Platelet antibodies have been demonstrated to cause platelet lysis, platelet aggregation, increased PF 3 availability, and serotonin release. These events can lead to platelet destruction, resulting in thrombocytopenia or acquired platelet defects.

Other conditions may be associated with an acquired qualitative platelet defect. Massive transfusion, defined as replacement of the majority of patient's blood volume, is often associated with severe trauma and results in many hemostatic defects. A large percentage of the massively transfused patients may acquire hemostatic defects as a result of the use of stored blood and blood components and dilutional effects. Platelets lose their viability when stored at 4 to 6°C and are considered nonfunctional. Massive transfusion of packed red cells or plasma dilutes the remaining platelets. This dilutional effect is somewhat proportional to the number of transfusions. Trauma and tissue injuries are believed to cause qualitative defects in platelet function.

QUANTITATIVE PLATELET DISORDERS

Platelets must be present in adequate numbers to maintain normal hemostasis. The average platelet count ranges from 150 to $400 \times 10^3/\mu l$ of whole blood. The platelet count is a routine screening test used to detect quantitative changes such as thrombocytosis (platelet counts greater than $400 \times 10^3/\mu l$) and thrombocytopenia (platelet counts less than $50 \times 10^3/\mu l$.) Quantitative changes in platelet counts may result from a primary disorder of the bone marrow or secondary to a variety of underlying conditions. Often the presence of qualitative defects may coexist with quantitative changes.

Thrombocytopenia

Decreased Platelet Production

Decreased platelet production resulting in thrombocytopenia may be associated with congenital or acquired disorders. These disorders generally affect the bone marrow, resulting in megakaryocytic hypoplasia. Concomitant anemia and leukopenia are also found in many patients in these disorders.

Many of the congenital disorders that produce hypoplasia of megakaryocytes include Fanconi's anemia, thrombocytopenia with absent radius (TAR baby syndrome), May-Hegglin anomaly, and fetal exposure to drugs and viral infections. A list of disorders associated with quantitative platelet changes is found in Table 26–3.

Replacement of marrow hemopoietic tissue occurs in association with infiltrative processes such as myelofibrosis, leukemia, metastatic tumors, Hodgkin's disease and non-Hodgkin's lymphoma, and tuberculosis. A myelophthisic anemia, characterized by nucleated red blood cells, teardrop cells, and immature granulocytes, is often found in the peripheral blood smear of patients with these disorders. Drugs, chemicals, radiation, and infections may result in injury to the marrow hematopoietic tissue causing anemia, leukopenia, and thrombocytopenia. Recognition of these disorders involves examination of the bone marrow to confirm a diagnosis and begin specific therapy if indicated.

Ineffective Thrombopoiesis

Ineffective thrombopoiesis is a state in which the number of megakaryocytes in the bone marrow is

Table 26-3. **CLASSIFICATION OF THROMBOCYTOPENIA**

Decreased production of platelets
  Leukemias
  Lymphomas
  Myelodysplastic syndrome
  Aplastic anemia
  Fanconi's anemia
  Metastatic carcinoma
  Myelofibrosis
  Chemotherapeutic and immunosuppressive agents
  Thrombocytopenia with absent radius (TAR baby syndrome)
  Osteoporosis
  Viral infections
  Drug ingestion
  May-Hegglin anomaly
  Bernard-Soulier syndrome
Ineffective thrombopoiesis
  Vitamin B_{12} deficiency
  Folic acid deficiency
  Alcohol ingestion
  Myelodysplastic syndrome
  Paroxysmal nocturnal hemoglobinuria
  Di Guglielmo syndrome
  Drug ingestion
Abnormal distribution of platelets
  Hypersplenism
Increased destruction of platelets
  Immune-mediated thrombocytopenia
    Idiopathic thrombocytopenic purpura
      Acute
      Chronic
      Recurrent
    Isoimmune neonatal
    Drug-induced thrombocytopenia
    Post-transfusion purpura
  Secondary immune-mediated
    Viral, bacterial, parasitic infections
    Lymphoproliferative disorders
    Collagen vascular disease (eg, SLE)
    HIV-1
    Drugs
    Transfusions
  Non-immune-mediated thrombocytopenia
    Disseminated intravascular coagulation
    Thrombotic thrombocytopenic purpura
    Hemolytic uremic syndrome
    Heparin
    Complications of pregnancy
    Viral, bacterial, mycotic infections

normal to increased, but maturation and release of platelets to the circulation is abnormal. Conditions that prevent normal maturation or platelet release result in ineffective thrombopoiesis.

Megaloblastic anemia associated with a vitamin B_{12} or folic acid deficiency is commonly associated with thrombocytopenia as a result of impaired deoxyribonucleic acid (DNA) synthesis. Thrombocytopenia is generally mild with clinical manifestations of purpura. Platelet lifespan has been reported as being normal to only slightly reduced. Ineffective thrombopoiesis has been reported in the myelodysplastic syndromes, Di Guglielmo syndrome, and PNH. Alcohol is thought to have a direct toxic effect on the marrow, thereby producing thrombocytopenia in the absence of a folic acid or vitamin B_{12} deficiency. The mild thrombocytopenia and acquired platelet defects appear to improve after stopping the use of alcohol. Drugs are also known to induce a thrombocytopenia (see section on acquired qualitative platelet defects and drug-induced thrombocytopenia).

Abnormal Distribution of Platelets

Normally the spleen pools approximately one third of all circulating platelets. Splenomegaly is associated with many conditions, causing increased pooling of circulating platelets thereby producing thrombocytopenia. Increased platelet destruction has been observed in splenomegaly.

Increased Destruction of Platelets

A sudden decrease in the platelet count without evidence of a hemorrhage suggests a condition of increased platelet sequestration by the spleen and liver or increased destruction of platelets in these organs, which reduces platelet lifespan. Increased sequestration or destruction of platelets is either immune- or non-immune-mediated. This section discusses the various disorders of non-immune-mediated thrombocytopenia.

Nonimmunologic Thrombocytopenia

Thrombotic Thrombocytopenic Purpura. First described in 1924 by Moschcowitz,[41] the hallmarks of this syndrome are thrombocytopenia, microangiopathic hemolytic anemia, fluctuating neurologic abnormalities, fever, and renal disease. The pathologic feature characteristic of TTP is the hyaline microthrombi composed of platelets and fibrin that occlude arterioles and capillaries in multiple organs **(see Color Plate 250)**. There is absence of localized fibrinolytic activity in the vessels occluded by these microthrombi. The microthrombi are not solely diagnostic for TTP; they occur in DIC as well. The composition of the thrombotic lesion, being predominantly platelets rather than fibrin, and the normal coagulation studies help to differentiate TTP from DIC.

The exact pathogenic mechanisms responsible for this disorder remain uncertain; however, four concepts help explain the pathogenesis and therapeutic response in TTP. These are (1) that TTP plasma is deficient in a platelet-aggregating factor inhibitor (an immunoglobulin normally found in plasma);[42] (2) that large vWF multimers promote platelet agglutination;[43,44] (3) that endothelial cell damage via a plasma factor results in platelet adhesion;[45] and (4) that as a consequence of endothelial cell damage there is a deficiency of PGI_2 synthesis and release, leading to platelet aggregation and thrombosis.[46]

The incidence of TTP is thought to be approximately one per million,[47] but increased awareness and diagnosis may change these statistics. Women appear to be affected twice as often as men with the peak incidence appearing at age 40. Patients who are pregnant, have viral infections, ingest drugs, or have autoimmune disorders appear to be predisposed to TTP.

Patients with TTP initially present with nonspecific symptoms of malaise, weakness, fatigue, often fever or abdominal pain, along with the hallmark neurologic complication and bleeding manifestations of thrombocytopenia. Clinical features of TTP are those of a severe microangiopathic hemolytic anemia with associated poikilocytosis (**see Color Plate 115**), reticulocytosis, and nucleated red blood cells indicating a compensatory marrow response. Signs of hemolysis are reflected by increases in serum lactate dehydrogenase (LDH), indirect bilirubin, and decreased haptoglobin levels. There is a severe thrombocytopenia and evidence of decreased platelet survival despite megakaryocytic hyperplasia in the bone marrow. Prothrombin time (PT), partial thromboplastin time (PTT), and fibrinogen levels are generally normal in patients with TTP, with slight elevations in fibrinogen degradation products (FDP) levels. Renal involvement is characterized by signs of hematuria, proteinuria, and acute renal failure. Neurologic abnormalities manifest as dysphasia or aphasia, headache, paresis, seizures, obtundation, and paresthesia. Abdominal pain, pancreatitis, and gastrointestinal bleeding may also be associated findings. Any organ system may show involvement; cardiac damage with arrhythmias is not unusual. Table 26–4 lists the common characteristics of TTP.

At present, there is no standard treatment for TTP. Although recovery from TTP has been reported as a result of numerous therapeutic modalities, the rarity of this disorder and its variable nature make evaluation of these therapies difficult. Prognosis of this disorder has improved considerably in the past 20 years. Early case histories were often fatal, with a term survival rate of less than 10 percent.[48] When used as the sole therapeutic agent, corticosteroid therapy is ineffective; however, corticosteroids in combination with other agents appear to have a greater efficacy. Splenectomy is considered in patients who fail to respond to other therapies. The majority of patients undergoing splenectomy have also received corticosteroids and blood products with an increase in response rate. Antiplatelet drugs such as aspirin, dipyridamole, dextran, and sulfinpyrazone have been used. Often these antiplatelet drugs are used in variable combinations, making their efficacy difficult to evaluate. Therapy involving dextran may be somewhat beneficial. Plasma exchange and the infusion of large amounts of plasma have met with a variable degree of success and are currently being used as the treatment of choice. Heparin therapy is discouraged because of its associated toxicity. Immunosuppressive drugs such as vincristine[49] have been used, as well as intravenous synthetic prostacyclin.[50] Both have been reported to induce remission. Most often, patients with TTP are treated by a combination of therapeutic modalities.

Hemolytic Uremic Syndrome. Hemolytic uremic syndrome is characterized clinically by microangiopathic hemolytic anemia, thrombocytopenia, and renal failure (**see Color Plate 124**). Renal vascular damage may initiate intravascular hemolysis with subsequent red cell ADP and platelet membrane phospholipid release. Renal damage may also promote coagulant activity, resulting in fibrin deposition and endothelial damage but no consumption of clotting factors.

Hemolytic uremic syndrome may clinically resemble TTP, but there is a difference in the age of the patients affected. Hemolytic uremic syndrome occurs primarily in children but has also been reported in adults. In women, HUS may occur with complications during pregnancy and childbirth. The prognosis in adults is more often worse than that of children with higher mortality rates and permanent renal damage. Following viral and bacterial infections HUS takes a mild course. The pathologic thrombi in HUS are almost always limited to the glomerular capillaries and afferent arterioles of the

Table 26–4. **COMPARISON OF TTP AND HUS**

Characteristics	TTP	HUS
Epidemiology		
Age	40 years — peak incidence	Childhood
Sex predilection	Female	Equal
Organ Involvement	Multiple	Limited to kidney
Hematologic		
Microangiopathic hemolytic anemia	Severe	Severe
Thrombocytopenia	Severe	Moderate
Neurologic	Common, severe	Uncommon, less severe
Renal Failure	Uncommon, mild	Common, severe

kidney. Fever, hypertension, and renal failure are common symptoms, whereas neurologic manifestations are less severe and less common. Severe neurologic problems or evidence of systemic thrombi are more likely to suggest the diagnosis of TTP (see Table 26–4). Following an infection HUS is generally less severe than the hereditary form, which is associated with a rather unfavorable prognosis.

Therapeutic management of HUS is usually conservative. Supportive therapy may include hemodialysis, antihypertensive therapy, anticoagulants, blood transfusions, antiplatelet drugs, steroids, and fibrinolytic agents.

Respiratory Distress Syndrome. This syndrome is characterized by excessive fibrin deposition localized in the lung of infants considered to be at high risk for this disorder. The fibrinolytic response is absent in these infants.

Severe cases of multiple trauma are also associated with pulmonary dysfunction, or adult respiratory distress syndrome subsequent to pulmonary vascular obstruction and numerous thrombi.

Heparin Therapy. Thrombocytopenia is a frequently observed complication of heparin therapy. Heparin administered intravenously has been reported to cause an immediate mild transient thrombocytopenia that reverses within 1 to 2 hours.[51] A mild to severe persistent thrombocytopenia may also occur, usually within 2 weeks of heparin therapy. Recovery from heparin-induced thrombocytopenia is not like that of drug immune purpura. Prior administration of heparin does not affect the frequency of developing thrombocytopenia. Mild persistent thrombocytopenia usually subsides within 1 to 5 days, or does not worsen, even during continued therapy. In severe persistent thrombocytopenia, platelet levels may return to normal within 1 to 10 days after stopping therapy, or may return to normal when heparin dosage is reduced. Thrombocytopenia seems to occur more often in patients given bovine heparin, as compared with porcine heparin. Thromboembolic complications may also occur with heparin therapy. Whether heparin-induced thrombocytopenia is an immune-mediated process is still uncertain. Complement-mediated platelet destruction brought about by an antibody to heparin has been reported in cases of severe persistent thrombocytopenia.[52]

Disseminated Intravascular Coagulation (Color Plates 257 and 258). A syndrome that results in the pathologic formation of thrombin and plasmin, DIC presents with clinical manifestations of hemorrhage and thrombosis. There is a significant thrombocytopenia seen in DIC as a result of increased platelet consumption. The hemorrhagic diathesis is attributed to the consumption of platelets coagulation factors, and increased fibrinolytic activity. In Chapter 28, DIC is discussed in greater detail.

Thrombocytopenia in Pregnancy. Various alterations in hemostasis have been seen in the obstetric population during pregnancy, the birthing process, and the postpartum period. Abruptio placentae and amniotic fluid embolism are generally associated with forms of acute intravascular coagulation leading to the consumption of plasma clotting factors. In pre-eclampsia and eclampsia, thrombocytopenia occurs as a result of platelet consumption. The nature of the mechanism for the associated thrombocytopenia is not clearly understood, but abnormal platelet to endothelial interaction has been reported.

Increased peripheral utilization and destruction of platelets resulting in thrombocytopenia is associated with various inherited and acquired disorders. Some mechanisms of platelet destruction are immune-mediated as in ITP, whereas increased platelet utilization such as in DIC and TTP is generally considered to be non–immune-mediated (see section on immunologic and nonimmunologic thrombocytopenia). Bone marrow examination of the patient shows a normal to increased number of megakaryocytes.

Clinically, thrombocytopenia is seen quite often as a symptom of an underlying disorder. Thrombocytopenic purpura is a common cause of bleeding resulting from thrombocytopenia. The hemorrhagic episodes associated with thrombocytopenia tend to be variable with mucocutaneous petechiae and ecchymoses as presenting features. Spontaneous bleeds do not occur unless the platelet count drops below $50,000/\mu l$. Serious bleeding complications such as epistaxis, gingival bleeds, menorrhagia, genitourinary, gastrointestinal, and intracranial bleeds are seen when the platelet count falls below 10,000 to $20,000/\mu l$.

Physical examination and family history are important to evaluate and properly manage the patient with thrombocytopenia. Patients with a positive history of bleeding require a different rationale to therapy than those patients with an underlying disease such as leukemia or prior exposure to viral infections.

Platelet transfusions are often effective when used to treat thrombocytopenia resulting from decreased platelet production. Transfusion brings about the increase in platelet count and controls the hemorrhage. The risk associated with repeated platelet transfusion is that of alloimmunization, causing decreased platelet survival and a decreased rise in the platelet count. Once patients become alloimmunized, the use of single-donor HLA-matched platelets have been associated with a better response.

The rationale for management of patients with thrombocytopenia as a result of increased destruction or utilization is somewhat more complex. Immune-mediated mechanisms are generally responsible for increased platelet destruction, as seen in ITP. The survival of transfused platelets in such patients is relatively short, and their use should be limited to life-threatening hemorrhages. Corticosteroids, splenectomy, plasma exchange, and immunosuppressive drugs have all been tried in an attempt to ameliorate the thrombocytopenia (see section on ITP for further discussion). In patients with TTP or DIC, in whom thrombocytopenia occurs as a result of increased platelet utilization from an underlying pathology, treatment involves a number of different therapeutic modalities.

Splenectomy was first used to treat thrombocytopenia in 1916. Now it is used to treat chronic ITP refractory to steroid therapy with partial or complete remission seen in approximately 40 to 80 percent of patients and in hematologic disorders associated with hypersplenism. Children are at increased risk of infection, particularly pneumococcus; therefore splenectomy may be contraindicated in this age group. When splenectomy is performed for states of hypersplenism, an associated rise in platelet count is not always observed.

Immunologic Thrombocytopenia

This group of thrombocytopenias all have an immune-mediated mechanism by which there is increased platelet sequestration and destruction.

Idiopathic Thrombocytopenic Purpura. This is one of the most common causes of thrombocytopenia as a result of immune-mediated platelet destruction. A clinical syndrome characterized by thrombocytopenia, ITP may arise by several different mechanisms or may have no known etiologic factor. The diagnosis of ITP is made by exclusion; the disease may occur in acute, chronic, or recurrent form.

Acute ITP occurs predominantly in young children, in the 2- to 5-year age group with no predilection for either sex. In as many as 84 percent of the cases, thrombocytopenia develops within 1 to 3 weeks following an acute viral illness.[53] The onset of bleeding is usually abrupt with initial platelet counts of less than 20,000/μl. This disorder is usually self-limiting and spontaneous remissions, with or without therapy, occur in a large majority of these patients (Table 26–5). Spontaneous remission rarely occurs after 1 year of onset. Patients who do not remit within 6 months are generally considered to have chronic ITP.

The bone marrow is characterized by megakaryocytic hyperplasia (**see Color Plate 246**), and young, abnormally large platelets with variation in shape are seen on the peripheral blood smear. Platelet lifespan is decreased.

Cases of acute ITP may range from mild to severe, with manifestations of scattered petechiae (**see Color Plates 245 and 248**) in milder cases and gastro-

intestinal bleeds, hematuria, retinal hemorrhage, and generalized purpura in more severe cases. Of all cases of ITP 3 to 4 percent are severe, with about one fourth to one half of these patients at risk for life-threatening intracranial hemorrhage. This complication accounts for the 1 to 2 percent morbidity for patients with acute ITP.[54]

Platelet-associated IgG (PAIgG)[55] and other platelet-associated proteins are increased in cases of acute ITP. In general, elevations of these platelet-associated proteins are a nonspecific consequence of platelet destruction. Platelets in acute ITP are thought to be destroyed by immune complexes or foreign antigens adsorbed by platelets following an infection. Serologic studies in cases of acute ITP are generally not considered diagnostic.

Most patients with acute ITP do not require treatment. Their clinical manifestations are mild, and spontaneous remissions are the general rule. Therapy is used in serious cases of ITP and may include intravenous gamma globulin, splenectomy, platelet transfusion, corticosteroids, plasma exchange, and immunosuppressive drugs. Intravenous gamma globulin (IVIgG) appears to be effective in most cases of childhood acute ITP when bleeding is rather severe. Splenectomy is considered for life-threatening intracranial hemorrhages. Splenectomy removes the primary site of platelet destruction and antibody production. Complications of sepsis in children with acute ITP have been reported following splenectomy. Corticosteroid therapy is considered ineffective in most cases of acute ITP. The shortened lifespan of transfused platelets makes their use effective only as a means of treating a severe hemorrhage. Plasma exchange appears to be more effective in treating acute ITP than chronic ITP.

Chronic ITP is most common in adults, 20 to 50 years of age, with a greater predilection for women between the ages of 20 and 50. The onset of bleeding is generally insidious, with variable platelet counts. Chronic ITP is characterized by a variable clinical course. Bleeding manifestations such as menorrhagia, recurrent epistaxis, or easy bruisability may persist for a few days or weeks with intermittent asymptomatic periods. Spontaneous remissions, as seen in acute ITP, are uncommon and no known associated findings can be attributed to the thrombocytopenia.

In chronic ITP, the bone marrow is characterized by megakaryocytic hyperplasia, as in the acute form

Table 26–5. **COMPARISON OF ACUTE AND CHRONIC ITP**

Characteristics	Acute	Chronic
Age of onset	Childhood	20–50 yr; females over males (2:1 to 3:1)
Previous infection	Common	Usually not associated
Platelet count	≤20,000/μl	Variable; 30,000–80,000/μl
Bleeding	Abrupt	Insidious
Duration of thrombocytopenia	Few weeks	Months to years
Spontaneous remissions	Occurs in majority of patients	Relatively rare

of ITP. Circulating platelets are young, as platelet lifespan is shortened, and appear more effective at maintaining hemostasis.

The differential diagnosis between acute and chronic ITP is not always possible at the onset, but platelet counts are usually lower in acute than in chronic ITP. Acute ITP and chronic ITP also differ in age of onset, prior infection, duration of thrombocytopenia, and method and response to therapy (see Table 26–5). Chronic ITP must also be differentiated from ITP-like syndromes. The diagnosis of ITP is always one of exclusion.

In some patients with chronic ITP, antiplatelet antibodies have been shown to react with specific platelet membrane glycoproteins, thus favoring the possibility of an immune mechanism involved in platelet sensitization.[56,57] Various methods have shown that PAIgG is elevated in thrombocytopenic patients with chronic ITP and that there is an inverse relationship between PAIgG levels and platelet counts.[58] Although a number of laboratory tests have been shown to detect antiplatelet antibodies, no established criteria for the laboratory diagnosis of ITP has yet been set forth.

In patients with chronic ITP, thrombocytopenia results from the destruction of platelets primarily through splenic sequestration rather than platelet lysis in circulation. Splenectomy and corticosteroids are the conventional therapies used to treat patients with chronic ITP. Patients with chronic ITP are initially treated with corticosteroids. Corticosteroids are thought to suppress splenic sequestration of moderately sensitized platelets, thereby increasing the platelet lifespan and ameliorating the thrombocytopenia. The aim of therapy is to give an initial dose of prednisone sufficient to obtain a satisfactory increase in the platelet count, and to reduce the dosage to a level that maintains the platelet count at hemostatic levels. Approximately 70 to 90 percent of patients treated respond favorably to steroids.[59]

Splenectomy is the treatment of choice for chronic ITP refractory to steroid therapy. Significant improvement following splenectomy is obtained in 70 to 90 percent of patients.[60] The benefit from splenectomy results from the removal of the organ responsible for the sequestration of moderately sensitized platelets. Splenectomy may be contraindicated in ITP in certain circumstances. Other, less frequently employed therapies used to treat chronic ITP include such drugs as vincristine, danazol, colchicine, immunosuppressive agents, plasma exchange, IVIgG, and epsilon aminocaproic acid (EACA).

A recurrent form of ITP also occurs, characterized by alternating intervals of thrombocytopenia and periods in which the platelet count is normal. This recurrent form is seen in children and adults.

Secondary Immune Thrombocytopenia. Lymphoproliferative disorders such as Hodgkin's disease and non-Hodgkin's lymphoma have been reported with an ITP-like thrombocytopenia associated with decreased platelet survival and increased PAIgG levels.[61] Chronic lymphocytic leukemia (CLL) is also associated with an ITP-like thrombocytopenia. In SLE, roughly 14 percent of the patients develop thrombocytopenia resembling ITP during the course of the disease. Thrombocytopenic purpura is often the presenting sign, preceding the other clinical manifestations of the disease. Bleeding in SLE due to thrombocytopenia responds well to corticosteroid therapy. Qualitative tests for antiplatelet antibodies and tests for PAIgG frequently are positive in disorders associated with immune-mediated thrombocytopenia.

Thrombocytopenia as a result of viral, bacterial, or parasitic infections has been well documented. An immunologic mechanism appears likely in the development of thrombocytopenia as a result of infection. Viral infections such as mumps and rubeola may be complicated by severe thrombocytopenia. As many as 25 percent of patients with human immunodeficiency virus-1 (HIV-1) infection present with thrombocytopenia during the course of the disease. Elevations in platelet-bound IgG and complement, as well as increases in serum immune complexes, have been documented;[62] however, little correlation exists between the degree of thrombocytopenia and the level of platelet-bound IgG.[63]

Bone marrow abnormalities seen in those with HIV-1 infection may also result in thrombocytopenia.[62] In patients with bacterial sepsis, thrombocytopenia is usually present with or without DIC. Malaria is frequently associated with thrombocytopenia as a result of increased destruction and splenic sequestration.

Drug-Induced Immune Thrombocytopenia. Quinine-induced thrombocytopenia was observed as early as 1928. It was noted that after discontinuing quinine therapy and after an initial recovery, thrombocytopenia could again be induced upon readministering the drug.[64] The drug appears to act as a hapten, eliciting an antibody response when complexed with a larger carrier molecule. The antibody-drug-platelet complex leads to thrombocytopenia. Antibody combining with drug appears to be the initial step in the formation of the complex. Cellular binding or adsorption of the antibody-drug complex to the platelet membrane results in platelet injury and splenic sequestration.

The list of drugs that can cause immune drug purpura is rather extensive. A few of the drugs most frequently implicated are quinine, quinidine, digitoxin, gold, thiazides, salicylates, and the various sulfa drugs.

Drug immune purpura appears to occur more frequently in the elderly population as a result of their increased usage of medication; however, cases have been reported in children and young adults. Purpura occurs approximately 7 days after first-time use of the drug but may occur within 3 to 5 days as in an anamnestic response on reexposure to the drug. It is estimated that 1 in 100,000 drug users per year will require hospitalization as a result of a drug-induced blood disorder.[65] The frequency for users of quinine and quinidine is roughly 1 in 1000.[65] The disorder is generally self-limiting, as the platelet count returns to normal once the drug has been removed from circulation. Readministration of a drug known to cause purpura should be avoided.

Several serologic techniques are used to detect drug-induced platelet antibodies such as platelet agglutination, complement fixation, platelet aggregation, inhibition of clot retraction, and platelet release of granular contents.

Post-transfusion Purpura. In this disorder, sudden onset of thrombocytopenia occurs 1 week after transfusion of blood or blood products containing platelets (**see Color Plate 249**). It is believed that post-transfusion purpura (PTP) results from an anamnestic response. In the cases that have been studied thus far, the antibody present in the patients sera has been directed against the platelet antigen PlA[1].[66] This antigen is found in approximately 97 percent of the normal population; the 3 percent of people who lack the PlA[1] antigen on their platelets are considered at risk for developing PTP. Most reported cases have been in middle-aged women who have had children. It is believed that primary immunization occurs in pregnancy; PlA[1]-positive fetal platelets sensitize a PlA[1]-negative mother (see section on isoimmune neonatal thrombocytopenia). Other mechanisms for the development of PTP have been suggested.[67]

Complement fixation and release of ^{51}Cr or ^{14}C-serotonin are some of the reliable laboratory tests used to detect and measure anti-PlA[1] antibodies in PTP. Currently direct and indirect laboratory tests have been developed to increase specificity and sensitivity in the detection of platelet antibodies. These tests employ some of the following techniques: enzyme-linked immunosorbent assay (ELISA), Western blot followed by ELISA or radioimmunoassay (RIA), platelet suspension immunofluorescence, and immunoprecipitation of radiolabeled GPIIa. To confirm the presence of a platelet-specific antibody, a panel with PlA[1]-positive cells should be run. The patient's platelets should also be phenotyped. In some cases of PTP, isosensitization to HLA antigens found on platelets occurs along with the appearance of platelet-specific antigens other than PlA[1],[68] making serologic typing difficult.

Exchange transfusion and the use of IVIgG have been effective means in treating the hemorrhagic complications associated with PTP. There have been a number of cases in which patients have had repeated episodes of PTP following reexposure to PlA[1]-positive blood.[69] PlA[1]-negative blood is indicated for all subsequent transfusions when possible, as all patients are considered at risk for recurrence of PTP.

Isoimmune Neonatal Thrombocytopenia. Similar to the pathogenesis of erythroblastosis fetalis, isoimmune neonatal thrombocytopenia results from immunization of the mother by fetal platelet antigens and placental transfer of maternal antibody. The PlA[1] antigen is most often associated with isoimmune neonatal thrombocytopenia and is con-

sidered to be strongly immunogenic. It is an uncommon disorder, generally affecting the first-born child. Based on gene frequency of the PlA[1] antigen in fathers, there is a high probability that a PlA[1]-negative mother will have a PlA[1]-positive child. Once isoimmune neonatal thrombocytopenia has developed, there appears to be an increased risk of the next child being affected, as most fathers are PlA[1]-homozygous.

A large percentage of PlA[1]-negative mothers give birth to an affected child that is phenotype-positive for the HLA-B8 antigen. It has been suggested that the HLA-B8 antigen serves to protect from immunization, which accounts for the relatively low incidence of isoimmune neonatal thrombocytopenia, despite the frequency of the PlA[1] antigen and the chance for maternal sensitization. ABO incompatibility and its relation to symptomatic isoimmune neonatal thrombocytopenia is unclear.

Infants who develop isoimmune neonatal thrombocytopenia appear normal at birth but within hours develop scattered petechiae and purpuric hemorrhages, with platelet counts below 30,000/μl. Intracranial hemorrhage is the primary cause of mortality in these infants.

Therapy is aimed at preventing intracranial hemorrhage and keeping platelet counts at hemostatically safe levels. Cesarean delivery is recommended to prevent birth trauma, thereby eliminating the potential for intracranial bleeds. Corticosteroids and IVIgG have recently been used as antenatal treatment. Postnatal treatment is not necessary as long as the infant remains asymptomatic and the platelet count stays above 30,000/μl. Characteristically, in this disorder the platelet count begins to decrease shortly after birth, reaching low levels several hours later. When the infant manifests clinical signs of bleeding and the platelet count falls below 10,000/μl, compatible platelet transfusion utilizing maternal platelets or PlA[1]-negative donor platelets are used. An effective hemostatic response is almost always seen when transfused platelets are compatible with maternal antibody.

Thrombocytosis

Increases in platelet counts indicate increased platelet production or proliferation of megakaryocytes. Thrombocytosis implies a moderate increase in platelet counts; however, counts of 500,000 to 1,000,000/μl may also be seen. Thrombocytosis may result from reactive transient stimuli to the bone marrow or may be associated with an underlying malignancy (Table 26–6).

Thrombocytosis Associated with Myeloproliferative Syndromes

The myeloproliferative syndromes, characterized by the autonomous proliferation of a pluripotent stem cell, are associated with thrombocytosis. Bleeding, thrombosis, platelet defects, and increases in platelet counts are seen in association with all the myeloproliferative syndromes. Essential thrombocythemia has platelet counts that often

Table 26-6. **CAUSES OF THROMBOCYTOSIS**

Myeloproliferative syndromes
    Essential thrombocythemia
    Polycythemia vera
    Agnogenic myeloid metaplasia
    Chronic myelocytic leukemia
Secondary (reactive) thrombocytosis
    Postsplenectomy
    Postoperative
    Acute blood loss
    Epinephrine
    Bone marrow recovery
        Vitamin B_{12} therapy
        Folic acid therapy
        Drug-induced thrombocytopenia
        Chemotherapy
    Iron-deficiency anemia
    Malignancy
        Hodgkin's disease
        Carcinoma
        Osteogenic sarcoma
    Chronic infections
        Osteomyelitis
        Tuberculosis
    Chronic inflammation
        Inflammatory bowel disease
        Collagen vascular disease

exceed 1 million/μl. Polycythemia vera and agnogenic myeloid metaplasia are also associated with thrombocytosis. Based on observations of patients with reactive thrombocytosis and normal platelet function in which bleeding and thrombotic complications are uncommon, thrombocytosis alone is not the sole factor in the development of bleeding and thrombosis in the myeloproliferative syndromes. These complications are suggested to result from qualitative platelet defects. (The MPDs as they relate to specific platelet defects, are further discussed in the section on acquired platelet defects, and Chapter 21.)

Reactive Transient Thrombocytosis

Thrombocytosis is seen following splenectomy. Within the first 2 weeks after surgery, platelet levels rise, returning to normal over a period of months after splenectomy. Platelet counts may increase as much as two to six times preoperative levels. Platelet survival has been documented to be normal. It has been suggested that the thrombocytosis seen after splenectomy is due to increased platelet production, as elimination of the splenic pool can account for no more than a 50 percent rise in the platelet count.[70] Regulation of thrombopoiesis is thought to be moderated by a humoral factor produced by the spleen. Thrombocytosis is also observed postoperatively as well. The nature of the mechanism is not clearly understood; however, hypoxia during anesthesia may be a cause.

Thrombocytosis is a common finding associated with acute hemorrhage. The platelet count is generally elevated within a day or so after hemorrhage as a result of increased marrow stimulation. Similar responses may be seen following therapeutic phlebotomy for PV.

Iron-deficiency anemia has classically been associated with thrombocytosis. Thrombocytosis is also associated with underlying malignancy and chronic inflammatory or infectious processes. In iron-deficiency anemia, the increased platelet count usually occurs in the initial stages of the disease. The process by which the platelet count increases in these disorders is poorly understood.

Patients with reactive thrombocytosis have elevated platelet counts as well. Bleeding and thrombosis are uncommon; platelet function is normal. Increased numbers of megakaryocytes are found in the marrow.

Administration of epinephrine will cause a transient thrombocytosis caused by platelet release from the spleen. Other causes of thrombocytosis are listed in Table 26-6.

VASCULAR DISORDERS

Because the hereditary and acquired vascular disorders are quite variable, the clinical manifestations also vary. The most common clinical and diagnostic finding of vascular disorders are petechiae and purpura (Table 26-7).

Inherited Vascular Disorders

Hereditary Hemorrhagic Telangiectasia (Osler-Weber-Rendu Disease)

This rather common disorder is inherited as an autosomal dominant trait. The classic telangiectatic lesions usually do not appear until the second or third decade of life and may be pinpoint, nodular, or

Table 26-7. **VASCULAR DISORDERS ASSOCIATED WITH BLEEDING**

Hereditary vascular disorders
    Hereditary hemorrhagic telangiectasia
    Ehlers-Danlos syndrome
    Marfan's syndrome
    Osteogenesis imperfecta
    Giant hemangioma
Acquired vascular disorders
    Paraproteinemias
    Amyloidosis
    Autoimmune disorders
    Henoch-Schönlein purpura
    Cushing's syndrome
    Diabetes mellitus
    Senile purpura
    Steroid purpura
    Drug ingestion
    Psychogenic purpura

spiderlike in appearance. They occur predominantly on the mucous membranes of the skin and sublingual and buccal areas. Bleeding in childhood is rare and does not appear until later in life. Hereditary hemorrhagic telangiectasia manifests as recurrent and severe epistaxis and gastrointestinal bleeds from telangiectatic lesions. The classic diagnostic triad is (1) an inherited trait, (2) presence of telangiectasia, and (3) bleeding from telangiectatic lesions. Coagulation test results, bleeding time, and platelet counts are usually normal. Therapy is directed at controlling localized epistaxis.

Ehlers-Danlos Syndrome

This syndrome is characterized by extreme vascular fragility, skin fragility, and hyperextensible joints. A rare connective tissue disorder, it is inherited as an autosomal dominant trait. Bleeding may clinically manifest as a result of increased fragility of subcutaneous vessels and is variable. Petechiae, purpura, and gastrointestinal and gingival bleeds are often present. Abnormal laboratory tests include prolonged bleeding time and a positive Rumpel-Leede tourniquet test. Abnormal platelet aggregation and adhesion has been described in association with this syndrome.

Marfan's Syndrome

This disorder is an inherited autosomal dominant trait characterized by skeletal and ocular defects, and cardiovascular abnormalities such as dissecting aneurysms. This vascular disorder is associated with abnormal collagen formation. Patients exhibit easy bruising and may bleed excessively during surgical procedures. Coagulation tests are usually normal. Poorly characterized platelet defects have been reported.

Pseudoxanthoma Elasticum

This very rare disorder, inherited as an autosomal recessive trait, is characterized by significant hemorrhages in which the elastic fibers of the entire arterial system are abnormal. Patients present with easy bruising and may develop life-threatening gastrointestinal bleeds. Intra-articular bleeds with hemarthrosis are common. Thrombosis affecting major arteries of the limbs may also be present.

Osteogenesis Imperfecta

This disorder is inherited as an autosomal dominant trait in which there is defective bone matrix. Easy and spontaneous bleeding, epistaxis, hemoptysis, and intracranial hemorrhages are associated with this disorder.

Giant Hemangiomas

This syndrome, characterized by tumorous masses composed of thin-walled blood vessels commonly found in the skin and subcutaneous tissue, is generally present at birth. The hemangiomatous lesions may be widespread, involving a single organ or multiple organs. The majority of patients present with chronic DIC, which may become acute. Treatments consist of surgical removal or radiation therapy in uncomplicated cases.

Acquired Vascular Disorders

The acquired vascular disorders are by far more common than the hereditary disorders previously discussed. Hemorrhagic and thrombotic tendencies manifest by petechiae, purpura, and thrombosis in the appropriate clinical setting characterize the acquired vascular disorders.

Paraproteinemia and Amyloidosis

Patients with paraprotein disorder and amyloidosis often develop a diffuse vascular disease with associated hemorrhage and thrombosis. It is believed that increased levels of complement-fixing immunoglobulins (IgM, IgG) cause release of histamine, platelet aggregation, and leukocyte chemotaxis, thereby increasing vascular permeability and small vein thrombosis. The associated hyperviscosity syndrome causes stasis and ischemia, which increases vascular permeability resulting in epistaxis, purpura, and petechiae, as well as organ hemorrhage. Patients with malignant paraproteins often have DIC due to endothelial damage.

In primary amyloidosis, hemorrhage is the classic hallmark as a result of deposition of amyloid on the endothelium. Petechiae, purpura, ecchymosis, easy bruisability, and spontaneous hemorrhages into organs are characteristic. In secondary amyloidosis, hemorrhagic as well as thrombotic tendencies are noted as a result of amyloid deposits along the endothelium as well as perivascular infiltration. The bleeding in amyloidosis is thought to be due to perivascular infiltration. Platelet function may be abnormal; rarely patients present with thrombocytopenia. A deficiency of factor X and other factors has been reported.[71] It is believed that factor X binds to the amyloid deposits. Amyloid purpura can be seen in **Color Plate 238** showing the characteristic periorbital distribution.

Autoimmune Disorders

Disorders associated with circulating immune complexes are associated with a diffuse vasculitis and hemorrhagic and thrombotic tendencies. Most often the circulating immune complexes attach to the endothelium, whereby they fix complement causing chemotaxis of leukocytes, increased vascular permeability, fibrin deposition, and vascular damage. A specific antibody directed against the endothelium is a rare mechanism of autoimmune induced vasculitis and is limited to the allergic purpuras such as Henoch-Schönlein purpura. **Color Plate 252** demonstrates this type of purpuric lesion located on the foot.

Infections

Many bacterial, viral, rickettsial, or protozoal infections have an associated vasculitis with hemorrhagic and thrombotic tendencies. Vascular damage occurs from the deposition of immune complexes

Table 26–8. **COMMON DRUGS THAT CAUSE VASCULITIS**

Aspirin	Digoxin	Methyldopa
Allopurinol	Estrogens	Penicillin
Atropine	Furosemide	Phenacetin
Belladonna	Indomethacin	Quinine
Chloramphenicol	Iodine	Quinidine
Chloral hydrate	Isoniazide	Sulfonamides
Coumarin	Meprobromate	Tolbutamide

within the vessel walls following infection or by endotoxin production. Characteristically, purpura develops symmetrically on the buttocks and posterior thighs. Diphtheria, septicemia from meningococcus or streptococcus, smallpox, measles, Rocky Mountain spotted fever, and malaria are infections commonly associated with purpura.

Drugs

Drug-induced vasculitis is a common cause of acquired vascular defects. An allergic mechanism has been described. Table 26–8 lists some of the drugs implicated in causing purpura in the face of a normal platelet count.

Psychogenic Purpura

This disorder is predominantly seen in middle-aged women with a positive psychiatric history and manifests by spontaneous painful ecchymoses. Characteristically, the ecchymoses are confined to the limbs, rarely affecting the trunk. The purpuric lesions are believed to develop from subcutaneous extravasation of red cells as a result of injury to the skin.[72]

Protein C Deficiency

During oral anticoagulant therapy, levels of protein C rapidly decline. It is believed that protein C may play a role in the development of the purpuric skin necrosis associated with this therapy.[73]

Miscellaneous Disorders

Malignant hypertension, diabetes mellitus, Cushing's disease, eclampsia, and senile purpura are disorders that cause vascular damage with increased vascular permeability and fibrin deposition. Ecchymoses, purpura, and a marked increase of thrombosis are common clinical manifestations seen in these disorders. In senile purpura (**see Color Plate 253**), in persons receiving prolonged corticosteroid therapy (**see Color Plate 254**), or in patients with Cushing's disease, purpura of the hands and forearms is common.

Table 26–9 summarizes the various qualitative and quantitative platelet and vascular disorders discussed.

Table 26–9. **PLATELET AND VASCULAR DISORDERS**

Disorder	Pathogenesis	Clinical	Laboratory
Platelet Disorders			
Alport's syndrome	Hereditary nephritis and deafness	Mild epistaxis; occasionally fatal CNS bleeding	Thrombocytopenia; giant platelets BT—abnormal Platelet aggregation—may be abnormal, often normal PF 3 release—may be abnormal
Bernard-Soulier syndrome (autosomal recessive)	Lack of glycoprotein Ib; platelets do not bind factors V, XI	Rather severe hemorrhagic diathesis	Thrombocytopenia; giant atypical platelets Platelet retention—abnormal Platelet adhesion—abnormal Ristocetin agglutination—abnormal Platelet aggregation—normal
Chédiak-Higashi syndrome (autosomal recessive)	Storage pool deficiency; large organelles, some with acid phosphatase	Increased susceptibility to pyogenic infections	BT—abnormal Platelet adhesion—abnormal Platelet aggregation—abnormal
Cyclo-oxygenase deficiency (inheritance undetermined)	Inability to activate prostaglandin pathway; aspirinlike defect	Moderate bleeding tendency Ecchymoses	BT—abnormal Platelet aggregation—abnormal
Essential athrombia		Mucosal bleeding Easy bruising	BT—abnormal Platelet count—normal Platelet aggregation—abnormal

(continued)

Table 26–9. **PLATELET AND VASCULAR DISORDERS** (*Continued*)

Disorder	Pathogenesis	Clinical	Laboratory
Fanconi's syndrome (autosomal recessive)	Inborn error of metabolism; megakaryocytic hypoplasia	Pancytopenia; dwarfism; microcephaly; hypogenitalism; strabismus; mental retardation; micro-ophthalmia; splenic atrophy; anomalies of thumbs, radial bones, kidneys	Thrombocytopenia
Glanzmann's thrombasthenia	Lack of glycoproteins IIb, IIIa	Severe bleeding—purpuric with spontaneous mucosal and cutaneous bleeding aggravated by trauma; occasional hemarthrosis; severity decreases with age	BT—abnormal Clot retraction—none Platelet adhesion—abnormal Platelet count—generally normal Platelet aggregation—abnormal Ristocetin agglutination—normal
Glycogen storage disease, type I (autosomal recessive?)	Storage pool deficiency; G6PD deficiency	Mild bleeding; corrects with treatment for enzyme deficiency	BT—abnormal Platelet aggregation—abnormal PF 3 activity—abnormal
Gray platelet syndrome (autosomal recessive?)	Storage pool deficiency; absence of alpha-granules; platelets appear amorphous; large platelets		BT—abnormal Platelet adhesion—abnormal Platelet aggregation—abnormal Thrombocytopenia
Hermansky-Pudlak syndrome (autosomal recessive)	Storage pool deficiency; absence of dense bodies	Oculocutaneous albinism Ceroidlike pigment in macrophages	BT—abnormal Platelet aggregation—abnormal Platelet adhesion—abnormal
May-Hegglin (autosomal dominant)	Ineffective thrombopoiesis	Giant platelets; Döhle bodies; generally asymptomatic; possible severe bleeding	Thrombocytopenia BT—abnormal
TAR baby syndrome (thrombocytopenia with absent radii) (autosomal recessive)	Storage pool deficiency; megakaryocytic hypoplasia	Skeletal, renal, and cardiac malformations; decreased dense bodies	BT—abnormal Platelet aggregation—abnormal
Thrombocythemia (essential/primary)		Associated with myeloproliferative disorders—polycythemia rubra vera, myeloid metaplasia, CML	Platelet count—high, may be >1,000,000/μl Large platelets Platelet retention—abnormal Platelet aggregation—abnormal BT—abnormal
Von Willebrand disease (autosomal dominant)	Low levels of plasma cofactor (VIII:vWF).	Variable clinical symptoms—may bleed; generally vascular and mucosal bleeding; severity depends on factor VIII levels	Lab testing variable BT—abnormal Platelet retention—abnormal Platelet aggregation—normal Ristocetin agglutination—abnormal VIII vWF: Ag—abnormal VIII—abnormal
Wiskott-Aldrich syndrome (sex-linked recessive)	Storage pool deficiency; immunologic disorders—B and T cell dysfunction; isohemagglutinins absent	Recurrent pyogenic infection; eczema; increased lymphoreticular malignancies; very small platelets; decreased or absent dense bodies; Mild-moderate bleeding—mucocutaneous bleeding, epistaxis, easy bruising	Thrombocytopenia—severe Shortened survival BT—abnormal Platelet aggregation—abnormal IgM—low IgG, IgA—normal

Table 26–9. **PLATELET AND VASCULAR DISORDERS (Continued)**

Disorder	Pathogenesis	Clinical	Laboratory
Hereditary hemorrhagic telangiectasia (Osler-Weber-Rendu) (autosomal dominant; most common vascular disorder associated with hemorrhagic diathesis)	Large capillaries; elastic fibers possibly missing; pinpoint, nodular, or spiderlike telangiectatic lesions in adults	Epistaxis in childhood; mucocutaneous bleeding; associated classic DIC-type syndrome	BT—normal or abnormal Tourniquet test—often abnormal Normal platelet function test results
Marfan's syndrome (autosomal dominant)	Collagen vascular disorder; skeletal defects—long extremities, arachnodactylia, "Lincolnesque" features; Cardiovascular abnormalities—diffuse or descending aortic aneurysm; ocular defects	Easy bruising	Large platelets Platelet adhesion—abnormal Platelet aggregation—abnormal
Osteogenesis imperfecta (autosomal dominant)	Collagen vascular disorder; brittle bone disease—lack of bone matrix; blue sclera	Skin and subcutaneous hemorrhages; easy bruising; epistaxis	BT—abnormal Tourniquet test—abnormal Platelet adhesion—abnormal Platelet aggregation—abnormal
Pseudoxanthoma elasticum (autosomal recessive; rare)	Abnormal elastic fibers throughout arterial system	Significant hemorrhage; easy, spontaneous bruising; petechiae; purpura; marked predisposition to thrombosis	
Homocystinuria (autosomal recessive)	Cystathione synthetase deficiency	Occasional mild bleeding; usually arterial and venous thrombosis	Possibly short platelet survival; unknown effect on platelet function
Kasabach-Merritt syndrome	Giant cavernous hemangioma	Mild bleeding at site of hemangioma; diffuse bleeding in association with DIC	Thrombocytopenia; low fibrinogen; high plasma fibrinopeptide A and FDP

Source: From Pittiglio, DH: Treating hemostatic disorders. A problem-oriented approach. In Hemostasis Overview. American Association of Blood Banks, Arlington, VA, 1984, pp. 19, 22.

BT = bleeding time.

REFERENCES

1. Nurden, AT, George, JN, and Phillips, DR: Human platelet membrane glycoproteins: Their structure, function and biological significance. In Phillips, DR and Shuman, MA: The Biology of Platelets. Academic Press, New York, 1986, p 159.
2. Ruggeri, ZM, et al: Platelets have more than one binding site for von Willebrand factor. J Clin Invest 72:1, 1983.
3. White, JG and Gerrard, JM: Ultrastructure features of abnormal platelets. Am J Pathol 85:590, 1976.
4. Weiss, HJ, et al: Decreased adhesion of giant (Bernard-Soulier) platelets to subendothelium: Further implications on the role of the von Willebrand factor in hemostasis. Am J Med 57:920, 1974.
5. George, JN and Reimann, TA: Inherited disorders of the platelet membrane: Glanzmanns thrombasthenia and Bernard-Soulier disease. In Coleman, RW, et al: Hemostasis and Thrombosis. JB Lippincott, Philadelphia, 1987, p 726.
6. Bray, PF, et al: Cell-free synthesis and membrane insertion of platelet membrane glycoproteins IIb and IIIa. Blood 64:243a, 1984.
7. Bai, Y, Durbin, H, and Hogg, N: Monoclonal antibodies specific for platelet glycoproteins that react with human monocytes. Blood 64:139, 1984.
8. Caen, JP and Michel, H: Platelet shape change and aggregation. Nature 240:148, 1972.
9. Malmsten, C, et al: Thromboxane synthesis and the platelet release reaction in Bernard-Soulier, Glanzmann's thrombasthenia and Hermansky-Pudlak syndromes. Br J Haematol 35:511, 1977.
10. Brown, CH, et al: Glanzmann's thrombasthenia: Assessment of the response to platelet transfusion. Transfusion 15:124, 1975.
11. White, JG: Ultrastructural studies of the gray platelet syndrome. Am J Pathol 95:445, 1979.
12. Weiss, HJ, et al: Heterogeneity in storage pool deficiencies: Studies on granule-bound substances in 18 patients including variants deficient in alpha granules, PF4, β-thromboglobulin and platelet derived growth factor. Blood 54:1296, 1979.
13. Lewis, JH, Zucker, MB, and Ferguson, JH: Bleeding tendency in uremia. Blood 11:1073, 1956.
14. Rabiner, SF and Hrodek, O: Platelet factor 3 in normal subjects and patients with renal failure. J Clin Invest 47:901, 1968.
15. Eknoyan, G, et al: Platelet function in renal failure. N Engl J Med 280:677, 1969.
16. Joist, HA, et al: Studies in the nature and etiology of uremic thrombocytopathy. Verh Dtsch Ges Inn Med 75:476, 1969.
17. Steiner, RW, Coggins, C, and Carvalho, AC: Bleeding time in uremia: A useful test to assess clinical bleeding. Am J Hematol 7:107, 1979.
18. Roa, AK: Uraemic platelets. Lancet 1:913, 1986.
19. Janson, PA, et al: Treatment of the bleeding tendency in uremia with cryoprecipitate. N Engl J Med 303:7318, 1980.
20. Mannucci, PM, et al: Deamino-8-D-arginine vasopressin

shortens the bleeding time in uremia. N Engl J Med 308:8, 1983.

21. Perkins, HA, McKenzie, MR, and Fundenberg, HH: Hemostatic defects in dysproteinemia. Blood 35:695, 1970.

22. Vigliano, EM and Horowitz, HI: Bleeding syndrome in a patient with IgA myeloma: Interaction of protein and connective tissue. Blood 29:823, 1967.

23. Silgals, RM and Sacher, RA: Quantitative and qualitative vascular and platelet disorders, both congenital and acquired. In Pittiglio, DH and Sacher, RA (eds): Clinical Hematology and Fundamentals of Hemostasis. FA Davis, Philadelphia, 1987, p 354.

24. Angelino, CA, Carvalho, AC, and Rao, AK: Acquired qualitative platelet defects. In Coleman, RW, et al: (eds): Hemostasis and Thrombosis: Basic Principles and Clinical Practice. JB Lippincott, Philadelphia, 1987, p 752.

25. Cortelazzo, S, Viero, P, and Barbui, T: Platelet activation in myeloproliferative disorders. Thromb Haemost 45:211, 1981.

26. Martinez, J, Shapiro, SS, and Holburn, RR: Metabolism of human prothrombin and fibrinogen in patients with thrombocytosis secondary to myeloproliferative states. Blood 42:35, 1973.

27. Boneu, B, et al: Platelets in myeloproliferative disorders. A comparative evaluation with certain platelet function tests. Scand J Haematol 25:214, 1980.

28. Hasegawa, DK, et al: Factor V deficiency in Philadelphia-positive chronic myelogenous leukemia. Blood 56:728, 1980.

29. Angelino, CA, Carvalho, AC, and Rao, AK: Acquired qualitative platelet defects. In Coleman, RW, et al: (eds): Hemostasis and Thrombosis: Basic Principles and Clinical Practice. JB Lippincott, Philadelphia, 1987, p 755.

30. Phadke, K, Dean, S, and Pitney, WR: Platelet dysfunction in myeloproliferative syndromes. Am J Hematol 10:57, 1981.

31. Zucker, S and Mielke, CH: Classification of thrombocytosis based on platelet function tests: Correlation with hemorrhagic and thrombotic complications. J Lab Clin Med 80:385, 1972.

32. Adams, T, Schultz, L, and Goldberg, L: Platelet function abnormalities in the myeloproliferative disorders. Scand J Haematol 13:215, 1974.

33. Walsh, PN, Murphy, S, and Barry, WE: The role of platelets in the pathogenesis of thrombosis and hemorrhage in patients with thrombocytosis. Thromb Haemost 38:1085, 1977.

34. Murano, G and Bick, RL: Basic Concepts of Hemostasis and Thrombosis. CRC Press, Boca Raton, FL, 1980, p 188.

35. Angelino, CA, Carvalho, AC, and Rao, AK: Acquired qualitative platelet defects. In Coleman, RW, et al (eds): Hemostasis and Thrombosis: Basic Principles and Clinical Practice. JB Lippincott, Philadelphia, 1987, p 758.

36. Solum, NO, et al: A quantitative evaluation of the inhibition of platelet aggregation by low molecular weight degradation products of fibrinogen. Br J Haematol 24:619, 1973.

37. Pareti, FI, Captianio, A, and Mannucci, PM: Acquired storage pool disease in platelets during disseminated intravascular coagulation. Blood 48:511, 1976.

38. Brown, CH, et al: Defective platelet function following the administration of penicillin compounds. Blood 47:949, 1976.

39. Silgals, RM and Sacher, RA: Quantitative and qualitative vascular and platelet disorders, both congenital and acquired. In Pittiglio, DH and Sacher, RA (eds): Clinical Hematology and Fundamentals of Hemostasis. FA Davis, Philadelphia, 1987, p 358.

40. Angelino, CA, Carvalho, AC, and Rao, AK: Acquired qualitative platelet defects. In Coleman, RW, et al (eds): Hemostasis and Thrombosis: Basic Principles and Clinical Practice. JB Lippincott, Philadelphia, 1987, p 761.

41. Moschcowitz, E: Hyaline thrombosis of the terminal arterioles and capillaries: A hitherto undescribed disease. Proc NY Pathol Soc 24:21, 1924.

42. Lian, EC-Y, Miu, PTK, and Siddiqui, FA: Inhibition of platelet-aggregating activity in thrombotic thrombocytopenic purpura plasma by normal adult immunoglobulin G. J Clin Invest 73:548, 1984.

43. Moake, JL, et al: Unusually large plasma factor VIII: von Willebrand factor multimers in chronic relapsing thrombotic thrombocytopenic purpura. N Engl J Med 307:1432, 1982.

44. Moake, JL, et al: Effects of fresh-frozen plasma and its cryosupernatant fraction on von Willebrand factor multimeric forms in chronic relapsing thrombotic thrombocytopenic purpura. Blood 65:1232, 1985.

45. Burns, ER and Zucker-Franklin, D: Pathologic effects of plasma from patients with thrombotic thrombocytopenic purpura on platelets and cultured vascular endothelial cells. Blood 60:1030, 1982.

46. Remuzzi, GR, et al: Thrombotic thrombocytopenic purpura—a deficiency of plasma factors regulating platelet-vessel-wall interaction. N Engl J Med 299:311, 1978.

47. Bukowski, RM: Thrombotic thrombocytopenic purpura: A review. Prog Hemost Thromb 6:287, 1982.

48. Amorsi, EC and Ultman, JE: Thrombotic thrombocytopenic purpura. Report of 16 cases and review of the literature. Medicine 45:135, 1966.

49. Gutterman, LA and Stevenson, TD: Treatment of thrombotic thrombocytopenic purpura with vincristine. JAMA 247:1433, 1982.

50. Fitzgerald, GA, Mass, RL, and Stern, R: Intravenous prostacyclin in thrombotic thrombocytopenic purpura. Ann Intern Med 96:227, 1982.

51. Gollub, S and Ulin, AW: Heparin-induced thrombocytopenia in man. J Lab Clin Med 59:430, 1962.

52. Coller, B: Disorders of platelets. In Ratnoff, OD and Forbes, CD (eds): Disorders of Hemostasis. Grune and Stratton, New York, 1984, p 73.

53. Lusher, JM and Iyer, R: Idiopathic thrombocytopenic purpura in children. Semin Thromb Hemost 3:3, 1977.

54. Lightsey, AS Jr, McMillan, R, and Koenig, HM: Childhood idiopathic thrombocytopenic purpura: Aggressive management of life threatening complications. JAMA 232:734, 1975.

55. Cheung, N-KV, et al: Platelet associated immunoglobulin G in childhood idiopathic thrombocytopenic purpura. J Pediatr 102:366, 1983.

56. Woods, VL Jr, et al: Autoantibodies against the platelet glycoprotein IIb/IIIa complex in patients with chronic ITP. Blood 63:368, 1984.

57. McMillan, R, et al: Evaluation of plasma antiplatelet antibodies (APA) in chronic ITP. Blood 66:293a, 1985.

58. Kernoff, LM, Blake, KCH, and Shackleton, D: Influence of the amount of platelet-bound IgG on platelet survival and site of sequestration in autoimmune thrombocytopenia. Blood 55:730, 1980.

59. Baldini, M: Idiopathic thrombocytopenic purpura. N Engl J Med 274:1245, 1966.

60. Picozzi, VJ, Roeske, WR, and Creger, WP: Fate of therapy failures in adult idiopathic thrombocytopenic purpura. Am J Med 69:690, 1980.

61. Kaden, BR, Rosse, WF, and Hauch, TW: Immune thrombocytopenia in lymphoproliferative diseases. Blood 53:545, 1979.

62. Spivak, JL, Bender, BX, and Quinn, TC: Hematologic abnormalities in the acquired immune deficiency syndrome. Am J Med 77:224, 1984.

63. Shulman, RN and Jordan, JV Jr: Platelet immunology. In Coleman, RW, et al (eds): Hemostasis and Thrombosis: Basic Principles and Clinical Practice. JB Lippincott, Philadelphia, 1987, p 491.

64. Rosenthal, N: The blood picture in purpura. J Lab Clin Med 13:303, 1928.

65. Schulman, RN and Jordan, JV Jr: Platelet immunology. In Coleman, RW, et al (eds): Hemostasis and Thrombosis: Basic Principles and Clinical Practice. JB Lippincott, Philadelphia, 1987, p 460.

66. Shulman, NR, et al: Immunoreaction involving platelets. V. Post-transfusion purpura due to a complement-fixing antibody against a genetically controlled platelet antigen: A proposed mechanism for thrombocytopenia and its relevance in "autoimmunity." J Clin Invest 40:1597, 1981.

67. Morrison, FS and Mollison, PL: Post-transfusion purpura. N Engl J Med 275:243, 1966.

68. Shulman, NR and Jordan, JV Jr: Platelet immunology. In Coleman, RW, et al (eds): Hemostasis and Thrombosis: Basic Principles and Clinical Practice. JB Lippincott, Philadelphia, 1987, p 473.
69. Bracey, AW and Shulman, NR: Effects of plasma exchange in an unusual case of post transfusion purpura. Transfusion 23:428a, 1983.
70. Shulman, NR and Jordan, JV Jr: Platelet kinetics. In Coleman RW, et al (eds): Hemostasis and Thrombosis: Basic Principles and Clinical Practice. JB Lippincott, Philadelphia, 1987, p 447.
71. Greipp, PR, Kyle, RA, and Bowie, EJW: Factor X deficiency in amyloidosis: A critical review. Am J Hematol 11:443, 1981.
72. Ratnoff, OD: The psychogenic purpuras: A review of autoerythrocyte sensitization, autosensitization to DNA, "hysterical" and factitial bleeding and religious stigma. Semin Hematol 17:192, 1980.
73. Branson, HE, et al: Inherited Protein C deficiency and coumarin-responsible chronic relapsing purpura fulminans in a newborn infant. Lancet 2:1165, 1983.

BIBLIOGRAPHY

Bailliere's Clinical Haematology, International Practice and Research. In Caen, JP (ed): Platelet Disorders 2:3, July 1989.
Hematology/Oncology Clinics of North America. In Coleman, RW and Rao, AK: Platelets in Health and Disease 4:1, Feb 1990.

QUESTIONS

1. Which factor decrease(s) is (are) characteristic of classic Von Willebrand's disease?
   a. Factor VIII
   b. Factor VIII:vWF, vWF:Ag
   c. Ristocetin cofactor
   d. All of the above

2. Which of the following is not characteristic for Bernard-Soulier syndrome?
   a. Prolonged bleeding time
   b. Absent platelet agglutination in response to bovine vWF or human vWF plus ristocetin
   c. Abnormal platelet aggregation in response to ADP, collagen, and epinephrine
   d. Abnormality in platelet membrane GPIb

3. Which of the following is not characteristic of Glanzmann's thrombasthenia?
   a. Prolonged bleeding time
   b. Giant platelets with decreased count
   c. Absent platelet aggregation to ADP, thrombin, collagen, and epinephrine
   d. Normal platelet aggregation to ristocetin and bovine vWF

4. Which of the following laboratory results would indicate a diagnosis of Von Willebrand's disease and not Glanzmann's thrombasthenia?
   a. Normal platelet aggregation to ADP; abnormal platelet agglutination by ristocetin
   b. Normal platelet aggregation to collagen; normal platelet agglutination by ristocetin
   c. Normal platelet aggregation to epinephrine; normal bleeding time
   d. Normal platelet aggregation to bovine vWF; normal factor VIII assay

5. What laboratory results are not normally associated with disorders of platelet secretion?
   a. Prolonged bleeding time
   b. Abnormal platelet morphology
   c. Abnormal aggregation response to ADP and epinephrine
   d. Normal platelet count

6. Which of the following disorders may be associated with acquired platelet defects?
   a. Uremia
   b. Malignant paraproteins
   c. Myeloproliferative syndromes
   d. Disseminated intravascular coagulation
   e. All of the above

7. Which of the following is not a cause for thrombocytopenia?
   a. Decreased platelet production
   b. Increased platelet destruction
   c. Proliferation of pluripotent stem cells
   d. Abnormal distribution of platelets

8. Which condition is classified as nonimmunologic thrombocytopenia?
   a. Disseminated intravascular coagulation
   b. Idiopathic thrombocytopenic purpura
   c. Storage pool deficiency
   d. Bernard-Soulier syndrome

9. Which condition is classified as immunologic thrombocytopenia? (Use answer choices for question 8.)

10. What type of disorders are usually associated with thrombocytosis?
    a. Myeloproliferative syndromes
    b. Autoimmune disorders
    c. Immunodeficiency syndromes
    d. Renal diseases

11. Which of the following is not an inherited vascular defect?
    a. Ehlers-Danlos syndrome
    b. Marfan's syndrome
    c. Amyloidosis
    d. Giant hemangiomas

12. Which disorder is an acquired vascular defect?
    a. Protein C deficiency
    b. Osteogenesis imperfecta
    c. Pseudoxanthoma elasticum
    d. Hemolytic uremic syndrome

ANSWERS

1. d (p. 441)
2. c (p. 443)
3. b (p. 444)
4. a (p. 444)
5. b (p. 444)
6. e (pp. 445–446)
7. c (pp. 448–449)
8. a (p. 451)
9. b (p. 452)
10. a (p. 454)
11. c (pp. 455–456)
12. a (p. 457)

CHAPTER 27

DAVID L. McGLASSON, M.S., C.L.S.(NCA)

Defects of Plasma Clotting Factors

OBJECTIVES

At the end of this chapter, the learner should be able to:
1. List defects that impair the coagulation system.
2. Name the factor deficiency of patients with hemophilia A.
3. Describe laboratory tests for the differential diagnosis of hemophilia A and von Willebrand's disease.
4. Name the factor deficiency of patients with hemophilia B.
5. Characterize various factor deficiencies.
6. Describe circulating anticoagulants-inhibitors.
7. Explain laboratory screening tests for the evaluation of coagulation abnormalities.

INTRODUCTION TO DEFECTS OF PLASMA CLOTTING FACTORS

Chapter 25 discusses the fibrin-forming (coagulation) system, the hemostatic function, physical properties, and the cascade theory of coagulation. This chapter discusses defects of plasma clotting factors and how these impairments can directly affect the hemostatic mechanism. Information is presented in some detail on each of the classic coagulation factors and these deficiencies[1] (see Tables 25–8 and 27–1), some of the acquired inhibitors of the coagulation system, and the laboratory testing used to detect the particular plasma clotting factor defects. The blood component of choice for treating each specific plasma clotting factor defect is briefly mentioned. A summary of the material presented and several case studies that illustrate the information are presented at the end of the chapter.

The plasma clotting factors are cofactors or precursors of serine proteases that circulate as inactive zymogens. Chapter 25 discussed the activation of these zymogens that participate in the coagulation cascade leading to the formation of an insoluble fibrin clot (see Tables 25–8 and 27–1).

Impairment of the coagulation system can occur because of defects in the individual plasma clotting factors. These defects can be produced by the following:

1. Decreased synthesis of the factors
2. Production of abnormal molecules that interfere with the coagulation cascade
3. Loss or consumption of the coagulation factors
4. Inactivation of these factors by inhibitors or antibodies[2]

Defects of the plasma clotting factors may be due to congenital sex-linked or autosomal hereditary disorders. They may be acquired conditions resulting from liver disease, vitamin K deficiency, or massive hemorrhage, or may be induced in response to blood component therapy or antibiotic treatment regimens.

COMMON HEREDITARY DISORDERS OF PLASMA CLOTTING FACTOR DEFECTS

The most common of the hereditary disorders of coagulation are the hemophilias A and B and von Willebrand's disease (vWD). A brief history of hemophilia can be found in *Laboratory Medicine*, edition 6, by J.B. Miale,[3] on which the following passages are based.

Hemophilia: History

Hemophilia is one of the oldest diseases known to humankind. One of the earliest references to the disorder was noted in the 5th century Talmud. A familial bleeding disorder was described that led to a rabbinic decree relating to circumcision.[4] The early scribes observed that the disease was transmitted through the mother. In the 16th century, Rabbi Joseph Kar noted that hemophilia could be transmitted through the male. He prohibited circumcision of the third son of a man whose son, born of a different mother, died of hemorrhage after circumcision. Modern rabbinic authority forbids circumcision of any child in whom the diagnosis of hemophilia can be ascertained.[3,4]

A newspaper obituary from the 1791 *Salem Gazette* (Massachusetts) describes what may have been the earliest account of hemophilia in America. The article relates the death of a 19-year-old man from a slight cut on the foot. The newspaper story related that his five brothers had died at different times in similar circumstances. The father of the brothers had two different wives and by each several children; those who died in these circumstances were all from the first wife.[5] Brinkhous[6] reviewed the history of hemophilia in 1975. He found what appears to be the first case of hemophilia in the medical literature recorded in 1793. Worldwide attention focused on a report of Otto in 1803 and led to other specific reports. The term hemophilia was introduced in 1828 by Hopff, who was a student of Schönlein. In 1893 Wright published his study on the determination of the clotting time, and reported that the abnormal coagulation in hemophilia could be measured.

Kunig, in 1892, established a relationship between hemophilia and hemarthrosis and warned against surgical intervention. He stated the question of "what to do for 'bleeders' joint is secondary to the question of what *not* to do."[6]

The demonstration of the abnormal clotting of blood generated speculation and research in this area. Morawitz,[7] in 1904, proposed that tissue thromboplastin or calcium may be deficient in hemophilia patients. Addis, in 1911, demonstrated the deficiency was not calcium but deficiency of a plasma globulin which he thought may be prothrombin. Platelets were even thought to be part of the link to hemophilia; however, this explanation was later refuted. This is easily explained by the fact that most hemophilia patients display normal bleeding times.

In 1936 and in later years Patek and Taylor[8] published evidence that the defect in hemophilia was due to a deficiency of a "globulin substance" that was called "antihemophilia globulin."

Later investigators such as Quick and Brinkhous conclusively demonstrated that prothrombin was normal in hemophilia. In 1947 the same investigators showed that the conversion of prothrombin to thrombin was dependent on the interaction of platelets and antihemophilia globulin. With the discovery of new factors of coagulation and the definition of the defect of classic hemophilia firmly established, it was possible to identify other hemophilia-like diseases caused by a deficiency of new coagulation factors IX, X, XI, and XII.[3]

Hemophilia influenced history to some extent. The disorder affected the Royal House of Stuart in Europe and Russia. Queen Victoria, a carrier of hemophilia, was the source of hemophilia in four sub-

Table 27-1. **FACTOR DEFICIENCIES**

Factor	Deficiency	Minimum for Hemostasis	Half-life	Laboratory	Clinical
I	Afibrinogenemia Autosomal recessive—homozygous Rare	50-100 mg	3.2-4.5 days	No clot formation <5 mg fibrinogen	Umbilical stump bleeding, easy bruising, ecchymosis, epistaxis, gingival oozing, hematuria, poor wound healing
	Hypofibrinogenemia Autosomal recessive—heterozygous Rare			Abn: PT APTT TCT Low fibrinogen	Mild bleeding, thrombotic episodes
	Dysfibrinogenemia Variable inheritance Uncommon—variants			Fibrinogen—qualitative abnormal; quantitative normal	Possible hemorrhage, possible thrombosis, possible asymptomatic
II	Hypoprothrombinemia Autosomal recessive Extremely rare	30-40%	2.8-4.4 days	Abn: PT APTT	Postoperative bleeding, epistaxis, menorrhagia, easy bruising
V	Parahemophilia Autosomal recessive 1/1,000,000—homozygote	10-25%	20 hr	Abn: PT APTT BT	Epistaxis, easy bruising, menorrhagia
VII	Hypoproconvertinemia Incomplete autosomal recessive—variable expression; 1/500,000	10-20%	100-300 min	Abn: PT Norm: APTT	Epistaxis, menorrhagia, cerebral hemorrhage
VIII	Hemophilia A (classic hemophilia); sex-linked recessive; 1/100,000	10-40%	9-18 hr	Abn: APTT Norm: PT BT	May be severe, moderate, or mild—spontaneous hemorrhage, hemarthroses, crippling, muscle hemorrhage, post-traumatic and postoperative bleeding
	von Willebrand's syndrome Variable inheritance—variants; autosomal dominant, variable penetrance; 1/80,000	20-40%	16-24 hr	Variable results: Platelet studies BT APTT	Mucous membrane bleeding, superficial wound bleeding—variable, depending on VIII:C levels
IX	Hemophilia B (Christmas disease) Sex-linked recessive; 1/100,000	20-50%	18-30 hr	Abn: APTT Norm: PT	May be severe, moderate, or mild—spontaneous hemorrhage, hemarthroses, crippling, ecchymoses, muscle hemorrhage, post-traumatic and postoperative bleeding
X	Stuart-Prower defect Autosomal recessive; <1/500,000—homozygous; 1/500—heterozygous	15-20%	32-48 hr	Abn: PT APTT	Menorrhagia, ecchymoses, central nervous system bleeding, excessive bleeding after childbirth

Table 27–1. **FACTOR DEFICIENCIES (Continued)**

Factor	Deficiency	Minimum for Hemostasis	Half-life	Laboratory	Clinical
XI	Hemophilia C Incomplete autosomal recessive-pseudodominant Rare	15–25%	40–84 hr	Abn: APTT Norm: PT	Mild bleeding, bruising, epistaxis, retinal hemorrhage, menorrhagia
XII	Hageman trait Autosomal recessive Rare	?	48–52 hr	Abn: APTT Norm: PT	Asymptomatic — rarely bleed, may thrombose
XIII	Factor XIII deficiency Autosomal recessive Rare	1%	12 days	Norm: PT APTT Clot soluble in 5M urea	Umbilical cord bleeding, delayed wound healing, minor injuries causing prolonged bleeding, fetal wastage, excessive fibrinolysis, male sterility, intracranial hemorrhage
PK	Fletcher trait Autosomal recessive Rare	?	?	Abn: APTT (normal after prolonged activation)	Asymptomatic
HMWK	Fitzgerald deficiency Autosomal recessive Rare	?	?	Abn: APTT	Asymptomatic
Plasminogen	Abnormal functional Plasminogen Autosomal Rare	?	2–2.5 days	Abnormal plasminogen function; normal clotting tests	Thrombosis
Protein C	Protein C deficiency Autosomal dominant	?	6–8 hr	Normal clotting tests	Thrombosis — thrombophlebitis, recurring pulmonary emboli

Source: From Pittiglio, DH, et al: Treating hemostatic disorders. A problem-oriented approach. In Pittiglio, DH: Hemostasis Overview. American Association of Blood Banks, Arlington, VA, 1984, p 28, with permission.
HMWK = high molecular weight kininogen.
TCT = thrombin clotting time.

sequent generations[3] (Fig. 27–1). (Note that the Russian line of the House of Stuart ended by extermination in the Russian Revolution.)

von Willebrand's Disease: History

In 1924 Dr. Erik von Willebrand was asked to evaluate a 5-year-old girl from the Aland Islands off the coast of Finland for a severe bleeding disorder.[9] After examining the patient and several other family members, Dr. von Willebrand submitted that his patient had a new bleeding disorder that differed from hemophilia. Instead of deep muscle hemorrhaging and hemarthroses, von Willebrand's patients had primarily mucocutaneous hemorrhaging. The inheritance was autosomal dominant instead of being sex-linked as in hemophilia. The affected persons also had prolonged bleeding times in contrast to the normal bleeding times usually seen in hemophilia. Noting that the affected persons had normal platelet counts, von Willebrand con-

cluded that the patients had a qualitative platelet functional disorder.[9] Later studies demonstrated that the hemostatic problems of patients with von Willebrand's disease resided in the plasma of these subjects and not in the platelets. This was done by a series of infusion experiments.[9] It was shown that plasma from normal healthy people corrected a prolonged bleeding time whereas plasma from persons with von Willebrand's disease did not. Infusion of normal platelets did not correct the prolonged bleeding time in von Willebrand's disease patients. Infusion of platelets from patients with von Willebrand's disease corrected thrombocytopenia in patients with aplastic anemia.[9]

FACTOR VIII (ANTIHEMOPHILIC FACTOR)

To understand factor VIII plasma clotting factor defects, a knowledge of the factor complex is necessary (see Chapter 25; see also Tables 27–1, 27–2, 27–3, and 27–4).

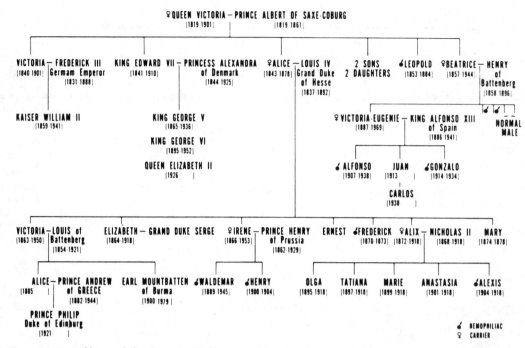

Figure 27-1. Transmission of hemophilia through the lineages of the Royal House of Stuart. (From Miale,[3] p 825, with permission.)

Table 27-2. **SELECTED PROPERTIES OF FACTOR VIII AND von WILLEBRAND FACTOR***

	Factor VIII	von Willebrand Factor
Cellular site of biosynthesis	Not certain	Endothelial cells and megakaryocytes
Plasma concentration	50–150 ng/ml	5–10 µg/ml
Molecular weight	265,000 (plus carbohydrate)	Polymers of 220 kDa subunit
Principal biologic activity	Procoagulant cofactor	Platelet adhesion to vessel wall
		Carrier for factor VIII in plasma
Assay		
Functional	PTT factor Xa formation	Bleeding time, platelet adhesion, platelet agglutination (e.g., ristocetin-induced)
Immunologic	IRMA, ELISA, immunoblot; inhibitor neutralization	Quantitative: IRMA, ELISA, electroimmunoassay (Laurell)
		Qualitative: Crossed immunoelectrophoresis, multimer analysis, immunoblot
Inheritance	X-linked recessive	Autosomal
Clinical disorder due to deficiency	Hemophilia A	von Willebrand's disease

Source: From Marder, VJ, et al: Standard nomenclature for factor VIII and von Willebrand factor: A recommendation by the International Committee on Thrombosis and Haemostasis. Thromb Haemost 54(4):871, 1985, with permission.

*In plasma, the two proteins are present as a biomolecular complex called the factor VIII–von Willebrand factor complex.

Table 27–3 **PROPOSED ABBREVIATIONS FOR FACTOR VIII AND von WILLEBRAND FACTOR***

Attribute	ABBREVIATION	
	Proposed	Outmoded
Factor VIII		
Protein	VIII	VIII:C
Antigen	VIII:Ag	VIIIC:Ag
Function	VIII:C	—
von Willebrand factor		
Protein	vWF	VIIIR:Ag, VIII/vWF, AHF-like protein
Antigen	vWF:Ag	VIIIR:Ag, AHF-like antigens
Function	—	VIIIR:RCo, VIIIR:vWFt

Source: From Marder, VJ, et al: Standard nomenclature for factor VIII and von Willebrand factor: A recommendation by the International Committee on Thrombosis and Haemostasis. Thromb Haemost 54(4):871, 1985, with permission.
*The two proteins form a bimolecular complex that can be abbreviated as VIII/vWF.
†These abbreviations have been used to indicate the ristocetin cofactor activity of von Willebrand factor. Bcause neither this test nor any other in vitro test completely reflects vWF activity, no abbreviation is recommended as representative of its function.

The site of factor VIII:C synthesis has not been established conclusively. It may originate in the liver, endothelial cells, and megakaryocytes. Factor VIII is a cofactor in the factor IX:A–mediated factor X activation. Factor VIII is not vitamin K dependent, is absent in serum, and is present in adsorbed plasma. It is extremely thermolabile. Unless the plasma is stored below − 70°C, it can lose activity rapidly.[10] In citrated plasma, 50 percent activity can be lost in 24 hours at 22°C.[11] One study cited a loss of 50.4 percent activity of VIII:C samples stored at −20°C for 5 days.[12]

There are two basic biologic functions of factor VIII:C–von Willebrand factor (vWF) complex. Factor VIII:C is the smaller protein subunit of the factor VIII complex and represents the procoagulant or clotting activity of the complex. The major protein portion of the complex is the factor VIII:vWF (formerly referred to as factor VIII:RAg) and represents von Willebrand activity and protein–mediated platelet adhesion. Factor VIII:vWF is the carrier protein of the factor VIII complex and serves to concentrate VIII:C present in small amounts to the site of the injury. The factor VIII:C portion of the molecule (the low molecular weight protein of factor VIII) has a molecular weight of approximately 150,000. The factor VIII:vWF protein (the carrier

Table 27–4. **LABORATORY DIAGNOSIS OF CLASSIC von WILLEBRAND'S DISEASE (TYPE IA) AND VARIANTS***

	AUTOSOMAL DOMINANT				AUTOSOMAL RECESSIVE	
	Type IA	Type IIA	Type IIB	Platelet-type	Type IIC	Type III
Bleeding time	Increased or normal	Increased	Increased	Increased	Increased	Increased
Platelet count	Normal	Normal	Normal or decreased	Low normal or decreased	Normal	Normal
VIII:C	Decreased	Normal or decreased	Normal or decreased	Normal or decreased	Normal	Markedly decreased
vWF:Ag	Decreased	Decreased or normal	Decreased or normal	Normal or decreased	Decreased or normal	Markedly decreased
Ristocetin cofactor	Decreased	Markedly decreased	Decreased or normal	Decreased or normal	Decreased	Markedly decreased
Crossed immuno-electrophoresis of plasma vWF	Normal	Abnormal	Abnormal	Abnormal	Abnormal	Variable
Multimeric structure of vWF						
Plasma	Normal	Absence of largest and intermediate multimers	Absence of largest multimers	Absence of largest multimers	Absence of largest multimers and abnormal band structure	Variable
Platelets	Normal	Absence of largest and intermediate multimers	Normal	Normal	Absence of largest multimers and abnormal band structure	Variable

(continued)

Table 27–4. **LABORATORY DIAGNOSIS OF CLASSIC von WILLEBRAND'S DISEASE (TYPE IA) AND VARIANTS* (Continued)**

	AUTOSOMAL DOMINANT				AUTOSOMAL RECESSIVE	
	Type IA	Type IIA	Type IIB	Platelet-type	Type IIC	Type III
Ristocetin-induced platelet aggregation in patient PRP	Decreased or normal	Markedly decreased	Increased	Increased	Decreased	Markedly decreased
Ristocetin-induced binding of vWF to platelets						
Patient plasma + normal platelets		Decreased	Increased	Normal or decreased		
Normal plasma + patient platelets		Normal	Normal	Increased		
vWF-induced aggregation of unstimulated patient platelets in PRP			Absent	Present		

Source: From Miller, JL: Blood coagulation and fibrinolysis. In Henry, JB (ed): Clinical Diagnosis and Management, 17 ed. WB Saunders, 1984, p 777, with permission.
VIII:C = VIII coagulant activity; vWF:Ag = von Willebrand factor antigen.
PRP = Platelet-rich plasma.

protein of the factor VIII complex) has a molecular weight greater than 10 million with multimers of 200,000 molecular weight subunits. The factor VIII:C portion of the molecule can be demonstrated by performing a one-stage activated partial thromboplastin time (APTT) factor assay to determine the level of factor VIII:C. The normal range of factor VIII:C is 50 to 200 percent activity. The VIII:vWF presence can be shown by the response of normal platelets in platelet rich plasma or normal washed platelets to aggregation by the antibiotic ristocetin (Fig. 27–2). The aggregation response is associated with the high molecular weight carrier portion of the factor VIII complex.[2,13,14]

Immunologic markers of factor VIII can also be measured. Antibodies directed toward the different parts of the factor VIII complex can recognize the antigenic expression of VIII:C-VIII:Ag or that of the higher molecular weight complex vWF:Ag. The factor vWF:Ag antibodies can be quantified by using Laurell rocket immunoelectrophoresis (Fig. 27–2).[15,16] The factor VIII:Ag can be measured by radioimmunoassays (RIAs) with human antibodies to factor VIII:C.[17] This assay is only performed in highly specialized laboratories. No commercial source of the test is yet available.

Hemophilia A

Hemophilia A is a sex-linked recessive disorder that, along with von Willebrand's disease, constitutes one of the most common coagulation defects.

Hemophilia disease affects approximately one male per 10,000 people in the whole population. The deficiency in factor VIII:C is determined by a defect of the X chromosome. Although found almost exclusively in males, there have been reports of female hemophiliacs. The mode of transmission of inheritance of the disease is as follows: the daughters of patients with hemophilia A are obligatory carriers, and sons of patients with hemophilia A are normal. The female carriers then transmit the disorder to half their sons and the carrier state to half their daughters. A female hemophiliac is possible if the mother was a carrier and the father had hemophilia.[18]

In approximately one third of newly diagnosed cases of hemophilia A there may be no previous family history of bleeding. This suggests that a mutation may be evident or there could be several generations of "silent carriers" of the sex-linked recessive trait.[19]

In patients with hemophilia A, factor VIII:C activity is impaired, whereas vWF function is normal. Patients may be divided into three groups according to their factor VIII:C activity: severe, less than 1 percent; moderate, 3 to 5 percent activity; and mild, 5 to 12 percent activity.[19] Further subgrouping of hemophilia A has been described in the results of immunologic studies on plasmas from hemophilia A patients. The studies displayed results that showed most hemophilia A patients were incapable of neutralizing naturally occurring human antibodies to factor VIII. These plasmas were then referred

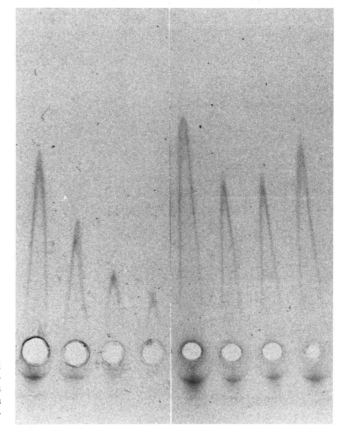

Figure 27–2. Quantitative immunoelectrophoresis of normal and hemophilic plasmas. Wells 1 through 4 contain serial dilutions of a standard plasma (Cutter Laboratories), wells 5 and 8 contain plasmas from two patients with severe hemophilia, wells 6 and 7 contain normal plasmas. (From Rock, G,[2] p 371, with permission.)

to as being cross-reacting material negative (CRM−). A small group of subjects with hemophilia A are capable of neutralizing human antibodies to the factor VIII molecule and are called CRM+.[17,19,20] This shows that some hemophilia A patients do have active antigenic forms of factor VIII that are functionally inactive. In both cases, however, the effect is still a deficiency of factor VIII:C and both groups are treated the same clinically.

Carriers of hemophilia A are usually asymptomatic. In some instances the factor VIII:C levels may be low enough for hemorrhaging to occur but these instances are rare. On the average, carriers are found to have half of the factor VIII:C activity when compared with healthy women.[19,21] The ratio comparing factor VIII:C with factor vWF:Ag in healthy women is usually 1.0. However, in carriers the ratio is usually 0.5 or lower. Using this ratio of both values, 70 to 90 percent of carriers of hemophilia A may be distinguishable from healthy women.[22] An in utero technique using fetal blood obtained at 18 to 20 weeks' gestation has also been developed to measure factor VIII:C and factor VIII:Ag.[23] More recently a procedure using DNA analysis to detect molecular defects of the factor VIII:C gene has shown a great deal of promise in giving an almost certain prediction of carrier status.[24] The latter two studies are performed only at a few research centers.

Clinical histories of patients with hemophilia A may indicate such symptoms as hemarthroses, easy bruising, mucous membrane hemorrhaging, severe postoperative bleeding, hematuria, gastrointestinal bleeding, and unexplained spontaneous hemorrhaging episodes.

Antibodies or inhibitors to factor VIII:C in hemophilia A occur in 10 to 15 percent of patients with hemophilia A.[25] The inhibitors are usually temperature dependent and are immunoglobulin (IgG) in nature. These inhibitors will neutralize factor VIII:C at 37°C.[26] The therapeutic administration of antihemophilic factor (AHF) may lead to a rise in antibody titer in patients who have developed antibodies to AHF.[26]

Treatment of hemophilia A can occur in many forms. Now that blood is screened for human immunodeficiency virus (HIV)–positive donors, it is somewhat safer to use concentrates of human plasma such as AHF. Most hemophilia A patients receive highly purified, heat-treated lyophilized preparations of factor VIII concentrates. Cryoprecipitate, which is also rich in factor VIII, can be administered. Unfortunately, the incidence of parenterally transmitted hepatitis C (formerly called non-A, non-B hepatitis) remains high. New ultra-pure preparations of AHF prepared from plasma by monoclonal antibody techniques are now licensed and a synthetic recombinant deoxyribonucleic acid (DNA) AHF may be significant in lowering the incidence of infection by blood products.[27,28] If inhibitors develop in response to factor VIII therapy, porcine plasma preparations are available. The porcine factor VIII concentrates usually do not have the cross-reacting inhibitor development that human factor VIII concentrates may produce.[2,26] In other extreme cases, factor IX concentrates of prothrombin complex may be used. The ideal therapeutic level to maintain hemostasis should be at least 30 percent of normal activity.

Laboratory Assessment

Patients with hemophilia A have extremely prolonged APTTs, normal prothrombin times (PT), and bleeding times that may be normal or slightly prolonged. The one-stage factor assay with the APTT method (see Chapter 30) shows a decrease of factor VIII:C. If inhibitors develop, they can cause the further prolongation of the APTT when incubated at 37°C for 2 hours. Mixing studies with normal plasma will show a correction of the APTT in a factor VIII:C deficiency. If an inhibitor is present, no correction will take place. Inhibitor activity is measured in terms of the capacity of an inhibitor to inactivate a quantity of a plasma clotting factor. Patient plasma is mixed with normal pooled plasma and incubated for 2 hours at 37°C. The presence of inhibitor activity is measured in a modified one-stage factor assay using the APTT test and quantitating the inhibitor in Bethesda units.[29] One unit of inhibitor is defined as the amount that will inactivate 50 percent of the specific factor during the incubation time.[29]

Patients with hemophilia should have normal vWF:Ag and platelet functional assays.

von Willebrand's Disease

In von Willebrand's disease (vWD) there is decreased or absent vWF activity and a decrease in factor VIII:C concentration secondary to the primary defect in vWF.[2] This disorder is autosomal in nature; therefore, it affects both sexes. The von Willebrand factor is extremely stable compared with the factor VIII:C portion of the factor VIII complex. Storage of plasmas for testing for the presence of vWF can be maintained at temperatures of −20°C with no loss of activity for long periods.[12]

Patients with vWD usually bleed from the mucous membranes and cutaneous sites. Frequent bouts of epistaxis, easy bruising, gastrointestinal bleeding, and excessive postoperative hemorrhaging following dental surgery and tonsillectomies can be observed.[18,19,30-32] The most frequent complaint from women with this disorder is heavy and prolonged menstrual bleeding.[32] Patients with vWD usually do not display the severe hemarthroses and deep muscle hematomas that may be seen in hemophilia A.[2,30,32]

The central role of von Willebrand's disease appears to be the inability of the patient's platelets to adhere to the subendothelial surfaces following injury to the blood vessel.[2,19,30-32]

Table 27–5 displays the laboratory diagnosis of classic vWD (type I) and its variants. Chapter 30 discusses the testing techniques and theory in some detail, with the exception of the crossed immunoelectrophoresis (CIE) procedure (Fig. 27–3)[33,34] and the technique for multimeric structure identification of vWF (Fig. 27–4).[35] These tests are usually performed in reference laboratories. The only direct test readily available to the laboratory clinician to demonstrate in vivo platelet response is the template type bleeding time. In vWD patients the bleeding time is usually prolonged.[2,18,19,31] Other tests available for diagnosis of vWD are mixed and varied. As mentioned, there are several variants of vWD that require specialized testing to identify properly the particular subgroup that responds to different types of treatment plans.

Table 27–5. **COMPARISON OF HEMOPHILIA A AND CLASSIC von WILLEBRAND'S DISEASE**

	Hemophilia A	von Willebrand's Disease
Deficiency	VIII:C, VIII:AHF	VIII:vWF
Inheritance	Recessive, X-linked	Dominant, autosomal
Clinical bleeding	Hemarthrosis, muscle, soft tissue, visceral	Gums, gastrointestinal tract, mucous membanes
Bleeding disorder	Moderate to severe (60% to severe)	Mild to moderate
Laboratory tests		
Bleeding time	N	A
Clot retraction	N	N
Glass bead retraction	N	A
Platelet count	N	N
Ristocetin aggregation	N	A
PT	N	N
PTT	A	A
VIII	A	A
vWF:Ag	N	A

Source: From Rock, G: Defects of plasma clotting factors. In Pittiglio, DH and Sacher, RA (eds): Clinical Hematology and Fundamentals of Hemostasis, ed 1. FA Davis, Philadelphia, p 373, with permission.
N = normal; A = abnormal.

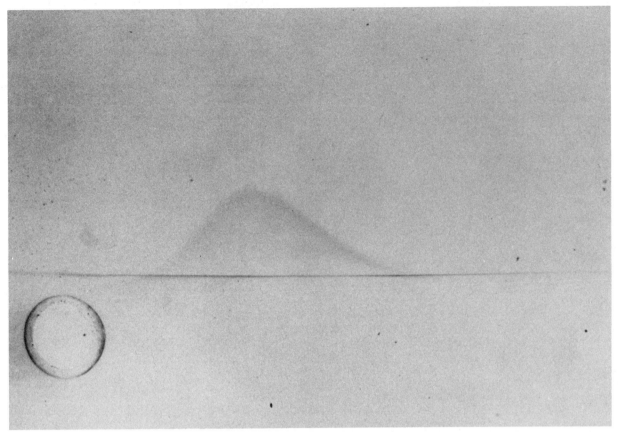

Figure 27–3. Crossed immunoelectrophoresis of vWF: Ag. Electrophoresis was performed on the plasma in the first dimension toward the anode. The agarose was then cut and the sample electrophoresed in the second dimension against rabbit antibody to vWF: Ag which was incorporated into the gel. The gels were stained with Coomassie blue to show the arc of immunoprecipitation. (From Rock, G,[2] p 372, with permission.)

Patients with vWD respond to treatment with either fresh frozen plasma or cryoprecipitate.[2,30,32] Factor VIII concentrates usually do not provide effective treatment in vWD. The vWF appears to be destroyed or removed during purification of cryoprecipitate to make the concentrates.[2,35] One drug, 1-deamino-8-D-arginine vasopressin (DDAVP), which is a synthetic analogue of the antidiuretic hormone, vasopressin, has been used extensively in recent years. Patients with some of the less severe forms of the disease may experience a rapid transient increase in VIII:C, vWF:Ag, and ristocetin cofactor, and a decrease in the prolonged bleeding time.[2,31,32] This drug has been administered both intravenously and intranasally.[2,36–38] The hemostasis level of VIII:C and vWF is usually 30 percent or greater.

Laboratory Assessment

In order to avoid confusion with hemophilia A, review Table 27–5 to compare test patterns for vWD and hemophilia A. All screening for vWD should include a PT, APTT, bleeding time, VIII:C, vWF:Ag (see Fig. 27–2), ristocetin cofactor, and ristocetin-induced platelet aggregation studies with normal platelets (Fig. 27–5). Specialty testing for CIE for vWF and abnormal multimeric structures may be necessary to identify a variant of the disorder. The glass bead adhesion test is rarely used anymore owing to the difficulty of standardization of test results.

Conditions presenting with disseminated intravascular coagulopathy can also cause decreases in factor VIII:C. Von Willebrand's disease can also be an acquired disorder. Decreased vWF similar to that found in congenital vWD has been described in a variety of autoimmune diseases, myeloproliferative disorders, lymphoproliferative diseases, and benign monoclonal gammopathies.[32]

Increased levels of factor VIII:C activity may be seen after exercise, during pregnancy, in renal disease or liver disease, or when taking oral contraceptives.[2,19] Women who are pregnant, taking oral contraceptives, or receiving other hormonal therapy may have vWD and yet be completely asymptomatic for the disorder while their condition exists.[30,39]

FACTOR IX (CHRISTMAS DISEASE OR PLASMA THROMBOPLASTIN COMPONENT)

Factor IX is a vitamin K–dependent factor that has a molecular weight of approximately 60,000. It is synthesized in the liver and is present in serum. Factor IX does not have the thermolabile qualities

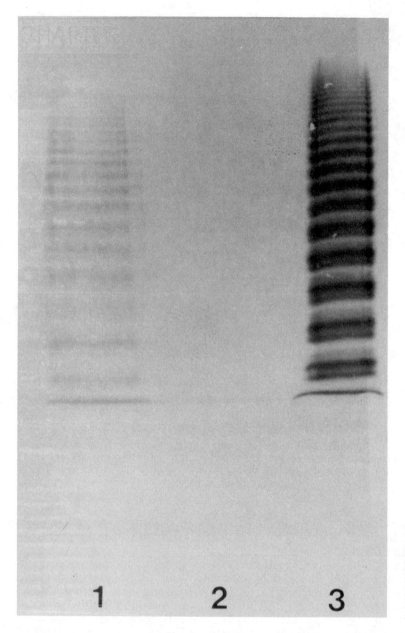

Figure 27–4. vWF: Ag multimers. Samples of (1) normal plasma, (2) von Willebrand plasma, and (3) cryoprecipitate underwent electrophoresis in SDS-agarose gel. A western blotting technique was performed. The gel on nitrocellulose paper was incubated first with a rabbit antihuman vWF: Ag antibody and then with goat antirabbit IgG; then it was stained. (From Rock, G,[2] p 371, with permission.)

that factor VIII possesses. Factor IX is present in serum but not in adsorbed plasma. Deficiencies of factor IX are seen in liver disease, in vitamin K deficiency, during oral anticoagulant therapy (Coumadin), and in hemophilia B.

Hemophilia B

Hemophilia B is a congenital disorder that is inherited through a sex-linked recessive gene with the same symptoms displayed in hemophilia A. Hemophilia B, like hemophilia A, occurs clinically as a mild to severe bleeding disorder. The severity of hemorrhaging in a patient with this disease is directly related to the level of factor IX clotting activity in the patient's plasma. The levels also correspond to those seen in hemophilia A.

Hemophilia B is rarer than hemophilia A with the incidence of occurrence in a normal population of approximately 1 per 100,000.[18,39] The incidence of inhibitor production against factor IX is very low when compared with those of hemophilia A, usually only 1 to 3 percent.[40,41]

Patients with hemophilia B have been divided into two groups based on the results of a PT in which ox brain thromboplastin is used. Those with a prolonged ox brain PT were said to be hemophilia Bm, the "m" refering to the family name of the original patient. Most hemophilia B patients have normal ox brain PTs.[42]

Carriers of hemophilia B transmit this sex-linked hereditary disorder in the same manner as occurs in hemophilia A. Screening for these subjects can be accomplished in the manner previously described

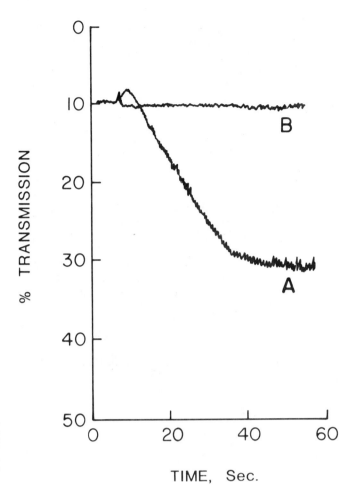

Figure 27–5. Factor VIII : vWF and platelet aggregation. Plasma is incubated with washed normal platelets and ristocetin. The aggregation slope is observed over 60 seconds after addition of (A) plasma containing a normal level of vWF and (B) plasma containing a low VIII : vWF level (patient with von Willebrand's disease). (From Rock, G,[2] p 370, with permission.)

in hemophilia A. These carriers also can exhibit bleeding disorders, but not as severe as those in individuals who are diagnosed with the hereditary bleeding condition.

Patients with hemophilia B are usually treated with prothrombin complex concentrates that have factors II, VII, IX, and X and fresh-frozen plasma (FFP). The development of inhibitors is treated in the same manner that hemophilia A is handled.[26]

Laboratory Assessment

In the laboratory, the detection of a factor IX deficiency is similar to that of a factor VIII : C defect. The bleeding time is usually normal. Prothrombin times are normal except that discussed earlier with ox brain thromboplastin. The APTT is prolonged and the one-stage APTT factor assay for factor IX is decreased for the presence of factor IX.

RARE DISORDERS OF PLASMA CLOTTING FACTOR DEFECTS

Factor I (Fibrinogen)

Fibrinogen is a large plasma protein of the keratin-myosin family with a molecular weight of 340,000. It is produced in the liver and is not vitamin K dependent. Fibrinogen is not present in serum, not adsorbed by barium sulfate, and therefore is found in adsorbed plasma. It functions in its active form as the clot structural protein.

Fibrinogen is the terminal substrate of the coagulation system which polymerizes into fibrin fibers upon the proteolytic action of thrombin. Thrombin converts fibrinogen to fibrin by splitting away the fibrinopeptides A and B from the terminal ends of the alpha and beta chains of the fibrinogen molecule. This forms soluble fibrin monomers. The fibrin monomers then undergo polymerization to form fibrin strands. Factor XIII, which is also activated by thrombin, acts as a fibrin-stabilizing factor to produce a covalently cross-linked, insoluble fibrin clot. This is the end-point of the plasma clotting factor process that assists in forming a stable hemostatic plug.[2,43,44]

Fibrinogen is present in the circulation of normal individuals' plasma at levels of 200 to 400 mg/dl.

Afibrinogenemia

By 1985 afibrinogenemia was reported in about 60 families.[2] This very rare inherited disorder results in a failure to synthesize adequate amounts of circulating fibrinogen. Two patterns of transmission have been reported: autosomal recessive and autosomal intermediate. These patients have many episodes of bleeding during their lifespan. Umbilical cord bleeding is the main symptom. Intracranial bleeding, easy bruising, epistaxis, gingival bleeding, gastrointestinal bleeding, menorrhagia, and rarely hemarthroses have been observed. The bleeding episodes usually decrease with age and there may be long periods without major bleeding episodes. Patients may be treated with FFP, cryoprecipitate, and even whole blood during bleeding episodes or before surgical procedures. Inhibitors have been reported in two cases.[2,45,46]

Laboratory Assessment. Table 27–6 presents a number of laboratory tests and results used to diagnose this condition. The thrombin time (TT), PT, APTT, and reptilase time (RT) are infinitely prolonged. Note that bleeding times may be prolonged even when the patient is not thrombocytopenic. This fact points out the importance of fibrinogen in the primary arrest of bleeding.[45] Fibrinogen levels using heat precipitation, chemical precipitation, and immunologic methods fail to detect any but very low levels of this clotting factor. Two studies failed to find fibrinogen present in platelets of patients with this disorder; therefore, platelet aggregation study results may also be abnormal.[2,45]

Hypofibrinogenemia

Hypofibrinogenemia is a congenital hereditary autosomal recessive disorder that may be autosomal dominant. The incidence of occurrence is lower than that of afibrinogenemia, but the condition itself is usually not as severe. Umbilical bleeding is again the first noted symptom. Some symptoms may develop that are similar to those of patients with afibrinogenemia but this condition may go unnoticed unless discovered before or during surgery. Treatment for this disorder is the same as that for afibrinogenemia.[2,44,45]

Laboratory Assessment. The laboratory tests for the diagnosis of this disorder are also listed in Table 27–6. Note that the levels for clottable fibrinogen and immunologic fibrinogen are from 20 to 100 mg/dl. The TT, PT, and APTT are all prolonged. The bleeding time is usually normal, and platelet functions are normal.

Dysfibrinogenemia

Dysfibrinogenemia is a qualitative abnormality rather than a quantitative problem as described in the previously discussed fibrinogen abnormalities. More than 100 reported cases of dysfibrinogenemia have been described in the literature to date. Most of these cases are autosomal dominant; only two cases have been acquired autosomal recessive. Dysfibrinogenemia may be associated with defects in the thrombin-fibrinogen reaction, forming an abnormal protein thereby causing defective formation of fibrin. The majority of patients with dysfibrinogenemia are asymptomatic.[45] The symptoms are similar to the two previously described disorders with some patients displaying arterial thrombosis. Treatment is the same as for the other two disorders.

Laboratory Assessment. Table 27–6 displays the common laboratory tests for diagnosing this condition. The RT in dysfibrinogenemia may be normal. Immunologic assays for fibrinogen usually present normal levels, whereas the clotting assays are decreased. Some effects of heparin are similar to those found in the fibrinogen disorders. The RT (see Chapter 30) is a test that is used to differentiate the presence of heparin from a fibrinogen abnormality. A normal RT and a prolonged TT suggest heparin, whereas a prolonged RT and TT suggest a fibrinogen disorder.

Table 27–6. **DIFFERENTIAL DIAGNOSIS OF AFIBRINOGENEMIA**

Test	Afibrinogenemia	Hypofibrinogenemia	Dysfibrinogenemia	Heparin
Bleeding time	P	N	N	N
Prothrombin time	P	P	P	P
Partial thromboplastin time	P	P	P	P
Thrombin time	P	P	P	P
Reptilase time	P	P	P(N)	N
Thrombin coagulase	P	P	N	N
Fibrinogen level (clotting assay)	10 mg/100 ml	20–100 mg/100 ml	10 mg/100 ml	N
Fibrinogen level (immunologic assay)	Absent	20–100 mg/100 ml	N	N
Platelet aggregation	ABN	N	N	N(ABN)
Fibrinolytic tests	N	N	N	N

Source: From Girolami, A, et al: Rare and quantitative and qualitative: Abnormalities of coagulation. Changes in Hematology 14(2):388, 1985, with permission.
N = normal; P = prolonged; ABN = abnormal.

Factor II (Prothrombin)

Factor II (prothrombin) is the immediate precursor to thrombin. It is synthesized in the liver, is vitamin K dependent, and has a molecular weight of approximately 70,000. Prothrombin is present in serum yet absent in adsorbed plasma. The biochemistry of factor II is similar to the other vitamin K–dependent coagulation factors of VII, IX, and X.

Congenital Hypothrombinemia

Congenital hypothrombinemia is very rare. Approximately 25 cases have been reported in the literature to date. Clinical symptoms are usually mild but hemarthroses have been reported.

Laboratory Assessment. The PT and APTT may feature a slight prolongation that corrects by the addition of normal plasma in mixing studies. The hereditary transmission is autosomal recessive.[45]

Acquired Dysprothrombinemias

Cases of acquired dysprothrombinemias have been reported but their incidence is even more rare than that of the congenital hypothrombinemias. The hereditary transmission is the same in both disorders. The clinical picture is of a mild nature similar to that of the congenital hypothrombinemias. The main laboratory discrepancy displays a decreased factor II activity in a one-stage factor assay and an immunologic level that is usually normal. The APTT and PT are moderately prolonged.[45]

Acquired defects of a single vitamin K–dependent coagulant factor are rare and usually come in relation to factors VII, IX, and X. Liver dysfunction, abnormal absorption of vitamin K in the intestinal tract, broad-spectrum antibiotic use over a prolonged period, and oral anticoagulant use (Coumadin) can cause a decrease of factor II.[2] There has been some evidence of lowered factor II levels in relation to lupus anticoagulants.[47]

Treatment of this deficiency includes the administration of FFP or prothrombin complex concentrates that contain factors II, VII, IX, and X. It is necessary to have 40 percent activity to achieve normal hemostasis.[45]

Laboratory Assessment. The PT and APTT are prolonged with a factor II deficiency. One-stage factor assays for factor II show a decrease in activity when using the prothrombin time assay. Mixing studies with normal plasma will correct the prolonged PT and APTT times. Mixing studies with adsorbed plasma and aged serum will not show a correction of the PT or APTT.

Factor V (Proaccelerin)

Factor V has a molecular weight of 350,000, is thermolabile, has a very short half-life, and is not vitamin K dependent. It is absent from serum and present in adsorbed plasma. Factor V participates in the coagulation cascade as a cofactor in the activation of prothrombin by Xa. Factor V is activated by thrombin and converted to a form that is able to bind to prothrombin. Factor V deficiencies were first described by Owren in 1947 as parahemophilia. The disorder is autosomal recessive, affecting both sexes. Heterozygotes with this disorder are usually asymptomatic.[45]

The clinical picture describes easy bruising, epistaxis, hemorrhaging of the mucous membranes, and, in females, menorrhagia. There have also been some documented cases of a combined defect of factor V and VIII activity that is controlled by the inhibitory activity of protein C.[48]

Acquired defects of factor V occur in patients with liver disease and disseminated intravascular coagulation (DIC). There are also a number of cases of acquired factor V inhibitors described in the literature, usually in response to antibiotic therapy. Two cases of a factor V deficiency have been cited in the literature that have the presence of an inhibitor and characteristics of a lupus anticoagulant.[49–51]

Treatment for a factor V problem is usually FFP. Platelet concentrates may be required when an inhibitor is present. The transfused platelets effects may include factor V provided by platelets; the platelet surface providing receptor sites for the factor V inhibitors or platelets participating in local hemostasis.[52] It should be noted that 80 percent of factor V is in circulation with 20 percent of body stores contained in normal platelets.[50,51]

Laboratory Assessment

Prothrombin times PT and APTT are usually prolonged and the platelet neutralization procedure (PNP) (see Chapter 30) may give abnormal results. The one-stage factor assay level of factor V with the PT method is decreased. Mixing studies with normal plasma will correct abnormal PT and APTT tests unless an inhibitor is present.

Factor VII (Proconvertin)

Factor VII is a vitamin K–dependent protein with a molecular weight of 48,000 in serum. It is produced in the liver. Factor VII is stable during storage of both serum and plasma.[2] It can be stored up to 4 days at 4°C with little loss of activity.[19] It is adsorbed by barium sulfate. The clinical picture may be variable (epistaxis, easy bruising, prolonged menstrual bleeding) and does not always correlate well with factor VII levels.[45]

Hereditary deficiency of factor VII is inherited in an autosomal recessive and has been described in approximately 100 cases. Acquired deficiencies of factor VII have been seen in patients with liver disease, receiving Coumadin therapy, and in vitamin K deficiency.

Treatment of a factor VII deficiency is with prothrombin complex concentrates and FFP. Five to 10 percent of normal activity is necessary to maintain hemostasis.

Laboratory Assessment

The laboratory features display a normal APTT and a prolonged PT corrected by normal serum in mixing studies. The PT is fully corrected by the use of Russell viper venom (see Chapter 30). One-stage factor assays using the PT method are usually abnormal.

Factor X (Stuart-Prower Factor)

Factor X is synthesized and produced in the liver. The factor is very stable during storage. Factor X is present in serum but absent in absorbed plasma. Factor X is also vitamin K dependent with a molecular weight between 50,000 and 100,000.

A factor X deficiency is one of the rarest congenital clotting defects. Through 1985 there were only 25 reported cases.[45] The hereditary transmission is autosomal recessive. In the normal population the deficiency occurs in one person per 500,000; however, the heterozygous state occurs in roughly 1 per 500. There are three variant forms of factor X deficiency and this can be a little confusing when using the Russell viper venom time (RVVT) as a diagnostic tool.[45] Usually the abnormal RVVT reflects a difference between a factor VII and a factor X deficiency. The variant forms of factor X are normal with the RVVT test.[45]

The clinical picture of factor X deficiency is not typical and may reflect epistaxis, gastrointestinal bleeding, and easy bruising. Hemarthroses have been reported.[2,45] During surgery, patients with the heterozygous state have displayed heavy bleeding.[45] Acquired defects of factor X usually correspond with other vitamin K–dependent disorder occurrences. Several reports have been cited of an isolated factor X deficiency that has occurred in connection with amyloidosis.[53]

Patients with factor X deficiency are treated with FFP or prothrombin complex factor concentrates rich in factor X. The disorder does not usually respond to vitamin K therapy. Hemostasis levels are maintained at 10 percent activity.[2]

Laboratory Assessment

The main laboratory features are a prolonged PT and APTT, which may be corrected by mixing studies with serum but not adsorbed plasma. This pattern is true for all of the factor X deficiencies including the variants. The RVVT may or may not be prolonged. The one-stage PT or APTT assay for factor X may be used for this assay with a marked decrease of factor X evident.

Factor XI (Plasma Thromboplastic Antecedent)

Factor XI is one of the contact factor plasma proteins involved in the early phases of coagulation. The molecular weight of the factor is approximately 124,000. It is found in serum and absorbed by kaolin but only partially absorbed by aluminum hydroxide and barium sulfate. Factor XI deficiency is transmitted by an autosomal recessive gene. Most cases of this disease have been found in people of Ashkenazi Jewish origin and consanguinous relationships.[45,54] Other people, however, may be affected. A factor XI

deficiency is the only contact factor defect in which a bleeding disorder may be evident.[45] There may be little correlation between bleeding episodes and the level of factor XI. Usually there is little spontaneous bleeding. Most cases of factor XI deficiencies remain undetected until the patient is screened for a surgical procedure. Abnormal bleeding has been seen in postoperative dental procedures, tonsillectomies, and urologic procedures. Excessive bleeding in postpartum deliveries has been seen. Factor XI deficiencies are usually treated with FFP. Heterozygotes have 10 to 20 percent of the normal mean level of factor XI. Factor XI levels are low in neonates (approximately 30 percent of adult values) and are also known to decline in women during pregnancy.

Acquired deficiency of factor XI is sometimes seen in DIC.[2] This is due to consumption following activation. The level required for hemostasis is 20 to 30 percent.[45]

Laboratory Assessment

The PT is normal. The APTT is prolonged and corrects upon mixing with normal plasma. The one-stage APTT factor assay displays a decreased level of factor XI.

Factor XII (Hageman Factor)

Factor XII is a member of the contact factor group of plasma clotting factors. Factor XII has a molecular weight of approximately 80,000. Its site of synthesis is unknown but is suspected to be produced in the liver. Factor XII is present in both serum and adsorbed plasma. The mode of inheritance is autosomal recessive. Deficiencies of factor XII usually do not cause hemorrhage; however, some of these patients may have thrombotic episodes.[45] It is not clear whether this means that patients with factor XII defect are more prone to thrombosis than is the general population or that no protection against thrombotic episodes is provided by the deficiency of factor XII.[45,55] The level of factor XII in normal healthy patients is between 70 and 140 percent activity. Heterozygotes show 40 to 60 percent of normal. The homozygotes for the defect usually have a level of 1 percent or less.[45]

Laboratory Assessment

The diagnosis of this disorder is usually made incidentally when the patient is being screened for a preoperative work-up. Factor XII can be activated by a variety of surfaces. In order to prevent a false shortening of an APTT by activation of factor XII by a nonsiliconized glass surface, care should be taken to use siliconized glassware or plastic for the collection of the blood samples.[2,56] The PT is normal; the APTT is prolonged, and the one-stage factor assay by APTT method for factor XII is decreased.

Factor XIII (Fibrin-Stabilizing Factor)

Factor XIII deficiency is inherited as an autosomal recessive trait. The molecular weight of factor XIII is approximately 320,000. Factor XIII may be produced in the liver, but at least 50 percent is associated with megakaryocytes. This factor acts as the stabilizer of the fibrin gel. The platelet fibrin-stabilizing factor portion of the molecule is activated by thrombin and acts much faster than the plasma fibrin-stabilizing factor which is activated by calcium. The net result is the formation of covalent cross-links between the polypeptide chains of the fibrin subunit.[2]

Factor XIII is composed of two subunits, subunit A and subunit B or S, respectively. Only subunit A displays fibrin-stabilizing activity. Subunit B's function is to carry subunit A into circulation. There are two types of factor XIII defects. In the first type, both subunit A and subunit B are immunologically decreased. In the other type only subunit A antigen is defective and subunit B is normal. The incidence of type I factor XIII deficiency is more rare than type II. Factor XIII activity is low and subunit A and B are absent immunologically. The factor XIII activity is again low in type II. The subunit A is absent but subunit B is present in normal or reduced amounts.[45,57]

The most common clinical symptom is bleeding from the umbilical stump. Most deaths with factor XIII deficiency occur at this stage of discovery of the plasma clotting factor defect. Rare cases of intracranial bleeding have been reported.[45,58] Keloid scar formation and retarded wound healing have been cited.[45] Initial stoppage of bleeding is normal but short-lived, with bleeding recurring 36 hours or longer after the initial trauma.[2]

Acquired defects of factor XIII may occur in patients who have leukemia.[2] Treatment of this disorder is usually accomplished with FFP or cryoprecipitate. The hemostatic level is approximately 1 to 2 percent.

Laboratory Assessment

All of the routine coagulation tests such as PT, APTT, bleeding time, and platelet functional assays are completely normal. Clot solubility in 5M urea or 1 percent monochloracetic acid is evident if factor XIII activity is less than 1 percent.[19,45,59] A device called the thromboelastograph has been used to determine a factor XIII deficiency, but this is primarily a research tool.[45]

Fletcher Factor Trait (Prekallikrein)

Fletcher factor behaves as a contact factor. It has a molecular weight of 80,000. In conjunction with Fitzgerald factor, the Fletcher factor works to activate factor XII.[45] Fletcher factor deficiency is inherited as an autosomal dominant trait.[45] A deficiency of this factor will cause a prolonged APTT, yet the patient is asymptomatic for bleeding. This factor along with factor XII and Fitzgerald factor is necessary for normal APTT results but can be bypassed in vivo.[59] Because the patient has no clinical symptoms of bleeding, no treatment is necessary.

Fletcher factor has also been studied in connection with its role in inflammation and chemotaxis.[2]

Laboratory Assessment

The laboratory evaluation of Fletcher factor can be a little perplexing. The PT, TT, and bleeding time are normal. The APTT is prolonged. There may be a borderline normal to normal correction of the APTT with mixing studies using fresh normal plasma, adsorbed plasma, and serum. Repeating the APTT using a prolonged incubation of 10 minutes at the activation step will usually normalize the prolonged APTT.[59] This is an excellent screening test for Fletcher factor deficiency. Confirmation of this deficiency should include one-stage APTT factor assays.

Fitzgerald Factor (High Molecular Weight Kininogen)

Site of synthesis for the Fitzgerald factor may be the liver. It has a molecular weight of 100,000. It functions primarily as a cofactor in plasma. Its role is one of activation of coagulation cascade.

Fitzgerald factor deficiency is a very rare asymptomatic disorder. This defect of the clotting system resembles closely the Fletcher factor.

Laboratory Assessment

A Fitzgerald factor deficiency can be investigated in a manner similar to that of Fletcher factor trait. The PT is normal and the APTT is prolonged. The APTT will correct with normal plasma, adsorbed plasma, and serum. Prolonged incubation of the APTT activation phase will remain prolonged. This will correct if the Fletcher factor is absent.[2,59] Confirmation should be with the one-stage APTT factor assay, which will show a decreased level.

Passovoy Trait

Patients with this trait have a moderate bleeding diathesis, which is transmitted as an autosomal dominant disorder.

Laboratory Assessment

The PT is normal and the APTT is slightly prolonged. The APTT is not corrected by prolonged incubation. The trait is the result of an abnormality in the intrinsic pathway of coagulation. Levels of all the known clotting factors are normal.[2,60]

CIRCULATING ANTICOAGULANTS-INHIBITORS

Circulating anticoagulants are inhibitors of the coagulation mechanism. They are endogeneously produced substances that interfere with various in vitro tests of coagulation.[61] These inhibitors present as acquired hemostatic defects and are usually immunoglobulins. Other materials such as heparin or fibrin degradation products can inhibit the hemostatic mechanism in vivo or in vitro.[62]

Specific Factor Inhibitors

Specific factor inhibitors are immunoglobulins with specificity for a single coagulation protein. The most common specific inhibitors are antibodies produced in relation to factor VIII:C. Identification of inhibitors to VIII:C is important because of the serious clinical bleeding that is associated with them.[62] Information discussed earlier in this chapter mentioned possible inhibitors related to each specific coagulation factor and the problems that could develop in testing and treatment.

Nonspecific Inhibitors – Lupus Anticoagulants

Nonspecific inhibitors like those of the lupus anticoagulant type are not specific for any single coagulation protein, are usually not associated with bleeding, and are usually not temperature dependent like those associated with factor VIII:C or factor V.[49,50,62]

The term lupus anticoagulant (LA) was suggested in 1972 by Feinstein and Rapaport.[63] The name was derived from an association of circulating anticoagulants originally reported by Conley and Hartmann in systemic lupus erythematosus (SLE).[64] Lupus anticoagulant is a misnomer owing to the fact that the majority of patients with an LA do not have SLE and, in the absence of other clinical hemostatic problems, do not bleed.[62] On the contrary, patients with an LA usually have a greater tendency toward thrombosis problems.[62]

Lupus anticoagulants are spontaneously occurring inhibitors that are immunoglobulins (IgG, IgM, IgA, or a combination) that directly react against anionic phospholipids in vitro. The LA inhibits the formation of the prothrombinase complex (factor Xa, factor Va, Ca^{2+}, prothrombin, and phospholipid surfaces). Therefore, the LA prolongs phospholipid-dependent coagulation tests (PT, APTT, RVVT, one-stage factor assays, and so on).[65-67]

Initially physicians and laboratory personnel viewed the presence of an LA as a nuisance.[62] Patients with a prolonged APTT needed to be evaluated for a possible bleeding tendency involving a long expensive work-up, requiring multiple factor assays, mixing studies, and other time-consuming tests.[62]

We are now aware that the presence of an LA can be associated with patients with autoimmune diseases such as SLE and acquired immunodeficiency syndrome (AIDS), infectious diseases (bacterial, viral, protozoal), following drug exposure (antibiotics, chlorpromazine, procainamide, and so on), strokes, spontaneous abortions, and lymphoproliferative disorders (Waldenström's macroglobulinemia, hairy-cell leukemia), and can occur even when no underlying disease is evident.[62]

Recently, enzyme-linked immunosorbent assay (ELISA) techniques have been developed to detect antibodies that react with cardiolipin.[68-72] The clinical conditions in which antibodies to cardiolipin — anticardiolipin antibodies (aCL or ACA) — are evi-

dent are very similar to those associated with LA.[68,70-75] Elevated IgG aCL levels seem to be more evident in patients with thrombotic tendencies.[76] Increased IgM aCL levels are seen in autoimmune disorders. Combinations of the two immunoglobulins present in aCL testing are not uncommon.[76] These assays are now being reported in units conforming to standards prepared by Dr. Nigel Harris of the Department of Rheumatology at the University of Louisville, in Kentucky. The units are reported as IgG phospholipid units (GPL) or IgM phospholipid units (MPL). Some patients with aCL antibodies display the presence of LA and others do not. Therefore, there may exist an overlap syndrome. A name suggested for this is antiphospholipid antibody syndrome (APA).[62,73] This group would include patients with phospholipid antibodies, whether or not an LA is present; patients who have tests evident for the presence of an LA only; and also a subset that have evidence of an LA and an APA. Thus, these antibodies should be considered as having overlapping reactivity rather than being different manifestations of the same antibody.[62,76]

The original classification for the presence of an LA, as suggested by the International Committee Communication for distinguishing LA in 1983,[77] is as follows:

1. APTT 5 seconds above the upper limits of normal range
2. APTT of a 1:1 mixture should be greater than 4 to 5 seconds over control
3. A decrease in at least two factors (VIII, IX, XI, XII) by one-stage factor assay
4. A sensitivity to dilution so that the apparent activity of the factor increases with dilution

These criteria have been found to be too restrictive and were not always valid. Better reagent systems and new procedures available made these criteria suspect in many cases. These guidelines were satisfactory for the classic LA, for which the Committee suggestions were originally proposed.

There is now a new set of proposed criteria that correlate clinical findings with laboratory results.[62] They are as follows:

1. Patients with APA syndrome should have at least one clinical and one laboratory finding during their disease.
2. An abnormality of phospholipid-dependent coagulation reaction(s) is found.
3. The abnormality is due to an inhibitor.
4. Inhibitor activity is directed at phospholipid rather than specific factors.

The laboratory findings should include APA detected by Venereal Disease Research Laboratories (VDRL) test, APTT, RVVT, PT, ELISA, RIA, platelet neutralization procedure (PNP), kaolin clotting time (KCT), and so on.

Laboratory Assessment

A number of tests are available to assist the laboratory clinician in confirming the presence of an LA/APA. These tests may be reviewed in Chapter 30. Tables 27–7 and 27–8 provide a complete listing

Table 27–7. **CONFIRMATORY TESTS FOR LUPUS ANTICOAGULANTS: DECREASED PHOSPHOLIPID**

| | TEST SYSTEM | | | SPECIFICITY | | | | |
Test	Nature of Phospholipid	Other Features	Sensitivity	Heparin	Oral Anticoagulant	Factor Deficiency	Specific Inhibitors	Comment
Tissue thromboplastin inhibition (TTI)	Simplastin diluted with saline 1:50 and 1:500	—	Sensitive but not specific; positive in 30% of normal subjects	False positive; 0.2 to 0.8 U/ml of heparin	False positive	False positive with factor VII, X, V, VIII, or IX deficiency	False positive with factors VIII, IX, or V inhibitors	May be negative with IgM drug-induced LA
Dilute Russell viper venom test (RVVT)	Thrombofax 1:8 TBS Correction: 0.1 ml (A23187) treated platelets	RVV diluted 1:200 TBS	Sensitive when compared with APTT and TTI	False positive	False positive, corrected by mixing studies	False positive with factor V or X deficiency	False positive with factor V inhibitor	Correction studies may use ionophore* platelets or PNP
KCT	No added phospholipid; KCT very sensitive to residual platelets	May use mixture of normal and patient plasma	Presence of platelets will significantly shorten KCT in presence of LA	—	—	—	—	Use of filtered plasma will increase sensitivity
Dilute phospholipid APTT (PL-APTT)	Thrombofax diluted 1:5, 1:10, 1:20, 1:40	Mixing patient and normal 1:1 and 0.5 silica	—	No effect if protamine added	No effect	No effect	Strong inhibitor (>10 Bethesda Units) may give false positive	

Source: From Triplett, DA and Brandt, JT: Confirmatory tests for lupus anticoagulants. Hematol Pathol 2(3):121, 1988, with permission.

*Ionophore: A 23187 (Eli Lilly)

Table 27–8. CONFIRMATORY TESTS FOR LUPUS ANTICOAGULANTS: INCREASED PHOSPHOLIPID*

	TEST SYSTEM			SPECIFICITY				
Test	Nature of Phospholipid	Other Features	Sensitivity	Heparin	Oral Anticoagulant	Factor Deficiency	Specific Inhibitors	Comment
Platelet neutralization procedure (PNP)	Outdated washed platelets, freeze-thawed	Use with sensitive APTT system	Sensitive in most cases with APTT 12 sec above upper limit of normal	False positive	False positive	—	Weak factor V inhibitor may be positive	Stored aliquots of platelets, stable for 3 mo at −20°C
High phospholipid APTT	Cephalin 1:200, 1:50, 1:25 (4–8 × normal conc)	Kaolin activator	—	—	—	—	—	In original study, time-dependent pattern noted
Rabbit brain neutralization procedure (RBNP)	Platelin high conc (use 4 × more lipid)	Kaolin, tilt tube	Original study 30/31 patients had positive test; only 18/30 had positive TTI	False positive	No effect	No effect	Slight shortening with factor VIII and XI inhibitors	—
PtdSer-liposome APTT	PtdSer vehicle final PS conc (24 × 10 moles/liter)	Kaolin, Manchester APTT reagent	—	False positive	No effect	No effect	No effect with factor VIII and IX inhibitors	Other lipids (PA, Phosphatidylserine PE, PG); no effect
Inside-out membrane absorption test	Washed fresh human red blood cells, lysed with phosphate buffer	Use APTT on mixture	—	No effect, as ECTEOLA† is used to absorb heparin	—	No effect	No effect with factor VIII inhibitor	—

Source: From Triplett, DA and Brandt, JT: Confirmatory tests for lupus anticoagulants. Hematol Pathol 2(33):121, 1988, with permission.
*The confirmatory tests for lupus anticoagulants may be divided into two categories. First is the use of test systems that seek to accentuate the effect of the anticoagulant by decreasing the amount of phospholipid in the test. Thus, the available phospholipid surfaces necessary for the assembly of the prothrombinase complex are limited and the presence of a low titer antiphospholipid antibody will prolong the coagulation time. The TTI and dilute RVVT are examples of this type of test system. The second group of tests rely on increased amounts of phospholipid to either neutralize or bypass the phospholipid antibodies and shorten the prolonged coagulation time (PNP).
†ECTEOLA = Cation ion exchange resin.

of procedures for determining the presence of an LA/APA. Unfortunately, a battery of tests must be used to classify this inhibitor properly. No single test is conclusive for the presence of an LA. Specimens being prepared for the presence of an LA/APA must be as free of platelets as possible.[78,79] The maximum platelet-poor plasma (PPP) count of residual platelets in plasma should be less than 15,000/μl.[79,80] Serum can be used for the aCL testing. When citrated plasma is used, the laboratory should take extra care in the centrifugation step. Platelets can cause inhibitor effects of their own on phospholipid-dependent tests. This is very evident when samples are frozen and thawed for further testing. Frequently this will cause a false shortening of the prolonged APTTs.[81]

SUMMARY

Tables 25–9 and 25–10 under laboratory evaluation of hemostasis in Chapter 25 should be reviewed at this time. This section of Chapter 25 gives an interpretation of screening for various coagulation abnormalities. Table 27–9 provides more reinforced information into the clotting factor defects and their laboratory diagnosis.

One of the most important parts of a work-up for a plasma clotting defect disorder is obtaining a good personal and family history from the patient. This should include a complete list of medications including both prescription medications and over-the-counter drugs.

A battery of screening tests for coagulation abnormalities should be performed to include:
1. A complete blood count (CBC) which should include a platelet count and differential smear to observe platelet morphology
2. Prothrombin time
3. Activated partial thromboplastin time
4. Bleeding time (BT)
5. Thrombin time

When the platelet count and morphology are normal, the results of the PT and APTT should be observed as follows:
1. Abnormal PT (could be due to deficiencies in fibrinogen; to deficiencies in factors II, V, VII, or X; or to an inhibitor to any of these factors, or to thrombin)
2. Abnormal APTT (could be due to deficiencies in factors II, V, VIII, IX, X, XI, XII, Fletcher, or Fitzgerald, or to inhibitors to these factors)
3. Normal PT, abnormal APTT (could be due to defects in factors VIII, IX, XI, XII, Fletcher, or Fitzgerald, or to inhibitors to these factors)
4. Abnormal PT, normal APTT (could be due to defects in factor VII)
5. Abnormal PT and APTT (may be due to defects of fibrinogen, factors II, VIII, IX, X, XI, or XII; or to a combined deficiency of factors V and VIII; or to the presence of inhibitors specific for the factors or the presence of an LA or heparin)

When testing for individual factor deficiencies, a factor assay specific for the suspected coagulation factor defects should be performed. Mixing studies using plasma or serum to the test plasma can help laboratorians narrow their search for the specific factor in question. When inhibitors are suspected, such as the LA or one that is specific for a certain factor, mixing studies and incubations should be performed. All specific factor inhibitors should be quantitated for the level of the inhibitor present. This is imperative because it lends valuable information to the physicians in their treatment plan.

The TT assesses thrombin-fibrinogen interaction and may be abnormal in patients who have hypofibrinogenemia or dysfibrinogenemia, and as a result of circulation inhibitors. In these cases, the PT and APTT both may be prolonged. Inhibitors such as fibrin-degradation products (FDPs) occurring in patients with DIC and following administration of heparin usually prolong the TT. The TT is the most sensitive index of heparin presence and of DIC.

CASE STUDIES

Case Study 1

A 10-year-old girl developed severe hemorrhaging after a puncture wound in the forearm following a bicycle accident. Patient had a prior history of easy bruising and frequent bouts of epistaxis. Her maternal grandmother and mother had experienced similar problems.

Upon physical examination, the patient was found to have several small bruises on her lower limbs and left upper forearm. She also had several small petechiae on her arms where her clothing was tight.

Laboratory findings included PT 11.0 sec; APTT 48.0 sec; BT 15.0 min; platelet count: 240,000/μl; VIII:C 30%; vWF:Ag 24%; ristocetin cofactor 38%; ristocetin-induced platelet aggregation decreased.

The prior history of bruising and frequent bouts of epistaxis, the prolonged APTT and bleeding time, and the decreased levels of VIII:C, vWF:Ag, ristocetin cofactor, and ristocetin-induced platelet aggregation are characteristic of von Willebrand's disease (type I).

Case Study 2

The patient, a 5-year-old girl, demonstrated a prolonged APTT during a severe bout of tonsillitis. There was no prior personal history or family history of bleeding. Her medications included penicillin, acetaminophen, and Dilantin.

The patient was found to have swollen lymph glands in her neck upon physical examination. No evidence of bruising, splenomegaly, or hemarthroses was present.

Laboratory findings were as follows: PT 12.0 sec; APTT 43.6 sec; TT 11.5 sec; BT 6.0 min; platelet count 300,000 μl.

Table 27–9. FACTOR DEFICIENCIES AND TEST RESULTS

	BT	PT	APTT	Adsorbed Plasma	Aged Serum	TT	Fibrinogen	Urea Solubility	Platelet Count	Protamine Sulfate	FDP
I	N	A	A	C	NC	A	A	N	N	—	—
II	N	A	A	NC	NC	N	N	N	N	—	—
V	A	A	A	C	NC	N	N	N	N	—	—
VII	N	A	N	NC	C	N	N	N	N	—	—
VIII : C	N	N	A	C	NC	N	N	N	N	—	—
VIII : vWF	A	N	A	C	C	N	N	N	N	—	—
IX	N	N	A	NC	C	N	N	N	N	—	—
X	N	A	A	NC	C	N	N	N	N	—	—
XI	N	N	A	C	C	N	N	N	N	—	—
XII	N	N	A	C	C	N	N	N	N	—	—
XIII	N	N	N	—	—	N	N	A	N	—	—
Prekallikrein	N	N	A*	C	C	N	N	N	N	—	—
HMWK	N	N	A	C	C	N	N	N	N	—	—
Plasminogen	N	N	N	—	—	N	N	N	N	—	—
Alpha-2-antiplasmin	N	N	N	—	—	N	N	N	N	—	—
Antithrombin-III	N	N	N	—	—	N	N	N	N	—	—
DIC	—	A	A	—	—	A	A	N	A	A	A
Fibrinolysis	—	N	A	—	—	A	A	N	N	N	A

Source: From Pittiglio, DH, et al: Treating hemostatic disorders. A problem-oriented approach. In Pittiglio, DH: Hemostasis Overview. American Association of Blood Banks, Arlington, VA, 1984, p 31, with permission.

N = normal; C = correction; A = abnormal; NC = no correction; BT = bleeding time; PT = prothrombin time; APTT = activated partial thromboplastin time; FDP = fibrin-degradation products.
*The APTT returns to normal after prolonged activation of the contact system.

APTT mixing studies:

1:1	39.0 sec patient + normal plasma (NP)
	30.5 sec NP
37°C (1:1)	48.5 sec patient
	35.6 sec NP
	46.0 sec patient + NP
KCT	114.1 sec patient
	80.0 sec NP
1:1	112.0 sec patient +NP
PNP	
Saline APTT	51.2 sec
Platelets APTT	42.0 sec
Correction	9.2 sec
Tissue-thromboplastin inhibition (TTI)	87.1 sec patient 59.0 sec NP
Ratio	1.48
Factor assays:	VIII:C 38.0%; corrects at 1:40 to 88.0%
	IX 41.5%; corrects
Anticardiolipin assay	IgG: Negative IgM: High positive

The negative clinical history of bleeding, accompanied by a prolonged APTT, abnormal mixing studies, a prolonged KCT, positive PNP, and TTI tests with reduced one-stage factor assays that correct upon dilution, is suggestive of the presence of acquired lupus anticoagulant. The high-positive IgM result of the anticardiolipin assay suggests there also exists an antiphospholipid antibody presence. Thus, the diagnosis would be evidence of an overlap syndrome or a LA/APA syndrome.

Case Study 3

A 55-year-old man with no prior history of bleeding developed a severe hemorrhaging problem after he was treated with cephalosporin (Cephalexin) for a bacterial infection of the groin region. The hemorrhaging occurred during surgery when the groin region was being drained.

The patient had no physical signs of bruising or hematomas prior to bleeding episode. His groin (right side) was swollen and slightly discolored prior to the postoperative hemorrhaging. He had to be given FFP and platelets to arrest the bleeding episode.

Laboratory findings included PT > 100 sec; APTT > 100 sec; platelet count 240,000; BT 6.0 min 30 sec; FDP [unable to assay; later results were greater than 320 and less than 640 μg/ml of FDPs (>320 < 640 μg/ml)].

APTT Mixing Studies:

1:1	87.2 sec patient + NP
	24.8 sec NP
37°C (1:1)	200 sec patient + NP
	31.6 sec NP

KCT	200.0 sec Patient
	85.1 sec NP
1:1	200 sec patient + NP
PNP	200 sec saline APTT
	94.1 sec platelets
Correction	100 sec

Platelet neutralization procedure with more than a 5.0 sec correction is usually indicative of a lupus anticoagulant. At first, coagulation factor assays were all abnormally low—factors II, V, VII, VIII, IX, X, XI, and XII were initially tested. Later assay showed a factor V of less than 1.0%, with a factor V inhibitor of greater than 1200 Bethesda units. The inhibitor type was IgG.

This patient was diagnosed as having an acquired factor V deficiency with a presence of a strong inhibitor to factor V. The PNP test result may be positive with a factor V deficiency, regardless of whether or not an inhibitor is present. This is due to the use of freeze-thawed platelets used in the PNP test to correct the APTT. Remember, 20 percent of factor V is contained on the platelet's surface membrane.[50-52]

REFERENCES

1. Pittiglio, DH: Introduction to hemostasis: An evaluation of hemostatic mechanism, platelet structure and function, and extrinsic and intrinsic systems. In Pittiglio, DH and Sacher, RA (eds): Clinical Hematology and Fundamentals of Hemostasis, ed 1. FA Davis, Philadelphia, 1987, p 324.
2. Rock, G: Defects of plasma clotting factors. In Pittiglio, DH and Sacher, RA (eds): Clinical Hematology and Fundamentals of Hemostasis, ed 1. FA Davis, Philadelphia, 1987, p 365.
3. Miale, JB: Hemostasis and blood coagulation: Hemophilia (factor VIII deficiency). In Laboratory Medicine: Hematology, ed 6. CV Mosby, St Louis, 1982, p 823.
4. Rosver, F: Hemophilia in the Talmud and rabbinic writings. Ann Intern Med 70:833, 1969.
5. McKusick, VA: The earliest record of hemophilia in America? Blood 19:243, 1962.
6. Brinkhous, KM: A short history of hemophilia with some comments on the word "hemophilia." In Brinkhous, KM and Hemker, HC (eds): Handbook of Hemophilia. American Elsevier Publishing, New York, 1975, p 3.
7. Morawitz, P: Die Chemie der Blutgerinnung. Erebn Physiol 4:307. Available in the English translation as: The Chemistry of Blood Coagulation, translated by Hartman, RC and Guenther, PF. Charles C Thomas, Springfield, IL, 1958.
8. Patek, AJ and Taylor, FHL: Hemophilia. II. Some properties of a substance detained from normal human plasma effective in accelerating the coagulation of hemophilic blood. J Clin Invest 16:113, 1937.
9. Coller, BS: von Willebrand Disease. In Colman, RW, Hirsh, J, Marder, VJ, and Salzman, EW (eds): Hemostasis and Thrombosis, ed 2. JB Lippincott, Philadelphia, 1987, p 60.
10. Palkuti, HS: Specimen collection and quality control. In Corriveau, DM and Fritsma, GA (eds): Hemostasis and Thrombosis in the Clinical Laboratory, ed 1. JB Lippincott, Philadelphia, 1988, p 67.
11. Rock, GA and Tittley, P: The effect of temperature variations on cryoprecipitate. Transfusion 19:86, 1979.
12. McGlasson, DL: Standardization of temperature handling and storage of plasma for coagulation testing. Tex J Med Tech 2:10, 1985.
13. Hoyer, LW: Factor VIII: Structure and function. In Biggs, R and Rizza, CR (eds): Human Blood Coagulation, Haemostasis and Thrombosis, ed 3. Blackwell Scientific, Oxford, 1984, p 57.

14. Weiss, HJ, Hoyer, LW, and Rickles, FR: Qualitative assay of plasma factor deficient in von Willebrand's disease, that is necessary for platelet aggregation. Relationship to factor VIII, procoagulant activity and antigen content. J Clin Invest 52:2708, 1973.

15. Zimmerman, TS, Ratnoff, DD, and Powell, AE: Immunologic differentiation of classic hemophilia (factor VIII deficiency) and von Willebrand's disease with observations on combined deficiencies of antihemophiliac factor and proaccelerin (factor V) and on an acquired circulating anticoagulant against antihemophiliac factor. J Clin Invest 50:244, 1971.

16. Laurell, CD: Electroimmunoassay. Scand J Clin Lab Invest 29 (Suppl 124): 21, 1972.

17. Lazarchick, J and Hoyer, LW: Immunoradiometric measurement of the factor VIII procoagulant antigen. J Clin Invest 62:1048, 1978.

18. Biggs, R: The inheritance of defects in blood coagulation. In Biggs, R and Rizza, CR (eds): Human Blood Coagulation, Haemostasis and Thrombosis, ed 3. Blackwell Scientific, Oxford, 1984, p 92.

19. Miller, JL: Blood coagulation and fibrinolysis. In Henry, JB (ed): Clinical Diagnosis and Management, ed 17. WB Saunders, Philadelphia, 1984, p 765.

20. Hoyer, LW and Breckenridge, RT: Immunologic studies of antihemophilic factor (AHF, factor VIII) II. Properties of cross reacting material. Blood 35:809, 1970.

21. Giddings, JC and Peake, IR: Laboratory support in the diagnosis of coagulation disorders. In Clinics in Hematology: Coagulation Disorders. Vol 14, no 2. WB Saunders, Philadelphia, 1985, p 571.

22. Graham, JB, et al: Statistical methods for carrier detection in haemophilias. In Bloom, AL (ed): Methods in Hematology: The Hemophilias. Churchill-Livingstone, Edinburgh, 1982, p 156.

23. Mihashan, RS, Rodeck, CH, and Thompston, JK: Prenatal diagnosis of the hemophilias. In Bloom, AL (ed): Methods in Hematology: The Hemophilias. Churchill-Livingstone, Edinburgh, 1982, p 176.

24. Antonarakis, SE, et al: Hemophilia A: Detection of molecular defects and of carriers by DNA analysis. N Engl J Med 313: 842, 1985.

25. Weiss, AE: Circulating inhibitors in hemophilia A and B: Epidemiology and methods of detection. In Brinkhous, KM and Henker, HC (eds): Handbook of Hemophilia. Excerpta Medica, Amsterdam, 1975, p 29.

26. Shapiro, SS: Hemorrhagic disorders associated with circulating inhibitors. In Ratnoff, OD and Forbes, CD (eds): Disorders of Hemostasis; Grune & Stratton, Orlando, FL, 1984, p 271.

27. Roberts, HR: The treatment of hemophilia: Past tragedy and future promise. N Engl J Med 321:1189, 1989.

28. White, GS, et al: Use of recombinant antihemophilic factor in the treatment of two patients with classic hemophilia. N Engl J Med 320:166, 1989.

29. Kasper, CK, et al: A more uniform measurement of factor VIII inhibitors. Thromb Diath Haemorrh 34:869, 1975.

30. Weiss, AE: The Hemophilias. In Corriveau, DM and Fritsma, GA (eds): Hemostasis and Thrombosis in the Clinical Laboratory, ed 1. JB Lippincott, Philadelphia, 1988, p 128.

31. Coller, BS: Von Willebrand's disease. In Ratnoff, OD and Farbes, CD (eds): Disorders of Hemostasis, Grune & Stratton, Orlando, FL 1984, p 241.

32. Holmborg, L and Nelson, IM: Von Willebrand's disease. In Clinics in Hematology: Coagulation Disorders. Vol 14, no 2. WB Saunders, Philadelphia, 1985, p 461.

33. Zimmerman, TS, Roberts, J, and Edgington, TS: Factor VIII, released antigen: Multiple molecular forms in human plasma. Proc Natl Acad Sci 72:5121, 1975.

34. Sultan, Y, Simeon, J, and Caen, JP: Electrophoretic heterogeneity of normal factor VIII/von Willebrand protein, and abnormal electrophoretic mobility in patients with von Willebrand's disease. J Lab Clin Med 87:185, 1976.

35. Ruggers, ZM and Zimmerman, TS: Variant von Willebrand's disease. Characterization of two subtypes by analysis of mul-

timeric composition of factor VIII/von Willebrand's factor in plasma and platelets. J Clin Invest 65:1318, 1980.

36. Manucci, PM, et al: Studies on the prolonged bleeding time in von Willebrand's disease. J Lab Clin Med 88:662, 1976.

37. Ludlam, CA, et al: Factor VIII and fibrinolytic response to deamino-8-D-arginine vasopressin in normal subjects and disassociate response in some patients with haemophilia and von Willebrand's disease. Br J Haematol 45:499, 1980.

38. Schmitz-Huebner, U, et al: DDAVP-induced changes of factor VIII related activities and bleeding time in patients with von Willebrand's syndrome. Haemostasis 9:204, 1980.

39. Forbes, CD: Clinical aspects of the hemophilias and their treatment. In Ratnoff, OD and Forbes, CD (eds): Disorders of Hemostasis. Grune & Stratton, Orlando, FL, 1984, p 204.

40. Shapiro, SS: Acquired inhibitors to the blood coagulation factors. Semin Thromb Hemost 1:336, 1975.

41. Eyster, ME, et al: The Pennsylvania hemophilia program 1973–1978. Am J Hematol 9:277, 1980.

42. McGraw, RL, et al: Structure and function of factor IX: Defects in haemophilia B. In Clinics in Hematology: Coagulation Disorders. Vol 14, no 2. WB Saunders, Philadelphia, 1985, p 359.

43. Lammle, B and Griffin, JH: Formation of the fibrin clot: The balance of precoagulant and inhibitory factors. In Clinics in Hematology: Coagulation Disorders. Vol 14, no 2. WB Saunders, Philadelphia, 1985, p 282.

44. Corriveau, DM: Plasma proteins: Factors of the hemostatic mechanism. In Corriveau, DM and Fritsma, GA (eds): Hemostasis and Thrombosis in the Clinical Laboratory, ed 1. JB Lippincott, Philadelphia, 1988, p 34.

45. Girolami, A, et al: Rarer quantitative and qualitative abnormalities of coagulation. In Clinics in Hematology: Coagulation Disorders, Vol 14, no 2. WB Saunders, Philadelphia, 1985, p 385.

46. Esnouf, MP: Thrombin-fibrinogen reaction and fibrin stabilization. In Biggs, R and Rizza, CR (eds): Human Blood Coagulation, Haemostasis and Thrombosis, ed 3. Blackwell-Scientific, Oxford, 1984, p 26.

47. Harrison, RL, Alperin, JB, and Dhruvik, K: Concurrent lupus anticoagulants and prothrombin deficiency due to phenytoin use. Arch Pathol Lab Med 3:719, 1987.

48. Brown, JM, et al: Combined factor V/VIII deficiency: A case report including levels of factor V and factor VIII coagulant and antigen as well as protein C inhibitor. Am J Hematol 20:401, 1985.

49. Brandt, JT, Britton, A, and Kraut, EA: Spontaneous factor V inhibitor with unexpected laboratory features. Arch Pathol Lab Med 110:224, 1986.

50. McGlasson, DL, et al: Acquired factor V inhibitor with laboratory features of a lupus anticoagulant. Proc Soc Armed Forces Med Lab Sci 17:20, 1988.

51. McGlasson, DL, et al: Platelet neutralization procedure (PNP): Atypical results seen with a factor V deficiency with and without the presence of an inhibitor. Clin Lab Sci 3:2, 1990, p 119.

52. Chediak, J, et al: Successful management of bleeding in a patient with factor V inhibitor by platelet transfusions. Blood 56:835, 1980.

53. Griep, PR, Kyle, RA, and Bowie, EJW: Factor X deficiency in amyloidosis: A critical review. Am J Hematol 11:443, 1981.

54. Rizza, CR and Matthews, JM: Clinical features of clotting factor deficiencies. In Biggs, R and Rizza, CR (eds) Human Blood Coagulation, Haemostasis and Thrombosis, ed 3. Blackwell-Scientific, Oxford, 1984, p 119.

55. Ratnoff, OD: A quarter century with Mr Hageman. Thromb Haemost 43:95, 1980.

56. Saito, H: Normal hemostatic mechanisms. In Ratnoff, OD and Forbes, CD (eds); Disorders of Hemostasis. Grune & Stratton, Orlando, FL, 1984, p 23.

57. Girolami, A, et al: A tentative classification of factor XIII deficiency in two groups. Acta Haematol 58:318, 1977.

58. Lorand, L, Losowski, MJ, and Miloszewski, KJM: Human factor XIII: Fibrin stabilizing factor. In Spret, T (ed): Progress in

Hemostasis and Thrombosis. Vol 5. Grune & Stratton, New York, 1980.

59. Fritsma, GA: Clot-Based assays of Coagulation: Disorders of Hemostasis. Grune & Stratton, Orlando, FL, 1984, p 123.

60. Houghie, C, McPherson, RA, and Aronson, L: Passovoy factor: A hitherto unrecognized factor necessary for haemostasis. Lancet 2:290, 1975.

61. Houghie, C: Circulating anticoagulants. In Pollen, L (ed): Recent Advances in Blood Coagulation. Vol 14. Churchill-Livingstone, Edinburgh, 1984, p 4.

62. Triplett, DA and Brandt, JT: Lupus anticoagulants: Misnomer paradox, riddle. Epiphenomenon. Hematol Pathol 2:121, 1988.

63. Feinstein, DI and Rapaport, SI: Acquired inhibitors of blood coagulation. In Spaet, T (ed): Progress in Hemostasis and Thrombosis, vol 1. Grune & Stratton, New York, 1972, p 75.

64. Conley, CL and Hartmann, RC: A hemorrhagic disorder caused by circulating anticoagulant in patients with disseminated lupus erythematosus. J Clin Invest 31:621, 1952.

65. Shapiro, SS and Thiagarajan, P: Lupus anticoagulants. In Spaet, T (ed): Progress in Hemostasis and Thrombosis. Vol 6. Grune & Stratton, New York, 1982, p 263.

66. Shapiro, SS, Thiagarajan, P, and DeMarco, L: Mechanism of action of the lupus anticoagulant. Ann NY Acad Sci 370:359, 1981.

67. Thiagarajan, P, Shapior, SS, and DeMarco, L: Monoclonal immunoglobulin M coagulation inhibitor with phospholipid specificity. Mechanism of a lupus anticoagulant. J Clin Invest 66:397, 1980.

68. Harris, EN, et al: Anticardiolipin antibodies: Detection by radioimmunoassay and association with thrombosis in systemic lupus erythematosus. Lancet 2:1211, 1983.

69. Triplett, DA, et al: Relationship between lupus anticoagulants and antibodies to phospholipid. JAMA 259:550, 1988.

70. Harris, EN, et al: Cross-reactivity of antiphospholipid antibodies. J Clin Lab Immunol 16:1, 1985.

71. Gharavi, AE, et al: Anticardiolipin antibodies: Isotype distribution and phospholipid specificity. Ann Rheum Dis 46:1, 1987.

72. Harris, EN, Gharavi, AE, and Hughes, GRV: Antiphospholipid antibodies. Clin Rheum Dis 11:591, 1985.

73. Hughes, GRV, Harris, NNR, and Gharavi, AE: The anticardiolipin syndrome. J Rheumatol 13:486, 1986.

74. Hughes, GRV: Editorial: The anticardiolipin syndrome. Clin Exp Rheum 3:285, 1985.

75. Asherson, RA, et al: Anticardiolipin antibody, recurrent thrombosis and warfarin withdrawal. Ann Rheum Dis 44:283, 1985.

76. Triplett, DA, et al: The relationship between lupus anticoagulants and antibodies to phospholipid. JAMA 259:550, 1988.

77. Green, D, et al: Report of the working party on acquired inhibitors of coagulation studies of the "lupus" anticoagulant. Thromb Haemost 49:144, 1983.

78. Exner, T: Comparison of two simple tests for the lupus anticoagulants. Am J Clin Pathol 83:215, 1985.

79. McGlasson, DL, et al: Differences in kaolin-clotting times and platelet counts resulting from variations in specimen processing. Clin Lab Sci 2:2, 1989.

80. Margolis, J: The kaolin clotting time: A rapid one stage method for diagnosis of coagulation defects. J Clin Pathol 11:406, 1958.

81. Triplett, DA, et al: Laboratory diagnosis of lupus inhibitors: A comparison of the tissue thromboplastin inhibition procedure with a new platelet neutralization procedure. Am J Clin Pathol 79:678, 1983.

QUESTIONS

1. *Which of the following can produce defects that lead to impairment of the coagulation system?*
   a. Decreased factor synthesis
   b. Interference of abnormal molecules
   c. Loss, consumption, or inactivation of factors
   d. All of the above

2. *Which of the following diseases show decreased activity of factor VIII:C?*
   a. Hemophilia A
   b. Hemophilia B
   c. Parahemophilia
   d. Passovoy trait

3. *Which disorder can display decreased activity of factor VIII:C vWF:Ag; ristocetin cofactor, and prolonged bleeding time?*
   a. Hypoprothrombinemia
   b. von Willebrand's disease
   c. Hemophilia A
   d. Hemophilia B

4. *Which disease shows severity directly comparable to the level of factor IX clotting activity? (Use answer choices for question 3.)*

5. *What coagulation factor deficiency shows clot solubility in 5M urea or 1 percent monochloracetic acid?*
   a. Factor XII
   b. Prekallikrein
   c. Factor XIII
   d. High molecular weight kininogen

6. *Which plasma clotting defect is not associated with bleeding?*
   a. Factor V
   b. Lupus anticoagulants
   c. Factor X
   d. Factor XI

7. *Which factor defect shows an abnormal PT, but normal APTT?*
   a. Factor VII
   b. Factor VIII
   c. Factor X
   d. Factor II

ANSWERS

1. d (p. 463)
2. a (p. 468)
3. b (p. 470)
4. d (p. 472)
5. c (p. 477)
6. b (p. 478)
7. a (p. 481)

CHAPTER 28

JOHN LAZARCHICK, M.D.
JOETTE KIZER, M.L.T.(ASCP)

Interaction of the Fibrinolytic, Coagulation, and Kinin Systems and Related Pathology

OBJECTIVES

At the end of this chapter, the learner should be able to:
1. List plasminogen activators and negative feedback clotting mechanisms.
2. Describe plasmin's action in forming the intermediate degradation product, D-dimer.
3. Name the primary inhibitor of the fibrinolytic system.
4. List mechanisms and clinical conditions associated with disseminated intravascular coagulation.
5. Define the three generalized clinical states of dissemi-

nated intravascular coagulation with regard to the typical laboratory abnormalities associated with each state.
6. Identify therapies for treatment of disseminated intravascular coagulation.
7. Describe the use of laboratory tests to distinguish primary fibrinolysis from disseminated intravascular coagulation.

Normal hemostasis is the result of the balanced interaction of the vascular endothelium and platelets with four biochemical systems:[1,2] the coagulation, the fibrinolytic, the kinin, and, to a lesser extent, the complement system. The interrelationship among these systems is illustrated in Figure 28–1. When a stimulus initiates activation of the coagulation system with resultant fibrin formation and the establishment of a hemostatic barrier, a series of enzymes composing the fibrinolytic system are simultaneously activated to lyse the fibrin thrombus and reestablish vessel lumen integrity and blood flow. This chapter deals with the biochemistry of the

components of this fibrinolytic system, its associated pathophysiologic disorders, and laboratory tests available to evaluate individual components and overall function.

MOLECULAR COMPONENTS: PHYSICOCHEMICAL AND FUNCTIONAL PROPERTIES

The molecular components of the fibrinolytic system consist of (1) the plasma protein plasminogen; (2) its active enzymatic form, plasmin; (3) a

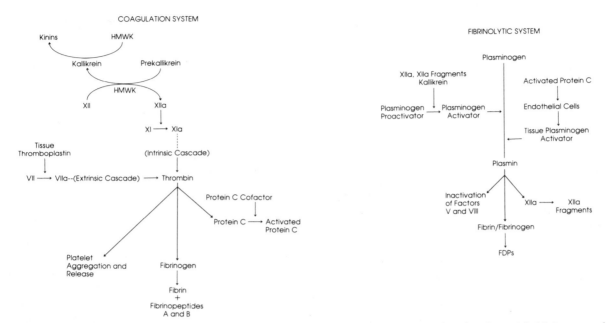

Figure 28–1. Diagrams of the interaction of the coagulation, fibrinolytic, and kinin systems. High molecular weight kininogen and prekallikrein catalyze the activation of factor XII to XIIa. Factor XIIa then promotes the conversion of prekallikrein to kallikrein. The latter liberates kinins from high molecular weight kininogen thus completing the positive feedback loops of the contact phase of coagulation. Thrombin formed through the extrinsic or intrinsic cascade systems converts fibrinogen to fibrin and induces platelet aggregation release. Thrombin bound to thrombomodulin on the endothelial surface activates protein C that indirectly promotes tissue plasminogen activator release from endothelial cells. A second point of interaction between these systems can also result in formation of plasminogen activator. Kallikrein in association with factor XIIa and XIIa fragments convert a plasmin proactivator to its activated state. Through either activating system, plasminogen can be proteolytically cleaved to form plasmin. Plasmin not only lyses fibrin and inactivates factors V and VIII but also degrades factor XIIa to inactivate fragments, which are a component of the second plasminogen activator system.

group of plasminogen activators that convert plasminogen to plasmin; (4) plasmin inhibitors, most prominently α_2-plasmin inhibitor; and (5) fibrin/fibrinogen, which serves as substrate for the active enzyme plasmin (Table 28–1).

Plasminogen

Native plasminogen is a single-chain plasma zymogen of approximately 90,000 daltons that circulates in two molecular forms, differing only in their carbohydrate content.[3] It is synthesized by the liver and has a half-life of 2 days. The plasma content is approximately 20 mg/dl. Each form of this molecule has an amino acid terminal glutamic acid (Glu-plasminogen) and is capable of undergoing limited proteolytic cleavage of this region to an incomplete molecule with lysine as the new terminal amino acid (Lys-plasminogen). This latter form is more readily converted to active plasmin by plasminogen activators than the Glu-plasminogen form and is probably of greater physiologic significance.

Table 28–1. **COMPONENTS OF THE FIBRINOLYTIC SYSTEM**

	Comments
1. Plasminogen	Circulating zymogen form with molecular weight of 90,000 daltons
2. Plasminogen activators	
Tissue activator	Endogenous activator liberated from endothelial cells by the action of protein C
Factor XIIa, kallikrein	Contact phase activator generated with the initiation of coagulation
Factor XIIa fragments	
Factor XIa	
Urokinase	Proteases produced in the kidney and secreted in the urine
Streptokinase	Bacterial cell product; forms complex with plasminogen which has intrinsic activating activity
3. Plasmin	Active serine protease of 70,000–75,000 daltons
4. α_2-Plasmin inhibitor	Primary inhibitor of plasmin; forms irreversible complex with plasmin
α_2-Macroglobulin	Serves as a plasmin inhibitor only when α_2-plasmin inhibitor binding sites are saturated
5. Fibrinogen, fibrin	Plasmin substrates; proteolytic cleavage results in the generation of degradation products

Plasminogen Activators

The conversion of either form to active plasmin can be initiated through a variety of direct or indirect mechanisms.[4] This group of activating proteins is collectively known as plasminogen activators. Regardless of the initiating mechanism, activation of plasminogen to yield plasmin proceeds through the cleavage of the same arginine 560 – valine 561 bond in the Glu and Lys forms of plasminogen. These activators are either endogenous or exogenous in origin. Endogenous activators are serine proteases present in the blood and a variety of other tissues, particularly the vascular endothelium. With the initiation of the contact phase of coagulation (see Chapter 25) factor XIIa, XIIa fragments, factor XIa, kallikrein, and high molecular weight kininogen interact to yield plasminogen-activating ability.[5] The exact biochemical steps involved in the formation of this intrinsic activator are not completely understood. The activator activity generated by this pathway slowly converts plasminogen to plasmin. A great deal of interest has been most recently directed toward the endogeneous activator system because of its potential for pharmacologic manipulation and its greater efficiency in thrombolytic therapy. This mechanism is probably the major physiologic activator of plasminogen. Tissue plasminogen activator (TPA) is an endothelial cell product with a molecular weight of approximately 68,000 daltons.[6] The mechanism controlling its release from vascular endothelium is unsettled, but protein C, a vitamin K–dependent serine protease, is a likely candidate. Thrombin generated during the coagulation binds to its receptor, thrombomodulin, on the endothelial surface. This complex then rapidly converts protein C to activated protein C. Activated protein C promotes clot lysis by indirectly liberating TPA from endothelial cells, thus initiating endogenous fibrinolysis. This function of activated protein C is probably due to its ability to inhibit plasminogen activator inhibitor 1 (PAI-1), an additional endothelial cell product. At the same time, protein C exerts a negative feedback control on the coagulation process by inactivating coagulant factors V and VIII, thus limiting further clot formation.[7,8] This latter function of activated protein C is accelerated by its formation of a complex with protein S, which serves as a cofactor. Tissue plasminogen activator has a high affinity for fibrin, and its adsorption to fibrin clots greatly enhances plasminogen conversion to plasmin. Because of a higher affinity of both the plasminogen activator and plasminogen for fibrin rather than fibrinogen, the effects of this reaction is accentuated on the surface of and within the clot. Release of TPA from endothelium is also responsive to a variety of other stimuli including venous occlusion, strenuous exercise, and treatment with vasoactive drugs including the vasopressin derivative 1-deamino-8-D-arginine vasopressin (DDAVP). Tissue plasminogen activator activity is increased severalfold under these conditions.[9]

Exogenous activators have been available for clinical use for a number of years. One of these, urokinase, is synthesized by the kidney and excreted in the urine.[10] It can also be identified in vitro using kidney cell cultures and is a potent direct activator of plasminogen. Its major drawbacks are its expense and its relatively lower affinity for fibrin compared with TPA. A consequence of the latter property is that the plasmin generated will digest not only fibrin but also circulating fibrinogen; therefore, the development of severe hypofibrinogenemia is not uncommon with its use. The other exogenous activator, streptokinase (SK), is a product of beta-hemolytic streptococci. It is not a serine protease and has no intrinsic proteolytic activity but is capable of forming a 1:1 stoichiometric complex with plasminogen. This interaction results in a conformational change of the plasminogen molecule and exposure of its active serine site.[11] The streptokinase-plasminogen complex can then undergo autocatalysis to yield other activators — namely, SK-Glu-plasmin and SK-Lys-plasmin. Any of these forms will readily convert free plasminogen to plasmin. Because streptokinase is a bacterial protein, a major limitation with its use in thrombolytic therapy is the induction of an immune response with resulting antibody development and an inhibition of its activity.

Plasmin

The pivotal serine protease generated through these complex biochemical processes is plasmin. This protein has a molecular weight of 77,000 to 85,000, depending on whether Lys-plasmin or Glu-plasmin is formed, and has a transient plasmin half-life measured in seconds.[12] Plasmin has the ability to proteolytically degrade both fibrin in clots and native fibrinogen in the circulation into a series of well-characterized end-products collectively known as fibrin/fibrinogen degradation products (FDPs). This process results in an asymmetrical, progressive breakdown of fibrin and fibrinogen.[13] The earliest recognized component is fragment X which is still capable of clotting. A recent finding has been the identification of a small peptide fragment from the B beta chain of fibrinogen which is released simultaneously with the formation of the X fragment. Measurement by radioimmunoassay of this B beta 15-42* related peptide may prove of value in the documentation of early fibrinolytic states.[14,15] The X fragment undergoes further plasmin attack to yield unclottable Y and D fragments. The Y fragment is further digested to yield an additional D fragment and a single E fragment. It is now realized that the proteolytic cleavage of cross-linked fibrin — that is, fibrin transamidated through the action of factor XIIIa and calcium — results in other intermediate degradation products such as D2E without the generation of fragment D or E. This proteolytic product is referred to as the D-dimer.

These breakdown products have specific inhibi-

---

*Amino acid sequence numbering of this peptide.

tory effects on the coagulation system and thereby suppress further clot formation. Fragment X is capable of clotting slowly and exerts an anticoagulant effect by competing with fibrinogen for thrombin. It also forms slowly polymerizing complexes with fibrin monomer. Fragment Y forms nonclottable complexes with fibrin monomer and inhibits the polymerization step. Fragment D forms abnormal complexes with fibrin monomers as it polymerizes. Fragment E is not known to have any specific anticoagulant effect. In high concentrations (greater than $100 \mu g/ml$), the degradation products are capable of inhibiting platelet aggregation and release. Plasmin also exerts a direct limiting effect on the coagulation process by being able to proteolytically cleave and render inactive factors V and VIII.

Plasmin Inhibitors

Although plasmin formation characteristically takes place in the area of fibrin deposition with little free plasmin circulating, this enzyme if unchecked by the presence of specific inhibitors would result in circulating fibrinogen being digested and the blood being rendered unclottable. The primary physiologic inhibitor of plasmin in vivo is α_2-plasmin inhibitor.[16,17] It rapidly and irreversibly binds to the lysine binding site on plasmin in a 1:1 molar ratio. Measurement of these plasmin: α_2-plasmin inhibitor complexes has been suggested as an indicator for activation of the fibrinolytic system. Plasmin adsorbed onto fibrin during the fibrinolytic process appears to be protected from this inhibitor because it binds to fibrin through the same lysine binding site. Because this binding site on plasmin is occupied, the inhibitor cannot bind and clot lysis can proceed. The overall effect is to ensure that plasmin activity is limited to the area of fibrin deposition and to prevent free plasmin from circulating. Other protease inhibitors in plasma include α_2-macroglobulin, C1 inactivator, and α_1-antitrypsin. Of these, only α_2-macroglobulin has a role in plasmin inhibition during normal hemostasis but only participates when α_2-plasmin inhibitor binding sites for plasmin are saturated.

CONGENITAL ABNORMALITIES

Congenital abnormalities of the fibrinolytic system are rare.[18] Only three cases of an abnormal plasminogen have been reported. Each patient in these reports had a history of recurrent thrombotic episodes. Low levels of TPA activity have been documented in two families and were associated with a similar thrombotic tendency. Deficiencies of α_2-plasmin inhibitor have been reported in four families to date and, in contrast, are associated with a severe hemorrhagic tendency. Acquired abnormalities of the fibrinolytic system are much more common and are discussed in the section on disseminated intravascular coagulation and related disorders.

In summary, an integrated system of serine pro-

teases is brought into play once the coagulation process is initiated in response to disruption of blood vessel integrity (Fig. 28-2). The response is balanced so that the same reaction that initiated thrombin formation and fibrin deposition also initiates a series of reactions to lyse the clot. Factor XII with other components of the contact phase of coagulation convert plasminogen to plasmin; protein C through its interaction with thrombin indirectly releases TPA with subsequent plasmin generation. Because of the high affinity of plasmin for fibrin, most of these fibrinolytic processes take place at the site of fibrin deposition within the damaged blood vessel. The presence of plasmin inhibitors further ensures that the proteolytic process is limited to this area.

DISSEMINATED INTRAVASCULAR COAGULATION

When there is damage to a blood vessel, an ordered, integrated series of reactions involving the coagulation, fibrinolytic, kinin, and complement systems occurs, as outlined in the previous chapters, with the initial formation and subsequent lysis of fibrin deposits. The initial formation of the fibrin clot prevents further hemorrhage and initiates vascular repair. The subsequent clot lysis serves to reestablish blood flow and vascular integrity. This process is normally self-limited and localized. Under certain pathologic stimuli, the coagulation response may be accentuated and the normal inhibitory mechanisms overwhelmed. Activation of the coagulation system under these circumstances causes consumption of the coagulation factors and platelets with subsequent formation of fibrin thrombi not only at the site of endothelial damage but also in a random manner throughout the microcirculation.[19] This hemorrhagic syndrome has been referred to as disseminated intravascular coagulation (DIC), defibrination syndrome, or consumptive coagulopathy. Simultaneous with and secondary to the activation of the coagulation cascade, the fibrinolytic system is activated. Regardless of the nature of the inciting stimulus, the pathophysiologic effect of this process is reflective of the balance between fibrin deposition (action of thrombin) and fibrinolysis (action of plasmin). The clinical manifestations thus can be one of diffuse hemorrhage (**see Color Plate 257**) owing to depletion of platelets and coagulation factors, ischemic tissue damage due to vascular occlusion, or the occurrence of both simultaneously in different areas of the microvasculature.

Triggering Mechanisms: Associated Clinical Disorders

The diverse stimuli that are capable of triggering the coagulation cascade in this manner all act through one or more of three mechanisms:[20] (1) activation of the extrinsic coagulation pathway by the release of tissue thromboplastin, (2) activation of the intrinsic coagulation pathway with factor XIIa for-

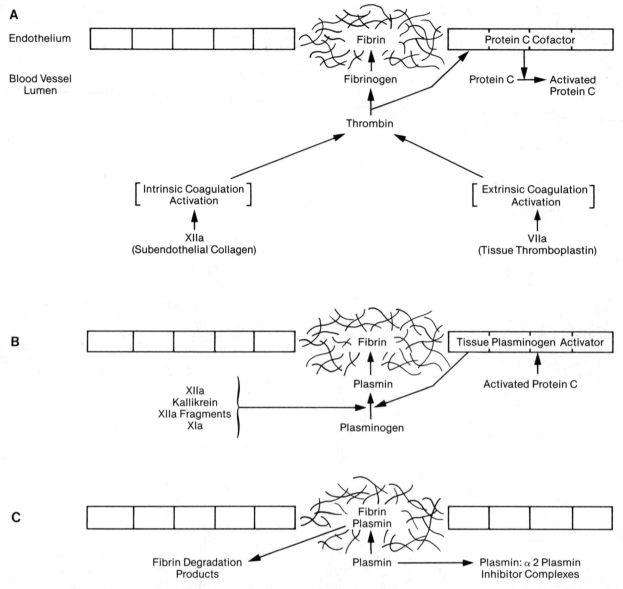

Figure 28-2. (*A*) Disruption of endothelial continuity results in platelet adherence, factor XIIa and VIIa formation, and the generation of thrombin at the damaged site. Thrombin then converts fibrinogen to fibrin to reestablish a temporary barrier. Secondarily and simultaneously thrombin complexes with thrombomodulin on the endothelial surface. Protein C once bound to this complex is rapidly converted to its activated state. (*B*) Activated protein C indirectly causes release of tissue plasminogen activator from endothelial cells. An additional plasminogen activator is formed through the interaction of the contact phase components. Both of these activators then convert plasminogen in and on the surface of the fibrin clot to plasmin. (*C*) Plasmin-induced proteolysis of the fibrin clot results in the formation of fibrin degradation products. Re-endothelialization of the damaged blood vessel begins as clot dissolution is occurring. Excess plasmin is irreversibly complexed with its inhibitor, alpha-2-plasmin inhibitor, preventing proteolysis of circulating fibrinogen.

mation, and (3) direct activation of factor X or II. The exact sequence of intermediary events by which certain of the stimuli initiate coagulation is well understood but with other stimuli this process is unknown. Disseminated intravascular coagulation due to direct activation of factor VII seen after massive injury or in certain obstetrical complications results from release of tissue thromboplastin from the injured tissue or from amniotic fluid entering the circulation. Certain tumors, particularly mucinous adenocarcinomas, are rich in thromboplastinlike material and may act through the same mechanism. The coagulopathy seen with red cell

lysis may be due to the release of thromboplastin-like activity from the stroma of these cells. All pathologic stimuli that result in activation of the intrinsic system probably do so indirectly by means of first inducing endothelial cell damage with subsequent exposure of the subendothelium. Platelet adherence and aggregation and factor XII activation can then occur. This is the proposed mechanism of DIC associated with sepsis, anoxia, and immune complex formation. Direct activation of coagulation factors can also occur in the presence of proteolytic enzymes. The venoms of certain snakes act through this mechanism; for example, Russell's viper venom

Table 28–2. **CLINICAL CONDITIONS ASSOCIATED WITH DIC**

Thromboplastin Release — Factor VII Activation	
Placental abruption	Promyelocytic leukemia
Trauma	Retained dead fetus syndrome
Fat emboli syndrome	Acute intravascular hemolysis*
Mucin-secreting adenocarcinoma	Amniotic fluid embolus*
Sepsis*	Cardiopulmonary bypass surgery
Endothelial Cell Damage — Factor XII Activation	
Immune complex disease	Burns
Intravascular hemolysis*	Vasculitis
Liver disease*	Anoxia
Heat stroke	Acidosis
Sepsis*	
Factor X/II Activation	
Snake venoms	Liver disease*
Acute pancreatitis	Fat emboli syndrome*

*More than one mechanism may be involved.

activates factor X, whereas venom from the sand rattlesnake causes direct conversion of prothrombin to thrombin. Certain malignancies have also been reported to have direct factor X–activating capability, which may account for the DIC seen in

these states. A list of clinical conditions associated with these triggering mechanisms is shown in Table 28–2.

Clinical Presentation

The clinical presentation depends to a great extent on which of the proteolytic processes (coagulant or fibrinolytic) is dominant. This allows for a wide spectrum ranging from an acute, severe hemorrhagic disorder to a low-grade disorder with predominantly thrombotic manifestations. A number of factors are important in determining the final clinical picture, including the magnitude and duration of the triggering stimulus; the functional ability of the reticuloendothelial system, particularly the liver, to remove from circulation activated coagulation factors, fibrin monomers, fibrin/fibrinogen products, as well as immune complexes; the compensatory ability of the liver and the bone marrow to accelerate clotting factor and platelet production; and finally the extent to which any particular organ is involved with hemorrhage or thrombus.[19]

Laboratory Diagnosis

The laboratory findings in patients with DIC reflect the direct or indirect effects of excess thrombin and plasmin generation (Table 28–3). The constellation of abnormalities in any particular patient, however, depends on the nature, magnitude, and

Table 28–3. **LABORATORY TESTS TO DETECT EXCESS THROMBIN AND/OR PLASMIN ACTIVITY**

Excess Protease	Effect	Laboratory Tests
A. Thrombin	Fibrinogen utilization	Fibrinogen concentration Thrombin/reptilase time PT and APTT
	Utilization of other coagulation factors	PT and APTT Coagulation factor assays
	Fibrin monomer generation	Ethanol gelation and protamine sulfate tests
	Fibrinopeptide A/B release	Radioimmunoassays for fibrinopeptides A/B
	Platelet aggregation	Platelet count Radioimmuno release assays for beta thromboglobulin and PF4
	Activation of protein C	TPA Activity Factor V/VIII assays
B. Thrombin/Plasmin	Proteolysis of fibrinogen/fibrin	FDPs D-dimer concentration B beta 15-42 peptide assay Fibrinopeptide A/B assays
	Indirectly activate plasminogen activators	Euglobulin lysis time
	Soluble fibrin Monomer/fibrinogen Monomer/fibrinogen/FDP complexes	Protamine sulfate precipitation Ethanol gelation test
C. Plasmin	Plasminogen utilization	Plasminogen concentration
	Proteolysis of fibrinogen/fibrin	FDPs Thrombin/reptilase times B beta 15-42 peptide assay Platelet aggregation and release tests
	Complexes with inhibitor	α_2-Plasmin inhibitor concentration; α_2-plasmin inhibitor: plasmin complexes
	Proteolysis of factors V/VIII	Factor assays

duration of the triggering stimulus; the compensatory capacity available; and the underlying disease state. Although the ultimate confirmatory test would be the direct demonstration of fibrin deposition in biopsy material from an involved blood vessel, this is not practical. As a result, a multitude of tests have been used by various laboratories to make this diagnosis.[15,21] It should be pointed out that no single test is diagnostic of DIC; however, in the appropriate clinical setting (patient history and the type of bleeding) a battery of tests can ensure a diagnosis of DIC. Indirect tests that lack specificity for thrombin action include the prothrombin time (PT), activated partial thromboplastin time (APTT), and thrombin/reptilase clotting times. Utilization and depletion of the clotting factors in the DIC process result in prolongation of each of these global tests. Because platelets are also consumed during the coagulation process and their contents released, the findings of thrombocytopenia and elevated plasma levels of the platelet-specific proteins beta thromboglobulin and platelet factor 4 (PF4) would be expected. The plasma inhibitor antithrombin III (AT-III) will complex with thrombin and activated factor X to result in diminished plasma levels of AT-III. If the fibrin deposition does not completely occlude the lumen of the damaged blood vessel, red cells may undergo a shearing effect as they traverse this area with resultant fragmentation and the development of a microangiopathic hemolytic anemia (**see Color Plate 258**).

Specific tests for direct evidence of thrombin activity relate to the action of thrombin on fibrinogen. Other than certain snake venoms, thrombin is the only enzyme that releases the specific peptides fibrinopeptide A and B from the fibrinogen molecule. Radioimmunoassays are available to measure each fibrinopeptide.[22] The major drawback to measuring these peptides, paradoxically, is the extreme sensitivity of the assay such that elevated levels can be seen in clinical conditions where thrombin is only transiently generated. As a consequence of fibrinopeptide release, soluble fibrin monomers are formed that are capable of forming complexes with intact fibrinogen molecules or with fibrin/fibrinogen degradation products. The ability to precipitate these complexes from plasma is the basis for two paracoagulation assays, the ethanol gelation test and the protamine sulfate test.[23] Positive test results are indirect indications that thrombin was generated; therefore, the coagulation system had to have been activated.

Tests for the secondary activation of the fibrinolytic system in DIC are directed primarily at demonstrating the action of plasmin on fibrin/fibrinogen. As already mentioned, a series of cleavage products are formed, the FDPs. The anticoagulant action of these fragments was noted previously. A number of immunologic tests are available to measure one or more of the fibrinogen fragments and can yield quantitative information on the degree of fibrinolysis. Because of its ease of performance and specificity (that is, evidence of plasmin action on cross-

linked fibrin), the D-dimer assay is gaining wide popularity as the immunologic assay of choice. One development has been the recognition of an early cleavage product of the B beta chain of the fibrinogen dimer, peptide B beta 1-42.[14] Clinical assessment of the utility of the B beta 15-42 radio-immunoassay for this peptide in diagnosing accelerated fibrinolysis is ongoing. Direct measurement of the plasminogen concentration in plasma can also be performed, and assays for measuring plasmin levels are being used. An indication of increased plasminogen activator activity seen in early stages of DIC can be obtained by performing a euglobulin lysis time.[24] The euglobulin fraction of plasma contains plasminogen, plasminogen activator, plasmin, and fibrinogen. The rapidity of lysis of the fibrin clot is directly related to plasminogen activator levels. Assays for α_2-plasmin inhibitor levels and for circulating plasma α_2-plasmin inhibitor complexes are under investigation for clinical use.

Table 28–4 summarizes laboratory tests available to diagnose DIC and the constellation of results possible in this syndrome, depending on the balance between thrombin and plasmin activities and the compensatory capacity of the patient. This table describes three generalized clinical states of DIC with the typical laboratory abnormalities associated with each. The decompensated DIC state refers to a condition in which active hemorrhage is evident and in which the consumption of the coagulation factors and platelets exceeds the capacity to increase the synthesis of these components. In the compensated state, laboratory evidence of an accelerated coagulation and fibrinolytic process is evident (increased fibrinopeptide A (FPA), positive protamine sulfate test, increased beta thromboglobulin, increased FDPs or D-dimer levels, presence of α_2-plasmin inhibitor complexes), but the rate of synthesis of the coagulation components is balanced with the rate of destruction. Because of this balance the PT, APTT, thrombin time (TT), and platelet count are usually normal. The hypercoagulable state is the result of excess thrombin present in the plasma with a delayed or lessened plasmin response. A characteristic finding in this form of DIC is a shortened APTT. It should be realized that these clinical states are not static, and it is not unusual for one state to evolve into another depending on the nature of the underlying disease process and response to therapy.

Therapy

Therapy of DIC is essentially twofold: treatment or removal of the underlying pathologic stimulus and maintenance of blood volume and hemostatic function.[19,20] Dramatic improvement in the patient's clinical status with abrupt cessation of bleeding and normalization of the coagulation abnormalities can be seen in certain cases of DIC with removal of the underlying pathologic stimulus alone, such as DIC associated with retained dead fetus. In cases of DIC associated with septicemia, ap-

Table 28–4. **LABORATORY TESTS TO DIAGNOSE DIC**

	Decompensated	Compensated	Hypercoagulability
Routine Test			
PT	I	N	N
APTT	I	N	D
TT/Reptilase time	I	N/I	N/I
Fibrinogen	D	N	I
Platelet count	D	N/D	N
FDPs	I	I	N/I
Euglobulin lysis test	N/I/D	N/D	N
Protamine sulfate test	P	P/Ng	P/Ng
Special Test			
Coagulation factor levels	D	N/D	I
Fibronopeptide A	I	I	I
D-dimer	I	I	N
Plasminogen	D	N/D	N
Plasmin: α_2-plasmin inhibitor complexes	I	I	N
Beta thromboglobulin/PF4 levels	I	I	I
AT-III	D	N/D	N/D

I = Increased; D = decreased; N = normal; P = positive; Ng = negative.

propriate antibiotic therapy is imperative in order to control the pathologic process—that is, bacterial or endotoxin-induced vascular damage. Blood component replacement therapy with transfusion of packed red blood cells, fresh frozen plasma, and platelets to maintain blood volume and to support hemostatic function is indicated in these patients with active bleeding or whose compensatory capacity is limited. In addition to fresh frozen plasma, cryoprecipitate (enriched in fibrinogen, factor VIII, and fibronectin), and prothrombin complex (enriched in vitamin K–dependent clotting factors) are often used as supplemental sources of blood component therapy. The administration of heparin in treatment of DIC has been advocated by a number of investigators, but its use is controversial. On the premise that the underlying pathologic basis for DIC is generation of excess thrombin, heparin should theoretically slow or stop the coagulation process by complexing with AT-III and thrombin or factor Xa. In control studies, however, it does not appear that heparin therapy influences the clinical outcome.[25] Its use can result in increased bleeding and, because heparin itself affects a number of coagulation tests, it is often difficult to monitor the effect of conventional therapy. Heparin should be used and is most effective in those cases of DIC that present with clinical evidence of a hypercoagulable state with evident vascular thrombosis. When major peripheral vessels are occluded as part of the hypercoagulable process, the use of fibrinolytic agents (streptokinase or urokinase) may be indicated as an initial management choice with subsequent heparinization, but clinical experience with this form of therapy is minimal. Table 28–5 summarizes the previously described profile of DIC.

RELATED DISORDERS

Primary fibrinolysis is an unusual situation in which plasmin is formed without coagulation taking place. The clinical presentation in this disorder is similar to that of DIC, with diffuse hemorrhage occurring as a result of increased plasma fibrinolytic activity. Several mechanisms can initiate this process. The presence of proteolytic enzymes in plasma which are capable of either directly or indirectly converting plasminogen to plasmin can occur in certain disease states. The genitourinary system is enriched in urokinases that can enter the systemic circulation following various urologic procedures. The fibrinolytic state seen with metastatic prostatic carcinoma is another example of this mechanism. The basis for the hemorrhagic state seen following cardiopulmonary bypass surgery is complex but activation of the plasminogen-plasmin systems with increased fibrinolytic activity is well documented. The failure of the hepatic clearance mechanism to remove plasminogen activator accounts for the increased fibrinolytic activity seen in a variety of hepatic disorders, particularly cirrhosis. Under normal circumstances the hepatic reticuloendothelial system removes not only activated clotting proteins but also plasminogen activator from the systemic circulation. When this function is impaired owing to hepatic disease or following portocaval shunting procedures, the removal of plasminogen activator is less than adequate and hyperplasminemia occurs with resultant hemorrhage.

The coagulation abnormalities seen in these fibrinolytic disorders are similar to those in DIC, with prolonged PT, APTT, and TT. These defects result from the hypofibrinogenemic state induced by the

Table 28–5. **PROFILE OF DIC**

Synonyms	Conditions Associated With DIC	Suggested Triggering Mechanisms	Clinical Manifestations	Clinical Laboratory Findings	Sequential Therapy

1. Consumptive coagulopathy
2. Defibrination syndrome
	Obstetric accidents
	Intravascular hemolysis
	Septicemia
	Viremia (varicella)
	Leukemias:
	  Acute
	  Promyelocytic
	  Other
	Solid malignancy
	Acidosis alkalosis
	Burns
	Crush injury and tissue necrosis
	Vascular disorders
		Amniotic fluid, which possesses thromboplastic activity
		Retained fetus, which possesses thromboplastic activity
		Byproduct of red cell hemolysis (phospholipid)
		Antigen/antibody complexes
		Endotoxin release
		Chronic stasis
		Complement activation
			1. *General signs:* significant hemorrhaging (usually from 3 unrelated sites: melena and hematemesis, epistaxis, or hemoptysis) fever, hypotension, acidosis, hypoxia, proteinuria, hematuria
			2. *Specific signs:* petechiae, purpura, gangrene, wound bleeding, venipuncture bleeding, subcutaneous hematomas
			3. *Microthrombi*
			4. *End-organ dysfunction*
				Hypofibrinogenemia
				Abnormal PT
				Abnormal PTT
				Abnormal thrombin time
				Abnormal platelet count
				Abnormal tourniquet test
				Abnormal clot retraction
				Abnormal factors V and VIII
				Positive fibrin(ogen)-split products
				Positive protamine sulfate test
				Positive ethanol gelatin test
				Antithrombin III consumption
				Leukocytosis
				Schistocytosis
				Thrombocytopenia
				Reticulocytosis
					1. Remove or treat triggering process
					2. Stop or slow coagulation process
					  a. Miniheparin
					  b. Heparin
					  c. Antiplatelet drugs
					  d. AT-III concentrates
					3. Blood component replacement
					  a. Platelets
					  b. Fibrinogen
					  c. Prothrombin complex
					  d. AHF
					4. Antifibrinolytic therapy*
					  a. Epsilon amino caproic acid (EACA)

Source: From Lazarchick, J and Kizer, J: Interaction of fibrinolytic, coagulation, and kinin systems and related pathology. In Pittiglio, DH and Sacher, RA (eds): Clinical Hematology and Fundamentals of Hemostasis, ed 1. FA Davis, Philadelphia, 1987, p 389, with permission.
*Sequential therapy used only after clotting is stopped (3% of patients may require this therapy).

proteolytic cleavage of fibrinogen by excess plasmin in addition to the catabolic effect of this enzyme on factors V and VIII. Fibrin degradation product concentrations are increased and, as previously noted, will further interfere with coagulation by acting as antithrombins. With the excess plasmin activity, the euglobulin lysis time is typically shortened. Because thrombin is not generated during this pathologic process, several laboratory tests can serve to readily distinguish primary fibrinolysis from DIC. The platelet count is typically normal, fibrinopeptides A and B levels are not elevated, and circulating fibrin monomer complexes and elevated D-dimer levels are absent in primary fibrinolysis, in contrast to the results in DIC.

Thrombotic thrombocytopenic purpura (TTP) is a syndrome of unknown etiology in which fibrin and platelet thrombi are formed diffusely throughout the microvasculature, in contrast to the localized thrombus formation seen in DIC.[26,27] The clinical picture consists of a pentad of findings: (1) fever, (2) microangiopathic hemolytic anemia, (3) thrombocytopenia, (4) azotemia, and (5) vacillating neurologic deficits. Despite fibrin and platelet deposition, this disorder is not typically associated with excessive activation of the coagulation system. Supportive evidence that this syndrome represents an abnormality of the fibrinolytic system is suggested by the finding of diminished or absent fibrinolytic activity, particularly of TPA, in plasma and blood ves-

Table 28–6. **OTHER CAUSES OF FIBRINOLYTIC ACTIVATION**

Clinical Condition	Mechanism	Clinical Manifestation	Other Hemostatic Alterations
1. Chronic liver disease	Abnormal fibrinolytic inhibitor (α_2-macroglobulin) Abnormal hepatic clearance of plasminogen activators	Often fulminant hemorrhage with massive hemoptysis, hematochezia, melena, or epistaxis May also demonstrate petechiae, purpura, spider telangiectasia, ecchymoses	1. Hypofibrinogenemia (due to lysis) 2. Elevated FDP (X, Y, D, and E) a. Defective fibrin monomer/ polymerization b. Platelet dysfunction 3. Proteolysis of factors V, VIII, IX, XI 4. Platelet defects a. Thrombocytopenia b. Platelet dysfunction (FDP, PF 3) 5. Coagulation protein defects a. Decreased synthesis of II, VII, IX, and X b. Decreased synthesis of Fletcher factor c. Decreased or dysfunctional synthesis of AT-III
2. Cardiopulmonary bypass (CPB)	Unclear; possibly direct activation of fibrinolysis by the oxygenation system of pump-induced accelerated flow rates may activate plasminogen to plasmin or may alter endothelial plasminogen activator activity	Hemorrhage; hematuria, petechiae/purpura, and oozing from intravenous site in conjunction with increased chest tube loss	1. Hyperfibrinolysis results in a. Elevated FDP b. Hypofibrinogenemia c. Low factors V and VIII 2. Functional platelet defect a. CPB-induced b. Drug-induced 3. Thrombocytopenia 4. Hyperheparinemia-heparin rebound(?) 5. DIC (?)
3. Malignancy	Poorly understood, in several instances tumor extracts possess the ability to activate directly or indirectly the fibrinolytic system (e.g., gastric carcinoma, sarcomas, and prostatic carcinoma)	Thrombosis/hemorrhage	1. Thrombocytopenia 2. Platelet function defects 3. Elevated FDP 4. Decreased AT-III 5. DIC(?)

Source: From Lazarchick, and Kizer, J: Interaction of fibrinolytic, coagulation, and Kinin systems and related pathology. In Pittiglio, DH and Sacher, RA (eds): Clinical Hematology and Fundamentals of Hemostasis, ed 1. FA Davis, Philadelphia, 1987, p 390, with permission.

sels affected with microthrombi. Therapy has not been standardized but antiplatelet drugs such as aspirin or dipyridamole, plasmapheresis, and exchange transfusion have been used either singularly or in combination with variable success. Table 28–6 summarizes the other causes of fibrinolytic activation.

CASE STUDY

A 32-year-old white woman, gravida 3, para 2, in her 36th week of pregnancy, experienced a sudden onset of lower abdominal pain and profuse vaginal bleeding. She was rushed to the emergency room. On examination she was hypotensive (blood pressure 70/40) and had a marked tachycardia. Large ecchymoses and continuous oozing of blood from venipuncture sites were evident. A fetal heart tone was barely audible. Births of her other children had been uncomplicated, and the family history was negative for a hemorrhagic diathesis.

Initial coagulation studies revealed PT 26 sec (normal 11 to 13 sec); APTT 84 sec (normal 24 to 30 sec); platelet count 20,000/μl (normal 140,000 to 440,000/μl); fibrinogen 85 mg/dl (normal 145 to 350 mg/dl); FDPs more than 40 μg/ml (normal, less than 10 μg/ml); protamine sulfate test positive (normal, negative). Peripheral blood smear showed presence of numerous red cell fragments.

A diagnosis of DIC was made based on the patient's clinical presentation and the supportive laboratory data. The patient was given intravenous fluids to maintain her blood pressure and 2 units of fresh frozen plasma and 10 units of platelets. She was taken to the operating room and underwent a cesarean section. Her bleeding abated postoperatively, and all coagulation parameters returned to normal within 36 hours.

This case is illustrative of an obstetrical complication, placental abruption, which resulted in an acute DIC syndrome. Several triggering mechanisms have been postulated as an explanation for the underlying coagulopathy in this disorder, including the release of thromboplastinlike material from the amniotic fluid and tissue necrosis in the area of the retroperitoneal hemorrhage. The laboratory parameters are consistent with a consumptive coagulopathy and secondary fibrinolysis. With the delivery and removal of the placenta the source of the triggering mechanism was removed and the pathologic process stopped. Normal hemostatic parameters are restored within hours postoperatively, and usually no further blood component replacement therapy is required.

REFERENCES

1. Kaplan, AP, et al: Interaction of the clotting, kinin forming, complement and fibrinolytic pathways. NY Acad Sci 389:25, 1982.
2. Sundsmo, JS and Fan, DS: Relationships among the complement, kinin, coagulation and fibrinolytic systems. Springer Semin Immunopathol 6:231, 1983.
3. Castellino, FJ: Recent advances in the chemistry of the fibrinolytic systems. Chem Rev 81:431, 1981.
4. Miller, JL: Normal fibrinolysis. In Henry, JB (ed): Clinical diagnosis and management by laboratory methods, ed. 17th. WB Saunders, Philadelphia, 1984, pp 769–771.
5. Mandle, RJ and Kaplan, AP: Hageman factor-dependent fibrinolysis: Generation of fibrinolytic activity by the interaction of human activated factor XI and plasminogen. Blood 54:850, 1979.
6. Bachman, F and Kruithof, IE: Tissue plasminogen activator: Chemical and physiological aspects. Semin Thromb Hemost 10:6, 1984.
7. Owen, WG: The control of hemostasis. Arch Pathol Lab Med 106:209, 1982.
8. Owen, WG and Esmon, CT: Functional properties of an endothelial cell cofactor for thrombin-catalyzed activation of protein C. J Biol Chem 256:5532, 1981.
9. Prowse, CV and Cash, JD: Physiologic and pharmacologic enhancement of fibrinolysis. Semin Thromb Hemost 10:51, 1984.
10. Rickli, EE: The activation mechanism of human plasminogen. Thromb Diath Haemorrh 34:386, 1975.
11. Brogden, RN, Speight, TM, and Avery, GS: Streptokinase: A review of its clinical pharmacology, mechanism of action and therapeutic uses. Drugs 5:357, 1973.
12. Gonzalez-Gronow, M, Violand, BN, and Castellino, FJ: Purification and some properties of the glu- and lys-human plasmin heavy chains. J Biol Chem 252:2175, 1977.
13. Marder, VJ, et al: High molecular weight derivatives of human fibrinogen produced by plasmin. I. Physicochemical and immunologic characterization. J Biol Chem 244:2111, 1969.
14. Kudryk, B, et al: Measurement in human blood of fibrinogen/fibrin fragments containing the B-beta 15-42 sequence. Thromb Res 25:277, 1982.
15. Ockelford, A and Carter, J: DIC: Application and utility of diagnostic tests. Semin Thromb Hemost 8:198, 1982.
16. Bini, A and Collen, D: Measurement of plasma alpha 2-antiplasmin coupled in human plasma. A comparison of latex agglutination inhibition and hemagglutination inhibition tests. Thromb Res 12:389, 1978.
17. Aoki, N and Harpel, PC: Inhibitors of the fibrinolytic enzyme system. Semin Thromb Hemost 10:24, 1984.
18. Kwaan, HC; Disorders of fibrinolysis. Med Clin North Am 56:163, 1972.
19. Brozovic, M: Disseminated intravascular coagulation. In Bloom, AL and Thomas, DP (eds): Haemostasis and Thrombosis. Churchill-Livingstone, New York, 1981, pp 415–422.
20. Muller-Berghaus, G: Pathophysiology of generalized intravascular coagulation. Semin Thromb Hemost 3:209, 1977.
21. Fareed, J, et al: Impact of automation on the quantitation of low molecular weight markers of hemostatic defects. Semin Thromb Hemost 9:355, 1983.
22. Hirsch, J: Blood tests for the diagnosis of venous and arterial thrombosis. Blood 57:1, 1981.
23. Jacobsen, CD and Southers, NJ: Ethanol gelation and protamine sulfate tests. Thromb Diath Haemorrh 29:130, 1973.
24. Buckell, H: The effect of citrate on euglobulin methods of estimating fibrinolytic activity. J Clin Pathol 11:403, 1958.
25. Mant, MJ and King, EG: Severe, acute disseminated intravascular coagulation. A reappraisal of its pathophysiology, clinical significance and therapy based on 47 patients. Am J Med 47:557, 1979.
26. Kwaan, HC, et al: The nature of the vascular lesion in thrombotic thrombocytopenic purpura. Ann Intern Med 68:1169, 1968.
27. Bukowski, RM: Thrombotic thrombocytopenic purpura: A review. Progr Hemost Thromb 6:287, 1982.

QUESTIONS

1. *Which of the following substances activates plasminogen and inhibits (by negative feedback) factors V and VIII?*
   a. XIIa, XIIa fragments, XIa
   b. Kallikrein and kininogen
   c. Activated protein C
   d. Urokinase and streptokinase

2. *What substance interacts with plasmin in the formation of D-dimers?*
   a. Fibrin monomer
   b. Cross-linked fibrin
   c. Fibrinogen
   d. FDPs

3. *What is the* primary *inhibitor of the fibrinolytic system?*
   a. Antithrombin III
   b. α_2-antiplasmin
   c. Protein C
   d. α_2-macroglobulin

4. *Which of the following is* not *a mechanism of a clinical condition associated with DIC?*
   a. Thromboplastin release, factor VII activation occurring in trauma
   b. Endothelial cell damage, factor XII activation occurring in burns
   c. Factor X/II activation occurring in venomous snake bite
   d. Fibrin activates plasmin release, occurring in anoxia

5. *Which coagulation time would be paradoxically shortened in DIC presenting clinically as a hypercoagulable state?*
   a. Activated partial thromboplastin time
   b. Reptilase time
   c. Euglobulin lysis time
   d. Thrombin time

6. *Which of the following treatments is* least *effective in the treatment of DIC?*
   a. Fresh frozen plasma
   b. Cryoprecipitate
   c. Heparin
   d. Prothrombin complex

7. *Which laboratory test will be abnormal in patients with primary fibrinolysis?*
   a. Platelet count
   b. D-dimer level
   c. Fibrin peptide A level
   d. Thrombin time

ANSWERS

1. c (p. 487)
2. b (p. 488)
3. b (p. 489)
4. d (p. 489–491)
5. a (p. 492)
6. c (p. 493)
7. d (p. 493–495)

CHAPTER **29**

MICHEL M. CANTON, PHARM.D.

Introduction to Thrombosis and Anticoagulant Therapy

OBJECTIVES

At the end of this chapter, the learner should be able to:
1. Name natural anticoagulants/inhibitors present in plasma.
2. Explain the action of thrombotic factors.
3. Name the most important serine-protease inhibitor and its cofactor.
4. Identify vitamin K–dependent inhibitors.
5. Identify components of plasminogen activation.
6. Recognize inhibitors known as serpins.
7. Describe the advantage of using functional assays instead of immunologic assays for evaluating thrombosis.
8. List similarities for deficiencies of antithrombin III, heparin cofactor II, protein C, and protein S.
9. Specify associated risks for patients with fibrinolytic defects.
10. Name laboratory tests for evaluation of antiphospholipid antibody syndrome.
11. Evaluate antithrombin III levels during heparin therapy.
12. State the association of thrombosis and pregnancy.
13. Recognize laboratory results associated with disseminated intravascular coagulation.
14. Explain the action of oral anticoagulants.
15. Name the most common laboratory test used to monitor oral anticoagulant therapy.
16. Explain the anticoagulant mechanism of heparin.
17. Name laboratory tests used to monitor heparin therapy.
18. List substances used as thrombolytic agents.
19. Name laboratory tests used for monitoring fibrinolytic therapy that are *not* affected by the presence of therapeutic heparin.

INTRODUCTION TO THROMBOSIS

Since the first description by Egeberg[1] in 1965 of a family with congenital deficiency of antithrombin III (AT-III) and a thrombotic diathesis, there was a rapidly increasing knowledge of the existing connections between alteration of coagulation inhibitors and thromboembolisms. Abnormalities of hemostasis, as observed in venous thrombosis, reflect disturbances in two regulatory mechanisms: the physiologic coagulation inhibitors and the fibrinolytic system. Hereditary deficiencies in AT-III, protein C, protein S, and defects of the fibrinolytic system, as well as the existence of antiphospholipid antibodies, are the abnormalities most directly associated with thromboembolic disease. The regulation of hemostasis is complex and involves interactions of many key components of the coagulation system. These components are able to bind to specific platelet receptors to form small amounts of thrombin. Natural anticoagulant mechanisms act to oppose the generation of the latter enzyme. Two types of natural anticoagulants or inhibitors are present in the plasma: (1) AT-III and heparin cofactor II (HC-II), which are serine-protease inhibitors, and (2) protein C, which, when activated in activated protein C (APC), is capable of degrading activated factors V (Va) and VIII (VIIIa) in the presence of its cofactor protein S.

If platelet activation occurs, prothrombin is brought into proximity with the prothrombinase complex, and significant amounts of thrombin can be generated. This overproduction of thrombin might overwhelm the natural anticoagulant mechanism. Therefore, the thrombotic accident can be defined as the result of an imbalance between the procoagulant and the anticoagulant systems.[2]

The fibrinolytic system is as complex as the coagulation system. The cause-and-effect relationship between the frequency of deficiencies in the physiologic fibrinolytic system and the occurrence of thromboembolism is yet to be established. However, it seems that the most common abnormality is the presence of an excess of plasminogen activator inhibitor 1 (PAI-1), leading indirectly to a decreased functional availability of the tissue plasminogen activator (TPA).[3]

REGULATION OF COAGULATION AND FIBRINOLYSIS

As mentioned before, in the normal healthy individual, procoagulant and anticoagulant systems are in equilibrium (Fig. 29–1). This balance may be tipped in either direction by a change in clinical circumstances. Because the levels of regulatory and procoagulant proteins vary, a patient may vacillate among a thrombotic, a prothrombotic, and a balanced state (Fig. 29–2).

Although the exact roles of platelets and other cells have still to be defined, blood cells, platelets, endothelial cells, subendothelial structures, and plasma components play important roles. The ex-

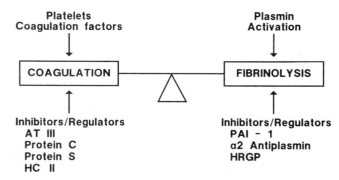

Figure 29–1. Physiological balance of hemostasis.
AT III = antithrombin III.
PAI-1 = plasminogen activator inhibitor-1.
HRGP = histidine-rich glycoprotein.

pression of these functions will be either a thrombotic factor or an antithrombotic reaction during the occurrence of thrombosis.

Thrombotic Factors

The Platelets

Thrombin generation in plasma is greatly accelerated by the presence of platelets. Indeed, the activated platelets have an enhanced capacity to catalyze interactions between the activated coagulation factors. This capacity is due to a rearrangement of the phospholipid structure of the platelet membrane that accompanies the platelet shape change, which offers support for the surface-dependent activation process of coagulation. The platelet release reaction also contributes to the thrombogenesis because, when platelets are exposed to various stimuli (e.g., thrombin), the alpha granule contents are released. These granules contain the platelet-specific proteins, platelet factor (PF) 4, beta thromboglobulin, platelet-derived growth factor, and a variety of other proteins including fibrinogen, factor V, von Willebrand factor (vWF).

Thrombin

Thrombin is one of the most fascinating enzymes in the coagulation system (Table 29–1). First, thrombin proteolytically cleaves fibrinogen to produce two molecules of fibrinopeptide A and two molecules of fibrinopeptide B from the $A\alpha$ and $B\beta$ fibrinogen chains, respectively—an event that converts fibrinogen to fibrin monomer. The released fibrin monomers may polymerize to form fibrin thrombi. Thrombin converts plasma and platelet factor XIII to an active transglutaminase, which, in turn, cross-links fibrin with covalent amide bonds that render the fibrin insoluble. Thrombin can "activate" the procoagulant factors, factors VIII and V, to participate in amplifying its own generation.

Thrombin participates in the activation of protein C, which serves as an anticoagulant to inactivate factors VIIIa and Va. Therefore, thrombin indirectly possesses some antithrombotic activities, limiting the extent of its own generation.

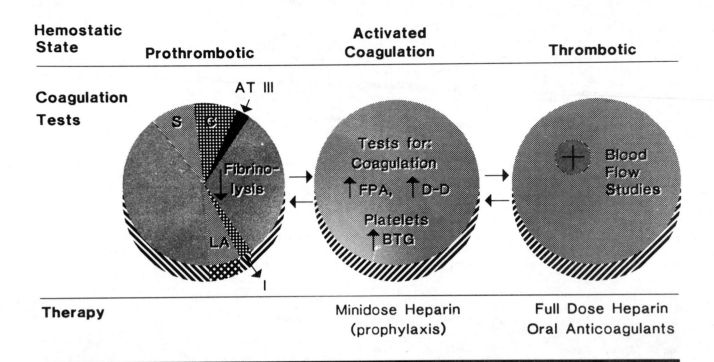

Figure 29-2. Continuum of hypercoagulability. With the new laboratory tests, approximately 55% of patients with recurrent thrombosis will be found to have demonstrable abnormalities. The relative proportion of each abnormality is shown in the prothrombotic category.
S = protein S.
C = protein C.
D-D = D-dimer.
βTG = beta-thromboglobulin.
LA = lupus anticoagulant.
I = fibrinogen.
FPA = fibrinopeptide A.
(From American Bioproducts Co., with permission.)

Thrombin also binds to platelets at low concentration and initiates shape change, aggregation, and secretion. Thrombin stimulates the platelets to make PF 3 available on the surface that accelerates the generation of more thrombin on the platelet surface.

Table 29-1. **ROLES OF THROMBIN**

Cleaves fibrinogen to form fibrinopeptides A and B and fibrin monomers
Activates factors V, VIII, and XIII and protein C
Activates platelets to aggregate and secrete
Contributes to the generation of platelet procoagulant activity
Induces endothelial release of PAF,* prostacyclin, vWF, interleukin-1, thrombospondin, TPA, and PAI-1
Induces granulocyte chemotaxis and adherence to endothelial monolayers to macromolecules
Depression of reticuloendothelial clearance of activated products of coagulation

*Platelet-activating factor.

Antithrombotic Factors

The normal plasma contains a sophisticated system of serine-protease inhibitors capable of inhibiting many of the activated proteases generated during coagulation (Fig. 29-3).

Antithrombin III

The most important of these inhibitors is AT-III. Antithrombin III is an α_2-glycoprotein with a molecular weight (MW) of 58,000 daltons (d). It is constituted of a single chain of 432 amino acids.[4] Its in vivo half-life is about 2 to 3 days. Normally, AT-III is a relatively weak inhibitor of the serine protease but it may be activated by various glucosaminoglycans —in particular heparin and the heparin sulfates.[5] Heparin, which is highly negatively charged, interacts with a domain in the AT-III molecule containing a high density of basic amino acids, particularly lysine. As a result, conformational changes occur in AT-III, making its active center containing arginine more available to the active serine residue of thrombin and other serine proteases. A complex is formed between AT-III and the serine protease,

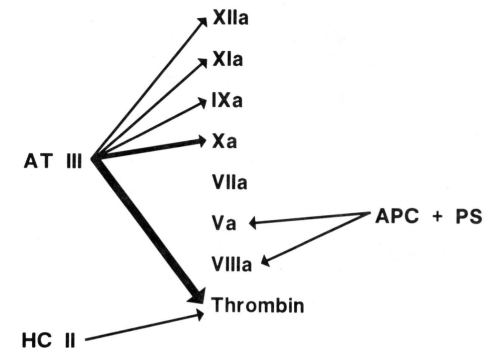

Figure 29-3. Physiological inhibitors of coagulation.
AT III = antithrombin III.
APC = activated protein C.
XIIa = activated factor XII.
HC II = heparin cofactor II.
PS = protein S.
(From Samama, MM: Hôtel-Dieu Hospital, Paris, personal communication, 1983.)

which possesses no enzyme and no inhibitor activity. As the complex forms, the heparin molecule falls off and is ready to react on another AT-III molecule. Therefore, heparin administered even in small doses converts AT-III from a slow, relatively ineffective inhibitor to a fast, effective one.

Heparin Cofactor II

Heparin cofactor II was first identified by Birginshaw in 1974[6] and isolated by Tollefsen in 1981.[7] The primary amino acid structure of HC-II is quite distinct from that of AT-III. Heparin cofactor II also possesses an affinity for heparin that is significantly less than that of AT-III. The specificity of HC-II is narrowly restricted to thrombin. The other mucopolysaccharides such as dermatan sulfate are able to accelerate dramatically the action of this protease inhibitor. Indeed, it appears likely that the observed anticoagulant effects of mucopolysaccharides other than heparin are primarily due to interactions with HC-II. Heparin cofactor II probably plays a minimal role when heparin is used clinically as an anticoagulant. Tollefsen has suggested that HC-II may function as a second-line inhibitor of thrombin after its activation by dermatan sulfate present on the surface of the vessel wall. Toulon and associates[8] also suggested that HC-II was present in a functional active form in human platelets and that platelet HC-II could play a role in the regulation of thrombin generated on the platelet surface.[9]

The Protein C System

Protein C, identified in 1960, is a vitamin K–dependent zymogen that, once activated by thrombin, proteolytically degrades factors VIIIa and Va,

two of the major cofactors involved in thrombin generation[10] (Fig. 29–4).

Protein C has a molecular weight of 62,000 d. It is a glycoprotein with heavy and light chains linked by a disulfide bond. Thrombin cleaves a specific Arg-Leu bond at the amino terminus of the heavy chain to release a 12–amino acid activation peptide resulting in activation of protein C.[11] A cofactor for thrombin-mediated activation of protein C was identified on the surface of the endothelial cells and designated thrombomodulin,[12] an integral membrane protein. Once thrombin binds to thrombomodulin, there appears to be a conformational change in thrombin as it loses its procoagulant activities. Thrombin bound to thrombomodulin no longer activates platelets or factors V, VIII, or XIII, nor does it cleave fibrinogen. Thrombin activation of protein C in the presence of thrombomodulin is modulated by activated factor V (Va). Low factor Va concentrations, which can be generated on and bound to endothelial cell surfaces, enhance the activation rate, whereas high concentrations of factor Va or light chain of factor V inhibit protein C activation. This mechanism provides a feedback control on the activation process of protein C. Protein C function is significantly enhanced in the presence of its cofactor, protein S, and phospholipids.[13] In the absence of adequate quantities of protein S, protein C function is inadequate to control the generation of thrombin. Factors VIIIa and Va appear to be relatively resistant to proteolysis in the presence of their associated serine proteases (factors IXa and Xa, respectively), suggesting that down-regulation of thrombin generation by protein C occurs in concert with decreasing quantities of factors IXa and Xa. Protein S is a vita-

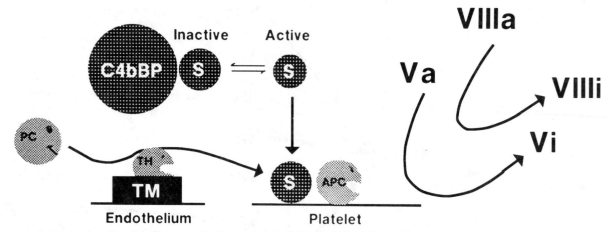

Figure 29–4. Activation of protein C system. In plasma protein S (S) is found both free and in complex with C4b binding protein (C4bBP). The free protein S is functionally active and serves on the membrane surface as cofactor for the degradation of factors Va and VIIIa by activated protein C (APC). The enzymatic degradation of V and VIII results in inhibition of the clotting cascade. The production of APC from protein C (PC) by the thrombin (TH)-thrombomodulin (TM) complex also occurs on the endothelial cell surface. (From Comp[41] p 178, with permission.)

min K–dependent protein that is produced in the liver, megakaryocytes, and endothelial cells.[14] Protein S is synthesized and released as a single chain with a molecular weight of 69,000 to 84,000. It is unique among the vitamin K–dependent coagulation proteins in that it is not the zymogen of a serine protease. Plasma protein S circulates in two forms, one bound to the C4b-binding protein (C4b-BP) from the complement, the other free.[15] Only the free form of protein S functions as protein C cofactor. Platelets contain protein S. Therefore, activation of platelets provides not only a surface for procoagulant reactions, but also a surface and a cofactor for eventual control of the thrombin generation (Fig. 29–4). In 1983, the presence of an inhibitor of APC in human plasma was described.[16] Initially, it was hypothesized that a deficiency of the protein C inhibitor (PCI) was the cause of the combined factor VIII/V deficiency.[17] Later this theory was refuted and the original results were explained as due to the repeated freezing and thawing of the test samples.[18] Suzuki and co-workers[19] described the purification and characterization of a plasma glycoprotein (MW 57,000) that neutralizes APC activity by forming a 1 : 1 stoichiometric complex. This inhibitor, PCI-I, was shown to be identical to the plasminogen activator inhibitor 3 (PAI-3). More recently a second inhibitor of protein C was described. Unlike PCI-I, this PCI-II is believed to be heparin independent and has a relatively high concentration.[20] The amino acid analysis revealed that PCI-II is identical to α_1-antitrypsin. Finally, analysis of the kinetics of APC inactivation in the plasma from a patient congenitally deficient in α_1-antitrypsin showed that there probably is a third inhibitor of APC in plasma different from PCI-I and from α_1-antitrypsin.[20]

Regulation of Fibrinolysis

Physiologic fibrinolysis results in the proteolytic degradation of polymerized fibrin.[2] The central reaction in this system is the conversion of a proenzyme, plasminogen, to the proteolytic enzyme plasmin. Plasminogen is a 90,000 d glycoprotein synthesized in the liver. Its half-life is 2 to 3 days. Plasminogen circulates free or bound to histidine-rich glycoprotein (HRGP), to α_2-antiplasmin and fibrinogen. The physiologic activation of plasminogen is achieved by the extrinsic pathway initiated by the TPA released from the endothelial cells after stimulation, and by the intrinsic pathway consisting of a factor XIIa–dependent activator and urokinase[21] (Fig. 29–5). A specific group of inhibitors has been described that controls the fibrinolytic process in the plasma. These serine protease inhibitors are members of the protein super-family called SERPINS. They are structurally homologous to many inhibitors of the serine proteases of the coagulation system (Table 29–2). Plasmin activity is regulated and inhibited by a number of plasma proteins such as α_2-antiplasmin, α_2-macroglobulin, α_1-antitrypsin, AT-III (especially in the presence of heparin), and C1 esterase inhibitor. Physiologically, α_2-antiplasmin is the main plasmin inhibitor. Alpha-2 antiplasmin is a 70,000 d glycoprotein, circulating in the plasma at a concentration of 1 micromole. Its properties include the immediate inhibition of plasmin, its interference with the absorption of plasminogen to fibrin, and its susceptibility to factor XIII–catalyzed cross-linking to fibrin. The combined effects of these three characteristics render α_2-antiplasmin much more specific and effective in inhibition of fibrinolysis than any of the other major inhibitors. Plasminogen activators (PAs) are inhibited by a number of specific proteins.[22] In recent years, research has revealed the existence of at least three different inhibitors of the extrinsic system[23]: PAI-1, PAI-2, and PAI-3 identified in plasma and urine[19] (Table 29–3). Plasminogen activator inhibitor 3 has also been described as one of the APC inhibitors, PCI-I. The most important inhibitor is PAI-1, a 50-kd plasma glycoprotein that is the primary fast-acting inhibitor of TPA and a member of the SERPIN protein super-family. The physiologic

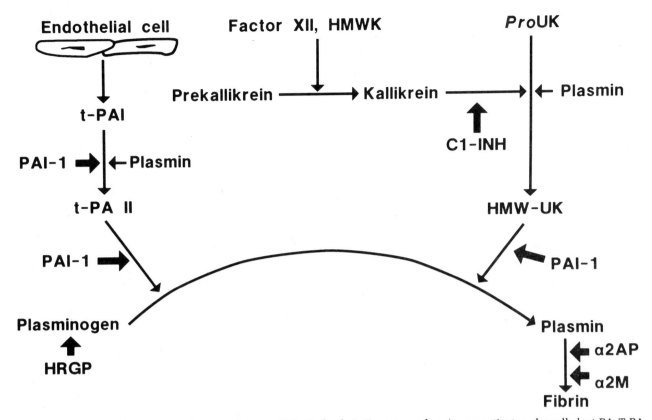

Figure 29–5. The fibrinolytic system of human plasma. t-PA I: single-chain tissue-type plasminogen activator, also called sct-PA; T-PA II: two-chain tPA (tct-PA); PAI-1: plasminogen activator inhibitor-1 (endothelial type); HMWK: high molecular weight kininogen; Pro-UK: pro-urokinase, also called single chain urinary-type PA (scu-PA); HMW-UK: high molecular weight urokinase, also called two chain u-PA (tcu-PA); C'1-INH: C1-inhibitor; α2AP: Alpha-2-antiplasmin; α2-M: Alpha-2-macroglobulin. (From Bachman,[21] p 194, with permission.)

Table 29–2. **INHIBITORY EFFECT OF THE SERINE-PROTEASE INHIBITORS**

SERPIN	Inhibitory Effects
α_2-Antiplasmin	Plasmin
α_2-Macroglobulin	Thrombin, plasmin, kallikrein
α_1-Antitrypsin	Thrombin, trypsin, chymotrypsin, factor XIa, elastase, activated protein C
AT-III	Thrombin; factors Xa, XIIa, IXa, and XIa; plasmin; kallikrein
C1 inhibitor	Kallikrein, plasmin, factors XIIa and XIa, C1 esterase
Antichymotrypsin	Chymotrypsin
HC-II	Thrombin
Protein C inhibitor	Activated protein C
PAI-1 and PAI-2	Plasminogen activators

plasma concentration of PAI-1 varies widely from 0 to 60 ng/ml with an average range of 5 to 20 ng/ml. The physiologic fibrinolytic activity seems to result primarily from the balance between TPA and its first inhibitor.

PATHOPHYSIOLOGY OF THROMBOSIS
Conditions Predisposing to Recurrent Thrombosis

Hereditary Disorders

Congenital or acquired changes in coagulation or fibrinolysis have been associated with an increased risk of thrombosis. The possibility of a hereditary defect predisposing to recurrent thrombosis should be entertained whenever a patient under the age of 40 presents with unexplained or recurrent thrombosis. The differential diagnosis includes evaluation of proteins C and S, SERPIN family, as well as the fibrinolytic system. Unfortunately there is no global test for these systems and each individual parameter has to be tested.

Functional assays (clotting or chromogenic assays) are always preferred because immunologic assays such as Laurell method, enzyme-linked immunosorbent assay (ELISA), and radial immunodiffusion (RID) may miss qualitative defects. A diagnosis should never be based on a single determination, particularly if the sample is obtained at the time of the thrombotic episode.

Table 29–3. **TPA INHIBITORS**

	PAI-1	PAI-2	PAI-3
Origin	Plasma	Placenta	Urine
	Platelets	Leukocytes	Plasma
	Endothelial cell	Macrophages	
	Granulocytes		
MW	54,000	47,000	50,000
Inhibitory Effect	TPA	TPA	UK
	UK	UK	APC
Concentration	0–1.3 nm	2 μm (3rd trimester)	—

UK = Urokinase.
APC = Activated protein C.

AT-III and HC-II Congenital Deficiencies. The prevalence of the AT-III deficiency is about 1 in 5000 in the normal population.[24] In the patients with antecedents of venous thrombosis, the frequency of the defect is about 2 to 3 percent. The trait is inherited in an autosomal dominant manner.[1] The clinical manifestations are essentially deep venous thrombosis (DVT), often complicated with pulmonary embolism. The occurrence of superficial thrombosis is relatively rare with AT-III. The AT-III deficiency seems to be also associated with arterial thrombosis.[25] It is important to mention that more than 90 percent of affected family members develop thrombotic episodes at some point in their life, usually before the age of 40.[26] These thrombotic episodes often occur after a triggering event such as surgery, confinement to bed, pregnancy, or even oral contraceptive use. The variants of the disease have been classified into two types and five subtypes,[27] as shown in Table 29–4.

The AT-III deficiencies are usually heterozygous and the AT-III levels are reported at about 50 percent (25 to 60 percent) of normal. The only cases of homozygous AT-III deficiencies belonged to the subtype IIc.

Autosomal dominant hereditary deficiency of HC-II has been described in several kindreds. At this point, it is unclear whether heterozygous deficiency of HC-II is associated with a thrombotic tendency.[26,28] Most of the affected family members described to date have been asymptomatic.

Table 29–4. **CLASSIFICATION OF AT-III CONGENITAL DEFICIENCIES**

Type I	Quantitative Defect
Subtype Ia	Reduced synthesis or increased turnover
Subtype Ib	Reduced synthesis or increased turnover with alteration of heparin-binding site
Type II	Qualitative Defect
Subtype IIa	Abnormalities of both active and heparin-binding sites
Subtype IIb	Abnormal active site
Subtype IIc	Abnormal heparin-binding site

Various methods have been described for the measurement of AT-III or HC-II. Functional assays are recommended that reflect the antithrombin activity. The end-point is measured using synthetic chromogenic substrates. These methods can be easily automated and standardized.

Protein C and Protein S Congenital Deficiencies. Several hereditary disorders of the protein C system have been identified and described.[29,30] Hereditary deficiency of protein C, whether heterozygous or homozygous, typically has an autosomal mode of inheritance. As with AT-III deficiency, the first thrombotic episode in these individuals classically occurs before they reach 40 years of age. The heterozygous deficiency is associated with DVT or pulmonary embolism, as well as with an increased risk of warfarin-induced skin necrosis. These episodes may occur when the deficient patient is receiving large doses of warfarin. The level of protein C in the heterozygous patient is typically found between 30 and 65 percent of the normal level.[31] The prevalence of this defect varies widely between 1 in 16,000 and 1 in 200 to 300 individuals. Indeed, Miletich[32] has screened almost 5000 asymptomatic blood donors, of which 79 had plasma levels of protein C under 65 percent of normal. None of these subjects had personal or familial thrombotic antecedents.[32]

Thus, it is suggested that some additional risk factors besides protein C deficiency may be necessary for the development of venous thrombosis. It is estimated that heterozygous protein C deficiency may account for 8 to 10 percent of all cases of recurrent DVT. Homozygous protein C deficiency is rare (1 in 500,000 births). In the classic form, affected newborn infants develop purpura fulminans and an acute form of disseminated intravascular coagulation (DIC) within the first 2 days of life.[33] As described with AT-III deficiency, several types of protein C defects have been reported.[31,34,35]

Subsequently, type I protein C deficiency is characterized with low antigenic and functional levels of the protein. In those with type II deficiency, the antigenic level of protein C is normal, and the structural abnormality of the protein is marked with a low functional activity of the molecule. Therefore, protein C deficiencies should be screened by using a protein C functional assay (clot-based[36,37] or chromogenic assay[38]), as this will detect both types I and II. Once a low protein C activity is determined, an immunologic assay should be performed to distinguish type I from type II protein C deficiency.[39] Recently, a low clot-based protein C level but normal chromogenic protein C level has been reported in a patient with DVT.[35]

Protein S differs significantly from deficiencies of the other vitamin K–dependent plasma proteins. The majority of individuals with protein S deficiency appear to have normal or moderately reduced levels of total protein S antigen, which suggests that the functional protein S deficiency involves the quantitative distribution of protein S between free and bound forms and not an abnormality of the protein S per se.[40] Comp[41] has proposed a classification of the congenital protein S deficiencies based on the free, total, and activity protein S levels (Table 29–5). The mode of inheritance of the type I defect is clearly autosomal dominant.[42] Although most of the protein S–deficient patients reported in the literature presented with DVT,[43] most recently several cases of severe cerebral arterial thrombosis were reported associated with protein S deficiency.[44–46] Immunologic assays (ELISA, Laurell) for both total and free protein S are commonly used.[47] However, functional assays have been described[48,49] that will be much preferable.

Fibrinolytic Defects. Impaired capacity to increase the catalytic concentration of TPA in plasma after stimulation (as from the venous occlusion test) has been associated with an increased risk of thromboembolism.[21] An impaired fibrinolytic potential has also been suggested to be an important risk factor in arterial thrombosis and atherosclerosis. More recently, it has been shown that the reduced TPA activity in patients with an inherited or acquired tendency to venous thrombosis as well as in patients with coronary artery disease may be related to a deficient release of TPA from the vessel wall,[50] an increased level of PAI-1,[3,51,52] or both.[53]

In support of a causative role of PAI-1 in thrombotic disease, an increased level of PAI-1 appears to constitute a risk factor for reinfarction in survivors of myocardial infarction and is the most commonly encountered abnormality in idiopathic DVT. However, it cannot be excluded that the increase in PAI-1 levels in septic shock merely reflect a nonspecific acute phase reactant behavior without direct pathogenic consequences.[54,55] The evaluation profile of the fibrinolytic system should consist of measurement of TPA and PAI-1 levels before and after venous occlusions. Plasminogen, α_2-antiplasmin, fibrinogen, and TPA–PAI-1 complex should also be determined.[56]

Acquired Thrombotic Disorders

Hospitalized patients may also present risk factors that are difficult to sort out and quite different from those found in young adults with recurrent thrombosis. In general, hospitalized patients show an activation state, frank thrombosis, or both. A particular case is the presence of antiphospholipid antibodies that have been recently linked to a variety of clinical findings, including arterial and venous thrombosis, recurrent spontaneous abortions, and fetal loss, as well as thrombocytopenia.[57,58]

Antiphospholipid Antibody Syndrome. The detection of the antiphospholipid antibodies (APA) is the biologic cornerstone in the diagnosis of this recently described syndrome[59] characterized by thrombotic episode or recurrent fetal loss. Beaumont[60] probably described the first case of association of recurrent pregnancy loss and a circulating anticoagulant; however, Laurell and Nilsson[61] received credit for the first report of such an association. Soulier and Boffa[62] reported a series of three women with histories of recurrent spontaneous abortion associated with previous thromboembolic events. The triad of recurrent fetal loss, thromboembolism, and lupus anticoagulant (LA) is called the Soulier-Boffa syndrome.

Finally, Hughes[63] was the first to propose the concept of an APA syndrome. The laboratory evaluation of APA is usually performed through two types of tests: (1) coagulation tests to identify a phospholipid dependent inhibitor of fibrin formation (platelet neutralization test,[64] dilute Russell viper venom time,[65] and so on), and (2) highly specific ELISA for APA.[66,67]

The criteria for diagnosis of a primary APA syndrome have been proposed as patients with at least two of the clinical manifestations that have been related to high titers of APA (DVT, arterial occlusion, thrombocytopenia, hemolytic anemia, recurrent fetal loss, leg ulcers, and livedo reticularis) but neither systemic lupus erythematosus (SLE) nor other connective tissue disorders.[68] The laboratory workup for diagnosis of APA syndrome is shown on Figure 29–6. Recently, a prospective study demonstrated an association between the presence of circulating APA and stroke.[69]

Drug-Induced Thrombotic Disorders. Because the major coagulation inhibitors and regulators may be affected by commonly used antithrombotic drugs or other medications such as L-asparaginase and oral contraceptives, it is essential to evaluate the possible effects of such medications in order to explain a low level of AT-III or protein C or protein S (Table 29–6). For its anticoagulant action, heparin requires the presence of AT-III. Heparin therapy was associated with a considerable progressive reduction in AT-III–binding capacity and antigenic

Table 29–5. **PROPOSED CLASSIFICATION OF HEREDITARY PROTEIN S DEFICIENCY**

	Free Protein S	Protein S Activity	Total Protein S
Type I	Low	Low	Low
Type IIa	Low	Low	Normal
Type IIb*	Normal	Low	Normal

*No cases reported to date.

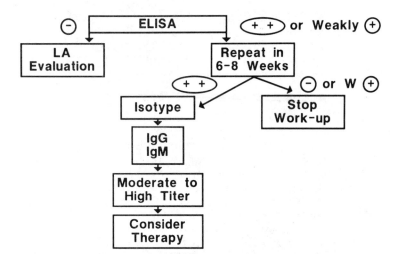

Figure 29–6. Antiphospholipid antibody (APA) syndrome, evaluation for APA.

protein. This decrease in AT-III is usually independent of its initial concentration. Plasma AT-III level returned to normal 2 to 3 days after the patient stopped receiving heparin. This finding is very relevant to the interpretation of clinical data in patients treated with heparin and may suggest that the decrease of AT-III may be related to the thrombotic complications sometimes encountered during heparin therapy. The level of AT-III during heparin therapy rarely drops below 70 percent of normal. Therefore, a level of less than 60 percent may be a real defect rather than an acquired one. In this case,

AT-III assay must be repeated 3 days after heparin administration was interrupted. Heparin cofactor II is not affected by anticoagulant therapies.[9]

Oral anticoagulants are known to affect the level of all vitamin K–dependent coagulation factors, including protein C and protein S.[70] Therefore, the interpretation of assays for these inhibitors may be difficult in those patients. Previously, the use of ratios of protein C antigen to factor X antigen or protein C to factor II antigen have been recommended. However, because factor VII has a half-life similar to that of protein C (6 to 7 hours), a ratio of protein C antigen to factor VII antigen may be more appropriate.[37] In this case, stable patients receiving oral anticoagulation yield similar values for both protein C and factor VII, provided that similar assay systems are used for determination of antigen ratios. Protein S is also depressed during oral anticoagulation. A considerable variation in plasma protein S levels is observed among individuals with similar intensity of anticoagulation.[71] Ratios between protein S antigen and factor II antigen may be useful to assess protein S status during warfarin and treatment. Oral contraceptives (OC) have been shown to affect protein S level.[72] Because protein S is distributed in plasma in two forms (free protein S and that bound to C4b-BP), a decrease of the total protein S due to OC may result in a more significant decrease of the active form, the free protein S.[14,73] In addition, the thromboembolic complications of OC use are often associated with periods of physiologic stress such as the postoperative period and during episodes of trauma and infection. Because C4b-BP is an acute-phase reactant, an elevated level of C4b-BP could shift the protein S to the complexed inactive form. This shift in protein S could further compromise the already reduced free protein S level found in OC users and thus might be a predisposing factor to thrombosis.[74] L-Asparaginase inhibits protein synthesis in leukemic cells. This accounts for its therapeutic effect in acute lymphoblastic leukemia but is also responsible for depression of a variety of proteins synthesized in the liver. The affected coagula-

Table 29–6. **CAUSES OF ACQUIRED DEFECTS OF COAGULATION INHIBITORS**

Inhibitors	Causes of Acquired Defects
AT-III	DIC
	Liver disease
	Nephrotic therapy
	Oral contraceptives
	L-Asparaginase
Protein C	Oral anticoagulant treatment
	DIC
	Vitamin K deficiency
	Newborn infants
	After plasma exchange
	Postoperative state
	L-Asparaginase
	Liver disease
Protein S	Oral anticoagulant treatment
	Pregnancy
	Oral contraceptives
	Vitamin K deficiency
	Liver disease
	Diabetes type I
	Acute inflammation
	Newborn infants

tion factors are fibrinogen, AT-III, protein C, and protein S.[75] These findings probably account for enhancement of thromboembolic risk in patients with predisposing factors such as immobilization, obesity, damage of vascular endothelium, or release of procoagulants from neoplastic cells.

Thrombosis and Malignancy. An association between cancer and the coagulation system was recognized by Trousseau more than a century ago. Activation of coagulation is a fundamental event in the pathogenesis of tumor growth and metastasis. Venous thrombosis may be the first indication of malignancy in an otherwise healthy individual. Among the most common coagulation abnormalities reported in several large series of cancer patients are elevation of fibrin(ogen) degradation products (FDPs) and an increase or a decrease of fibrinogen, factors V and VIII, and other clotting factors. Several studies have revealed elevated levels of plasma fibrinopeptide A in almost all patients with acute leukemia.[75,76] It should be emphasized that none of the clotting tests currently available is specific for cancer. More recently, a study postulated the possible role of thrombospondin, a large platelet-secreted protein that promotes platelet aggregation and cell adhesion, in the mediation of tumor cell metastasis.[77] This study suggested that thrombospondin may play a role in the development of human metastatic colorectal carcinoma.

Thrombosis and Pregnancy. A number of thrombogenic factors operate during normal pregnancy and delivery, including a decrease in fibrinolytic activity, an increase of plasma fibrinogen and factor VIII, a release of tissue thromboplastin into the circulation at the time of placental separation. The hemostatic capacity appears to increase progressively during normal pregnancy. This may represent a physiologic adaptation to ensure efficient control of bleeding at the time of placental separation. A parallel reduction in TPA increase in PAI activities can be observed during normal pregnancy, with rapid return to nonpregnant levels postpartum. D-Dimer level will be elevated during the third trimester.[78] Although protein C and AT-III levels remain normal during pregnancy, both are decreased during pre-eclampsia.[72,79] In normal pregnancy and pre-eclampsia, both free and total forms of protein S are decreased (Table 29–6). A decrease in functional protein S activity during early puerperium may be connected with the risk of developing thrombotic episodes during the postpartum period.[80] Fibronectin may be a valuable marker for the detection of pre-eclamptic states.[81]

Disseminated Intravascular Coagulation. Recognition of the simultaneous formation of thrombin and plasmin in the appropriate clinical setting is the definition of the diagnosis of DIC. The pathogenesis of DIC in most instances is the generation of procoagulant material with secondary fibrinolysis. Using a specific hemagglutination assay for fibrin monomers (FS Test), results of this assay will remain positive in most cases of DIC, thus showing that thrombin is being generated during the early activation stage of DIC.[82] Whereas an acute DIC is usually characterized with a hemorrhagic syndrome, the diagnosis of subacute or chronic DIC is suggested by the presence of unexplained thrombosis in patients suspected or proven to have an underlying malignancy or who have mucin-producing adenocarcinomas. Chronic DIC develops in as many as one quarter of pregnant women in whom a dead fetus has been retained for more than 5 weeks. Whatever the etiology and the severity of the DIC must be, AT-III, protein C, fibronectin, and other plasma protein levels are decreased. Although depressed levels are probably not helpful in the diagnosis of DIC, recognition of their presence may be important in the pathogenesis and may suggest modes of therapy.[83,84] Other laboratory findings associated with DIC include an acquired aberrant decrease of α_1-antitrypsin, perhaps reflecting the inhibition of activated protein C.

Suggested Test Panel for Recurrent Thrombosis

When a thrombotic disorder is suspected in a young patient, the coagulation laboratory can aid the clinician in (1) assessing the prothrombotic or prethrombotic state; (2) detecting an activated coagulation state; and (3) monitoring anticoagulant therapy. A particular area of concern for both clinicians and laboratories is the proper interpretation of the test results, especially when there is a familial history of thrombotic events. Labeling a patient with a hereditary disease such as protein C or S deficiency has significant ramifications. Because these disorders are autosomal dominant, 50 percent of the family members may potentially be affected. Therefore, the laboratory and physician must be absolutely sure that the diagnosis is correct. Two factors are critical: drawing an appropriate blood sample and doing family studies for substantiation. The laboratory studies and tests should follow the panel shown on Table 29–7.

Table 29–7. **SUGGESTED TEST PANEL FOR RECURRENT THROMBOSIS**

Test	Recommended Methodology
Protein C	Functional and antigenic assay
Protein S	Antigenic assay for total and free forms (functional assay preferable when available)
AT-III	Functional assay
Fibrinogen	Clauss method (clot-based assay)
Plasminogen	Functional assay
LA test	Increased phospholipid: PNP
	Decreased Phospholipid: dRVVT
APA	ELISA for APA IgG and IgM
PAI-1 and TPA	Functional and antigenic assay (before and after venous occlusion)
TPA–PAI-1 complexes	Antigenic assay

dRVVT = Russell viper venom time.

ANTITHROMBOTIC THERAPIES AND MONITORING

Administration of intravenous heparin, followed by long-term oral anticoagulants is the therapy of choice for most patients with DVT. In 1916, McLean isolated heparin from the liver and demonstrated its anticoagulant properties. Following the severe winter of 1921, a previously undescribed hemorrhagic disorder in cattle resulted from the ingestion of spoiled sweet-clover silage. In 1939, Link identified the responsible agent as dicumarol. Warfarin sodium, a dicumarol derivative, is now the most popular vitamin K antagonist used in the United States.

Vitamin K Antagonists: Oral Anticoagulants

Mechanism of Action

All the vitamin K–dependent coagulation proteins, factors II, VII, IX, and X, protein C, and protein S are characterized in their structure by a specific chain where some glutamic acid residues undergo a gamma-carboxylation. This gamma-carboxylation is vitamin K dependent. The presence of these carboxylated groups is necessary for the binding of calcium ions, required for the formation of the various activation complexes during the activation of the coagulation. The classic oral anticoagulants present a structural similarity with vitamin K. Therefore, these anticoagulants are able to inhibit the regeneration step of reduced vitamin K (Fig. 29–7). Because the reduced vitamin K, together with a carboxylase activity, is needed to convert the precursors of the vitamin K–dependent coagulation factors into the zymogens that are further activated to form the active coagulation enzymes, the inhibition of the reduced vitamin K by dicumarol-type anticoagulants blocks the final synthesis step of these vitamin K–dependent proteins. The peak effect of the vitamin K antagonists does not occur until 36 to 72 hours after drug administration. Indeed, the effect of the drug is delayed until the normal clotting factors are cleared from the circulation. The rate of disappearance of the coagulation factors depends on their in vivo half-life (Fig. 29–8). Factor VII and protein C have similar half-lives (6 to 7 hours).[37] Their respective levels fall during the initiation of the therapy, whereas the levels of functionally active factors II, IX, X, and protein S remain normal. That explains why, during the initiation of oral anticoagulation, the drug has the potential to be thrombogenic. This is due to the fact that the low level of factor VII is counteracted by the low level of protein C, with almost normal levels of procoagulant factors II, IX, and X. These factors will drop after 72 to 96 hours, and then the anticoagulant properties of the anticoagulant drug can be expressed. This justifies the need for an overlapping of oral anticoagulant therapy with heparin therapy for 3 to 4 days.

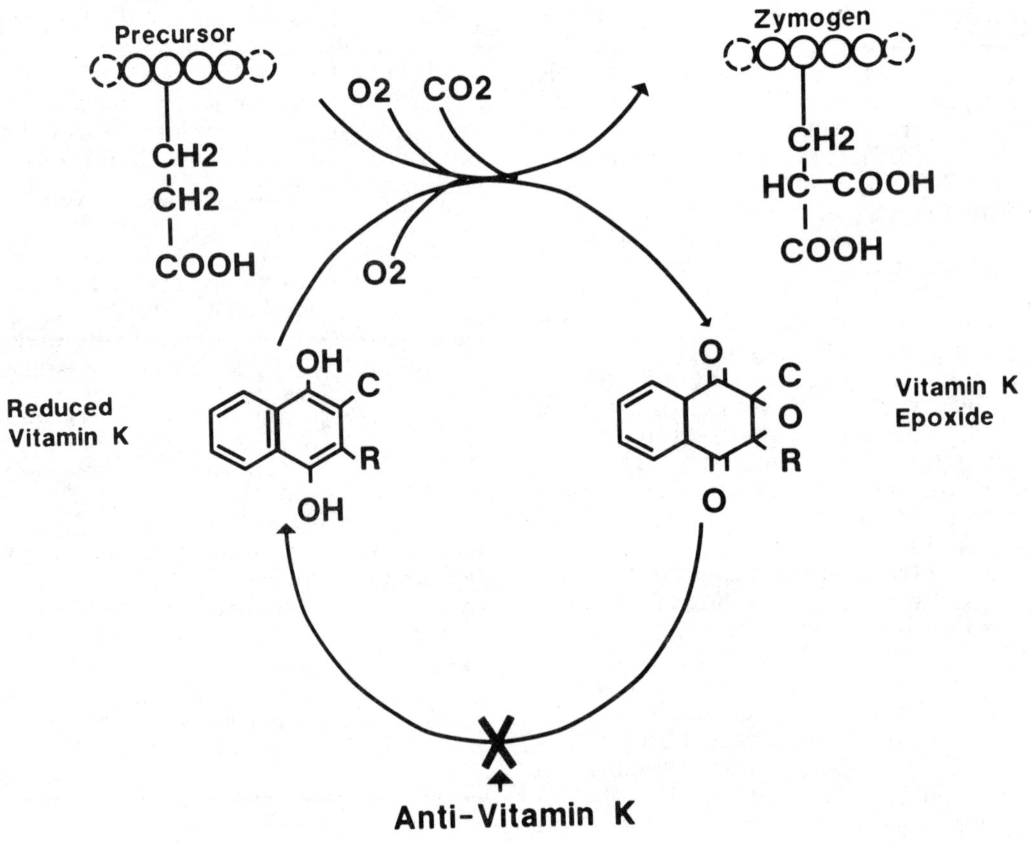

Figure 29–7. Mechanism of action of anti-vitamin K.

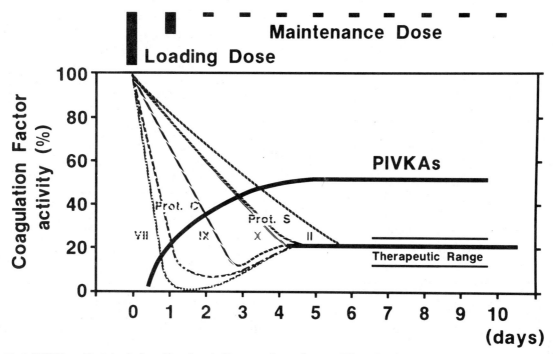

Figure 29-8. PIVKAs = Proteins induced by vitamin K antagonist or absence: Effect of oral anticoagulants on plasma activity of vitamin K–dependent coagulation factors. (From Loeliger, EA: In AMHP van der Besselaar, et al., eds: Thromboplastin Calibration and Oral Anticoagulant Control. Martinus Nijhoff, Boston, 1984, p 2, with permission.)

Clinical Applications

The clinical use of warfarin has been established in (1) prevention of DVT (warfarin is effective for DVT prophylaxis following hip fractures, hip surgery, and possibly other forms of general abdominal surgery); (2) long-term use following pulmonary embolism and DVT; (3) prevention of arterial emboli originating from the heart; and (4) acute myocardial infarction.

Laboratory Monitoring

The most common laboratory test used to monitor oral anticoagulant therapy is the conventional prothrombin time (PT). The PT evaluates the extrinsic pathway of the coagulation. Therefore, it is sensitive to the decrease of factors II, VII, and X. However, the PT does not reflect the effect of the drug on factor IX.

Further confusion about the appropriate therapeutic range has occurred because the available reagents used for the determination of the PT may vary in sensitivity to the vitamin K–dependent factors and in response to the drug. Numerous international trials have shown that considerable differences may exist in the same plasma, depending not only on the origin of the reagent but also on the method used to read the test. Therefore, each reagent should have its own therapeutic range defined, using the World Health Organization (WHO)–recommended standardization protocol.[85] The target value corresponding to the best balance between the prevention of thrombosis and the hemorrhagic risk is function of the therapeutic indication and the clinical context. The desired anticoagulation degree, usually low in presurgical situation or for prophylaxis of thrombosis, is expected to be higher in the prevention or the treatment of recurrent venous thrombosis, and even more so in arterial thrombosis or after implant of heart valves (Table 29-8).

Table 29-8. **RECOMMENDED THERAPEUTIC RANGE FOR ORAL ANTICOAGULANT TREATMENT**

Condition	INR	Patient/Control PT Ratio
Prophylaxis of venous thrombosis in high-risk medical or surgical patients	2.0–3.0	1.2–1.5
Treatment of venous thrombosis	2.0–3.0	1.2–1.5
Prevention of embolism	2.0–3.0	1.2–1.5
Prevention of recurrent embolism, or patients with mechanical prosthetic intravascular valves	3.0–4.5	1.5–2.0

In order to promote standardization of the PT for monitoring oral anticoagulant therapy, the WHO has developed an international reference thromboplastin from human brain tissue and has recommended that the PT ratio be expressed as the international normalized ratio (INR).[86] The INR value for a plasma depends on the international sensitivity index (ISI) of the reagent used.[87] In order to determine the sensitivity of a given reagent, PTs obtained with it are graphed against values obtained on the same specimens using the WHO standard. A linear plot is usually obtained, the slope of which is defined as the ISI. The INR is calculated from the following formula:

$$INR = \left(\frac{\text{Patient Value, in seconds}}{\text{Control Value, in seconds}} \right)^{ISI}$$

Heparin Therapy

Structure and Heterogeneity of Standard Heparin

Heparin consists of unbranched oligosaccharide chains of varying lengths (and thus molecular weights).[88] This natural oligosaccharide is present in mastocytes and is industrially extracted from ox lung and pork intestine. Heparin is composed of alternating units of D-glucosamine and either D-glucuronic acid or L-iduronic acid (Fig. 29–9). A variety of substitutions may occur at various sites on these basic sugars. These substitutions include the following:

For R1 : —H or —OSO3
For R2 : —SO3 or —COCH3

The molecular weight of heparin varies from 3000 to 30,000 d with a distribution peak of about 13,000 to 15,000. Although the length of polysaccharide chains varies, a pentasaccharide structure has been identified and then synthesized,[89] which is randomly distributed along the polysaccharide chains of heparin. In the heparins used in therapy, only one third of the polysaccharide chains carries the pentasaccharide sequence responsible for the binding to AT-III. This fraction of high affinity for AT-III is responsible for most of the anticoagulant and antithrombotic functions of heparin.[90]

Anticoagulant Activity of Heparin

Classically, the coagulation factors are bound on the phospholipid surface of platelets or tissue. The enzymatic cascade leads to the generation of thrombin which is then released from the phospholipid environment. In this environment, the other coagulation factors are protected from the inhibition by heparin–AT-III complex.[91] Therefore, thrombin, the only free coagulation enzyme, is preferentially inhibited by the heparin–AT-III complex, whereas the phospholipid-bound factors IXa and Xa are little inhibited.[92]

Thrombin participates in its own formation by activating the platelets and the cofactors V and VIII. Any inhibition of thrombin has an impact on these feedback mechanisms and leads to more thrombin inhibition.[93] However, during the platelet activation by thrombin, the PF4 is released from the PF4 platelets and inhibits heparin.[94]

Thus, the complexity of the anticoagulant mechanism of heparin is related to its initial target, which is thrombin inhibition. At low doses, heparin inhibits the first traces of thrombin generated, then slows down the thrombin generation.[95,96] At high doses, heparin inhibits the thrombin entirely, making the blood uncoagulable.

In addition, many other actions of heparin are known, apart from its effects on the blood coagulation, such as enzyme inhibition, tumor growth inhibition, and antibacterial activity.

Pharmacokinetics of Heparin

After intravenous (IV) administration, heparin is cleared from the blood through two distinct mechanisms. The first system is composed of the reticuloendothelial cells that bind heparin with a high affinity, then internalize before degrading heparin by desulfatation and depolymerization. The second mechanism is renal filtration. If used at therapeutic doses, heparin is principally cleared through the cellular system, which is extremely effective. At higher doses, the clearance capacity of the reticuloendothelial system (RES) mechanism is saturated, and the excess of heparin present in the blood is passively filtrated by the kidney. These features explain why the half-life of heparin increases with the dose administered and why, above a certain dose, the clearance curve of heparin loses its linearity and

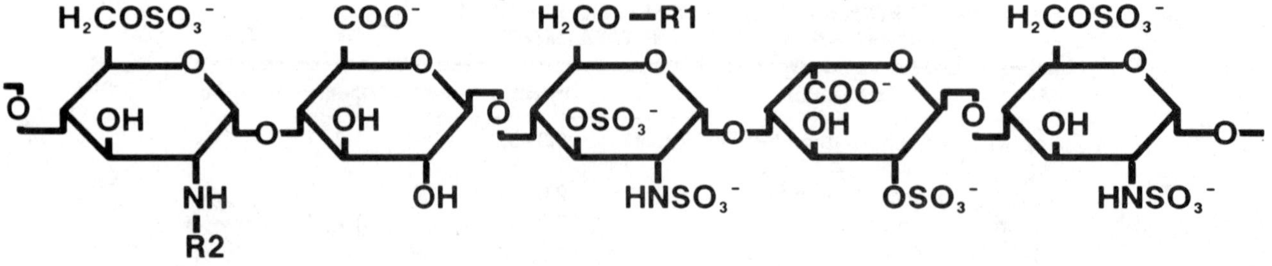

Figure 29–9. Heparin structure.

becomes concavoconvex.[97] As an indication, the half-life of heparin after an IV injection of 60 IU/kg is about 1 hr with a wide intersubject variability (30 to 90 min).[98] Standard heparin can be administered subcutaneously (SC). In this case the activity peak is obtained 2 to 4 hours after the time of the injection. The half-life depends on the level of the peak. It is classically admitted that the bioavailability of SC heparin is 30 percent of what is obtained with IV heparin. However, it has been shown that during curative heparinotherapy of DVT, the total heparin levels required to treat the patients are equivalent, whatever the route of administration of the drug is. Thus, the bioavailability of the SC heparin increases with the dose administered and can reach 100 percent with the doses used for a curative therapy.

In 1982, Bjornsson and Wolfrom[99] showed the intersubject variability in the anticoagulant response to heparin in vitro. Several other authors have described the in vivo intersubject and circadian variability in heparin sensitivity with obvious implications in the method of choice for the monitoring of heparin.[98]

Clinical Applications

Although the use of long-term warfarin therapy for the treatment of venous thromboembolism is well established, heparin has been proposed as the therapy of choice in treatment of DVT[100] 30 years after its discovery. Later it was suggested that it might be of use in prevention of thrombotic complications following vascular surgery,[101] myocardial infarction,[102] and extracorporeal circulation.[103] It must be emphasized that all treatment with heparin is prophylactic — either primary (to prevent thromboembolism) or secondary (to limit previous thromboembolism).[104] The administration of heparin postoperatively in full therapeutic dose is often accompanied by bleeding complications. Subsequently, administration of small doses of heparin has been shown to prevent venous thrombosis and pulmonary embolism. A large number of clinical trials have been conducted to establish the efficacy of low-dose heparin therapy. Further studies suggested that the combined administration of low-dose heparin with dihydroergotamine may have greater efficacy than low-dose heparin alone.

In regard to the prevention of arterial thromboembolism, a renewed interest for heparin came from the observation that arterial thrombosis is not totally a platelet-driven event but is also coagulation factor dependent.[105] This concept was emphasized after the results of treating coronary thrombosis with thrombolytic agents.[106]

Other studies have examined the use of heparin in patients with unstable angina. When used to treat patients with active thrombosis, heparin should be administered in doses large enough to prolong results of an appropriate coagulation test to within a defined anticoagulant level. The anticoagulant effect is usually achieved by an initial IV bolus injection of heparin, which is then followed by continuous infusion, intermittent IV injection, or SC

Table 29–9. **INDICATION FOR HEPARIN THERAPY**

Heparin Regimens	Clinical Use
Full therapeutic dose	Treatment of acute thromboembolism
	DVT
	Pulmonary embolism
	Acute myocardial infarction
	Arterial thrombosis
Low-dose	Prophylaxis of venous thromboembolism
	Postsurgery
	Stroke, acute myocardial infarction
	Pregnancy
	Thrombotic tendency
Adjusted dose	DIC
	Extracorporeal circulation
	Hemodialysis
	Pregnancy
	Prosthetic heart valves

injection. The efficiency and safety of heparin given by either one or the other administration route have been compared in various prospective, randomized studies. It is possible that the incidence of bleeding during heparin therapy is related more to the total daily dose of heparin given than to its method of administration.[107] The indications for heparin therapy are summarized in Table 29–9.

Low Molecular Weight Heparins

The low molecular weight heparins (LMWHs) are defined as products that have been developed from standard heparin by extraction processes or by chemical or enzymatic depolymerization. The molecular weight of these fragments ranges from 3000 to 9000 d, with a mean of 5000. The LMWHs have antithrombin (anti-IIa) activity that is low, compared with their anti-Xa activities. They are very efficiently absorbed from SC injection and have a longer half-life than standard heparins. The LMWHs bind to AT-III and they do not interact with platelets to the same degree as standard heparin. Therefore, they may be less likely to cause bleeding in the treated patients. The LMWHs are effective as antithrombotic agents, particularly in prevention of DVT.[108]

Monitoring of Heparin Therapy

Owing to the potent in vivo anticoagulant activity of heparin, monitoring is justified in order to improve the antithrombotic efficacy of heparin and to reduce the risk of bleeding. Another implication of the laboratory monitoring in heparin treatment should be adjustment of dose according to the result of the treatment.

Influence of Sample Collection and Storage. However accurate may be the assay of heparin in plasma, its partial inactivation during the time lapse between blood collection and laboratory assay decreases the reliability of the methods for monitoring heparin therapy. This inactivation of heparin is mainly due to PF4 or to other heparin-binding proteins.[109] Various options have been proposed for preventing heparin inactivation during blood centrifugation and storage. Current recommendation is not to chill specimen until after the plasma is separated so that PF4 (platelet factor 4) is not released by platelets agglutinated by exposure to cold temperatures. The blood collection in a combination of citric acid, theophylline, adenosine, dipyridamole—CTAD mixture—was found to reduce greatly the heparin loss during blood centrifugation and storage.[111]

Laboratory Tests for Heparin Monitoring. The development of new heparins by manufacturers, as well as the need for more clinical trials, led to a dramatic evolution of the methods used by the control authorities and subsequently by the clinical laboratories for assessment of the heparinization level in patients.

The most popular test remains the activated partial thromboplastin time (APTT). In 1973, specific methods based on the heparin ability to neutralize factor Xa (anti-Xa assay) or factor IIa (anti-IIa assay) in plasma were developed. The introduction of chromogenic substrates methodology then opened the way for standardization of the methods and to the pharmacologic approach of monitoring of heparin therapy (Table 29–10).

Activated Partial Thromboplastin Time. The sensitivity to heparin of the various commercially available APTT reagents shows considerable variation. The logic of the APTT system and its simplicity all contribute to its popularity. However, for heparin monitoring, the response of the particular APTT reagent used must be known.[112] Individual variation in the APTT response to heparin may reflect variation in coagulation factor levels. Classically, high factor VIII levels in an acute phase reaction is the main cause of shortening of APTT. This short APTT may be misinterpreted as a low response to heparin. Presence of abnormal inhibitors such as LA may lead to prolonged baseline APTT.

Thrombin Time. Heparin prolongs the coagulation of plasma in the presence of thrombin. Modified thrombin times have been used for heparin monitoring. However, this test may also respond to the existence of low fibrinogen, the presence of FDPs. One may note that antithrombin level influences the thrombin clotting time, particularly at low heparin concentration.

Anti-Xa Assay: Clot-Based Method. The assessment of the anti-Xa effect of heparin by this method gives a high sensitivity in detecting low heparin level.[113] This assay is influenced by the level of AT-III and FDPs. However, this method is less sensitive to individual variation than is the popular APTT. This assay is easily automated. It is standardized and may also be used to monitor LMWH therapy or low-dose heparin therapy.

Anti-Xa Assay: Chromogenic Substrates. The introduction of synthetic substrates in the evaluation of coagulation began a new era in monitoring of heparin. The end-point is read by instrument, and the precision is higher than for clotting assays. The assay that follows is a modification of the original amidolytic assay proposed by Teien and Lie[109]:

1. $\text{Heparin} + \text{AT-III} \longrightarrow \text{Heparin–AT-III complex}$
2. $\text{Heparin–AT-III} + \text{Xa} \longrightarrow \text{Heparin–AT-III-Xa} + \text{residual Xa}$
3. $\text{R-pNA} + \text{residual Xa} \longrightarrow \text{R—COOH} + \text{pNA*}$ (yellow)

If the test plasma is the only source of AT-III, a combined heparin–AT-III activity is measured. It would be reasonable to monitor heparin therapy in venous thrombosis by either the heparin level or global tests such as APTT. If the heparin level is used, it should be maintained above 0.2 to 0.3 IU/ml at all times, with an upper limit of 0.5 IU/ml. If the APTT is used, it should be adjusted to 1.5 to 2 times the mean of the normal laboratory control subject.

Thrombolytic Therapy

In recent years, thrombolytic therapy has become the treatment of choice for eligible patients with acute myocardial infarction.[114] As a consequence, the clinical use of thrombolytic therapy has increased rapidly from the small number of patients treated with these agents for DVT, pulmonary embolism, and blocked arteriovenous shunts. Monitoring of effectiveness and of bleeding complications has been the primary focus of most of the

Table 29–10. **ASSAYS FOR MONITORING HEPARIN**

Test	Comment
APTT	Most commonly used test
	Inaccurate at fibrinogen level <75 mg/dl
Thrombin time	Evaluates anti-IIa* effect of heparin
	Extremely sensitive to heparin, but also to elevated FDPs and to hypofibrinogenemia
	Not commonly used in US for heparin monitoring
Heparin assays	Residual added Xa or IIa is measured by
Anti-Xa† clotting assay	clotting assay or by cleavage of chromogenic substrate; clotting time or color development is inversely proportional to heparin concentration
Anti-IIa or anti-Xa chromogenic assay	Easy to automate or standardize
	Anti-Xa chromogenic or clotting assay may be monitoring assays of choice for LMWH

Source: Courtesy of American Bioproducts Co.
*IIa = thrombin.
†Xa = activated factor X.

*pNA = para-Nitroaniline.

studies related to thrombolytic therapy. Several thrombolytic agents have been made available for clinical use. The aim of these drugs is to activate plasminogen into the active form, plasmin. The exact mechanism of activation of plasminogen differs depending on the thrombolytic agent.

Thrombolytic Agents

These agents may be classified into two groups according to their mechanism of action: (1) non–fibrin-specific plasminogen activators, which cause the conversion of plasminogen to plasmin (in this group, streptokinase and urokinase are the most widely used); and (2) fibrin-specific agents such as TPA, pro-urokinase, and acylated streptokinase-plasminogen complex (APSAC).

Streptokinase forms a stoichiometric complex with plasminogen leading to a modification of plasminogen, allowing the complex to activate plasminogen to plasmin. Therefore, streptokinase infusion to patients is usually associated with a systemic fibrinolytic state characterized by a plasminogen activation, a depletion of α_2-antiplasmin (the circulating physiologic inhibitor of plasmin), and fibrinogen breakdown. This mechanism implies that the streptokinase-plasminogen complex activates circulating plasminogen and fibrin-associated plasminogen equally and thus lacks significant fibrin specificity. Streptokinase is antigenic for humans. In contrast, urokinase is a human protein and is therefore non-antigenic. Like streptokinase, urokinase also has a minimal fibrin specificity. Its mode of action is a direct activation of plasminogen.[2]

Tissue plasminogen activator is a fibrin-specific lytic agent. It forms a ternary complex with plasminogen on the fibrin surface. Thus, plasmin is generated directly on the surface of the fibrin clot to be lysed. Basically, fibrin increases the local plasminogen concentration by creating the interaction between TPA and plasminogen. The plasmin produced on the fibrin surface is protected from its inhibitor, α_2-antiplasmin.[2]

Laboratory Monitoring during Fibrinolytic Therapy

The goal for monitoring of thrombolytic therapy is twofold:

1. To predict which patients are at greatest risk for bleeding and to guide therapy
2. To assess the status of the hemostatic system before coronary artery bypass grafting in the patient who has recently received lytic therapy.

A baseline study of the hemostatic functions is always indicated regardless of the underlying clinical condition being treated and the lytic agent of choice (Table 29–11). Classically, this baseline study consists of the evaluation of PT, APTT, complete blood count (CBC) in all patients, and fibrinogen assay, using the Clauss method (clotting method) or thrombin time. Then, during the therapy, it is useful to determine the extent of the coagulopathy for patients who are demonstrating signifi-

Table 29–11. BASELINE STUDIES FOR MONITORING OF FIBRINOLYTIC THERAPY

All patients
  PT
  APTT
  CBC (with platelet count)
Patients receiving non–fibrin-specific agents
  Thrombin time or fibrinogen assay

Source: Courtesy of American Bioproducts Co.

cant hemorrhage. This information may guide the clinician to decide whether or not to transfuse with substitutive products. Thrombin time and APTT show a prolongation in these patients with persistent lytic state. However, because thrombin time, as well as APTT, is affected by the presence of therapeutic heparin in the patients, it has been recently emphasized that reptilase time may be a more adequate method to evaluate the patients at risk of hemorrhagic complication.[115] The Clauss fibrinogen assay is also preferred because heparin levels in the therapeutic range do not affect the test.

In summary, the only useful routine monitoring of thrombolytic therapy consists of pretreatment baseline studies and evaluation of the presence of a lytic state in patients treated with more or less non–fibrin-specific agents.

REFERENCES

1. Egeberg, O: Inherited antithrombin deficiency causing thrombophilia. Thromb Diath Hemorrh 13:516, 1965.
2. Stump, D and Mann, KG: Mechanisms of thrombus formation. Ann Emerg Med 17:1138, 1988.
3. Almer, LO and Ohlin, H: Elevated levels of the rapid inhibitor of plasminogen activator (t-PAI) in acute myocardial infarction. Thromb Res 47:335, 1987.
4. Abildgaard, U: Antithrombin and related inhibitors of coagulation. In Poller, L (ed): Recent Advances in Blood Coagulation. Churchill-Livingstone, New York, 1981, p 151.
5. Yin, ET: Effect of heparin on the neutralization of factor Xa and thrombin by the plasma alpha-2-globulin inhibitor. Thromb Diath Haemorrh 33:43, 1974.
6. Birginshaw, GF and Shanberg, JN: Identification of two distinct cofactors in human plasma. Inhibition of thrombin and activated factor X. Thromb Res 4:463, 1974.
7. Tollefsen, DM, Majerus, DW, and Blank, MK: Heparin cofactor II. Purification and properties of a heparin-dependent inhibitor of thrombin in human plasma. J Biol Chem 257:2162, 1982.
8. Toulon, P, Aiach, M, and Gianese, F: In vitro study of a new potential antithrombotic drug MF 701 (dermatan sulfate). Ann NY Acad Sci 556:486, 1989.
9. Toulon, P, et al: Heparin cofactor II in patients with deep venous thrombosis under heparin and oral anticoagulant therapy. Thromb Res 49:497, 1988.
10. Seegers, WH, McCoy, LE, and Groben, HD: Purification and some properties of autoprothrombin II-A: An anticoagulant perhaps also related to fibrinolysis. Thromb Res 1:443, 1972.
11. Fernlund, P and Stenflo, J: Amino acid sequence of protein C. In Suttie, JW (ed): Vitamin K Metabolism and Vitamin K–Dependent Proteins. University Park Press, Baltimore, 1980, p 84.

12. Esmon, NL: Thrombomodulin. In Coller, BS (ed): Progress in Hemostasis and Thrombosis. WB Saunders, Philadelphia, 1989, p 55.
13. Walker, RJ: Protein S and the regulation of activated protein C. Semin Thromb Hemost 10:131, 1984.
14. DiScipio, RG, et al: A comparison of human prothrombin, factor IX (Christmas factor), factor X (Stuart factor), and protein S. Biochemistry 16:698, 1977.
15. Dahlback, B, Smith, CA, and Muller-Eberhard, HJ: Visualization of an C4b-binding protein and its complexes with vitamin K–dependent protein S and complement protein C4b. Proc Natl Acad Sci USA 80:3461, 1983.
16. Suzuki, K, Nishioka, J, and Hashimoto, S: Protein C inhibitor. Purification from human plasma and characterization. J Biol Chem 258:163, 1983.
17. Marlar, RA and Griffin, JH: Deficiency of protein C in combined factor V/VIII deficiency disease. J Clin Invest 66:1186, 1980.
18. Canfield, WM and Kiesel, W: Evidence of normal functional levels of activated protein C inhibitor in combined V/VIII deficiency disease. J Clin Invest 70:1260, 1982.
19. Suzuki, K, et al: Protein C inhibitor: Structure and function. Thromb Haemost 61:337, 1989.
20. Van der Meer, FJM, et al: A second plasma inhibitor of activated protein C: Alpha 1-antitrypsin. Thromb Haemost 62:763, 1989.
21. Bachmann, F: Laboratory diagnosis of impairment of fibrinolysis in patients with thromboembolic disease. Semin Thromb Hemost 16(2):193, 1990.
22. Bachman, F: Fibrinolysis. In Verstraete, M, et al (eds): Thrombosis and Haemostasis. ISTH-University Press, Leuven, Belgium, 1987, p 227.
23. Thorsen, S and Philips, M: Plasminogen activator inhibitors. In Castellino, FJ, et al (eds): Fundamental and Clinical Fibrinolysis. Elsevier, Amsterdam, 1987, p 83.
24. Shapiro, SS and Anderson, DB: Thrombin inhibitor in normal plasma. In Lundbald, PL, et al (eds): Chemistry and Biology of Thrombin. Science Publishing, Ann Arbor, 1977, p 361.
25. Johnson, EJ, Prentice, CRM, and Parapia, LA: Premature arterial disease associated with familial antithrombin III deficiency. Thromb Haemost 63:13, 1990.
26. Tollefsen, DM: Laboratory diagnosis of antithrombin and heparin cofactor II deficiency. Semin Thromb Hemost 16:162, 1990.
27. Finazzi, G, Caccia, R, and Barbui, T: Different prevalence of thromboembolism in the subtypes of congenital antithrombin III deficiency: Review of 404 cases. Thromb Haemost 58:1090, 1987.
28. Bertina, RM, et al: Hereditary heparin cofactor II deficiency and the risk of development of thrombosis. Thromb Haemost 57:196, 1987.
29. Bertina, RM: Hereditary protein S deficiency. Haemostasis 15:241, 1985.
30. Rick, ME: Protein C and protein S. Vitamin K–dependent inhibitors of blood coagulation. JAMA 263:701, 1990.
31. Marla, RA and Adcock, DM: Clinical evaluation of protein C: A comparative review of antigenic and functional assays. Hum Pathol 20:1040, 1989.
32. Miletich, JP: Laboratory diagnosis of protein C deficiency. Semin Thromb Hemost 16:169, 1990.
33. Tuddenham, EGD, et al: Homozygous protein C deficiency with delayed onset of symptoms at 7 to 10 months. Thromb Res 53:475, 1989.
34. Sala, N, et al: Dysfunctional activated protein C (PC Cadiz) in a patient with thrombotic disease. Thromb Haemost 57:183, 1987.
35. Vasse, M, Borg, JY, and Monconduit, M: Protein C: Rouen, a new hereditary protein C abnormality with low anticoagulant but normal amidolytic activities. Thromb Res 56:387, 1989.
36. Martinoli, JL and Stocker, K: Fast functional protein C assay using PROTAC, a novel protein C activator. Thromb Res 43:253, 1986.
37. Triplett, DA, Sandquist, DS, and Musgrave, KA: Clinical application of a functional assay for protein C. Hematol Pathol 1:239, 1987.
38. Walker, PA, Bauer, KA, and McDonagh, J: A simple, automated functional assay for protein C. Am J Clin Pathol 92:210, 1989.
39. Marlar, RA, Montgomery, RR, and Broekmans, AW: Report on the diagnosis and treatment of homozygous protein C deficiency. Report of the working party on homozygous protein C deficiency of the ICTH-subcommittee on protein C and protein S. Thromb Haemost 61:529, 1989.
40. Comp, PC, et al: Familial protein S deficiency is associated with recurrent thrombosis. J Clin Invest 74:2082, 1984.
41. Comp, P: Laboratory evaluation of protein S status. Semin Thromb Hemost 16(2):178, 1990.
42. Broekmans, AW, et al: Hereditary protein S deficiency and venous thrombo-embolism. A study in three Dutch families. Thromb Haemost 53:273, 1985.
43. Engesser, L, et al: Hereditary protein S deficiency: Clinical manifestations. Ann Intern Med 106:677, 1987.
44. Sie, P, et al: Arterial thrombosis and protein S deficiency. Thromb Haemost 62:1040, 1989.
45. Girolami, A, et al: Severe arterial cerebral thrombosis in a patient with protein S deficiency (moderately reduced total and markedly reduced free protein S): A family study. Thromb Haemost 61:144, 1989.
46. Schäfer, HP and Von Felten, A: Protein S deficiency in younger patients with cerebral arterial thrombosis. Protein-S-Mangel bei jungen Patienten mit thrombotischen Hirn-infarkten. Schweiz Med Wochenschr 119:489, 1989.
47. Amiral, J, et al: Immunoassays for the measurement of protein S. In Gaffney, PJ (ed): Fibrinolysis: Current Prospects. John Libbey, London, 1988, p 125.
48. Kobayashi, I, et al: Functional activity of protein S determined with use of protein C activated by venom activator. Clin Chem 35:1644, 1989.
49. Wolf, M, et al: A new functional assay for human protein S activity using activated factor V as substrate. Thromb Haemost 62:1144, 1989.
50. Gram, J and Jespersen, J: A selective depression of tissue plasminogen activator (tPA) activity in euglobulins characterises a risk group among survivors of acute myocardial infarction. Thromb Haemost 57:137, 1987.
51. Hamsten, A, et al: Increased plasma levels of a rapid inhibitor of tissue plasminogen activator in young survivors of myocardial infarction. N Engl J Med 313:1557, 1985.
52. Jorgensen, M and Bonnevie-Nielsen, V: Increased concentration of the fast-acting plasminogen activator inhibitor in plasma associated with familial venous thrombosis. Br J Haematol 65:175, 1987.
53. Juhan-Vague, I, et al: Deficient t-PA release and elevated PA inhibitor levels in patients with spontaneous or recurrent deep venous thrombosis. Thromb Haemost 57:67, 1987.
54. Pralong, G, et al: Plasminogen activator inhibitor 1: A new prognostic marker in septic shock. Thromb Haemost 61:459, 1989.
55. Engesser, L, et al: Elevated plasminogen activator (PAI), a cause of thrombophilia? — A study in 203 patients with familial or sporadic venous thrombophilia. Thromb Haemost 62:673, 1989.
56. Amiral, J, et al: Measurement of tPA and tPA-PAI-1 complexes by ELISA, using monoclonal antibodies: Clinical relevance. Thromb Res (Suppl VIII):99, 1988.
57. Triplett, DA: Antiphospholipid antibodies and recurrent pregnancy loss. Am J Reprod Immunol 20:52, 1989.
58. Alarcon-Segovia, D, Cardiel, MH, and Reyes, E: Antiphospholipid arterial vasculopathy. J Rheumatol 16:762, 1989.
59. Harris, EN: Antiphospholipid antibodies (annotation). Br J Haematol 74:1, 1990.
60. Beaumont, JL: Syndrome hemorragique acquis du a un anticorps circulant. Sangr 25:1, 1954.
61. Laurell, AB and Nilsson, IM: Hypergamma-globulinaemia, circulating anticoagulant and biologic false positive Was-

serman reaction: A study of 2 cases. J Lab Clin Med 49:694, 1957.

62. Soulier, JP and Boffa, MC: Avortements a repetition, thromboses et anticoagulant circulant anti-prothrombinase. Nouv Presse Med 9:859, 1980.

63. Hughes, GVR: Thrombosis, abortion, cerebral disease and the lupus anticoagulant. Br Med J 287:1088, 1983.

64. Triplett, DA, et al: Laboratory diagnosis of lupus inhibitors: A comparison of the tissue thromboplastin inhibition procedure with a new platelet neutralization procedure. Am J Clin Pathol 79:678, 1983.

65. Thiagarajan, P, Pengo, V, and Shapiro, SS: The use of the diluted Russel viper venom time for the diagnosis of lupus anticoagulants. Blood 68:869, 1986.

66. Amiral, J, Minard, F, and Laroche, P: Assay of anti-phospholipid antibodies (APA) and clinical significance (abstr). Thromb Haemost 62:593, 1989.

67. Canton, M and Gennevois, D: Evaluation of the antiphospholipid antibody syndrome. Clin Hemost Rev 4:9, 1990.

68. Alarcon-Segovia, D and Sanchez-Guerrero, J: Primary antiphospholipid syndrome. J Rheumatol 16:482, 1989.

69. Kushner, MJ: Prospective study of anticardiolipin antibodies in stroke. Stroke 21:295, 1990.

70. Weiss, P, et al: Decline of proteins C and S and factors II, VII, IX and X during the initiation of warfarin therapy. Thromb Res 45:783, 1987.

71. Takahashi, H, et al: Behavior of protein S during long-term oral anticoagulant therapy. Thromb Res 51:241, 1988.

72. Gilabert, J, et al: Physiological coagulation inhibitors (protein S, protein C and antithrombin III) in severe preeclamptic states and in users of oral contraceptives. Thromb Res 49:319, 1988.

73. Boerger, LM, et al: Oral contraceptives and gender affect protein S status. Blood 69(2):692, 1987.

74. Huisveld, IA, et al: Oral contraceptives reduce total protein S, but not free protein S. Thromb Res 45:109, 1987.

75. Rodeghiero, F, Castaman, G, and Dini, E: Fibrinopeptide A changes during remission induction treatment with L-asparaginase in acute lymphoblastic leukemia: Evidence for activation of blood activation. Thromb Res 57:31, 1990.

76. Rocha, E, et al: Clotting activation and impairment of fibrinolysis in malignancy. Thromb Res 54:699, 1989.

77. Tuszinski, GP, et al: Thrombospondin mediates tumor cell metastasis (abstr). Thromb Haemost 62:22, 1989.

78. Wright, JG, et al: Fibrinolysis during normal human pregnancy: Complex inter-relationships inhibitors and the euglobulin clot lysis time. Br J Haematol 69:253, 1988.

79. Friedman, KD, Borok, Z, and Owen, J: Heparin cofactor activity and antithrombin III antigen levels in preeclampsia. Thromb Res 43:409, 1986.

80. Fernández, JA, et al: Functional and immunologic protein S in normal pregnant women and in full-term newborns. Thromb Haemost 61:474, 1989.

81. Mombaerts, P, et al: Fibrinolytic response to venous occlusion, and fibrin fragment D-Dimer and fibronectin levels in normal and complicated pregnancy (abstr). Thromb Haemost 58:98, 1987.

82. Largo, R, Heller, V, and Straub, PW: Detection of soluble intermediates of the fibrinogen-fibrin conversion using erythrocytes coated with fibrin monomers. Blood 47:991, 1976.

83. Bick, RL and Dukes, ML: Antithrombin III (AT III) as a diagnostic aid in disseminated intravascular coagulation. Thromb Res 10:721, 1977.

84. Spero, JA, Lewis, JH, and Hasiba, U: Disseminated intravascular coagulation: Findings in 346 patients. Thromb Haemost 43:28, 1980.

85. Van den Besselaar, AMHP, Gralnick, HR, and Lewis, SM (eds): Thromboplastin Calibration and Oral Anticoagulant Control. Martinus Nijhoff, Boston, 1984.

86. WHO Expert Committee on Biological Standardization. Thirty-Third Report: Technical Report Series 687. WHO, Geneva, 1983, p 81.

87. Peters, RHM, Van den Besselaar, AMHP, and Olthuis,

FMFG: A multicentre study to evaluate method dependency of the international sensitivity index of bovine thromboplastin. Thromb Haemost 61:166, 1989.

88. Casu, B: Structure of heparin and heparin fragments. Ann NY Acad Sci 556:1, 1989.

89. Choay, J, et al: Structure activity relationship in heparin: A synthetic pentasaccharide with high affinity for antithrombin III and eliciting high anti-factor Xa activity. Biochem Biophys Res Comm 116:492, 1983.

90. Van Boeckel, CAA, et al: Synthesis of a pentasaccharide corresponding to the antithrombin III fragment of heparin. J Carbohydrate Chem 4:293, 1985.

91. Marciniak, E: Factor Xa inactivation by antithrombin III: Evidence for biological stabilization of factor Xa by factor V phospholipid complex. Br J Haematol 24:391, 1973.

92. McNeely, TB and Griffith, MJ: The anticoagulant mechanism of action of heparin in contact activated plasma. Blood 65:1226, 1985.

93. Ofosu, DA, et al: The inhibition of thrombin-dependent positive feed-back reactions is critical to the expression of the anticoagulant effect of heparin. Biochem J 243:579, 1987.

94. Barber, AJ, et al: Characterization of a chondrointin-sulphate proteoglycan carrier for heparin neutralizing activity (platelet factor 4) released from human blood platelets. Biochem Biophys Acta 286:312, 1972.

95. Hull, R, Delmore, T, and Genton, E: Warfarin sodium versus low-dose heparin in the long-term treatment of venous thrombosis. N Engl J Med 301:855, 1979.

96. Kakkar, VV: Low-dose heparin in the prevention of venous thromboembolism. Thromb Diath Haemorrh 33:87, 1974.

97. De Swart, CAM et al: Kinetics of intravenously administered heparin in normal humans. Blood 60:1251, 1982.

98. Scully, MF, et al: Measurement of heparin in plasma: Influence of inter-subject and circadian variability in heparin sensitivity according to method. Thromb Res 46:447, 1987.

99. Bjornsson, TD and Wolfrom, KM: Intersubject variability in the anticoagulant response to heparin in vitro. Eur J Clin Pharmacol 21:491, 1982.

100. Murray, G: Heparin in surgical treatment of blood vessels. Arch Surg 40:307, 1940.

101. Jaques, LB: Heparins—Anionic polyelectrolyte drugs. Pharmacol Rev 31:99, 1980.

102. Wright, IS, Marple, CD, and Beck, DF: Report of the committee for the evaluation of heparin in the treatment of coronary thrombosis with myocardial infarction: A progress report on the statistical analysis of the first 800 cases by this committee. Am Heart J 36:801, 1948.

103. Best, CH, Cowan, C, and MacLean, DL: Heparin and the formation of white thrombi. J Physiol 92:20, 1938.

104. Ware, JA and Salzman, EW: Use of Heparin in Treatment of Thromboembolic Disorders. In Lane, AL and Lindahl, U (eds): Heparin. Chemical and Biological Properties. Clinical Applications. CRC Press, Boca Raton, FL, 1989, p 475.

105. Mitchell, JRA: Theory and practice in prevention of arterial thrombosis. Br Heart J 48:417, 1982.

106. TIMI Study Group: The thrombolysis in myocardial infarction trial. N Engl J Med 312:932, 1985.

107. Mant, MJ, et al: Hemorrhagic complications of heparin therapy. Lancet 1:1133, 1977.

108. Holm, HA, et al: Subcutaneous heparin treatment of deep venous thrombosis: A comparison of unfractionated and low molecular weight heparin. Haemostasis (Suppl)16:30, 1986.

109. Teien, AN and Lie, M: Evaluation of an amidolytic heparin assay method. Increased sensitivity by adding purified antithrombin III. Thromb Res 10:399, 1977.

110. Godal, HC: The antiheparin effect of platelets. Scand J Clin Lab Invest 14:223, 1962.

111. Contant, G, Gouault-Heilmann, M, and Martinoli, JL: Heparin inactivation during blood storage: Its prevention by blood collection in citric acid, theophylline, adenosine, dipyridamole—CTAD mixture. Thromb Res 31:365, 1983.

112. Brandt, JT and Triplett, DA: Laboratory monitoring of heparin. Effect of reagents and instruments on the activated par-

tial thromboplastin time. Am J Clin Pathol (Suppl) 76:530, 1981.

113. Yin, ET, Wessler, S, and Butler, JV: Plasma heparin: A unique, practical, submicrogram-sensitive assay. J Lab Clin Med 81:298, 1973.

114. Naylor, CD, et al: Guidelines for the use of intravenous thrombolytic agents in acute myocardial infarction. Can Med Assoc J 140:1289, 1989.

115. Sane, DC, et al: Bleeding during thrombolytic therapy for acute myocardial infarction: Mechanisms and management. Ann Intern Med 111:1010, 1989.

QUESTIONS

1. Which of the following is not a natural anticoagulant/inhibitor?
   a. Antithrombin III
   b. Heparin cofactor II
   c. Factor Va
   d. Protein C
   e. Protein S

2. What is not true concerning the action of thrombin?
   a. Converts fibrinogen to fibrin
   b. Inactivates protein C
   c. Binds to platelets and stimulates release of platelet factors
   d. Activates factors VIII and V

3. What is the most important serine-protease inhibitor?
   a. Antithrombin III
   b. Protein C and protein S
   c. Factors IXa and Xa
   d. PCI-I and α_1-antitrypsin

4. Which inhibitors are vitamin K dependent? (Use answer choices for question 3.)

5. How are TPA and urokinase-type plasminogen activator classified in the plasminogen activation mechanism?
   a. Intrinsic
   b. Extrinsic
   c. Exogenous

6. Which of the following is not classified as a SERPIN?
   a. α_2-antiplasmin
   b. α_2-macroglobulin
   c. α_1-antitrypsin
   d. Protein S

7. Why are functional assays preferred to immunologic assays when evaluating thrombosis?
   a. Easier to perform
   b. Easier to interpret
   c. Detects qualitative defects
   d. Detects small quantitative defects

8. Which of the following characteristics are similar for deficiencies of antithrombin III, heparin cofactor II, protein C, and protein S?
   a. Onset before age 40
   b. Deep venous thrombosis
   c. Pulmonary embolism
   d. All of the above

9. What are associated risks for patients with fibrinolytic defects?
   a. Thromboembolism, arterial thrombosis, and arteriosclerosis
   b. Fetal loss and lupus anticoagulant
   c. Neoplastic cell development and tumor cell metastasis
   d. Hemorrhagic syndrome and chronic DIC

10. What laboratory tests are performed for evaluation of APA syndrome?
    a. Nontreponemal (cardiolipin) tests for syphilis
    b. Coagulation tests such as Russell viper venom time
    c. ELISA for APA
    d. All of the above

11. Which level of AT-III would suggest a real defect rather than a defect acquired during heparin therapy?
    a. Below 80% of normal
    b. Below 75% of normal
    c. Below 60% of normal
    d. Below 50% of normal

12. Which factors may be decreased during preeclampsia?
    a. Fibrinogen and factor VIII
    b. Protein S and D-dimer
    c. Protein C and AT-III
    d. α_1-antitrypsin and PAI

13. Which laboratory test result would not be associated with DIC?
    a. Decreased AT-III
    b. Decreased protein C
    c. Positive for fibrin monomers
    d. Increased α_1-antitrypsin

14. What is the action of oral anticoagulants?
    a. Degrades clotting factors
    b. Blocks vitamin K
    c. Inhibits binding of calcium
    d. Replaces activated zymogens

15. What laboratory test is most commonly used to monitor oral anticoagulant therapy?
    a. PT
    b. APTT
    c. Platelet count
    d. Protein C and protein S levels

16. What is the anticoagulant mechanism of heparin?
    a. Inhibits PF4
    b. Inhibits thrombin by complexing with AT-III
    c. Degrades AT-III
    d. Complexes with HC-II

17. Which laboratory tests are used to monitor heparin therapy?
    a. APTT
    b. Anti-Xa heparin assay
    c. Thrombin time
    d. All of the above

18. Which of the following are thrombolytic agents?
    a. Streptokinase
    b. Urokinase
    c. TPA
    d. All of the above

19. What laboratory tests are not affected by the presence of therapeutic heparin?
    a. PT and APTT
    b. Thrombin time
    c. Reptilase time
    d. Whole blood clotting time and heparin assay

ANSWERS

1. c (p. 499)
2. b (p. 499–500)
3. a (p. 500)
4. b (p. 501–502)
5. b (p. 502)
6. d (p. 503)
7. c (p. 503)
8. d (p. 504)
9. a (p. 505)
10. d (p. 505)
11. c (p. 506)
12. c (p. 507)
13. d (p. 507)
14. b (p. 508)
15. a (p. 509)
16. b (p. 510)
17. d (p. 512)
18. d (p. 513)
19. c (p. 513)

PART **FIVE**

LABORATORY METHODS

CHAPTER 30

Laboratory Methods in Hematology and Hemostasis

SECTION I

Routine Hematology Methods

JANIS WYRICK-GLATZEL, M.S., M.T.(ASCP)
SANDRA GWALTNEY-KRAUSE, M.A., M.T.(ASCP)

SECTION II

Principles of Automated Differential Analysis

ELLEN HOPE, M.S., S.H.(ASCP)H
ELLINOR I. B. PEERSCHKE, Ph.D.

SECTION III

Special Stains/Cytochemistry

MARY LORING PERKINS, M.S., M.T.(ASCP)S.H.

SECTION IV

Coagulation

JANIS WYRICK-GLATZEL, M.S., M.T.(ASCP)
SANDRA GWALTNEY-KRAUSE, M.A., M.T.(ASCP)

Routine Hematology Methods

MANUAL BLOOD CELL COUNTS
HEMATOCYTOMETER
MANUAL CELL COUNTING USING THE HEMACYTOMETER
BLOOD DILUTION VIALS
DILUTING PIPETTES
RBC COUNT USING THE HEMATOCYTOMETER
WBC COUNT USING THE HEMATOCYTOMETER
MANUAL DETERMINATION OF THE PLATELET COUNT
EOSINOPHIL COUNT
RETICULOCYTES
RBC INDICES

OTHER ROUTINE HEMATOLOGY METHODS
ERYTHROCYTE SEDIMENTATION RATE
HEMATOCRIT

TESTS FOR HEMOGLOBINS
HEMOGLOBINOMETRY
HEMOGLOBIN ELECTROPHORESIS
CITRATE AGAR HEMOGLOBIN ELECTROPHORESIS
HEMOGLOBIN A_2 BY COLUMN
DIFFERENTIAL SOLUBILITY TEST FOR HEMOGLOBIN S
  (SICKLEQUIK BY GENERAL DIAGNOSTICS)
SODIUM METABISULFITE SLIDE TEST

ACID ELUTION FOR HEMOGLOBIN F
STAINING FOR HEINZ BODIES
HEINZ BODY INDUCTION TEST

TESTS FOR HEMOLYTIC ANEMIAS
OSMOTIC FRAGILITY

**ACIDIFIED SERUM TEST (HAM TEST) FOR
  PAROXYSMAL NOCTURNAL HEMOGLOBINURIA**
SUGAR-WATER TEST FOR PNH
AUTOHEMOLYSIS TEST

**PREPARATION OF BLOOD SMEARS AND GROSS
  EXAMINATION**
PREPARATION OF THE PERIPHERAL BLOOD SMEAR
SLIDE-TO-SLIDE METHOD
COVERSLIP-TO-COVERSLIP METHOD
COVERSLIP-TO-SLIDE METHOD
AUTOMATIC SPINNER TECHNIQUE
EXAMINATION OF THE PERIPHERAL BLOOD SMEAR

PRINCIPLES OF AUTOMATED CELL COUNTING
COULTER COUNTER MODEL S-PLUS
COULTER COUNTER MODEL S-PLUS STKR
TECHNICON H*1 SYSTEM

OBJECTIVES

At the end of this section, the learner should be able to:
1. Calculate a manual white blood cell count.
2. Calculate a manual red blood cell count.
3. Calculate a manual platelet count.
4. Calculate percent of reticulocytes.
5. Calculate absolute reticulocyte count.
6. Calculate a corrected reticulocyte count.
7. Calculate a reticulocyte production index.
8. List errors in the performance of a centrifugal microhematocrit.
9. Calculate mean corpuscular volume.
10. Calculate mean corpuscular hemoglobin.
11. Calculate mean corpuscular hemoglobin concentration.
12. Classify red blood cells based on the value of mean corpuscular volume.
13. Classify red blood cells based on the value of mean corpuscular hemoglobin concentration.
14. Identify factors that affect the erythrocyte sedimentation rate.
15. Identify hemoglobins separated at alkaline and acid pH in hemoglobin electrophoresis.
16. Name a method for quantitating hemoglobin A_2.
17. Describe the differential solubility test for hemoglobin S.
18. Describe the acid elution test for hemoglobin F.
19. Name tests that measure Heinz bodies.
20. Identify conditions that show increased and decreased osmotic fragility.
21. Describe the basic principle for the ham test and the sugar-water test for paroxysmal nocturnal hemoglobinuria.
22. Calculate a platelet estimate from values for a peripheral blood smear count.
23. Calculate a corrected white blood cell count for a smear containing more than 1 nucleated red blood cell per 1000 white blood cells.
24. Explain the principle of automated cell counting.
25. Identify cell parameters directly measured by automated cell (Coulter) counters.
26. Identify cell parameters calculated by automated cell (Coulter) counters.
27. Explain the basic principle of the cyanmethemoglobin method for hemoglobin determinations.

HEMACYTOMETER

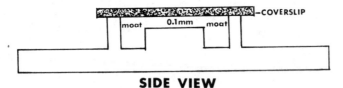

SIDE VIEW

Figure 30–I–1. Hemacytometer: side view.

Our goal in this chapter is to present the student with basic hematologic and coagulation procedures. Emphasis is placed on interpretation as well as on procedure. At the end of some of the procedures we have included a comment section, which serves as a potpourri highlighting general points of information concerning the procedure, its limitations, and its interpretation.

The intention was never to make this section all-inclusive. We realize that with a rapid expansion of automation, some of these procedures have become antiquated. We believe, however, that an understanding of these basic procedures will serve as a sound building block for the application of more advanced technology.

MANUAL BLOOD CELL COUNTS
Hemacytometer

The *hemacytometer* counting chamber is used for cell counting. It is constructed so that the distance between the bottom of the *coverslip* and the surface of the counting area of the chamber is 0.1 mm (Fig. 30-I-1). The surface of the chamber contains two square ruled areas separated by an H-shaped moat (Fig. 30-I-1). These two squares are identical, allowing the technologist to duplicate the count, and each has a total area of 9 mm² (3 mm on each side). These squares are divided into nine primary squares (Fig. 30-I-2), each with an area of 1 mm² (1 mm on each side). The four corner primary squares are used when counting leukocytes. The four corner primary squares are further divided into 16 smaller secondary squares to aid in counting leukocytes. The center primary square, however, is divided into 25 secondary squares, each with an area of 0.04 mm². The four corner and center secondary squares of the center primary square (Fig. 30-I-2) are used to count erythrocytes. All 25 secondary squares of the center primary square are used to count platelets, and each of these 25 squares is further divided into 16 smaller tertiary squares.

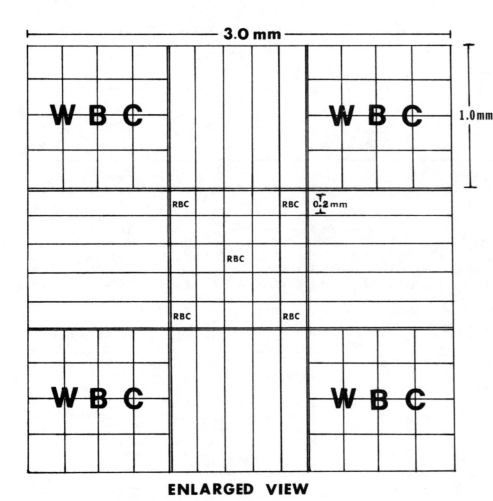

ENLARGED VIEW

Figure 30–I–2. This represents an enlarged view of one of the two ruled squares of the hemacytometer. The four corner primary squares are used for counting white cells. Five secondary squares labeled ("RBC") of the center primary square are used in counting platelets.

The boundary lines of the central primary square are either double or triple. When the boundary line is double, all the cells within the squares and those touching the innermost line are counted. If the boundary line is triple, all the cells within the squares and those touching the middle line inward are counted.

Hemacytometers and coverslips should meet the specifications of the National Bureau of Standards and are so marked by the manufacturer. Always use the coverslip that accompanies the hemacytometer; it has been ground to fit the specifics of the hemacytometer in order to ensure a uniform depth and therefore a constant volume. A regular coverslip cannot be used.

Manual Cell Counting Using the Hemacytometer

With the introduction of sophisticated electronic equipment such as the Coulter counter into the field of hematology, there is a diminished need for manual cell counting. However, a knowledge of this method is still important in the field of hematology. Manual cell counts are often performed in patients with extreme cases of thrombocytosis, thrombocytopenia, leukocytosis, and leukocytopenia. Perhaps the most clearcut use for manual cell counts is for measuring body fluids such as cerebral spinal fluid (CSF) and pleural fluid, as these can be counted only manually.

Blood Dilution Vials

Dilution of blood samples may be performed by using prepackaged blood dilution vials available from manufacturers, such as the UNOPETTE kit by Becton Dickinson Vacutainer Systems. Each vial is filled with premeasured diluent and capillary pipettes appropriate for the necessary dilutions. A wide variety of test vials are available including those for white blood cells (WBCs), platelets, red blood cells (RBCs), eosinophils, and hemoglobin. With the implication of infectious diseases such as hepatitis and acquired immunodeficiency syndrome (AIDS), mouth section pipettes are no longer advocated as proper procedure for making dilutions with micropipettes. Once the dilutions are made, the manual counts may be performed as described on p. 526. Any changes in dilution factors that may vary with manufacturer must be kept under consideration.

Diluting Pipettes

Dilution of the blood sample may be accomplished by the use of a cell-diluting pipette. Both the RBC and WBC pipettes are composed of a stem that is divided into 10 equal parts and a mixing chamber containing a red, white, or clear bead, which aids in mixing the diluent and blood.

When the WBC pipette is used, blood is drawn to either the 0.5 or the 1.0 mark and the diluent to the 11 mark, making dilutions of 1:20 and 1:10, respectively.

When the RBC pipette is used, blood is drawn to the 0.5 and the 1.0 mark and the diluent to the 101 mark, making dilutions of 1:200 and 1:100, respectively.

In calculating the dilution, only the volume contained in the bulb is considered, as the stem will contain only diluent and its contents will be discarded before charging the chambers. The *dilution factor*, used in calculating the cells/mm³, is the reciprocal of the dilution and therefore can be calculated using the following formula.

$$\text{Dilution} = \frac{\text{Amount of Blood}}{\text{Total Volume}}$$

WBC Pipette

$$\frac{0.5 \text{ (Blood)}}{10 \text{ (Volume)}} = \frac{1}{20} \text{ (Dilution)}$$

RBC Pipette

$$\frac{1.0 \text{ (Blood)}}{100 \text{ (Volume)}} = \frac{1}{100} \text{ (Dilution)}$$

RBC Count Using the Hemacytometer

Definition

The RBC count is the determination of the number of erythrocytes in 1 mm³ or 1 μl of blood.

Principle

Using an RBC diluting pipette, venous or capillary blood is mixed with a diluting fluid. The hemacytometer then is charged with this dilution and the cells counted with a microscope.

For RBC counts, the solution that is used is isotonic with the erythrocytes. The diluting fluids used do not lyse the leukocytes. Normally, the leukocytes are too few to interfere with the RBC count. In cases of leukocytosis, however, the leukocytes are easily identified and are not counted.

Reagents

The following diluents can be used in counting RBCs: Gower's, Hayem's, and isotonic saline. In our laboratory we prefer using isotonic saline owing to its accessibility.

Equipment

RBC diluting pipettes
Hemacytometer and coverslip
Pipette suction apparatus
Alcohol pads
Lint-free wipes
Hand counter
Microscope

Procedure

1. Clean the hemacytometer and its coverslip with an alcohol pad and then dry with a wipe. Clean the pipettes with pipette washers.

2. The blood specimen must be mixed just prior to use to ensure even cell suspension; mixing is accomplished by gentle inversion of the tube 10 to 20 times. Never vigorously shake the sample, as this could cause cell lysis and produce erroneous results.

3. After attaching the pipette suction apparatus to the pipette, aspirate blood to the 0.5 mark without letting any bubbles into the pipette.

4. Clean the outside of the pipette with a wipe, being careful not to contact the bore of the pipette. If the wipe contacts the bore, fluid and not cells will be pulled out of the pipette, causing a false increase in cell concentration.

5. If the blood overshoots the 0.5 mark by no more than 1 to 2 mm, remove the excess blood by tapping the pipette tip with any nonabsorbent material, but not a wipe. If you overshoot the 0.5 mark by more than 2 mm, clean the pipette and start over.

6. When the specimen is at the 0.5 mark, quickly and carefully aspirate the diluting solution to the 101 mark, with a steady suction and rotation of the pipette between your fingers, without overshooting the mark or letting any bubbles into the pipette.

7. Again carefully wipe clean the outside of the pipette, without contacting the bore of the pipette with the wipe.

8. If the 101 mark is overshot by no more than 1 to 2 mm, you may correct it by tapping the pipette tip with any nonabsorbent material.

9. The aspirator tubing is removed from the pipette by rolling it off—not by pulling or pinching, as this will expel fluid, changing the dilution.

10. While wearing gloves, place a finger over each end of the pipette and vigorously shake the pipette for 2 to 3 minutes, or shake the pipette on a mechanical shaker for 45 seconds. When manually shaking the pipette, do not shake it in an end-to-end fashion but rather in a figure-8 pattern or by rotating between the fingers.

11. Discard 4 to 5 drops from the pipette before charging the hemacytometer chamber, to expel any undiluted diluent.

12. Charge the two chambers on the hemacytometer by touching the tip of the pipette to the coverslip edge where it meets the chamber floor. To aid in charging the hemacytometer, hold the pipette at a 45-degree angle. The chamber will fill by capillary action if the hemacytometer and coverslip are clean. Overcharging the hemacytometer will result in fluid flowing into the moat, requiring you to clean and recharge the hemacytometer.

13. You may keep the remaining fluid in the pipette should you need to repeat a count. Place the pipette in a horizontal position when not in use. To reuse, shake the pipette as stated before, again discarding 4 to 5 drops prior to charging the chambers.

14. Mount the hemacytometer on the microscope and lower its condenser.

15. Let the hemacytometer rest for 1 to 2 minutes to allow the cells to settle.

16. Procedure for counting RBCs:
    a. Cells are scanned under a 10× objective to ensure even distribution.
    b. Use a 40× objective to count the erythrocytes in the four corner and center secondary squares of the center primary square. This counting procedure is repeated on the opposite side of the hemacytometer (Fig. 30-I-2).
    c. To count the cells in the tertiary squares, use the following pattern:
       (1) Count cells starting in the upper left corner square; continue counting to the right hand square; drop down to the next row; continue counting from the right hand square to the left square. Continue in this fashion until the total area in that secondary square has been counted.
       (2) Count all cells that touch any of the upper and left lines. Do not count any cell that touches a lower or right line.
    d. The difference between the highest and lowest number of cells of the 10 squares should be no greater than 25.

17. Calculate the RBCs per mm³ on the basis of the number of cells counted, area, and the dilution made, as previously outlined.

Calculations

The following formula may still be used to calculate the RBC count:

$$\text{Count (cells/mm}^3) = \text{Cells/mm}^2 \times 10 \times \text{Dilution}$$

In the case of a normal RBC count, the factor can be determined by the following calculation:

$$\begin{aligned}
\text{Factor} &= 1/\text{area} \times \text{Depth factor} \times \text{Dilution factor} \\
&= 1/0.2 \text{ mm}^2 \times 10 \times 200 \\
&= 10,000
\end{aligned}$$

Note: Depth factor equals depth of chamber, which is 0.1 mm. You must multiply by 10 to get 1 mm³.

Example

Blood is drawn to the 0.5 mark of the RBC pipette, and the number of cells counted in the four corner and center secondary squares equals 300 RBCs.

$$\begin{aligned}
\text{Cells/mm}^3 &= \text{Cells/mm}^2 \times \text{Depth factor} \\
&\quad \times \text{Dilution factor} \\
&= (300/0.2 \text{ mm}^2) \times 10 \times 200 \\
&= 3.0 \times 10^6/\text{mm}^3
\end{aligned}$$

In this example, the area equals 0.2 mm², because the length of each of the small squares counted is equal to 0.2 mm. Thus, the area of each square is

0.04 mm². Because five of these squares were counted, the total area counted is 0.04 times 5, or 0.2 mm².

Interpretation

Normal values:

Newborn	4.4–5.8 million/mm³
Infant/Child	3.8–5.5 million/mm³
Adult male	4.7–6.1 million/mm³
Adult female	4.2–5.4 million/mm³

WBC Count Using the Hemacytometer

Definition

The WBC or leukocyte count is the determination of the number of WBCs in 1 mm³ or 1 μl of blood.

Principle

Using a WBC diluting pipette, mix venous or capillary blood with a diluting fluid. Charge (fill) the hemacytometer with this dilution, and count the cells with a microscope.

For WBC counts, Turk's solution is used. This diluting fluid contains an acid solution that lyses the non-nucleated RBCs and a stain that stains the nuclei of the WBCs and allows for easy identification and counting.

Reagents

The preferred diluent for counting WBCs is Turk's solution. A useful formula for this reagent is as follows:

Glacial acetic acid	1 ml
Gentian violet (1% aqueous)	2 ml
Distilled water to	100 ml

Equipment

WBC diluting pipette
Hemacytometer and coverslip
Aspirator tubing and mouthpiece
Alcohol pads
Lint-free wipes
Hand counter
Microscope

Procedure

1. Clean the hemacytometer and its coverslip with an alcohol pad and then dry with a wipe. Clean the pipettes using pipette washers.
2. Mix the blood specimen just prior to use to ensure even cell suspension. Mixing is accomplished by gentle inversion of the tube 10 to 20 times. Never vigorously shake the sample, as this could cause cell lysis and give erroneous results.
3. After attaching the aspirator tubing and mouthpiece to the pipette, aspirate blood to the 0.5 mark without letting any bubbles into the pipette.
4. Clean the outside of the pipette with a wipe, being careful not to contact the bore of the pipette. If the wipe contacts the bore, fluid and not cells will be pulled out of the pipette, causing a false increase in cell concentration.
5. If blood overshoots the 0.5 mark by no more than 1 to 2 mm, remove the excess blood by tapping the pipette tip with any nonabsorbent material, but not a wipe. Overshooting the 0.5 mark by more than 2 mm will necessitate cleaning the pipette and starting over.
6. When the specimen is at the 0.5 mark, quickly and carefully aspirate Turk's solution to the 11 mark, with a steady suction and rotation of the pipette between the fingers, without overshooting the mark or letting any bubbles into the pipette.
7. Carefully wipe clean the outside of the pipette again, without contacting the bore of the pipette with the wipe.
8. If the 11 mark is overshot by no more than 1 to 2 mm, you may correct it by tapping the pipette tip with any nonabsorbent material.
9. Remove the aspirator tubing from the pipette by rolling it off—not by pulling or pinching, as this will expel fluid, changing the dilution.
10. With a finger over each end of the pipette, vigorously shake the pipette for 2 to 3 minutes or use a mechanical shaker for 45 seconds. When manually shaking the pipette, do not shake it in an end-to-end fashion but rather in a figure-8 pattern or by rotating it between the fingers.
11. Discard 4 to 5 drops from the pipette before charging the hemacytometer chamber to expel any undiluted diluent.
12. The two chambers on the hemacytometer are charged by touching the tip of the pipette to the coverslip edge where it meets the chamber floor. To aid in charging the hemacytometer, hold the pipette at a 45-degree angle. The chamber will fill by capillary action, if the hemacytometer and coverslip are clean. Overcharging the hemacytometer will result in fluid flowing into the moat, requiring you to clean and recharge the hemacytometer.
13. You may keep the remaining fluid in the pipette in case you need to repeat a count. Place the pipette in a horizontal position when not in use. To reuse, shake the pipette as stated before, again discarding 4 to 5 drops prior to charging the chambers.
14. Mount the hemacytometer on the microscope and lower its condenser.
15. Let the hemacytometer sit for 1 to 2 minutes to allow the cells to settle.
16. Procedure for counting WBCs:
    a. Cells are scanned under a 10× objective to ensure even distribution.
    b. Use the 40× objective to count the WBCs in each of the four corner secondary squares on both sides of the chamber.
    c. In counting the cells in the secondary squares use the following pattern:

(1) Count cells starting in the upper left corner square; continue counting to the right hand square; drop down to the next row; continue counting from the right square to the left square. Continue in this fashion until the total area in that primary square has been counted.

(2) Count all cells that touch any of the upper and left lines. Do not count any cell that touches a lower or right line.

d. The difference between the highest and lowest number of cells of the eight squares should be no greater than 15.

17. Calculate the WBCs per mm³ on the basis of the number of cells counted, area, and the dilution made, as previously outlined.

Calculations

There are several ways to calculate direct cell counts. The preferred method is to convert the number of cells counted in 1 mm² to cells in 1 mm³ by correcting for the dilution made and the area counted. The following formula is used to calculate any type of cell count:

$$\text{Count (cells/mm}^3) = \text{Cells/mm}^2 \times 10 \times \text{Dilution}$$

In this equation:

$$\text{Cells/mm}^2 = \frac{\text{Cells counted}}{\text{Area counted (mm}^2)}$$

The number of cells per mm² is multiplied by 10 (the reciprocal of the depth of the chamber, 0.1), giving the cells in 1 mm³, and then multiplied by the dilution, thus giving the number of cells/mm³. The count per cubic millimeter is then multiplied by a factor of 10^6 to yield cells per liter (10^9).

The second method of calculating direct cell counts involves a factor dependent on the area counted and the dilution of the sample. The factor is then multiplied by the total number of cells counted, yielding the number of cells per mm³. The determination of a factor is not the method of choice, especially in situations involving severe leukopenia, leukocytosis, or for use with body fluids where variations in the dilution as well as the area counted are made. In the case of a normal WBC count, however, the factor can be determined by the following calculation:

$$
\begin{aligned}
\text{Factor} &= 1/\text{Area} \times \text{Depth factor} \times \text{Dilution factor} \\
&= 1/4 \text{ mm}^2 \times 10 \times 20 \\
&= 50
\end{aligned}
$$

Example

Blood is pipetted to the 1.0 mark of the WBC pipette and the number of cells counted in the four large corner primary squares equals 100 WBCs.

$$
\begin{aligned}
\text{Cells/mm}^3 &= \text{Cells/mm}^2 \times \text{Depth factor} \\
&\quad \times \text{Dilution factor} \\
&= (100/4) \times 10 \times 10 \\
&= 2500 \text{ WBC/mm}^3
\end{aligned}
$$

Interpretation

Normal values:

Newborn	9,000–30,000/mm³
1 wk	5,000–21,000/mm³
1 mo	5,000–19,500/mm³
6–12 mo	6,000–17,500/mm³
2 yr	6,200–17,000/mm³
Child/Adult	4,800–10,800/mm³

Comments

1. Discard any damaged pipettes (such as those with chipped tips), to avoid inaccurate counts.
2. The hemacytometer, coverslip, and pipette must be clean and dry prior to use. Errors are introduced by fingerprints, lint, and dirt. Check the diluting fluid to ensure that it is free from contamination.
3. Never aspirate blood into the pipette unless using the aspirator tubing.
4. Use the coverslip that accompanies the hemacytometer.
5. When counting cells, follow the procedure as outlined before. This will prevent counting the same cell more than once or missing a cell that should be counted, thereby producing erroneous results.
6. Allow the cells to settle in the counting chamber for 1 to 2 minutes prior to counting to ensure accurate counts.
7. When using anticoagulated blood, ensure proper mixing of specimen before sampling.
8. In cases of leukopenia, with a count below 4000/mm³, the dilution factor is 10.
9. In cases of leukocytosis, with a count in excess of 11,000/mm³, an RBC pipette is used and the dilution factor is 100 or even 200 (depending on the degree of leukocytosis).
10. There are physiologic variations to consider when performing WBC counts. Higher counts are seen following exercise, emotional stress, anxiety, and food intake. Blacks generally show slightly lower WBC counts than whites.

Manual Determination of the Platelet Count

Principle

The reference method for determining manual platelet counts uses the phase contrast microscope. When whole blood is added to 1 percent ammonium oxalate, mature red cells are hemolyzed. Platelets, leukocytes, and reticulocytes, however, are preserved. By use of phase microscopy, platelets can easily be counted in a special counting chamber, as described by Brecher and Cronkite.[1]

Equipment

Phase contrast microscope equipped with a
  40× annulus,
  40× phase objective, and
  10× oculars (total of 400×)
Special thin flat-bottom counting chamber
No. 1 glass coverslip

RBC diluting pipettes
1% ammonium oxalate (W/V)
Petri dish and cover with moist filter paper

To prepare 1 percent ammonium oxalate, weigh 10 g ammonium oxalate (reagent grade) in a weighing boat. Transfer to a 1000-ml volumetric flask. Add about 500 ml distilled water and mix to dissolve. Fill the flask to mark and mix. Store in the refrigerator to prevent growth of microorganisms. Filter before use.

Procedure

1. Use thoroughly mixed venous blood collected in ethylenediaminetetraacetic acid (EDTA), or peripheral blood from a freely flowing skin puncture.
2. Fill duplicate RBC pipettes to the 1 mark with blood and dilute to the 101 mark with 1 percent ammonium oxalate.
3. Shake the two pipettes for 2 to 3 minutes and fill the chamber. Fill one side of the chamber with each pipette.
4. Place the counting chamber in a petri dish containing a moistened filter paper and let stand for 15 minutes, but no more than 20 minutes.
5. Using the phase contrast microscope set at 400×, count the platelets in the entire center square millimeter (center primary square) on both sides of the chamber. Duplicate counts or a sample (for example, both sides of the hemacytometer) should agree within 10 percent for the counts to be acceptable. Platelets appear as dense, dark bodies and can be round, oval, or rod shaped, with a diameter of about 2 to 4 μm.
6. Calculate the number of platelets per cubic millimeter using the following factor formula:

Cells/mm³

$$= \frac{\text{No. cells counted} \times \text{Dilution} \times \text{Depth factor}}{\text{No. squares counted} \times \text{Area } (0.04 \text{ mm}^2)}$$

Interpretation

Normal values: 150,000 to 450,000/mm³

Comments

1. Platelets appear round, oval, or rodlike, sometimes showing dendritic processes. Their internal granular structure and pearlescent sheen allows the platelets to be distinguished from debris, which is often refractile. Red blood cells will appear as ghost cells. Use caution when RBCs have inclusions present, so as not to confuse the inclusions with platelets.
2. If platelet clumping is observed, redilute count. If clumping is still present, obtain a fresh specimen. Because of the adhesive quality of platelets, fingerstick specimens are least desirable.
3. The phase platelet determination should be compared with a review of the blood film for correction of count and morphology.
4. Ethylenediaminetetraacetic acid is the anticoagulant of choice when performing phase platelet counts. The student should be aware of the phenomenon of "platelet satellitosis" when using this anticoagulant.[2] Platelet satellitosis appears as neutrophils ringed with adhering platelets. Obtain correct platelet counts by collecting a fresh specimen with sodium citrate as the anticoagulant. When sodium citrate is used as an anticoagulant, make the correction for the dilution by multiplying by 1.1.
5. Ordinary light microscopy may be used; however, in this method differentiation and enumeration are more difficult.
6. In cases of thrombocytopenia (less than 100,000/mm³) the count should be repeated with a 1:20 dilution of blood using a WBC pipette.

Eosinophil Count

The absolute number of eosinophils per cubic millimeter of blood can be calculated by two methods. The first is an estimate using the number of eosinophils from the differential and the total leukocyte count. The second is by a direct hemacytometer count. The former is the least accurate, owing to the nature of a 100 WBC differential count.

The absolute eosinophil count uses a stain in which the RBCs are lysed and the eosinophils stained. In this method eosinophils can be directly counted in a hemacytometer.

Reagents and Equipment

WBC diluting pipettes
Hemacytometer and coverslip
Eosinophil diluting fluid (Pilot's solution)

Propylene glycol	50 ml
Distilled water	40 ml
Phloxine, 1% aqueous solution	10 ml
Sodium carbonate, 10% aqueous solution	1 ml

Filter and store at refrigerator temperature. Discard after 1 month.

Procedure

1. Aspirate blood to the 1.0 line in the WBC diluting pipette. Place the tip of the pipette in diluting fluid, and aspirate until it reaches the 11 line.
2. Shake the pipette briefly and let it stand for 15 minutes.
3. Shake again for 30 seconds in a mechanical shaker.
4. Load the hemacytometer chamber and allow it to stand for 2 minutes to permit cells to settle.
5. Scan for an even distribution prior to counting.
6. Count the eosinophils in all nine of the large secondary squares (1 mm² each) on both sides of the hemacytometer, using the 10× objective. If the eosinophil count is extremely low, fill and count several chambers. Count at least 50 eosinophils.
7. Calculate the absolute eosinophil count using the following equation:

Cells/mm³

$$= \frac{\text{Cells counted} \times \text{Dilution} \times \text{Depth factor}}{\text{Area}}$$

Interpretation

Normal values: The eosinophil count of normal blood ranges from 50 to 400 cells/μl.

Comments

1. It is important to note that eosinophils will stain deep-red with Pilot's solution.
2. A good quality control point would be to check the eosinophil count obtained from the leukocyte and differential counts. To check the accuracy of the hemacytometer count, take the percentage of eosinophils counted on the differential smear and multiply by the total WBC count. This is the relative eosinophil count.

For example:

WBC count: 7500
Differential: 4%

$$7500 \times 0.04 = 300 \text{ cells}/\mu l$$

Allow for one more or one fewer eosinophil on the differential (for example, if the count had been 3 or 5, the estimated count from the differential smear would have been 225 to 375). A differential count of 3, 4, or 5 eosinophils giving a relative range of 225 to 375 would be a good verification of accuracy.

Reticulocytes

Principle

Reticulocytes are immature RBCs that contain remnant cytoplasmic ribonucleic acid (RNA) and organelles such as mitochondria and ribosomes. Reticulocytes are visualized by staining with vital dyes (such as new methylene blue) that precipitate the RNA and organelles, forming a filamentous network of reticulum. The reticulocyte count is a means of assessing erythropoietic activity of the bone marrow.

Reagents

New Methylene Blue

1. Dissolve 0.5 g of new methylene blue and 1.6 g of potassium oxalate in distilled water and Q.S. to 100 ml.
2. Filter before use. Store at room temperature.

Equipment

Whole blood anticoagulated with EDTA
6-in capillary tubes
Microscope slides
12 × 75 test tubes

Procedure

1. Mix equal amounts of blood and new methylene blue staining solution in a test tube.
2. Draw the blood-dye mixture up into a capillary pipette. Allow the mixture to stand for 10 minutes at room temperature.
3. Prepare thin wedge smears of blood-dye mixture using 1 small drop. Air dry. Do not fix or counterstain slides.

4. Under oil immersion, count all red cells in each field where the cells do not overlap, inclusive of reticulocytes. The Miller eyepiece[3] will facilitate counting.
5. Count 1000 red cells in consecutive oil immersion fields. Record the number of reticulocytes seen.
6. Calculate the percent of reticulocytes as follows:

$$\frac{\text{Reticulocyte count}/1000 \text{ RBCs}}{10} = \% \text{ Reticulocytes}$$

Note: Counting 1000 red cells is sufficient for normal or increased reticulocyte counts; however, for decreased reticulocyte counts, 2000 or more red cells should be counted.

Interpretation

Normal values:
Newborn (falls to
  normal adult values in 2 wk)   2.5 to 6.0%
Adult   0.5 to 2.0%

Absolute reticulocyte count
$$= \frac{\text{Reticulocytes} (\%) \times \text{RBC count (mm}^3)}{100}$$

Calculate the absolute reticulocyte count by this formula. The absolute reticulocyte count expresses the number of reticulocytes in 1 mm³ of whole blood; it is not a percentage of RBCs. The normal value is 60,000/mm³.

The reticulocyte count is most often expressed as a percentage of total red cells. In states of anemia the reticulocyte percentage is not a true reflection of reticulocyte production. A correction factor must be used so as not to overestimate marrow production, as each reticulocyte is released into whole blood containing fewer RBCs—a low hematocrit (Hct)—thus relatively increasing the percentage. The corrected reticulocyte count may be calculated by the following formula:

Corrected reticulocyte count
$$= \text{Reticulocytes} (\%) \times \frac{\text{Patient Hct}}{45 \text{ (average normal Hct)}}$$

For example, if a patient presents with a reticulocyte count of 12 and a hematocrit of 24, the corrected reticulocyte count would be 12 (percent) times (24/45), or 6.4 percent. In other words, the patient who presents with a reticulocyte count of 12 and a hematocrit of 24 would have the equivalent of a reticulocyte count of 6.4 percent in a patient with a hematocrit of 45.

Estimating RBC production by using the corrected reticulocyte count may yield erroneously high values in patients when there is a premature release of younger reticulocytes from the marrow (owing to increased erythropoietin stimulator). These premature reticulocytes are called stress or shift reticulocytes. These result when the reticulocytes of the bone marrow pool are shifted to the circulatory pool to compensate for anemia. The younger stress reticulocytes present with more filamentous reticulum. The mature reticulocyte may present with granular dots representing reticulum. Normally, reticulocytes lose their reticulum within 24 to 27 hours after entering the peripheral circulation. The premature stress reticulocytes have increased reticulum and require 2 to 2½ days to lose their reticulum, resulting in a longer peripheral blood maturation time. The peripheral smear should be carefully reviewed for the presence of many polychromatophilic macrocytes, thus indicating stress reticulocytes and the need for a correction for both the RBC count and the presence of stress reticulocytes. The value obtained is called the reticulocyte production index (RPI). To calculate the RPI the following formula is used:

$$RPI = \frac{\% \text{ Reticulocytes}}{\text{Reticulocyte maturation time}} \times \frac{\text{Hematocrit}}{45}$$

Comments

The reticulocyte count is elevated (1) in patients with hemolytic anemia, (2) in those with hemorrhage (acute and chronic), (3) following treatment of iron-deficiency anemia and the megaloblastic anemias, and (4) in patients with uremia (Fig. 30-I-3).

The reticulocyte count is decreased in cases of (1) aplastic anemia, (2) aplastic crises of hemolytic anemias, and (3) ineffective erythropoiesis as seen in thalassemia, pernicious anemia, and sideroblastic anemia.

Reticulocytopenia in the presence of a suggested hemolytic anemia may often make diagnosis difficult. The diagnosis of a hemolytic anemia can be made because the combination of both hemolysis and reticulocytopenia results in a rapidly falling hemoglobin and hematocrit.

By convention, single-dot reticulocytes are not counted. A reticulocyte must contain two or more discrete blue granules. The granular reticulum of the reticulocyte may be confused with Heinz bodies. Heinz bodies stain as light blue-green granules present at the periphery of the red cell.

According to the pattern of reticulum and the degree of maturation, reticulocytes can be divided into four categories, from the youngest to the most mature.

There is a high degree of inaccuracy in the reticulocyte count owing to error (±2 percent in low counts and ±7 percent in high counts) and lack of reproducibility. Because of the inaccuracy of the blood film, flow microfluorometry has been adapted to count reticulocytes automatically. The principle is based on staining of the RNA by an acridine orange dye, which fluoresces when exposed to ultraviolet (UV) light.

RBC Indices

Principle

The values obtained for the erythrocyte count, hematocrit, and hemoglobin concentration can be further used to calculate RBC indices, which define the size and hemoglobin content of the average RBC in a given specimen of blood. The values for the RBC

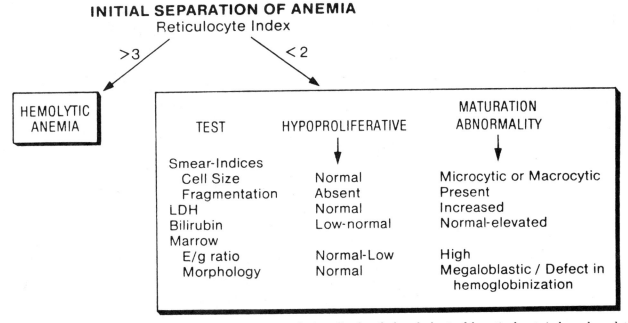

INITIAL SEPARATION OF ANEMIA
Reticulocyte Index

Test	HYPOPROLIFERATIVE	MATURATION ABNORMALITY
Smear-Indices		
Cell Size	Normal	Microcytic or Macrocytic
Fragmentation	Absent	Present
LDH	Normal	Increased
Bilirubin	Low-normal	Normal-elevated
Marrow		
E/g ratio	Normal-Low	High
Morphology	Normal	Megaloblastic / Defect in hemoglobinization

Figure 30–I–3. The initial separation of anemia. Anemias may be broadly classified on the basis of the reticulocyte index as hemolytic (index greater than 3) or impaired production, either a hypoproliferative or maturation abnormality (index less than 2). Further tests are required to separate the latter two functional defects as shown.

indices are useful tools in the classification of anemias.

The three most commonly used RBC indices are (1) mean corpuscular volume (MCV), (2) mean corpuscular hemoglobin (MCH), and (3) mean corpuscular hemoglobin concentration (MCHC).

Definitions

Mean Corpuscular Volume. This is the average volume of the RBC, in cubic microns (μ^3) or femtoliters (fl). Normal erythrocytes have an MCV of 80 to 98 fl (replaces old units, μ^3). Results below 80 fl indicate a smaller than normal MCV; that is, the cells are on the average microcytic. Similarly, an MCV of greater than 100 fl indicates the cells are macrocytic.

It is imperative to interpret the value for MCV along with a careful inspection of the peripheral blood smear, as the MCV is only a mean volume measurement. It is possible, for example, to have a wide variation in cell size — from cells that are microcytic to some that are macrocytic — and still have an MCV within the normal range. This may be true if there is a large number of reticulocytes in the peripheral blood because reticulocytes usually have a larger volume than adult cells have.

$$MCV = \frac{Hematocrit~(\%) \times 10}{RBC~count~(in~millions/mm^3)}$$

OR

$$MCV = \frac{Hematocrit~(liter/liter) = n \times 10-15/liter = fl}{RBC~count~(\times 10^{12}/liter)}$$

This value is reported in fl (μ^3) to the nearest whole number.

Mean Corpuscular Hemoglobin. This is the average weight of hemoglobin, in absolute units, in the RBC. The result gives the average content of hemoglobin per erythrocyte in picograms (pg) or micromicrograms ($\mu\mu g$). The normal MCH in adults is 27 to 31 pg. This value is generally higher in newborns and infants, because their MCV is higher than in adults.

$$MCH = \frac{Hemoglobin~(g/100~ml) \times 10}{RBC~count~(millions/mm^3)}$$

OR

$$MCH = \frac{Hemoglobin~(g/liter)}{RBC~count~(\times 10^{12}/liter)}$$

Mean Corpuscular Hemoglobin Concentration. This is the average concentration of hemoglobin in each individual RBC. It is a ratio of the weight of hemoglobin to the volume of the RBC.

$$MCHC = \frac{Hemoglobin~(g/100~ml) \times 100}{Hematocrit}$$

OR

$$MCHC = \frac{Hemoglobin~(g/liter)}{Hematocrit~(liter/liter)}$$

This value is reported to the nearest 10th of a percent. The normal MCHC is 32.0 to 36.0 g/liter (Fig. 30-I-4).

RBC Distribution Width (RDW). This is the coefficient of variation of the red cell volume distribution. It is provided by automated hematology instruments and is used as an indication of anisocytosis. The normal value for RDW is 11.5 to 14.5. An elevated RDW may be seen on blood smears with varying degrees of anisocytosis.

$$RDW = \frac{Standard~deviation~of~RBC~volume}{Mean~MCV}$$

Comments

Determination of the MCV, MCH, and MCHC gives valuable information that helps to characterize RBCs. According to the MCV, erythrocytes may be classified as normocytic, microcytic, or macrocytic. Based on the MCHC, erythrocytes may be classified as normochromic or hypochromic. The MCH only expresses the mean weight of hemoglobin per erythrocyte.

OTHER ROUTINE HEMATOLOGY METHODS

Erythrocyte Sedimentation Rate

Principle

When anticoagulated blood is allowed to stand undisturbed, the RBCs will normally settle out to the bottom of the tube. This principle is the basis for the erythrocyte sedimentation rate (ESR). By definition, the ESR is the distance in millimeters that RBCs fall per unit of time, which is usually 1 hour. Various factors will affect the ESR, such as RBC size and shape, plasma fibrinogen, and globulin levels, as well as mechanical and technical factors.

The ESR is directly proportional to the RBC mass and inversely proportional to plasma viscosity. In normal whole blood, RBCs do not form rouleaux; the RBC mass is small and therefore the ESR is decreased (cells settle out slowly). In abnormal conditions when RBCs can form rouleaux, the RBC mass is greater, thus increasing the ESR (cells settle out faster).

Historically there have been two methods to perform an ESR — the Westergren method[4] and the Wintrobe and Landsberg method.[5]

Stages of Sedimentation

1. Initial period of aggregation: Rouleaux are formed with minimal sedimentation. This phase lasts about 10 minutes.
2. Period of fast settling: At this stage the settling rate is constant and lasts about 40 minutes.

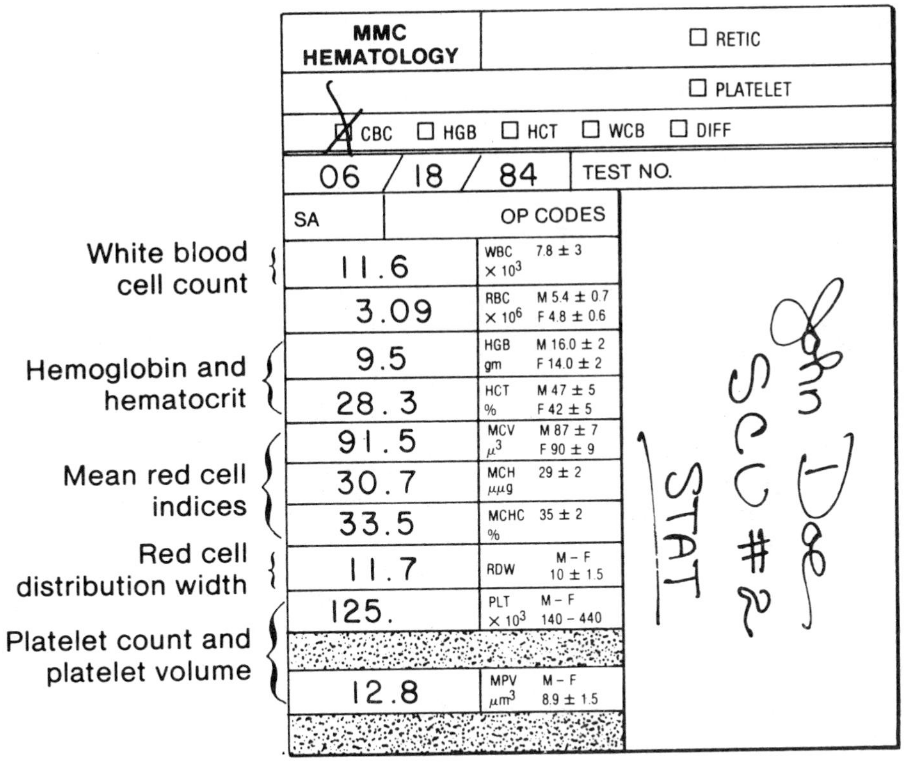

Figure 30-I-4. The results of blood cell counts and indices.

3. Final stage: The remaining amount of time is a period of packing at the bottom of the tube.

Reagents and Equipment

Wintrobe tubes, disposable
Sedimentation tube rack
Patient EDTA specimen

ESR Determinations

1. Collect blood with proper anticoagulant in proportion to volume of blood to avoid shrinkage of erythrocytes. EDTA is suggested.
2. Thoroughly mix blood with anticoagulant immediately before filling tube.
3. Using a 9-inch Pasteur pipette that will reach the bottom of the tube, slowly fill the tube with blood, avoiding air bubbles in the column.
4. Adjust the meniscus of the specimen to the 0 line at the top of the tube.
5. Place tube in upright position, in rack that will maintain the tube in this position.
6. At the end of 1 hour read the fall of erythrocytes by recording the level of erythrocytes in the tube. Read the ESR on the same side of the tube as the 0 line. Going from the top downward, read the ESR as the fall of cells in mm per hour.
7. If the demarcation between plasma and RBC column is hazy, take the level where the full density is first apparent.

Rapid sedimentation will occur with large bore tubes and tall columns of blood. Keep the position of the tube vertical at all times. Slight degrees of tilting will accelerate the ESR.

Normal values:

Adult men	0–9 mm/hr
Adult women	0–15 mm/hr

Comments

The ESR is not a very specific or diagnostic test. Despite the time constraints and the lack of specificity among disorders that can cause an abnormal ESR, this test is still used in many institutions as a screening test.

Perhaps the usefulness of this test lies in its ability to differentiate among diseases with similar symptoms or to monitor the course of an existing disease. For example, early in the course of an uncomplicated viral infection the ESR is usually normal, but it may rise later with a superimposed bacterial infection. Within the first 24 hours of acute appendicitis, the ESR is not elevated, but in the early stage of acute pelvic inflammatory disease or ruptured ectopic pregnancy it is elevated. The ESR is elevated in established myocardial infarction but normal in angina pectoris. It is elevated in rheumatic fever, rheumatoid arthritis, and pyogenic arthritis but not in osteoarthritis. The ESR can be an index to disease severity. In many cases it can be an index of the activity of pulmonary tuberculosis. In general, there is no direct correlation between fever and the ESR.

Interpretation

Factors that Affect ESR

Plasma Factors. Increased plasma concentration of fibrinogen, and immunoglobulin, will result in rouleaux formation and an increased ESR. It can therefore be expected that disease states that are characterized by hyperfibrinogenemia or elevated immunoglobulin levels will result in an increased ESR.

Extreme increases in plasma viscosity slow down the ESR, thus resulting in a decreased ESR.

RBC Factors. When rouleaux formation cannot occur, owing to the shape or size of the RBC, a decreased or low ESR is expected. This is observed with sickle cells and spherocytes. The ESR is of little diagnostic value in severe anemia or in hematologic states noted by poikilocytosis.

Anticoagulants. Sodium citrate or EDTA can be used without an effect on the ESR. Sodium or potassium oxalate can cause RBC shrinkage. Heparin causes only a slight amount of shrinkage but a falsely elevated ESR. Our anticoagulant of choice is EDTA because of its routine use in the hematology laboratory.

Mechanical Factors. Different normal values are given for various methods owing to variations in the caliber of the tube and height of the column of blood.

A number of years ago Wintrobe and Landsberg[6] proposed a method of correcting the ESR for anemia, based on the patient's hematocrit level. The significance of a corrected ESR is still debatable because the hematocrit can vary according to the type and severity of anemia present and therefore may influence the corrected ESR. As a result, we do not correct the ESR for anemia in our laboratory.

Hematocrit

Principle (Centrifugal Microhematocrit Method)

Hematocrit is defined as the volume occupied by erythrocytes (RBCs) in a given volume of blood and is usually expressed as a percentage of the volume of the whole blood sample.

The hematocrit is usually determined by spinning a blood-filled capillary tube in a centrifuge. The Coulter counter series of analyzers provide an indirect measurement of hematocrit (see section on automated cell counting).

Reagents and Equipment

Capillary tubes, heparinized or plain (75 mm)
Microhematocrit centrifuge
Microhematocrit reader (needed only if centrifuge does not have one incorporated in the tube holder)

Procedure

1. Draw venous blood from an antecubital vein and into potassium EDTA. Take care to avoid tourniquet stasis, as this can elevate venous hematocrit results. Carefully mix the blood, preferably on a mechanical rotator. Venous blood may also be obtained through capillary puncture using a heparinized capillary tube to collect the specimen.

2. Once adequately mixed, place the unmarked end of a plain capillary tube in the blood and let it fill rapidly to approximately three quarters of its length. Tipping the tube horizontally will speed filling. Then remove the tube from the blood and wipe it clean of excess blood.

3. Plug the unmarked end with modeling clay and place it in the centrifuge, clay-filled end against the rubber gasket (that is, against the peripheral rim). For accuracy, each determination should be done in duplicate or triplicate.

4. Centrifuge for 5 minutes at a set speed (force is approximately 14,500 rpm). This separates RBCs from plasma and leaves a band of buffy coat at the interface consisting of WBCs and platelets.

5. Allow the centrifuge to stop on its own; *do not hand brake.*

6. Read the hematocrit as the percent of whole venous blood occupied by RBCs. Using a constant bore capillary tube, obtain a distance ratio on a microhematocrit reader. Set the reader first with the clay-red cell interface at 0 percent. Next, shift the ruled scale or etched line to 100 percent and align it with the plasma meniscus. Read down to the percent spiral line that intersects with the RBC-WBC interface. This percent is the hematocrit value. Do not include the buffy coat layer in this value. If it exceeds 2 percent it should be recorded and noted as volume of packed WBCs (VPW).

7. Results should duplicate within 1 percent.

Interpretation

Normal values:

	Percent	Standard International (SI) (liter/liter)
Newborn	53–65	0.53–0.65
Infant/Child	30–43	0.30–0.43
Man	42–52	0.42–0.52
Woman	37–47	0.37–0.47

Comments

1. Incomplete sealing of the capillary tubes will give falsely low results because in the process of spinning, RBCs and a small amount of plasma will be forced from the tube.

2. Shortened spin time or slowed centrifugation speed may yield falsely elevated results.
3. If the buffy coat is included in the RBCs when reading the result, the hematocrit will be falsely elevated.
4. The microhematocrit centrifuge should never be forced to stop by applying pressure to the metal cover plate. This will cause the RBC layer to "sling" forward and results in a falsely elevated value.
5. The hematocrit is usually three times the hemoglobin value.
6. The Standard International (SI) unit (liter/liter) of reporting expresses the hematocrit as the volume of packed RBCs in relation to volume of whole blood.

TESTS FOR HEMOGLOBINS
Hemoglobinometry

Principle

Hemoglobin, the main component of the RBC, transports oxygen to and CO_2 from the body's tissues. Hemoglobin in circulating blood is a mixture of hemoglobin, oxyhemoglobin, carboxyhemoglobin, and minor amounts of other forms of this pigment. It is necessary to prepare a stable derivative involving all forms of hemoglobin in the blood in order to measure this compound accurately. The cyanmethemoglobin (HiCN) derivative can be conveniently and reproducibly prepared and is widely used for hemoglobin determination. All forms of circulating hemoglobin are readily converted to HiCN except for sulfhemoglobin, which is rarely present in significant amounts. Cyanmethemoglobin can be measured accurately by its absorbance in a colorimeter.

The basic principle of the cyanmethemoglobin (HiCN, hemoglobin-cyanide method) is that blood is diluted in a solution of potassium ferricyanide and potassium cyanide. The potassium ferricyanide oxidizes hemoglobin to methemoglobin (Hi, hemoglobin) and the potassium cyanide converts methemoglobin to the stable cyanmethemoglobin, which is read on a spectrophotometer at 540 nm.

Reagents and Equipment

Hemoglobin Calibrators

Cyanmethemoglobin reagent (Drabkin's reagent)
5-ml pipettes
Spectrometer
Cuvettes
Test tubes
20-μl pipette

Cyanmethemoglobin reagent (Drabkin's reagent)

Sodium bicarbonate	1.00 g
Potassium cyanide	0.05 g
Potassium ferricyanide	0.02 g
Distilled water	1000 ml

Procedure

Standard Curve. Prepare a standard curve by diluting the hemoglobin standard with cyanmethemoglobin reagent. Measure the absorbance of each dilution at 540 nm. The dilutions should be made to yield a linear curve.

The hemoglobin concentration of a blood sample is determined by diluting 0.02 ml of blood with 5.0 ml of cyanmethemoglobin reagent. The absorbance of the formed cyanmethemoglobin solution is measured at 540 nm and blood concentration is derived from the corresponding absorbance on the linear standard curve.

For example, 5 ml of a standard solution with a concentration of 80 mg/dl has the same number of milligrams of cyanmethemoglobin as 0.02 ml of a solution with a concentration of 20 g/dl.

$$\frac{80 \text{ mg}}{1 \text{ dl}} \times 5 \text{ ml} = \frac{20 \text{ grams}}{\text{dl}} \times 0.02 \text{ ml}$$

Concentration × Volume = Concentration × Volume
of standard   of blood

Since 1 dl = 100 ml, we can substitute 100 ml for 1 dl.

$$\frac{80 \text{ mg}}{100 \text{ ml}} \times 5 \text{ ml} = \frac{20 \text{ grams}}{100 \text{ ml}} \times 0.02 \text{ ml}$$

$$4 \text{ milligrams} = 0.004 \text{ grams}$$

Setting Up a Standard Calibration Curve. Each time a new bottle of reagent is opened, a new calibration curve must be made for the reagent. The standard cyanmethemoglobin solution represents 20 g/dl and is also diluted to represent 5, 10, and 15 g/dl for additional points on the curve.

1. Label five clean and dry cuvettes: blank, 5, 10, 15, and 20 g/dl.
2. Use a volumetric or transfer pipettes to dispense reagents into the appropriate cuvettes according to the following chart:

TUBE	REAGENT	STANDARD (80 mg/dl)
Blank	5.0 ml*	—
5	4.5 ml	1.5 ml
10	3.0 ml	3.5 ml
15	1.5 ml	4.5 ml
20	—	5.0 ml

*Only 3 ml is necessary if the spectrophotometer has a minimum requirement of 2 ml for an accurate reading.

3. Cover and invert to mix well.
4. Use a spectrophotometer that has been set at 540 nm.

5. Use the blank to set the absorbance on "zero."
6. Read and record the absorbance for each tube.
7. Use linear graph paper to make the curve. Plot the concentration (g/dl) on the abcissa (bottom line) and the absorbance on the ordinate (vertical line).[6a]

Specimen Testing

1. Prepare tubes containing 5 ml of the cyanmethemoglobin reagent and label them for the controls (high and low) and one for each unknown sample. Use the same blank as above or just prepare an extra tube for the blank.
2. Using a 20-μl pipette, add 20 μl (0.02 ml) of mixed whole blood (EDTA) to the reagent, rinsing the pipette at least three times.
3. Mix thoroughly by vortexing or inversion with parafilm, and allow the tube to stand at least 10 minutes before reading.
4. Using cyanmethemoglobin reagent as a blank, adjust the spectrophotometer to read 100 percent transmittance at wavelength 540 nm. Invert sample to be analyzed and aspirate into a cuvette. Read percent transmittance.
5. Determine hemoglobin values of the test sample and control from the standard curve.

Normal values (in g/100 ml blood):

Man	14–17
Woman	12.5–15
Newborn	17–23
3 month old	9–14
10 yr old	12–14.5

Special Considerations and Comments

Before the test sample is read, the solution should be clear:

1. A high WBC count: Centrifuge specimen and use the supernatant for reading.
2. Hemoglobin S (HbS) and hemoglobin C (HbC). Dilute the mixture 1:1 with distilled water and then read in the colorimeter; multiply the reading by 2.
3. Abnormal globulins: Add 0.1 g of potassium carbonate to the solution.

Hemoglobin Electrophoresis

Principle

Electrophoresis is defined as the movement of charged particles in an electric field. The different normal and abnormal hemoglobins show different mobilities or migration patterns in an electric field at a fixed pH. The usual support medium is cellulose acetate at an alkaline pH of 8.5. The procedure that follows is from Helena Laboratories, and all reagents and apparatus are available from them.

Reagents

1. Hemolysate reagent
2. Controls A_1FSC; normal A_1A_2 patient
3. Buffer: SupreHeme buffer (one envelope is dissolved in distilled water and diluted to 980 ml tris-EDTA–boric acid buffer, pH 8.4)
4. Ponceau S stain
5. Destain: 5 ml glacial acetic acid per 100 ml distilled water, a 5 percent solution
6. Dehydrating agent: Absolute methanol
7. Clearing solution: 150 ml glacial acetic acid, 350 ml absolute methanol, and 20 ml Clear Aid
8. Titan III-H cellulose acetate plates.

Equipment

All are available from Helena Laboratories.
1. Cliniscan
2. Helena Titan Power Supply
3. Incubator-oven-dryer
4. Electrophoresis chamber
5. Super Z sample well plate
6. Super Z aligning base
7. Applicator
8. Zip-zone chamber wicks

Procedure

1. Preparation of hemolysate: Spin EDTA blood for 20 minutes at 3000 rpm to pack the RBCs. Remove the plasma and buffy coat. Add 6 drops of hemolysate reagent to 1 drop of packed RBCs. Let stand for 1 minute; then vortex for 1 minute. Hemolysate may be frozen and then thawed to ensure complete hemolysis.
2. Preparation of electrophoretic chamber: Pour 100 ml of buffer into each outer compartment. Soak a wick in each compartment, and then drape it over the bridge, making sure it contacts the buffer. Cover the chamber.
3. Preparation of cellulose acetate plates: Number the plates on the bottom right of the glossy side. Wet the plates by slowly lowering the rack into a container of buffer. Allow to soak for at least 5 minutes.
4. Preparation of sample well plates: Clean with distilled water and dry each well with a cotton swab. Prepare two rinse plates by filling the wells with distilled water. Prepare the patient samples by using a 5-lambda microdispenser to fill the wells on clean dry plates. Patient samples should be run in duplicate, and a normal A_1A_2 and A_1FSC control should be run on each plate. Cover with glass slide to prevent evaporation.
5. Loading of cellulose acetate plates:
   a. Prime the applicator by depressing several times into the same well plate and then depressing once on a blotter.
   b. Remove the cellulose acetate plate from the

buffer; blot once firmly; place on the aligning base with the number at the bottom left.
   c. Load the applicator by depressing three times into the sample well plate; then transfer the applicator to the aligning base, and depress the bar firmly for 5 seconds.
   d. Place the plate, glossy side up, across the bridge in the electrophoresis chamber.
6. Electrophorese at 350 volts for 25 minutes.
7. Staining:
   a. Apply Ponceau S for 5 minutes. Drain 5 to 10 seconds.
   b. Four successive washes of 5 percent glacial acetic acid are used to destain. Leave in each for 2 minutes, draining for 5 seconds between each wash.
   c. Use two successive washes of absolute methanol to dehydrate. Leave for 2 minutes in each, draining for 5 seconds between each wash.
   d. Apply clearing solution for 5 minutes.
   e. Dry vertically for 1 to 2 minutes.
   f. Dry in the oven for 3 to 4 minutes, acetate side up.
8. Scan the plate with the Cliniscan using a 525-nm filter, slit size 5, and optics filter wheel V-2 O.D.
9. Label the plate and store in a plastic envelope as a permanent record.

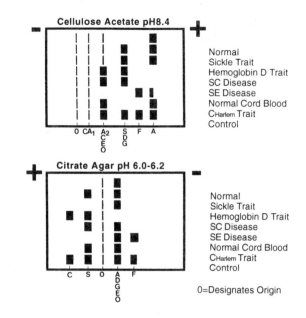

Figure 30–I–5. Comparative hemoglobin electrophoresis. Hemoglobin electrophoresis on cellulose acetate and citrate agar indicating patterns of mobility. The width of the band is not indicative of hemoglobin concentration.

Results

Variant hemoglobins are reported in relative percentages.

Hemoglobin A_1 (HbA$_1$)	96.0–98.6%
Hemoglobin A_2 (HbA$_2$)	1.5–4.0%
Hemoglobin F (HbF)	
At birth	60.0–90.0%
After 1 yr old	1.0–2.0%

Comments

At an alkaline pH, hemoglobins S and D have the same mobility, as do hemoglobins A_2, C, E, and O Arab. These hemoglobins may be separated by electrophoresing on citrate agar at an acid pH (Fig. 30-I-5). Hemoglobin A_2 may also be quantitated by column. It should be kept in mind that HbA$_1$ and HbF cannot be separated on cellulose acetate. The procedure for separation and quantitation of HbF is based on acid and/or alkali resistance (see HbF denaturation).

Citrate Agar Hemoglobin Electrophoresis

Principle

As mentioned earlier, electrophoresis is the movement of charged particles in an electric field.

Using citrate agar at an acid pH facilitates the separation of hemoglobins that migrate together on other media (cellulose acetate) at a different pH (alkaline). The following procedure is that of Helena Laboratories, and all reagents and apparatus are available from them.

Reagents

1. Hemolysate reagent
2. Controls A$_1$FSC; normal A$_1$A$_2$
3. Buffer: Citrate buffer. Dissolve one package in distilled water and dilute to 1 liter.
4. Stain:
   a. 10 ml of 5 percent glacial acetic acid
   b. 5 ml of toluidine in methanol
   c. 1 ml of sodium nitroferricyanide in water
   d. 1 ml of 3 percent hydrogen peroxide
   e. Prepare fresh on day of use.
5. Titan IV citrate agar plates

Equipment

All are available from Helena Laboratories.
1. Helena Titan Power Supply
2. Electrophoresis chamber
3. Sample well plate
4. Aligning base

5. Applicator
6. Sponge wicks

Procedure

1. Preparation of hemolysate: Spin EDTA blood for 20 minutes at 3000 rpm to pack the red cells. Remove the plasma and buffy coat. Add 10 drops of hemolysate reagent to 1 drop of packed RBCs. Let stand for 1 minute, then vortex for 1 minute. Hemolysate may be frozen and then thawed to ensure complete hemolysis.
2. Preparation of electrophoresis chamber: Pour 100 ml of buffer into each outer compartment. Soak a sponge wick in each compartment, then place it so that the top of the sponge protrudes over the inner ridge of the compartment. Cover the chamber.
3. Preparation of sample well plates: Clean all wells with distilled water and dry with cotton swabs. Prepare the patient samples by using a 5-lambda microdispenser to fill the wells. Patient hemolysates should be run in duplicate, plus an A_1FSC and an A_1A_2 control should be run on each plate. Cover the plate with a glass slide to prevent evaporation.
4. Loading of citrate agar plates:
   a. Prime the applicator by pressing several times into the sample well plate, and then dispensing once on a blotter.
   b. Place the Titan IV citrate agar plate on the aligning base.
   c. Load the applicator by pressing three times into the sample well plate; then transfer applicator to the aligning base.
   d. Depress the applicator onto the gel surface using no pressure, and allow hemolysate to absorb for 1 minute.
5. Place the plate gel side down across the inner ridges of the electrophoresis chamber with the application point near the anode.
6. Electrophorese for 40 minutes, at 40 milliamps per plate and 50 volts per plate.
7. Staining:
   a. Place the plate in a staining dish and puddle the stain over the surface. Let stand for 5 to 10 minutes.
   b. Rinse with distilled water for 10 minutes.
   c. Cover with another gel plate and seal with tape to store.

Results

With this procedure, hemoglobins S and D can be separated. Hemoglobin D, instead of migrating with HbS as in an alkaline buffer, will migrate with HbA. This procedure also separates hemoglobins A_2 and E from HbC, as hemoglobins A_2 and E will migrate with HbA, leaving HbC by itself. The pattern distributes thus from anode to cathode: hemoglobins C, S, A_1, A_2, D, E, and F (Fig. 30-I-5).

Hemoglobin A₂ by Column

Principle

This is an anion exchange chromatography method. The anion exchange resin is a preparation of cellulose covalently coupled to small positively charged molecules, which will attract negatively charged molecules. Hemoglobins have positive or negative charges, owing to properties of their component amino acids. Here buffer and pH favor net negatively charged hemoglobins, which are attracted and bound to the resin. Once bound, the hemoglobins can be selectively eluted and measured on a spectrophotometer. This procedure (the Sickle-Thal column method) is that of Helena Laboratories.

Reagents

1. Control: Quik column control
2. Sickle-Thal Quik column
3. Hemoglobin A_2 developer
4. Hemoglobin S developer
5. Hemolysate Reagent-C

All are available in a kit from various manufacturers.

Equipment

1. Column rack and collection tubes
2. Spectrophotometer

Procedure

1. Preparation of hemolysate: Add 50 lambda EDTA blood plus 200 lambda Hemolysate Reagent-C to a small test tube. Vortex vigorously and allow to stand 5 minutes before use.
2. Preparation of columns:
   a. Allow to come to room temperature.
   b. Turn each column upside down twice, place it in the rack, remove top cap, and resuspend with a pipette.
   c. Remove the bottom cap and allow the buffer to drain out.
   d. After the resin repacks, remove any buffer remaining at the top, being careful not to disturb the resin.
3. Slowly apply 100 lambda of patient hemolysate to the column and allow to absorb into the resin.
4. Put 100 lambda of patient hemolysate in a large collection tube and Q.S. to 15 ml with distilled water. Label this tube "total fraction."
5. Elution of HbA_2:
   a. Slowly apply 3 ml of HbA_2 developer and allow to pass through the column into the small collection tube (approximately 30 minutes).
   b. Q.S. the tube to 3 ml with distilled water.
6. Elution of HbS (optional):
   a. Slowly add 10 ml of HbS developer to the column in aliquots of 3 ml, 3 ml, and 4 ml.
   b. Allow it to pass through the column into a large collection tube (approximately 1½ to 2 hours).

c. Q.S. the tube to 15 ml with distilled water.
7. Using the spectrometer at 415 nm, record the absorbance of the HbA$_2$ eluate, the HbS eluate, and the total fraction.

Results

$$\% \text{ HbA}_2 = \frac{\text{OD HbA}_2 \text{ eluate}}{5 \times \text{OD total fraction}} \times 100$$

$$\% \text{ HbS} = \frac{\text{OD HbS eluate}}{\text{OD total fraction}} \times 100$$

$$\text{OD} = \text{optical density}$$

The HbS eluate is optional, as it can be picked up on alkaline electrophoresis.

The normal range for HbA$_2$ is 1.5 to 4.0 percent. This can be used to separate HbA$_2$ and HbC or HbE. Elevated levels of HbA$_2$ may be useful in diagnosing a β-thalassemia.

Differential Solubility Test for Hemoglobin S (Sicklequik by General Diagnostics)

Principle

This particular test is a rapid, self-contained tube test manufactured by General Diagnostics as a modification of the solubility test. It is a biphasic (that is, two-layer) system, with an upper organic layer of toluene and a lower aqueous layer of phosphate buffer, saponin, and reducing agents. When whole blood is added and mixed, the RBCs are lysed by toluene and saponin, and the hemoglobin is reduced by sodium hydrosulfite. If any insoluble HbS is present, it rises to the top of the aqueous layer and forms a dark interface between the layers.

Reagents

None are required. A ready-to-use tube comes from General Diagnostics.

Procedure

1. Add 0.1 ml EDTA blood to the tube.
2. Shake vigorously for 10 seconds.
3. Let the tube stand for 5 minutes.
4. Centrifuge for 5 minutes at 3400 rpm.
5. Run a positive and a negative control.

Results

A negative result (indicating no sickling hemoglobin) shows a gray-pink interface with a dark-red aqueous layer.

A positive result (indicating the presence of a sickling hemoglobin) will show one of two patterns. The homozygous state shows a dark-red interface with a pale straw-colored aqueous layer. All of the hemoglobin is abnormal and is picked up at the interface. The heterozygous state shows a dark-red interface with an aqueous layer of varying shades of pink to red, depending on the amount of nonsickling hemoglobin.

Sodium Metabisulfite Slide Test

Principle

The addition of a reducing agent (sodium metabisulfite) to cells containing hemoglobin S causes them to sickle.

Reagents

Sodium metabisulfite solution: Dissolve 200 mg of sodium metabisulfite in 10 ml distilled water. This solution is stable for 24 hours.

Procedure

1. Make a very dilute suspension of EDTA blood in the sodium metabisulfite solution on a slide. The tip of an applicator stick swirled through a drop of the solution is sufficient.
2. Coverslip the drop and seal with permount.
3. Examine the slide immediately, then every 15 minutes for 1 hr, and again at 2 hours.

Results

In patients with sickle-cell disease, the sickling process will be immediate with obvious sickled, elongated, and holly-leaf shapes. In those with sickle-cell trait or a combination, the process will be slower. This test cannot be used to differentiate the homozygous and heterozygous states and is used only to show the presence of a sickling hemoglobin.

Acid Elution for Hemoglobin F

Principle

Hemoglobin F in RBCs is resistant to acid elution; therefore, it can be precipitated and stained. Hemoglobin A will be eluted from the RBCs. This is a modification of the original Kleihauer stain.

Reagents

1. Fetal cell fixing solution: 80 percent reagent alcohol
2. Fetal cell buffer solution: citrate buffer 0.027 M
3. Fetal cell stain: erythrosin B
4. Control: 0.1 ml of cord blood plus 0.9 ml of normal adult blood

Procedure

1. Add 2 drops of EDTA blood to 3 drops of 0.85 percent saline.
2. Prepare a monolayer film of this suspension. Allow to air dry.
3. Immerse film in fixing solution for 5 minutes at room temperature.
4. Rinse in distilled water and allow to air dry.
5. Immerse in buffer solution for 8 to 10 minutes at room temperature.
6. Immediately immerse in staining solution for 3 minutes at room temperature.
7. Rinse in distilled water and allow to air dry.
8. Examine for the presence of cells staining for fetal hemoglobin.

Results

Cells containing HbF will stain bright pink-red. Those containing only HbA will be very light pink. The stain may be useful in distinguishing hereditary persistence of fetal hemoglobin (HPFH), in which most RBCs show an even distribution of HbF, from a high level of HbF in a patient with thalassemia minor (in which the distribution of HbF is uneven). The percentage of fetal cells may be calculated if this stain is to be used to assess fetal cells in maternal circulation.

Staining for Heinz Bodies

Principle

Heinz bodies are denatured hemoglobulin precipitated in the RBC and attached to the RBC membrane. They are not visible with Wright's stain but show up with vital staining and phase microscopy.

Reagents

1. Crystal violet solution: 1.0 g of crystal violet dissolved in 50 ml of a 0.85 percent saline solution, which is shaken for 5 minutes and filtered before storage.
2. Methyl violet solution: 0.5 g of methyl violet dissolved in 100 ml of a 0.85 percent saline solution, which is shaken for 5 minutes and filtered before storage.

Note: A 0.75 percent saline solution may be used. This slightly hypotonic solution swells the cells slightly.

Procedure

1. Mix equal volumes of EDTA blood and stain in a small test tube. Either stain may be used.
2. Incubate for 20 minutes at room temperature.
3. Remix the blood/stain solution and transfer 1 drop to a slide.
4. Place a coverglass on the slide and examine for Heinz bodies under oil immersion.

Results

Heinz bodies appear as irregular, refractile, purple inclusions, 1 to 3 μm in diameter, located on the periphery of the cell. They may even seem to be outside the cell. Reticulocytes should not stain.

The presence of Heinz bodies indicates exposure of the RBCs to various oxidizing agents or the presence of an unstable hemoglobin.

Heinz Body Induction Test

Principle

Heinz bodies can be induced in great numbers in susceptible individuals by incubating the blood in various reducing substances. Susceptible individuals such as those with glucose-6-phosphate dehydrogenase (G6PD) deficiency are those who would hemolyze following administration of aniline derivatives such as primaquine, phenacetin, or sulfanilamides.

Reagents

1. Buffer solution:
   a. Dissolve 0.908 g of KH_2PO_4 in 100 ml of distilled water.
   b. Dissolve 0.824 g of Na_2HPO_4 in 87 ml of distilled water.
   c. Mix 13 ml of the KH_2PO_4 solution with 87 ml of the Na_2HPO_4 solution.
2. Acetylphenylhydrazine solution: Dissolve 0.1 g of acetylphenylhydrazine in 100 ml of the buffer solution. Make fresh on day of use and use within 1 hour.
3. Crystal violet solution: Dissolve 1.0 g of crystal violet in 50 ml of a 0.85 percent saline solution. Shake for 5 minutes and filter before use. A 0.75 percent saline solution may be used. This is slightly hypotonic and swells the cells a little.

Procedure

1. Add 0.1 ml of EDTA blood to 2 ml of acetylphenylhydrazine solution. Mix on a vortex so that air will enter suspension.
2. Incubate at 37°C for 2 hours.
3. Mix again and incubate an additional 2 hours at 37°C.
4. Mix equal volumes of cell suspension and crystal violet in a small tube. Incubate for 10 minutes.
5. Make a wet prep (a drop of stained suspension plus a coverslip) and let settle. Examine and count under oil immersion.

Results

A normal control subject will have at least one Heinz body in each RBC. A susceptible patient (such as one with G6PD deficiency, defects of glutathione reductase enzyme, or unstable hemoglobins) will have five or more Heinz bodies in 40 percent or more of the RBCs. The Heinz bodies appear as irregular, refractile purple inclusions, 1 to 3 μm in diameter, and located either on the periphery or bulging out of the RBC.

TESTS FOR HEMOLYTIC ANEMIAS
Osmotic Fragility

Principle

Whole blood is added to a series of saline dilutions. The presence or absence of hemolysis is an effective measure of erythrocyte susceptibility to hypotonic damage. This test is more than just an index of cell shape; it is also a measure of the surface-to-volume ratio. When an RBC's membrane surface decreases and its volume remains the same or increases, the cell becomes more turgid and less deformable. This is because the RBC membrane is flexible but not elastic. The result of this loss of surface-to-volume ratio is similar to what happens to a small plastic bag that is filled with more and more water—a rupture of the cell membrane.

Spherocytes, which have a decreased surface-to-volume ratio, demonstrate an increased osmotic fragility. This is due to their inability to swell in a hypotonic medium before leaking hemoglobin. Sickle cells, target cells, and other poikilocytes are relatively resistant to osmotic change and therefore demonstrate a decreased fragility.

Reagents and Equipment

1. Twenty-four 12 × 75 mm test tubes
2. Two 5-ml serologic pipettes (TD); one 3-ml pipette
3. Parafilm squares
4. One heparinized normal control sample
5. One heparinized patient sample
6. Linear graph paper
7. One percent NaCl Solution: Weight 1.0 g NaCl crystals on an analytical balance. Place crystals in a 100-ml volumetric flask and fill to the mark with distilled water. Stir to completely dissolve NaCl.

Procedure can also be performed using UNO-PETTE Erythrocyte Fragility Test Kit by Becton Dickinson Vacutainer Systems. When using this kit, note that saline dilutions are packaged in individual reservoirs.

Procedure

1. Arrange two series of 12 tubes in the rack. Label both sets of tubes 1 through 12. The first series of tubes 1 through 12 is for the patient and the second series is for the control.
2. With a 5-ml pipette add 1 percent NaCl solution, and with the other 5-ml pipette add distilled water into the series of patient tubes according to the following schedule:

Tube	1% NaCl (ml)	Distilled Water (ml)	NaCl%, Final Concentration
1	4.25	0.75	0.85
2	3.50	1.50	0.70
3	3.25	1.75	0.65
4	3.00	2.00	0.60
5	2.75	2.25	0.55
6	2.50	2.50	0.50
7	2.25	2.75	0.45
8	2.00	3.00	0.40
9	1.75	3.25	0.35
10	1.50	3.50	0.30
11	1.25	3.75	0.25
12	0.75	4.25	0.15

3. Thoroughly mix the contents of each tube by covering with parafilm and inverting several times.

4. With a 3-ml pipette, transfer 2.5 ml of solution from the first set of tubes to the corresponding second set. Only one pipette is necessary if you start to transfer with the most dilute solution.
5. Draw blood into a tube containing heparin. Immediately add 50 μl of blood into each tube of the first set. The blood should drop directly into the solution. Do not allow the blood to drop onto the sides of the tube. Cover each tube with parafilm and invert gently.
6. Add 50 μl of known normal blood, collected in the same manner, to each tube in the second set.
7. Let the tubes sit at room temperature for half an hour.
8. Mix gently and centrifuge at 2000 rpm for 5 minutes.
9. When interpreting results, note which tubes show initial and complete hemolysis. Initial hemolysis is recognized by a faintly pink supernatant and a cell button at the bottom of the tube. Complete hemolysis is seen as a red supernatant with possibly a button of cell stroma at the bottom of the tube.
10. This test may be quantitated by measuring each tube on the spectrophotometer. To do this, two additional tubes are necessary. The first is a blank containing 50 μl of blood to which 2.5 ml of 0.9 percent NaCl is added, which will result in no hemolysis. The second blank is for complete (100 percent) hemolysis and is obtained by adding 50 μl of blood to 2.5 ml of distilled water.
11. These blanks are run in parallel with the other tubes.
12. After centrifugation, the supernatant of each tube is removed, and its optical density (OD) is read in a spectrophotometer using a 540-nm filter. The percentage of hemolysis in each tube is calculated using the following equation:

$$\% \text{ Hemolysis} = \frac{OD_{(x)} - OD\ 0.85\%}{OD_{(o)} - OD\ 0.85\%} \times 100$$

An osmotic fragility curve may be drawn by plotting the percent hemolysis in each tube against the corresponding concentration of NaCl solution, as shown (Fig. 30-I-6). It is helpful to plot the normal control with the patient so that any difference can be seen more clearly.

Interpretation

1. Patient values are always reported with the value of the control. With the normal samples, initial hemolysis is generally around 0.45 percent, with complete hemolysis occurring at 0.30 percent or 0.35 percent.
2. Examples of initial and complete hemolysis in various conditions follow:

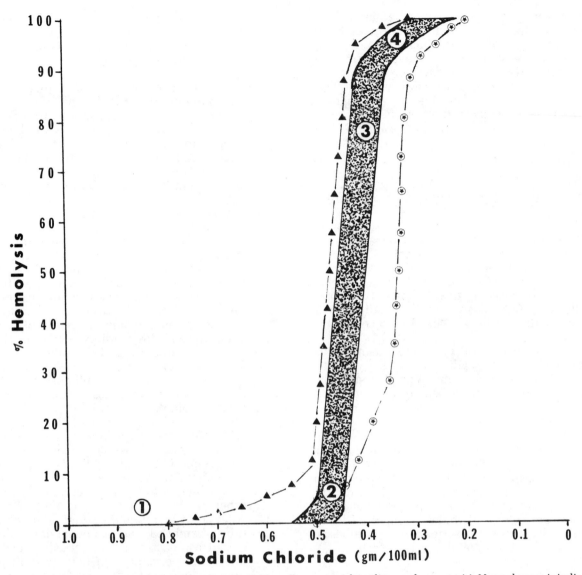

Figure 30–I–6. Comparative osmotic fragility curve (⊛ Sickle-cell anemia; ▲ hereditary spherocytosis). Normal range is indicated by shaded area: 1 = normal biconcave disc; 2 = disc-to-sphere transformation; 3 = disc-to-sphere transformation; 4 = lysis.

	Initial Hemolysis (% NaCl)	Complete Hemolysis (% NaCl)
Normal	0.45	0.35
Hereditary spherocytosis	0.65	0.45
Acquired hemolytic anemia	0.50	0.40
Hemolytic disease of the newborn	0.55	0.40
Thalassemia	0.35	0.20
Sickle-cell anemia	0.35	0.20

It may be necessary in some cases to incubate the patient's heparinized blood for 24 hours at 37°C. This will enhance increased osmotic fragility, which may reveal a subtle but abnormal osmotic fragility not apparent upon initial testing.

Comments

1. Fresh heparinized blood is recommended, but defibrinated blood may be used. Oxalate, EDTA, or citrate should not be used because of the additional salts present.
2. Perform this test immediately because cell shape and osmotic conditions change with time.
3. Osmotic fragility can be altered by pH and temperature.
4. If the plasma is significantly jaundiced, replace the plasma with isotonic saline before testing to prevent interference.
5. Hemolytic organisms in a blood specimen can cause erroneous results owing to hemolysis, which is not attributed to test conditions.
6. If the patient has a low hemoglobin level, wash

patient and control cells once with isotonic saline and resuspend with equal volumes of RBCs and saline for both specimens. This will correct for the anemia.
7. In some anemias, when poikilocytosis accompanies a low hemoglobin level, decreased osmotic fragility may be seen. This may be due in part to the decreased hemoglobin concentration and not to the presence of poikilocytes.

Acidified Serum Test (Ham Test) for Paroxysmal Nocturnal Hemoglobinuria

Principle

Confirmation of diagnosis of paroxysmal nocturnal hemoglobinuria (PNH) is dependent on a positive acidified serum test result. The RBCs of patients with PNH are complement sensitive. In this test, complement will affix to the RBCs at a slightly acidic pH, become activated by the alternate pathway, and result in lysis of the RBCs.

Reagents and Equipment

1. Venous patient specimen
2. Venous normal control (ABO compatible)
3. Five 12 × 75 test tubes
4. 0.2 N HCl
5. 1-ml serologic pipettes
6. Two Erlenmeyer flasks
7. Glass beads

Procedure

1. Collect venous specimens from patient and control in a plastic syringe and defibrinate by swirling in an Erlenmeyer flask that contains glass beads.
2. Centrifuge the defibrinated blood and separate serum from cells. Save the normal control serum, the patient's serum, and RBCs.
3. Wash the RBCs from the patient and control three times with isotonic saline, and dilute to a 50 percent cell suspension.
4. Label test tubes 1 through 5.
5. Add the reagents to the five tubes in numerical order, as shown below.

6. Cover with parafilm and incubate all tubes for 1 hour at 37°C.
7. Centrifuge and examine supernatant for hemolysis.

Interpretation

1. Patients with PNH will demonstrate hemolysis in tubes 2 and 3. Tube 3 was run in the event the patient had decreased complement levels.
2. Little or no hemolysis will be seen in tubes 1 and 4.
3. No hemolysis should be seen in the control, tube 5.

Comments

1. The optimum pH for this test is 6.5 to 7.0.
2. Blood containing a large number of spherocytes, as seen in hereditary spherocytosis, may result in a false-positive result.
3. The test result may be positive also in hereditary erythroblastic multinuclearity with positive acidified serum (HEMPAS) test. There are, however, two differentiating features; in HEMPAS the RBCs are not lysed by the patient's own acidified serum, and the sugar-water test result is negative for patients with this condition.

Sugar-Water Test for PNH

Principle

In patients with PNH, the sucrose solution provides a low ionic strength environment that allows complement to bind to the RBCs. These abnormal cells are extremely complement sensitive, which results in complement-mediated lysis.

Reagents and Equipment

1. Sugar-water solution: Dissolve 10 g table sugar in 100 ml distilled water. Prepare fresh daily.
2. Patient and control, venous
3. Test tubes, 12 × 75
4. 1-ml serologic pipettes

Reagents	TUBES				
	1	2	3	4	5
Patient serum	0.5 ml	0.5 ml			
Normal serum			0.5 ml	0.5 ml	0.5 ml
0.2 N HCl		0.5 ml	0.5 ml		0.05 ml
Patient's RBCs (50%)	1 drop	1 drop	1 drop	1 drop	
Normal RBCs (50%)					1 drop

Procedure

1. Obtain clotted specimens, centrifuge, and separate serum from clot.
2. Prepare 50 percent RBC suspensions.
3. In separate labeled tubes, add 0.85 ml of sugar solution, 0.5 ml of autologous serum, and 0.1 ml of the corresponding RBC suspensions. Mix thoroughly but gently.
4. Incubate at 37°C for 30 minutes. Centrifuge for 1 to 2 minutes at 3400 rpm.
5. Examine the supernatant for any hemolysis.

Interpretation

1. The presence of marked hemolysis in the patient tube is indicative of PNH. No hemolysis should be evident in the control.
2. Slight hemolysis is not usually indicative of PNH and is considered questionable.

Comments

1. Fresh samples must be used in order to retain complement activity.
2. The sugar-water solution must be made fresh daily; otherwise false-negative results will occur.
3. This is a screening test and is considered diagnostic only when used in conjunction with the acidified serum (Ham) test.

Autohemolysis Test

Principle

When defibrinated blood is incubated at 37°C for 48 hours, only minimal hemolysis will occur. In patients with hereditary spherocytosis (HS), autohemolysis is increased. The addition of glucose or adenosine triphosphate (ATP) to the incubation state will decrease the percentage of the abnormal hemolysis seen in the spherocytes of HS patients.

Reagents and Equipment

1. Ammonia water: Add 0.4 ml concentrated ammonium hydroxide to 1 liter of deionized water.
2. 0.239 M ATP: Weigh out 121 mg of ATP, dilute with 1 ml saline, and carefully neutralize to pH 7.5 to 8.0 with 1 M NaOH. This solution must be sterilized through a 0.45-μm pore filter unit syringe.
3. Sterile 10 percent dextrose in 0.85 percent NaCl solution.
4. Sterile 125-ml Erlenmeyer flasks with approximately 25 glass beads (4 mm)
5. Sterile polypropylene tubes with caps (12 × 75 mm)
6. Sterile 5-ml pipettes
7. Sterile 3-ml syringes
8. Spectrophotometer set to read at 540 nm
9. Assorted volumetric flasks, test tubes, and Pasteur pipettes

Procedure

Day 1

1. Draw 25 ml of blood from the patient, and carefully defibrinate by swirling blood in a sterile 125-ml Erlenmeyer flask with glass beads. Repeat the same procedure for a control sample.
2. Prelabel six sterile 12 × 75 polypropylene tubes for each patient, and control and dispense the appropriate reagents as follows:

Tubes 1 and 2	Plain
Tubes 3 and 4	0.1 ml of 10% dextrose in saline
Tubes 5 and 6	0.1 ml of 0.239 M ATP

3. Add 2 ml of the appropriate defibrinated blood to each tube and gently rotate to mix.
4. Incubate for 24 hours in a 37°C incubator.
5. Prepare a 1:100 dilution of defibrinated blood by pipetting 0.5 ml of whole blood into a 50-ml volumetric flask, and bring it to volume with ammonia water. This is done for both the control and the patient blood.
6. Centrifuge remaining defibrinated blood, and remove serum.
7. Prepare a reagent blank by making a 1:10 dilution of serum with 4.5 ml ammonia water. This is done for both the control and the patient serum.
8. Refrigerate serum for use on day 3.
9. Read the OD of the whole blood dilutions against the serum blanks at 540 nm. Record these results.

Day 2

1. Rotate incubated samples gently, and reincubate for an additional 24 hours.

Day 3

1. Gently mix incubated samples, and pool pairs.
2. Perform a spun hematocrit on each sample (total three hematocrits per patient and control). Record results.
3. Pour each sample into a tube, and centrifuge for 5 minutes at 2500 rpm.
4. Remove the serum from each tube, and prepare a 1:10 dilution of each serum with ammonia water (0.5 ml serum with 4.5 ml ammonia water).
5. Make a 1:10 dilution of original serum saved from day 1. This will be your serum blank.
6. Read the OD of the serum samples made in step 4 at 540 nm using the sample prepared in step 5 as the reagent blank.

Calculations

The percentage of hemolysis for each tube is calculated as shown here:

$$\% \text{ Hemolysis} = \frac{(100 - \text{Hct of tube}) \times \text{OD of serum sample}}{\text{OD of whole blood} \times 10}$$

Normal values: Lysis at 48 hours

	Lysis at 48 hours
Without added dextrose	0.2–2.0%
With added dextrose	0–0.9%
With added ATP	0–0.8%

Comments

When normal blood is incubated for 48 hours under sterile conditions, the amount of hemolysis is relatively small. If dextrose or ATP is added, hemolysis is further slowed.

Increased autohemolysis occurs in many types of hemolytic anemia. The patterns that may be observed, according to Dacie and Lewis,[7] are as follows:

1. Type I—Patients whose red cells show slight autohemolysis, corrected by dextrose, as seen in those with G6PD deficiency, hexokinase deficiency, and acquired nonspherocytic hemolytic anemia.
2. Type II—Patients with moderate autohemolysis without dextrose and in whom correction with dextrose does not take place, as seen in those with pyruvate kinase deficiency and acquired spherocytic hemolytic anemia.
3. The third type they observe demonstrates marked autohemolysis without dextrose correction; seen in patients with HS and in those with triose phosphate isomerase deficiency (Fig. 30-I-7).

The autohemolysis test is no longer used in the differential diagnosis of nonspherocytic congenital hemolytic anemia, because specific enzymatic assays are now available that are considerably more accurate. It is, however, a useful screening test for some RBC enzyme deficiencies to hemolysis.

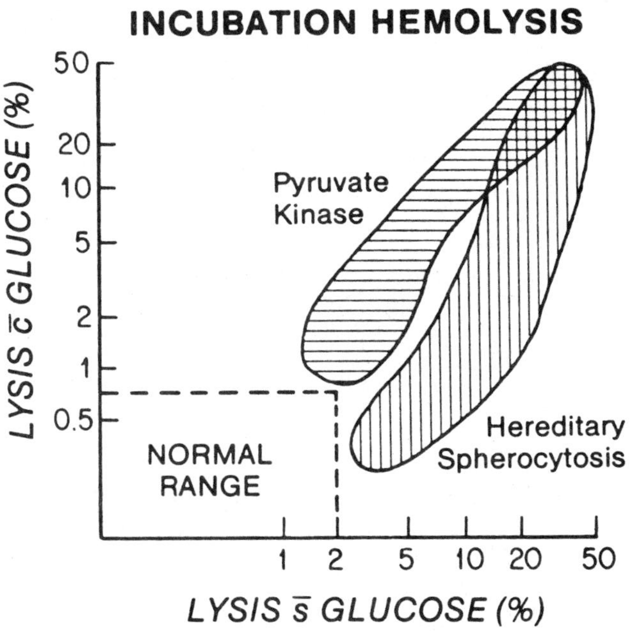

PREPARATION OF BLOOD SMEARS AND GROSS EXAMINATION

Preparation of the Peripheral Blood Smear

The preparation and examination of a peripheral blood smear is one of the most frequently requested tests in the hematology laboratory. This procedure is requested not only for the diagnosis of hematologic disorders but also to provide information for diagnosis of nonhematologic diseases, for indicating side effects in chemotherapy, and for monitoring patient therapy. Reasons such as these make it essential that a blood smear be prepared correctly and examined in such a way as to provide the physician with an accurate interpretation.[8]

There are four methods used to prepare blood smears:

1. Slide-to-slide
2. Coverslip-to-coverslip
3. Coverslip-to-slide
4. Automatic spinner

Figure 30–I–7. Incubation hemolysis test. This test provides a further measure of cell resistance to hemolysis. Pyruvate kinase–deficient blood demonstrates an abnormal rate of hemolysis that is independent of the presence or absence of glucose in the incubation media. In contrast, the blood from a patient with hereditary spherocytosis shows more marked hemolysis when glucose is absent.

Blood smears are prepared with EDTA-anticoagulated blood to minimize degenerative changes in the blood cells. The collection tube must be completely filled with the appropriate amount of blood so that it can mix with the anticoagulant. If there is an excess of anticoagulant, artifacts will occur. To ensure good preservation of cellular morphology, differential smears should be made as soon as possible and no later than 3 hours after collection.[7]

Slide-to-Slide Method

Principle

A small drop of blood is placed near the frosted end of a clean glass slide. A second slide is used as a spreader. The blood is streaked in a thin film over the slide. The slide is allowed to air dry and is then stained.

Equipment

1. Glass slides, 3 × 1 inch (precleaned with frosted edge)
2. Capillary tubes, plain

Procedure

1. Fill a capillary tube three-quarters full with the anticoagulated specimen.
2. Place a drop of blood, about 2 mm in diameter, approximately ⅓ inch from the frosted area of the slide.
3. Place the slide on a flat surface, and hold the

narrow side of the nonfrosted edge between your left thumb and forefinger.

4. With your right hand, place the smooth clean edge of a second (spreader) slide on the specimen slide, just in front of the blood drop.
5. Hold the spreader slide at a 30-degree angle, and draw it back against the drop of blood.
6. Allow the blood to spread almost to the edges of the slide.
7. Push the spreader forward with one light, smooth, and fluid motion. A thin film of blood in the shape of a bullet with a feathered edge will remain on the slide.
8. Allow the blood film to air dry completely before staining (Fig. 30-I-8).

Comments

1. A good blood film preparation will be thick at the drop end and thin at the opposite end.
2. The blood smear should occupy the central portion of the slide and should not touch the edges.
3. The thickness of the spread when pulling the smear is determined by the (1) angle of the spreader slide (the greater the angle, the thicker and shorter the smear),[8] (2) size of the blood drop; and (3) speed of spreading.
4. This is one of the easiest and most popular methods for producing a blood smear, but it does not produce quality smears. The WBCs are unevenly distributed, and RBC distortion is seen at the edges. Smaller WBCs such as lymphocytes tend to reside in the middle of the feathered edge. Large cells such as monocytes, immature cells, and abnormal cells can be found in the outer limits of this area.

Coverslip-to-Coverslip Method

Principle

A drop of blood is placed in the middle of a clean glass coverslip. A second coverslip is placed over the first coverslip to form an octagon. The blood drop is allowed to spread between the two coverslips and quickly pulled apart horizontally.

Equipment

1. Coverslips, clean, 22 × 22 mm
2. Capillary tubes, plain

Procedure

1. Hold a coverslip by two sides between the thumb and forefinger of your right hand. Place a drop of blood from a capillary tube in the center of the coverslip.
2. With your left hand pick up a second coverslip at one corner, holding the slide with the thumb and forefinger.
3. Quickly place the second coverslip over the first so that they are superimposed to form an octagon. Allow 2 to 4 seconds for the blood drop to spread; then quickly pull them apart in a rapid, smooth, and horizontal motion. Lifting either coverslip during this process will ruin the smear, owing to an uneven distribution of cells.
4. Allow the coverslips to air dry, smear side up.
5. Wright-stain the smear, using staining jars instead of an automatic stainer.
6. Mount on a 3 × 1 glass slide.

Comments

1. This method, when performed correctly, results in an even distribution of WBCs. However, this method is difficult to master, and technologists find it awkward to work with fragile coverslips.
2. An advantage to this method is that one can end up with two smears on the same glass slide, if they are mounted side by side.
3. A disadvantage is that an automatic slide stainer cannot be used. It is more time consuming to stain the smears by hand and therefore less efficient for a high-volume laboratory.

Coverslip-to-Slide Method

Principle

This method is similar to the coverslip-to-coverslip method. It differs in that two drops of blood are placed approximately 1 inch apart on a slide. A coverslip is placed, with three of its corners touching the slide, on top of one drop of blood and allowed to spread. The coverslip is quickly pulled off the slide in a quick horizontal motion. The coverslip is then immediately turned over, and the same sequence is repeated on the other drop of blood. As with the coverslip-to-coverslip method, two smears are obtained for evaluation.

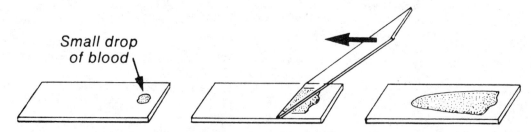

Figure 30-I-8. Preparation of a peripheral blood smear; slide-to-slide technique.

Equipment

1. Glass slides, 3×1 inch, precleaned and without a frosted edge
2. Coverslips, 22×22 mm
3. Capillary tubes, plain

Procedure

1. Hold a 3×1 inch glass slide lengthwise between the thumb and forefinger of your left hand. Hold a capillary tube with the blood sample in your right hand and place two drops of blood approximately 1 inch apart on the slide.
2. Pick up a coverslip by one edge with the thumb and forefinger of your right hand, and place it on top of the blood drop. Three corners of the coverslip should cover the blood drop, and the fourth corner should extend slightly from the edge of the slide.
3. Allow the blood to spread evenly, and then grasp the extended corner of the coverslip between the thumb and forefinger and pull it from the slide in a quick, smooth, horizontal motion.
4. Turn the coverslip over and repeat the procedure on the adjacent blood drop.
5. Allow both smears on the slide to air dry and stain.

Comments

1. This procedure yields an even distribution of WBCs and two blood smears on one slide, which can facilitate evaluation.
2. If an automatic stainer is used, take care not to place one of the blood drops too close to the edge of the slide. If this slide happens to be toward the bottom of the staining plate, the stain may not cover it sufficiently. This would result in only one smear being completely stained.

Automatic Spinner Technique

Principle

Although there are several automatic slide spinners on the market, their basic principle remains the same. A small quantity of patient blood is placed in the middle of a 3×1 inch glass slide. The slide is held in a horizontal position by a platen. The motor of the spinner is activated and accelerates rapidly to a predetermined speed. When the slide has spun for its predetermined time, the motor quickly stops.

A slide with a monolayer of cells is produced, which is suitable for evaluation. An even distribution of cells over the entire slide makes this preparation ideal for performing differentials on samples with low WBC counts, as well as normal and abnormal specimens. One disadvantage is that the slides must be extremely clean to prevent the shearing and spreading of cells as they are spun. The main disadvantage to this method is the hazard of blood aerosols from the spinner. Unfortunately this disadvantage has lead to the decline in the use of this method.

Examination of the Peripheral Blood Smear

There are several necessary steps in the examination of a peripheral blood smear.

Low-Power ($\times 10$) Scan

1. Determine the overall staining quality of the blood smear.
2. Determine if there is a good distribution of cells on the smear.
   a. Scan the edges and center of the slide to be sure there are no clumps of RBCs, WBCs, or platelets.
   b. Scan the edges for abnormal cells.
3. Find an optimal area for the detailed examination and enumeration of cells.
   a. The RBCs should not quite touch each other.
   b. There should not be areas containing large amounts of broken cells or precipitated stain.
   c. The RBCs should have a graduated central pallor.

High-Power ($\times 40$) Examination

1. Determine the WBC estimate.
2. Correlate the WBC estimate with the WBC count per mm³.
3. Evaluate the morphology of the WBCs and record any abnormalities such as toxic granulation or Döhle bodies.

Oil Immersion ($\times 100$) Examination

1. Perform a 100 WBC differential count.
   a. All WBCs are to be included.
2. Evaluate RBC anisocytosis, poikilocytosis, hypochromasia, polychromasia, and inclusions.
3. Perform a platelet estimate and evaluate platelet morphology.
   a. Count the number of platelets in 10 oil immersion fields.
   b. Divide by 10.
   c. Multiply by 15,000/mm³ if smear was prepared by an automatic slide spinner; multiply by 20,000/mm³ for all other blood smear preparations.
4. Correct any total WBC count per mm³ that has greater than one nucleated red blood cell (NRBC) per 100 WBCs.
   a. When performing the WBC differential, do not include NRBCs in your count, but report them as the number of NRBCs per 100 WBCs.
   b. Use the following formula to correct a WBC count:

$$\frac{\text{WBC/mm}^3 \times 100}{100 + \text{no. of NRBCs/100 WBCs}}$$

$$= \text{Corrected WBCs/mm}^3$$

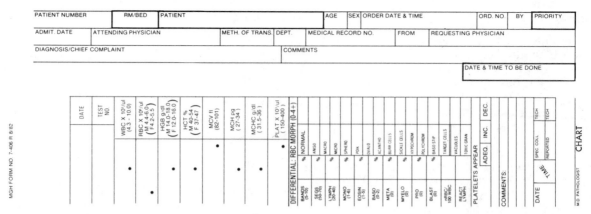

Figure 30-I-9. Hematology laboratory report sample form illustrating the complete blood count (CBC).

The examination of the peripheral blood smear is performed as part of the hematologic laboratory work-up called the complete blood count (CBC) (Fig. 30-I-9).

PRINCIPLES OF AUTOMATED CELL COUNTING

Coulter Counter Model S-Plus

Over the past two decades, the hematology laboratory has witnessed the evolution of the Coulter Counters from the Model A to the sophisticated Model S-Plus series. Despite the technologic advances, the principles of these instruments remain the same: one-by-one, nonoptical particle counting based on volumetric impedance. The Coulter principle of volumetric impedance uses the principle that the measure of volume displacement is directly proportional to cell size (Fig. 30-I-10). An electric current exists between two electrodes immersed in a conductive (saline) solution and contained in an aperture tube. Blood cells are also suspended in this fluid and are directed through an orifice in the aperture tube. As a blood cell passes through the orifice, it displaces its own volume of solution. This displacement increases the resistance between the electrodes, which results in an electrical pulse. The pulse, or signal, is a precise measurement of cell volume. Pulses are then electronically amplified and transmitted to a scaling circuit with adjustable threshold levels (Fig. 30-I-11). Particles with counts (volumes) below a selected size are separated out from the cell counts. In the Coulter S-Plus series, each cell count is performed in triplicate, compared, and, if in agreement, averaged for the best result. Whenever three counts are not in agreement the operator is alerted to the problem.

The Coulter S-Plus series directly measures RBCs, WBCs, and platelets. Hematocrit, MCH, and MCHC are electronically computed from the other data. Hemoglobin concentration is measured photometrically after lysis for the WBC determination (see section on Hemoglobinometry). The MCV is directly measured from the amplitude of the pulse signals from the second and third RBC aperture tubes.

Coulter Counter Model S-Plus STKR

The Coulter Model S-Plus STKR uses the same Coulter principles as earlier models but incorporates computer technology with a data terminal. This model also provides a histogram differential with a CBC and analysis of quality control results. The STKR has two operating modes—primary and secondary. Primary mode operation uses a bar code reader to process automatically as many as 144 tubes with pierceable caps that have been loaded into cassettes. Results are displayed and printed out in less than a minute from time of sampling. In the secondary mode, the open sample vials are manually aspirated by the aspirator tip. The entire cycle for one sample is less than a minute and uses a total volume of 200 μl in the primary mode or 100 μl in the secondary mode. Table 30-I-1 shows the determinations provided by the STKR.

A three-part differential is performed based on the variation in size of the three WBC populations. The lysing reagent, which is added to the WBC segment, rapidly lyses RBCs, releasing the hemoglobin and reducing the size of the cellular debris so that it does not interfere with WBC counts. As the WBC nucleus passes through the aperture, the pulse size and volume of electrolyte solution displaced will vary with cell size. Both the pulse size and the volume displaced are correlated to the corresponding cell type (Table 30-I-1).

Platelet counts are based on the premise that cells in the RBC bath that are 2 to 20 fl in size are classified as platelets. Mean platelet volume (MPV) is derived from the platelet histogram in the same manner as MCV is derived from the RBC histogram.

Coulter has also employed the technology of volume conductivity, and light scatter (VCS) in the differential analysis of the Coulter STKS. Volume is determined by the volume of electrolyte displaced by leukocytes, and the resulting voltage pulse is proportional to volume. Conductivity of the cellular

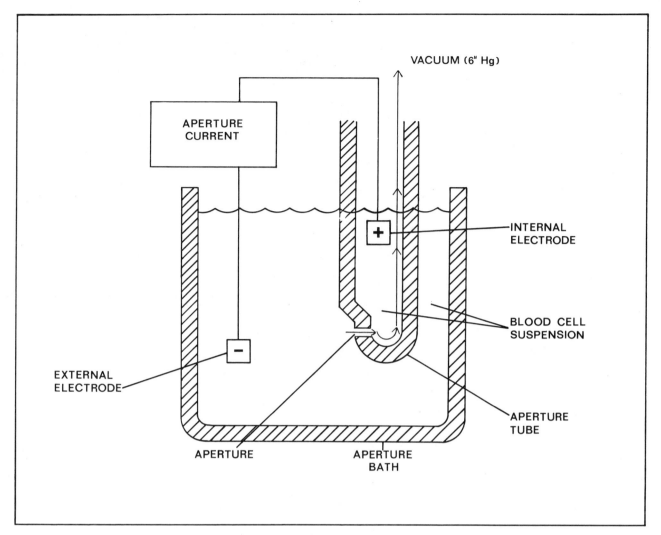

Figure 30–I–10. Coulter method of counting and sizing.

internal contents is measured using a high-frequency electromagnetic probe. Light scatter is a result of each cell being scanned with a monochromatic light from a laser. The amount of light scattered and the resulting patterns are useful in differentiating the types and quantity of granules in a cell. These additions to cell analysis enable eosinophils and basophils to be added to the differential. Scatterplots can be viewed and are color coded to represent population density of the different cell types. Suspect messages are provided to flag atypical cells such as blasts, immature granulocytes, and NRBCs. User-defined messages can also be used to flag samples demonstrating abnormalities such as leukopenia, anemia, anisocytosis, and other qualitative and quantitative anomalies.

Technicon H*1 System

The Technicon H*1 System is a continuous flow laser instrument that generates CBCs and a WBC differential from a 100-μl sample of whole blood.

The Technicon H*1 is a modular instrument with three main components: the electronic module, the analytical module, and the data handler.

The CBC includes the following test results: WBC, RBC, hemoglobin (Hgb), Hct, MCV, MCH, MCHC, RDW, platelets, MPV, and the hemoglobin distribution width (HDW). The WBC differential assays the percentage and count of neutrophils, lymphocytes, eosinophils, monocytes, basophils, and large unstained cells (LUC) and generates a lobularity index (LI) and a mean peroxidase index (MPI). Morphology flags alert the instrument operator to cellular abnormalities that may require further laboratory testing such as microscopic evaluation of the patient's blood smear.

These results are produced from four analytic channels: hemoglobin, RBC/platelet, peroxidase, and basophil/lobularity. A brief description of the methodology used to assay each parameter is given here, but the reader is referred to the Technicon H*1 System Operator's Guide for greater detail.

The Technicon H*1 assays hemoglobin using a

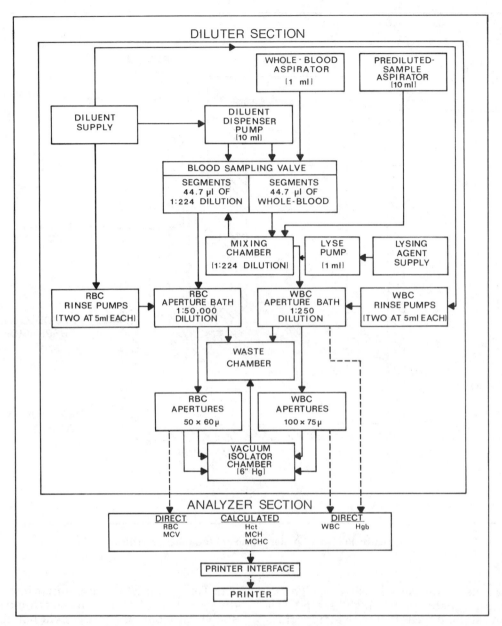

Figure 30–I–11. Flow diagram of the Coulter S-Plus Counter: diluter, analyzer, power unit, pneumatic power supply, printer.

modification of the manual cyanmethemoglobin method. Red blood cells and platelets are counted from the signals received by a detector with two different gain settings and analyzed by an optical cytometer after a dilution factor. The method of sizing RBCs uses the simultaneous measurement of laser light scattered in two different angles. This method eliminates the effect of variation in hemoglobin concentration on the measurement of cell volume. Platelet size is evaluated by measurement of laser light scattered in a single angle. The RBC count, platelet count, MCV, HDW, and Hgb are directly measured. The MCH, MCHC, and Hct are mathematically derived.

The Technicon H*1 uses the cytochemical stain peroxidase to classify leukocytes. When treated with peroxidase, specific cellular organelles demonstrate characteristic staining properties, thus allowing for their classification, Neutrophils, eosinophils, and monocytes stain peroxidase positive to varying degrees, whereas lymphocytes and large unstained cells contain no peroxidase activity. In performing the WBC differential, RBCs are lysed and the WBCs are stained with peroxidase. A small constant portion of the peroxidase channel is applied to a flow cell where the absorbance and forward light scatter characteristics of each cell are measured.

The basophil/lobularity channel allows for accurate basophil counts as well as a measure of cellular

Table 30–I–1. **COULTER MODEL S-PLUS STKR, CBC PARAMETERS, METHODS, CALCULATIONS, AND CONVERSIONS TO SI UNITS**

Parameter	Method	Calculation	Conventional Units	SI Units
WBC	Direct count; particles >35 fl	$n \times 10^3$ cells/μl	10^3 cells/μl	10^9 cells/liter
RBC	Direct count; cells >36 fl	$n \times 10^6$ cells/μl	10^6 cells/μl	10^{12} cells/liter
Hgb	Directly measured; cyanide-pigment	Concentration	g/dl	g/liter
Hct	Computed; relative volume of RBCs	RBC × MCV ÷ 10	%	liter/liter
MCV	Derived from RBC histogram	Average volume of one RBC in blood	fl	fl
MCH	Computed from Hgb and RBC	Hgb ÷ RBC × 10	pg	pg
MCHC	Computed from Hgb and Hct	Hgb ÷ HCT × 100	g/dl	g/liter
RDW	Derived from RBC histogram	Coefficient of variation (CV) of RBC distribution	%	None
Platelets	Direct count; RBC bath, cells 2–20 fl	$n \times 10^3$ cells/μl	10^3 cells/μl	10^9 cells/liter
MPV	Derived from platelet histogram	Average volume of platelets	fl	fl
Lymph %	Derived from WBC histogram	Particles 35–90 fl; % of WBCs	%	None
Mono %	Derived from WBC histogram	Particles 90–120 fl; % of WBCs	%	None
Gran %	Derived from WBC histogram	Particles 160–450 fl; % of WBCs	%	None
Lymph No.	Computed from lymph % and WBC	Absolute no. = lymph %/100 × WBC	10^3 cells/μl	10^9 cells/liter
Mono No.	Computed from mono % and WBC	Absolute no. = mono %/100 × WBC	10^3 cells/μl	10^9 cells/liter
Gran No.	Computed from gran % and WBC	Absolute no. = gran %/100 × WBC	10^3 cells/μl	10^9 cells/liter

lobularity. When whole blood enters this channel, it reacts with an acid and a surfactant, thereby hemolyzing the RBCs and rupturing the cytoplasm of all WBCs except for basophils which are resistant to lysis. The sample is then analyzed by a double-angle laser light-scattering module that separates the leukocytes into three classes: mononuclear cells, polymorphonuclear cells, and basophils. The cellular lobularity index is measured by a ratio of the signals from two nuclear classes. This measurement is a means of assessing the presence of a left shift.

The differential and CBC performed by this instrument has proved both accurate and precise. By means of computer analysis of RBC volume and hemoglobin concentration, histograms and RBC parameters are reproducible, thereby eliminating variability when evaluating RBC abnormalities. This new technology has made performing the differential more precise.

REFERENCES

1. Brecher, G and Chronkite, EP: Morphology and enumeration of human blood platelets. J Appl Physiol 3:365, 1958.
2. Dale, NL and Schumacher HR: Platelet satellitism—new spurious results with automated instruments. Lab Med 13:5, 1982.
3. Brecher, G and Schneiderman, BS: A time saving device for the counting of reticulocytes. Am J Clin Pathol 20:1079, 1950.
4. Westergren, A: Die Senkungsreaction. Ergeb Inn Med Kinderheilkd 5:531, 1924.
5. Wintrobe, MM and Landsberg, JW: A standardized technique for blood sedimentation test. Am J Med Sci 189:102, 1935.
6. Wintrobe, MM and Landsberg, JW: A standardized technique for blood sedimentation test. Am J Med Sci 189:102, 1935.
6a. Henry, JB: Clinical Diagnosis and Management by Laboratory Methods. WB Saunders, Philadelphia, 1984.
7. Dacie, JV and Lewis, SM: Practical Hematology, ed 4. Grune & Stratton, New York, 1968.
8. O'Connor, BH: A Color Atlas and Instruction Manual of Peripheral Blood Cell Morphology. Williams & Wilkins, Baltimore, 1984.

BIBLIOGRAPHY

Technicon H*1 System Operator's Guide, North American Ed. Technicon Instruments Corporation, Tarrytown, NY, 1985.

QUESTIONS

Section I: Routine Hematology Methods

1. *Calculate the WBC count if blood is drawn to the 1.0 mark in a WBC diluting pipette and a total of 150 WBCs are counted in 4 large squares.*
   a. $37 \times 10^3/\mu$l
   b. $375 \times 10^3/\mu$l
   c. $3.75 \times 10^3/\mu$l
   d. $0.375 \times 10^3/\mu$l

2. *Blood is drawn to the 0.5 mark in an RBC diluting pipette. In five small squares of the center square in a Neubauer hemocytometer, 210 cells are counted. What is the RBC count?*
   a. $2.1 \times 10^6/\mu$l
   b. $210 \times 10^9/\mu$l
   c. $0.21 \times 10^6/\mu$l
   d. $2.1 \times 10^{12}/\mu$l

3. *Blood is drawn to the 0.5 mark in an RBC diluting pipette. In 10 small squares of the center square in a Neubauer hemocytometer, 75 platelets are counted. What is the platelet count?*
   a. $187,000 \times 10^3/\mu$l
   b. $3.75 \times 10^3/\mu$l
   c. $375 \times 10^3/\mu$l
   d. $750 \times 10^3/\mu$l

4. *The reticulocyte count is 20 per 1000 RBCs. Calculate the percentage of reticulocytes.*
   a. 20 percent
   b. 2 percent
   c. 200 percent
   d. 0.2 percent

5. *The reticulocyte count is 3.5% with an RBC count of $4.1 \times 10^6/\mu l$. What is the absolute reticulocyte count?*
   a. 143,500
   b. 14,350
   c. 1435
   d. 1,435,000

6. *If a patient has a reticulocyte count of 8% with a hematocrit of 18, what is the corrected reticulocyte count?*
   a. 20 percent
   b. 2.3 percent
   c. 3.2 percent
   d. 8 percent

7. *Calculate a RPI for a corrected reticulocyte count of 3 and a maturation time of 1.5 days.*
   a. 1
   b. 4.5
   c. 2.1
   d. 2

8. *Which of the following errors will cause falsely elevated results for a centrifugal microhematocrit?*
   a. Reading of buffy coat with red cells
   b. Incomplete sealing of capillary tubes
   c. Allowing the centrifuge to stop without braking
   d. All of the above

Use the following values for questions 9–13.
RBC 5.0×10^{12}/liter
Hgb 14 g/dl
Hct 0.45 liter/liter

9. *Calculate the MCV.*
   a. 90 fl
   b. 9.0 fl
   c. 11 fl
   d. 25 fl

10. *Calculate the MCH.*
    a. 35 pg
    b. 31 pg
    c. 28 pg
    d. 25 pg

11. *Calculate the MCHC.*
    a. 13 g/dl
    b. 29 g/dl
    c. 42 g/dl
    d. 31 g/dl

12. *Based upon the previously calculated MCV, how would the RBCs be classified?*
    a. Microcytic
    b. Normal
    c. Macrocytic

13. *Based upon the previously calculated MCHC, how would the RBCs be classified?*
    a. Hypochromic
    b. Normochromic to slightly hypochromic
    c. Impossible to determine

14. *Which of the following factors affect the ESR?*
    a. Increased fibrinogen
    b. Extreme poikilocytosis
    c. Use of heparin as an anticoagulant
    d. All of the above

15. *What type of hemoglobin electrophoresis would be best to separate hemoglobins S and D?*
    a. Cellulose acetate at alkaline pH
    b. Citrate agar at acid pH
    c. Either cellulose acetate or citrate agar may be used

16. *Which method is best to quantitate HbA_2?*
    a. Cellulose acetate electrophoresis
    b. Citrate agar electrophoresis
    c. Anion exchange chromatography
    d. Differential solubility test

17. *What test is based on a reducing agent, sodium metabisulfite, causing HbS to sickle? (Use answer choices for question 16.)*

18. *What is the principle for the acid elution test for HbF?*
    a. HbF is resistant to acid elution; it can be precipitated and stained.
    b. HbF is susceptible to acid elution; it can be dissolved and measured photometrically.
    c. HbF is resistant to acid elution; it can be separated by aspirating the acid from the remaining hemoglobin.
    d. HbF is susceptible to acid elution; it can be destroyed and the denatured hemoglobin can be detected by a color reaction.

19. *Which test(s) measure Heinz bodies?*
    a. Staining for Heinz bodies
    b. Heinz body induction test
    c. Both staining and induction test
    d. Not given

20. *Which condition shows decreased osmotic fragility?*
    a. Hereditary spherocytosis
    b. Sickle-cell anemia
    c. Acquired hemolytic anemia
    d. Hemolytic disease of the newborn

21. *What is the basic principle of both the Ham test and the sugar-water test for PNH?*
    a. Complement-mediated RBC lysis
    b. Precipitation of abnormal RBCs
    c. Vital staining of affected RBCs
    d. Differential agglutination of RBCs

22. *Calculate the platelet count based on the following result: number of platelets in 10 oil immersion fields equals 150 (smear was prepared manually).*

a. 150,000
b. 300,000
c. 450,000
d. 15,000

23. Calculate the corrected WBC count for a smear containing 20 NRBCs (WBC count = 4500/μl).
    a. 4500/μl; no need to correct
    b. 375/μl
    c. 4480/μl
    d. 3750/μl

24. What is the principle of automated cell counting?
    a. Size referencing
    b. Volumetric impedance
    c. Photometric displacement
    d. None of the above

25. Which cell parameters are directly measured by automated cell (Coulter) counters?
    a. RBCs, WBCs, and platelets
    b. RBCs, WBCs, platelets, Hct, Hgb, MCV, MCH, and MCHC

    c. RBCs, WBCs, platelets, Hgb, and MCV
    d. Hct, MCH, and MCHC

26. Which cell parameters are calculated? (Use answer choices for question 25.)

27. What is the principle of the cyanmethemoglobin method in the colorimetric determination of hemoglobin?
    a. Potassium ferricyanide oxidizes hemoglobin to methemoglobin; potassium cyanide converts methemoglobin to cyanmethemoglobin.
    b. Potassium cyanide oxidizes hemoglobin to methemoglobin; potassium ferricyanide converts methemoglobin to cyanmethemoglobin.
    c. Potassium ferricyanide oxidizes hemoglobin to cyanmethemoglobin; cyanmethemoglobin degenerates to form potassium cyanide.
    d. Potassium cyanide reduces hemoglobin to cyanmethemoglobin.

Answers to Section I study questions are on p. 617.

Principles of Automated Differential Analysis

OBJECTIVES

At the end of this section, the learner should be able to:
1. Explain the main use of the leukocyte histogram differential.
2. Decide when to accept an automated leukocyte histogram differential or perform a conventional manual differential.

3. Determine the correct action to be taken when a result is flagged.
4. Interpret a WBC histogram.

The differential analysis of peripheral blood smears consists of the examination and identification of leukocyte subpopulations, an evaluation of red blood cell (RBC) morphology, and an estimation of platelet sufficiency. It represents one of the most frequently ordered and most time-consuming hematology test procedures. Differential analysis of peripheral blood has been considered the single laboratory test from which the most information regarding patient disease status can be derived.[1] Examination of peripheral blood smears, for example, can reveal hematologic abnormalities such as anemia and leukemia, aid in the identification of infectious conditions including mononucleosis and para-

sitemia, monitor the progress of disease, and follow a patient's response to therapy.[2]

In the past decade, reliable automated methods for analyzing peripheral blood cell populations have emerged. In addition to providing complete blood count (CBC) parameters such as white blood cell (WBC), RBC, hemoglobin (Hgb), hematocrit (Hct), platelets (PLT), and RBC indices, current instruments also quantify WBC subpopulations, and identify samples with abnormalities for further review. Many instruments also determine parameters such as red cell and platelet distribution widths (RDW and PDW) and mean platelet volume (MPV).

The accuracy of the automated leukocyte differential has been compared with that of the manual, microscopic differential in a variety of studies.[3-6] The data suggest good correlations between instrument and manual-derived granulocyte and lymphocyte counts, but poorer correlations for monocyte counts. This most likely reflects the decreased precision of counting monocytes during traditional 100 or 200 cell differential analysis owing to their low prevalence[7] rather than to instrument inaccuracies. The automated leukocyte analysis eliminates statistical variations associated with 100 or 200 cell manual differential counts based on the increased number of cells (several thousand) that are analyzed. This has also contributed to the increased sensitivity of automated leukocyte differentials to abnormalities such as the clumping of platelets and the presence of nucleated red blood cells (NRBCs) and leukemic blasts.[8,9] Moreover, a number of studies suggest that the automated differential is more efficient and cost-effective than the manual procedure.[10,11]

Despite advantages of using the automated differential to evaluate hematologically normal patients, automated methods should not replace the manual procedure,[5] particularly in evaluating blood samples from oncology patients[12,13] and neonatal intensive care populations.[14] Ideally, the automated leukocyte differential should be used in conjunction with careful screening of a Wright-stained peripheral blood smear. To enhance the utility, reliability, and cost-effectiveness of automated differential analysis, each laboratory must establish criteria for manual review of automated results that are appropriate for specific patient populations.

Automated differential analysis is currently based on the quantitation and evaluation of cell volume, cell light scattering, and cytochemistry, used alone or in combination. Applications of cell volume analysis, will be illustrated by the Coulter three-part screening differential which provides information about granulocytes, lymphocytes, and mononuclear cell fractions.[15,16] The leukocyte differential, available from Technicon systems, demonstrates cell analysis based on light-scattering events and cytochemistry.[17]

EVALUATION OF BLOOD SPECIMENS BY CELL VOLUME ANALYSIS: THE COULTER DIFFERENTIAL

The Coulter automated differential generates three histograms representing WBC, RBC, and platelet volume distributions, expressed in femoliters (fl). The histograms display cells as small as 30 fl, but only those greater than 35 fl are counted. Histograms of WBCs, RBCs, and platelets are displayed simultaneously with CBC information.

Leukocyte Histogram Analysis

Leukocytes in ethylenediaminetetraacetic acid (EDTA)–anticoagulated peripheral blood are separated into three major cell fractions by cell volume analysis (Fig. 30–II–1). Using an isotonic saline solution and lysing reagent to dilute and differentially shrink WBCs, the instruments differentiate between lymphocytes (lymphocytes and atypical lymphocytes), granulocytes (segmented neutrophils, bands, metamyelocytes, eosinophils, and basophils) and mononuclear cells (monocytes, promyelocytes, myelocytes, plasma cells, and blasts) based on differences in nuclear size and cytoplasmic complexity. Cells with a volume of approximately 35 to 90 fl are defined as lymphocytes. Those with volumes ranging from 160 to 450 fl are classified as granulocytes and those ranging from 90 to 160 fl are identified as mononuclear cells. Results are expressed in absolute and relative numbers for each cell category.[5]

To highlight results that are out of range, the Coulter instrument backlights the offending number. Backlighting occurs in the presence of abnormal cells or interferences to alert the operator to the possibility of erroneous or abnormal results. Region flag indicators or R flags (R1, R2, R3, R4) indicate the specific location(s) of abnormalities in the WBC size distribution (Fig. 30–II–2). They may also denote overlapping of two or more of the cell populations at the four designated threshold/valley regions (35, 90, 160, and 450 fl) of the WBC size distribution his-

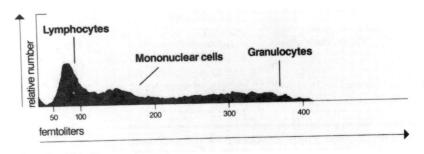

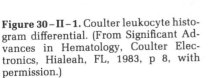

Figure 30–II–1. Coulter leukocyte histogram differential. (From Significant Advances in Hematology, Coulter Electronics, Hialeah, FL, 1983, p 8, with permission.)

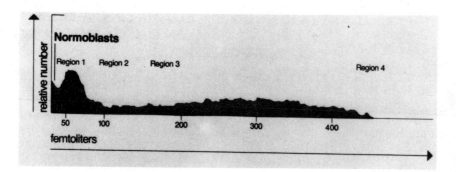

Figure 30–II–2. Region flags, *R flags*, superimposed on Coulter WBC histogram. (From Significant Advances in Hematology, Coulter Electronics, Hialeah, FL, 1983, p 9, with permission.)

togram. Common abnormalities associated with each flag[18] are listed in Table 30–II–1.

The presence of backlighting and/or flagging of the results suggests that a manual differential count or careful microscopic scanning of a stained peripheral blood smear is indicated. The decision to perform a manual differential should be based on the individual laboratory's established criteria for manual review of automated, histogram differential analysis. Examples of criteria for manual review and reference values for the automated histogram differential, established at a tertiary care hospital, appear in Tables 30–II–2 and 30–II–3.

Red Cell Histogram Analysis

Particles with a volume of greater than 36 fl and less than or equal to 360 fl are identified as RBCs. The RBC histogram displays particles with a vol-

Table 30–II–2. CRITERIA FOR MANUAL REVIEW OF THE COULTER HISTOGRAM DIFFERENTIAL ESTABLISHED AT A TERTIARY CARE HOSPITAL

WBC count	$<4.0 \times 10^9$/liter
	$>15.0 \times 10^9$/liter
Monocytes	$>1.5 \times 10^9$/liter
Lymphocytes	$>50\%$
Granulocytes	$<50\%$
All Backlighting	
All R Flags	
All Incomplete Computations	

ume greater than 24 fl, but the mean corpuscular volume (MCV) is calculated from the area under the curve of the RBC histogram, depicted in Figure 30–II–3. Deviations in the shape and position of the RBC histogram indicate changes in RBC size and/or shape.

The availability of red cell parameters such as RBC, Hgb, Hct, MCV, mean corpuscular hemoglobin (MCH), and mean corpuscular hemoglobin concentration (MCHC), in conjunction with information derived from RBC histograms, may provide valuable information for assessing erythrocytic disorders. The RDW represents a new parameter that quantifies relative anisocytosis. It is calculated as the coefficient of variation (CV) of the MCV (Table 30–II–4). Its usefulness in the early detection of iron deficiency (increased RDW) and in distinguishing between iron deficiency and β-thalassemia (normal RDW) has been suggested.[19]

Table 30–II–1. ABNORMALITIES ASSOCIATED WITH SPECIFIC FLAGGING REGIONS OF THE COULTER WBC HISTOGRAM

R Flag	Region	Abnormality
R1	Far left	Erythrocyte precursors
		Cryoglobulins
		Nonlysed erythrocytes
		Giant and/or clumped platelets
R2	Between lymphocytes and monocytes	Blasts
		Basophilia
		Eosinophilia
		Plasma cells
		Abnormal/variant lymphocytes
R3	Between monocytes and granulocytes	Abnormal cell populations
		Eosinophilia
		Immature granulocytes
R4	Far right	Increased absolute granulocytes
RM		Multiple flags

Source: Pierre, RV: Seminar and Case Studies: The Automated Differential. (From Coulter Electronics, Hialeah, FL, 1985, p 9, with permission.)

Table 30–II–3. REFERENCE VALUES FOR SELECTED BLOOD CELL PARAMETERS ESTABLISHED AT A TERTIARY CARE HOSPITAL

Granulocytes	50–75%
Lymphocytes	25–40%
Monocytes	4–10%

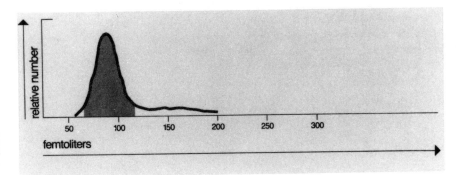

Figure 30–II–3. Normal Coulter RBC histogram. (From Significant Advances in Hematology, Coulter Electronics, Hialeah, FL, 1983, p 11, with permission.)

Platelet Histogram Analysis

The PLT histogram displays native platelet size. Particles with volumes ranging from 2 to 20 fl are counted. The raw data are fit to a log normal distribution (Fig. 30–II–4) from which the reported platelet count is calculated.

The MPV and PDW are additional parameters describing platelet size. The MPV is equivalent to the MCV and is inversely proportional to the platelet count (Fig. 30–II–5).[20] The PDW measures uniformity of platelet size and is equivalent to the RDW. In combination with the platelet histogram, the MPV and PDW provide greater distinction between normal and abnormal platelet populations.

ADVANCES IN COULTER LEUKOCYTE DIFFERENTIAL ANALYSIS: VCS TECHNOLOGY

The Coulter WBC differential has recently been expanded to include enumeration of eosinophils and basophils, by combining measurements of cell volume with conductivity and light-scatter data. Light-scattering characteristics provide additional information about cell structure and shape. This technology is particularly useful for identifying eosinophils. Conductivity measurements are made using a high-frequency electromagnetic probe and reflect the nuclear, granular, and chemical properties of cells. Conductivity measurements aid in dif-

Table 30–II–4. **CALCULATION OF THE RDW AS DETERMINED BY COULTER**

$$RDW = \frac{SD}{MEAN} \times 100$$

Normal Range = 11.5–14.5%

Source: Pierre, RV: Seminar and Case Studies: The Automated Differential. (From Coulter Electronics, Hialeah, FL, 1985, p 38, with permission.)

ferentiating between cells of similar size, such as lymphocytes and basophils which differ in internal structure.

An example of WBC analysis by volume conductivity scattering (VCS) technology is provided in Figure 30–II–6. Individual cells are depicted as points on a scatterplot, reflecting cell volume and light-scattering characteristics. Clusters of cells are identified as monocytes, eosinophils, lymphocytes, and neutrophils based on their relative position on the scatterplot. Separate scatterplots comparing cell volume and conductivity properties are generated to quantify basophils.

Floating discriminators examine areas between different cell populations. Abnormalities are identified by specific region flags. The VCS flagging system is enhanced by providing specific alphanumeric codes. For example, suspect messages include "nucleated red blood cells, platelet clumps, blasts, variant lymphocytes, and immature granulocytes."

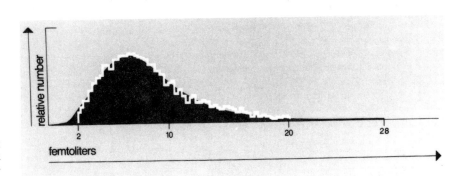

Figure 30–II–4. Normal Coulter platelet histogram. (From Significant Advances in Hematology, Coulter Electronics, Hialeah, FL, 1983, p 13, with permission.)

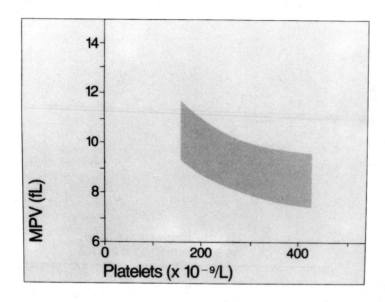

Figure 30–II–5. Coulter MPV nomogram. (From Significant Advances in Hematology, Coulter Electronics, Hialeah, FL, 1983, p 14, with permission.)

EVALUATION OF BLOOD SPECIMENS BY LIGHT SCATTERING AND CYTOCHEMICAL ANALYSIS: THE TECHNICON DIFFERENTIAL

Enumeration and identification of blood cells by the Technicon automated blood analyzer is based on optical flow cytometry, cytochemistry, and light scattering. The instrument's sampling mechanism divides blood samples into aliquots that are treated in four separate reaction chambers: the red cell and platelet reaction chamber, hemoglobin reaction chamber, basophil/lobularity reaction chamber, and peroxidase reaction chamber. Cells are counted as they pass through a flow cell. A laser beam is located on one side of the flow cell. As the cells pass in front of the beam, they are counted by a light-scatter detector.

Red Cell and Platelet Histogram Analysis

Red cells and platelets are identified based on their light-scattering properties. A buffered reagent isovolumetrically fixes and spheres platelets and red cells, while light scattered at high and low angles concurrently measures cell volume and optical density. Red cell and platelet histograms are generated based on light-scatter measurements translated into cell volume. Additional parameters such as the RDW and platelet cell volume (PCV) are derived from these histograms. The instrument's interpretive report identifies and grades (1+ to 4+) various RBC abnormalities including microcytosis, macrocytosis, hypochromia, hyperchromia, and anisocytosis.

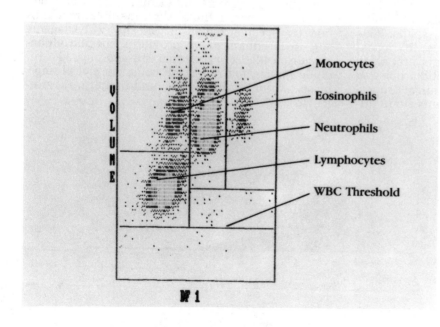

Figure 30–II–6. White blood cell analysis by Coulter VCS technology. (From Coulter VCS Technology Casebook, Coulter Electronics, Hialeah, FL, 1989, p 62, with permission.)

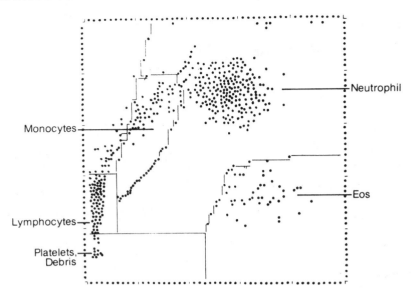

Figure 30–II–7. Technicon WBC/peroxidase scattergram. Cell size is indicated on the abscissa axis, peroxidase activity is presented on the ordinate. (From Brown,[22] p 388, with permission.)

Technicon's RDW reference range of 10.2 to 11.8 percent is different from the Coulter range of 11.5 to 14.5 percent.[21] The difference is likely due to each instrument's individualized mathematical trimming of the data. Because the absolute value reported for the CV of RBC size is variable based on the program of each standardized analyzer, each laboratory should determine its own normal ranges.[19]

Leukocyte Analysis

White blood cells are fixed with formaldehyde and stained with peroxidase in the peroxidase reaction chamber. The chamber is heated to a relatively high temperature which lyses PLTs and RBCs and causes the WBC to be fixed and dehydrated. Narrow forward-angle light scatter and tungsten light optics are used to measure WBC size and peroxidase activity, respectively. Myeloperoxidase is a granulocyte enzyme marker that is present to varying degrees in neutrophils, eosinophils, and monocytes but absent from basophils, lymphocytes, and blasts.[22]

A peroxidase scattergram depicting peroxidase staining intensity on the abscissa and cell size on the ordinate is generated (Fig. 30–II–7). Each point in the scattergram characterizes the peroxidase activity and size of a single cell. Clusters of points represent distinct leukocyte subpopulations.

A specific basophil count is determined separately in the basophil/lobularity chamber. Whole blood is exposed to an acid buffer that selectively lyses all cells except basophils. The resulting particles are subsequently sorted, and their forward angle and light-scattering properties quantified. Because basophils are resistant to lysis, they appear larger than the bare nuclei of other leukocytes, scatter more light, and appear higher on the vertical axis of the scattergram (Fig. 30–II–8). A fixed horizontal

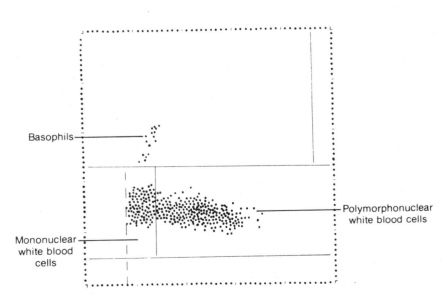

Figure 30–II–8. Technicon cytogram for basophil/lobularity. (From Brown,[22] p 389, with permission.)

threshold separates the nuclei of other WBCs from basophils.

The WBC differential report generated by Technicon instruments not only includes the relative percentages and absolute values for neutrophils, lymphocytes, monocytes, eosinophils, and basophils but also provides additional interpretive data to signal the presence of abnormalities. The differential report defines the proportion of leukocytes with high myeloperoxidase content, designated the high peroxidase (HPX) fraction, and the percentage of large unstained cells (LUC). Increased myeloperoxidase activity may be associated with reactive states, megaloblastic anemia, or hyperproliferative granulopoiesis,[17] whereas increased numbers of LUCs may reflect the presence of atypical lymphocytes or blasts.[23] Normal ranges of 0 to 3.7 percent for LUCs and 0 to 5.4 percent for HPX have been established.[24]

QUALITY CONTROL AND QUALITY ASSURANCE

Quality control measures for the automated screening differential consist of performing daily, monthly, and annual instrument maintenance procedures as specified by the manufacturer, and evaluating instrument accuracy and precision on a daily or per shift basis with stabilized controls for which target values—mean ± standard deviation (SD)—have been established.[25] Usually three levels of control material are analyzed to evaluate instrument performance over the spectrum of clinically relevant values. In addition, establishing action limits for manual review of automated results is essential. Separate criteria for review of automated results should be established for adult and pediatric patient populations, as well as for oncology, acquired immunodeficiency syndrome (AIDS), and transplant patients. Action limits on RDW, Hgb, and RBC count and indices may be included to trigger a morphologic evaluation of blood films for RBC abnormalities. Similarly, action limits on platelet counts should be established to verify manually low automated platelet counts.

Participation in external quality assurance programs provided by manufacturers of quality control materials and the American Society of Clinical Pathologists should be included in a comprehensive quality control program.[26] Comparison of laboratory performance with that of other laboratories evaluating aliquots of the same specimen by the same method (intralaboratory quality control) provides an independent assessment of instrument accuracy. Comparison of laboratory values with those reported by other institutions should include not only a comparison of the test result but also, when applicable, a comparison of the standard deviation. An increased standard deviation may indicate problems in instrument performance, resulting in decreased precision. In evaluating any changes in instrument performance, comprehensive instrument control, maintenance, and problem logs can provide valuable information.

CASE STUDIES: LEUKOCYTE HISTOGRAM/SCATTERGRAM ANALYSIS

The following cases are selected to illustrate automated differential analysis of whole blood by Coulter (S + IV) and Technicon (H-6000 and H-1) instruments.

Case 1: Granulocytosis/Neutrophilia (Fig. 30–II–9)

The Coulter WBC histogram depicts a large granulocyte population spanning the region between 200 and 400 fl, a small lymphocyte population, and few mononuclear cells. The shaded area represents the normal WBC distribution. An elevated WBC count is consistent with a shift to the left. Manual differential analysis revealed 56 percent bands, 35 percent neutrophils, 8 percent lymphocytes, and 1 percent monocytes.

Case 2: Acute Lymphoblastic Leukemia (Fig. 30–II–10)

Examination of the Coulter WBC histogram reveals a single WBC peak spanning the region between 50 and 150 fl. The shaded area represents the normal WBC distribution. An R2 flag alerts the operator to the skewed patient WBC distribution to the right of the normal lymphocyte peak. The R3 flag reflects the absence of a normal granulocyte peak. Manual differential analysis revealed the presence of 11 percent lymphoblasts, 50 percent lymphocytes, 32 percent neutrophils, 1 percent metamyelocytes, and 6 percent myelocytes.

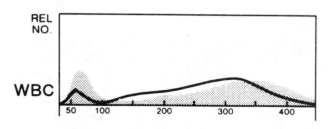

WBC	16.8
LY %	8.2
MO%	7.2
GR%	84.6
LY #	1.4
MO #	1.2
GR #	14.2

Figure 30–II–9. Coulter WBC histogram depicting granulocytosis and neutrophilia. The shaded area represents the normal WBC distribution. (From Pierre,[18] p 23, with permission.)

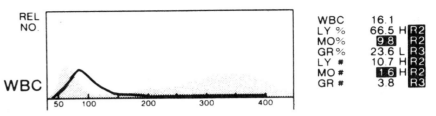

Figure 30-II-10. Coulter WBC histogram depicting acute lymphoblastic leukemia. The shaded area represents the normal WBC distribution. (From Pierre,[18] p 16, with permission.)

Case 3: Acute Lymphoblastic Leukemia (Fig. 30-II-11)

Examination of the Technicon WBC/peroxidase scattergram reveals a marked increase in LUCs (66 percent). Note the vertical band of lymphoid blasts extending upward from the lymphocyte region.

Case 4: Chronic Lymphocytic Leukemia (Fig. 30-II-12)

The Coulter WBC histogram reveals abnormal cell populations both to the left and right of the normal lymphocyte peak indicated by the shaded region between 50 and 100 fl. The peak to the right represents lymphocyte doublets that were counted coincidentally owing to the extremely elevated WBC count (more than 99×10^6/liter). Dilution of the blood sample to achieve a WBC count of less than $50 \times$ 10^6/liter eliminated this peak. The abnormal cell population on the left side of the normal lymphocyte peak is consistent with a pattern of B cell chronic lymphocytic leukemia.

Case 5: Chronic Lymphocytic Leukemia (Fig. 30-II-13)

The Technicon scattergram reveals a major concentration of cells in the lymphocyte region and a small granulocyte component.

Case 6: Acute Myeloblastic Leukemia (Fig. 30-II-14)

Examination of the Coulter WBC histogram shows a broadening and shift to the right of the lymphocyte peak. An R2 flag suggests an increased mononuclear

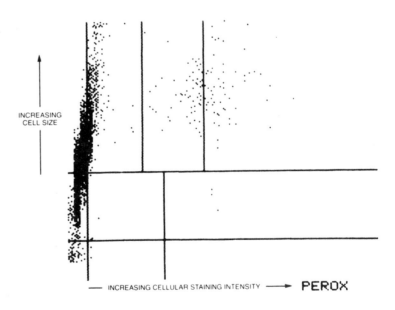

Figure 30-II-11. Technicon WBC/peroxidase scattergram illustrating a case of acute lymphoblastic leukemia. (From Simmons,[23] p 370, with permission.)

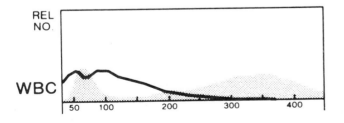

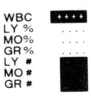

Figure 30-II-12. Coulter WBC histogram illustrating a case of chronic lymphocytic leukemia. The shaded area represents the normal WBC distribution. (From Pierre,[18] p 32, with permission.)

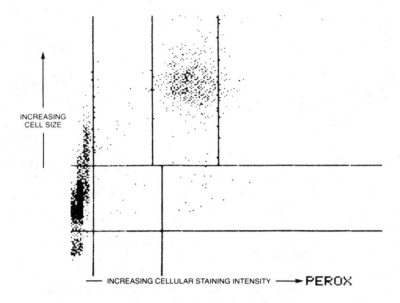

INCREASING CELL SIZE

— INCREASING CELLULAR STAINING INTENSITY ——▶ PEROX

Figure 30–II–13. Technicon WBC/peroxidase scattergram illustrating a case of chronic lymphocytic leukemia. (From Simmons,[23] p 371, with permission.)

cell population. Examination of the blood film indicated the presence of 82 percent blasts.

Case 7: Acute Myeloblastic Leukemia (Fig. 30–II–15)

Examination of the Technicon WBC/peroxidase scattergram reveals a large cluster of LUCs representing blasts.

Case 8: Chronic Myelocytic Leukemia (Fig. 30–II–16)

The Coulter WBC histogram demonstrates a broadened curve extending through the mononuclear and immature granulocyte regions, and an elevation at the right of the normal lymphocyte peak. This irregularity is characteristic of the lymphopenia and granulocytosis associated with granulo-

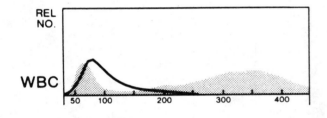

REL NO.

WBC

50 100   200   300   400

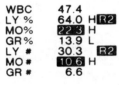

WBC	47.4	
LY %	64.0	H R2
MO%	22.3	H
GR %	13.9	L
LY #	30.3	R2
MO #	10.6	H
GR #	6.6	

Figure 30–II–14. Coulter WBC histogram depicting acute myeloblastic leukemia. The shaded area represents the normal WBC distribution. (From Pierre,[18] p 27, with permission.)

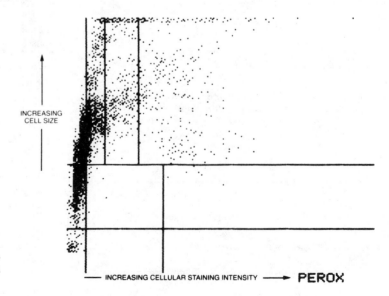

INCREASING CELL SIZE

Figure 30–II–15. Technicon WBC/peroxidase scattergram depicting acute myeloblastic leukemia. (From Simmons,[23] p 367, with permission.)

— INCREASING CELLULAR STAINING INTENSITY ——▶ PEROX

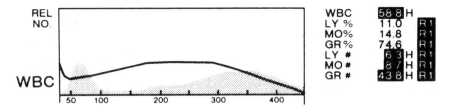

Figure 30-II-16. Coulter WBC histogram illustrating a case of chronic myelocytic leukemia. The normal WBC distribution is depicted by the shaded area. (From Pierre,[18] p 25, with permission.)

cytic immaturity, often seen in chronic myeloproliferative disorders. An R1 flag suggests the presence of nucleated RBCs and/or clumped platelets.

Case 9: Chronic Myelocytic Leukemia (Fig. 30-II-17)

Cells are spread diagonally across the Technicon WBC/peroxidase scattergram. An increase in the number of cells with high peroxidase activity is depicted in the upper right section of the scattergram. This pattern is typical of the increased numbers of immature granulocytes seen in this malignancy.

Case 10: Infectious Mononucleosis (Fig. 30-II-18)

The Coulter WBC histogram reveals an abnormal WBC distribution with a lymphocyte peak that was shifted to the right of normal, suggesting the presence of an abnormal lymphocyte/mononuclear population. The R2 flag is consistent with the presence of large atypical lymphocytes. Note the similar WBC distribution in Case 6, acute nonlymphocytic leukemia, emphasizing the importance of manual review of automated differential results.

Case 11: Nucleated Red Blood Cells (Fig. 30-II-19)

The Coulter WBC, RBC, and PLT histograms all show abnormal cell distributions. The RBC histogram shows a left-shifted curve with interference below 35 fl. The WBC histogram depicts an extremely high peak to the left of the normal lymphocyte region, accompanied by an R1 flag. The platelet histogram failed to return to baseline near 20 fl. These patterns are consistent with the presence of NRBCs (affecting the WBC histograms) and RBC fragments (affecting RBC and PLT histograms).

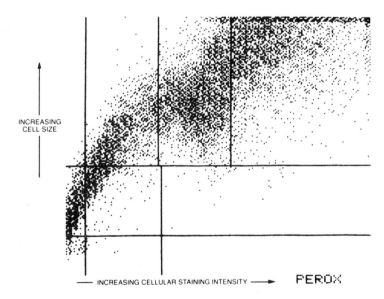

Figure 30-II-17. Technicon WBC/peroxidase scattergram illustrating a case of chronic myelocytic leukemia. (From Simmons,[23] p 367, with permission.)

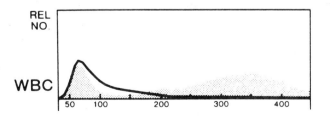

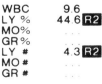

Figure 30-II-18. Coulter WBC histogram depicting infectious mononucleosis. The shaded area represents the normal WBC distribution. (From Pierre,[18] p 12, with permission.)

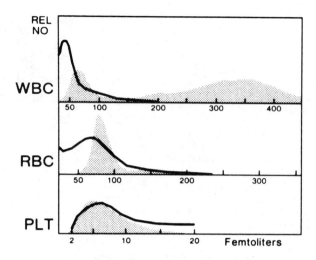

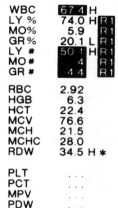

WBC	67.4	H
LY %	74.0	H R1
MO%	5.9	R1
GR%	20.1	L R1
LY #	50.1	H R1
MO #	.4	R1
GR #	4.4	R1

RBC	2.92
HGB	6.3
HCT	22.4
MCV	76.6
MCH	21.5
MCHC	28.0
RDW	34.5 H *

PLT	. . .
PCT	. . .
MPV	. . .
PDW	. . .

Figure 30–II–19. Coulter WBC, platelet, and RBC histograms depicting abnormalities associated with the presence of nucleated RBC. The shaded areas represent normal cell volume distributions. (From Pierre,[18] p 51, with permission.)

CASE STUDIES: RED CELL AND PLATELET ANALYSIS

Because RBC and PLT histograms generated by Coulter and Technicon instruments are not significantly different, Coulter case studies are provided to depict some of the more frequently encountered abnormalities.

Case 12: Iron-Deficiency Anemia (Fig. 30–II–20)

The RBC histogram shows an RBC distribution curve that is shifted to the left, which is characteristic of microcytosis. The slightly elevated RDW is consistent with iron deficiency and is flagged for review.

Case 13: Folic Acid Deficiency (Fig. 30–II–21)

The RBC histogram demonstrates an abnormal shift to the right, suggesting macrocytosis. Note the extremely elevated MCV and RDW, reflecting marked macrocytosis and anisocytosis, respectively.

Case 14: Cold Agglutinins (Fig. 30–II–22)

The Coulter RBC histogram appears relatively normal except for a slight elevation at the far right of the curve. Red cell indices, however, are flagged with the letter "H," emphasizing marked elevations in the MCH and MCHC. In addition, RBC parameters show discrepancies among the RBC count, Hgb, and Hct, which normally differ by a factor of 3.[25] Characteristic of cold agglutinins, the Hct and the RBC count are disproportionately low.

RBC	3.05
HGB	5.8
HCT	19.9
MCV	65.4
MCH	19.0 L
MCHC	29.1
RDW	16.8 *

Figure 30–II–20. Coulter RBC histogram illustrating a case of iron-deficiency anemia. The shaded area represents normal RBC volume distribution. (From Pierre,[18] p 43, with permission.)

Figure 30–II–21. Coulter RBC histogram depicting folic acid deficiency. The shaded area represents normal RBC volume distribution. (From Pierre,[18] RV, p 45, with permission.)

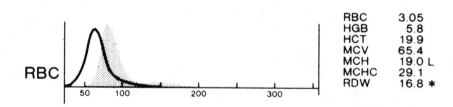

RBC	1.05 L
HGB	5.9
HCT	16.7
MCV	158.7 H
MCH	56.2 H
MCHC	35.4
RDW	31.5 H*

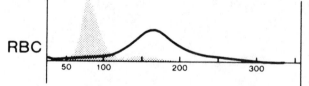

RBC	1.79 L
HGB	9.7
HCT	17.3
MCV	96.8
MCH	54.2 H
MCHC	56.0 H
RDW	16.6

Figure 30–II–22. Coulter RBC histogram depicting abnormalities associated with the presence of cold agglutinins. The shaded area represents normal RBC volume distribution. (From Pierre,[18] p 55, with permission.)

Case 15: Sickle-Thalassemia (Fig. 30–II–23)

The Coulter RBC histogram demonstrates an abnormal shift to the left of the RBC volume distribution, representing a moderate microcytosis. The RBC parameters are consistent with microcytic anemia (decreased MCV) and anisocytosis (increased RDW). In addition to iron deficiency, an increased RDW has been reported in patients with hemoglobin SS, hemoglobin SC, and S-Beta thalassemia.[26]

Case 16: Platelet Clumping (Fig. 30–II–24)

The Coulter PLT histogram appears normal. A PLT count, however, is not computed, based on dis-

agreement among simultaneous independent automated PLT count determinations. The WBC histogram depicts interference at approximately 35 fl. This is confirmed by an R1 flag. Careful examination of the peripheral blood smear reveals the presence of PLT clumps. The RBC histogram is unremarkable.

Case 17: Giant Platelets (Fig. 30–II–25)

The Coulter PLT histogram is grossly abnormal and fails to return to baseline near 20 fl. The R1 flag reflects the high left shoulder of the WBC histogram. Examination of a stained peripheral blood film reveals the presence of giant platelets. The RBC histogram is unremarkable.

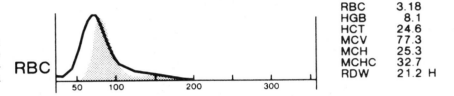

RBC	3.18
HGB	8.1
HCT	24.6
MCV	77.3
MCH	25.3
MCHC	32.7
RDW	21.2 H

Figure 30–II–23. Coulter RBC histogram depicting a case of sickle thalassemia. The shaded area represents normal RBC volume distribution. (From Pierre,[18] p 50, with permission.)

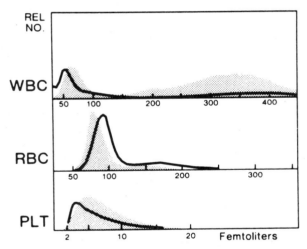

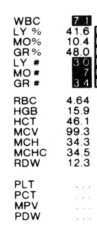

WBC	7.1	
LY %	41.6	R1
MO%	10.4	R1
GR%	48.0	R1
LY #	3.0	R1
MO #	.7	R1
GR #	3.4	R1

RBC	4.64
HGB	15.9
HCT	46.1
MCV	99.3
MCH	34.3
MCHC	34.5
RDW	12.3

PLT	. . .
PCT	. . .
MPV	. . .
PDW	. . .

Figure 30–II–24. Coulter histograms depicting abnormalities associated with platelet clumping. The shaded area represents normal platelet volume distribution. (From Pierre,[18] p 71, with permission.)

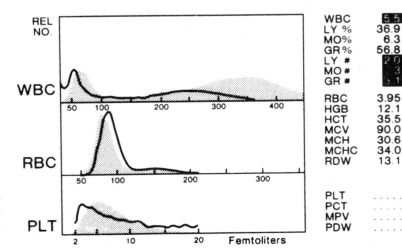

WBC	5.5	
LY %	36.9	R1
MO%	6.3	R1
GR%	56.8	R1
LY #	2.0	R1
MO #	.3	R1
GR #	3.1	R1

RBC	3.95
HGB	12.1
HCT	35.5
MCV	90.0
MCH	30.6
MCHC	34.0
RDW	13.1

PLT	. . . . .
PCT	. . . . .
MPV	. . . . .
PDW	. . . . .

Figure 30–II–25. Coulter histograms reflecting the presence of giant platelets. The shaded area represents normal platelet volume distribution. (From Pierre,[18] p 73, with permission.)

Although examples in this section have focused only on Coulter and Technicon analyzers, a number of other automated hematology analyzers perform CBCs and histogram/scattergram differentials. Some of these include Sysmex systems (Toa Medical Electronics, Los Alamitos, CA); CELL-DYN systems (Sequoia-Turner, Mountain View, CA); HC-1020 (Danam, Dallas, TX); and ABX series (ABX, Horsham, PA). We do not endorse any particular model. Owing to the abundance of hematology analyzers and publication delay factors, it is not feasible to identify and individually discuss all of these systems. Information, instrument manuals, and descriptions of upgraded models are usually available from the manufacturers.

CONCLUSION

Future trends point to increased hematology testing, requiring automated specimen processing, multitest analysis, and advances in data processing. Thus, in addition to the improved accuracy and precision of automated whole blood differential analysis, new advances in hematology analyzers are directed at improving laboratory safety, productivity, efficiency, and work flow. Because current automated analyzers with histogram differential capabilities generate comprehensive interpretive reports containing detailed information about abnormalities, careful evaluation of the data can provide an efficient screening tool.

A review of the literature, however, underscores the importance of the smear differential for confirming and reviewing automated results.[3-5,27] Confirmatory evaluation of blood smears, to identify abnormalities can be considerably more efficient and less labor-intensive with the help of automated differential results. Automated results can direct the technologist to focus on specific problems.

Improved features such as user-friendly software, bar code sample identification, closed tube sampling, and greater sample throughput enhance overall laboratory safety, efficiency, and productivity. Moreover, these advanced features contribute to cost-effective laboratory operations and efforts to preserve quality patient care despite the current shortages in qualified laboratory personnel.

In the past, automated hematologic analysis of bone marrow aspirates and body fluids has not been feasible due to limitations associated with samples with very low cell counts, the presence of microclots and extraneous debris, decreased sample volume, and interferences by heparin anticoagulants. Recent advances in instrumentation have overcome such obstacles, and automated procedures for analyzing body fluids and bone marrow specimens are being investigated.

REFERENCES

1. Hyun, BH, Ashton, JK, and Dolan, K: Practical Hematology. WB Saunders, Philadelphia, 1975, p 193.
2. O'Connor, BH: A Color Atlas and Instruction Manual of Peripheral Blood Cell Morphology. Williams and Wilkins, Baltimore, 1984, p 1.
3. Watson, JS and Davis, RA: Evaluation of the Technicon H-1 hematology system. Lab Med 18(5):316, 1987.
4. Miers, MK, et al: Evaluation of the Coulter S-Plus IV three-part differential as a screening tool in a tertiary care hospital. Am J Clin Pathol 87:745, 1987.
5. Griswold, DJ and Champagne, VD: Evaluation of the Coulter S-Plus IV three-part differential in an acute care hospital. Am J Clin Pathol 84(1):49, 1985.
6. Greendyke, RM, et al: A comparison of differential white blood cell counts using manual technic and the Coulter S-Plus IV. Am J Clin Pathol 84:348, 1985.
7. Rumpke, CL: Statistical reflections on finding atypical cells. Blood Cells 11:141, 1985.
8. Cox, CJ, et al: Evaluation of the Coulter Counter Model S-Plus IV. Am J Clin Pathol 84(3):297, 1985.
9. Bollinger, P: The Technicon H-1 hematology analyzer: Sensitivity and specificity of blast identification in peripheral blood. In Simson, E, et al (eds): Proceedings of the Technicon H-1 Hematology Symposium. Technicon Instruments Corp, New York, 1985, p 39.
10. Kalish, RJ and Becker, K: Evaluation of the Coulter S-Plus V three-part differential in a community hospital, including criteria for its use. Am J Clin Pathol 86:751, 1986.
11. Gauvin, GP, et al: Evaluation of the SYSMEX CC-800/PDA-410 system with trimodal histogram for white cell differential analysis. Lab Med 18(6):373, 1987.
12. Lai, AP, et al: Automated leucocyte differential counts in acute leukemia: A comparison of the Hemalog D, H600 and Coulter S-Plus IV. Clin Lab Haematol 8(1):33, 1986.
13. Drewinko, B: Utility of the Technicon H-1 system in malignant disease. In Simson, E, et al (eds): Proceedings of the Technicon H-1 Hematology Symposium, Technicon Instrument Corporation, New York, 1985, p 23.
14. Nelson, L, et al: Laboratory evaluation of differential white blood cell count information from the Coulter S-Plus IV and Technicon H-1 in patient populations requiring rapid "turnaround" time. Am J Clin Pathol 91:563, 1989.
15. Payne, BA and Pierre, RV: Using the three-part differential: Part I. Investigating the possibilities. Lab Med 17(8):459, 1986.
16. Payne, BA and Pierre, RV: Using the three-part differential: Part II. Implementation of the system. Lab Med 17(9):517, 1986.
17. Ross, DW and Bentley, SA: Evaluation of an automated hematology system (Technicon H-1). Arch Pathol Lab Med 110:803, 1986.
18. Pierre, RV: Section One: WBC case studies. In Pierre, RV: Seminar and Case Studies: The Automated Differential, Coulter Electronics, Hialeah, FL, 1985, p 7.
19. Bessman, JD: Red cells. In Bessman, JD: Automated Blood Counts and Differentials. Johns Hopkins University Press, Baltimore, 1988, p 5.
20. Bessman, JD: Platelets. In Bessman, JD: Automated Blood Counts and Differentials. Johns Hopkins University Press, Balimore, 1988, p 57.
21. Dito, WR, Gray, G, and Acosta, E: Red cell distribution width as an indicator of abnormal erythrocyte morphology. In Simson, E (ed): Hematology Beyond the Microscope. Technicon Instrument Corp, New York, 1984, p 147.
22. Brown, BA: Special hematology procedures. In Brown, BA: Hematology: Principles and Procedures, ed 5. Lea & Febiger, Philadelphia, 1988, p 123.
23. Simmons, A: Apparatus and automation. In Simmons, A: Hematology: A Combined Theoretical and Technical Approach. WB Saunders, Philadelphia, 1989, p 351.
24. Drewinko, B: Flow cytochemical patterns in human hematopoietic malignancies. In Simson, E, (ed): Hematology Beyond the Microscope. Technicon Instruments Corp, New York, 1984, p 36.
25. Rickets, C: Intralaboratory quality control using control samples. In Cavill, I (ed): Methods in Hematology Quality Control. Churchill-Livingstone, New York, 1982, p 151.

26. Ward, PG, Wardle, F, and Lewis, SM: Standardization for routine blood counting—the role of interlaboratory trials. In Cavill, I (ed): Methods in Hematology Quality Control. Churchill-Livingstone, New York, 1982, p 102.
27. Cornbleet, PJ and Kessinger, S: Evaluation of Coulter S-Plus three-part differential in population with a high prevalence of abnormalities. Am J Clin Pathol 84(5):620, 1985.

BIBLIOGRAPHY

Bessman, JD, Gilmer, PR Jr, and Gardner, FH: Improved classification of anemias by MCV and RDW. Am J Clin Pathol 80:322, 1983.
Coulter Hematology Education Series: Significant Advances in Hematology. Coulter Electronics, Hialeah, FL, 1983.
Coulter Hematology Education Series: Coulter VCS Technology Casebook. Coulter Electronics, Hialeah, FL, 1989.
Hillman, RS and Finch, CA: Red Cell Manual, ed 5. FA Davis, Philadelphia, 1985.

QUESTIONS

1. *What is the main use of the leukocyte histogram differential?*
   a. Diagnostic laboratory test for hematologic diseases
   b. Research tool for the routine hematology laboratory
   c. Replacement for the conventional manual differential
   d. Screening tool for hematologic diseases

2. *What should be the basis for the decision to accept an automated leukocyte histogram differential or to perform a conventional manual differential?*
   a. Each individual laboratory's established criteria for manual review of automated differential analysis
   b. Availability of qualified technologists
   c. Laboratory workload
   d. Manufacturer's recommendation

3. *A 47-year-old woman was admitted to the hospital for elective surgery. Her bleeding history was unremarkable. Results from her admission CBC revealed normal RBC parameters, an increased WBC count, and a decreased PLT count. The Coulter WBC histogram revealed a large shoulder to the left of the lymphocyte region accompanied by an R1 flag. The letter "H" appeared next to the WBC count. What should be done first, to verify these results?*
   a. Examine the patient's blood smear for the presence of blasts and immature granulocytes, shift to the left.
   b. Request another sample from the patient and repeat the automated CBC and differential on the new sample.
   c. Notify the hematologist.
   d. Examine the patient's stained peripheral blood smear for platelet clumps and/or NRBCs.

4. *Which area of the cell size distribution WBC histogram from a Coulter analyzer illustrated below is appropriate for a mononuclear population curve?*
   a. a
   b. b
   c. c
   d. d

a. a
b. b
c. c
d. d

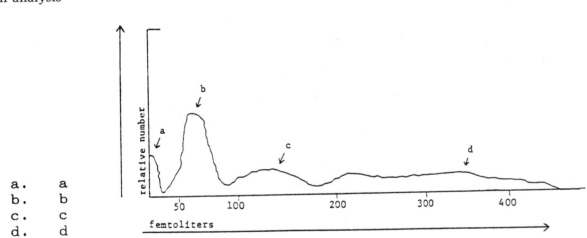

Answers to Section II study questions are on p. 617.

Special Stains/Cytochemistry*

---

*Staining of bone marrow smears by Milka Monteil, M.D.

OBJECTIVES

At the end of this section, the learner should be able to:

1. Correlate a leukocyte alkaline phosphatase score with clinical diagnosis.
2. Explain the purpose of a peroxidase stain.
3. Name the types of cells that are stained by the Sudan black B stain.
4. Name the types of cells that are stained by the specific esterase stain.
5. Name the cells that are differentiated by the combined esterase stain.
6. Explain the diagnostic value of the acid phosphatase/TRAP stain.
7. Describe the conditions under which the periodic acid–Schiff stain can aid in diagnosis.
8. Describe the conditions that are suggested by positive terminal deoxynucleotidyl transferase activity.
9. Explain the principle underlying the E-rosette test for evaluating T cells.
10. Name the type of cell detected by the immunofluorescent method for cytoplasmic immunoglobulin.
11. Explain the principle of flow cytometry.

SPECIAL STAINS (SEE ALSO CHAPTER 19)
Cytochemistry

Leukocyte Alkaline Phosphatase Stain

Alkaline phosphatase is located in the specific granules of neutrophils. It is combined with the substrate at an alkaline pH. A colored precipitate is formed at the site of hydrolysis of the substrate.

The purpose of this procedure is to distinguish the cells of a leukemoid reaction from those of chronic myelocytic leukemia (CML). One hundred mature neutrophils are counted on the blood smear and are scored on the following basis:

0	Colorless
1	Diffuse, slight positivity or occasional granules
2	Diffuse positivity and moderate number of granules
3	Strongly positive (granules fill cell)
4	Very deep staining, nucleus almost obscured

The score values for various disease states may vary, and each laboratory must establish its own limits. The chart below is a general guide.

Purpose. This stain is used to describe cytoplasmic leukocyte alkaline phosphatase (LAP) enzyme activity, which is decreased in patients with CML and increased in those with leukemoid reactions.

Principle. The LAP within the cell hydrolyzes the substrate naphthol AS-BI phosphate. The hydrolyzed substrate then couples with the dye (fast red-violet salt L.B.) and precipitates out at the site of enzyme activity.

Specimen. Fingerstick specimens are ideal. Heparinized blood may be used. Do not use ethylenediaminetetraacetic acid (EDTA)–anticoagulated blood. If staining is to be delayed, fix slides and store at $-20°C$ within 2 hours of specimen collection. Smears should be thin.

LAP Control. Establishing limits for LAP control:

1. Obtain fresh, heparinized blood from an individual who has an elevated LAP score (such as a pregnant woman in last trimester or person with leukemoid reaction). The control is usually stable for 12 months.
2. Make smears, dry, fix with LAP fixative, and rinse. Allow fixed smears to air dry, then store at $-22°C$.
3. Run a new control with an old control at least

	Leukemoid Reaction	Chronic Granulocytic Leukemia	Acute Granulocytic Leukemia	Polycythemia Rubra Vera (PRV)	Myelofibrosis	Paroxysmal Nocturnal Hematuria	Pregnancy
Leukocyte alkaline phosphatase score	↑	↓	Varies	↑	Varies	↓	↑

Source: From procedures by Mary Loring Perkins, M.T.(ASCP), S.H., and Joe Marty, M.S., M.T.(ASCP).

five times. Calculate the mean LAP score and set control limits at ±15 percent.

4. When LAP control is outside the acceptable range (a mean of ±15 percent), the following action should be taken:
   a. Have a second technologist count. If still out of limits, then:
   b. Repeat LAP stain on patient and control. If this action fails to bring control to within acceptable limits, new reagents may be necessary.

Reagents. Control: Heparinized blood with score close to 200. Fix and store at −20°C.

1. Fixative: Store at room temperature. Expires in 90 days, pH 4.2 to 4.5.

Sodium citrate (formula weight 294.10)	0.282 g
Citric acid (F.W. 210.14)	1.058 g
Deionized water	200 ml
Acetone	300 ml

Allow dry reagents to dissolve in water before adding acetone.

2. Substrate solution: Aliquots of 45 ml are stored at −20°C. Expires in 8 months.

2-amino-2-methyl-1,3-propanediol	13.15 g
0.1 N HCl	125 ml

Check the pH (9.5 to 9.7) before adding 0.2 g naphthol AS-BI phosphate dissolved in 10 ml N,N-dimethylformamide. Q.S. with deionized water to 2500 ml.

3. Dye: 40 mg aliquots of fast red-violet salt L.B. are stored at −20°C.
4. Hematoxylin: See hematoxylin counterstain procedure.
5. Glycerol-Gelvatol mounting media: Good for 5 months at 4°C.
   a. Dissolve 996 mg Trizma 9.0 in 160 ml deionized water.
   b. Add 40 g of Gelvatol and stir overnight.
   c. Add 80 ml of glycerol and stir overnight.
   d. Spin at 10,000g for 30 minutes and store in syringes.

Procedure

1. Allow smears to dry for 30 minutes. (This helps to keep the cells from falling off the slides when rinsing after fixation.)
2. Fix smears in fixative for 30 seconds at room temperature.
3. Rinse with distilled water.
4. Thaw substrate solution to room temperature (22 to 24°C); check with thermometer.
5. Add dye to substrate solution, agitate, filter, and use immediately.
6. Place slides, including control, in mixture for 15 minutes at room temperature.
7. Rinse slides in deionized water.
8. Counterstain with hematoxylin for 2 minutes.
9. Rinse slides in deionized water.
10. Air dry and mount with Gelvatol.

Interpretation. Score 100 cells from 0 to 4+, and add the scores on the sample

0	No staining
1+	Faint staining
2+	Moderate staining
3+	Strong staining (some cytoplasm background visible)
4+	Brilliant (no cytoplasm background visible)

Report patient score if control is within previously established limits, and report normal value.

Normal values:

Males	22–124
Females	33–149

Leukocyte alkaline phosphatase activity is decreased in patients with CML, paroxysmal nocturnal hematuria (PNH), and hereditary hypophosphatasia. Increased activity is seen in those with polycythemia vera, myelofibrosis, and leukemoid reactions.

Comments

1. Controls are obtained from blood smears of patients in the third trimester of pregnancy. Control slides are stable for 1 year at −40°C. Repeat stain if control values are not within ±15 percent of control average.
2. Blood smears should be made thin so that white blood cells (WBCs) do not touch erythrocytes. Thick smears may falsely elevate results.
3. The control used should score high. If it does not score as high as previous runs, the test should be repeated after new reagents are made.
4. Only segmented and band form neutrophils are scored. Do not include other cells. Monocytes and eosinophils do not stain.
5. Leukocyte alkaline phosphatase slides need to be scored as quickly as possible. The dye tends to fade, especially if Permount is used as a mounting media.

Peroxidase Stain

Purpose. The peroxidase reaction is positive for myeloid cells and negative for lymphoid and erythroid cells. It is, therefore, useful in identifying granulocytic leukemias.

Principle. The enzyme peroxidase is present in the primary granules of myeloid cells. These primary granules first appear in the early promyelocyte and persist through subsequent stages. In the presence of hydrogen peroxide, the enzyme peroxidase oxidizes the substrate 3-amino-9-ethylcarbazole to a red-brown color. Some of the oxidized substrate remains at the site of enzyme activity.

Specimen. Smears or imprints may be used. Fresh capillary blood is best for smears; however, smears made from EDTA, heparinized, or oxalated blood are adequate. The fresher the specimen, the more reliable the results.

Reagents

1. Fixative (buffered formalin acetone pH 6.6). Store at 4 to 10°C. Good for 90 days.

a. Na_2HPO_4 anhydrous (F.W. 141.96)   0.2 g
   KH_2PO_4 anhydrous (F.W. 136.09)   1.0 g
   Deionized water   300 ml
b. Add 250 ml reagent-grade formalin 37 percent.
c. Add 450 ml reagent-grade acetone.
d. The pH should be 6.6. If necessary, adjust the pH with appropriate buffer salt.
2. 0.02 M acetate buffer pH 5.2. Store at 4 to 10°C. Good for 90 days.
   a. 900 ml distilled water
   b. 2.72 g sodium acetate (F.W. 136.08)
   c. Adjust the pH to 5.2 with dilute acetic acid.
   d. Bring the volume to 1000 ml with distilled water.
3. Hydrogen peroxide 30 percent
4. 3-amino-9-ethylcarbazole (AEC)
5. Dimethylsulfoxide (DMSO)
6. Mayer's hematoxylin
7. Glycerol-Gelvatol mounting media. Good for 5 months at 4°C.
   a. Dissolve 996 mg Trizma 9.0 in 160 ml deionized water.
   b. Add 40 g of Gelvatol and stir overnight.
   c. Add 80 ml of glycerol and stir overnight.
   d. Spin at 10,000g for 30 minutes and store in syringes.

Procedure

1. Fix smears or imprints for 15 seconds.
2. Rinse with deionized water.
3. Incubate smears for 8 minutes at room temperature in a freshly made filtered mixture containing the following:

   AEC   10   mg
   DMSO   6   ml
   Acetate buffer   50   ml
   Hydrogen peroxide 30 percent 0.005 ml
4. Rinse with deionized water.
5. Stain with Mayer's hematoxylin for 2 minutes. (Do not differentiate.)
6. Rinse in deionized water.
7. Air dry and mount with glycerol-Gelvatol.

Interpretation

1. Red-brown peroxidase positive granules are found in promyelocytes, myelocytes, metamyelocytes, neutrophils, eosinophils, and monocytes. Monocytes stain less intensely than neutrophils and eosinophils. Auer's rods are peroxidase positive.
2. Early myeloblasts, lymphoblasts, lymphocytes, basophils, and plasma cells are peroxidase negative.
3. In acute and chronic leukemia, some mature neutrophils may be peroxidase negative.

Comments

1. Peroxidase enzyme is sensitive to light. Smears should be stained immediately or kept in the dark. Smears that are older than 2 weeks or that have been exposed to excessive light should not be reported as peroxidase negative. If smears are to be stained at a later date, they should be fixed, air dried, and stored in an envelope in the freezer.
2. Permount must not be used for mounting. Color usually fades before microscopic observation can be made. In addition, xylene should not be used to clean unmounted slides.
3. A 2-minute stain with 1 percent methyl green may be used instead of Mayer's hematoxylin.
4. Test should be run on a healthy individual as a positive control.
5. If some of the red blood cells (RBCs) are peroxidase positive, the incubation period was too long.
6. Handle DMSO with care.

Alternative Method — Peroxidase Stain

Purpose. The peroxidase reaction is positive for myeloid cells and negative for lymphoid and erythroid cells. It is, therefore, useful in identifying granulocytic leukemias. Use this alternative method only when the regular procedure does not stain blasts that are still suspected to be myeloid. This procedure requires approval by a hematopathologist.

Principle. The enzyme peroxidase is present in the primary granules of myeloid cells. These primary granules first appear in the early promyelocyte and persist through subsequent stages. In the presence of hydrogen peroxide, the enzyme peroxidase oxidizes the substrate benzidine dihydrochloride to a black crystal. The oxidized substrate essentially remains at the site of the enzyme activity.

Specimen. Smears or imprints may be used. A fresh specimen is best. Capillary blood is best when staining smears; however, EDTA, heparinized, or oxalated blood are adequate.

Reagents

1. Fixative (store at room temperature, good for 90 days).
   Formaldehyde (37 percent)   10 ml
   Absolute ethyl alcohol   90 ml
2. Zinc sulfate solution
   Zinc sulfate ($ZnSO_4 \cdot 7H_2O$)   0.38 g
   Deionized water   10 ml
3. Substrate solution: Filter and store at room temperature, good for 6 months. Add reagents in order, mixing well after each addition.
   Ethyl alcohol (30 percent)   100   ml
   Benzidine dihydrochloride   0.3   g
   Zinc sulfate solution   1.0   ml
   Sodium acetate (F.W. 136.1)   1.0   g
   Hydrogen peroxide (30 percent)   0.005 ml
   Sodium hydroxide (1.0 N)   1.5   ml
   Safranin O   0.2   g
   Note: Benzidine is a potential carcinogen, and the following precautions should be taken when handling the reagent or its solutions.
   a. Wear protective clothing including gloves,

laboratory coat, and mask when weighing out powders.

b. Use mechanical aids for all pipetting.
c. Clean up spills immediately.
d. Wash hands after completion.
e. Weigh benzidine in hood.

The 30 percent alcohol may be warmed with hot tap water to help dissolve the benzidine.

Procedure

1. Fix smears or imprints for 60 seconds.
2. Rinse with deionized water.
3. Incubate for 30 seconds in substrate solution at room temperature.
4. Rinse with deionized water.
5. Air dry and mount with Permount.

Interpretation. Peroxidase positive granules are black.

Sudan Black B Stain

Purpose. Sudan black B stain is the most sensitive stain for granulocytic precursors.

Principle. Sudan black B stains phospholipids and other lipids. This is believed to be due to physical solubility of the dye in the lipid particles. These lipid particles occur in both primary and secondary granules. They also occur to some extent in monocytic lysozomal granules. They may rarely occur in lymphocytes.

Specimen. Smears or imprints may be used. Fresh capillary smears are best; however, smears made from EDTA or heparinized blood are also adequate.

Reagents

1. Polyvinyl pyrrolidone (K-29-33)
2. Phosphate buffer, pH 7.2
   0.15 M Na_2HPO_4 (21 g/l)   7.0 ml
   0.15 M $Na_2H_2PO_4 \cdot H_2O$ (20.7 g/liter) 3.0 ml
   Distilled water   30.0 ml
3. Fixative, pH 5.5; store at room temperature in amber bottle; good for 90 days.
   a. Dissolve 10 g of Plasdone in 400 ml of absolute ethanol.
   b. Add 75 ml of 37 percent formaldehyde.
   c. Add 10 ml phosphate buffer pH 7.2.
   d. Add 15 ml liquefied phenol.
4. Sudan black B solution, good for 1 year.
   a. Dissolve 1.5 g of Sudan black B in 500 ml of absolute ethanol.
   b. Stir with a magnetic stirrer for 60 minutes; filter before use.
5. Phosphate: Phenol buffer; good for 6 months.
   a. Dissolve 0.48 g anhydrous Na_2HPO_4 (F.W. 141.96) in 400 ml of distilled water.
   b. Dissolve 64 g of crystalline phenol (or 72.8 ml of liquified phenol) in 120 ml of absolute ethanol and mix with the phosphate.
6. Nuclear counterstain, good for 1 year.
   a. 1 percent aqueous cresyl violet
7. Background stain, good for 1 year.
   a. 0.2 percent aqueous light-green to which 2 drops of glacial acetic acid have been added

Procedure

1. Fix slides or coverslip smears for 60 seconds.
2. Rinse three times with tap water.
3. Incubate slides in the following mixture for 60 minutes (prepare daily):
   a. 20 ml phosphate-phenol buffer
   b. 30 ml Sudan black B solution
   c. Filtering solution is not necessary.
4. Rinse in 70 percent ethanol.
5. Air dry.
6. Counterstain for 10 seconds in 1 percent violet. Wash three times in tap water. Air dry.
7. Counterstain for 10 seconds in 0.2 percent light-green. Wash three times in tap water. Air dry, and mount in Permount.

Interpretation. Lymphoid cells rarely stain. Brownish-black cytoplasmic granules occur in myelocytic precursors. Monocytes have a few small brownish-black granules. Eosinophilic granules are brown and usually show central pallor.

Comments

1. The peroxidase reaction parallels the Sudan black B stain except that the peroxidase enzyme is found only in primary granules.
2. Mayer's hematoxylin or Giemsa stain may be used as counterstains.
3. Normal blood smears should always be run as a control.
4. Ideally smears should be made and stained as soon as possible.

Specific Esterase (Naphthol AS-D Chloroacetate)

Purpose. This is used to aid in differentiation of granulocytes, lymphocytes, and monocytes.

Principle. The esterase enzyme within the cell hydrolyzes the substrate naphthol AS-D chloroacetate. The hydrolyzed substrate then couples with the diazo salt (hexazotized pararosaniline). The diazo dye precipitates out at the site of enzymatic activity.

Specimen. This consists of paraffin sections, smears, and imprints. For smears, fresh capillary blood is best; however, anticoagulated blood is acceptable.

Reagents

1. Esterase fixative, pH 6.6; store at 4°C; good for 90 days.
   a. In 120 ml of deionized water dissolve:
   Na_2HPO_4 (F.W. 141.96)   0.08 g
   KH_2PO_4 (F.W. 136.09)   0.40 g
   Formaldehyde 37 percent   100 ml
   Acetone   180 ml
   b. Adjust pH to 6.6 if necessary with appropriate buffer salt.
2. Phosphate buffer, 0.1 M pH 6.5; store at 4°C; good for 90 days. Discard if mold develops.
   NaH_2PO_4 H_2O (F.W. 137.99)   9.45 g
   Na_2HPO_4 (F.W. 141.96)   4.47 g
   Deionized water   1000 ml

Check pH, and adjust to 6.5 if necessary with appropriate buffer salt solution.

3. Substrate solution. Store in glass (*not plastic*) stoppered bottle at 4°C. Good for 1 month.
   a. Dissolve 100 mg of naphthol AS-D chloroacetate in 10 ml of N,N-dimethylformamide (F.W. 73.1).
4. Pararosaniline solution: Store in brown bottle at 4 to 10°C. Good for 3 months.
   Caution: Pararosaniline is a potential carcinogen.
   a. Dissolve 1.0 g pararosaniline HCl (F.W. 323.8) in 20 ml distilled water plus 5 ml concentrated HCl. Solution may be gently heated to dissolve pararosaniline.
   b. Filter.
5. Sodium nitrite solution. Prepare daily.
   a. Dissolve 1.0 g NaNO$_2$ (F.W. 69.0) in distilled water to a volume of 25 ml.
6. Mayer's hematoxylin
7. Acid alcohol working solution

70 percent ethanol	5	ml
Deionized water	995	ml
Concentrated HCl	0.05	ml

8. Blueing agent

NaHCO$_3$	1	g
Deionized water	100	ml

Procedure

1. Deparaffinize and hydrate sections. The fixative B5 can be used if the fixation time is short and if the mercury precipitate is not removed with iodine.
2. For blood smears and imprints, fix in esterase fixative and wash well with deionized water at 4°C for 30 seconds.
3. Incubation mixture:
   a. To 40 ml of buffer add 1.0 ml of substrate solution.
   b. In a separate test tube add 0.1 ml of sodium nitrite solution to 0.1 ml of pararosaniline solution. Wait 1 minute and add buffer substrate solution.
   c. Filter.
4. After 30 minutes at room temperature, check control slide microscopically. If the reacting cells are not red enough, refilter the solution and replace slides for 15 to 30 minutes.
5. Wash slides in running tap water for 5 minutes.
6. Counterstain for 2 minutes in Mayer's hematoxylin.
7. Rinse well with deionized water.
8. Dip in blueing solution until counterstain turns from purple to blue (approximately 10 dips).
9. Wash, dry, and mount smears with Permount. Tissue sections must be dehydrated and cleared in xylene before mounting with Permount.

Interpretation. The cytoplasm of granulocytes and tissue mast cells appears red. Nuclei are counterstained blue.

Comments. Esterase is inhibited to varying degrees by mercury, acid solutions, heat, and iodine. Poor or false-negative results occur under the following conditions:

1. Slides are overheated when drying.
2. Mercury crystals are removed from tissues with an iodine solution.
3. Tissues are fixed in an acid fixative such as Zenker's (formalin or acetic) or Bouin's fixative.
4. Tissues are decalcified in an acid solution. Use EDTA.
5. Using solutions that are too old.
6. Tissue may be dezenkerized after incubation in substrate solution.

Nonspecific Esterase (Alpha-Naphthol Butyrate)

Purpose. The purpose of nonspecific esterase is to aid in differentiation of granulocytes, lymphocytes, and monocytes.

Principle. The esterase enzyme within the cell hydrolyzes the substrate alpha-naphthol butyrate. The hydrolyzed substrate then couples with the diazo salt (hexazotized pararosaniline). The diazo dye formed precipitates out at the site of enzymatic activity.

Specimen. Smears or imprints may be used. A fresh specimen is best. Capillary blood is preferred when staining smears; however, EDTA, heparinized, or oxalated blood is adequate.

Reagents

1. Esterase fixative, pH 6.6; store at 4°C; good for 90 days.
   a. In 300 ml of deionized water dissolve:

Na$_2$HPO$_4$ (F.W. 141.96)	0.2 g
KH$_2$PO$_4$ (F.W. 136.09)	1.0 g
Formaldehyde 37 percent	250 ml
Acetone	450 ml

   b. Adjust pH to 6.5 if necessary with appropriate buffer salt. (*Note:* pH has tendency to increase if allowed to sit. If pH is near 6.5, allow to stand overnight, and then test new fixative on known positive.)
2. Phosphate buffer 0.15 M, pH 6.3; store at 4°C; good for 90 days. Discard if mold growth is observed.

NaH$_2$PO$_4$ · H$_2$O (F.W. 137.99)	8.02 g
Na$_2$HPO$_4$ (F.W. 141.96)	2.4 g
Deionized water	1000 ml

   Check the pH and adjust to 6.3 if necessary with appropriate buffer salt.
3. Substrate solution: Store in glass stoppered bottle at 4 to 10°C. Good for 1 month. Dissolve 250 mg alpha-naphthol butyrate in 12.5 ml ethylene glycol monomethyl ether (Eastman Kodak). If alpha-naphthol butyrate is in liquid form, then use 0.225 ml/12.5 ml of solvent.
4. Sodium nitrite solution. Prepare daily.
   a. Dissolve 1.0 g NaNO$_2$ (F.W. 69.0) in distilled water to a volume of 25 ml.

5. Pararosaniline solution (possible carcinogen; see under comments). Store in brown bottle at 4 to 10°C; good for 90 days.
   a. Dissolve 1.0 g pararosaniline HCl (F.W. 323.8) in 20 ml distilled water plus 5 ml concentrated HCl. Solution may be gently heated to dissolve pararosaniline.
6. Mayer's hematoxylin
7. Acid alcohol working solution
   70 percent ethanol   5   ml
   Deionized water   995 ml
   Concentrated HCl   0.05 ml
8. Blueing agent
   NaHCO$_3$ 1   g
   Deionized water   100 ml

Procedure

1. Fix smears for 30 seconds at 4 to 10°C in esterase fixative.
2. Wash three times with deionized water.
3. Air dry smears and place in Coplin jar.
4. a. To 40 ml of buffer (pH 6.3) add 2 ml of substrate solution.
   b. In a separate container, add 0.2 ml sodium nitrite solution to 0.2 ml pararosaniline solution. Wait 1 minute and add to buffer substrate solution.
   c. Filter into Coplin jar.
5. Incubate for 45 minutes at room temperature.
6. Wash well with deionized water.
7. Counterstain with hematoxylin for 2 minutes.
8. Wash well with deionized water.
9. Place slides in blueing reagent for 30 seconds.
10. Wash well with deionized water.
11. Air dry and mount with Permount.

Interpretation. Megakaryocytes, histiocytes, macrophages, and monocytes stain brick-red. Lymphocytes have punctate staining. Granulocytes have little or no activity. Histiocytes are fluoride resistant, and monocytes are fluoride sensitive.

Comments

1. Pararosaniline is a possible carcinogen and the following precautions should be taken when handling the reagent or its solutions.
   a. Wear protective clothing: gloves, laboratory coat, smock. Wear a mask when weighing out powders.
   b. Use mechanical pipetting aids for all pipetting.
   c. Immediately clean up all spills.
   d. Wash hands after completion.
2. A control must be run to be sure reagents are working.
3. Hexazotized reagents are unstable and must be used immediately.
4. Fixation keeps the enzyme from washing out of the cell during staining and improves the morphologic preservation of the cells.
5. Smears should be fixed after drying, even if staining is to be performed at a later date.
6. Because this stain depends on an enzymatic re-

action, take care to preserve the enzyme activity by avoiding light, heat, and aging. Store fixed smears in freezer.
7. For sodium fluoride inhibition studies, add NaF 1.5 mg/ml to incubation mixture.

Combined Esterase

Purpose. The purpose of combined esterase is to aid in differentiation of granulocytes, lymphocytes, and monocytes. It is especially valuable when a limited number of smears are available.

Principle. The esterase enzymes within the cell hydrolyze the substrate alpha-naphthol butyrate and naphthol AS-D chloroacetate. The hydrolyzed substrate then couples with the dye, fast blue BB, or pararosaniline, and the colored complex formed precipitates out at the site of enzymatic activity.

Specimen. This may be a fresh smear or an imprint. For smears, fresh capillary blood is best; however, anticoagulated blood is acceptable.

Reagents

1. Esterase fixative pH 6.6. Store at 4°C. Good for 3 months.
   a. In 120 ml of deionized water dissolve:
      Na$_2$HPO$_4$ (F.W. 141.96)   0.08 g
      KH$_2$PO$_4$ (F.W. 136.09)   0.40 g
   b. Formaldehyde 37 percent   100   ml
   c. Acetone   180   ml
   d. Adjust pH to 6.6 if necessary with appropriate buffer salt.
2. Phosphate buffer pH 7.4. Store at 4°C. Good for 90 days. Discard if any mold is observed.
   a. NaH$_2$PO$_4$ · H$_2$O (F.W. 137.99)   1.67 g
   b. Na$_2$HPO$_4$ (F.W. 141.96)   7.74 g
   c. Deionized water   1000 ml
   d. Adjust pH to 7.4 if necessary with appropriate buffer salt solution.
3. Naphthol AS-D chloroacetate. Store at 0°C.
4. Substrate solution. Store at 4°C in glass stoppered bottle. Good for 30 days.
   a. Naphthol AS-D chloroacetate   20 mg
   b. N,N-dimethylformamide (F.W. 73.1) 10 ml
5. Fast blue BB salt. Store at 0°C.
6. Mayer's hematoxylin
7. Blueing agent
   NaHCO$_3$ 1   g
   Deionized water   100 ml
8. See nonspecific esterase procedure for reagents needed for step 1 of this combined esterase procedure.

Procedure

1. Perform as for a nonspecific esterase procedure, but do not counterstain.
2. Incubate slides in the following filtered mixture for 20 minutes:
   Buffer   38 ml
   Substrate solution   2 ml
   Fast blue BB   20 mg
3. Wash well with deionized water.
4. Counterstain with hematoxylin for 2 minutes.

5. Wash well with deionized water.
6. Place slides in blueing reagent for 30 seconds.
7. Wash, air dry, and mount with Permount.

Interpretation. Monocytes, histiocytes, macrophages, and mesothelial cells stain diffusely brick-red. T cells usually stain with a punctate red granule. Mast cells, early promyelocytes, and later granulocytes stain a granular blue.

Acid Phosphatase Stain/Tartrate Resistant Acid Phosphatase (TRAP) for Smears, Imprints, and Frozen Sections

Purpose. This procedure is useful for making a diagnosis of leukemic reticuloendotheliosis (hairy-cell leukemia). It may also be of use in T-cell identification and in multiple myeloma.

Principle. The acid phosphatase within the cell hydrolyzes the substrate naphthol AS-BI phosphoric acid. The hydrolyzed substrate then couples with the dye (hexazotized pararosaniline), and because the colored complex is insoluble, it precipitates out at the site of enzymatic activity. Tartaric acid, when added to the incubation mixture, will not inhibit the enzyme fraction found in hairy-cell leukemia (isoenzyme 5).

Specimen. Smears, imprints, or frozen sections may be used. Fresh capillary smears are best; however, smears made from EDTA or heparinized blood are also adequate.

Reagents

1. Acid phosphatase fixative, pH 5.4; store at 4 to 10°C; good for 90 days. Discard if RBC morphology is poor.
   a. Dissolve 0.63 g citrate acid (F.W. 210.14) in 30 ml of deionized water.
   b. Add 10 ml of methanol and 60 ml of acetone.
   c. Mix and adjust the pH to 5.4 with concentrated NaOH solution.
2. 0.1 N acetate buffer, pH 5.2; store at 4°C; good for 90 days.
   a. 600 ml distilled water
   b. 13.6 g sodium acetate (F.W. 136.1)
   c. Adjust the pH to 5.2 with 1.0 M acetic acid. Bring the volume to 1000 ml with distilled water.
3. Tartrate sodium acetate buffer, pH 5.2; store at 4 to 10°C; good for 3 months.
   a. Dissolve 3.75 g of L-(+)-tartaric acid in 490 ml of 0.1 N acetate buffer.
   b. Adjust the pH to 5.2 with concentrated NaOH.
   c. Bring the volume to 500 ml with distilled water.
4. 0.1 M acetic acid
   a. 200 ml distilled water
   b. 1.25 ml glacial acetic acid (F.W. 60.05, 16N)
5. L-(+)-tartaric acid
6. Substrate solution: Store in glass-stoppered bottle at 4 to 10°C; good for 30 days. Discard if it turns pink.

a. Dissolve 100 mg naphthol AS-BI phosphoric acid in 10.0 ml N,N-dimethylformamide.
b. When used infrequently, make up fresh by adding 10 mg naphthol AS-BI phosphoric acid in 1.0 ml N,N-dimethylformamide.
7. 4 percent sodium nitrate solution: prepare daily.
   a. Dissolve 1.0 g $NaNO_2$ (F.W. 69.0) in distilled water to a volume of 25 ml.
8. 4 percent pararosaniline solution (possible carcinogen; see comments under nonspecific esterase). Store in brown bottle at 4 to 10°C; good for 90 days.
   a. Dissolve 1.0 g pararosaniline HCl (F.W. 323.8) in 20 ml distilled water plus 5 ml concentrated HCl. Solution may be gently heated to dissolve pararosaniline. Filter.
9. Mayer's hematoxylin
10. Acid alcohol solution
    Concentrated HCl   0.05 ml
    100 percent ethanol   3.5 ml
    Deionized water   996.5 ml
11. Blueing reagent
    $NaHCO_3$ 1 g
    Deionized water   100 ml

Procedure

1. Fix smears, imprints, or frozen section for 30 seconds with cold fixative.
2. Wash three times with deionized water. Air dry.
3. Incubate smears or imprints at 37°C in the appropriate filtered mixture:
   a. Acid phosphatase stain
      Acetate buffer   50 ml
      Stock substrate solution 2 ml
   In a separate container add 0.2 ml of 4 percent sodium nitrate solution to 0.2 ml of 4 percent pararosaniline solution. Wait 1 minute, and then add to buffer substrate solution.
   b. TRAP stain
      Acetate-tartrate buffer   50 ml
      Stock substrate solution   2 ml
   In a separate container add 0.2 ml of 4 percent sodium nitrate solution to 0.2 ml of 4 percent pararosaniline solution. Wait 1 minute, and then add to buffer substrate solution.
4. Incubate for 60 minutes at 37°C.
5. Wash three times in tap water.
6. Counterstain with hematoxylin for 2 minutes.
7. Rinse well with deionized water.
8. Place in blueing solution for 30 seconds.
9. Wash, dry, and mount with Permount. Frozen tissue sections must be dehydrated and cleared in xylene before mounting with Permount.

Interpretation. Acid phosphatase activity is shown by an orange-red precipitate with pararosaniline. The test result is considered positive when two or more cells are found with 4+ activity. Seven acid phosphatase isoenzymes have been identified in various blood cells. The fraction found in leukemic reticuloendotheliosis is resistant to the addition of L-(+)-tartaric acid (isoenzyme 5). In addition, when acid phosphatase is present in a localized (dotlike) fashion — that is, in the Golgi zone — there is evidence that this may be a marker for T lymphocytes. Increased activity is seen in myeloma cells.

Comments

1. A control must be run to be sure reagents are working.
2. Hexazotized reagents are unstable and must be used immediately.
3. Fixation keeps the enzyme from washing out of the cell during staining and improves the morphologic preservation of the cells.
4. Because these stains depend on enzymatic reactions, take care to preserve the enzyme activity by avoiding light, heat, and aging.
5. Smears can be kept at room temperature for at least 2 weeks without apparent loss of enzymatic activity.
6. After a couple of weeks, reaction products may precipitate out (salting-out phenomenon). This false-positive result should not be confused with the original stain.
7. Controls should be fixed, air dried, and stored at $-20°C$.
8. Increasing the temperature beyond $37°C$ causes inactivation of the enzyme and decomposition of the azo dye, resulting in nonspecific precipitation.
9. Mayer's hematoxylin as a counterstain gives a light gray tint to the cytoplasm of the leukocytes, which at times may mask some weak enzymatic activity. Methyl green gives poor nuclear detail, but it does not mask weak enzymatic activity in the cytoplasm.

Periodic Acid–Schiff Reaction

Purpose. Periodic acid–Schiff (PAS) stain is used in identifying M6 leukemias, and the reaction is negative in Burkitt's lymphoma.

Principle. Periodic acid–Schiff stains glycogen. Periodic acid oxidizes glycols to aldehydes. The aldehydes react with Schiff's reagent.

Specimen. Smears or imprints may be used. Anticoagulants do not inhibit activity. Paraffin tissue sections may also be used but sections must first be hydrated.

Reagents

1. Fixative: Store at room temperature. Expires in 1 year.
37 percent reagent-grade formalin	50 ml
Absolute ethanol	450 ml
2. 1 percent periodic acid: Store at room temperature. Expires in 3 months.
Periodic acid	5 g
Deionized water	500 ml
3. Schiff's reagent: Store at $4°C$. Expires in 3 months.
Basic fuschin Cl 42500	2.5 g
Deionized water	500 ml
Sodium metabisulfite	5 g
1 N HCl	50 ml

   Stir all ingredients for 2 hours, or until solution turns yellow (light amber). Add 4.0 g of activated charcoal. Filter until all charcoal is removed from solution. Do not use solution if it turns pink.
4. 0.5 percent sodium metabisulfite ($Na_2S_2O_5$): Store at room temperature. Expires in 3 months.
Sodium metabisulfite	2.5 g
Deionized water	500 ml
5. Hematoxylin (see hematoxylin counterstain)
6. Acid alcohol solution: Store at room temperature. Expires in 6 months.
1 percent HCl in 70 percent ethanol	2.5 ml
Deionized water	497.5 ml
7. 1 percent sodium bicarbonate solution. Store at room temperature. Expires in 6 months.
Sodium bicarbonate	5 g
Deionized water	500 ml

Procedure

1. Fix smears for 15 minutes. Paraffin tissue sections need to be hydrated if they have already been fixed.
2. Rinse gently in deionized water. Take extra care to rinse gently to avoid causing the smear partially to lift off the slide.
3. Place in periodic acid for 10 minutes.
4. Rinse in deionized water and dry.
5. Place dried smears in Schiff's reagent for 30 minutes.
6. Place in three 10-minute changes of metabisulfite solution.
7. Wash in deionized water for 10 minutes.
8. Counter stain with hematoxylin for 2 minutes.
9. Rinse in deionized water.
10. Place in sodium bicarbonate (blueing) solution for 30 seconds.
11. Rinse in deionized water, dry (tissue needs to be dehydrated), and mount with Permount.

Interpretation. Material that stains PAS positive appears bright-red. If neutrophils are present, they serve as a good auto positive control. The staining pattern may be granular, diffuse, or block. Lymphocytes, granulocytes, monocytes, and megakaryocytes may be positive. Normal erythroid precursors are negative. In M6 leukemia, the normoblasts usually stain positive, but normoblasts may also be positive in sideroblastic anemia, iron deficiency, thalassemia, and severe hemolytic anemias. Burkitt's lymphoma cells stain PAS negative. Ewing's sarcoma cells are PAS positive. Lymphocytic leukemia cells may or may not stain with a block pattern. Because PAS positivity may occur in acute lymphoblastic leukemia (ALL) and acute myeloblastic leukemia (AML), the PAS stain should not be used to distinguish AML from ALL.

Terminal Deoxynucleotidyl Transferase Test

Purpose. Terminal deoxynucleotidyl transferase (TdT) is an enzyme marker for primitive lymphocytic cells.

Principle. Terminal deoxynucleotidyl transferase is a deoxyribonucleic acid (DNA) polymerase, present in lymphocytic cells. Fluorescein isothiocyanate (FITC)–labeled goat antirabbit antibody is then incubated with the cells. If TdT is present in the nucleus of the cells, the positive cells will fluoresce.

Specimen. A nonheparinized bone marrow aspirate or one in which the cells have been separated and washed three times with culture media (RPMI-1640) and 2 percent fetal calf serum may be used. Peripheral blood may also be used; however, it requires special specimen collection. Store the slides at 4°C in the dark. Slides should be stained within a few days of preparation.

Reagents

1. Antiserum, Kit No. 9311 SB (Bethesda Research Laboratories)
2. Rabbit anticalf TdT, affinity purified IgG
3. Goat antirabbit IgG, FITC conjugated
   a. Every time a new batch of antisera is received, the plateau end-point of antibody activity should be determined. This is the highest dilution at which optimum staining occurs. If the antibody concentration is the same as the previous batch, it is usually acceptable to run one higher and one lower dilution, in addition to the regular one.
   b. Dilute antisera at optimum dilution using diluting media. An 8- to 10-fold dilution is recommended for the rabbit anticalf TdT, and a 70- to 100-fold dilution for the goat antirabbit TdT.
   c. Store anti-TdT at 4°C. Aliquot antirabbit antisera (20 lambda) and store at −20°C.
5. Diluting media: RPMI with 2 percent fetal calf serum and 0.1 percent sodium azide.
6. Phosphate buffered solution (PBS), pH 7.4

$NaH_2PO_4 \cdot H_2O$	0.4 g
Na_2HPO_4	1.6 g
NaCl	8.0 g

7. Mounting media (buffered glycerol)

Glycerol	90 ml
0.05 M Trizma 9.0	10 ml

8. Control
   a. Make cytopreps from a known ALL with a positive TdT.
   b. Air dry cytopreps.
   c. Wrap with plastic wrap.
   d. Freeze and store at −70°C.
   e. Bring to room temperature before unwrapping.
   f. Follow test procedure and treat as unknown sample.

Procedure

1. Circle an area rich in nucleated cells on the side with a diamond scribe. Fix slides in methanol at 4°C for 30 minutes.
2. Rinse well in PBS to remove all fixative. Do not air dry.
3. Hydrate the fixed slides in PBS for 5 minutes at room temperature.
4. Carefully wipe off all the sample on the slide outside the circle. Apply 10 μl of primary antibody (rabbit, anticalf TdT) onto this area and distribute it over the circle. Incubate for 30 minutes at room temperature in a humid chamber. It is very important that the slide does not dry out.
5. Wash slides with three changes of PBS over a period of 15 minutes to remove excess antibody. Wipe off all the excess PBS around the circle, being especially careful not to let the sample dry out.
6. Apply 15 μl of secondary antibody [FITC F(ab')$_2$ goat, antirabbit IgG] to the circled area of the slide and incubate for 30 minutes at room temperature in a humid chamber.
7. Repeat wash as in step 5.
8. Apply a small drop of mounting media and cover with a coverslip.
9. Examine the nuclei for fluorescence at 495 nm excitation with a Barrier filter. Record the intensity of fluorescence, 0 to 4+, and the percentage of cells that are positive. The preparation can be stored in the dark in the refrigerator for several days.

Interpretation. The majority of patients with T-cell and precursor B-cell ALL and lymphoma will have positive TdT activity. In addition, 50 percent of patients with acute undifferentiated leukemia, and 30 percent of patients in CML blast crisis will also have TdT activity. Approximately 5 percent of patients with AML will have TdT activity. In summary, TdT is a marker for primitive lymphoid cells.

Comments

1. Peripheral blood, bone marrow aspirate smears, or touch preps can be examined for TdT activity. The slides should be stored no longer than 7 days at room temperature. It is best to stain them as soon as possible.
2. A control slide should be run periodically and with each new lot number of reagents.

Cytochemical Stains

Table 30-III-1 describes the reactions of normal cells, leukemic blasts, and immature cells to cytochemical stains.

Immunologic Surface Markers

E Rosettes for Evaluation of T Cells

Purpose. E rosettes are to identify T cells that have receptors for sheep red blood cells (SRBCs).

Principle. Washed lymphocytes are incubated

Table 30–III–1. **CYTOCHEMICAL REACTIONS**

	Px	SBB	PAS	"Specific" Esterase (NCA)	"Nonspecific" Esterase (NA or NB)	αNA with NaF	αNA or αNB with NaFl
Normal Cells							
Granulocytes	4+	4+	4+*	4+	(+/−)	(+/−)	
Monocytes	2+	2+	2+*	−	4+	−	
Lymphocytes	−	−	−/+	−	−/+("dot")	−/+("dot")	
Platelets or megakaryocytes	−	−	2+	−	+/−		
Erythroid cells	−	−	−	−	−	−	
Leukemic Blasts and Immature Cells							
ALL	−	−	−/+*	−	−/+("dot")		−/+("dot")
AML	+	+	+*	+	(+/−)		(+/−)
AMML	+	+	+*	+	+		(+/−)
AMoL	+	+	+*	−	+		−
EL	−	−	+	−	−		−

Source: Mary Jo Fackler, B.Sc., M.T.(ASCP), S.H., with permission.
Px = peroxidase; SBB = Sudan black B; PAS = periodic acid–Schiff; NCA = naphthol AS-D chloroacetate; NA = α naphthol acetate; NB = α-naphthol butyrate; NaF = sodium fluoride; ALL = acute lymphoblastic leukemia; AML = acute myelogenous leukemia; AMML = acute myelomonocytic leukemia; AMoL = acute monocytic leukemia; El = erythroleukemia.
*Diffuse background staining of cytoplasm and fine PAS granulation.
"dot" = staining reaction confined to small circular area of cytoplasm.

with washed sheep red blood cells. The percentage and population of cells forming rosettes is determined.

Specimen. This includes blood, bone marrow aspirates, or fluids that have been anticoagulated with heparin or EDTA. The specimen should be less than 48 hours old.

Reagents

1. Culture media (RPMI 1640)
2. Heat-inactivated fetal calf serum. Thaw, dispense into 1-ml aliquots, and store −20°C.
3. Sheep red blood cells (SRBCs) (must be less than 2 weeks old)
4. Trypan blue solution stock solutions
   a. Trypan blue 0.2 percent
      1.0 g trypan blue
      500 ml deionized water
   b. NaCl 4.25 percent
      21.25 g NaCl
      500 ml deionized water
   c. Working solution: Make fresh.
   Add 100 μl 4.25 percent NaCl to 400 μl 0.2 percent trypan.

Procedure

1. Wash SRBCs with culture media three times.
2. Add 50 μl of SRBC pellet to 5 ml of culture media. Mix suspension.
3. Add an equal volume of SRBC suspension to an equal volume of a 4000 cell/mm³ lymphocyte suspension. (When there is ample lymphocyte suspension, use 0.5 ml of SRBCs and 0.5 ml of lymphocyte suspension.)
4. Incubate at 37°C for 15 minutes.
5. Centrifuge for 10 minutes at 1000 rpm.
6. Remove half of the supernatant, replace with an equal amount of heat-inactivated fetal calf serum. Do not disturb the cell button.
7. Incubate for 2 hours or overnight in refrigerator at 4°C.
8. Gently resuspend the button with a Pasteur pipette. Stop resuspension while there are still small visible clumps of cells present.
9. Add 100 μl of cell suspension to 100 μl of fresh trypan solution. Gently make a wet prep and record the percentage of viable cells that have three or more SRBCs attached.
10. Take 2 drops of the resuspended button (not trypan) and make a cytocentrifuge prep for a Wright's stain. Make extra preps if special stains are needed.

Comments

1. The Wright-stained cytocentrifuge prep is valuable in determining what population of cells is rosetting.
2. On a cytocentrifuge prep, true rosettes will be surrounded by SRBCs that have a stretched appearance.
3. Specimens from healthy individuals should be run as controls. They should have 60 to 80 percent T cells.
4. Viable cells do not stain with trypan. Dead cells cannot exclude trypan and stain blue.

Cytoplasmic Immunoglobulin (Immunofluorescent Method)

Purpose. The purpose of this procedure is to detect cytoplasmic immunoglobulin (CIg). Some lymphocytes lack surface immunoglobulins and SRBC receptors but do contain CIg. These cells are believed to be pre-B cells. Plasma cells also contain CIg.

Principle. Cells are fixed to expose CIg. Fluorescein-conjugated F(ab')$_2$ fragment antihuman IgM (or other immunoglobulin chain) is incubated with fixed cells and examined for the presence of cytoplasmic fluorescence.

Specimen. Use a fresh smear, tissue imprint, or cytocentrifuge preparation (cytoprep) of cells. A cytoprep made from a washed cell suspension is best, giving less background staining. Smears must be fresh. As the specimen ages, background fluorescence becomes a problem.

Reagents

1. Fluorescein conjugated antisera, produced in goat, F(ab')$_2$ fragment: Antihuman IgM, IgG, IgA, IgD, IgE, kappa, lambda.
   a. Determine optimal dilution with each new lot (usually between 1:10 and 1:20).
   b. Make appropriate dilution using culture media, with 0.1 percent sodium azide, and 2 percent fetal calf serum.
   c. Aliquot (150 to 200 μl) and store at $-20°$C.
2. Culture media (RPMI 1640)
3. Heat-inactivated fetal calf serum (FCS)
4. Culture media with 2 percent FCS and 0.1 percent azide
Culture	500 ml
FCS	10 ml
Sodium azide	500 mg
5. Fixative: Make fresh
Absolute ethanol	47.5 ml
Acetic acid	2.5 ml
6. PBS, 0.14 M, pH 7.4
NaH$_2$PO$_4$ · H$_2$O (F.W. 137.99)	4 g
Na$_2$HPO$_4$ (F.W. 141.96)	16 g
NaCl	80 g
Deionized water	10 l
7. Glycerol-Gelvatol mounting media; good for 5 months at 4°C.
   a. Dissolve 1.5 g Trizma 9.0 in 240 ml deionized water.
   b. Add 60 g of Gelvatol and stir overnight to dissolve.
   c. Add 120 ml glycerol and stir overnight.
   d. Spin at 10,000g for 30 minutes, and store in syringes.

Procedure

1. With a diamond marker, etch a circle around the cells to be stained. Wipe off extra cells with a Kimwipe.
2. Fix smear for 10 minutes at 4°C.
3. Rinse smear in PBS.
4. Do not allow smear to air dry.
5. Wash smear for 10 minutes with PBS.
6. Distribute 100 μl of antiserum onto the inside of circle. Incubate for 30 minutes at room temperature in a humid chamber.
7. Wash smear for 15 minutes with PBS.
8. Apply a small drop of mounting media and coverslip smear.
9. Using the 63 oil objective, and epifluorescence with FITC filter, examine the cytoplasm of the cells for fluorescence. Do not mistake the autofluorescence of eosinophilic granules for cytoplasmic fluorescence.
10. Report the degree and pattern of fluorescence, and the percentage of cells positive.

Comments. Smears should be fresh. As the smear ages, background fluorescence becomes a problem. Immediately after fixation, it is important to rinse smears before they are allowed to dry.

Surface Immunoglobulins

Purpose. This procedure is to identify B cells that have surface-bound immunoglobulins.

Principle. Monospecific fluorescein-conjugated F(ab')$_2$ antisera are incubated at 4°C to detect surface-bound immunoglobulins.

Specimen. Blood, bone marrow aspirates, or fluids that have been anticoagulated with heparin or EDTA. The specimen should be less than 48 hours old.

Reagents

1. Antiserum:
   a. Antihuman IgG, fluorescein-conjugated antisera, produced in goat F(ab')$_2$ fragment
   b. Antihuman IgA, fluorescein-conjugated antisera, produced in goat F(ab')$_2$ fragment
   c. Antihuman IgM, fluorescein-conjugated antisera, produced in goat F(ab')$_2$ fragment
   d. Antihuman IgD, fluorescein-conjugated antisera, produced in goat F(ab')$_2$ fragment
   e. Antihuman albumin, fluorescein-conjugated antisera, produced in goat.
   f. Antihuman kappa (κ) light chain, fluorescein-conjugated antisera, produced in goat F(ab')$_2$ fragment.
   g. Antihuman lambda (λ) light chain, fluorescein-conjugated antisera, produced in rabbit (may substitute goat). F(ab')$_2$ fragment.
   h. Fluorescein-conjugated antiserum to total human gamma globulins. Produced in goat F(ab')$_2$ fragment.
   i. Normal rabbit serum, 2.5-ml vial.
2. Ficoll-Hypaque, density gradient media
3. Culture media (RPMI 1640)
4. Fetal calf serum (FCS), heat-inactivated. Keep at 20°C for long-term storage.
5. Diluting media: Culture media with 2 percent FCS, 0.1 percent azide, store at 4°C.
Culture media	500 ml
FCS (heat-inactivated)	10 ml
Sodium azide	500 mg
6. Mounting media (buffered glycerol); store at 4°C.

Glycerol	90 ml
Trizma 9.0, 0.05 M	10 ml

7. Culture media with 0.5 percent sodium azide; store at 4°C.

Culture media	500 ml
Sodium azide	250 mg

Procedure

1. Separate cells by using Ficoll-Hypaque density gradient procedure.
2. Incubate the cell suspension in culture media at 37°C on rocket for 45 minutes to remove cytophilic antibodies.
3. Spin down cell suspension at 1000 rpm for 10 minutes and pour off supernatant. Adjust cell count 4.0×10^6/ml with 37°C culture media.
4. Place 500 μl of the cell suspension in microfuge tubes. Centrifuge for 5 seconds. Remove the supernatant. (The pellicles will contain approximately 2.0×10^6 cells.) Centrifuge antiserum for 4 minutes before using.
5. Add 100 μl of supernatant of a 1:10 dilution of fluorescein-conjugated antiserum to the cell button and gently resuspend the cells. (Antiserum is diluted with culture media and aliquots of 200 μl are stored frozen at -20°C.)
6. Cap the tubes and incubate at 4°C for 45 minutes. [For patients known to have chronic lymphocytic leukemia (CLL), incubate for 60 minutes.]
7. Make cytoprep of the cell suspension for Wright's and special stains.
8. Following incubation, wash the cells three times with cold culture media containing 0.05 percent sodium azide (25 mg azide/50 ml culture media).
9. After the last wash, remove all of the supernatant and add 1 drop of buffered glycerol.
10. Resuspend the cells and make a wet mount.
11. Examine the preparation under a fluorescent microscope. (Xenon epifluorescence is recommended.) If wet prep is not to be looked at immediately, store slides on slide tray in refrigerator.

Comments

1. Avoid excessive exposure of antiserum to light.
2. For best results, the slides should be read immediately.
3. The Wright's stain cytoprep should be examined and a differential done.
4. By using F(ab')$_2$ fragment antiserum, the nonspecific binding of lymphocytes and monocytes for the Fc portion of the antibody can be eliminated.
5. Immunoglobulin bearing lymphocytes (B cells) have a stippled or dusty stained pattern (apple-green fluorescence) around the circumference of the cell. Some cells, especially lymphoma cells, may show prominent capped staining.

Indirect Immunofluorescence Using Monoclonal Antibodies (for Evaluation of Lymphocyte Subsets)

Purpose. This procedure is used to recognize lymphocyte cell types by identifying specific antigens on the surface of the cells.

Principle. Cells are separated from blood or tissue and incubated with monoclonal antibodies produced by mouse hybridoma cell lines. Indirect immunofluorescence and phase microscopy or a flow cytometer are used to identify the cell types.

Specimen. Bone marrow aspirate or peripheral blood with adequate numbers of the cells in question may be used. A cell suspension is prepared using the Ficoll-Hypaque method of cell separation to obtain a mononuclear cell population.

Reagents

1. Antisera
   a. Becton Dickinson monoclonal antisera
      OKT antisera
      CALLA antiserum
   b. Coulter clone antisera (Coulter Immunology)
   c. Secondary antibody, FTC-conjugated anti-mouse IgG
2. Culture media (RPMI 1640)
3. FCS, heat-inactivated
4. Sodium azide
5. Diluting media: Culture media with 2 percent FCS and 0.1 percent sodium azide. After optimal dilutions are determined, the remaining concentrated antisera may be diluted, aliquoted, and stored at -20°C. For dilution of all antisera, the following diluting media should be used:

Culture media	500 ml
FCS, heat-inactivated	10 ml
Sodium azide	500 mg

6. Antisera dilutions
   a. Every time a new batch of antisera is received, the plateau end-point of antibody activity should be determined. This is the highest dilution at which optimum staining occurs. If the antibody concentration is the same as the previous batch, it is usually acceptable to run one higher and one lower dilution in addition to the regular one.
   b. Protocol for freezing reconstituted Coulter clone monoclonal antibody
      (1) Reconstitute the antibody with 500 μl of distilled water.
      (2) Dilute the reconstituted antibody solution prior to freezing according to manufacturer's directions.
      (3) Aliquot 110 to 120 μl of antibody solution into micro Eppendorf centrifuge tubes. Store at -20°C.
      (4) To use this material, allow the solution to return to room temperature. Centrifuge for 4 minutes at 4000 rpm.

Procedure

1. Follow the cell separation procedure and adjust cell concentration to 4×10^6 cells per ml.
2. Place 0.5 ml of the cell suspension in microfuge tubes. Centrifuge for 15 seconds and remove supernatant.
3. Add 0.100 ml of the thawed monoclonal aliquot. Resuspend cells and incubate at 4°C for 30 minutes. (Note: If antiserum is stored at −20°C, it should be centrifuged for 4 minutes after thawing.)
4. Wash cells once with 4°C culture media.
5. Add 0.100 ml of the secondary antibody to each monoclonal that was set up. Resuspend cells and incubate at 4°C for 30 minutes.
6. Wash cells three times with 4°C culture media.
7. After last wash, remove all of the supernatant and add 1 drop of buffered glycerol to cell button.
8. Resuspend the cells and make a wet mount.
9. Examine the preparation with a fluorescent microscope (blue light excitation). If the wet prep is not to be examined immediately, store the slides in the refrigerator.

Interpretation. Positive cells stain green with a granular appearance on the surface of the cell. Dead cells fluoresce diffusely and should not be included in the count. It is important to use phase microscopy in addition to fluorescent microscopy to determine what population of cells is positive. This is especially important when working with cell suspensions that have more than one cell type (for example, suspensions from CLL patients with low WBC counts generally contain a higher percentage of normal lymphocytes than do those from CLL patients with high WBC counts). Low counts generally make it more difficult to assess the surface marker phenotype of the malignant cells. Correlate all findings.

Comments

1. Avoid excessive exposure of antiserum to light.
2. For best results, the slides should be read immediately.

LASER-BASED FLOW CYTOMETRY

Flow cytometry (FCM) is an automated method used to measure cells or particles as they flow single-file through a sensing area. Sensing can be accomplished electronically, as done by the Coulter principle, or optically. The term flow cytometry is commonly used to denote the optical type. Optical sensing is done with an intense light source, usually a laser or mercury-arc lamp. These instruments measure light scatter and fluorescent signals generated as cells pass through a light beam. This review will focus on the main components of laser-based FCM and its clinical applications.

Flow Cytometry Components

The four main components of FCM (Fig. 30-III-1) include the fluidics (or cell transportation system), a laser for cell illumination, photodetectors for signal detection, and a computer-based management system. The fluidics are regulated by pressurized gas, usually nitrogen. Cells suspended in fluid are transported to a flow tip where the sample is surrounded by a liquid sheath. The sheath and sample stream both exit the flow chamber through a small orifice (usually 75 μm). This laminar flow design confines cells to the center of the sheath and can be adjusted to obtain single-file alignment of cells.

As a cell enters the laser beam, light is scattered through 360 degrees. Forward-angle light scatter (FALS, 2 to 10 degrees) provides information relevant to the cell size. Light scattered at 90 degrees (90° LS) reflects cellular structure or granularity. In addition to light scatter, fluorescent signals can also be measured when cells are tagged with appropriate dyes. Fluorescence occurs when a chemical absorbs light, causing its electrons to be excited briefly to a higher, less-stable energy state. As the electrons return to their resting state, light at a longer wavelength (lower energy) than the initial exciting light is emitted. Laser-based FCM is well adapted for measurement of fluorescence because it provides a stable source of coherent monochromatic light. Proper alignment of this intense light beam with the sample stream is required for optimal signal production. Many flow systems use argon gas, which generates a strong laser line at 480 nm. Fluorescein isothiocyanate (FITC), phycoerythrin (PE), and propidium iodide (PI) are popular dyes for these systems, because they are excited at 488 nm.

Detection and conversion of light signals into electrical signals are accomplished by a series of photodetectors and photomultiplier tubes (PMTs). The PMTs also serve to amplify the light signals. An assembly of filters and mirrors directs the light to various detectors. A clinical FCM system typically has a photodetector for FALS, a PMT for 90LS, and one or two PMTs for fluorescence detection. These photodetectors can be adjusted to manipulate the intensity of single output. The filter assembly used in conjunction with the photodetection system can also be adjusted for sensitivity to different fluorescent emissions.

The heart of the FCM system is the computer, which controls the instrument's operation, data collection, storage, and analysis. The computer capabilities vary among different instruments, and computer software is in a constant state of development. The beauty of FCM lies in the user's ability, through computer control, to create different test systems or profiles for the analysis of multiple sample types. Different combinations of parameters can be measured as needed. For example, simultaneous evaluation of FALS and 90LS allows for separation of peripheral blood leukocytes on the basis of size and internal cell structure (such as granularity). Lymphocytes, monocytes, and granulocytes fall

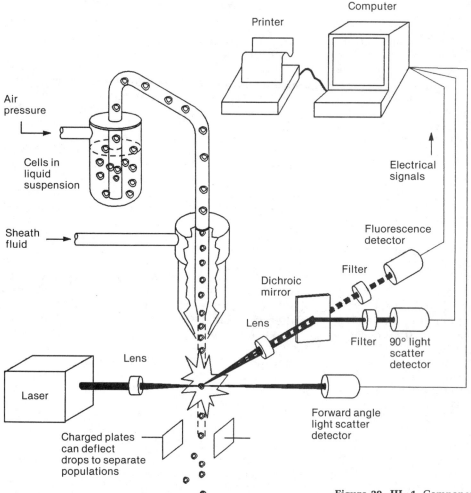

Figure 30–III–1. Components of a laser-based flow cytometer.

into three separate populations by these criteria (Fig. 30-III-2). Further manipulation can be done by placing "electronic gates" around the population of interest. In this way, fluorescence of just lymphocytes, or of another population, can be measured. Other combinations of parameters and gating can be used, depending on the needs of the investigator.

Some FCM systems have the additional option of cell sorting. Cells flow through the laser beam, where they produce light scatter and fluorescent signals, and then continue their movement downstream. Vibration of the sample stream causes droplets to form that contain single cells. Those droplets that have cells meeting the sorting criteria are electronically charged and deflected in an electromagnetic field. In this way, purified cell populations can be collected for further studies.

Clinical Applications

Laser-based FCM is relatively new to the clinical laboratory. Its greatest contribution has been in the detection of lymphocyte cell surface markers and DNA analysis. Other clinical uses of flow technology include assessment of phagocytosis, reticulocyte counts, human leukocyte antigen (HLA) crossmatching, detection of platelet autoantibodies,

evaluation of spermatogenesis, cell kinetic studies, and rare event analysis such as detection of small numbers of lymphoma cells in the peripheral blood. This is only a partial list and one that is still growing.

The basis of cell surface marker studies is the ex-

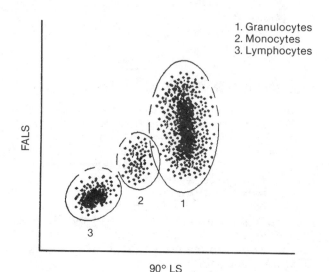

Figure 30–III–2. Peripheral blood leukocyte analysis by simultaneous evaluation of FALS and 90°LS.

istence of specific proteins on the surface of cells that distinguish one cell line from another. Evaluation of lymphocyte subsets most clearly exemplifies this. Helper and suppressor lymphocytes have glycoproteins on their surface that are unique to each. Through the use of monoclonal antibodies against these proteins coupled with fluorescent dyes, it is possible to distinguish and quantitate these subsets. Lymphocyte subset evaluation is useful for investigating a number of immunologic conditions and disorders, including leukemias and lymphomas, acquired immunodeficiency syndrome (AIDS) and other immunodeficiencies, transplant rejection, and autoimmune diseases.

Cells for evaluation of surface markers can be obtained from whole blood, Ficoll-Hypaque separation, bone marrow aspirates, body fluids, or solid tissue such as lymph nodes that are disrupted to release cells into suspension. Samples can be evaluated rapidly (up to 10,000 cells per second) and quantitatively, eliminating some of the human subjectivity encountered with the microscope.

Flow cytometric DNA analysis is accomplished by exposing cellular DNA to dyes such as PI that stoichiometrically bind to DNA. The more DNA present, the stronger the fluorescent signal produced. Cells at different stages of the cell cycle have different but predictable amounts of DNA. Thus, a normal resting cell will produce a 2 N peak (diploid); whereas a cell in mitosis, just before cell division, will have twice as much DNA (4 N, or tetraploid). Malignant cells tend to have abnormal amounts of DNA (aneuploidy). Measurement of DNA ploidy and cell proliferation in tumors has been applied to cancer detection and attempts to grade some cancers. Frequency of aneuploidy varies with the type of neoplasm, and its detection depends on the resolving power of the FCM system.

In summary, laser-based FCM systems provide a versatile and powerful tool for laboratory studies. Any particle that can be put into suspension and tagged with a fluorescent marker is fair game for analysis by this technique. Clinical laboratories are currently using these systems for a vast array of studies. Undoubtedly, as more laboratories gain access to these new instruments, the number of clinical uses will grow.

QUESTIONS

1. A 57-year-old woman has a LAP score of 22. What is a possible clinical correlation for this score?
   a. Normal
   b. Leukemoid reaction
   c. Chronic granulocytic leukemia
   d. Myelofibrosis

2. In which condition would the majority of cells stain positive with myeloperoxidase and Sudan Black B?
   a. Acute lymphocytic leukemia
   b. Chronic myelogenous leukemia
   c. Chronic lymphocytic leukemia
   d. Erythroleukemia

3. Which of the following cells would stain positive using Sudan black B?
   a. Myeloblast
   b. Monocyte
   c. Promyelocyte
   d. All of the above

4. Which of the following cells would stain positive using the specific esterase stain?
   a. Megakaryocytes
   b. Macrophages
   c. Neutrophils
   d. Lymphocytes

5. Which cell would stain diffusely positive using the nonspecific esterase stain?
   a. Monocyte
   b. Histiocyte
   c. Lymphocyte
   d. Myelocyte

6. For which of the following diseases would the acid phosphatase/TRAP stain have diagnostic value?
   a. Hairy-cell leukemia
   b. Burkitt's lymphoma
   c. Lymphocytic leukemia
   d. Erythroleukemia

7. Which condition(s) show(s) positive TdT activity?
   a. T-cell ALL
   b. Null-cell ALL
   c. Pre-B ALL
   d. All of the above

8. What is the principle of the E-rosette test for detecting T cells?
   a. Sheep red cells will lyse in the presence of T cells and complement
   b. T cells have receptors for sheep red cells
   c. Sheep red cells have receptors for T cells
   d. Sheep red cells bind all white cells except T cells

9. What type of cell(s) is/are detected by the immunofluorescent method for cytoplasmic immunoglobulin (CIg)?
   a. Pre-B and plasma cells
   b. T cells
   c. T cells and B cells
   d. Null cells

10. Which methodology uses fluorescent-labeled monoclonal antibodies to detect lymphocyte subsets by measuring light scatter and fluorescent signals generated as cells pass through a laser light beam?
    a. Automated leukocyte differential
    b. Flow cytometry
    c. Electromagnetic conductivity
    d. None of the above

Answers to Section III questions are found on page 617.

Coagulation

OBJECTIVES

At the end of this section, the learner should be able to:
1. Explain the diagnostic use of a bleeding time.
2. Explain the principle of platelet retention.
3. List some basic requirements for platelet aggregation as an in vitro means of evaluating platelet function.
4. Correlate platelet aggregation results with clinical conditions.
5. Explain the use of the whole blood clotting time.
6. Explain the use of the activated partial thromboplastin time.
7. Explain the use of the prothrombin time.
8. Describe the basis for one-stage quantitative factor assays.
9. Explain the use of the Stypven time test (Russell's viper venom time test).
10. Explain the indications for use of the prothrombin consumption test.
11. Explain the use of the thrombin time.
12. Characterize the reptilase time.
13. List conditions having low and high fibrinogen levels.
14. Interpret a factor XIII screening test.
15. Relate clinical conditions to measurements of factor VIII–related antigen.
16. List methods employed for measuring the natural anticoagulant antithrombin III.

17. Identify methods for laboratory diagnosis of protein C deficiency.
18. Define pathologic anticoagulants.
19. Identify an activated partial thromboplastin time result that indicates presence of circulating anticoagulants.
20. List criteria for the laboratory detection of lupus inhibitors.
21. Name confirmatory tests for lupus anticoagulants.
22. Explain the use of the latex agglutination test in the diagnosis of disseminated intravascular coagulation.
23. Name a test for measuring plasmin's action on the fibrin clot.
24. Name a test that evaluates fibrinolytic activity by measuring plasminogen activator concentration.

GENERAL POINTS REGARDING COAGULATION PROCEDURES

1. Most coagulation procedures are performed on plasma, thereby requiring the addition of calcium in order to perform the tests.
2. Testing is performed at $37°C \pm 1°$.
3. Each laboratory should develop its own normal values reflective of the methodology, reagents, instrumentation, and patient population.
4. Sodium citrate (3.2 percent or 3.8 percent) is the anticoagulant used for routine coagulation procedures. Other anticoagulants such as ethylenediaminetetraacetic acid (EDTA), heparin, and oxalate are unacceptable.
5. The ratio of blood to anticoagulant should be 9:1. This may vary as long as the final concentration of sodium citrate remains 3.2 percent or 3.8 percent of the final blood mixture. The disproportion of anticoagulant to blood is seen in patients with polycythemia and those with moderate to severe anemia.
6. Immunologic assays are currently available for several coagulation factors, inhibitors, and proteins involved in fibrinolysis. Because these assays determine the presence or absence of these proteins and not their biologic activity, the tests should be performed in conjunction with various clotting tests.
7. Enzyme-specific synthetic substrates: In the past, evaluation of hemostasis has relied upon the traditional procedures based upon the detection of a clot. The innovation of enzyme-specific synthetic substrates has had a great impact on the field of hemostasis. With the knowledge of the molecular structures for different enzymes and their cleavage points at their corresponding substrate factors, it has been possible to develop synthetic substrates that are cleaved by a single factor enzyme. Synthesis of synthetic substrates occurs when the amino acids of the substrate on the molecule fit into the active sites and the binding sites of the enzyme. All the synthetic substrates rely on cleavage of the peptide by their specific enzymes, releasing a chromogenic complex such as paranitroaniline or a fluorogenic complex such as aminoisophthalic acid dimethyl ester (AIE), which may be detected and measured by means of a spectrophotometer or fluorimeter. Various synthetic chromogenic and fluorogenic assays exist for the evaluation of plasmin, plasminogen activator, α_2-antiplasmin, kallikrein, antithrombin III (AT-III), factor Xa, thrombin, and several other serine proteases, making these assays applicable for routine laboratory testing.

Procedures using synthetic substrates have numerous advantages over the traditional clot formation techniques. They are rapid and sensitive, have a greater degree of standardization, require smaller sample volumes, and are well suited for automation. Synthetic substrates allow for the activity of clotting factors as well as their inhibitors to be measured. Often individual stages of a reaction can be assayed without having to observe the entire cascade of the clotting process. As the field of blood coagulation continues to undergo major technical advancement, the use of synthetic substrates will certainly gain increasing significance and may replace many of the time-honored clotting tests currently used in the routine clinical laboratory.

PLATELET FUNCTION TESTS
Bleeding Time

Principle. Bleeding time is defined as the time taken for a standardized skin wound to stop bleeding. Upon vessel injury, platelets adhere and form a hemostatic platelet plug. Bleeding time measures the ability of these platelets to arrest bleeding and therefore measures platelet number and function. Capillary contractility, as well as both the intrinsic and the extrinsic systems of coagulation, functions in a minor capacity in the bleeding time. Bleeding time is measured as a screening procedure used to detect both congenital and acquired disorders of platelet function. The bleeding time assesses in vivo platelet function.

There are several methods of measuring the bleeding time. The Duke method[1] is performed by puncturing the earlobe with a lancet, making a 3-mm deep incision. This method is not easily standardized and is rather insensitive. Prolonged bleeding times occur in severe platelet disorders. In recent years a new device to perform bleeding time tests has been introduced in the coagulation laboratory. The Surgicutt device by International Technidyne Corporation is gaining popularity because it causes less pain for the patient and tends to give a more uniform cut. The pros and cons of each method and device for measuring the bleeding time should be weighed by each laboratory when choosing a procedure.

Duke Method

Reagents and Equipment

Sterile disposable lancet
Filter paper disc (Whatman No. 1)
Stopwatch
Alcohol wipes

Procedure

1. Cleanse the site (earlobe) with alcohol. Allow it to dry.
2. Pierce the earlobe with the lancet, making the incision 3 mm deep. Start the stopwatch.
3. Blot the blood with the filter paper at regular 30-second intervals. Move the filter paper so that each drop of blood touches a clean area. Do not touch the incision with the filter paper.
4. When the filter paper no longer shows signs of blood, stop the stopwatch and record the time.

Interpretation. Normal values range from 0 to 6 minutes.

Comments. If the patient continues to bleed after 15 minutes, stop the test and apply pressure to the wound.

Ivy Method

Reagents and Equipment

Sphygmomanometer
Sterile, disposable lancet
Stopwatch
Filter paper disc (Whatman No. 1)
Alcohol wipes

Procedure

1. Place a blood pressure cuff on the patient's arm above the elbow. Inflate the cuff and maintain pressure at 40 mmHg.
2. Cleanse the outer surface of the patient's forearm with alcohol. The area should be free of all superficial veins.
3. Holding the skin tightly, make three small punctures about 3 mm deep and 1.5 cm apart. Start the stopwatch.
4. Blot the blood at regular 30-second intervals with the filter paper. Move the filter paper so that each drop of blood touches a clean area. Do not touch any of the incisions with the filter paper.
5. When the filter paper no longer shows signs of blood, stop the stopwatch.
6. The average of the times for bleeding to stop

from the three puncture sites is recorded as the bleeding time.

Interpretation. Normal values range from 1 to 6 minutes.

Comments. If the patient continues to bleed after 15 minutes, terminate the test and apply pressure to the wound. If a superficial vein is punctured during the procedure, the bleeding time will be falsely prolonged. Repeat the test. Should bleeding not cease at any one of the puncture sites, average the bleeding time of the two other sites.

Simplate Method[3]

This is a standardized bleeding time procedure that is a modification of the template procedure employing a commercially available device, Simplate.

Caution: Each patient should be informed that with any bleeding time procedure, the possibility of faint scarring exists. Keloid formation, although rare, may occur with certain patients.

Materials

1. Simplate is a sterile disposable device used to make uniform incisions. When the spring-loaded blade is triggered on the forearm, an incision 5 mm by 1 mm is made. Simplate II makes duplicate incisions.
2. Sphygmomanometer
3. Timer (stopwatch) with sweep second hand
4. Filter paper disc (Whatman No. 1)
5. Alcohol sponge
6. Butterfly bandage and covering bandage

Procedure

1. The preferred site for the bleeding time test is the muscular area over the lateral aspect of the forearm approximately 5 cm below the antecubital crease. Take care to avoid surface veins, scars, and bruises. Place a sphygmomanometer cuff on the upper arm, cleanse the site with an alcohol sponge, and allow the area to air dry at least 30 seconds. If the patient has marked hair, lightly shave the area.
2. Remove the Simplate II from the blister pack, and twist off the white, tear-away tab on the side of the device. Do not push the trigger or touch the blade slot. Inflate the sphygmomanometer cuff to 40 mmHg. The time between inflation of cuff and incision should be 30 to 60 seconds. Monitor pressure frequently to ensure maintenance of pressure during test procedure.
3. Place Simplate II firmly on the forearm parallel to the fold of the elbow. Do not press.
4. Depress the trigger and simultaneously start the timer. Remove the Simplate II approximately 1 second after triggering.
5. At 30 seconds, blot the flow of blood with filter paper. Bring the filter paper close to the incisions without touching the edges of the wounds. (Do not disturb either platelet plug.) Blot in a similar manner every 30 seconds until

blood no longer stains the filter paper. Stop timer.

6. Remove cuff, clean arm with water. (Do not use alcohol sponge; alcohol on open incisions will increase scarring tendency.) Apply both a butterfly and a covering bandage across the incision. Ask the patient to keep the bandages in place for 24 hours. Record the bleeding time to the nearest 30 seconds and average test results. Return the device to the opened blister pack and discard in a biohazard container.

Hints on Technique

1. The pressure placed on the Simplate will affect the bleeding time.
2. The incision(s) may be made either parallel or perpendicular to the fold of the elbow. Results will vary depending on the direction of the incision; therefore, one direction should be used consistently.
3. If two incisions are made, the results should be recorded within 1½ minutes of each other.
4. Blood should flow freely within 20 seconds after incision is made.

Interpretation. Normal values range from 2.3 to 9.5 minutes. Owing to variations in technique and patient population, it is recommended that each laboratory establish its own "normal" values.

Surgicutt Method[2]

This is a standardized bleeding time procedure that is a modification of the template procedure employing a commercially available device.

Caution: Each patient should be informed that with any bleeding time procedure, the possibility of faint scarring exists. Keloid formation, although rare, may occur with certain patients.

Materials

1. Sterile Surgicutt device
2. Stopwatch, with seconds available
3. Sphygmomanometer
4. Filter paper disc (Whatman No. 1)
5. Alcohol swab
6. Butterfly bandage and covering bandage

Procedure. Before a bleeding time is measured, it is important that a platelet count from within the past 24 hours be available. Bleeding time should be measured only if the patient has a platelet count of greater than 100,000 per mm³.

1. Place the patient's arm on a steady support with the muscular area over the lateral aspect of the forearm exposed. The preferred site for the procedure is 5 cm below the antecubital crease. Take care to avoid surface veins, scars, and bruises. If the patient has a notable amount of hair, lightly shave the area first.
2. Place the sphygmomanometer to 40 mmHg. The time between inflation of the cuff and the incision should be between 30 and 60 seconds. Hold at this pressure for the duration of the test.
3. Cleanse the arm with an appropriate swab and allow it to air dry.
4. Remove the Surgicutt device from the blister pack, being careful not to contaminate the instrument by touching or resting the blade-slot end on any unsterile surface.
5. Remove the safety clip.
6. Hold the Surgicutt device securely between thumb and middle finger.
7. Gently rest the device horizontally on the patient's forearm and apply minimal pressure so that both ends of the instrument are lightly touching the skin.
8. Push the trigger and start the stopwatch simultaneously. The blade will make an incision 5 mm long by 1 mm deep.
9. Remove the Surgicutt device from the patient's forearm immediately after making the incision.
10. After 30 seconds, blot the flow of blood with filter paper. Bring the filter paper close to the incision, but do not touch the paper directly to the incision, so as not to disturb the formation of a platelet plug.
11. Blot the blood every 30 seconds thereafter until blood no longer stains the paper. Stop the timer. Bleeding time is determined to the nearest 30 seconds. If the bleeding continues after 15 minutes, terminate the test and apply pressure to the incision site. Report the bleeding time as greater than 15 minutes.
12. Remove the blood pressure cuff and carefully cleanse around the incision site with alcohol. Apply butterfly bandage vertically and keep in place for 24 hours to prevent scarring.

Interpretation

1. Normal values are from 2.5 to 9.5 minutes. Owing to variations in technique and patient population, it is recommended that each laboratory establish its own "normal" values.
2. Prolonged bleeding times are found in the following situations:
   a. Thrombocytopenia: Platelet counts less than 100,000 per mm³
   b. Platelet dysfunction
   c. After the administration of aspirin or aspirin-containing drugs
   d. After the administration of other drugs that inhibit platelet function such as antihistamines

Notes

1. If the incision fails to bleed or if a small vein is cut, disregard the bleeding time of the incision and repeat test.
2. The bleeding time should be measured in the diagnostic work-up of a qualitative platelet disorder, not for the evaluation of a coagulation factor deficiency.

General Comments Regarding Bleeding Time

Prolonged bleeding times are seen in patients with platelet counts of less than 100,000 per mm³. With platelet counts below this level, the bleeding time increases proportionately to the decrease in platelet count. The use of aspirin, aspirin-containing drugs, and antihistamines causes a prolonged bleeding time. The patient should be instructed not to take any aspirin or drugs containing aspirin for 1 week prior to the test. The bleeding time should be measured in the diagnostic work-up of a qualitative platelet disorder.

Clot Retraction

Principle. In a normal blood specimen, a clot after the first hour should be firm and retract from the walls of the test tube. The process of retraction is influenced by platelet number and activity, fibrinogen concentration, packed red cell volume, and excessive fibrinolytic activity.

Reagents and Equipment

37°C waterbath
Plastic syringe
21-gauge needle
13 × 100 test tube

Procedure

1. A blood sample is allowed to clot in a test tube.
2. The clotted specimen is incubated at 37°C, and inspected at 1 and 24 hours.
3. Clot retraction should be recorded as normal or defective. Complete retraction occurs when about half the total volume is serum and the other half clot. Clot retraction may also be recorded as normal or defective, based on a normal retraction of about 50 percent.

Interpretation. Normal clot retraction starts in 1 hour and is complete in 24 hours.

Comments. Clot retraction is poor in patients whose platelet count is less than 100,000 per mm³ (0.10 × 10¹² /liter) and in those with Glanzmann's thrombasthenia. Erythrocytosis results in increased red blood cell (RBC) fallout. Anemia facilitates clot retraction resulting in a small clot. In hypofibrinogenemic conditions, the clot is small with evidence of increased RBC fallout. In states of disseminated intravascular coagulation (DIC) the clot appears small and ragged with evidence of RBC fallout. Rapid dissolution of the clot is evidence of increased fibrinolytic activity.

Platelet Retention/Adhesion

Principle. This in vitro test is designed to measure the ability of platelets to adhere to glass surfaces. When anticoagulated blood is passed through a column of glass beads at a constant rate, some platelets will be retained by the glass beads. The percentage of platelets retained by the glass beads is calculated from the difference between platelet counts before and after passage through the glass bead column. It is not certain what aspects of platelet function are involved; however, it is probable that both adhesion to the glass beads and the formation of platelet aggregates cause platelet retention.[4]

Reagents and Equipment. All necessary reagents and equipment used in the Bowie and Owens[5] modification of platelet retention are available though Pacific Hemostasis Laboratories, Los Angeles.

Procedure

1. Draw 12 ml of blood from a clean venipuncture into a 20-ml plastic syringe. To prevent thrombin generation and the loss of platelet function and platelet count, the time taken to draw the sample should be no longer than 60 seconds.
2. Immediately aliquot 1.0 ml of whole blood into an EDTA tube.
3. Label this tube as the control.
4. Connect the syringe to the column. Insert the syringe into the perfusion pump.
5. Start the pump at a rate of 5.8 ml of blood per minute.
6. Collect the first 1 ml of blood after passage through the column into an EDTA tube. Label 1. Collect the second 1-ml aliquot of blood into an EDTA tube labeled 2. Collect the third 1-ml aliquot of blood into an EDTA tube labeled 3.
7. Perform platelet counts on tubes 1, 2, 3, and control.
8. Properly discard the rest of the blood, syringe, and column.
9. Calculate platelet retention (PR) as shown here (PC = platelet count):

$$PR = \frac{\text{Control tube PC} - \text{Tube 3 PC}}{\text{Control tube PC}} \times 100$$

Interpretation. Normal range is 75 to 95 percent platelet retention.

Comments. Decreased platelet retention is seen in patients with hereditary disorders such as Glanzmann's thrombasthenia, von Willebrand's disease, Bernard-Soulier syndrome, and Chédiak-Higashi syndrome. The acquired disorders associated with decreased platelet retention include some of the myeloproliferative disorders, plasma cell dyscrasias, uremia, and ingestion of aspirin and other drugs. Increased platelet retention has been reported in individuals with thrombotic disorders such as venous thrombosis, pulmonary emboli, hyperlipidemia, and carcinomas. It also occurs in patients taking oral contraceptives and those who are pregnant. Normal platelet retention is seen in patients with a factor deficiency and in those receiving anticoagulant therapy.

Factors that influence platelet retention are the size of the glass beads, the length of the column, the type of plastic used in the column, the degree of packing of the column, the rate of blood flow, and the packed cell volume. The value of platelet retention in the diagnosis of von Willebrand's disease is still questionable, as different methods yield varying results.[6]

It is quite important that each laboratory determine its own range of normal values, as minor differences in technique yield varying results.

Platelet Aggregation

Principle. Platelets function in primary hemostasis by forming an initial platelet plug at the site of vascular injury. The phenomenon occurs in part by the ability of platelets to adhere to one another, a process known as aggregation. Substances that can induce platelet aggregation include collagen, adenosine diphosphate (ADP), epinephrine, thrombin, serotonin, arachidonic acid, the antibiotic ristocetin, snake venoms, antigen-antibody complexes, soluble fibrin monomer complexes, and fibrin-(ogen)olytic degradation products (FDPs). These aggregating agents induce platelet aggregation or cause platelets to release endogenous ADP, or both. Platelet aggregation is an essential part of the investigation of any patient with a suspected platelet dysfunction.

Platelet aggregation is studied by means of a platelet aggregometer, a photo-optical instrument connected to a chart recorder. Platelet-rich plasma, which is turbid in appearance, is placed in a cuvette, warmed to 37°C in the heating block of the instrument, and stirred by a small magnetic bar. Light transmittance through the platelet-rich plasma, relative to the platelet-poor plasma, is recorded. The addition of an aggregating agent causes the formation of larger platelet aggregates with a corresponding increase in light transmittance, owing to a clearing in the platelet-rich plasma. The change in light transmittance is converted to electronic signals and recorded as a tracing by the chart recorder.

Note: There are some basic requirements for platelet aggregation as an in vitro means of evaluating platelet function:

1. In performing platelet aggregation studies, a clean venipuncture is crucial. Hemolyzed samples should not be studied, because RBCs contain ADP.
2. It is preferred to test plasma from fasting patients. Lipemic samples may obscure changes in optical density owing to platelet aggregation.
3. Sodium citrate is the anticoagulant used in aggregation studies. Keep in mind that in vitro aggregation is dependent on the presence of calcium ions. The concentration of calcium even after anticoagulation may be sufficient for aggregation to occur.
4. Fibrinogen must be present in the test sample for aggregation to occur.
5. The plasma sample should not come in contact with a glass surface unless siliconized. Platelets adhere to glass.

6. Aggregation studies should be performed at 37°C and a sample pH of 6.5 to 8.5. To help maintain pH values, all samples once collected should be capped to prevent CO_2 loss.
7. Test samples should be maintained at room temperature during processing. Cooling inhibits the platelet aggregating response. Just prior to performing the test, the plasma is incubated at 37°C in the heat block of the aggregometer.
8. Stirring is necessary to bring the platelets in close contact with one another to allow aggregation to occur.
9. All aggregation studies should be performed within 3 hours of sample collection
10. It is essential that the patient refrain from taking any anti-inflammatory drugs 1 week prior to the test. These drugs inhibit the platelets' release reaction.
11. Thrombocytopenia makes evaluation of the aggregation responses difficult.
12. Aggregating agents should be prepared fresh daily and brought to room temperature prior to use. They must be of known potency and added in small volumes.
13. Control tests using platelet-rich plasma from a known donor must be performed with the test samples.

Reagents and Equipment

Control and test platelet-rich plasma
Aggregometer and cuvettes
Aggregating agents
Magnetic stirring bar
Pipettes
1. ADP: adenosine-5'-phosphate, grade 1, sodium salt. Dissolve 4.93 mg of trisodium salt or 4.71 mg of the disodium salt in 10 ml of saline pH 5.8. Makes 1 mmol/liter stock solution. Freeze in 0.5-ml aliquots in plastic vials at −20°C until use. For aggregation testing, prepare 100 μmol/liter, 50 μmol/liter, 25 μmol/liter, and 10 μmol/liter solutions in saline from the stock solution.
2. Collagen: a 1 mg/ml stock solution. Store at 4°C until use. For aggregation testing, dilute the stock solution with buffer supplied to obtain 40 μg/ml and a 20 μg/ml working concentration.
3. Ristocetin: antibiotic. Each vial contains 100 mg of ristocetin. Dissolve in 5 ml of saline. Freeze in 0.5-ml aliquots at −20°C until use. For aggregation testing prepare 15 mg/ml, 12 mg/ml, and 10 mg/ml working solutions.
4. Arachidonic acid: sodium salt 99 percent pure. Dissolve 4.10 mg in 25 ml of 0.1 mol/liter Na_2CO_3 to prepare a 0.50 mmol/liter stock solution. Freeze in 0.5-ml aliquots at −20°C until use. Use undiluted in aggregation testing.
5. Epinephrine: epinephrine tartrate. Dissolve 3.33 mg in 10 ml of deionized water containing 0.1 percent sodium metabisulphite, pH 3.5 This will yield a 1 mmol/liter stock solution.

Freeze in 0.5-ml aliquots at −20°C until use. For aggregation testing, prepare 20 μmol/liter and 200 μmol/liter solutions in 0.1 percent sodium metabisulphite.

Procedure

1. Centrifuge the citrated venous blood sample at room temperature (18 to 25°C) at 150 to 200 g for 10 to 15 minutes. Dilute the platelet-rich plasma with platelet-poor plasma to obtain a platelet count of 250×10^9/liter. Plasma may be left at room temperature in capped plastic tubes for up to 2 hours before testing. Repeat procedure for control sample.
2. Turn on heating block of the aggregometer 30 minutes before tests are to be run.
3. Pipette into a cuvette the appropriate volume of plasma and place into the 37°C heat block for 1 minute to warm the test plasma.
4. Place a magnetic stirring bar into the cuvette and turn on the motor. Adjust the speed of the stirring bar to between 800 and 1100 rpm (the speed that yields optimal platelet aggregation when strong concentrations of ADP are added to normal plasma). Adjust the absorbance of the plasma to 0.40, and adjust the chart recorder so that the difference in absorbance between platelet-rich and platelet-poor plasma causes the pen to cover the width of the paper.
5. Pipette 0.1 ml of aggregating agent to the plasma. Observe the aggregation curve for 3 minutes.
6. Tests are usually performed with three dilutions of ADP, collagen, ristocetin, and epinephrine for patient and normal plasma samples.

Interpretation. Low concentrations of ADP induce biphasic aggregation (that is, both a primary and a secondary wave of aggregation); very low concentrations of ADP induce a primary wave followed by disaggregation; and high concentrations of ADP induce a single, broad wave of aggregation.[7] A biphasic aggregation response to ADP is not seen in patients with platelet release disorders. Patients with Glanzmann's thrombasthenia show incomplete aggregation with ADP regardless of the final concentration. Platelet aggregation induced by collagen is characterized by a lag period prior to aggregation, followed by only a single wave of aggregation.[8] A biphasic aggregation response is seen with the antibiotic ristocetin; however, often only a single, broad wave of aggregation will occur. In patients with severe von Willebrand's disease, aggregation to ristocetin characteristically is absent. Decreased to normal aggregation to ristocetin can be seen in patients with mild von Willebrand's disease. Correction of the abnormal ristocetin aggregation curves can be seen by the addition of normal, platelet-poor plasma to the patient's platelet-rich plasma.

Abnormal ristocetin-induced platelet aggregation may occur in patients with Bernard-Soulier syndrome, platelet storage pool defects, and idiopathic thrombocytopenia purpura. Platelet aggregation induced with arachidonic acid causes a rapid secondary wave of aggregation. Biphasic aggregation is observed with epinephrine. One third to one half of normal, healthy patients will produce a primary wave of aggregation with epinephrine.[9] The aggregating agent thrombin induces a biphasic wave of aggregation. Platelet aggregation induced by serotonin will normally produce a wave of aggregation with a maximum of 10 to 30 percent transmittance followed by disaggregation (Figs. 30–IV–1 and 30–IV–2).[10]

Comments. When evaluating patients with suspected platelet disorders, the aggregating agents most commonly used are ADP in various concentrations, collagen, epinephrine, and ristocetin.

Aspirin, aspirin compounds, and anti-inflammatory drugs inhibit the secondary wave of aggregation by inhibiting the release reaction of the platelet. Reduced or absent aggregation as well as disaggregation curves may be observed in patients taking aspirin medication.

The intensity of platelet aggregation may be estimated by recording the change in absorbance as a percentage of the difference in absorbance between platelet-rich and platelet-poor plasma. This has limited usefulness, as absorbance is dependent on the size and density of platelet clumping and the number of platelets that aggregate. A more complex analysis of aggregation related to the rate of aggregation may also be obtained. However, visual interpretation of the aggregation curves suffices and can establish whether aggregation is abnormal or normal.

Platelet Factor 3 Availability

Principle. Platelets serve as templates on which activation of coagulation proteins can occur by releasing a phospholipid (platelet factor 3) that acts as a partial thromboplastin, which is necessary for the intrinsic conversion of prothrombin to thrombin. Platelet factor 3 (PF3) is not available in normal intact circulating platelets. It is released when platelets are activated by a stimulus such as celite or kaolin, which are contact activators. The recalcification time of platelet-rich plasma (PRP) will be shortened when plasma is incubated with celite before the addition of calcium. Celite causes the release of PF3 from the patient's platelets and activation of intrinsic coagulation. Platelet-rich plasma, a source of PF3, and platelet-poor plasma (PPP), which is low in PF3 activity, are compared with an activated partial thromboplastin reagent for activity.

Reagents and Equipment

Celite 505, 1 percent suspension in 0.85 percent NaCl
0.025 M $CaCl_2$
Platelet plus activator
Activated partial thromboplastin time (APTT) assay equipment
Plastic tubes and pipettes

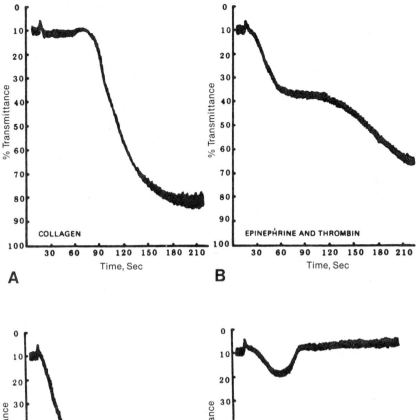

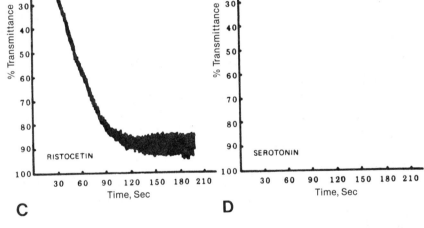

Figure 30-IV-1. Aggregation curves with various aggregating agents. (*A*) Aggregation curve induced by collagen. Note the lag time before aggregation followed by a single wave of aggregation. (*B*) Aggregation curve induced with epinephrine and thrombin. Note the biphasic wave of aggregation. (C) Aggregation curve induced by ristocetin. A biphasic wave of aggregation as well as a single wave of aggregation may be seen. (*D*) Aggregation curve induced by serotonin. Generally a single wave of aggregation followed by disaggregation is seen.

Preparation of Plasma Samples

1. Obtain 9.0 ml of blood with a plastic syringe and place in a plastic tube containing 1.0 ml of 3.8 percent sodium citrate and mix thoroughly. Generally, hemolyzed samples are not satisfactory. The phospholipid in the membrane of the red cells may act like PF3 and yield questionable results.
2. Platelet-rich plasma: Spin the citrated sample at 1500 rpm for 5 minutes. Do not use the centrifuge brake; gently remove sample from the centrifuge. Remove as much of the plasma as possible using a plastic pipette and place in a plastic tube labeled PRP.
3. Platelet-poor plasma: Re-spin the blood sample for 10 to 15 minutes at 1500 rpm. Remove as

much plasma as possible with a plastic pipette and place in a plastic tube labeled PPP.

Procedure

Determine the clotting time for the following three assays:

1. Control: Add 0.1 ml platelin plus activator to 0.1 ml PPP and incubate for 5 minutes at 37°C. Add 0.1 ml of 0.025 M $CaCl_2$. Obtain clotting time.
2. PRP: Add 0.1 ml of 1 percent celite suspension to 0.1 ml PRP and incubate for 5 minutes at 37°C. Add 0.1 ml of 0.025 M $CaCl_2$. Obtain clotting time.
3. PPP: Add 0.1 ml 1 percent celite suspension to 0.1 ml PPP and incubate for 5 minutes at 37°C.

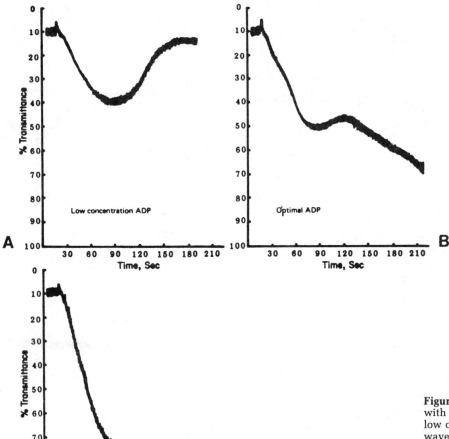

Figure 30–IV–2. Aggregation curves induced with various concentrations of ADP. (*A*) Very low concentrations of ADP induce a primary wave of aggregation followed by disaggregation. (*B*) The optimal concentration of ADP induces a biphasic wave of aggregation. (*C*) High concentrations of ADP induce a broad wave of aggregation.

Add 0.1 ml of 0.025 M $CaCl_2$. Obtain clotting time.

Results. The PRP and celite should have a clotting time close to that of the control. In vitro platelin acts like PF3, so by recalcifying the PRP and control, the test systems and results are similar.

The PPP will have a prolonged clotting time because of a lack of platelets and PF3. If the PRP clotting time is prolonged, close to the PPP time, there is reduced PF3 activity in the patient sample.

TESTS TO MEASURE THE INTRINSIC SYSTEM

Whole Blood Clotting Time

Principle. The whole blood clotting time is the length of time required for blood to clot in a glass test tube and measures the activity of the intrinsic system of coagulation. It is an insensitive test and not satisfactory for use as a screening procedure. It is an outdated test which was utilized in the past as a means of monitoring heparin therapy; however, other tests such as the APTT and thrombin time (TT) are preferred for monitoring heparin. Despite the insensitivity of the test, visual inspection of the clot may reveal useful information.

Reagents and Equipment

37°C waterbath
Plastic syringe (glass or siliconized syringes)
21-gauge needles
Three 13 × 100 test tubes
Stopwatch

Procedure

1. Label three 13 × 100 test tubes 1, 2, and 3.
2. Using a plastic syringe, draw 4 ml of blood. If blood has been drawn with difficulty or a poor venipuncture has been performed, the specimen is unsatisfactory for this test.
3. When using a glass syringe, the stopwatch is started as blood enters the syringe. If a siliconized or plastic syringe is used, the stopwatch is started as blood is dispersed into test tube 3.
4. Remove the needle from the syringe and dispense 1 ml of blood into each tube. Fill tube 1 first, then tube 2, and then tube 3 last. Start the stopwatch as the blood is dispensed into tube 3.

5. Place the tubes in the 37°C waterbath.
6. Tilt tube 3 at 30-second intervals until the blood clots. Then tilt tube 2 in the same manner until the blood clots. Finally tilt tube 1 at 30-second intervals until the blood clots. Stop the watch when the blood in tube 1 clots.
7. The whole blood clotting time is the length of time required for the blood in tube 1 to clot. Visually inspect the clot in each tube at the end of 1 hour and again 24 hours later.

Interpretation. The normal value obtained by this method is between 7 and 15 minutes. A time of less than 7 minutes may be the result of poor technique. When using a siliconized syringe and test tubes, the clotting time is usually prolonged to about 30 minutes.

Comments. Many uncontrollable variations occur when performing the whole blood clotting time, making this a rather insensitive test. Prolongation of the whole blood clotting time occurs in patients with marked factor deficiencies, with the use of heparin, and in the presence of circulating anticoagulants.

Activated Partial Thromboplastin Time

Principle. The APTT is a screening test used to measure the intrinsic pathway of coagulation more precisely, to assay all the plasma coagulation factors with the exception of factors VII and XIII and platelet factor. The formation of fibrin occurs at a normal rate only if the factors involved in the intrinsic pathway (factors XII, XI, IX, and VIII) and the common pathway (factors I, II, V, and X) are present in normal concentrations. In the APTT, variables of plasma recalcification have been removed in modifications to the test. Optimal activation is achieved by the addition of a platelet phospholipid substitute, which eliminates the test's sensitivity to platelet number and function, as well as the addition of activators such as kaolin, celite, and ellagic acid, which eliminates the variability of activation by glass contact. The APTT is also used to monitor heparin therapy.

Reagents and Equipment

Fibrometer
Fibrometer cups and tips
Commercial activated cephaloplastin
$CaCl_2$, 0.02 M
Citrated plasma (test plasma and control)
Stopwatch
Pipettes
37°C heat block

The Fibrometer coagulation timer (BBL-Microbiology Systems) is a semi-automated procedure for coagulation testing which determines the presence of a fibrin clot. Two metal electrodes make contact with the reaction mixture. There is a moving and a stationary electrode. A small hook on the tip of the moving electrode will detect the initial fibrin strand. The stationary electrode is responsible for creating an electric potential between the electrodes. When a fibrin strand is formed between the two electrodes, the circuit is complete, stopping the timing device. (Please refer to the operator's manual for a complete description.)

Procedure

1. Obtain 4.5 ml of blood by means of clean venipuncture. Mix by gentle inversion with 0.5 ml of 0.109 M sodium citrate. Oxalate is not recommended.
2. Centrifuge for 5 minutes at 1500 rpm. Collect plasma and store at 4°C until use. Testing should be performed within 4 hours.
3. Reconstitute activated cephaloplastin reagent according to directions.
4. Prewarm a small amount of activated cephaloplastin at 37°C. Prewarm a small amount of control plasma at 37°C for 3 to 5 minutes but no longer than 10 minutes. Place a tube of $CaCl_2$ into the heat block. (The major concerns are those of evaporation and contamination.)
5. With reagent, $CaCl_2$, and control plasma prewarmed at 37°C, pipette 0.1 ml of activated cephaloplastin into number of cups for tests to be performed. (Assays are to be run in duplicate.)
6. Pipette 0.1 ml of control plasma into activated cephaloplastin. Allow the cephaloplastin plasma mixture to warm and activate for 3 minutes.
7. Transfer cup containing cephaloplastin-plasma mixture to the reaction well. Pipette 0.1 ml $CaCl_2$ into the cup in the reaction well and simultaneously start the stopwatch. (The fibrometer system will start automatically when test plasma is added with the automatic pipette switched on, and will stop when fibrin web is formed.)
8. Record time for fibrin formation.
9. Repeat procedure with test plasma.
10. All testing, both on control and test plasma, must be performed in duplicate. (Normal duplicate results should be within ±0.5 second of each other; therapeutic results within ±1.0 second.) Calculate the mean plotting time and report results in seconds to the nearest 10th. *Note:* the exact procedure will vary depending on the methodology used to measure fibrin formation.

Interpretation. We consider less than 35 seconds to be a normal value (each laboratory should develop its own normal range). The test result is abnormal in patients with deficiencies of all factors involved in the intrinsic pathway. The APTT is prolonged with levels of factors IX and VIII 30 to 40 percent below normal. Hypofibrinogenemia (levels less than 100 mg/dl) will prolong the APTT. When the APTT is used to monitor heparin therapy, it is prolonged 1.5 to 2.5 times the control level.

Comments. Both the APTT and the prothrombin time (PT) should be performed as screening procedures, since together the tests evaluate the intrinsic, extrinsic, and common pathways of coagulation.

TESTS TO MEASURE THE EXTRINSIC SYSTEM
One-Stage Prothrombin Time (Quick)

Principle. The PT is the time required to form a fibrin clot when plasma is added to a thromboplastin-calcium mixture. The test is a measure of the extrinsic pathway of coagulation involving factors II, V, VII, and X (as well as fibrinogen). Tissue thromboplastin activates factor VII, which proceeds through the cascade, ultimately generating thrombin. The thrombin thus formed converts fibrinogen to fibrin. The rate of fibrin formation therefore depends on the level of factors II, V, VII, and X, and fibrinogen, and thus measures the overall activity of these factors.

The test is a valuable screening procedure used to indicate possible factor deficiencies of the extrinsic pathway. The PT test is sensitive to the vitamin K–dependent factors of the extrinsic pathway (factors II, VII, and X) and therefore is used as a means of monitoring oral anticoagulant therapy. (The fourth vitamin K–dependent factor, factor IX, is measured by the APTT.)

Reagents and Equipment

Fibrometer
Fibrometer cups and tips
Commercial thromboplastin $CaCl_2$ reagent
Citrated plasma (test plasma and control)
Stopwatch
Pipettes
37°C heat block

Procedure

1. Obtain 4.5 ml of blood by means of a clean venipuncture. Mix by gentle inversion with 0.5 ml of 0.109 M sodium citrate. (Becton-Dickinson vacutainer tubes containing sodium citrate may be used.) Oxalate is recommended.
2. Centrifuge for 5 minutes at 1500 rpm. Collect plasma and store at 4°C until use. Testing should be performed within 4 hours.
3. Reconstitute thromboplastin-$CaCl_2$ reagent according to directions.
4. Prewarm a small amount of thromboplastin-$CaCl_2$ mixture at 37°C. Prewarm a small amount of control plasma at 37°C for 3 to 5 minutes, but no longer than 10 minutes.
5. With reagent and control plasma prewarmed at 37°C, pipette 0.2 ml of thromboplastin-$CaCl_2$ mixture into the cup in the reaction well. Pipette 0.1 ml of control plasma into the cup in the reaction well and simultaneously start stopwatch. (The fibrometer system will start automatically when test plasma is added with the automatic pipette switched on, and will stop when fibrin web is formed.)

6. Record time for fibrin formation.
7. Repeat procedure with test plasma.
8. All testing on both control and test plasma must be performed in duplicate. (Normal duplicate results should be within ±0.5 second of each other; therapeutic results within ±1.0 second.) Calculate the mean clotting time and report results in seconds to the nearest 10th.

Interpretation. Normal prothrombin time is 12 to 14 seconds. (It is recommended that each laboratory develop its own "normal" range.) *Note:* There are many acceptable methods of reporting the patient's clotting time. The preferred method reports the patient's clotting time in seconds and compares that with normal control time, also reported in seconds. Another method is to report percent activity as compared with a prothrombin activity curve using normal pooled plasma.

The PT is prolonged in individuals with a factor deficiency involving a single factor (as in those with a congenital deficiency) or involving multiple factors (as in patients with acquired deficiencies, such as those with liver disease receiving coumarin therapy, or with vitamin K deficiency) and in the presence of circulating anticoagulants such as FDPs and heparin.

In patients with polycythemia, the PT is prolonged as a result of a change in the ratio of anticoagulant to plasma.

Coagulation Factor Assays
One-Stage Quantitative Assay Method for Factors II, V, VII, and X

Principle. The PT is the basis of this test system, with specific factor-deficient plasmas being used instead of a correction plasma or serum. The percentage of factor activity is determined by the amount of correction detected when specific dilutions of patient plasma are added to a factor-deficient plasma. These results are obtained from an activity curve made from dilutions of normal reference plasma and specific factor-deficient plasma.

Reagents and Equipment

Simplastin
Specific factor-deficient plasma (II, V, VII, X)
Imidazole buffered saline, pH 7.3 ± 0.1
Normal reference plasma (commercial reference plasma with known factor levels)
Equipment used for PT assay

Procedure

1. Preparation of activity curve
   a. Prepare 1:10, 1:20, 1:40, 1:80, 1:160, 1:320, 1:640, and 1:1280 serial dilutions of the normal reference plasma with imidazole buffered saline. The 1:10 dilution is considered 100 percent factor activity.
   b. Warm Simplastin to 37°C.

PREPARATION OF TEST DILUTIONS FOR REFERENCE PLASMA IN THE ONE-STAGE ASSAY FOR FACTORS

Tube No.	Amount of Plasma	Imidazole Buffered Saline	Dilution	% of Factor
1	0.1 ml	0.9 ml	1 : 10	100.00
2	0.5 ml of 1	0.5 ml	1 : 20	50.00
3	0.5 ml of 2	0.5 ml	1 : 40	25.00
4	0.5 ml of 3	0.5 ml	1 : 80	12.50
5	0.5 ml of 4	0.5 ml	1 : 160	6.25
6	0.5 ml of 5	0.5 ml	1 : 320	3.13
7	0.5 ml of 6	0.5 ml	1 : 640	1.56
8	0.5 ml of 7	0.5 ml	1 : 1280	0.78

c. Perform the following test procedure on each dilution:
  (1) Add 0.1 ml of specific factor-deficient plasma to 0.1 of diluted normal reference plasma and warm to 37°C for allotted time.
  (2) Add 0.2 ml Simplastin to the sample and determine the clotting time.
  (3) Repeat procedure on duplicate sample and average results.
d. Plot results on 2 × 3 cycle log graph paper, with percent factor activity on the X axis and seconds on the Y axis. Draw a best-fit line. The curve will demonstrate a plateau at the least concentrated dilutions and should be plotted as such demonstrating the end of sensitivity for the assay.
2. Procedure for testing patient plasma
  a. Prewarm Simplastin to 37°C.
  b. Prepare a 1 : 10 dilution of citrated patient plasma with imidazole buffered saline. It is important to keep samples and dilutions refrigerated until they are to be tested.
  c. Add 0.1 ml of specific factor-deficient plasma to 0.1 ml of diluted patient plasma. Warm for allotted time at 37°C.
  d. Add 0.2 ml Simplastin to sample and determine the clotting time.
  e. Repeat procedure on a duplicate sample and average results.
  f. Read the percent activity directly from the activity curve (Fig. 30–IV–3). A 35-second result on a 1 : 10 dilution of plasma would be interpreted as 8.3 percent activity.

Results. A range of 40 to 150 percent is considered normal, but each laboratory should define its own range.

Comments

1. If the result is greater than 100 percent, dilute the test sample with buffered saline until re-

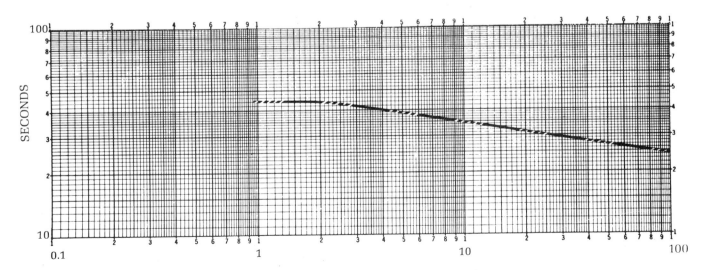

Percent Factor V Activity

Figure 30–IV–3. Percent factor V activity curve.

sults fall within the sensitivity range of the curve.

2. Calculate the percent activity of the dilution tested, and multiply by the dilution factor for the percent activity of the patient sample.

3. These tests require the same considerations as the APTT and PT assay with regard to quality control, specimen handling, reagent preparation, and points of procedure importance. The assay should be performed on the same equipment and in the same manner as all other coagulation assays in your laboratory.

One-Stage Quantitative Assay Method for Factors VIII, IX, XI, and XII

Principle. The APTT is the basis of this test system. This method is also based on the ability of patient plasma to correct specific factor-deficient plasma. Results in percent activity are obtained from an activity curve.

Reagents and Equipment

APTT reagent
0.025 M $CaCl_2$
Specific factor-deficient plasma (VIII, IX, XI, and XII)
Normal reference plasma (with known factor levels)
Imidazole buffered saline, pH 7.3 ± 0.1
Equipment for APTT assay

Procedure

1. Preparation of activity curve:
   a. Prepare a 1:10, 1:20, 1:40, 1:80, 1:160, 1:320, 1:640, 1:1280 serial dilution of the normal reference plasma with imidazole buffered saline (see previous table). The 1:10 dilution is considered 100 percent in factor activity.
   b. Prewarm the $CaCl_2$ and APTT reagent to 37°C.
   c. Perform the following test procedure on each dilution.
      (1) Add 0.1 ml of specific factor-deficient plasma and 0.1 ml of diluted normal reference plasma to 0.1 ml APTT reagent. Mix well and incubate for the specified time.
      (2) Add 0.1 ml $CaCl_2$ into the mixture at the specified time, and determine the clotting time.
      (3) Repeat the procedure on a duplicate sample and average results.
   d. Plot results on 2×3 cycle log graph paper, with percent factor on the X axis and seconds on the Y axis. Draw a best-fit line. The curve will demonstrate a plateau at the least concentrated dilutions and should be plotted as such, demonstrating the end of sensitivity for the assay.
2. Procedure for testing patient plasma:
   a. Prewarm $CaCl_2$ and APTT reagent to 37°C.
   b. Prepare a 1:10 dilution of citrated patient plasma with imidazole buffered saline. It is important to keep samples and dilutions refrigerated until they are to be tested.
   c. Add 0.1 ml of specific factor-deficient plasma and 0.1 ml of diluted patient plasma to 0.1 ml APTT reagent. Mix well and incubate for the allotted time.
   d. Add 0.1 ml $CaCl_2$ into the mixture at the specified time, and determine the clotting time.
   e. Repeat the procedure on a duplicate sample and average the results.
   f. Read the percentage of activity directly from activity curve (see Fig. 30-IV-3).

Results. A range of 40 to 150 percent is considered normal, but each laboratory should define its own range.

Stypven Time Test (Russell's Viper Venom Time Test)

Principle. This test is performed to differentiate a deficiency of factor VII from a deficiency of factor X, as both of these disorders present with a prolonged PT. Russell's viper venom (Stypven) has thromboplastic activity and can be substituted for tissue thromboplastin in the one-stage PT. The thromboplastic activity of the venom is dependent on factor X, factor V, prothrombin, platelets, and phospholipid. The venom does not require factor VII for activity.[12] The Stypven time is also a useful means of measuring prothrombin plus factor V when tested on platelet-rich nonlipemic plasma.[13]

Reagents and Equipment

Stypven: Dilute 1:10,000 with distilled water according to package directions
0.02 M $CaCl_2$
Platelet-rich plasma (test plasma and control)
Equipment as needed for one-stage prothrombin time

Procedure

1. Obtain 4.5 ml of blood by means of a clean venipuncture. Mix by gentle inversion with 0.5 ml of 0.109 M sodium citrate. (Beckton-Dickinson vacutainer tubes containing sodium citrate may be used.)
2. Centrifuge for 5 minutes at 1500 rpm. Collect the platelet-rich plasma.
3. With all reagents prewarmed at 37°C, pipette 0.1 ml of control plasma and 0.1 ml of venom into the reaction well. Pipette 0.1 ml of 0.02 M $CaCl_2$ into the cup in the reaction well, and simultaneously start stopwatch.
4. Record the clotting time.
5. Repeat procedure with test plasma.

Interpretation. The normal value is that obtained with tissue thromboplastin in the one-stage PT. A deficiency of factor X, factor V, and prothrombin will prolong the Stypven time. In factor VII deficiency, the Stypven time will be normal.

Comments. The use of platelet-rich plasma makes the Stypven time sensitive to both quantitative and qualitative platelet deficiencies.

TESTS TO MEASURE FIBRIN FORMATION
Prothrombin Consumption Test (Serum Prothrombin Time)

Principle. When normal whole blood coagulates, prothrombin is converted to thrombin by the interaction of plasma thromboplastin. Only small amounts of prothrombin will remain in the serum after clotting has occurred, and virtually all of the prothrombin will be consumed if the serum is tested 1 hour after whole blood has clotted. When there is a deficiency in any of the factors required for thromboplastinogenesis (that is, all the intrinsic factors that activate factor X), prothrombin will have been incompletely consumed, and more than the normal amount will be present in the serum 1 hour after clotting. The prothrombin consumption test (PCT) measures this residual prothrombin by a one-stage PT test. Essentially, it is a serum PT assay. In the test system, Simplastin A supplies fibrinogen, factor X, calcium, and thromboplastin, which are needed to form a fibrin clot in serum. This test is sensitive to plasma thromboplastin precursors, platelet dysfunction, and thrombocytopenia.

Reagents and Equipment

Simplastin A
Patient and control sera
Coagulation equipment used for determining one-stage PT assay

Procedure

1. Draw the patient's blood sample using a two-syringe technique in a nontraumatic manner.
2. Add exactly 1 ml of blood to a glass (not siliconized) tube, and allow the blood to clot undisturbed for 1 hour at 37°C.
3. After the sample has incubated for 1 hour, spin for 1 minute at 3000 rpm. Transfer serum to a clean test tube; warm to 37°C.
4. Reconstitute Simplastin A and warm 0.2 ml at 37°C for designated amount of time.
5. Add 0.1 ml of serum and simultaneously start the timer.
6. Record the time for fibrin formation.

Results. Normal serum PT is greater than 20 seconds. A range for this assay should be determined by each laboratory based on its test system and normal population.

Interpretation

1. The concentration of prothrombin in serum is inversely proportional to the thromboplastinogenesis activity of coagulation. Because normal serum is prothrombin depleted, a normal serum PT is prolonged.
2. A shortened or quick PCT is indicative of defects in phase I and/or phase II of coagulation.

In patients with defective plasma thrombogenesis, less of the prothrombin will be converted to thrombin and is subsequently measured by supplying fibrinogen and thromboplastin (Simplastin A) to the test system.

3. The serum PT or PCT is an indicator of the entire intrinsic clotting system, platelets, and factor X.
4. The following conditions negate the need for determining the PCT:
   a. Thrombocytopenia and platelet function abnormalities will result in an abnormal PCT, as normal platelet function is necessary for thromboplastinogenesis.
   b. A patient who has a prolonged one-stage plasma PT will also have an abnormal PCT because of the inadequate amount of prothrombin complex.

Thrombin Time

Principle. The TT is the time required for thrombin to convert fibrinogen to an insoluble fibrin clot. Fibrin formation is triggered by the addition of thrombin to the specimen and therefore bypasses prior steps in the coagulation cascade. The TT does not measure defects in the intrinsic or extrinsic pathways. The test is affected by the levels of fibrinogen, dysfibrinogenemia, and the presence of circulating anticoagulants (antithrombins) such as heparin, plasmin, and FDPs.

Reagents and Equipment

Fibrometer
Fibrometer cups and tips
100-ml pipette and tips
1.0-ml disposable serologic pipette
13 × 75 mm plastic test tubes
Thrombin-50 NIH thrombin units 1 ml
0.85 percent NaCl
Normal control plasma
NaOH-IN
ACl-IN
TRIS base
TRIS base stock solution: Weigh 72.9 g TRIS base; Q.S. to 3 liters with deionized water. Stable at room temperature for 1 year.
Working TRIS buffer, 0.05 pH 7.4: Add 42.0 ml 1 N HCl to 250 ml TRIS base stock solution in a 1-liter volumetric flask.
TRIS CaCl$_2$ 0.05 M: 1.38 g anhydrous CaCl$_2$: Q.S. to 500 ml with working TRIS buffer. Stable at room temperature for 1 year.
Thrombin solution, 10 NIH units thrombin per ml: To one vial of thrombin 50 NIH units, add 5 ml of physiologic saline. Mix. Aliquot 1 ml into each of four plastic test tubes. Store at −15°C. Stable for 2 weeks.
Working thrombin reagent: Thaw a 1-ml aliquot of thrombin solution at room temperature. Add 1 ml of TRIS buffered CaCl$_2$. Mix. Stable for 8 hours at room temperature.

Procedure

1. Prepare platelet-poor plasma. Separate plasma and immediately refrigerate at 4°C or store on ice. Test should be performed as soon as possible; however, stoppered refrigerated plasmas are stable for 4 hours.
2. Perform all tests in duplicate. Deliver 0.1 ml of working TRIS buffer into a fibrometer cup and incubate at 37°C for a minimum of 3 minutes, but not more than 10 minutes.
3. Add 0.1 ml of test plasma to the fibrometer cup containing 0.1 ml of working TRIS buffer. Start the stopwatch.
4. Incubate at 37°C. Prior to 1 minute transfer the fibrometer cup containing the plasma-TRIS buffer mixture to the reaction well.
5. Exactly at 1 minute, add 0.1 ml of thrombin reagent.
6. Measure the clotting time.
7. If the patient's average clotting time greatly exceeds the average control time, the test should be repeated using a 1:1 mixture of patient's plasma and normal or control plasma (see Interpretation).

Interpretation. Normal value is approximately 15 seconds. The TT is prolonged in patients with hypofibrinogenemia (usually less than 100 mg/dl), in those with dysfibrinogenemia, and in the presence of circulating anticoagulants.

If the mixing test results in a clotting time that approximates that of the control plasma, a deficiency or a molecular abnormality of fibrinogen is most likely indicated. If the mixing tests fail to correct the TT, the presence of a circulating inhibitor is indicated.

The TT does not differentiate a state of DIC from primary fibrinolysis; however, it is a sensitive test for determining the presence of DIC.

Reptilase Time

Principle. The reptilase time is similar to the TT, except that with the former technique clotting is initiated with the snake venom enzyme, reptilase. Reptilase, thrombinlike in nature, hydrolyzes fibrinopeptide A from the intact fibrinogen molecule in contrast to thrombin, which hydrolyzes fibrinopeptide A and B from fibrinogen. The clot that forms by the action of reptilase on fibrinogen is more fragile than that formed by thrombin's action on fibrinogen. The reptilase time is not inhibited by heparin. There is only a minimum effect on the reptilase time by FDPs.

Reagents and Equipment

Fibrometer
Fibrometer cups and tips
Reptilase-R
Platelet-poor citrated plasma (control and test plasma)
37°C heat block
Stopwatch

Procedure

1. Obtain 4.5 ml of blood by means of a clean venipuncture. Mix by gentle inversion with 0.5 ml of 0.109M sodium citrate. Reject any specimens that are hemolyzed.
2. Prepare platelet-poor plasma by centrifugation at 1500 rpm for 10 to 15 minutes.
3. Reconstitute a vial of reptilase-R with 1.0 ml of deionized water. Stable for 28 days at 4°C.
4. Pipette 0.3 ml of reptilase-R reagent into a fibrometer cup. Incubate at 37° for 5 minutes.
5. Pipette 0.3 ml of control plasma into a fibrometer cup. Start the stopwatch.
6. Prior to 2 minutes, transfer the fibrometer cup to the reaction well. At exactly 2 minutes, add 0.1 ml of prewarmed reptilase-R reagent. (The fibrometer system will start automatically when reagent is added with the automatic pipette on, and will stop when fibrin web forms.)
7. Record time for clot formation.
8. Repeat procedure with test plasma.
9. All testing, both on control and test plasma, must be performed in duplicate. (Duplicate results should agree within ±0.5 second.) Calculate the average clotting time and report results in seconds.

Interpretation. Normal values are 18 to 22 seconds. Except for fibrinogen Oklahoma and fibrinogen Oslow, all the congenital dysfibrinogenemias have an infinite reptilase time. The reptilase time is also infinitely prolonged in cases of congenital afibrinogenemia. In states of hypofibrinogenemia the reptilase time may be variable, dependent on the levels of fibrinogen present. The reptilase time is moderately prolonged in the presence of FDPs and is unaffected by heparin (see *test comparison* below).

Comments. In the presence of heparin, thrombin is inhibited by way of AT-III. However, heparin does not interfere with reptilase's ability to cleave fibrinopeptide A from fibrinogen. A comparison of both TT and reptilase time will aid in detecting the presence of thrombin inhibitors such as heparin.

TEST COMPARISON

Thrombin Time	Reptilase Time	Defect
Infinitely prolonged	Infinitely prolonged	Dysfibrinogenemia
Infinitely prolonged	Infinitely prolonged	Afibrinogenemia
Prolonged	Equally prolonged	Hypofibrinogenemia
Prolonged	Normal	Heparin
Prolonged	Slight to moderately prolonged	FDPs

Fibrinogen

Principle. Fibrinogen can be quantitatively measured by a modification of the TT because the thrombin clotting time of dilute plasma is inversely proportional to the concentration of fibrinogen. This method involves clotting dilutions of both patient's test plasma and control plasma with an excess of thrombin.[14] Results are calculated from a calibration curve.

Reagents and Equipment

Fibrometer
Fibro-cups and tips
12 × 75 test tubes
Data-Fi Fibrinogen Determination Kit (Baxter Healthcare Corp., Dade Division)

1. Thrombin, 100 NIH units per ml bovine lyophilized: Reconstitute with 1.0 ml distilled water.
2. Fibrinogen standard: Fibrinogen concentration is standardized by the macro-Kjeldahl method. Reconstitute with 1.0 ml distilled water. Mix by gentle inversion; do not shake.
3. Owren's Veronal buffer, pH 7.35
4. Control (with a known fibrinogen concentration)

Procedure

1. Mix nine parts of freshly collected blood to one part 3.8 percent sodium citrate.
2. Centrifuge for 15 minutes at 1500g. Collect plasma.

Preparation of Calibration Curve

3. Make dilutions of the fibrinogen standard with Owren's Veronal buffer as follows: 1:5, 1:15, and 1:40. Make all transfers from the first test tube.
   a. 1:5 dilution (first tube): 1.6 ml buffer to 0.4 ml fibrinogen standard
   b. 1:15 dilution (second tube): 0.8 ml buffer to 0.4 ml mixture from the first test tube
   c. 1:40 dilution (third tube): 2.8 ml buffer to 0.4 ml mixture from the first test tube.

Fibrometer

4. Perform duplicate determinations on each dilution of fibrinogen standard as follows:
   a. Incubate 0.2 ml fibrinogen standard dilution at 37°C for at least 2 minutes but no more than 5 minutes.
   b. Add 0.1 ml thrombin reagent.
   c. Measure the clotting time. Average the values.

Calibration Curve

5. Using the graph paper furnished, plot the clotting time in seconds on the vertical axis versus the concentration of fibrinogen standard dilutions on the horizontal axis. Depending on the known concentration of fibrinogen in the standard, the points on the horizontal axis will approximate the three vertical lines marked 1:5, 1:15, and 1:40. Connecting the plotted points usually approximates a straight line. The calibration curve may be extended to a minimum of 50 mg/ml and a maximum of 800 mg/ml.

Sample Assay

6. Make a 1:10 dilution of test plasmas and control using Owren's Veronal buffer as follows: 0.1 ml plasma to 0.9 ml buffer.
7. Perform duplicate determinations on each dilution of test sample.
   a. Incubate 0.2 ml sample dilution at 37°C for at least 2 minutes but no more than 5 minutes.
   b. Add 0.1 ml thrombin reagent.
   c. Measure the clotting time. Average the values.
8. Read results from calibration curve and record in mg/dl (Fig. 30-IV-4).

Interpretation. Normal values range from 200 to 400 mg/dl.

Comments. Prolonged clotting times may indicate either a low fibrinogen concentration or the presence of inhibitors such as heparin or circulating FDPs. The effect of heparin may be excluded by performing the TT using reptilase in place of thrombin because reptilase is unaffected by heparin. A comparison of clotting times using both TT and reptilase may help to distinguish a fibrinogen deficiency from a dysfibrinogenemia.

If a prolonged clotting time is obtained using a 1:10 dilution of patient plasma, this may indicate low fibrinogen levels of 50 mg/dl or less. Retest sample using a 1:5 or a 1:2 dilution.

If a short clotting time is obtained using a 1:10 dilution of patient plasma, this may indicate high fibrinogen levels of 800 mg/dl or more. Retest sample using a 1:20 dilution.

Low fibrinogen levels are seen in infants and children and in those with congenital afibrinogenemia or hypofibrinogenemia. Acquired deficiencies are seen in states of liver disease, DIC, and fibrinolysis.

High fibrinogen levels are seen in pregnancy and in women taking oral contraceptives. Fibrinogen is considered an acute phase reactant, and therefore high levels may be seen in states of acute infection, neoplasms, collagen disorders, nephrosis, and hepatitis.

Other tests are available to assay fibrinogen. The classic assay measures fibrinogen concentrations by adding thrombin or calcium chloride to plasma, washing the clot, and determining the protein content by the biuret or Folin-Ciocaltea method.[15] This assay is both tedious and time consuming; however, it yields reliable fibrinogen determinations. Semiautomated instruments such as the Bio/Data Coagulation Profiler may yield fibrinogen determinations based on maximum change in optical density. The automated Dupont ACA also determines fibrinogen concentrations. The assay is based on changes in optical density (OD) after the addition of thrombin.

Fibrinogen levels may also be assayed by means of single radial immunodiffusion (RID). The protein (antigen) solution is applied to a well in a gel matrix containing a standardized concentration of mono-

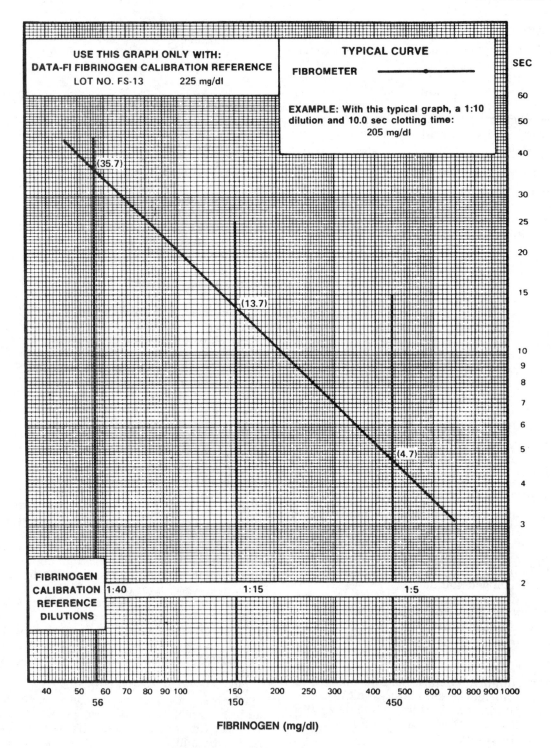

Figure 30–IV–4. Fibrinogen calibration curve.

specific antisera to fibrinogen. The antigen diffuses radially, producing a precipitin ring. Because antibody is present in excess, after incubation an end-point is reached and the diameter of the precipitin ring remains constant. Precipitin rings can be read following incubation or at end-point. Results are quantitated by comparing precipitin rings of the test sample to precipitin rings of standards or by reading from a table of precalibrated reference values.

Simple observation of the clot retraction also may yield information regarding the fibrinogen concentration of the blood. The higher the concentration of fibrinogen, the larger the fibrin web resulting in less RBC fallout.

Factor XIII Screening Test

Principle. Stabilization of the fibrin clot depends on plasma factor XIII, which converts hydrogen bonds to covalent bonds by transamidation. In the absence of factor XIII, the hydrogen-bonded fibrin polymers are soluble in 5 M urea or 1 percent monochloroacetic acid.

Reagents and Equipment

5 M urea or 1 percent monochloroacetic acid
Bovine thrombin (200 NIH units/ml)
0.15 M NaCl
Patient plasma
37°C waterbath

Procedure

1. Add 0.5 ml of patient plasma and 0.1 ml thrombin solution to a 12 × 75 mm test tube.
2. Incubate at 37°C for 30 minutes.
3. Remove the clot from the test tube with a glass rod.
4. Wash the clot with cold saline.
5. Place the clot in a clean 12 × 75 mm test tube containing 1 ml of 5 M urea or 1 ml of 1 percent monochloroacetic acid.
6. The tube is incubated at room temperature for 24 hours.

Interpretation. After 24 hours the presence of a formed clot indicates a plasma factor XIII concentration of greater than 1 percent of normal.

Comments. A deficiency of factor XIII is not detected by other coagulation tests; therefore, hemostatic evaluation is not complete without a factor XIII assay. Because the minimum level of factor XIII is about 5 percent, this assay will reliably detect those individuals with a rare factor XIII deficiency.[16]

Those patients who present with a homozygous deficiency of factor XIII show dissolution of a fibrin clot, usually within 1 hour.

TESTS FOR von WILLEBRAND'S DISEASE

Measurement of Factor VIII – Related Antigen

Principle. Factor VIII antigen, the high molecular weight component of the factor VIII molecule, is measured by Laurell rocket electrophoresis. Factor VIII antigen is electrophoresed through agar containing antisera to factor VIII. The rocketlike immunoprecipitate that forms is measured, the length of which is directly proportional to the amount of antigen present.

Equipment

Electrophoresis chamber and power supply
3¼ × 4 inch Kodak glass slides precoated with 0.1 percent agarose
5-μl pipette
Wicks—telfa strips
Well cutter

Template: Single row of 14 holes, 3 mm in diameter; 3 mm apart; 2 cm from edge of plate

Reagents

1. TRIS barbital buffer, pH 8.8
   TRIS barbital buffer   17 g
   Deionized H_2O 2000 ml
   Dissolve buffer in deionized H_2O. Q.S. to 2000 ml.
2. Destaining solution
   Glacial acetic acid   200 ml
   Methyl alcohol   1000 ml
   Distilled H_2O 1000 ml
   Mix together well.
3. Coomassie brilliant blue R 250 (Gelman Instrument Co.)
   Stain   0.25 g
   Destaining solution   1000 ml
   Dissolve stain in destaining solution. Q.S. to 1000 ml.
4. Antisera to human factor VIII – associated protein (Calbiochem-Behring Corp.)
5. Patient's platelet-poor plasma
6. Pooled normal serum
7. Physiologic saline

Procedure

1. Agarose gel slides
   a. Wash and dry the number of glass slides needed. Precoat with a thin layer of 0.1 percent agarose. Allow to air dry.
   b. Dissolve 0.15 g agarose in 15 ml of TRIS barbital buffer for agar. Heat to boiling, constantly stirring with a magnet stirring bar.
   c. When the solution is clear and the agarose dissolved, place in a 55°C waterbath.
   d. When the solution is at 50 to 55°C, add 0.5 ml of factor VIII antiserum to the solution.
   e. Mix thoroughly by swirling the solution.
   f. Place a warm precoated slide on a level work area and pour the agarose-antiserum mixture onto the slide. Allow to cool for 10 to 15 minutes at 22 to 25°C.
   g. Store overnight at 4°C in a moist chamber. Do not make slides more than 3 days prior to use.
   h. By following the pattern of the template, cut wells in the agar. Remove the agar from the wells with a pipette attached to a suction. Wells should not be cut in the agar until just prior to use.
2. Electrophoresis
   a. Pour 500 ml of TRIS barbital buffer for electrophoresis into each side of the electrophoresis chamber. Cool in refrigerator.
   b. Wet two wicks by soaking in buffer in the chamber for several minutes.
   c. Prepare dilutions of frozen normal plasma pool with TRIS buffer as follows: undiluted (100 percent), 1:2 (50 percent), 1:4 (25 percent), and 1:8 (12.5 percent).

d. Prepare dilutions of patient plasma with TRIS buffer as follows: undiluted (100 percent) and 1:2 (50 percent).

e. Place 5 μl of each dilution in each of the wells. Do not perform this step until the electrophoretic apparatus is ready. All samples must be applied and electrophoresis begun within 5 minutes to minimize radial diffusion.

f. Place the slide in the chamber with the sample wells toward the cathode.

g. Place the wet wicks on both the cathode and anode ends of the slide. Be sure the wicks lie flat against the agar with the other end immersed in buffer.

h. Run at 4°C for 18 hours at 8 to 10 mA.

i. When run is complete, wash slide with physiologic saline overnight.

3. Staining

a. Remove slides from saline and place on filter paper. Cover slide with 8 to 10 layers of filter paper. Place a glass slide over filter paper and place a 1-pound weight over glass slide for 15 minutes. This sandwich effect will remove excess water from the slide.

b. At the end of 15 minutes, remove weight and filter paper and allow the slide to air dry.

c. Stain the slide for 10 minutes.

d. Destain slide in several changes of destaining solution until background is almost clear.

Interpretation

1. Measure in millimeters the length of the rockets from the center of the wells to the apex.

2. Make a reference curve using the pooled normal plasma control. Plot the lengths of the rocket for the control dilutions against their concentrations expressed in percent of normal on log-log paper.

3. Draw a best-fit line.

4. Determine the percent of factor VIII–related antigen in the patient's sample from the reference curve. Values for sample dilutions are multiplied by the corresponding dilution factor.

Normal values are 70 to 150 percent. Patients with hemophilia A show normal levels of factor VIII–related antigen. Female carriers of hemophilia A show normal or slightly elevated levels of factor VIII-related antigen. All patients with von Willebrand's disease were originally thought to show decreases in factor VIII–related antigen. It is now recognized that about two thirds of the patients with von Willebrand's show a decrease in the VIII antigen.[17] The remaining patients may show slightly reduced to normal VIII antigen levels.

Comments. Some patients may show variable levels of activity. To accommodate this, undiluted plasma samples should be assayed. This test measures antigenic activity, not biologic activity.

von Willebrand Factor Assay

Patients with von Willebrand's disease (vWD) show abnormal platelet aggregation with ristocetin. The aggregation defect in vWD is due to a humoral factor known as von Willebrand factor (vWF). Supporting evidence is obtained by demonstrating that the abnormal ristocetin aggregation is corrected upon the addition of normal platelet-poor plasma or factor VIII–rich plasma to the platelet-rich plasma prior to testing. Von Willebrand factor is thought to be a required plasma cofactor for the normal adhesion of platelets to the subendothelium at sites of vascular injury. Absence of the vWF results in abnormal platelet adhesion and prolonged bleeding time. The test is based on the concept of a receptor, possibly a glycoprotein, for the vWF on the platelet membrane surface. Washed human platelets will aggregate with ristocetin when normal vWF is present and binds to its receptor.

Principle. In this test, normal washed formalin-fixed platelets are mixed with dilutions of plasma. Ristocetin is added and the rate of aggregation is quantitated. The rate of aggregation is proportional to von Willebrand factor activity.[18] The activity of unknown test samples are extrapolated from a reference graph obtained by testing dilutions of normal pooled plasma.

Reagents and Equipment

Aggregometer
37°C waterbath
Refrigerated centrifuge
16 × 150 mm plastic screw-cap test tubes
Plastic centrifuge tubes
Micropipettes
Formalin fixed platelets

1. TRIS buffered saline, pH 7.3 to 7.4: Mix two parts 0.85 percent NaCl to one part TRIS buffer.
2. NaCl 0.15 M
3. Ristocetin: Dissolve ristocetin in TRIS buffer to a final concentration of 10 mg/ml. Freeze at −30°C in 0.5-ml aliquots.

Procedure

1. Obtain EDTA anticoagulated blood from both patients and normal donors. At least 10 normal donors should be drawn for reference pooled plasma. (Women should not be pregnant or taking oral contraceptives.)

2. Centrifuge at 3000 Gs for 10 minutes. Remove plasma. Do not disturb the buffy coat.

3. Prepare dilutions of reference pooled plasma in TRIS buffer as follows: 1:2, 1:4, 1:8, and 1:16. The dilution of 1:2 represents 100 percent.

4. Prepare dilutions of patient's test plasma in TRIS buffer as follows: 1:2 and 1:4.

5. Prepare the reference blank as follows: 0.25 ml fixed-platelet suspension is added to 0.25 ml of TRIS buffer in an aggregometer cuvette and mixed.

6. To a second aggregometer cuvette, pipette 0.4

ml fixed-platelet suspension. Add 0.05 ml of 1:2 reference-pool dilution to the curvette. Incubate at 37°C for 2 minutes.

7. Add a magnetic stirring bar to the cuvette.
8. Set the baselines for 0 percent and 100 percent for the aggregometer.
9. When the 0 percent baseline has stabilized, add 0.05 ml of ristocetin. Note the point of ristocetin addition on the chart paper.
10. Observe aggregation until point of completion.
11. Repeat steps 4 through 10 on each serial dilution of reference plasma.
12. Repeat steps 4 through 10 on each serial dilution of patient's test plasma.

Interpretation

1. The slope of the aggregation curve for each serial dilution is measured. The slope is defined as the change in OD expressed in millimeters. The slope is determined on the steepest part of the aggregation curve measured down the middle of the curve.
2. Using log-log paper, the slope in millimeters is plotted on the vertical axis for each of the four reference dilutions, while the percent activity is plotted on the horizontal axis.
3. Draw a best-fit line through the points.
4. To determine the percent activity for both dilutions of the patient's test plasma, locate the points where the slope values intersect the reference curve. Average the results.

Normal values are 50 to 150 percent activity (compared with normal pooled plasma as reference). Patients with von Willebrand's disease range from 0 to 50 percent activity.

Comments. There is a high degree of correlation between the activity of von Willebrand factor in vitro and its activity in vivo, as assayed by means of the bleeding time.[19] The results also correlate well with factor VIII:Ag. Von Willebrand factor activity may become normal in those with vWD, during inflammation, pregnancy, or following transfusion with components rich in factor VIII despite the prolonged bleeding times.[20,21] Patients who present with a variant form of vWD may show prolonged bleeding times in the face of decreased to normal vWF levels but increased activity to ristocetin.[22,23]

Normal or increased levels of vWF are found in patients with hemophilia A and in those with Bernard-Soulier syndrome.

Certain disease states such as diabetes mellitus, hyperthyroidism, liver disease, chronic renal failure, pregnancy, endothelial cell damage, and disorders of the myeloproliferative syndrome may cause an increase in the level of vWF activity. Because of these variations, it is suggested that "two or three" separate assays be performed prior to making a diagnosis.

When vWF is assayed by immunologic methods, the protein detected is measured as VIII:Ag. When it is assayed through its interaction with ristocetin and platelets, it is measured as ristocetin cofactor or VIII:vWF.

TESTS FOR NATURAL AND PATHOLOGIC CIRCULATING ANTICOAGULANTS
AT-III Assay

Antithrombin III is a naturally occurring inhibitor of blood coagulation and serves an important role in maintaining blood in the fluid state. It is an α_2-globulin synthesized in the liver, circulating in the plasma, and is the major plasma inhibitor responsible for neutralizing the activity of thrombin, factors IXa, Xa, and plasmin. Antithrombin III slowly, progressively, and irreversibly inhibits the action of thrombin by forming a 1:1 stoichiometric complex with thrombin. This complex forms when the active serine site of thrombin binds with the arginine site of antithrombin. The inhibition of thrombin by AT-III is greatly accelerated by heparin.

Antithrombin III can be measured by a variety of techniques. The most frequently employed assays are (1) a clotting time based on thrombin neutralization, (2) Laurell rocket electroimmunoassay, (3) Mancini radial immunodiffusion, and (4) chromogenic substrate assays.

Assays for AT-III based on thrombin neutralization are not entirely specific for AT-III, as it composes only 75 percent of the blood's antithrombotic activity.[24]

The use of serum instead of plasma may make the clotting tests somewhat more specific for AT-III because its activity is considered progressive. However, some AT-III is thought to be consumed during the clotting process, so that AT-III assays using plasma rather than serum yield higher levels. As a result of these variables, a carefully standardized technique is critical with normal values established for each laboratory.

Assays for AT-III based on immunologic techniques appear to be more sensitive as long as the antiserum employed is specific for AT-III.

Thrombin Neutralization

Principle. By measurement of the neutralization of the clotting activity of a standard solution of thrombin, AT-III is assayed.

Reagents and Equipment

Thrombin
Lyophilized normal human serum
Physiologic saline
Fibrometer
Fibrometer cups and tips
Pipettes

Procedure

1. Draw at least 5 ml of blood in a plastic syringe by means of a clean venipuncture.

2. Aliquot 5 ml of blood into a plain glass tube and allow to clot.
3. Keep the clotted sample at room temperature for exactly 2 hours.
4. Collect the serum by centrifugation. Keep at constant room temperature.
5. Prepare a solution of thrombin in saline that will yield a TT of 15 to 16 seconds with normal plasma (0.2 ml normal plasma added to 0.1 ml thrombin).
6. Warm at 37°C.
7. Deliver 0.2 ml normal plasma into a fibrometer cup and incubate at 37°C.
8. Add 0.1 ml of test serum to 0.9 ml of standard thrombin solution. Mix well. Incubate at 37°C for exactly 3 minutes.
9. Move the fibrometer cup containing 0.2 ml normal plasma to the reaction well of the fibrometer.
10. Immediately at the end of the 3-minute incubation, deliver 0.1 ml of thrombin test serum solution to the 0.2 ml normal plasma and activate the fibrometer.
11. Record the clotting time.

Interpretation. In individuals with normal antithrombin levels, the TT is 33 ± 3 seconds. In patients with decreased antithrombin levels, the TT is less than 26 seconds.

Laurel Rocket Electroimmunoassay

Principle. Plasma or serum containing AT-III is electrophoresed through an agarose gel containing antiserum to AT-III. Precipitation of the antigen with the antibody in the gel results in a rocketlike immunoprecipitate, the length of which is directly proportional to the concentration of antigen in the well.

Equipment

Electrophoresis chamber and power supply
$3\frac{1}{4} \times 4$ inch Kodak glass slides precoated with 0.1 percent agarose
5-μl micropipette
Wicks-telfa strips
Well cutter, 3 mm deep
Template; single row of 14 holes; 3 mm in diameter; 3 mm apart; 2 cm from side of slide

Reagents

1. Barbital buffer for agar, pH 8.6
   Diethylbarbituric acid   1.04 g
   Sodium diethylbarbiturate   6.57 g
   Na$_2$ EDTA   1.0 g
   In 100 ml of warm distilled H$_2$O dissolve barbituric acid. Add remaining salts and 850 ml of distilled H$_2$O. With 1 N NaOH adjust pH to 8.6 Q.S. with distilled H$_2$O to 1 liter.
2. Barbital buffer for electrophoresis, pH 8.6
   Diethylbarbituric acid   2.07 g
   Sodium diethylbarbiturate   13.14 g
   Na$_2$ EDTA   1.0 g
   In 100 ml of warm distilled H$_2$O dissolve barbituric acid. Add remaining salts and 850 ml of distilled H$_2$O. With 1 N NaOH adjust the pH to 8.6. Q.S. with distilled H$_2$O to 1 liter.
3. Agarose
4. Destaining solution
   Glacial acetic acid   200 ml
   Methyl alcohol   1000 ml
   Distilled H$_2$O   1000 ml
   Mix together well.
5. Amido black
   Amido black stain   2 g
   Destaining solution   1000 ml
   Dissolve amido black in destaining solution. Mix well.
6. AT-III antiserum
7. Pooled normal serum frozen in aliquots at −20°C. This control is run on each slide undiluted (100 percent), diluted 1:2 (50 percent), and diluted 1:4 (25 percent). All dilutions are made using barbital buffer.
8. Reference plasma
9. Frozen or fresh patient EDTA plasma or serum. Patient samples are run undiluted (100 percent) and diluted 1:2 (50 percent) as with pooled normal plasma.
10. Physiologic saline

Procedure

1. Agarose gel slides
   a. Wash and dry the number of glass slides needed. Precoat with a thin layer of 1 percent agar. Allow to air dry.
   b. Dissolve 0.115 g agarose in 15 ml of barbital buffer for agar. Heat to boiling, constantly stirring with a magnetic stirring bar.
   c. When the solution is clear and the agarose dissolved, place in a 55°C waterbath.
   d. When the solution is at 50 to 55°C, add 0.6 ml of AT-III antiserum to the solution.
   e. Mix thoroughly by swirling the solution.
   f. Place a warm precoated slide on a level work area and pour the agarose-antiserum mixture onto the slide. Allow to cool for 10 to 15 minutes at 25°C.
   g. Store overnight at 4°C in a moist chamber. Do not make slides more than 3 days prior to use.
   h. By following the pattern of the template, cut wells in the agar. Remove the agar from the wells with a pipette attached to a suction. Wells should not be cut in the agar until just prior to use.
2. Electrophoresis
   a. Pour 500 ml of barbital buffer for electrophoresis into each side of the electrophoretic chamber. Cool in the refrigerator.
   b. Wet two wicks by soaking in buffer in the chamber for several minutes.
   c. Prepare a dilution of frozen normal serum pool as a control: undiluted (100 percent), 1:2 (50 percent), and 1:4 (25 percent).
   d. Prepare dilutions of patient's serum: undiluted (100 percent), 1:2 (50 percent).

e. Place 5 µl of each dilution in each of the wells. Do not perform this step until the electrophoretic apparatus is ready. All samples must be applied and electrophoresis begun within 5 minutes to minimize radial diffusion.
f. Place the slide in the chamber with the sample wells toward the cathode.
g. Place the wet wicks on both the cathode and anode ends of the slide. Be sure the wicks lie flat against the agar with the other end immersed in buffer.
h. Run at 4°C for 6 hours at 7 to 10 mA.
i. When run is complete, wash slide with physiologic saline for several hours or overnight.
3. Staining
a. Remove slides from saline and place on filter paper (No. 1). Cover slide with 8 to 10 layers of filter paper. Place a glass slide over filter paper and place a 1-pound weight over glass slide for 15 minutes. This sandwich effect will remove excess water from the slide.
b. At the end of 15 minutes, remove weight and filter paper and allow the slide to air dry.
c. Stain slide for 5 minutes.
d. Destain slide in several changes of destaining solution until the background is almost clear.

Interpretation

1. Measure in millimeters the length of the rockets from the center of the well to the apex.
2. Make a reference curve using the pooled normal serum control. Plot the lengths of the rocket for the control dilutions against their concentrations expressed in percent of normal on log-log paper.
3. Draw a best-fit line.
4. Determine the percent AT-III in patient sample from reference curve. Values for sample dilutions are multiplied by the corresponding dilution factor.
Normal values range from 88 to 140 percent.

Radial Immunodiffusion

Equipment

3¼ × 4 inch Kodak glass slides precoated with 0.1 percent agarose
5-µl pipette
Well cutter
Template
Agarose, stain, destaining solution, AT-III antiserum, control serum, and patient serum (all the same as for AT-III electroimmunoassay)

Reagents

Phosphate buffer	pH 6.5
K_2HPO_4	0.56 g
KH_2PO_4	0.93 g

Na_2EDTA	1.0 g

Mix salts with 1000 ml of distilled H_2O.

Procedure

1. Using the procedure as described in AT-III rocket assay, prepare the precoated slides with 1 percent agarose in phosphate buffer pH 6.5. Add 0.25 ml of AT-III antiserum to agar.
2. Make a template with 20 wells 3 mm in diameter.
3. By following the pattern of the template, cut 20 wells 3 mm in diameter in the agar. Lift the agar from the wells with suction.
4. Prepare dilutions of control serum: undiluted (100 percent), 1:2 (50 percent). Dilutions are made with phosphate buffer.
5. Place 5 µl of each dilution in each well. The 200 percent reference well receives 10 µl of serum.
6. Place the slide in a moist chamber and incubate at 37°C for 18 hours.
7. Dry and stain, as described for AT-III rocket assay.

Interpretation

1. Measure the diameter of the circles in two directions that are perpendicular to one another.
2. Use the mean diameter of each control sera to make a standard curve. Plot on log-log paper.
3. Determine the percent AT-III in each patient sample from the standard curve.

AT-III Synthetic Substrate Assay

Plasma AT-III activity is determined indirectly by incubation of thrombin with patient plasma and heparin. Residual thrombin activity is used to calculate the percent thrombin inhibited according to a formula. Release of the fluorescent molecule AIE from the substrate by thrombin is measured kinetically using a fluorometer (see package insert for procedural details).

Protein C Assay

Protein C is a vitamin K–dependent serine protease that functions as a major regulatory protein in the control of coagulation. Activated protein C is a potent anticoagulant and mediates this activity by proteolytically inactivating cofactor V and factor VIII, and also elicits fibrinolytic activity in plasma. Cofactors Va and VIIIa are important in accelerating the activation of prothrombin and factor X.

Components of the protein C system include proteins C and S, C4b-binding protein, thrombomodulin, activated protein C inhibitor, and factor V. Protein S, a second vitamin K–dependent factor, is a necessary cofactor in the reaction in which factor Va is inactivated by protein C.

Protein C deficiency is inherited as an autosomal dominant disorder, with three recognizable clinical states: homozygous, heterozygous, and double heterozygous. Patients present with venous thrombosis at an early age of which superficial thrombophlebitis is the most common clinical feature. Some patients with recurrent venous thrombosis have abnormal functional levels of protein C but normal levels of protein C antigen. Plasma protein C levels are decreased in patients with liver disease, in those receiving coumarin, in some patients with DIC, and in some postoperative patients.

Laboratory diagnosis of a protein C deficiency is by means of antigenic or functional assays. Antigenic assays use radioimmunoassays (RIAs), Laurell rocket immunoelectrophoresis, and an enzyme-linked immunosorbent assay (ELISA) method. Laurell rocket assay and ELISA appear to be somewhat more sensitive than RIAs. In patients who present with venous thrombosis in the face of normal antigenic levels, functional protein C assays should be performed. The APTT and the PT are not sensitive to decreases in protein C levels. One functional assay extracts protein C by barium citrate or aluminum hydroxide, activates it by means of thrombin-thrombomodulin complex, and measures activated protein C with a synthetic chromogenic substrate. This assay is capable of detecting low levels of protein C in both acquired and congenital deficiencies. Heparin may interfere with the test system. An alternate method of separation uses polyclonal antibodies to human protein C. In this method, protein C is activated in recalcified plasma with thrombin-thrombomodulin complex. Protein Ca (activated) is then immunoabsorbed with anti-human protein C. The immunoadsorbed protein C retains the ability to hydrolyze chromogenic substrates. After washing, to remove unbound plasma proteins, the bound activated protein C is quantitated by incubation with a synthetic substrate. The advantage of this method is that functional defects of protein C, in which activation or amidolytic activity is lost, may be detected. Heparin interferes with this test system. Recently, an assay has been developed that measures the anticoagulant and amidolytic activity of protein C in the presence of heparin and in patients receiving oral anticoagulants. The method uses a Ca^{2+}-dependent monoclonal antibody to human protein C. Protein C is adsorbed from recalcified heparinized plasma and then eluted. Activation of protein C is by either thrombin or the thrombin-thrombomodulin complex. Protein Ca is then measured by both amidolytic and anticoagulant assays. This assay is used to monitor changes in functional protein C activity during oral anticoagulant therapy.

Protein S Assay

Protein S, a second vitamin K–dependent factor, is required for activated protein C anticoagulant activity. Both functional and antigenic assays exist for protein S. Because protein S exists in two states, bound and free, interpretation of laboratory tests are more complex than those for protein C. Protein S bound to C4b-binding protein (C4b-BP) has little or no cofactor activity; free protein S is functional. It is recommended that both free protein S and total protein S be determined. Total protein S can be determined by means of Laurell rocket electrophore-

sis performed at 25°C. Higher temperatures dissociate the complex, whereas reduced temperatures make interpretation difficult. Distribution of free and bound protein S is determined by crossed immunoelectrophoresis in which free protein S migrates faster than C4b-BP–bound protein S. Semiquantitative information about protein S distribution is obtained by comparing normal plasma patterns with those in the patients. The functional protein S assay is based on the observation that activated protein C will not anticoagulate plasma in the absence of protein S. Protein S–deficient plasma is clotted by factor Xa in a one-stage assay that uses cephalin. Activated protein C is then added. A linear relationship exists between the concentration of protein S and the prolonged clotting time. Normal plasma added to protein S–deficient plasma causes a prolonged clotting time proportional to the amount of normal plasma added. Functional protein S determinations are obtained by comparing the clotting time response of normal plasma with that of the patient. Presence of heparin and factor Va interferes with this assay, as will oral anticoagulants.

Screening Test for the Detection of Circulating Anticoagulants

Circulating anticoagulants are acquired pathologic plasma proteins that inhibit normal coagulation. Circulating anticoagulants differ from naturally occurring inhibitors such as AT-III, α_2-macroglobulin, α_2-antitrypsin, and C1 esterase and must be differentiated from anticoagulants such as heparin and coumarin analogues. The majority of these pathologic anticoagulants are inhibitors or autoantibodies of the IgG class whose inhibitory effects are directed against certain coagulation factors or demonstrate specific activity against phospholipids (such as factor VIII and the prothrombin complex).

Some of the circulating anticoagulants that have been detected thus far have been encountered in patients with the following conditions: hemophilia A, Christmas disease, DIC, pregnancy, systemic lupus erythematosus (SLE), the plasma cell dyscrasias, Waldenström's macroglobulinemia, advanced age, and others.

The circulating anticoagulant directed against the factor VIII molecule is the most common specific factor inhibitor. It is seen in patients with hemophilia A and may be related to repeated therapeutic transfusions of antihemophilic factor (AHF) but is also seen in nonhemophiliac patients (for example, women following childbirth or abortion, elderly individuals, and those with immunologic disorders such as rheumatoid arthritis). Antibodies to factor VIII may also be seen in those patients known to have the severe form of von Willebrand's disease.

Other specific inhibitors have been reported against factor IX, factor XI, factor XII, factor V, factor XIII, and inhibitors of fibrin formation.

Some patients with SLE develop an acquired circulating anticoagulant. This inhibitor demonstrates specific activity against phospholipids and thus interferes with phospholipid-dependent complexes that involve factors V and VIII.[27]

Principle. The APTT is useful as a screening test for all types of circulating anticoagulants. The test is based on the ability of normal plasma to correct an abnormal clotting time with a factor deficiency. The addition of normal plasma will not correct the clotting time in the presence of a circulating anticoagulant.

Reagents and Equipment

APTT reagent
$CaCl_2$ (0.025 M)
Test plasma
Normal plasma

Procedure

1. Collect citrated plasma from patients and from a normal control.
2. Mix patient's plasma with normal control plasma in a series of six 12 × 75 test tubes, as follows:

Tube No.	Patient's Plasma	Normal Control Plasma
1	0.20 ml	—
2	0.15 ml	0.05 ml
3	0.10 ml	0.10 ml
4	0.05 ml	0.15 ml
5	0.02 ml	0.18 ml
6	—	0.20 ml

Tube 6 is the control; tube 1 is 100 percent patient's plasma; tube 2 is 75 percent patient's plasma; tube 3 is 50 percent patient's plasma; tube 4 is 25 percent patient's plasma; and tube 5 is 10 percent patient's plasma.

3. Incubate each tube for 1 hour at 37°C.
4. Measure APTT for each tube.

Interpretation. If the APTT is corrected by normal plasma, a factor deficiency is indicated. The addition of normal plasma supplies the coagulation factor or factors that are deficient, and thus corrects the APTT. When a factor deficiency is present, there should be correction of the abnormal APTT by only 10 to 25 percent normal plasma[28] (tubes 5 and 4).

If the APTT is not corrected by the addition of normal plasma in most of the mixtures, a strong circulating anticoagulant is indicated.

A weak circulating anticoagulant is indicated by a prolonged APTT following incubation at 37°C for 1 hour. Upon incubation, a weak inhibitor progressively inactivates the coagulation factor, thus prolonging the APTT. This pattern is most typical of a factor VIII inhibitor.

Comments. The circulating anticoagulant that inhibits factor VIII is a specific IgG antibody.[29] These antibodies are often present as weak circulating anticoagulants but are temperature and time dependent, thus causing only a slightly prolonged clotting time on fresh patient plasma. Mixing tests may yield APTT results intermediate between the clotting times of patient and normal control. Upon incubation at 37°C, both the patient plasma and mixing plasmas will show prolonged times, but the normal control plasma will show no change. Owing to the nature of the factor VIII inhibitor, the mixture of test plasma and normal control plasma must be incubated for a period of 30 to 120 minutes to allow for the inhibitor's progressive activity.

If a factor VIII inhibitor is present, it is important to determine the level of activity periodically because the development of an inhibitor complicates the management of a patient with hemophilia when therapy involves AHF concentrates.

The TT is also of value in the detection of circulating anticoagulants.

Screening Tests for the Detection and Confirmation of Lupus Anticoagulants

Lupus anticoagulants (LA) are antibodies (IgG, IgM, IgA, or a mixture) reactive against phospholipids, thereby prolonging in vitro phospholipid-dependent coagulation tests. First recognized in patients with SLE, lupus anticoagulants have been identified in a variety of disorders including malignancies, infections, and autoimmune disorders, as well as following drug therapy. The presence of an LA is usually not associated with a bleeding problem unless accompanied by thrombocytopenia, platelet dysfunction, or drug administration (that is, aspirin). The LA, however, has been associated with a risk factor for venous and arterial thrombosis and recurrent spontaneous abortions.[25]

The laboratory diagnosis of a lupus inhibitor is critical in terms of distinguishing it from other specific factor inhibitors and to identify patients at potential risk for thrombotic problems. Triplett and Brandt[26] have established criteria for the laboratory detection of these inhibitors. They include (1) an abnormal phospholipid dependent coagulation test result (APTT and/or PT), (2) demonstration that the abnormal test is due to an inhibitor, and (3) proof that the inhibitor is directed against phospholipids. Suspicion of an LA is most often aroused by an unexplained prolongation of the APTT that is not corrected by the addition of an equal volume of normal plasma. Confirmatory tests to identify an LA include those that decrease the phospholipid in the test system, thereby increasing the LA effect, such as the tissue thromboplastin inhibition (TTI) test, dilute Russell's viper venom time (dRVVT), and the kaolin clotting time (KCT), or those that increase the phospholipid, thereby neutralizing the LA effect, such as the platelet neutralization procedure (PNP).

Tissue Thromboplastin Inhibition Test

The LA inhibits coagulation at the prothrombin complex (factor Xa-V-PF 3-Ca^{2+}), thereby interfering in the activation of prothrombin. The TTI test may be used to detect the presence of an LA. The test is not specific for LAs; false-positive results have been noted in patients with factor deficiencies, with factor inhibitors, and receiving anticoagulant therapy.

Dilute Russell's Viper Venom Test

The dRVVT is used as a confirmatory test for the presence of LA. The test system uses a dilute solution of Russell's viper venom and a dilute solution of phospholipid. If the dRVVT result is abnormal, a 1 : 1 mixing test using patient plasma and normal plasma is performed to differentiate a factor deficiency from an LA. The mixing test will remain abnormal in the presence of an LA.

Kaolin Clotting Time

Kaolin activates coagulation by means of the contact factors. The KCT of platelet-poor plasmas with no added phospholipid is a sensitive test for the detection of LA. The test may be performed on patient plasma or on mixtures of patient plasma and normal plasma.

Platelet Neutralization Procedure

Principle. The PNP is based on the ability of platelets to correct significantly in vitro coagulation abnormalities. The disrupted platelet membranes present in the freeze-thawed platelet suspension neutralizes phospholipid antibodies present in the plasma of patients with LA. After mixing the patient plasma with the freeze-thawed platelet suspension, the APTT will be "corrected" when compared with the original baseline APTT.

Reagents and Equipment

TRIS buffered saline (pH 7.4 ± 0.1)
CaCl$_2$ (0.02 M)
Washed freeze-thawed platelet suspension
APTT reagent
37°C heat block
Control (TRIS buffered saline)
Patient sample

Procedure for Washed Freeze-Thawed Platelet Suspension

1. Add 20 ml of recently expired platelet concentrate into a large plastic test tube with a cap.
2. To this, add 20 ml of cold TRIS buffered saline. Mix.
3. To remove any contamination by RBCs, centrifuge for 15 minutes at 1000 rpm.
4. Transfer the platelet-rich supernatant to a new plastic test tube.

5. Centrifuge for 10 minutes at 3000 rpm.
6. Discard supernatant, resuspend platelets in 5 ml of TRIS buffered saline.
7. Repeat steps 5 and 6 twice. Platelet suspension should be washed a total of three times.
8. After the last wash, resuspend platelets in a volume of TRIS buffered saline to adjust the platelet count to 200,000 to 300,000 per mm^3. Adjust the platelet count (PC) using the formula at the bottom of the page.
9. Make 1-ml aliquots of the platelet suspension and place in plastic tubes. Freeze at −20°C.

Control. Substitute 0.1 ml of TRIS buffered saline for the washed freeze-thawed platelet suspension in the Procedure.

Procedure

1. Thaw platelet suspension at room temperature.
2. Warm of 0.02 M CaCl$_2$ at 37°C.
3. In a 12 × 75 mm glass test tube add:
   0.1 ml patient plasma
   0.1 ml platelet suspension
   0.1 ml APTT reagent
4. Incubate for 5 minutes at 37°C.
5. Add 0.1 ml prewarmed CaCl$_2$. Start the stopwatch.
6. Record the time it takes to form a clot.
7. Run control as in test plasma substituting, 0.1 ml of TRIS buffered saline for platelet suspension.
8. All testing, both on controls and on test plasma, must be performed in duplicate.

Interpretation. A correction of the baseline APTT of 5 seconds or more by the platelet suspension as compared with the control is indicative of the presence of an LA.

Comments. Specimen collection, centrifugation, and processing are critical when testing for the presence of an LA. Coagulation assays that have a phospholipid-dependent reaction are affected by the presence of platelets in platelet-poor plasma. Lupus anticoagulants are directed against phospholipids, and therefore the relative concentration of phospholipid affects the sensitivity of the assay for detection of the LA.

Previously considered as indicative of factor VIII inhibitors, time-dependent inhibition has been seen in lupus anticoagulants and factor V inhibitors.

Lupus anticoagulants demonstrate considerable heterogeneity and show variable differences in sensitivity and responsiveness to various reagents. Laboratory recognition of these inhibitors depends on the sensitivity and responsiveness of the reagent, as well as on the selection of an appropriate confirmatory test. Despite the differences in testing methodology and reagents currently available, the majority of these anticoagulants can be detected and identified.

$$\underset{\text{(count obtained)}}{PC_1} \times V_1 = \underset{\text{(final concentration)}}{PC_2} \times \underset{\text{(total volume 5 ml)}}{V_2}$$

Anticardiolipin Assay

Principle. Anticardiolipin antibodies (ACAs) and LAs are antiphospholipid immunoglobulins (IgG, IgM, or a combination). Several studies have shown that patients with the LA and the closely related ACA are prone to recurrent venous and arterial thrombosis, recurrent spontaneous abortions, and thrombocytopenia.[30] Some patients with anticardiolipin antibodies have been reported to show an LA. The concept of an antiphospholipid antibody syndrome has been proposed. This would include patients with antiphospholipid antibodies (APAs), whether or not an LA is present; patients who have a confirmed LA only; and those who show evidence of both APA and an LA.

An ELISA assay for anticardiolipin antibodies has recently been developed. The commercial kits use cardiolipin or a mixture of negatively charged phospholipids as antigen (see Chapter 28).

TESTS FOR THE FIBRINOLYTIC SYSTEM

Tests for FDPs

Plasmin proteolytically cleaves fibrin(ogen) into fragments X and Y, known as early degradation products, and fragments D and E, known as late degradation products. These FDPs share antigenic determinants with both fibrin and fibrinogen, thus allowing for detection by immunologic methods by the use of antisera to highly purified preparations of human fibrinogen fragments D and E. Measurement of FDPs provides an indirect assay of fibrinolysis.

Thrombo-Wellcotest: Latex Agglutination Test

Principle. This test is a direct latex agglutination slide test for the detection and semiquantitation of FDPs. Latex particles in glycine buffer are coated with specific antibodies to human fibrinogen fragments D and E. The presence of FDPs, either in the serum or in the urine, causes the latex particles to clump, yielding macroscopic agglutination. An approximate concentration of FDPs in the sample can be determined by testing the sample at different dilutions. Thrombin is added to the test sample to ensure complete clotting and complete removal of fibrinogen. The addition of a proteolytic inhibitor—soybean trypsin—prevents in vitro activation of the fibrinolytic system.

Reagents and Equipment. Thrombo-Wellcotest kit (Burroughs-Wellcome and Co., Triangle Park, NC).

Procedure[31] (Serum Sample)

1. Collect 2 ml of venous blood in a special FDP sample vacutainer tube (provided with test kit). Mix immediately by gentle inversion several times.
2. Ring the clot to allow retraction to occur. Keep the sample tube at 37°C for 30 minutes or centrifuge to separate serum.
3. If the sample is obtained from a heparinized patient, reptilase (Abbott Laboratories, North Chicago, IL) should be added to the blood. Reptilase-R, an enzyme isolated from snake venom, will clot fibrinogen in the presence of heparin and other such antithrombins. Reptilase-R 0.1 ml will clot 1.0 ml of blood.
4. Label two 12 × 75 test tubes. Prepare dilutions of the serum as follows:

	Tube 1	Tube 2
Glycine buffer	0.75 ml	0.75 ml
Serum	5 drops	1 drop
Final dilution	1:5	1:20

To aliquot the buffer, use the graduated dropper provided. To deliver the sample, use the disposable pipette and bulb provided in the kit. Mix well.

5. Label two rings on the glass slide provided as 1 and 2.
6. Transfer 1 drop of the dilution from test tube 2 to position 2 on the glass slide and 1 drop from test tube 1 to position 1. Deliver the dilutions in this order.
7. Thoroughly mix the latex suspension. Add 1 drop to each position on the slide.
8. Stir the latex-serum mixture. Start with position 2 on the slide, then mix position 1. When stirring the mixture, spread to fill the circles.
9. Gently rotate the slide for 2 minutes and no longer. Observe the slide for macroscopic agglutination by viewing against a dark background.

Controls

1. Label two of the rings on the glass test slide (+) and (−) for positive and negative controls.
2. Place one drop of the appropriate control and one drop of latex suspension on the slide and mix as described earlier.
3. Read results. Failure of the controls to react as described indicates deterioration of at least one of the reagents or an improperly performed test.

Interpretation. The test is sensitive to values of 2 μg of FDP per ml. The presence of agglutination in position 1 indicates the presence of FDPs in a final concentration greater than 10 μg/ml. The presence of agglutination in position 2 indicates the presence of FDPs in a final concentration of greater than 40 μg/ml. For the test to be valid, if agglutination is present in position 2 it must also be present in position 1 on the slide. Agglutination in tube 1 and lack of agglutination in tube 2 indicates FDPs greater than 10 μg/ml but less than 40 μg/ml.

Lack of agglutination indicates an FDP concentration of less than 2 μg/ml. The mean normal level of serum is 4.9 ± 2.8 μg FDP per ml. The normal value may be elevated during exercise and stress.

The latex agglutination assay has been documented to give false-positive results with sera from patients with rheumatoid arthritis. Trace amounts of FDPs occur in the blood of normal healthy adults and children as a result of physiologic fibrinolysis.

Procedure[32] (Urine Sample)

1. Obtain a fresh urine sample.
2. Add 2 ml of urine to a special FDP sample vacutainer tube. Mix immediately by gentle inversion several times. If the urine sample has been contaminated with blood, do not accept for testing.
3. Filter the urine through a membrane filter with a pore size of less than or equal to 8 μm and freeze at $-20°C$ overnight. Centrifuge the sample upon thawing. If the assay must be run immediately, use the urine sample after filtering.
4. Label a 12 × 75 test tube. Prepare a dilution of the urine as follows: Add 0.75 ml of glycine buffer to the test tube; add 4 drops of urine to the buffer in the test tube. Mix thoroughly. This yields a 1:5 dilution.
5. On the glass slide provided, label two rings as 1 and 2.
6. Transfer 1 drop of diluted urine to position 2 on the glass slide and 1 drop of undiluted urine to position 1.
7. Thoroughly mix the latex suspension. Add 1 drop to each position on the slide.
8. Stir the latex-urine mixture. Start with position 2 on the slide, then mix position 1. When stirring the mixture spread to fill the circles.
9. Gently rotate the slide for 2 minutes and no longer. Observe the slide for macroscopic agglutination by viewing against a dark background.

Interpretation. The test is sensitive to values of 2 μg of FDP per ml. The presence of agglutination in position 1 indicates the presence of FDPs in a final concentration greater than 2 μg/ml. The presence of agglutination in position 2 indicates the presence of FDPs in a final concentration greater than 10 μg/ml. For the test to be valid if agglutination is present in position 2, it must also be present in position 1 on the slide. Lack of agglutination indicates an FDP concentration of less than 2 μg/ml. Urine normally contains less than 0.25 μg FDP per ml.

Comments. Generally, elevated levels of FDP are associated with thrombotic episodes such as myocardial infarcts, pulmonary emboli, and deep vein thrombosis, as well as with certain complications of pregnancy.

The assay is of value in the differential diagnosis of patients with certain kidney diseases. Quantitation of urine FDP levels provides a useful clinical means of monitoring glomerulonephritis and kidney rejection following transplantation.

The detection of FDPs is of great clinical value in assessing patients with DIC. A positive test result, accompanied by an elevated PT and APTT and a decrease in platelet count and fibrinogen concentration, is suggestive of DIC.

There are other tests that can be used to detect the presence of FDPs. A test that is used to screen for FDPs is the TT. The TT is prolonged in the presence of a low fibrinogen concentration, as well as antithrombins such as FDPs or heparin, or both. To differentiate a prolonged TT due to the presence of heparin or of FDPs, the reptilase time is used. The reptilase time is prolonged in the presence of FDPs but normal in the presence of heparin.

The test generally thought of as the reference method of assaying FDPs is the tanned red cell hemagglutination inhibition immunoassay (TRCHII). This test, performed as a microtiter procedure, is sensitive to fragments X, Y, D, and E. Patient's serum is mixed with antiserum to fibrinogen and then with fibrinogen-coated tanned red cells. If the patient's serum contains FDPs, the FDPs will complex with the antisera and will not agglutinate. If the patient's serum does not contain FDPs, the antisera will complex with the fibrinogen-coated red cells and will agglutinate. Results with the latex method closely correlate with TRCHII. The TRCHII is suitable if a precise quantitation for FDP is required.

The staphylococcal clumping test uses a strain of staphylococcus that clumps in the presence of fragments X and Y, fibrinogen, and fibrin monomers. The test is insensitive to the late degradation products, fragments D and E.

Other immunologic means of assaying FDPs include immunodiffusion, immunoelectrophoresis, counterelectrophoresis, and radioimmunoassay.

D-Dimer (D-DI Test)

Principle. Under the action of thrombin, fibrinogen is cleaved to give rise to fibrin monomers. These monomers form polymers, which are stabilized by factor XIII, forming covalent cross-linkages in the D domain to produce an insoluble fibrin clot. Plasmin, a potent clot-lysing enzyme, attacks fibrin clots as well as fibrinogen in the body. Unlike plasmin's action on fibrinogen, which produces FDPs, its action on the fibrin clot leads to the generation of cross-linked fibrin containing D-dimer. The latex particles provided in the D-DI test are coated with mouse antihuman D-dimer monoclonal antibodies. Test samples containing D-dimers when mixed with the latex particle suspension make the particles agglutinate.

Reagents and Equipment

D-DI Test Kit (American Bioproducts Company, Parsippany, NJ)

Specimen: Citrated plasma; EDTA or heparinized plasmas can also be used. Samples must be collected with the appropriate amount of blood-to-anticoagulant ratio.

20-μl pipette

Procedure (Qualitative)[33]

1. Centrifuge samples at 3000 rpm for 10 minutes. Plasmas are good at room temperature (18 to 25°C) for 4 hours, at 2 to 8°C for 8 hours.

2. Allow reagents from the kit to come to room temperature.
3. Label the test slide with the identification of the patient(s) undiluted and 1:2 dilution plasma and label the positive and negative controls.
4. Prepare the 1:2 dilution of each patient's plasma by placing 100 μl of glycine buffer in a test tube, and then add 100 μl of the patient's plasma. Mix well.
5. Place 20 μl of patient's undiluted plasma and 20 μl of the 1:2 dilution in their respective circles. Place the same amount of the positive and negative controls in the appropriately labeled circles.
6. Invert the latex suspension vial several times to mix and dispense 20 μl in each circle on the slide that contains test samples. Use separate mixing rods to mix the contents of each circle.
7. Rock the slide gently for 2 minutes.
8. Examine for agglutination and compare with the positive and negative controls.

Procedure (Semiquantitative)

1. If dilutions are requested, perform the test as follows:

Transfer	μl of Glycine Buffer	Dilution
100 μl of 1:2	100	1:4
100 μl of 1:4	100	1:8
100 μl of 1:8	100	1:16
100 μl of 1:16	100	1:32

2. Perform qualitative procedure steps 3 through 8.

Results. Use the following table to interpret patterns.

Undiluted Plasma	1:2 Dilution	D-Dimer μg/ml
0	0	<0.5
+	0	0.5–1.0
+	+	>1.0

Semiquantitative DILUTIONS					Approximate
1:2	1:4	1:8	1:16	1:32	D-Dimer Level
++	+	0	0	0	1.0–2.0
+	+	+	0	0	2.0–4.0
+	+	+	+	0	4.0–8.0
+	+	+	+	+	8.0–16.0

Interpretation

1. Normal values are less than 0.5 μg/ml.
2. A positive D-DI test result is usually seen in DIC, deep vein thrombosis, and pulmonary embolism.

3. The presence of rheumatoid factor (RF) may cause false-positive results with the D-DI test.

Paracoagulation Tests

Principle. The formation of soluble fibrin monomer complexes occurs through the action of thrombin on fibrinogen. Thrombin cleaves fibrinopeptides A and B from fibrinogen, resulting in the formation of fibrin monomer. Fibrin monomers are capable of polymerizing to form insoluble fibrin. During intravascular coagulation the fibrin monomers generated remain in solution by complexing with fibrinogen, FDPs, or cold insoluble globulins. When plasma is cooled to 40°F, soluble fibrin monomer-fibrinogen complexes will precipitate as cryofibrinogen. Paracoagulants, such as protamine sulfate, ethanol, and products from staphylococci, will convert soluble fibrin monomer complexes into insoluble fibrin. Ethanol as well as protamine sulfate will dissociate the soluble fibrin monomer complexes, allowing the fibrin monomers to polymerize, becoming insoluble and resulting in the formation of visible fibrin strands.

Soluble fibrin monomer complexes may be detected by gelation or paracoagulation as with ethanol or protamine sulfate, by cooling as in the formation of cryofibrinogens, or by the formation of a precipitate as in the staphylococcal clumping test.

Ethanol Gelation Test

Principle. When ethanol is added to plasma containing soluble fibrin monomers, a visible gel is formed.

Reagents and Equipment

Ethyl alcohol 50 percent (v/v)
Platelet-poor citrated plasma from patient and normal donor as "control" (perform test within 1 hour of blood collection)
Test tube, 12 × 75 mm
Pipettes

Procedure

1. Add 0.5 ml of plasma to a 12 × 75 mm test tube. To this add 0.15 ml of 50 percent ethyl alcohol.
2. Mix gently. Leave at room temperature undisturbed for exactly 10 minutes. Tilt tube to check for gel formation.
3. Run a normal donor as control.

Interpretation. A positive test result causes visible gel formation. A granular precipitate is read as a negative result.

Comments. The presence of soluble fibrin monomers is seen in patients with DIC, in some patients with acute myocardial infarction, and in patients with pulmonary emboli or with extensive deep vein thrombophlebitis. Five to 10 percent of patients who present with acute DIC have negative paracoagulation test results.[34] The test result is negative in patients with primary fibrinolysis.

False-negative results may occur in patients with severe cases of hypofibrinogenemia. False-positive results may be seen in those with dysproteinemias or hyperfibrinogenemia. The diagnosis of DIC should be supported by other clinical and laboratory findings.

Protamine Sulfate Test

Principle. When protamine sulfate is added to plasma containing soluble fibrin monomer complexes and FDPs, visible fibrin formation occurs.

Reagents and Equipment

Protamine sulfate, 1 percent solution
Platelet-poor plasma, patient and control
37°C incubator
Test tubes 12 × 75 mm
Pipettes

Procedure

1. Pipette 1.0 ml of plasma to a test tube. Place in 37°C incubator. To this add 0.1 ml of protamine sulfate solution.
2. Mix gently. Incubate at 37°C for 15 minutes.
3. Remove tube and inspect for clot formation.
4. Run normal control.

Interpretation. A positive test result shows definite fibrin strands. A negative result is indicated by no precipitated material in the test tube.

Comments. A positive test result is suggestive of DIC. The result is negative in those with primary fibrinolysis. The diagnosis of DIC should be supported by other clinical and laboratory findings.

Euglobulin Lysis Time

Principle. Most tests that evaluate fibrinolytic activity are based on fibrin formation in the presence of plasminogen and its activators. Under normal circumstances the dissolution of a clot occurs slowly, for the plasminogen activators must diffuse into or adsorb onto the clot and mediate lysis. The euglobulin test evaluates fibrinolytic activity and therefore is a measure of plasminogen activator concentration. The euglobulin fraction of plasma contains fibrinogen, plasminogen, and plasminogen activators, with only trace amounts of antiplasmins. In the presence of increased plasminogen activators, the lysis time is shortened.

Reagents and Equipment

Equipment for the collection of blood
37°C waterbath
Centrifuge
Centrifuge tubes, 12-ml graduated and 10-ml tubes
Serologic pipettes
Sodium citrate, 0.11 M
Buffered physiologic saline (1 part sodium barbital acetate buffer pH 7.42 and 4 parts of 0.85 percent NaCl)
Thrombin (1000 NIH units in 5 ml 50 percent glycerol)
CO_2—a tank fitted with a valve to control flow rate

Procedure

1. Add 0.5 ml of 0.11 M sodium citrate to a 12-ml graduated centrifuge tube. To this, add 4.5 M of venous blood.
2. Mix blood and anticoagulant by gentle inversion. Centrifuge immediately for 4 minutes at 1000gs.
3. Transfer plasma to a clean test tube.
4. To a 50-ml Erlenmeyer flask containing 15 ml of distilled water, add 1 ml of plasma. Mix thoroughly.
5. Bubble a stream of CO_2 over the surface of the plasma water mixture for 4 minutes. Slowly swirl the flask for the entire 4-minute period. This may be done by hand or with a magnetic stirrer. Avoid excessive foaming.
6. Transfer the mixture to a 40-ml centrifuge tube and spin for 3 minutes at 1000gs.
7. Discard the supernatant. Invert the tube and allow to drain for 2 to 4 minutes.
8. Without disturbing the euglobulin fraction, wipe the inside walls of the tube clean.
9. Add 1 ml of buffered saline solution to the euglobulin fraction. Stir the mixture with a siliconized glass rod. Within 1 minute the euglobulin fraction dissolves. The remaining procedure must be performed quickly to avoid spontaneous clotting of the euglobulin fraction.
10. Transfer 0.3 ml of the mixture into two 10 × 75-mm test tubes.
11. Blow 0.01 ml of thrombin into each tube. Invert the tubes once. Clotting will occur in a few seconds.
12. Stopper the test tubes and incubate in a 37°C waterbath. Observe at 15-minute intervals for lysis. The end-point is complete dissolution of the clot with no remaining residue.

Interpretation. Normal euglobulin lysis time is greater than 2 hours. Complete lysis in less than 2 hours is evidence of increased fibrinolytic activity.

Comments. States of hypofibrinogenemia or afibrinogenemia will yield results that are difficult to interpret, because dissolution of the clot may occur faster than normal. The test is most useful as a means of monitoring urokinase and streptokinase therapy.[35] A loss of fibrinolytic activity is seen in stored and frozen plasma; therefore, the test should be performed as soon as the blood is drawn.[36]

REFERENCES

1. Davidson, I and Henry, JB: Clinical Diagnosis by Laboratory Methods, ed 15. WB Saunders, Philadelphia, 1974.
2. Surgicutt Brochure. International Technidyne Corporation, Edison, NJ, 1986.
3. Lenahan, JG and Smith, K: Hemostasis, ed 16. General Diagnostics, Division of Warner-Lambert Co, Morris Plains, NJ, 1982.
4. Dacie, JV and Lewis, SM: Practical Hematology, ed 4. Grune & Stratton, New York, 1968.
5. Bowie, EJW and Owens, CA Jr: The value of mesuring platelet "adhesiveness" in the diagnosis of bleeding diseases. Am J Clin Pathol 60:302, 1973.

6. Dacie, JV and Lewis, SM: Practical Hematology, ed 4. Grune & Stratton, New York, 1968.

7. Born, GVR: Aggregation of blood platelets by adenosine diphosphate and its reversal. Nature 194:927, 1962.

8. Wilner, AD, Nossel, HL, and LeRoy, EC: Aggregation of platelets by collagen. J Clin Invest 47:2616, 1968.

9. Triplett DA, et al: Platelet Function: Laboratory Evaluation and Clinical Application. American Society of Clinical Pathologists, Chicago, 1978.

10. Triplett, DA, et al: Platelet Function: Laboratory Evaluation and Clinical Application. American Society of Clinical Pathologists, Chicago, 1978.

11. Quick, AJ, Stanley-Brown, M, and Bancroft, FW: A study of the coagulation defect in hemophilia and jaundice. Am Med Sci 190:501, 1935.

12. Prentice, CMR and Ratnoff, OD: The action of Russell's viper venom on factor V and the prothrombin-converting principle. Br J Haematol 16:29, 1969.

13. Bauer, JD: Clinical Laboratory Methods, ed 9. CV Mosby, St Louis, 1982.

14. Clauss, A: Gerinnungsphysiologishe Schneliomethode zur Bestimmung des Fibrinogens. Acta Haematol 17:237, 1957.

15. Quick, AJ: Hemorrhagic Diseases and Thrombosis, ed 2. Lea & Febiger, Philadelphia, 1966.

16. Kitchens, CS and Newcomb, TF: Factor XIII. Medicine 58:413, 1979.

17. Gralnick, HR, Sultan, Y, and Coller, BS: von Willebrand's disease. Combined qualitative and quantitative abnormalities. N Engl J Med 296:1024, 1977.

18. Weiss, HJ, et al: Quantitative assay of a plasma factor, deficient in von Willebrand's disease, that is necessary for platelet aggregation. Relationship to factor VIII procoagulant activity and antigen content. J Clin Invest 52:2708, 1973.

19. Weiss, HJ, et al: Quantitative assay of a plasma factor, deficient in von Willebrand's disease, that is necessary for platelet aggregation. Relationship to factor VIII procoagulant activity and antigen content. J Clin Invest 52:2708, 1973.

20. Ratnoff, OD and Saito, H: Bleeding in von Willebrand's disease. N Engl J Med 290:420, 1974.

21. Weiss, HJ: Relation of von Willebrand's factor to bleeding time. N Engl J Med 291:420, 1974.

22. Ruggeri, ZM, et al: Heightened interaction between platelets and factor VIII/von Willebrand's factor in a new subtype of von Willebrand's disease. N Engl J Med 302:1047, 1980.

23. Ruggeri, ZM and Zimmerman, TS: Variant von Willebrand's disease. Characterization of two subtypes by analysis of multimeric composition of factor VIII/von Willebrand's factor in plasma and platelets. J Clin Invest 65:131a, 1980.

24. Miale, JB: Laboratory Medicine: Hematology, ed 6. CV Mosby, St Louis, 1982.

25. Carreras, LO, et al: Arterial thrombosis, intrauterine death, and "lupus anticoagulant": Detection of immunoglobulin interfering with prostacyclin formation. Lancet 1:244, 1981.

26. Triplett, DA and Brandt, JT: Lupus anticoagulant: Misnomer, paradox, riddle, epiphenomenon. Hematol Pathol, 1988.

27. Schleider, MA, Nachman, RL, Jaffe, EA, et al: A clinical study of the lupus anticoagulant. Blood 48:499, 1976.

28. Sirridge, MS and Shannon, R: Laboratory Evaluation of Hemostasis and Thrombosis, ed 3. Lea & Febiger, Philadelphia, 1983, p 124.

29. Sirridge, MS and Shannon, R: Laboratory Evaluation of Hemostasis and Thrombosis, ed 3. Lea & Febiger, Philadelphia, 1983.

30. Harris, NE, et al: Thrombosis, recurrent fetal loss and thrombocytopenia: Predictive value of the anticardiolipin antibody test. Arch Intern Med 146:2153, 1986.

31. Detection of fibrinogen degradation products and fibrinogen. Wellcome Reagents Division, Burroughs-Wellcome Co, Research Triangle Park, NC, 1977.

32. Detection of fibrinogen degradation products and fibrinogen. Wellcome Reagents Division, Burroughs-Wellcome Co, Research Triangle Park, NC, 1977.

33. D-DI Test Kit. American Bioproducts Company, Parsippany, NJ, test revised 1988.

34. Murano, G amd Bick, RL: Basic Concepts of Hemostasis and Thrombosis. CRC Press, Boca Raton, FL, 1980.

35. Williams, JW, et al: Hematology, ed 2. McGraw-Hill, New York, 1977.

36. von Kaulla, KN and Schultz, RL: Methods for the evaluation of human fibrinolysins. Am J Clin Pathol 29:104, 1952

BIBLIOGRAPHY

Abildgard, CF, et al: Serial studies in von Willebrand's disease: Variability versus "variants." Blood 56:4, 1980.

Alami, SY, et al: Fibrin stabilizing factor (Factor XIII). Am J Med 44:1, 1968.

Ambruso, DR, et al: Antithrombin III deficiency: Decreased synthesis of a biochemically normal molecule. Blood 60:1, 1982.

Automated APTT, package insert. General Diagnostics, Morris Plains, NJ, 1977.

Bauer, JD: Clinical Laboratory Methods, ed 9. CV Mosby, St Louis, 1982.

Beck, WS: Hematology, ed 3. MIT Press, Cambridge, MA, 1981.

Benavides, I and Catovsky, D: Myeloperoxidase cytochemistry using 2,7-fluorenediamine. J Clin Pathol 31:1114, 1978.

Bessis, M: Blood Smears Reinterpreted. Springer International, New York, 1977.

Bessman, J: New parameters on automated hematology instruments. Lab Med 14:8, 1983.

Beutler, E: Red Cell Metabolism: A Manual of Biochemical Methods, ed 2. Grune & Stratton, New York, 1975.

Biggs, R and Rizza, CR: Human Blood Coagulation: Hemostasis and Thrombosis, ed 3. Blackwell Scientific, Boston, 1984.

Bloom, AL: The von Willebrand syndrome. Semin Hematol 27:4, 1980.

Bollum, FJ: Terminal deoxynucleotidyl transferase: Biological studies. In Meister, A (ed): Advances in Enzymology. Vol 47. John Wiley & Sons, New York, 1979, p 347.

Bowie, EJW, et al: Platelet adhesiveness in von Willebrand's disease. Am J Clin Pathol 52:69, 1969.

Boyum, A: Isolation of lymphocytes, granulocytes, and macrophages. Scand J Immunol 5:9, 1976.

Brecher, G: New methylene blue as a reticulocyte stain. Am J Clin Pathol 19:895, 1949.

Brown, BA: Hematology: Principles and Procedures, ed 4. Lea & Febiger, Philadelphia, 1984.

Coleman, MS, et al: Terminal deoxynucleotidyl transferase in human leukemia. Proc Natl Acad Sci (USA) 71:4404, 1974.

Coleman, MS, et al: Serial observations on terminal deoxynucleotidyl transferase activity and lymphoblastic surface markers in acute lymphoblastic leukemia. Cancer Res 36:120, 1976.

Comp, PC, Nixon, RR, and Esmon, CT: Determination of functional protein C, and antithrombotic protein, using thrombin-thrombomodulin complex. Blood 63(1):15, 1984.

Cotter, DA: The safe use of dimethyl sulfoxide in the laboratory. Am J Med Tech 41:63, 1975.

Coulter Electronics: Coulter Counter Model S-Plus Operators Manual. Coulter Electronics, Inc., Hialeah, FL, 1977.

Dacie, JV and Lewis, SM: Practical Hematology, ed 4. Grune & Stratton, New York, 1975.

Dacie, JV and Lewis, SM: Practical Hematology, ed 6. Grune & Stratton, New York, 1984.

Data-Fi Fibrinogen Determination Kit, package insert. American Dade, Division of American Hospital Supply Corporation, Miami, 1978.

Eliman, L, et al: The Thrombo-Wellcotest as a screening test for disseminated intravascular coagulation. N Engl J Med 288:633, 1973.

Ellas, JM: A rapid, sensitive myeloperoxidase stain using 4-chloro-l-naphthol. Brief scientific reports. Am J Clin Pathol 73:797, 1980.

Epstein, DJ, et al: Radioimmunoassay for protein C and factor X. Am J Clin Pathol 82:573, 1983.

Esmon, CT: The Protein C Anticoagulant Pathway. American Dade Monograph, Miami, 1986.

Ewing, NP and Kasper CK: In vitro detection of mild inhibitors to factor VIII in hemophilia. Am J Clin Pathol 77:6, 1982.

Fannon, M, Thomas, R, and Sawyer, L: Effects of staining and storage times on reticulocytes. Lab Med 13:7, 1982.

Fischbach, DP and Fogdall RP: Coagulation: The Essentials. Williams & Wilkins, Baltimore, 1981.

Francis, RB and Thomas, W: Behavior of protein C inhibitor in intravascular coagulation and liver disease. Thromb Haemost 52:71, 1984.

Funk, A, et al: Reptilase-R, a new reagent in blood coagulation. Br J Haematol 21:43, 1971.

Gilmer, PR Jr and Koepke, JA: The reticulocyte: An approach to definition. Am J Clin Pathol 66:262, 1976.

Godal, HC and Abildgaard, U: Gelation of soluble fibrin in plasma by ethanol. Scand J Haematol 3:432, 1966.

Gomori, G: Microchemical demonstration of phosphatase in tissue sections. Proc Soc Exp Biol Med 42:23, 1939.

Graham, RCJ, Lundholm, U, and Karovsky, MJ: Cytochemical demonstration of peroxidase activity with 3-amino-9-ethyl-carbazole. J Histochem Cytochem 13:150, 1965.

Gupta, S and Good, RA: Markers of human lymphocyte subpopulations in primary immunodeficiency and lymphoproliferative disorders. Semin Hematol 17(1):1, 1980.

Harker, L and Thompson, AR: Manual of Hemostasis and Thrombosis, ed 3. FA Davis, Philadelphia, 1983.

Hayhoe, FGI: The cytochemical demonstration of lipids in blood and bone marrow cells. J Pathol Bacteriol 65:413, 1953.

Hellem, AJ: Platelet adhesiveness. Semin Haematol 1:2, 1968.

Henry, JB: Clinical Diagnosis and Management by Laboratory Methods, ed 17. WB Saunders, Philadelphia, 1984.

Higgy, KE, Burns, GF, and Hayhoe, FGJ: Discrimination of B and null lymphocytes by esterase cytochemistry. Scand J Hematol 18:437, 1977.

Hoyer, LW: The factor VIII complex: Structure and function. Blood 58:1, 1981.

Hutton, JJ, et al: Terminal deoxynucleotidyl transferase as a tumor cell marker in leukemia and lymphoma: Results from 1000 patients. In Mihich, E and Baserga, R (eds): Tumor Markers. Pergamon Press, Oxford, 1979.

Hyun, BH, Ashton, JK, and Dolan, K: Practical Hematology: A Laboratory Guide with Accompanying Filmstrip. WB Saunders, Philadelphia, 1975.

Janckila, A, et al: The cytochemistry of tartrate-resistant acid phosphatase. Am J Clin Pathol 70:45, 1978.

Kaplow, LS: Cytochemistry of leukocyte alkaline phosphatase. Use of complex naphthol HS phosphates in azo dye — coupling technics. Am J Clin Pathol 39:439, 1963.

Kaplow, LS: Simplified myeloperoxidase stain using benzidine dihydrochloride. Blood 26:215, 1965.

Kaplow, LS: Substitute for benzidene in myeloperoxidase stains. Am J Clin Pathol 63:451, 1974.

Kaplow, LS: Special stains for blood cells. MEDCOM, New York, 1975.

Kelly, PA and Penner, JA: Anticoagulants: Heparin and Coumadin. Dade, Division of American Hospital Supply Corporation, Miami, 1974.

Kennedy, J: Fibrinogen, Fibrin and Fibrinolysis. Dade, Division of American Hospital Supply Corporation, Miami, 1974.

Koepke, JA, et al: The prediction of prothrombin time system using secondary standards. Am J Clin Pathol 68:191, 1977.

Kowalski, E: Fibrinogen derivatives and their biologic activity. Semin Hematol 5:45, 1968.

Kung, PC and Goldstein, G: Functional and developmental compartments of human T lymphocytes. Vox Sang 39:121, 1980.

Kung, PC, et al: Terminal deoxynucleotidyl transferase in the diagnosis of leukemia and malignant lymphoma. Am J Med 64:788, 1978.

Latallo, ZS and Teisseyre, E: Evaluation of Reptilase-R and thrombin clotting time in the presence of fibrinogen degradation products and heparin. Scand J Haematol (Suppl 13)4:261, 1971.

Laurell, CB: Quantitative estimation of proteins by electrophoresis in agarose gel containing antibodies. Ann Biochem 15:45, 1966.

Laurrell, CB: Electroimmunoassay. Scand J Clin Lab Invest 29 (Suppl 124):21, 1972.

Leder, LD: The selective enzymocytochemical demonstration of neutrophil myeloid cells and tissue mast cells in paraffin sections. Klinische Wochenschrift 42(11):553, 1964.

Lee, RL and White, PD: A clinical study of the coagulation time of blood. Am J Med Sci 145:495, 1913.

Lehmann, H and Huntsman, RG: Man's Hemoglobins, ed 2. JB Lippincott, Philadelphia, 1974.

Lenahan, JG and Smith, K: Hemostasis, ed 16. General Diagnostics, Division of Warner-Lambert Company, NJ, 1982.

Li, CY, Lam, KW, and Yam, LT: Esterase in human leukocytes. J Histochem Cytochem 21(1)1, 1973.

Li, CY, Yam, LT, and Crosby, WH: Histochemical characterization of cellular and structural elements of the human spleen. J Histochem Cytochem 20(12):1049, 1972.

Losowsky, MA, Hall, R, and Goldie, W: Congenital deficiency of fibrin stabilizing factor. Lancet 2:156, 1965.

Macfarlane, RG: A simple method for measuring clot retraction. Lancet 1:1199, 1939.

Mammen, EF: Congenital abnormalities of the fibrinogen molecule. Semin Thromb Hemost 1:184, 1974.

Mancini, G, Carbonara, AO, and Heremans, JF: Immunochemical quantitation of antigens by single radial immunodiffusion. Immunochemistry 2:235, 1965.

McGann, MA and Triplett, DA: Interpretation of antithrombin III activity. Lab Med 13:12, 1982.

Melvin, L: Comparison of techniques for detecting T-cell acute lymphocytic leukemia. Blood 54(1):210, 1979.

Miale, JB: Laboratory Medicine: Hematology, ed 6. CV Mosby, St Louis, 1982.

Mielke, CH, et al: The standardized normal Ivy bleeding time and its prolongation by aspirin. Blood 34:204, 1969.

Moloney, WC, McPherson, K, and Fliegelman, L: Esterase activity in leukocytes demonstrated by the use of napthol AS-D chloroacetate substrate. J Histol Chem Cytochem 8:200, 1960.

Murano, G and Bick, RL: Basic Concepts of Hemostasis and Thrombosis. CRC Press, Boca Raton, FL, 1980.

National Committee for Clinical Laboratory Standards: Tentative guidelines for the standardized collection, transport, and preparation of blood specimens for coagulation testing and performance of coagulation assays. Vol 2, p 4, Villanova, PA, 1982.

Nor-Partigen Fibrinogen kit, package insert. Behring Diagnostics, LaJolla, CA, 1988.

O'Connor, BH: A Color Atlas and Instruction Manual of Peripheral Blood Cell Morphology. Williams & Wilkins, Baltimore, 1984.

Olson, JD, et al: Evaluation of ristocetin-Willebrand's factor assay and ristocetin-induced platelet aggregation. Am J Clin Pathol 63:210, 1975.

Ortho Diagnostics Systems, Inc: Ortho ELT-8 Training Manual. Westwood, MA, 1984.

Ortho Diagnostics Systems, Inc: Ortho ELT-8 Hematology Analyzer Operator Manual. Westwood, MA, 1984.

Parpart, AK, et al: The osmotic resistance (fragility) of human red cells. J Clin Invest 26:636, 1947.

Patterson, BB: Clot observation — A review of an important but neglected coagulation test. Lab Med 7:12, 1976.

Platelet Neutralization Procedure. Department of Air Force, Lackland AFB, TX, 1989.

Protein C Antigen Rocket EID Method, package insert. Helena Laboratories, Beaumont, TX, 1989.

Protopath Proteolytic Enzyme Detection System: Antithrombin III Synthetic Substrate Assay for determination of AT-III activity in plasma, package insert. American Dade, Division of American Hospital Supply Corp, Miami, 1986.

Quagliano, D and Hayhoe, FGJ: Periodic acid–Schiff positivity in erythroblasts with special reference to di Guglielmo's disease. Br J Haematol 6:26, 1960.

Ramsey, R and Evatt, BL: Rapid assay for von Willebrand's factor activity using formalin-fixed platelets and microtitration technique. Am J Clin Pathol 72:996, 1979.

Ray, M and Noteboom, G: A modification of the erythrocyte osmotic fragility test. Am J Clin Pathol 54:711, 1970.

Reich, PR: Hematology: Physiopathologic Basis for Clinical Practice, ed 3. Little, Brown, Boston, 1984.

Reptilase-R, package insert. Abbott Laboratories, Diagnostics Division, IL, 93-4260, 1974.

Royston, I: Monoclonal antibodies for human T lymphocytes: Identification of normal and malignant T cells. Blood 54(Suppl 1):106, 1979.

Rozenszajin, L, et al: The esterase activity in megaloblasts, leukaemic and normal haemopoietic cells. Br J Haematol 14:605, 1968.

Russell's Viper Venom Reagent for Factor X Assays, package insert. General Diagnostics, Morris Plains, NJ, 1976.

Sala, N, Owen, WG, and Collen, D: A functional assay of protein C in human plasma. Blood 63(3):671, 1984.

Salzman, ER: Measurement of platelet adhesiveness: A simple in vitro technique demonstrating an abnormality in von Willebrand's disease. J Lab Med 62:724, 1963.

Schaefer, HE and Fischer, R: Peroxidase detection in smear preparations and tissue sections after decalcification and paraffin embedding. Klin Wochenschr 46:1228, 1968.

Schmidt, RM and Brocious, EM: Basic Laboratory Methods of Hemoglobinopathy Detection. HEW Pub (CDC) 75-8296, US Department of Health and Centers for Disease Control, Atlanta, 1975.

Seaman, AJ: The recognition of intravascular clotting: The plasma protamine paracoagulation tests. Arch Intern Med 125:1016, 1970.

Shafer, JA and Stein, BL: Blood smear observation workshop manual. University of Rochester, NY, 1975.

Shafer, JA: Hematology morphology workshop manual. University of Rochester, NY, 1981.

Shapiro, SS and Hultin, M: Acquired inhibitors to the blood coagulation factors. Semin Thromb Hemost 1:366, 1975.

Shapiro, SS and Hultin, M: Acquired inhibitors to the blood coagulation factors. Clin Haematol 8:207, 1979.

Sheehan, HL and Storey, GW: An improved method of staining leukocyte granules with Sudan black B. J Pathol Bacteriol 19:336, 1947.

Shitamoto, BS, Leslie, KO, and Galloway, WB: Postpartum hemophilia. Am J Clin Pathol 78:5, 1982.

Sicklequik, package insert. General Diagnostics, Morris Plains, NJ, 1977.

Sickle-Thal Quick Column Method, package insert. Helena Laboratories, Beaumont, TX, 1981.

Simmler Fetal Cell Stain Kit, package insert. Simmler, St Louis, 1979.

Simmons, A: Technical Hematology, ed 2. JB Lippincott, Philadelphia, 1976.

Sirridge, MS and Shannon, R: Laboratory Evaluation of Hemostasis and Thrombosis, ed 3. Lea & Febiger, Philadelphia, 1983.

Spero, JA, Lewis, JH, and Hasiba, V: Disseminated intravascular coagulation: Findings in 346 patients. Thromb Haemost 43:28, 1980.

Super Z and Zip Zone Hemoglobin Electrophoresis Procedure, package insert. Helena Laboratories, Beaumont, TX, 1978.

Super Z and Zip Zone Titan IV Hemoglobin Electrophoresis Procedure. Helena Laboratories, Beaumont, TX, 1978.

Sussman, LN: The clotting time — An enigma. Am J Clin Pathol 60:5, 1973.

The Fibrometer Precision Coagulation Timer, Instructions and Technical Information, BBl Division of Becton, Dickinson and Company, Cockeysville, MD, 1977.

Thomson, JM: Blood Coagulation and Hemostasis: A Practical Guide, ed 2. Churchill Livingstone, New York, 1980.

Thrombo-Wellcotest, package insert. Wellcome Research Laboratories, Breckenham, England, 1974.

Triplett, DA and Brandt, JT: Lupus anticoagulant: Misnomer, paradox, riddle, epiphenomenon. Hematol Pathol 1988 (in press).

Triplett, DA, et al: Platelet Function: Laboratory Evaluation and Clinical Application. American Society of Clinical Pathologists, Chicago, 1978.

Triplett, DA and Harms, CS: Procedures for the Coagulation Lab-

oratory, American Society of Clinical Pathologists, Chicago, 1981.

von Kaulla, E and von Kaulla, N: Deficiency of antithrombin III activity associated with hereditary thrombosis tendency. J Med 3:349, 1972.

WHO Report, 1974: Identification, enumeration and isolation of B and T lymphocytes from human peripheral blood. Scand J Immunol 3:521, 1974.

Williams, J, et al: Hematology, ed 2. McGraw-Hill, New York, 1977.

Winchester, RJ and Ross, G: Methods for enumerating lymphocyte populations. In Rose, NR and Friedman, H (eds): Manual of Clinical Immunology. American Society for Microbiology, Washington, DC, 1976, p 64.

Wintrobe, MM, et al: Clinical Hematology, ed 8. Lea & Febiger, Philadelphia, 1982.

Wintrobe Sedimentation Tubes, package insert. American Dade, Division of American Hospital Supply Corporation, Miami.

Wislocki, GB, Rheingold, JM, and Dempsey, EW: The occurrence of the periodic acid Schiff reaction in various normal cells of blood and connective tissue. Blood 4:562, 1949.

Wolf, PL: Practical Clinical Hematology Interpretations and Techniques. John Wiley & Sons, New York, 1973.

Yam, LT, Li, CY, and Crosby, WH: Cytochemical identification of monocytes and granulocytes. Am J Clin Pathol 55(3):283, 1971.

Yam, LT, Tavassoli, M, and Jacobs, P: Differential characterization of the "reticulum cell" in lymphoreticular neoplasms. Am J Clin Pathol 64:171, 1974.

QUESTIONS

1. *What is measured by a bleeding time?*
   a. Platelet number
   b. Platelet function
   c. Intrinsic and extrinsic coagulation systems
   d. All of the above

2. *What is the principle of the platelet retention test?*
   a. Blood is allowed to clot slowly in a glass tube as platelet counts are made every 15 minutes.
   b. Platelet count is taken on an anticoagulated sample; blood is passed through a column of glass beads and a second platelet count is taken.
   c. Platelet count is taken on an anticoagulated sample and the sample is then agitated in a glass tube and a second platelet count is taken.
   d. Platelet count is taken and then the blood sample is allowed to clot in a tube with glass beads; the beads are then washed and a platelet count is performed on the washings.

3. *Which of the following represent basic requirements for measuring in vitro platelet aggregation?*
   a. The anticoagulant should be sodium citrate.
   b. The sample should not be hemolyzed or lipemic.
   c. Samples should be kept at 37°C.
   d. Patient should not have taken anti-inflammatory drugs for 1 week.
   e. All of the above.

4. *Which platelet aggregation result would be characteristic for patients with Bernard-Soulier syndrome?*

a. Incomplete aggregation with ADP
b. Primary wave of aggregation in response to collagen
c. Abnormal ristocetin-induced platelet aggregation
d. Primary wave of aggregation with epinephrine

5. *What is measured by the whole blood clotting time?*
   a. Intrinsic system; may be used for monitoring heparin therapy
   b. Extrinsic system; may be used for assessing platelet function
   c. Both intrinsic and extrinsic systems; may be used for measuring factor deficiency
   d. All coagulation systems; may be used for measuring both congenital and acquired coagulation disorders

6. *Which of the following tests measures the intrinsic pathway of coagulation and is used to detect factor deficiencies and hypofibrinogenemia and to monitor heparin therapy?*
   a. Activated partial thromboplastin time
   b. Prothrombin time
   c. Quantitative factor assay
   d. Stypven time test (Russell's viper venom time test)

7. *Which test measures the extrinsic pathway of coagulation and is used to measure factor deficiencies and monitor oral anticoagulant therapy?*
   a. Activated partial thromboplastin time
   b. Prothrombin time
   c. Quantitative factor assay
   d. Stypven time test (Russell's viper venom time test)

8. *Which test is based upon the ability of patient plasma to correct specific factor deficient plasma?*
   a. Activated partial thromboplastin time
   b. Prothrombin time
   c. Quantitative factor assay
   d. Stypven time test (Russell's viper venom time test)

9. *Which test is used to differentiate a deficiency of factor VII from factor X and to measure prothrombin plus factor V when tested on platelet-rich, nonlipemic plasma?*
   a. Activated partial thromboplastin time
   b. Prothrombin time
   c. Quantitative factor assay
   d. Stypven time test (Russell's viper venom time test)

10. *Which test measures the entire intrinsic clotting system, platelets, and factor X?*
    a. Thrombin time
    b. Prothrombin consumption test
    c. Reptilase time
    d. Fibrinogen

11. *Which test does not measure defects in intrinsic or extrinsic pathways and is affected by the levels of fibrinogen and dysfibrinogenemia, as well as the presence of circulating anticoagulants?*
    a. Thrombin time
    b. Prothrombin consumption test
    c. Reptilase time
    d. Fibrinogen

12. *Which of the following characteristic(s) is (are) true of the reptilase time?*
    a. Clotting is initiated with the snake venom enzyme, reptilase.
    b. The test result is not inhibited by heparin.
    c. Reptilase time is prolonged in most congenital dysfibrinogenemias/afibrinogenemias.
    d. All of the above

13. *Which of the following conditions would show a short clotting time indicating high fibrinogen levels?*
    a. Disseminated intravascular coagulation
    b. Liver disease
    c. Pregnancy
    d. Fibrinolysis

14. *Which test result would indicate a factor XIII defect?*
    a. Presence of a formed clot after 24 hours
    b. Dissolution of a fibrin clot within 1 hour
    c. Presence of a formed clot after 48 hours
    d. Dissolution of a fibrin clot within 72 hours

15. *Which condition would most likely show a decrease in factor VIII antigen?*
    a. Hemophilia A
    b. Female carriers of hemophilia A
    c. Myeloproliferative syndrome
    d. von Willebrand's disease

16. *Which of the following techniques are used to measure AT-III?*
    a. Clotting time based on thrombin neutralization
    b. Radial immunodiffusion
    c. Chromogenic substrate assay
    d. All of the above

17. *What type of tests are used in the laboratory diagnosis of protein C deficiency?*
    a. Primarily antigenic assays
    b. Primarily functional assays
    c. Both antigenic and functional assays

18. *What type of anticoagulants are inhibitors or autoantibodies of the IgG class whose effects are directed against coagulation factors?*
    a. Naturally occurring inhibitors
    b. Therapeutically administered inhibitors
    c. Pathologic anticoagulants
    d. All of the above

19. *Which APTT result would indicate the presence of a strong circulating anticoagulant?*
    a. APTT not corrected by the additional of normal plasma
    b. Prolonged APTT (more than 1 hour)
    c. APTT corrected by the addition of normal plasma
    d. Any of the above results

20. Which of the following are criteria for the laboratory detection of lupus inhibitors?
    a. Abnormal APTT and/or PT
    b. Demonstration that an abnormal APTT/PT is due to inhibitors
    c. Proof that the inhibitor is directed against phospholipids
    d. All of the above

21. Which test is not a confirmatory test for lupus anticoagulants?
    a. Thromboplastin inhibition test
    b. Dilute Russell's viper venom time
    c. APTT
    d. Kaolin clotting time
    e. Platelet neutralization procedure

22. Which test result, using the FDPs test, would be indicative of a patient having DIC? (Assume fibrinogen concentration is indicative of DIC.)
    a. Positive FDP test result; increased PT and APTT; decreased platelet count
    b. Positive FDP test result; decreased PT and APTT; increased platelet count
    c. Negative FDP test result; increased PT, decreased APTT; decreased platelet count
    d. Negative FDP test result; decreased PT, increased APTT; increased platelet count

23. Which test measures plasmin's action on the fibrin clot?
    a. FDP test
    b. D-Dimer test
    c. Ethanol gelatin test
    d. Euglobulin lysis time

24. Which test evaluates fibrinolytic activity by measuring the concentration of plasminogen activators?
    a. FDP test
    b. D-Dimer test
    c. Ethanol gelatin test
    d. Euglobulin lysis time

ANSWERS

Section I

1. c (p. 528)
2. a (p. 526)
3. c (p. 529)
4. b (p. 530)
5. a (p. 530)
6. c (p. 530)
7. d (p. 531)
8. a (pp. 534–535)
9. a (p. 532)
10. c (p. 532)
11. d (p. 532)
12. b (p. 532)
13. b (p. 532)
14. d (p. 534)
15. b (p. 536)
16. c (p. 538)
17. d (p. 539)
18. a (p. 539)
19. c (p. 540)
20. b (p. 543)
21. a (p. 543)
22. b (p. 547)
23. d (p. 547)
24. b (p. 548)
25. c (p. 548)
26. d (p. 548)
27. a (p. 535)

Section II

1. d (p. 555)
2. a (p. 555)
3. d (p. 556)
4. c (p. 555)

Section III

1. c (p. 569)
2. b (pp. 572 and 578)
3. d (pp. 572 and 578)
4. c (pp. 573 and 578)
5. a (pp. 574 and 578)
6. a (p. 576)
7. d (p. 577)
8. b (p. 578)
9. a (p. 579)
10. b (p. 581)

Section IV

1. d (p. 585)
2. b (p. 588)
3. e (p. 589)
4. c (p. 590)
5. a (p. 592)
6. a (p. 593)
7. b (p. 594)
8. c (p. 594)
9. d (p. 596)
10. b (p. 597)
11. a (p. 597)
12. d (p. 598)
13. c (p. 599)
14. b (p. 601)
15. d (p. 602)
16. d (p. 603)
17. c (p. 606)
18. c (p. 606)
19. a (p. 607)
20. d (p. 607)
21. c (p. 607)
22. a (p. 610)
23. b (p. 610)
24. d (p. 612)

Glossary

Abruptio placenta: Premature detachment of normally situated placenta.

Acanthocyte: An abnormal red cell that is slightly reduced in size and that possesses 3 to 12 spicules of uneven length distributed along the periphery of the cell membrane.

Achlorhydria: Absence of free hydrochloric acid in the stomach.

Acholuria: Absence of bile pigments in urine, occurring when unconjugated bilirubin does not pass through the glomerular filter.

Acrocyanosis: Bluish tinge to the extremities.

Activated partial thromboplastin time (APTT): A test to evaluate the overall integrity of the clotting system that involves factors XII, XI, IX, VIII, X, V, II, and I. Usually a means of evaluating the intrinsic system of coagulation.

Acute phase reactant: Plasma protein, the concentration of which increases in response to a variety of stimuli.

Adenopathy: Swelling and morbid change in lymph nodes; glandular disease.

Adenosine diphosphate (ADP): A substance used to induce platelet aggregation that may be derived from injured tissues, erythrocytes, or platelets.

Adhesion: The molecular attraction exerted between the surfaces of bodies in contact (for example, platelets to connective tissue structures).

Afibrinogenemia: A rare blood disease characterized by the absence of fibrinogen in the plasma; may be congenital or acquired.

Agammaglobulinemia: A rare disorder in which there is a virtual absence of gamma globulins.

Agglutination: The clumping together of red blood cells or any particulate matter resulting from interaction of antibody and its corresponding antigen.

Aggregation: A clustering or clumping together (for example, platelet aggregation plays a critical role in hemostasis).

Agnogenic dyspoiesis: Preleukemic disorder of unknown origin that is characterized by hypercellular marrow and abnormal cell maturation.

Agranulocytosis: An acute disease in which the white cell count is markedly reduced and neutropenia becomes pronounced.

Alkaline phosphatase: An enzyme that is found in a number of tissues but is chiefly used in connection with diagnosis of bone and liver disease. The granules of normal granulocytic cells contain alkaline phosphatase; patients with chronic myelogenous leukemia (CML) have decreased phosphatase activity.

Alkalosis: Excessive alkalinity of body fluids, owing to accumulation of alkalies or to the reduction of acids.

Alloantibody: An antibody produced by an immune response that was stimulated by a foreign antigen.

Alloimmunization: The process in which a patient develops antibodies to foreign and/or white blood cell antigen(s) through transfusion or pregnancy.

Allograft: A tissue transplant between individuals of the same species.

Alpha chain: A type of globin chain found in hemoglobin and coded for by the alpha gene.

Alpha methyldopa (Aldomet): A common drug used to treat hypertension; frequently the cause of a positive direct Coombs' test result.

Amaurotic: Caused by the atrophying of optic nerve or vision centers.

Ameliorate: Moderate, improve.

Amniocentesis: Transabdominal puncture of the amniotic sac, using a needle and syringe, in order to remove amniotic fluid. The material may then be studied to detect genetic disorders or maternal-fetal blood incompatibility.

Amphophilic: Having an affinity for acid and/or basic dyes.

Amyloidosis: A metabolic disorder marked by extracellular deposition of amyloid (an abnormal protein) in the tissues; this usually leads to loss of function and organ enlargement.

Anamnestic (response): An accentuated antibody response following a secondary exposure to an antigen. Antibody levels from the initial exposure are not detectable in the patient's serum until the secondary exposure, when a rapid rise in antibody titer is observed.

Anaphylaxis: An allergic hypersensitivity reaction of the body to a foreign protein or drug.

Ancillary: Auxiliary, supplementary.

Androgenic: Causing masculinization.

Anemia: A condition in which there is reduced oxygen delivery to the tissues. It may result from increased destruction of red cells, excessive blood loss, or decreased production of red cells.

    Aplastic a.: Anemia caused by aplasia of bone marrow or its destruction by chemical agents or physical factors.

    Autoimmune hemolytic a.: Acquired disorder characterized by premature erythrocyte destruction owing to abnormalities in the individual's own immune system.

    Hemolytic a.: Anemia caused by hemolysis of red blood cells resulting in reduction of normal red cell lifespan.

    Iron-deficiency a.: Anemia resulting from a demand on stored iron greater than can be met.

    Megaloblastic a.: Anemia in which megaloblasts are found in the blood; usually due to a deficiency of folic acid or vitamin B_{12}.

    Microangiopathic hemolytic a.: A hemolytic process associated with thrombotic thrombocytic purpura (TTP), prosthetic heart valve, and burns. It is visualized in the peripheral blood smear by fragmentation of the red cells and other bizarre morphology.

Pernicious a.: A type of megaloblastic anemia due to a deficiency of vitamin B$_{12}$ that is directly linked to absence of intrinsic factor (IF).

Sickle-cell a.: See **Sickle-cell anemia.**

Aneuploidy: Having an abnormal number of chromosomes.

Angina pectoris: Severe pain and constriction about the heart caused by insufficient supply of blood to the heart.

Anisochromia: Not of uniform color.

Anisocytosis: Variation in the size of erythrocytes when observed on a peripheral blood smear.

Anoxia: Without oxygen.

Antenatal: Occurring before birth.

Antibody: A protein substance developed in response to, and interacting specifically with, an antigen. In blood banking, it is found in serum, from either a commercial manufacturer or a patient. It is secreted by plasma cells.

Cross-reacting a.: An antibody that reacts with antigens functionally similar to its specific antigen.

Maternal a.: An antibody produced in the mother and transferred to the fetus in utero.

Naturally occurring a.: An antibody present in a patient without known prior exposure to the corresponding red cell antigen.

Antibody screen: Testing the patient's serum with group O reagent red cells in an effort to detect atypical antibodies.

Anticoagulant: An agent that delays or prevents blood coagulation.

Antigen: A substance that is recognized by the body as being foreign and that therefore can elicit an immune response.

Antiglobulin test (AGT) or antihuman globulin (AHG) test: Test to ascertain the presence or absence of red cell coating by immunoglobulin (IgG) and/or complement.

Direct AGT (DAT): Used to detect in vivo cell sensitization

Indirect AGT (IAT): Used to detect antigen-antibody reactions that occur in vitro.

Antihemophilic factor (AHF): A commercially prepared source of factor VIII. (See also Hemophilia A.)

Antihuman serum: An antibody prepared in rabbits or other suitable animals that is directed against human immunoglobulin or complement or both. It is used to perform the AGT or Coombs' test. The serum may be either polyspecific (anti-IgG plus anticomplement) or monospecific (anti-IgG or anticomplement).

Antiplasmin: Plasma proteins that are known to neutralize free plasmin: α_2-antiplasmin, α_2-macroglobulin.

α_2-a.: The major inhibitor of plasmin.

Antipyretic: An agent that reduces fever.

Antiseptic: Preventing decay, putrefaction, or sepsis.

Antithrombin: A substance that opposes the action of thrombin and thus prevents or inhibits coagulation of blood.

Antithrombin III (AT-III): A naturally occurring inhibitor of coagulation responsible for neutralizing the activity of thrombin; factors IXa, Xa, and XIa; and plasmin. (Also known as the heparin cofactor.)

Anuria: Absence of urine formation.

Apheresis: A method of blood collection in which whole blood is withdrawn, a desired component separated and retained, and the remainder of the blood returned to the donor. (See also **Plateletpheresis; Plasmapheresis.**)

Aplasia: Failure of an organ or tissue to develop normally.

Ascites: The accumulation of serous fluid in the peritoneal cavity.

Asphyxia: Condition caused by insufficient intake of oxygen.

Asthenic: Weak; caused by a muscular or cerebellar disease.

Asynchrony: The failure of events to occur in time with each other as they usually do. In hematology, nuclear and cytoplasmic development are mismatched.

Atypical lymphocyte: A benign reactive change in the morphologic appearance of the lymphocyte, which is frequently secondary to a viral disease (for example, infectious mononucleosis).

Auer's rod: Rod-shaped alignment of primary granules that are present only in the cytoplasm of myeloblasts and monoblasts in leukemic states.

Autohemolysis: Hemolysis of an individual's blood corpuscles by his or her own serum.

Autoimmune: The production of antibodies directed against one's own tissues, usually in association with a disease state.

Autoimmune hemolytic anemia (AIHA): Abnormality of the immune system resulting in production of antibodies against self, which occurs due to failure of the mechanism regulating the immune response.

Autologous: Of the self.

Autosomal: Relating to any of the chromosomes other than the sex (X and Y) chromosomes.

Autosplenectomy: Formation of a fibrotic, nonfunctioning spleen caused by restrictive blood flow to the organ; often seen in sickle-cell anemia.

Azotemia: Presence of increased amounts of urea in the blood.

Babesiosis: A rare, often severe and sometimes fatal disease of humans caused by the protozoal parasite of the red blood cells, *Babesia microti*, and perhaps other *Babesia* species.

Band: An immature neutrophilic granulocyte with a horseshoe- or sausage-shaped nucleus (also called a stab). Composes 2 to 6 percent of the normal differential count.

Basophil: A mature white blood cell whose cytoplasmic granules stain deep blue-purple with basic dyes like methylene blue. Composes 0 to 2 percent of the normal differential count.

Basophilia: An absolute increase in basophils.

Basophilic normoblast: An immature red cell precursor found only in the bone marrow that is characterized by a vivid blue cytoplasm and a high nuclear-to-cytoplasmic ratio. (Synonym: **Prorubricyte.**)

Basophilic stippling: Red blood cell inclusion that consists of precipitated ribonucleoprotein and mitochrondrial remnants. Stippling may be fine, coarse, or punctate and is seen in toxic states such as metal poisoning, severe bacterial infection, drug exposure, and so forth.

Bernard-Soulier syndrome: A congenital bleeding disorder characterized by the presence of large platelets, thrombocytopenia of varying degrees, and a prolonged bleeding time.

Beta chain: A type of globin chain found in hemoglobin that is coded for by the beta gene.

Betke-Kleihauer technique: An acid elution test used to quantitate the amount of fetal hemoglobin present. Fetal hemoglobin is more resistant than adult hemoglobin to elution at acid pH during this procedure, and stains red.

Bilirubin: The orange or yellowish pigment in bile, which is carried to the liver by the blood. It is produced from hemoglobin of red blood cells by reticuloendothelial cells in the bone marrow, spleen, and elsewhere.

    Direct b.: The conjugated water-soluble form of bilirubin.

    Indirect b.: The unconjugated water-insoluble form of bilirubin.

Bilirubinemia: Pathologic condition in which excessive destruction of red blood cells occurs, increasing the amount of bilirubin found in the blood.

Blackwater fever: Hemoglobinuria following chronic falciparum malaria infection.

Bleeding time: A test used to evaluate the hemostatic role of platelets in vivo.

Bradykinin: A plasma kinin.

Buffy coat: The layer of leukocytes and platelets lying directly on top of the red cell layer seen after sedimentation or centrifugation.

Burr cells (echinocytes): Red cells with approximately 10 to 30 spicules evenly distributed over the surface of the cell.

Burst-forming unit committed to erythropoiesis (BFU-E): A primitive stem cell committed to erythropoiesis and thought to be a precursor to the CFU-E.

C1 esterase inhibitor: A protein in the blood that inhibits the activity of plasmin as well as the activity of C1 esterase in the complement pathway.

C3a: A biologically active fragment of the C3 molecule, which demonstrates anaphylactic capabilities upon liberation.

C3b: A biologically active fragment of the complement C3 molecule, which is an opsonin and promotes immune adherence.

C3d: A biologically inactive fragment of the C3b complement component formed by inactivation by the C3b inactivator substance present in serum.

C4: A component of complement present in serum, which participates in the classic pathway of complement activation.

C5a: A biologically active fragment of the C5 molecule, which demonstrates anaphylactic capabilities as well as chemotactic properties upon liberation. This fragment has also been reported to be a potent aggregator of platelets.

Cabot's rings: A red blood cell inclusion resembling a figure 8. It is usually found in heavily stippled cells.

Cachexia: A condition that may result from chronic disease or certain malignancies whereby a state of malnutrition, weakness, and muscle wasting exists.

Calmodulin: A cytoplasmic calcium-binding protein.

Carcinoma: A new growth or malignant tumor that occurs in epithelial tissue. A neoplasm can infiltrate or metastasize to any tissue or organ of the body.

Cardiac output: The amount of blood discharged from the left or right ventricle per minute.

Catecholamines: Biologically active amines, epinephrine, and norepinephrine, derived from the amino acid tyrosine. They have a marked effect on nervous and cardiovascular systems, metabolic rate, temperature, and smooth muscle.

Celiac: Related to the abdominal regions.

Celite: A substance that acts as a contact activator causing the release of PF 3 and the activation of the intrinsic system.

Central venous pressure: The pressure within the superior vena cava reflecting the pressure under which the blood is returned to the right atrium.

Centripetal: Moving toward the center.

Cerebriform: A word that is used to describe the brainy convolutions of some nuclear chromatin material.

Chédiak-Higashi inclusions: Gigantic, fused lysosomal deposits seen in the cytoplasm of leukocytes.

Chelation: Combining of metallic ions with certain heterocyclic ring structures so that the ion is held by chemical bonds from each of the participating rings.

Chemotactic: Referring to the ability of white cells to move nondirectionally toward an attractant.

Chemotaxis: Describes movement toward a stimulus, particularly that displayed by phagocytic cells toward bacteria and sites of cell injury.

Cholecystectomy: Excision of a gallbladder.

Cholecystitis: Acute or chronic inflammation of the gallbladder.

Christmas factor: Plasma thromboplastin component (PTC); factor IX. Functions in the intrinsic system of coagulation.

Chromatin: A darkly staining substance located in the nucleus of the cell that contains the genetic material composed of deoxyribonucleic acid (DNA) attached to a protein structure.

Chromogenic: Pigment-producing.

Circulating anticoagulants: Acquired pathologic plasma proteins that inhibit normal coagulation. The majority of these pathologic anticoagulants are inhibitors or autoantibodies of the IgG class whose inhibitory effects are directed against a specific factor or a complex of coagulation factors.

Coagulation: The process of stopping blood flow from a wound. This process involves the harmonious relationship of the blood-clotting factors, the blood vessels, and the fibrin-forming and fibrin-lysing system.

Coagulopathy: A disease affecting the blood-clotting process.

Collagen: A fibrous insoluble protein found in the connective tissue, including skin, bone, ligaments, and cartilage; represents about 30 percent of the total body protein.

Colony-forming unit committed to erythropoiesis (CFU-E): A stem cell that is committed to forming cells of the red blood cell series.

Colony-forming unit–culture (CFU-C): Generation of stem cells using tissue culture methods. Current synonym is CFU-GM, which is a colony-forming unit committed to the production of myeloid cells (granulocytes and monocytes).

Complement: A series of proteins in the circulation that, when sequentially activated, cause disruption of bacterial and other cell membranes. Activation occurs via one of two pathways, and once activated, the components are involved in a great number of immune defense mechanisms including anaphylaxis, chemotaxis, and phagocytosis. Red cell antibodies that activate complement may be capable of causing hemolysis.

Complement fixation (CF): An immunologic test.

Congenital: Present at birth.

Consanguinous: Relationship by blood (that is, being descended from a common ancestor).

Contiguous: In contact or closely associated with.

Convulsion: Involuntary muscle contraction and relaxation.

Cord cells: Fetal cells obtained from the umbilical cord at birth. They may be contaminated with Wharton's jelly.

Corticosteroid: Any of a number of hormonal steroid substances obtained from the cortex of the adrenal gland.

Coumarin drugs (Warfarin, Coumadin, Dicumarol): Oral anticoagulants that act as vitamin K antagonists and result in depression of the concentration of prothrombin and factors VII, IX, and X.

Counterelectrophoresis (CEP): An immunologic procedure.

Cryoglobulin: An abnormal protein in the blood that forms gels at low temperatures.

Cryoglobulinemia: An increase in the concentration of cryoglobulins in the blood.

Cryoprecipitate: A concentrated source of coagulation factor VIII that has been prepared from a single unit of donor blood. The product also contains fibrinogen, factor XIII, and von Willebrand factor.

Cryoprotein: A protein circulating in the plasma or demonstrable in serum testing that precipitates on exposure to cold temperature.

Cyanosis: Slightly bluish or grayish discoloration of the skin caused by accumulation of reduced hemoglobin or deoxyhemoglobin in the blood caused by oxygen deficiency or carbon dioxide buildup.

Cytochemistry: The microscopic study of the chemical constituents in cells, the purpose of which includes differentiation of cell types and assistance in the diagnosis of hematologic diseases.

Cytogenetics: The study of cytology in relation to genetics, especially the chromosomal behavior in mitosis and meiosis.

Cytomegalovirus (CMV): One of a group of species-specific herpes viruses.

Cytopheresis: A procedure using a machine by which one can selectively remove a particular cell type normally found in peripheral blood of a patient or donor.

Cytotoxicity: Ability to destroy.

Dactylitis: Painful swelling of the feet and hands.

Dacrocyte: See **Teardrop cell**.

Defibrinated: Deprived of fibrin (the conversion of fibrinogen into fibrin is the basis for the clotting of blood).

Delayed hemolytic transfusion reaction (DHTR): A hemolytic reaction that occurs when previously sensitized individuals have antibody levels that are undetectable and are once again exposed to the offending antigen(s). In most cases of DHTR the antibodies implicated are IgG.

Delta: A type of globin chain found in hemoglobin coded for by the delta gene.

Desferrioxamine: Substance obtained from certain bacteria that is used to chelate iron. This substance is used orally or parenterally in treating iron poisoning.

Diagnosis: The use of scientific and skillful methods to establish the cause and nature of a disease process.

Diapedesis: The journey of the blood cells (that is, leukocytes) through the unruptured walls of a capillary.

Diaphoresis: Profuse sweating.

Differential: Microscopic examination of a stained blood smear to determine relative number of each type of white blood cell; an estimate of white cell, red cell, and platelet counts; and an inspection of the morphology of red cells, white cells, and platelets.

Dimorphism: Existence of a two-cell population in the peripheral blood smear (for example, few microcytes, few macrocytes; few hypochromic, few normochromic).

2,3-Diphosphoglycerate (2,3-DPG): An organic phosphate in red blood cells that alters the affinity of hemoglobin for oxygen. Blood cells stored in a blood bank lose 2,3-DPG, but once infused the substance is resynthesized or reactivated.

Disseminated intravascular coagulation (DIC): A pathologic form of coagulation that is diffuse rather than localized, and is characterized by generalized bleeding and shock.

Diuresis: Secretion and passage of large amounts of urine.

Diuretic: An agent that increases the secretion of urine. Action is in one of two ways; by increasing glomerular filtration or by decreasing reabsorption from the tubules.

Diurnal: Occurring during the daytime.

Diverticulosis: Outpouching of the colon without inflammation or symptoms. There are many locations of diverticula but all are saccular dilatations protruding from the wall of a tubular organ.

Döhle bodies: Single or multiple, round or oval, blue cytoplasmic inclusions (with Romanowsky stain) seen in neutrophils, usually associated with toxicity.

Donath-Landsteiner antibody test: A test usually performed in the blood bank to detect the presence of the Donath-Landsteiner antibody, which is a biphasic IgG antibody with anti-P specificity found in patients suffering from paroxysmal cold hemoglobinuria.

Dyscrasia: An old term now used as a synonym for disease.

Dyserythropoiesis: Changes in erythroid cell nuclear chromatin pattern; some of these changes are bizarre.

Dysfibrinogenemia: A congenital disorder characterized by the synthesis of abnormal fibrinogen molecules with different functional characteristics.

Dyshematopoiesis: Abnormalities in the maturation, division, or production of blood cells.

Dyskeratosis: Any alteration in the keratinization of the epithelial cells of the epidermis.

Dysostosis: Defective ossification.

Dyspnea: Labored or difficult breathing.

Dyspoiesis: Nuclear-cytoplasmic dissociation, especially in red cells.

Early degradation products: The large fragments X and Y that result from the proteolytic action of plasmin on fibrin or fibrinogen. Fragments X and Y have antithrombin activity

Ecchymosis: A form of macula appearing in large, irregularly formed hemorrhagic areas of the skin, originally blue-black and changing to greenish brown or yellow.

Eclampsia: An acute disorder of pregnant and puerperal women, associated with convulsions and coma.

Edema: A local or generalized condition in which the body tissues contain an excessive amount of tissue fluid.

Edematous: Pertaining to swelling of body tissues.

Electrophoresis: The movement of charged particles through a medium (paper, agar, gel) in the presence of an electrical field. Useful in the separation and analysis of proteins.

Elliptocyte: See **Ovalocyte.**

Elution: A process whereby cells that are coated with antibody are treated in such a manner as to disrupt the bonds between the antigen and the antibody. The freed antibody is collected in an inert diluent such as saline or 6 percent albumin. This serum can then be tested to identify its specificity using routine methods. The mechanism to free the antibody may be physical (heat, shaking) or chemical (ether, acid), and the harvested antibody-containing fluid is called an eluate.

Embolism: Obstruction of a blood vessel by foreign substances or by a blood clot.

Embolus: A mass of undissolved matter present in a blood or lymphatic vessel brought there by the blood or lymph circulation.

Endemic: A disease that occurs continuously in a particular population but has a low mortality rate, such as measles; used in contrast to epidemic.

Endocarditis: Inflammation of the lining membrane of the heart. May be due to invasion of microorganisms or an abnormal immunologic reaction.

Endogenous: Produced or arising from within a cell or organism.

Endoplasmic reticulum: A connecting network of microcanals or tubules running through the cytoplasm of a cell that serves in intracellular transport.

Endothelium: A form of squamous epithelium consisting of flat cells that line the blood and lymphatic vessels, the heart, and various other body cavities. It is derived from the mesoderm.

Endotoxemia: The presence of endotoxin in the blood (endotoxin is present in the cells of certain bacteria, such as gram-negative organisms).

Eosinophil: A mature type of granulocyte in which cytoplasmic granules are large, round, and refractile and stain orange or red with Wright's stain. Composes 0 to 4 percent of the normal differential count.

Epistaxis: Hemorrhage from the nose; nosebleed.

Epsilon: A type of globin chain found in embryonic hemoglobins.

Epsilon aminocaproic acid (EACA): A synthetic inhibitor of plasminogen activation.

Erythroblastosis fetalis: See **Hemolytic disease of the newborn (HDN).**

Erythrocyte: A mature red blood cell or corpuscle.

Erythrocyte sedimentation rate (ESR): The rate at which red blood cells settle per hour; affected by three factors: erythrocytes, plasma, and mechanical factors.

Erythrocytosis: Abnormal increase in the number of red blood cells in circulation, secondary to many disorders.

Erythroid hyperplasia: As seen in the bone marrow, an increase in the number of immature red cell forms; usually a response to anemic stress.

Erythropoiesis: The production and maturation of erythrocytes.

Erythropoietin: A hormone that regulates red blood cell production.

Etiology: The study of the causes of disease.

Euglobulin: The fraction of plasma containing fibrinogen, plasminogen, and plasminogen activators with only trace amounts of antiplasmins.

Euglobulin lysis time: Coagulation procedure testing for fibrinolysins.

Exocytosis: Secretion of the contents of cytoplasmic granules.

Exogenous: Originating outside an organ or part.

Extracorporeal: That which exists outside of the body.

Extramedullary hematopoiesis: Formation of blood cells in sites other than the bone marrow (that is, liver, spleen).

Extravascular: Outside of the blood vessel.

E. hemolysis: Hemolysis occurring within the cells of the reticuloendothelial system.

Factor VIII antigen: The high molecular weight component of the factor VIII molecule.

Factor assay: Coagulation procedure to assay the concentration of specific plasma coagulation factors.

Factor VIII concentrate: A commercially prepared source of coagulation factor VIII.

Favism: An inherited condition resulting from sensitivity to the fava bean, usually seen in people of Mediterranean origin who have a deficiency in the enzyme glucose-6-phosphate dehydrogenase, which may result in a severe hemolytic episode.

Femto-: A prefix used in the metric system to signify 10^{-15} of any unit. Femtoliter (fl) is used in reporting mean corpuscular volume (MCV) of erythrocytes.

Ferritin: The storage form of iron in the tissues, which is found principally in the reticuloendothelial cells of the liver, spleen, and bone marrow.

Fibrin: A whitish filamentous protein or clot formed by the action of thrombin or fibrinogen, converting it to fibrin.

Fibrin monomer: The altered molecule that results from thrombin splitting fibrinopeptides A and B from two of the three paired chains of the fibrinogen molecule.

Fibrinogen: A protein produced in the liver that circulates in plasma. In the presence of thrombin, an enzyme produced by the activation of the clotting mechanism, fibrinogen is cleaved into fibrin, which is insoluble protein that is responsible for clot formation.

Fibrinogen-degradation products (FDPs): The polypeptide fragments X, Y, D, and E that result from the proteolytic action of plasmin on fibrinogen or fibrin.

Fibrinolysin: The substance, also called plasmin, that has the ability to dissolve fibrin.

Fibrinolysis: Dissolution of fibrin by fibrinolysin caused by the action of proteolytic enzyme system that is continually active in the body but that is increased greatly by various stress stimuli.

Fibrinopeptides: Peptides released when fibrinogen is

converted to fibrin by thrombin. The fibrinopeptides released by thrombin are designated A and B.

Fibrin-split products: Those products that result from fibrin digestion.

Fibrin-stabilizing factor (FSF): Factor XIII.

Fibrosis: Excessive formation of fibrous tissue.

Fitzgerald factor: High molecular weight kininogen (HMWK).

Fletcher factor: Prekallikrein.

Fractures: The sudden breaking of bones.

Fragility: Liability to break, burst, or disintegrate as erythrocytes are prone to do when exposed to varying concentrations of hypotonic salt solutions.

Fresh frozen plasma (FFP): A frozen plasma product (from a single donor) that contains all clotting factors, especially the labile factors V and VIII. Useful for clotting factor deficiencies other than hemophilia A, von Willebrand's disease, and hypofibrinogenemia.

Friable: Easily broken or pulverized.

Gallops: Relating to cardiac rhythms, an abnormal third or fourth heart sound in a patient experiencing tachycardia. Gallops are indicative of a serious heart condition.

Gamma: A type of globin chain found in fetal hemoglobin. Two types exist: G gamma contains glycine at position 13 of the amino acid sequence, and A gamma contains alanine at the same position.

Gamma globulin: A protein found in plasma and known to be involved in immunity.

Gammopathy: Abnormalities of the immune or gamma system arising in a single disordered clone of cells that is able to synthesize immunoglobulin.

Gastrectomy: Surgical removal of part or all of the stomach.

Gastritis: Inflammation of the stomach, characterized by epigastric pain or tenderness, nausea, vomiting, and systemic electrolyte changes if vomiting persists. The mucosa may be atrophic or hypertrophic.

Gestation: In mammals, the length of time from conception to birth.

Gigantism: Excessive development of part or all of the body.

Glanzmann's thrombasthenia: A congenital bleeding disorder characterized by impaired or absent clot retraction and a failure of the platelets to aggregate with most aggregating agents, particularly with ADP.

Globin: A protein constituent of hemoglobin. There are four globin chains in the hemoglobin molecule.

Glossitis: Inflammation of the tongue.

Glucose-6-phosphate dehydrogenase (G6PD): An intracellular red cell enzyme important in the hexose monophosphate pathway.

Glycolysis: Hydrolysis of sugar by an enzyme in the body.

Glycophorin: The principal integral blood cell protein, containing 60 percent carbohydrate and giving the red cell its negative charge. It appears on the external surface of the red cell.

Golgi apparatus: A lamellar membranous structure near the nucleus of almost all cells. The structure is best seen by electron microscopy. It contains enzymes that add terminal sugar sequences to protein moieties.

Gout: Hereditary metabolic disease that is a form of acute arthritis and is marked by inflammation of the joints.

The affected joint may be at any location, but gout usually begins in the knee or foot.

Graft-versus-host (GVH) disease: A disorder in which the grafted tissue attacks the host tissue.

Granulocyte: A mature granular leukocyte; refers to band or polymorphonuclear neutrophil, eosinophil, or basophil.

Granulocytopenia: Abnormal reduction of granulocytes in the blood.

Granulomas: A granular tumor or growth usually of lymphoid and epithelial cells. It occurs in various infectious diseases such as leprosy, cutaneous leishmaniosis, yaws, and syphilis.

Granulopoiesis: The production and maturation of granulocytes.

Hageman factor: Synonym for coagulation factor XII.

Haplotypes: A term used in human leukocyte antigen (HLA) testing to denote the five genes (HLA-A, B, C, D, and DR) on the same chromosome.

Hapten: The portion of an antigen containing the grouping on which the specificity is dependent.

Haptoglobin: An α_2-glycoprotein produced in the liver, having three phenotypes with differing abilities to bind hemoglobin.

Heinz bodies: Large red blood cell inclusions that are formed as a result of denatured or precipitated hemoglobin. May be seen in the thalassemia syndromes, G6PD deficiency, or any of the unstable hemoglobin conditions.

Hemangioma: A benign tumor of dilated blood vessels.

Hemarthrosis: Bloody effusion into the cavity of a joint.

Hematemesis: Vomiting of blood.

Hematocrit: The proportion of red blood cells in whole blood expressed as a percentage.

Hematoma: A swelling or mass of blood confined to an organ, tissue, or space and caused by a break in a blood vessel.

Hematopoiesis: Formation and development of blood cells, normally in the bone marrow. (Synonym: **Hemopoiesis.**)

Hematuria: Blood in the urine.

Heme: The iron-containing protoporphyrin portion of the hemoglobin wherein the iron is in the ferrous (Fe^{2+}) state.

Hemochromatosis: A disease of iron metabolism in which iron accumulates in body tissues, causing complications and tissue damage.

Hemoconcentration: An increase in the number of red cells, resulting from a decrease in the volume of plasma.

Hemodialysis: Removal of chemical substances from the blood by passing it through tubes made of semipermeable membranes. This procedure is used to cleanse the blood of patients in whom one or both kidneys are defective or absent; and remove excess accumulation of drugs or toxic chemicals in the blood.

Hemoglobin: The iron-containing pigment of the red blood cells that functions to carry oxygen from the lungs to the tissues. Consists of approximately 6 percent heme and 94 percent globin.

    H. A: The major portion of adult hemoglobin (95 percent), composed of two alpha and two beta chains.

    H. A A_2: A small portion of adult hemoglobin (2 to 4 percent), composed of two alpha and two delta chains.

H. Bart's: An abnormal hemoglobin composed of four gamma chains. Formed in α-thalassemia major, the most severe form of thalassemia occurring in anemic, edematous stillborn infants whose hemoglobin composition is almost all hemoglobin Bart's.

H. F: The major fetal hemoglobin, composed of two alpha and two gamma chains.

H. Gower 1: A type of hemoglobin found in the embryo, composed of two zeta and two epsilon chains.

H. Gower 2: A type of hemoglobin found in the embryo composed of two alpha and two epsilon chains.

H. H inclusions: Red cell inclusions that are formed in the α-thalassemia in which hemoglobin (four beta chains) is in high concentration.

H. Lepore: A type of abnormal hemoglobin that is the product of a fused delta and beta gene formed by an unequal crossing over resulting in a hemoglobin with fused delta/beta chains; a form of thalassemia.

H. Portland: A type of hemoglobin found in the embryo, composed of two zeta and two gamma chains.

Hemoglobinemia: Presence of hemoglobin in the blood plasma.

Hemoglobinopathies: The group of diseases caused by or associated with the presence of one of several forms of abnormal hemoglobin in the blood.

Hemoglobin-oxygen dissociation curve: The relationship between the percent saturation of the hemoglobin molecule with oxygen and the environmental oxygen tension.

Hemoglobinuria: The presence in the urine of hemoglobin freed from lysed red blood cells. Occurs when the amount of hemoglobin from disintegrating red blood cells, rapid hemolysis, or when red cells exceeds the ability of the blood proteins to combine the hemoglobin.

Hemolysin: An antibody that activates complement, leading to cell lysis.

Hemolysis: The destruction of red blood cells.

Intravascular h.: The disruption of the red cell membrane and release of hemoglobin into the surrounding fluid within the vasculature.

Extravascular h.: The phagocytosis of erythrocytes by the reticuloendothelial system, primarily in the spleen and liver.

Hemolytic: Pertaining to, characterized by, or producing hemolysis.

H. anemia: Anemia caused by increased destruction of erythrocytes.

H. disease of the newborn (HDN): A disease characterized by anemia, jaundice, enlargement of the liver and spleen, and generalized edema (hydrops fetalis), owing to the maternal IgG antibodies that cross the placenta and attack fetal red cells when there is a fetomaternal blood group incompatibility. Usually caused by ABO or Rh antibodies. (Synonym: **Erythroblastosis fetalis.**)

Hemolytic uremic syndrome (HUS): A disorder that usually affects young children and is characterized by the combination of severe hemolytic anemia and renal failure. Reticulocytosis and schistocytes are the morphologic findings of this microangiopathic hemolytic anemia.

Hemopexin: A β_1-globulin that has the capacity to bind hemoglobin when haptoglobin has been depleted.

Hemophilia: A hereditary blood disease characterized by impaired coagulability of the blood and a strong tendency to bleed.

H. A: A sex-linked hereditary bleeding disorder characterized by greatly prolonged coagulation time owing to a deficiency of factor VIII.

H. B: Christmas disease, a hereditary bleeding disorder caused by a deficiency of factor IX.

H. C: A hereditary bleeding disorder caused by a deficiency of factor XI.

Hemoptysis: Coughing and spitting of blood as a result of bleeding from any part of respiratory tract.

Hemorrhage: Abnormal internal or external bleeding. May be venous, arterial, or capillary from blood vessels into the tissues, or into or from the body.

Hemorrhagic diathesis: Predisposition to spontaneous bleeding from a trivial trauma caused by a defect in clotting or in the structure or function of blood vessels.

Hemosiderin: An iron-containing pigment derived from hemoglobin upon disintegration of red cells; one method whereby iron is stored until needed for making hemoglobin.

Hemosiderinuria: The excretion of hemosiderin from disintegrated red blood cells into the urine.

Hemosiderosis: A condition in which the iron content of blood is increased.

Hemostasis: The process in which blood clots and bleeding are arrested.

Hemotherapy: Blood transfusion as a therapeutic measure.

Heparin: A sulfonated mucopolysaccharide that acts as a powerful anticoagulant at several sites in the coagulation sequence: (1) inhibition of thrombin, (2) inhibition of factor Xa, (3) inhibition of factor IXa, and (4) inhibition of factor XIIa. Used therapeutically in the treatment of thromboembolic disease.

Hepatitis: Inflammation of the liver.

Hepatosplenomegaly: Enlargement of the liver and the spleen.

Hereditary: Transmitted from parent to offspring.

Hereditary angioneurotic edema: A disease state in which there is no inhibition of C1 enzyme activity. There are increased levels of plasmin and complement activator.

Hereditary erythrocytic multinuclearity with a positive acid serum (HEMPAS): A type II congenital dyserythropoietic anemia (CDA), also known as Ham's test.

Hereditary elliptocytosis (HE): An inherited (autosomal dominant) intracorpuscular defect of the red cell membrane that is characterized by the presence of greater than 40 percent elliptical red cells on the peripheral blood smear. The condition is generally asymptomatic. There is a biochemical and genetic relationship to hereditary pyropoikilocytosis (HPP).

Hereditary hemorrhagic telangiectasia: A congenital hemorrhagic abnormality of the vascular system characterized by localized dilation and convolution of capillaries and venules giving rise to the characteristic telangiectases.

Hereditary persistence of fetal hemoglobin (HPFH): A group of conditions characterized by the persistence of fetal hemoglobin synthesis into adult life.

Hereditary pyropoikilocytosis (HPP): A relatively rare and severe autosomal recessive hemolytic anemia characterized by striking bizarre micropoikilocytosis in which the red cells bud, fragment, and form microspherocytes. In addition, the red cells are thermally unstable when heated to 45°C and strikingly fragmented in comparison to normal red cells which fragment only at 49°C.

Hereditary spherocytosis (HS): An inherited (autosomal dominant) intracorpuscular defect of the red cell membrane (altered spectrin) that results in the most common hereditary hemolytic anemia found in whites. The morphologic hallmark of hereditary spherocytosis is the presence of spherocytes on the peripheral blood smear.

Hereditary stomatocytosis (hereditary hydrocytosis): A heterogenous group of rare red cell membrane disorders inherited in an autosomal dominant fashion that are characterized by the presence of stomatocytes on the peripheral blood smear and alterations in the permeability of the red cell membrane to cations.

Hereditary thrombophilia: Antithrombin III deficiency; an autosomal dominant disorder in which there is an increased tendency toward thrombosis.

Heterozygous: Possessing different alleles in regard to a given characteristic.

Histamine: A substance normally present in the body that is released by the mast cells and basophils. It exerts a pharmacologic action when released from injured cells.

Histiocyte: A large fixed macrophage. (See also **Macrophage.**)

Hodgkin's disease: A disease of unknown etiology producing enlargement of lymphoid tissue, spleen, and liver, with invasion of other tissues.

Homozygous: Possessing identical alleles in regard to a given characteristic.

Howell-Jolly bodies: Red cell inclusions that develop in periods of accelerated or abnormal erythropoiesis. They represent nuclear remnants containing DNA.

Humoral: Pertaining to body fluids or substances contained in them.

Hybridization: The production of hybrids by crossbreeding.

Hybridoma: A neoplastic cell.

Hydrops fetalis: Erythroblastosis fetalis. A hemolytic disease of the newborn characterized by anemia, jaundice, enlargement of liver and spleen, and generalized edema.

Hypercoagulability: A condition in which activated coagulation factors are found intravascularly; may or may not be associated with increased incidence of thromboembolus.

Hyperkalemia: Excessive amounts of potassium in the blood.

Hyperplasia: Excessive proliferation of normal cells in the normal tissue arrangement of an organ.

Hypersegmentation: An increase in the number of nuclear lobes or segments (more than 6) in segmented neutrophils; especially characteristics in vitamin B_{12} or folate deficiencies.

Hypersplenism: A condition arising as a result of an enlarged spleen. Red cell survival is significantly shortened.

Hypertension: Increase in blood pressure to above normal.

Hyperviscosity: Excessive viscosity or exaggeration of adhesive properties seen in anemias and inflammatory disease.

Hypochromia: Increased area of central pallor in red cells.

Hypofibrinogenemia: A congenital disorder characterized by low levels of fibrinogen, usually without any bleeding tendencies.

Hypogammaglobulinemia: Decreased blood levels of gamma globulins seen in some disease states.

Hypogonadism: Defective internal secretion of the gonads.

Hyposplenism: Decreased or improper splenic function. There are a variety of conditions and splenic sizes associated with hyposplenism; however, all have in common hematologic manifestations that suggest loss of many or all of the vital splenic functions (for example, Howell-Jolly bodies, Pappenheimer's bodies, poikilocytes, increased platelet count).

Hypotension: Decrease in blood pressure to below normal.

Hypothermia: Having a body temperature below normal.

Hypothyroidism: A condition due to deficiency of the thyroid secretion, resulting in a lowered basal metabolism.

Hypovolemia: Diminished blood volume.

Hypoxia: Deficiency of oxygen.

Icterus: A condition characterized by yellowish skin, eyes, mucous membranes, and body fluids owing to deposition of excess bilirubin.

Idiopathic: Pertaining to conditions without clear pathogenesis or to disease without recognizable cause, as of spontaneous origin.

Idiopathic thrombocytopenia purpura (ITP): Bleeding due to a decreased number of platelets: the etiology is unknown, with most evidence pointing to platelet autoantibodies.

Idiothrombocythemia: An increase in blood platelets with unknown etiology.

Immune response: The reaction of the body to substances that are foreign or are interpreted as being foreign. Cell-mediated or cellular immunity pertains to tissue destruction mediated by T cells such as graft rejection and hypersensitivity reactions. Humoral immunity pertains to cell destruction response during the early period of the reaction.

Immune serum globulin: Gamma globulin protein fraction of serum containing antibodies.

Immunoblast: A mitotically active T or B cell.

Immunodeficiency: A decrease in the normal concentration of immunoglobulins in serum.

Immunogenicity: The ability of an antigen to stimulate an antibody response.

Immunoglobulin (Ig): One of a family of closely related, yet not identical, proteins that are capable of acting as antibodies: IgA, IgD, IgE, IgG, and IgM. The principal immunoglobulin in exocrine secretions such as saliva and tears is IgA. Immunoglobulin D may play a role in antigen recognition and the initiation of antibody synthesis. Immunoglobulin E is produced by the cells lining the intestinal and respiratory tracts and is important in forming reagin. The main immunoglobulin in human serum is IgG. A globulin formed in almost every immune response during the early period of the reaction is IgM.

Immunologic memory: The development of T and B memory cells that have been sensitized by exposure to an antigen and respond rapidly under subsequent encounters with the antigen.

Immunologic unresponsiveness: Development of a tolerance to certain antigens that would otherwise evoke an immune response.

Immunoprecipitin: An antigen-antibody reaction that results in precipitation.

Inflammation: Tissue reaction to injury. The succession of changes that occurs in living tissue when it is injured.

Inhibitor: A chemical substance that stops enzyme activity.

Insidious: Without warning.

Insomnia: Inability to sleep, or sleep prematurely ended or interrupted by periods of wakefulness.

Interferon: A protein or proteins formed when cells are exposed to viruses. Noninfected cells exposed to interferon are protected against viral infection.

Intravascular hemolysis: Hemolysis occurring within the blood vessels. (See **Hemolysis**.)

Intrinsic factor (IF): A protein secreted by the parietal cells of the stomach that is necessary for vitamin B_{12} absorption.

Intrinsic system: Initiation of blood clotting that occurs through a surface-mediated pathway.

In utero: Within the uterus.

In vitro: In glass, as in a test tube.

In vivo: In the living body or organism.

Ischemia: Local and temporary deficiency of blood supply caused by obstruction of the circulation to a part.

Isoagglutinins: A term used to denote the ABO antibodies anti-A, anti-B, and anti-A,B.

Isoimmune: An antibody produced against a foreign antigen in the same species.

Jaundice: A condition characterized by yellowing of the skin and the whites of the eyes. One cause is excess hemolysis, which results in increased circulating bilirubin. Another cause is liver damage caused by hepatitis.

Juvenile: A common-usage term that is a synonym for neutrophilic metamyelocyte.

Kaolin: A surface-activated substance.

Karyorrhexis: A necrotic stage with fragmentation of the nucleus whereby chromatin is distributed irregularly throughout the cytoplasm.

Karyotype: A photomicrograph of a single cell in the metaphase stage of mitosis that is arranged to show the chromosomes in descending order of size.

Keratocytes: Synonymous with **Burr cells**.

Kernicterus: A form of icterus neonatorum occurring in infants. Develops at 2 to 8 days of age. Prognosis is poor if untreated.

Ketosis: The accumulation in the body of the ketone bodies: acetone, beta hydroxybutyric acid, and acetoacetic acid.

Kinin: A general term for a group of polypeptides that have considerable biologic activity (for example, vasoactivity).

Koilonychia: A disorder of the nails, which are abnormally thin and concave from side to side, with the edges turned up.

Late degradation products: The terminal fragments D and E that result from the proteolytic action of plas-

min on fibrin or fibrinogen. Fragments D and E are known to inhibit fibrin polymerization.

Lepore: See **Hemoglobin Lepore**.

Leptocyte: Synonymous with **Target cell**.

Lethargic: Sluggish; having a lack of energy.

Leukemia: A chronic or acute disease of unknown etiologic factors characterized by unrestrained growth of leukocytes and their precursors in the tissues.

Leukemic hiatus: A phase of leukemia in which the normal maturation series of white cells is not seen because blast cells crowd out normal cells.

Leukemoid reaction: A moderate or advanced degree of leukocytosis in the blood that is not a result of a leukemic disease. These reactions are frequently observed as a feature of infectious disease, drug and chemical intoxication, or secondary to nonhematopoietic carcinoma.

Leukoagglutinins: Antibodies to white blood cells.

Leukocytosis: Increase in number of leukocytes (more than 10,000 cells/mm³) in the blood.

Leukoerythroblastosis: The presence of immature white cells and nucleated red cells on the blood smear; frequently denotes a malignant or myeloproliferative process.

Leukopheresis: Withdrawal of leukocytes from the circulation; may be used to obtain leukocytes for administration to patients with severe granulocytopenia.

Lymphadenitis: Inflammation of the lymph nodes.

Lymphadenopathy: Disease of the lymph nodes.

Lymphocyte: A white blood cell formed in lymphoid tissue throughout the body, generally described as nongranular and including small and large varieties. Composes approximately 20 to 45 percent of the total leukocyte count.

Lymphocytosis: An increase in lymphocytes within the blood.

Lymphoma: Asymmetrical enlargement of a group of lymph nodes, which destroys the normal histologic lymph node architecture.

Lysosomes: Part of an intracellular digestive system that exists as separate particles in the cell. Even though their importance in health and disease is certain, all the precise ways lysosomes affect changes are not understood.

Lysozyme (muramidase): A hydrolytic enzyme destructive to cell walls of certain bacteria. It is present in body fluids and found in high concentration within granulocytes.

Macrocephaly: Enlargement of the head.

Macrocyte: A red cell 9 μl in diameter or larger.

α_2-Macroglobulin: A protease inhibitor present in the blood that inhibits the activity of plasmin.

Macroglobulinemia: Abnormal presence of high molecular weight immunoglobulins (IgM) in the blood.

Macrophage: Cells of the reticuloendothelial system having the ability to phagocytose particulate substances and to store vital dyes and other colloidal substances. They are found in loose connective tissues and various organs of the body.

Major histocompatibility complex (MHC): Present in all mammalian and ovarian species (analogous to human HLA complex); HLA antigens are within the MHC at a locus on chromosome 6.

Malabsorption syndrome: Disordered or inadequate absorption of nutrients from the intestinal tract. May be due to a disease that affects the intestinal mucosa such as infections, tropical sprue, gluten enteropathy, or pancreatic insufficiency or due to antibiotic therapy.

Malaria: An acute and sometimes chronic infectious disease due to the presence of protozoan plasmodium parasites within red blood cells.

Mast cell: A tissue basophil. (See **Basophil.**)

Mastoiditis: Inflammation of the air cells of the mastoid process.

Mean corpuscular hemoglobin (MCH): A measure of hemoglobin content of red corpuscles. It is reported in picograms.

$$MCH = \frac{\text{Hemoglobin in g/100 ml} \times 10}{\text{RBC count, millions of cells/}\mu l}$$

Mean corpuscular hemoglobin concentration (MCHC): A measure of concentration of hemoglobin in the average red cell.

$$MCHC = \frac{\text{Hemoglobin in g/100 ml} \times 100}{\text{Hematocrit, \%}}$$

Mean corpuscular volume (MCV): A measure of the volume of red corpuscles expressed in cubic micrometers or femtoliters.

$$MCV = \frac{\text{Hematocrit, \%} \times 10}{\text{RBC count, millions of cells/}\mu l}$$

Mediastinal: Related to the mediastinum

Mediastinum: A septum or cavity between two principal portions of an organ.

Medullary: Concerning marrow or medulla.

Megakaryocyte: The intermediate platelet precursor cell in the bone marrow, not normally present in peripheral blood. It is a large cell, usually having a multilobed nucleus, that gives rise to blood platelets owing to a pinching off of the cytoplasm.

Megaloblast: A large, nucleated, abnormal red cell precursor, 11 to 20 μm in diameter, oval and slightly irregular, resulting from a nuclear/cytoplasmic maturation asynchrony characteristic of vitamin B_{12} or folate deficiency.

Megaloblastoid: Term used to describe changes in the bone marrow that are morphologically similar to, yet etiologically different from, megaloblastic change.

Meiosis: Type of cell division of germ cells in which two successive divisions of the nucleus produce cells that contain half the number of chromosomes present in somatic cells.

Melena: Black tarry feces due to the action of intestinal juices on free blood.

Menorrhagia: Menstrual bleeding that is excessive in number of days or amount of blood, or both.

Menstruation: The periodic discharge of a bloody fluid from the uterus, occurring at more or less regular intervals during the life of a woman from age of puberty to menopause.

Metamyelocyte: An immature neutrophilic granulocyte with a kidney-bean-shaped nucleus or an indent, with the presence of specific granules (neutrophilic, eosinophilic, or basophilic) in the cytoplasm (such as neutrophilic metamyelocyte, eosinophilic metamyelocyte, basophilic metamyelocyte).

Metaphyseal dysostosis: Defective bone formation in the metaphysis—the portion of a developing long bone between diaphysis or shaft and epiphysis.

Metaplasia: Conversion of one kind of tissue into a form that is not normal for that tissue.

Metarubricyte: Synonymous with **Orthochromic (orthochromatophilic) normoblast**.

Metastasis: Movement of bacteria or body cell, especially cancer cells, from one part of the body to another. Change in location of a disease or of its manifestations or transfer from one organ or part to another not directly connected. Spread is by the lymphatics or bloodstream.

Metastatic: Pertaining to metastasis, which is a manifestation of a malignancy as a secondary growth in a new location. Spread is by the lymphatics or bloodstream.

Methemoglobin: A form of hemoglobin wherein the ferrous ion (Fe^{2+}) has been oxidized to ferric ion (Fe^{3+}), possibly owing to toxic substances such as aniline dyes, potassium chlorate, or nitrate-contaminated water.

Microaggregates: Aggregates of platelets and leukocytes that accumulate in stored blood.

Microcephaly: Abnormal smallness of the head, often seen in mental retardation; it is congenital.

Microspherocytes: Small, sphere-shaped red blood cells seen in certain kinds of anemia.

Mitochondria: Slender microscopic filaments or rods 0.5 μm in diameter that can be seen in cells by using phase contrast microscopy or electron microscopy. They are a source of energy in the cell and are involved in protein synthesis and lipid metabolism.

Mitosis: Type of cell division in which each daughter cell contains the same number of chromosomes as the parent cell. All cells except sex cells undergo mitosis.

Mixed field: A type of agglutination pattern in which there are numerous small clumps of cells amid a sea of free cells.

Mixed lymphocyte culture (MLC): A technique for typing cells in which lymphocytes of different individuals are co-cultured.

Mixed lymphocyte reaction (MLR): A method of tissue typing that exploits the fact that T lymphocytes are stimulated to grow in the presence of cells carrying foreign histocompatibility class II antigens.

Monoclonal: Antibody derived from a single ancestral antibody-producing parent cell.

Monocyte: A white blood cell that normally constitutes 2 to 10 percent of the total leukocyte staining count. This cell is 9 to 12 μl in diameter and has an indented nucleus and an abundant pale blue-gray cytoplasm containing many fine red-staining granules.

Morbidity: The number of sick persons or cases of disease in relationship to a specific population.

Mortality: The death rate; ratio of number of deaths to a given population.

Multiparous: Having borne more than one child.

Multiple myeloma: A neoplastic proliferation of plasma cells, characterized by very high immunoglobulin levels of monoclonal origin.

Mutant: A variation of genetic structure that breeds true.

Mutation: A change in a gene potentially capable of being transmitted to offspring.

    Frameshift m.: A change in which a message is read incorrectly because either a base is missing or an extra base is added. This results in an entirely new polypeptide because the triplet sequence has been shifted one base.

Point m.: A change in a base in DNA that can lead to a change in the amino acid incorporated into the polypeptide. The change is identifiable by analyzing the amino acid sequences of the original protein and its mutant offspring.

Myeloblast: The first recognizable "mother cell" (precursor) of the granulocytic cell line.

Myelocyte: An immature neutrophilic granulocyte characterized by an eccentrically located round nucleus and specific granules—neutrophilic, eosinophilic, or basophilic (such as neutrophilic myelocyte, eosinophilic myelocyte, basophilic myelocyte).

Myelodysplasia: Abnormal division; maturation and production of erythrocytes, granulocytes, monocytes, and platelets.

Myelodysplastic syndrome (MDS): A group of primary hematologic disorders associated with abnormal division, maturation, and production of erythrocytes, granulocytes, monocytes, and platelets; also referred to as preleukemic myelodysplastic syndrome.

Myelofibrosis: Replacement of the bone marrow by fibrous tissue.

Myeloid-to-erythroid (M:E) ratio: Differential count of bone marrow obtained by dividing the number of granulocytes and their precursor cells by the number of nucleated red cells.

Myeloperoxidase: An enzyme that is present in the primary (azurophilic) granules of polymorphonuclear neutrophils, eosinophils, and monocytes-macrophages.

Myelophthisic: The process that occurs primarily in the bone marrow as a result of the crowding out of normal elements by a neoplasm, histiocytic type cells, and so on. A consequent reduction in normal marrow cells and release of immature hematopoietic cells (especially nucleated red cells) into the blood occurs.

Myeloproliferative: A group of disorders characterized by autonomous proliferation of one or more hematopoietic elements in the bone marrow. In many cases, the liver and spleen are enlarged.

Necrosis: The pathologic death of one or more cells of a portion of tissue or organ.

Neonatal: Pertaining to the first 6 weeks after birth.

Neoplasm: A new and abnormal formation of tissue such as a tumor or growth.

Neuraminidase: An enzyme that cleaves sialic acid from the red cell membrane.

Neutralization: Inactivating an antibody by reacting it with an antigen against which it is directed.

Neutropenia: The presence of abnormally small numbers of neutrophils in the circulating blood.

Neutrophil: A medium-sized mature leukocyte, with a three- to five-lobed nucleus, and cytoplasm containing small lilac-staining granules. Normally constitutes 50 to 70 percent of leukocytes in the blood.

Nondisjunction: Failure of a pair of chromosomes to separate during meiosis.

Nonresponder: An individual whose immune system does not respond well in antibody formation to antigenic stimulation.

Nuclear-to-cytoplasmic (N:C) ratio: The proportion of nucleus to cytoplasm found in nucleated cells; often used in identification of cell maturity.

Obstetric: Referring to the branch of medicine that concerns itself with the management of women during pregnancy, childbirth, and puerperium.

Oculocutaneous: Relating to the eyes and the skin.

Oliguria: Diminished amount of urine formation.

Oncogenic: Tumor-forming.

Opisthotonus: Extreme aching in the spine.

Opsonin: Substance in the blood serum that acts upon microorganisms and other cells, facilitating phagocytosis.

Organomegaly: Enlargement of any of the specific organs of the body.

Orthochromic (orthochromatophilic) normoblast: An immature red cell precursor characterized by pink cytoplasm and a small round pyknotic nucleus. This stage of maturation normally is found only in the bone marrow.

Orthodontic: Referring to the branch of dentistry that deals with the prevention and correction of irregularities of the teeth.

Orthostatic hypotension: Decreased blood pressure in an erect position.

Osmolality: The osmotic concentration of a solution determined by the ionic concentration of dissolved substances per unit of solvent.

Osmotic fragility: The ability of the red cells to withstand different salt concentration; this is dependent on the volume, surface area, and functional state of the red blood cell membrane.

Osteoclast: Giant multinuclear cell formed in the bone marrow of growing bones.

Osteomyelitis: Inflammation of the bone—especially the marrow—caused by a pathogenic organism.

Osteoporosis: Increased porosity of the bone, seen most often in the elderly.

Ovalocyte: An abnormal red cell that is egg shaped or elliptical. (Synonym: **Elliptocyte.**)

Oxyhemoglobin: The combined form of hemoglobin and oxygen.

P_{50}: The partial pressure of oxygen or oxygen tension at which the hemoglobin molecule is 50 percent saturated with oxygen.

Pagophagia: The craving to eat ice.

Pallor: Paleness; lack of color.

Panagglutinin: An antibody capable of agglutinating all red blood cells tested, including the patient's own cells.

Pancytopenia: A depression of each of the normal bone marrow elements: white cells, red cells, and platelets in the peripheral blood.

Panel: A large number of group 0 reagent red cells that are of known antigenic characterization and are used for antibody identification.

Panmyelosis: Increase in all the elements of the bone marrow.

Papilledema: Edema and inflammation of the optic nerve at its point of entrance into the eyeball.

Pappenheimer's bodies: Basophilic inclusions in the red blood cell that are clusterlike. They are believed to be iron particles: confirmation is made by Prussian blue stain.

Parachromatin: The portions of the nuclear chromatin that are nonstained or lightly stained.

Paracoagulants: A variety of substances capable of converting soluble fibrin monomer complexes into insoluble fibrin. These include protamine sulfate, ethanol, and material from staphylococci.

Paracoagulation tests: Coagulation procedures used to indicate the presence of soluble fibrin monomer complexes, which is indirect evidence of the action of thrombin on fibrinogen.

Paraproteinemia: A general term for abnormalities of the immunoglobulins, associated with one of several disease states.

Parenchymal: Relating to parenchyma, the essential parts of an organ that are concerned with its function in contradistinction to its framework.

Parenteral: Entry into the body through the intravenous (IV) or intramuscular (IM) route rather than the alimentary route.

Paresis: Partial or incomplete paralysis.

Paresthesia: Numbness.

Paroxysm: A sudden, periodic attack or recurrence of symptoms of a disease.

Paroxysmal cold hemoglobinuria (PCH): A type of cold autoimmune hemolytic anemia usually found in children suffering from viral infections in which a biphasic IgG antibody can be demonstrated with anti-P specificity. (See also **Donath-Landsteiner antibody test.**)

Paroxysmal nocturnal hemoglobinuria (PNH): An uncommon acquired form of hemolysis caused by an intrinsic defect in the red blood cell membrane, rendering it more susceptible to hemolysins in an acid environment, and characterized by hemoglobin in the urine following periods of sleep.

Pathogenesis: Origination and development of a disease.

Pathognomonic: Specifically distinctive or characteristic of a disease or pathologic condition.

Perfusion: Supplying an organ or tissue with nutrients and oxygen by passing blood or other suitable fluid through it.

Perioral paresthesia: Tingling around the mouth, occasionally experienced by apheresis donors, resulting from the rapid return of citrated plasma which contains citrate-bound calcium and free citrate.

Peroxidase: An enzyme that hastens the transfer of oxygen from peroxide to a tissue that requires oxygen; essential to intracellular respiration.

Petechiae: Pinpoint hemorrhages from arterioles, venules.

Phagocytosis: Ingestion and digestion of bacteria and particles by phagocytes.

Pharmacologic: Relating to the study of drugs and their origin, natural properties, and effects on living organisms.

Phlebotomy: Surgical opening of a vein to withdraw blood.

Phosphoglyceromutase (PGM): A red cell enzyme.

Photodermatitis: Lesion development upon exposure to sunlight.

Phototherapy: Exposure to sunlight or artificial light for therapeutic purposes.

Pica: A perversion of appetite associated with ingestion of material not fit for food such as starch, clay, ashes, or plaster.

Pico-: A prefix used in the metric system to signify 10^{-12}; picogram is used in reporting the mean corpuscular hemoglobin.

Pinguecula: A yellowish discoloration near the corneal-scleral junction of the eye.

Pinocytosis: Process by which cells absorb or ingest nutrients and fluid.

Plaques: Small flat growths.

Plasma: The liquid portion of whole blood containing water, electrolytes, glucose, fats, proteins, and gases. Contains all the clotting factors necessary for coagulation but in an inactive form. Once coagulation occurs, the fluid is converted to serum.

Plasma cell: A B lymphocyte–derived cell that secretes immunoglobulins or antibodies.

Plasma protein fraction (PPF): Also known as Plasmanate. Sterile pooled plasma stored as a fluid or freeze-dried. Used for volume replacement.

Plasma thromboplastin antecedent (PTA): See **Christmas factor**.

Plasmacytomas: Localized or generalized tumor masses of plasma cells.

Plasmapheresis: Removal of blood, separation of plasma by centrifugation, and reinjection of the cells into the body. Used as a means of obtaining plasma and in the treatment of certain pathologic conditions.

Plasmin: Fibrinolytic enzyme derived from its precursor plasminogen.

Plasminogen: A protein found in many tissues and body fluids. It is important in preventing fibrin clot formation.

Plasmodium: See **Malaria**.

Platelet: A round or oval disc, 2 to 4 μm in diameter, that is derived from the cytoplasm of the megakaryocyte, a large cell in the bone marrow. Plays an important role in blood coagulation, hemostasis, and blood thrombus formation.

Platelet adhesion: The interaction of platelet surface glycoproteins with connective tissue elements of the subendothelium, requiring von Willebrand factor as a plasma cofactor.

Platelet aggregation: Platelet-to-platelet interaction dependent on calcium.

Platelet concentrate: Platelets prepared from a single unit of whole blood or plasma and suspended in a specific volume of the original plasma. Also known as random donor platelets.

Platelet factor (PF) 3: A phospholipid found within the platelet membrane required for coagulation. Platelet factor 3 assays are used to evaluate platelet disorders.

Platelet plug: Platelets that function in arresting bleeding by "plugging" any damage in the vessel wall and providing phospholipids essential for blood coagulation. The development of a hemostatic platelet plug depends on adhesion, aggregation, and consolidation.

Platelet-rich plasma (PRP): Plasma that is derived from a citrated blood sample span at 1500 rpm for 5 minutes.

Plateletpheresis: A procedure using a machine by which one can selectively remove platelets from a donor or patient.

Platelin: A substance that acts in vitro like PF3.

Plethoric: Congestion causing distention of the blood vessels.

Pleural effusion: Fluid in the pleural space.

Pneumonitis: Inflammation of the lung.

Poikilocytosis: Variation in shape of red cells.

Polyacrylamide gel: A type of matrix used in electrophoresis upon which substances are separated.

Polyagglutination: A state in which an individual's red cells are agglutinated by all sera regardless of blood type.

Polychromasia: Describes the blue-gray color of some younger red cells in evaluation of red blood cell morphology. Increased polychromasia is a sign of a very active bone marrow.

Polychromatophilic normoblast: An immature red cell precursor characterized by blue-gray cytoplasm and round, eccentrically located nucleus with a distinct chromatin/parachromatin pattern of staining, and normally only found in the bone marrow. (Synonym: **Rubricyte.**)

Polyclonal: Antibodies derived from more than one antibody-producing parent cell.

Polycythemia: An excess of red blood cells in the peripheral blood.

P. vera: A chronic life-shortening myeloproliferative disorder involving all bone marrow elements, characterized by an increase in red blood cell mass and hemoglobin concentration.

Polymorphism: A genetic system that possesses numerous allelic forms, such as a blood group system.

Polymorphonuclear neutrophil (PMN): A mature granulocyte with neutrophilic granules and a segmented nucleus (also called segmented neutrophil). (See **Neutrophil**).

Polyspecific Coombs' sera: A reagent that contains antihuman globulin sera against IgG and C3d.

Porphyria: A group of inherited disorders caused by excessive production of porphyrins in the bone marrow or the liver. Two types are recognized: erythropoietic and hepatic.

Portal hypertension: Increased pressure in the portal vein as a result of obstruction of the flow of blood through the liver.

Postpartum: Occurring after childbirth.

Precipitation: The formation of a visible complex (precipitate) in a medium containing soluble antigen (precipitinogen) and the corresponding antibody (precipitin).

Precipitin: An antibody formed in the blood serum of an animal by the presence of a soluble antigen, usually a protein. When added to a solution of the antigen, it brings about precipitation. The injected protein is called the antigen and the antibody produced is the precipitin.

Preleukemia (myelodysplastic syndrome): A clinical syndrome in which the bone marrow shows marked hypocellularity with clusters of immature cells that in many cases evolve into true nonlymphocytic leukemia.

Priapism: Abnormal, painful, and continued erection of the penis owing to disease, accompanied by loss of sexual desire.

Primary fibrinolysis: Activation of the fibrinolytic system that is not secondary to coagulation.

Primary hemostasis: The interaction of platelets and the vascular endothelium to stop bleeding following vascular injury.

Proaccelerin: Factor V; functions in the common pathway of coagulation as a cofactor.

Proband: The initial subject presenting a mental or physical disorder; the heredity of this individual is studied in order to determine if other members of the family have had the same disease or carry it. (Synonym: **Propositus/proposita.**)

Proconvertin: Factor VII, functions in the extrinsic system of coagulation.

Prodrome: A symptom indicative of an approaching disease.

Progranulocyte: An immature white blood cell precursor found only in the bone marrow that is the characteristic stage of maturation where azurophilic non-specific granules first appear in the cytoplasm of the granulocytic cell line.

Pronormoblast: The first recognizable "mother cell" (precursor) of the erythrocytic cell line. (Synonym: **Rubriblast.**)

Prophylaxis: Any agent or regimen that contributes to the prevention of infection and disease.

Propositus/Proposita: The initial individual whose condition led to investigation of a hereditary disorder or to a serologic evaluation of family members. (Synonym: **Proband.**)

Proprioception: The awareness of posture movement and change in equilibrium and the knowledge of position, weight, and resistance of objects in relation to the body.

Prorubricyte: See **Basophilic normoblast**.

Prostaglandins: A group of fatty acid derivatives present in many tissues, including prostate gland, menstrual fluid, brain, lung, kidney, thymus, seminal fluid, and pancreas.

Prosthesis: Replacement of a missing part by an artificial substitute, such as an artificial extremity.

Prostration: Absolute exhaustion.

Protamine sulfate: A substance used to detect the presence of soluble fibrin monomer complexes. It is also used to neutralize the effects of heparin. (See also **Paracoagulants.**)

Prothrombin: Factor II; functions in the common pathway of coagulation.

Prothrombin complex: A commercially prepared concentrate of the vitamin K–dependent factors, prothrombin, and factors VII, IX, and X in lypholized form. Preparations of prothrombin complex are used therapeutically to treat acquired and congenital hemorrhagic disorders.

Prothrombin consumption test (PCT): A test that measures prothrombin activity in serum after coagulation has taken place.

Prothrombin time (PT): A test to evaluate the overall integrity of the clotting system that involves factors VII, X, V, II, and I. Commonly referred to as a means of evaluating the extrinsic system of coagulation.

Protoporphyrin: A porphyrin whose iron complex forms the heme of hemoglobin and the prosthetic groups of myoglobin and certain respiratory pigments.

Pulmonary artery wedge pressure: Pressure measured in the pulmonary artery at its capillary end.

Pulse pressure: The difference between the systolic and the diastolic blood pressures.

Punctate: Having pinpoint punctures or depressions on the surface; marked with dots.

Purpura: A condition with various manifestations and diverse causes characterized by hemorrhages into the skin, mucous membranes, internal organs, and other tissues.

Pyelogram: A roentgenogram of the ureter and renal pelvis.

Pyknosis (pyknotic): Condensation and shrinkage of cells through degeneration.

Pyoderma: Any acute inflammatory skin disease of unknown origin. Bacteria may be cultured from the lesions, but there are normal resident flora.

Pyogenic: Producing pus (for example, pyogenic infection).

Pyroprotein: A serum protein that precipitates upon exposure to hot temperatures.

Raynaud's disease: A peripheral vascular disorder characterized by abnormal vasoconstriction of the extremities upon exposure to cold or during emotional stress. A history of symptoms for at least 2 years is necessary for diagnosis.

Recessive: In genetics, incapable of expression unless carried by both members of a set of homologous chromosomes; not dominant.

Recipient: A patient who is receiving a transfusion of blood or a blood product.

Red cell distribution width (RDW): This measurement is included on some instrumentation as part of the complete blood count. It measures the distribution of red blood cell volume and is equivalent to anisocytosis on the peripheral blood smear. It is calculated as the coefficient of variation of the red cell volume and is expressed as a percentage (normal 11.5 to 14.5 percent).

Refractory: Not responsive to therapy.

Reniform—kidney bean shape: Characteristic shape of the nucleus of metamyelocytes; often used to distinguish metamyelocytes from myelocytes and neutrophilic bands; may also be used to characterize the appearance of reactive lymphocytes.

Reptilase: An enzyme, thrombinlike in nature, derived from the venom of *Bothrops atrox*. Predominantly hydrolyzes fibrinopeptide A from the fibrinogen molecule, in contrast to thrombin, which hydrolyzes fibrinopeptides A and B.

   R. time: A coagulation procedure similar to the thrombin time except that clotting is initiated with the snake venom enzyme reptilase.

Respiratory distress syndrome (RDS): A condition, formerly known as hyaline membrane disease, accounting for more than 25,000 infant deaths per year in the United States. Clinical signs, including delayed onset of respiration and low Apgar score, are usually present at birth.

Reticulocyte: A red blood cell containing a network of granules or filaments representing an immature stage in development. Normally compose about 1 percent of circulating red blood cells.

Reticuloendothelial system (RES): Term applied to those cells scattered throughout the body that have the power to ingest particulate matter. Includes histiocytes of loose connective tissue; reticular cells of lymphatic organs; Kupffer's cells of the liver; cells lining blood sinuses of spleen, bone marrow, adrenal cortex, and hypophysis; and other cells.

Retinopathy: Any disorder of the retina.

Rh immune globulin (RhIg): A passive form of anti-D given within 72 hours of delivery to all Rh-negative mothers delivering an Rh-positive fetus.

Ribonucleic acid (RNA): A nucleic acid that controls protein synthesis in all living cells. There are three different types, and all are derived from the information encoded in the DNA of the cell. Messenger RNA (mRNA) carries the code for specific amino acid sequences from the DNA to the cytoplasm for protein synthesis. Transfer RNA (tRNA) carries the amino acid groups to the ribosome for protein synthesis. Ribosomal RNA (rRNA) exists within the ribosomes and is thought to assist in protein synthesis.

Ribosome: A cellular organelle that contains ribonucleoprotein and functions to synthesize protein. Ribosomes may be single units or clusters called polyribosomes or polysomes.

Rickettsia: Any of the microorganisms belonging to the genus *Rickettsia*.

Ristocetin: Drug used in platelet aggregation studies.

Rouleaux: A group of red blood corpuscles arranged like a roll of coins, owing to an abnormal protein coating on the cells' surfaces; seen in multiple myeloma and Waldenström's macroglobulinemia.

Rubriblast: See **Pronormoblast**.

Rubricyte: See **Polychromatophilic normoblast**.

Russell's viper venom (Stypven): Snake venom with thromboplastic activity.

Sarcoidosis: A disease of unknown etiology characterized by widespread granulomatous lesions that may affect any organ or tissue of the body.

Sarcoma: Cancer arising from connective tissue such as muscle or bone. It may affect the bones, bladder, kidneys, liver, lungs, parotids, and spleen.

Schistocyte: An abnormal red cell that is formed when pieces of the red cell membrane become fragmented. Whole pieces of the red cell membrane appear to be missing, causing bizarre-looking red cells.

Sclera: A tough, white fibrous tissue that covers the so-called white of the eye. It extends from the optic nerve to the cornea.

Scleroderma: A chronic disease of unknown etiology that causes sclerosis of the skin and certain organs, including the gastrointestinal tract, lungs, heart, and kidneys. The skin feels tough and leathery, may itch, and later becomes hyperpigmented.

Screening cells: Group O reagent red cells that are used in antibody detection or screening tests.

Scurvy: A deficiency disease characterized by hemorrhagic manifestations and abnormal formation of bones and teeth.

Senescence: The aging process of the red cells.

Sensitization: A condition of being made sensitive to a specific substance (such as an antigen) after the initial exposure to that substance. Results in the development of immunologic memory that evokes an accentuated immune response with subsequent exposure to the substance.

Sepsis: Pathologic state, usually febrile, resulting from the presence of microorganisms or their poisonous products in the bloodstream.

Septicemia: Presence of bacteria in the blood. The microorganisms may multiply and cause overwhelming infection and death.

Sequestration: An increase in the quantity of blood within the blood vessels, occurring physiologically or produced artificially.

Serine protease inhibitors: The activity of the various enzymes (serine proteases) involved in the coagulation sequence is controlled to a variable extent primarily by plasma proteins generally known as inhibitors (such as antithrombin III).

Serine proteases: A family of proteolytic enzymes with the amino acid serine at the active site.

Serositis: Inflamed condition of a serous membrane.

Serotonin: A chemical present in platelets that is a potent vasoconstrictor.

Serum: The fluid that remains after plasma has clotted.

Sex linkage: A genetic characteristic located on the X or Y chromosome.

Sézary syndrome: Skin disease characterized by infiltration with atypical Sézary cells. The exfoliative dermatitis is considered a variant form of mycosis fungoides.

Shift to the left: An abnormal cell maturation situation that occurs when increased bands, less mature neutrophils, and smaller average number of lobes are found in segmented cells; may be caused by infection, hematologic disorders, or physiologic factors.

Shift to the right: An abnormal cell maturation situation that occurs when more than one hypersegmented cell is seen; indicative of vitamin B_{12} or folate deficiency.

Shock: A clinical syndrome in which the peripheral blood is inadequate to return sufficient blood to the heart for normal function, particularly transport of oxygen to all organs and tissues.

Sickle cell: An abnormal red cell seen in patients who possess high quantities of hemoglobin S, an abnormal hemoglobin. The red cell is crescent- or sickle-shaped.

   S.-c. anemia: Hereditary, chronic anemia in which abnormal sickle- or crescent-shaped erythrocytes are present. It is due to the presence of hemoglobin S in the red blood cells. (The gene that causes this disease occurs with high frequency in African and Mediterranean populations.)

Sickle trait: Blood that is heterozygous for the gene coding for the abnormal hemoglobin of sickle-cell anemia.

Sideroblast: A ferritin-containing normoblast in the bone marrow. Composes from 20 to 90 percent of normoblast in the marrow.

Siderocyte: A non-nucleated red blood cell containing iron in a form other than hematin, and confirmed by a specific iron stain such as the Prussian blue reaction.

Siderosis: A form of pneumoconiosis resulting from inhalation of dust or fumes containing iron particles.

Sodium dodecyl sulfate (SDS): An anionic detergent that renders a net negative charge to substances it solubilizes.

Somatic: Pertaining to nonreproductive cells or tissues.

Specificity: The affinity of an antibody and the antigen against which it is directed.

Spectrin: A large molecule found on the inner surface of red blood cell membrane, that is responsible for the biconcave shape of the red cell as well as for its deformability.

Spectrophotometer: Device for measuring amount of color in a solution by comparison with the spectrum.

Spherocyte: An abnormal red blood cell shape. These are smaller than the normal red cell, have a concentrated hemoglobin content, and have a decreased surface to volume ratio.

Splenomegaly: Enlargement of the spleen seen in several blood disorders.

Sprue: A disease endemic in many tropical regions and occurring sporadically in temperate countries, characterized by weakness, loss of weight, steatorrhea, and various digestive disorders.

Spurious: Not true or genuine; adulterated; false.

Stab: See **Band**.

Staphylococcal clumping test: A coagulation procedure used to detect the presence of fibrin-fibrinogen degradation products. The test uses a strain of staphylococcus that clumps in the presence of fibrinogen, fibrin monomers, or X and Y fragments.

Steatorrhea: Increased secretion of sebaceous glands; fatty stools.

Stenosis: Constriction or narrowing of a passage or orifice.

Steroid hormones: Hormones of the adrenal cortex and the sex hormones.

Stertorous: Pertaining to laborious breathing.

Stomatocyte: An abnormal red cell shape; this shape appears as having a slitlike area of central pallor.

Strabismus: Disorder of the eye in which optic axes cannot be directed to same object. Strabismus can result from reduced visual activity, unequal ocular muscle tone, or an oculomotor nerve lesion.

Streptokinase: A product of beta-hemolytic streptococci capable of liquefying fibrin.

Stroma: The red cell membrane that is left after hemolysis.

Stuart-Prower factor: Factor X; functions in the common pathway of coagulation.

Stypven time test: A coagulation procedure used to distinguish between a deficiency of factor VIII and a deficiency of factor X.

Supernatant: Floating on surface, as oil on water.

Supervention: The development of an additional condition as a complication to an existing disease.

Syncytial: Of the nature of a syncytium, which is a group of cells in which the protoplasm of one cell is continuous with that of adjoining cells, such as the mesenchyme cells of the embryo.

Systemic: Pertaining to a whole body rather than to one of its parts.

Systemic lupus erythematosus (SLE): A disseminated autoimmune disease characterized by anemia, thrombocytopenia, increased IgG levels, and the presence of four IgG antibodies: antinuclear antibody, antinucleoprotein antibody, anti-DNA antibody, and antihistone antibody. Believed to be caused by suppressor T-cell dysfunction.

Systolic pressure: Maximum blood pressure that occurs at ventricular concentration. The upper value of a blood pressure reading.

Tachycardia: Abnormal rapidity of heart action, usually defined as a heart rate greater than 100 per minute.

Tachypnea: Abnormal rapidity of respiration.

Tanned red cell hemagglutination inhibition immunoassay (TRCHII): A test that is the reference method for the asay of fibrinogen degradation products.

Target cell: This abnormal red cell looks like a "bull's eye" with hemoglobin concentrated in the center and on the rim of the cell.

Teardrop cell: This abnormal red cell is seen with frequency in the myeloproliferative disorders, it is shaped like a tear. (Synonym: **Dacrocyte**.)

Telangiectasia: The presence of small, red focal lesions, usually in the skin or mucous membrane, caused by dilation of capillaries, arterioles, or venules.

Template bleeding time: The elapsed time it takes for a uniform incision made by a template and blade to stop bleeding; a test of platelet function in vivo assuming a normal platelet count.

Tertian malaria: Malaria in which sporulation occurs every 48 hours. Symptoms are more common during the day; paroxysms divided into chill, fever, and sweating stages. Benign tertian malaria is caused by *Plasmodium vivax*, malignant tertian malaria by *Plasmodium falciparum*.

Tetany: A nervous affection characterized by intermittent spasms of the muscles of the extremities.

Thalassemia: A group of hereditary anemias produced by either a defective production rate of alpha or the beta hemoglobin polypeptide. This disorder is inherited in homozygous or heterozygous state.

   T. major: The homozygous form of deficient beta chain synthesis, which is very severe and presents itself during childhood. Prognosis varies, however—the younger the child when the disease appears, the more unfavorable the outcome.

Thermal amplitude: The range of temperature over which an antibody demonstrates serologic or in vitro activity or both.

Thrombin: An enzyme that converts fibrinogen to fibrin so that a soluble clot can be formed.

Thrombin time: A coagulation procedure that measures the time required for thrombin to convert fibrinogen to an insoluble fibrin clot.

Thrombocytopathies: Inherited disorders of platelets.

Thrombocytopenia: Decreased numbers of platelets.

Thrombocytosis: Increased numbers of platelets.

Thromboembolism: An embolism; the blocking of a blood vessel by a thrombus (blood clot) which has become detached from the site of formation.

Thrombopoiesis: The formation of platelets.

Thrombosis: The formation or development of a blood-clot or thrombus.

Thrombotic thrombocytopenic purpura (TTP): A severe condition characterized by thrombocytopenia, microangiopathic hemolytic anemia, renal dysfunction, neurologic abnormalities, and fever.

Thymidine: An essential ingredient used in DNA synthesis and incorporated by T lymphocytes undergoing blast transformation in response to foreign HLA-D antigens in the mixed lymphocyte culture test.

Thyromegaly: Enlargement of the thyroid gland.

Tinnitus: Buzzing in the ears.

Tissue plasminogen activator (TPA): A clotting factor produced by vascular endothelial cells that selectively binds to fibrin as it activates fibrin-bound plasminogen.

Tissue thromboplastin: Factor III; functions in the extrinsic system of coagulation.

Titer score: A method used to evaluate more precisely than simple dilution by comparing the titers of an antibody. Agglutination at each higher dilution is graded on a continuous scale; the total is the titer score.

Total iron-binding capacity (TIBC): The amount of iron that transferrin can bind; normal range is 250 to 360 μl/dl. TIBC = unsaturated iron-binding capacity (UIBC) or amount of additional iron that transferrin can bind above that which is already complexed + serum Fe.

Toxic granulation: Medium to large metachromatic granules that are evenly distributed throughout the cytoplasm. May be seen in severe bacterial infections, severe burns, and other conditions.

Trait: A characteristic that is inherited.

Transcription: The process of RNA production from DNA, which requires the enzyme RNA polymerase.

Transferase: An enzyme that catalyzes the transfer of atoms or groups of atoms from one chemical compound to another.

Transferrin: A glycoprotein synthesized in the liver, with the primary function of iron transport.

Transfuse: To perform a transfusion.

Transfusion: The injection of blood, a blood component, saline, or other fluids into the bloodstream.

   T. reaction: An adverse response to a transfusion.

Translation: The production of protein from the interactions of the RNAs.

Translocation: Transfer of a portion of one chromosome to its allele.

Transplacental: Through the placenta.

Transposition: The location of two genes on opposite chromosomes of a homologous pair.

Ubiquitous: Existing everywhere at the same time.

Urokinase: A trypsinlike protease, found in the urine and synthesized by the kidney, that activates plasminogen by proteolytic cleavage. Differs from tissue plasminogen activators in that urokinase reacts with plasminogen in the fluid phase of blood.

Urticaria: A vascular reaction of the skin similar to hives.

Vaccine: A suspension of infectious organisms or components of them that is given as a form of passive immunization to establish resistance to the infectious disease caused by that organism.

Valvular: Relating to or having a valve.

Variable region: Portion of the immunoglobulin light and heavy chains in which amino acid sequences vary tremendously. These amino acid variations permit the different immunoglobulin molecules to recognize different antigenic determinants. In other words the variable region determines the antigen against which the antibody will react, thus providing each antibody molecule with its unique specificity. The variable region is located at the amino terminal region of the molecule.

Vascular: Pertaining to or composed of blood vessels.

Vasculitis: Inflammation of a blood or lymph vessel.

Vasoconstriction: Constriction of blood vessels.

Vasodilatation: Dilatation of blood vessels, especially small arteries and arterioles.

Vaso-occlusive: Obstruction of the vasculature by some pathologic process that seriously impedes blood flow.

Vasovagal syncope: Syncope resulting from hypotension caused by emotional stress, pain, acute blood loss, fear, or rapidly rising from a recumbent position.

Venipuncture: Puncture of a vein for any purpose.

Venom: A poison excreted by some animals such as insects or snakes and transmitted by bites or stings.

Venule: A tiny vein continuous with a capillary.

Verrucous: Wartlike, with raised portions.

Vertigo: Dizziness.

Vitamin K: A fat-soluble vitamin required for maintenance of normal blood levels of the vitamin K–dependent factors: prothrombin and factors VII, IX, and X. Vitamin K is necessary for carboxylation of specific glutamic acid residues in the postprotein synthesis of the vitamin K–dependent factors.

von Willebrand's disease (vWD): A congenital bleeding disorder inherited as an autosomal dominant trait and characterized by a decreased level of factor VIII:C and a prolonged bleeding time.

von Willebrand factor (vWF): A component of the factor VIII molecule that mediates platelet interaction with subendothelium.

WAIHA: Warm autoimmune hemolytic anemia
Whole blood clotting time: A test that evaluates the overall activity of the intrinsic system of coagulation.

Xerocyte: A dehydrated red blood cell having a peculiar morphologic appearance (that is, hemoglobin concentration at one pole of the red cell).

Zeta: A type of globin chain found in embryonic hemoglobin.

Index

A number in *italics* indicates a figure; a number followed by a "t" indicates a table.

DETERMINATION	REFERENCE RANGE		NOTES
	Conventional	SI*	
HEMATOLOGY *(continued)*			
Hemoglobin Studies			Collect with anticoagulant
Electrophoresis			Use oxalate as anticoagulant
A_1 hemoglobin	96.0–98.6%		Anion exchange chromatog-
A_2 hemoglobin	1.5–4.0%	0.015–0.040	raphy
A_2 hemoglobin	1.7–3.3%		
Hemoglobin F (fetal hemoglobin)	Newborn: 60–90% After 1 year of age: less than 2%	<0.02	Collect with anticoagulant
Hemoglobin, met- and sulf-	0	0	Use heparin as anticoagulant
Serum hemoglobin	2–3 mg/100 ml	1.2–1.9 umol/liter	
Thermolabile hemoglobin	0	0	Any anticoagulant
SYSTEMIC LUPUS ERYTHEMATOSUS (SLE) PREPARATION:			
Method I	0	0	Use heparin as anticoagulant
Method II	0	0	Use defibrinated blood
Vitamin B_{12}	205–876 pg/ml	150–674 pmol/liter	
Borderline	140–204 pg/ml	102.6–149 pmol/liter	
Leukocyte alkaline phosphatase (LAP)	Males: 22–124 Females: 33–149		Isolated blood leukocytes
Acid phosphatase	<2 cells with 4+ activity		
Muramidase	Serum, 3–7 mg/liter Urine, 0–2 μg/ml	0–2 mg/liter	
Peroxide hemolysis	Less than 10%	0.10	Use EDTA as anticoagulant
BODY FLUIDS			
Spinal fluid (CSF) Colorless	0–10 lymphocytes/mm³ 0 RBC/mm³ Rare ependymal cell		
Synovial fluid Pale yellow to colorless Crystals—none No clot formation	200–600 WBC/mm³ 0 RBC/mm³ Few synovial cells Differential: PMN 0–25% Mononuclear 0–75%		
Pleural and peritoneal fluid Yellow	≤1000 cells/mm³ 0 RBC/mm³ Differential: PMN ≤25% Mononuclear 0–75%		
Seminal fluid White, gray	Total volume 1.5–5.0 ml Total count 60–100 mil/ml		
COAGULATION			
Platelet count	150,000–450,000/mm³		Hemacytometer
Platelet function tests:			
Clot retraction	50–100%/2 hr	0.50–1.00/2 hr	Collect in plastic tubes with 3.8% sodium citrate
Platelet aggregation	Full response to ADP epinephrine, and collagen	1.0	Collect in plastic tubes with 3.8% sodium citrate